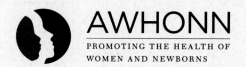

AWHONN
PROMOTING THE HEALTH OF
WOMEN AND NEWBORNS

Perinatal Nursing

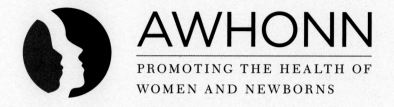

Perinatal
Nursing

FOURTH EDITION

Kathleen Rice Simpson, PhD, RNC, FAAN

Perinatal Clinical Nurse Specialist
Mercy Hospital
St. Louis, Missouri

Patricia A. Creehan, MSN, RNC

Manager of Clinical Operations Labor and Delivery
Advocate Christ Medical Center
Oak Lawn, Illinois

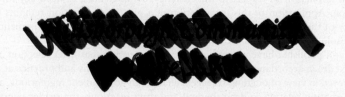

Wolters Kluwer | Lippincott Williams & Wilkins
Health
Philadelphia · Baltimore · New York · London
Buenos Aires · Hong Kong · Sydney · Tokyo

Senior Acquisitions Editor: Shannon Maqee
Developmental Editor: Lisa Marshall
Product Manager: Ashley Fischer
Production Project Manager: Marian Bellus
Design Coordinator: Joan Wendt
Manufacturing Coordinator: Beth Welsh
Production Services / Compositor: Absolute Service, Inc
Printer: RR Donnelley-Shenzhen

4th edition

Library of Congress Cataloging-in-Publication Data

Perinatal nursing / [edited by] Kathleen Rice Simpson, Patricia A. Creehan.
  – 4th ed.
     p. ; cm.
  At head of title: AWHONN, Association of Women's Health, Obstetric and
Neonatal Nurses
  Includes bibliographical references and index.
  ISBN 978-1-60913-622-2
  I. Simpson, Kathleen Rice. II. Creehan, Patricia A. III. Association of
Women's Health, Obstetric, and Neonatal Nurses. IV. Title: AWHONN,
Association of Women's Health, Obstetric and Neonatal Nurses.
  [DNLM: 1. Maternal-Child Nursing. 2. Neonatal Nursing. 3. Perinatal
Care. WY 157.3]
  RG951
  618.2'0231–dc23
                              2013004566

To
the perinatal nurses at Mercy Hospital in St. Louis, Missouri
and the mothers and babies they care for every day

and

my parents, William and Dorothy; my husband, Dan; and my children,
Daniel, Katie, Michael, John, and Elizabeth

—KRS

To
the perinatal nurses at Advocate Christ Medical Center in Oak Lawn, Illinois, and
the mothers and babies they care for every day

and

To Patrick, Sean, Melissa, and Kelly Mitchell

—PAC

Contributors

Julie Arafeh, RN, MSN
Simulation Specialist
The Simulation Center
Texas Children's Hospital
Houston, Texas
Chapter 9: Cardiac Disease in Pregnancy

Suzanne McMurtry Baird, DNPc, MSN, RN
Assistant Director, Clinical Practice
Texas Children's Hospital Pavilion for Women
Houston, Texas
Chapter 10: Pulmonary Complications in Pregnancy

Mary Lee Barron, PhD, APRN, FNP-BC
Associate Professor
Director, Advanced Nursing Practice Programs
Saint Louis University
St. Louis, Missouri
Chapter 4: Antenatal Care

Susan Tucker Blackburn, RN, PhD, FAAN
Professor Emeritus, Department of Family and Child
  Nursing
University of Washington
Seattle, Washington
Chapter 3: Physiologic Changes of Pregnancy

Nancy A. Bowers, BSN, RN, MPH
Education Specialist
American Society for Reproductive Medicine
Birmingham, Alabama
Chapter 11: Multiple Gestation

Carol Burke, MSN, RNC, APN
Perinatal Clinical Nurse Specialist
Northwestern Memorial Hospital—Prentice Women's
  Hospital
Chicago, Illinois
*Chapter 16: Pain in Labor: Nonpharmacologic and
  Pharmacologic Management*

Lynn Clark Callister, RN, PhD, FAAN
Professor Emerita
Brigham Young University
Provo, Utah
*Chapter 2: Integrating Cultural Beliefs and Practices
  When Caring for Childbearing Women and
  Families*

Annette Carley, RN, MS, NNP-BC, PNP-BC
Clinical Professor, Department of Family Health Care
  Nursing
University of California, San Francisco School of
  Nursing
San Francisco, California
Chapter 21: Common Neonatal Complications

Julie M. Daley, RN, MS, CDE
Senior Diabetes Nurse Clinician
Women and Infants Hospital
Providence, Rhode Island
Chapter 8: Diabetes in Pregnancy

Debbie Fraser, MN, RNC-NIC
Associate Professor, Faculty of Health Disciplines
Athabasca University
Athabasca, Alberta
Chapter 18: Newborn Adaptation to Extrauterine Life

Dotti C. James, PhD, RNC-OB, C-EFM
Director, Mercy East Communities
Talent Development and Optimization
Mercy Hospital
Chesterfield, Missouri

Jill Janke, RN, WHNP, PhD
Professor
University of Alaska Anchorage
Anchorage, Alaska
Chapter 20: Newborn Nutrition

Betsy B. Kennedy, MSN, RN
Assistant Professor of Nursing
Faculty Development Coordinator
Vanderbilt University School of Nursing
Nashville, Tennessee
Chapter 10: Pulmonary Complications in Pregnancy

Audrey Lyndon, PhD, RNC, CNS-BC
Assistant Professor
Director, Perinatal Clinical Nurse Specialist Program
Department of Family Health Care Nursing
University of California, San Francisco
San Francisco, California
Chapter 15: Fetal Assessment during Labor

Mary Ann Maher, MSN, RNC-OB, C-EFM
Advanced Nurse Clinician
Labor and Delivery/Women's Evaluation Unit
Mercy Hospital St. Louis
St. Louis, Missouri
Chapter 12: Obesity in Pregnancy

Nancy O'Brien-Abel, MN, RNC
Perinatal Clinical Nurse Specialist
Perinatal Consulting, LLC
Bellevue, Washington
Chapter 14: Labor and Birth
Chapter 15: Fetal Assessment during Labor

Judith H. Poole, PhD, MBA/MHA, RNC-OB,
    C-EFM, NEA-BC
Assistant Professor
Blair College of Health Presbyterian School of
    Nursing
Queens University
Charlotte, North Carolina
Chapter 5: Hypertensive Disorders in Pregnancy

Nancy Jo Reedy, RN, CNM, MPH, FACNM
Adjunct Assistant Professor
Georgetown University School of Nursing &
    Health Studies
Georgetown University
Washington, District of Columbia
Chapter 7: Preterm Labor and Birth

Joan Renaud Smith, PhD(c), RN, NNP-BC
Neonatal Nurse Practitioner, Newborn Intensive
    Care Unit
St. Louis Children's Hospital
St. Louis, Missouri
Chapter 21: Common Neonatal Complications

Mary Ellen Burke Sosa, RNC, MS
President, Perinatal Resources
Per Diem Staff Nurse, Labor/Delivery/Recovery
Women and Infants Hospital
Providence, Rhode Island
Chapter 6: Bleeding in Pregnancy

Lyn Vargo, PhD, RN, NNP-BC
Clinical Assistant Professor
Stony Brook University
University of Missouri—Kansas City
Stony Brook, New York/Kansas City, Missouri
Chapter 19: Newborn Physical Assessment

Judy Wilson-Griffin, RN-C, MSN
Perinatal Clinical Nurse Specialist
SSM St. Mary's Health Center
St. Louis, Missouri
Chapter 13: Maternal–Fetal Transport

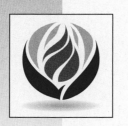

Reviewers

Susan Bakewell-Sachs, PhD, RN, PNP-BC
Interim Provost and Vice President for Academic
  Affairs, Professor of Nursing, Pediatric Nurse
  Practitioner
The College of New Jersey
Ewing Township, New Jersey

Ocean Berg, RN, MSN, CNS
Perinatal Clinical Nurse Specialist
San Francisco General Hospital and Trauma Center
San Francisco, California

Mary Campbell Bliss, RN, MS, CNS
Perinatal Clinical Nurse Specialist
Sutter Medical Center, Sacramento
Sacramento, California

Cathy Collins-Fulea, MSN, CNM, FACNM
Division Head Midwifery, Women's Health Services
Henry Ford Health System
Detroit, Michigan

Phyllis Lawlor-Klean, MS, RNC, APN/CNS
Clinical Nurse Specialist
Advocate Christ Medical Center/Hope Children's
  Hospital
Oak Lawn, Illinois

Audrey Lyndon, PhD, RNC, CNS-BC
Assistant Professor
Director, Perinatal Clinical Nurse Specialist Program
Department of Family Health Care Nursing
University of California, San Francisco
San Francisco, California

Mary Ann Maher, MSN, RNC-OB, C-EFM
Advanced Nurse Clinician
Labor and Delivery/Women's Evaluation Unit
Mercy Hospital St. Louis
St. Louis, Missouri

Nancy O'Brien-Abel, MN, RNC
Perinatal Clinical Nurse Specialist
Perinatal Consulting, LLC
Bellevue, Washington

Mary Ellen Burke Sosa, RNC, MS
President, Perinatal Resources
Per Diem Staff Nurse, Labor/Delivery/Recovery
Women & Infants Hospital
Providence, Rhode Island

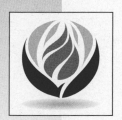

Preface

This fourth edition reflects 20 years of working together on this textbook. We began the first edition in 1993. It has been an amazing process. We hope the text has well served perinatal nurses and the mothers and babies in their care over the years. It has been our privilege to be part of this resource offered by the Association of Women's Health, Obstetric and Neonatal Nurses. We attempted to involve the most expert nurses from across the county who were willing to volunteer their time to contribute to this book. It is only through their collective generosity that this book was possible. We have strived to present up-to-date information based on the most rigorous evidence and offer suggestions for best practices as appropriate. The goal was to provide useful clinical information for practicing perinatal nurses, and we hope we have succeeded.

Kathleen Rice Simpson, PhD, RNC, FAAN
Patricia A. Creehan, MSN, RNC

Contents

CHAPTER 21
COMMON NEONATAL COMPLICATIONS 662
Joan Renaud Smith and Annette Carley

APPENDIX

CHAPTER 1

Perinatal Patient Safety and Professional Liability Issues

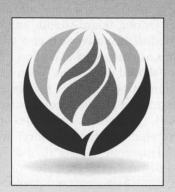

Kathleen Rice Simpson

CREATING a safe clinical environment during labor and birth requires effective leadership, a shared philosophy, interdisciplinary collaboration, professional behavior, and excellence in key clinical practices. When unit operations and clinical care are based on "What is best (safest) for the mother and baby?", quality is a natural outcome. Ideally, there are established criteria for ongoing monitoring of quality of care that include structure, process, and outcome measures. This chapter offers recommendations for creating conditions that provide the safest care possible for mothers and babies using a framework for perinatal high reliability that includes each of these essential criteria. Suggestions to minimize risk of professional liability are also provided. The recommendations are based on data concerning the most common causes of preventable injuries to mothers and babies during labor and birth. Data include the Joint Commission (TJC) sentinel event alerts *Preventing Infant Death and Injury During Delivery* (Joint Commission on Accreditation of Healthcare Organizations [JCAHO], 2004) and *Preventing Maternal Death* (TJC, 2010), *Summary Data of Sentinel Events Reviewed by the Joint Commission* (TJC, 2011b), the American College of Obstetricians and Gynecologists' (ACOG, 2009a) *2009 ACOG Survey on Professional Liability*, the Jury Verdict Research (2009) report *Current Award Trends in Personal Injury*, reports from reviews of professional liability insurance company claims (Clark, Belfort, Dildy, & Meyers, 2008; Crico Strategies, 2010; Greenwald & Mondor, 2003), and experience working with hospitals and healthcare systems to reduce risk of perinatal patient harm and to promote patient safety.

Inpatient obstetric care results in more than 50% of obstetrics and gynecology claims (White, Pichert, Bledsoe, Irwin, & Entman, 2005). In a review of over 800 obstetric malpractice cases from the medical malpractice company owned by the Harvard medical community, the average payment in obstetric-related malpractice claims was more than twice that of other clinical areas, with birth asphyxia, shoulder dystocia, intrauterine fetal death, and maternal hemorrhage accounting for the majority of cases (Crico Strategies, 2010). Contributing factors to the adverse events were noted to be inappropriate management of pregnancy, failure to timely diagnose and treat "fetal distress," and inappropriate management of the second stage of labor via operative vaginal birth. The number and severity of successful obstetric liability claims and jury awards have steadily increased over the years (Crico Strategies, 2010). Based on a review of 1,213 closed obstetric cases, 44% resulted in payment with the average payment nearly 1 million dollars and 12% over 1 million dollars (Crico Strategies, 2010). Although the number of obstetric claims typically represents only about 5% of all malpractice claims, the dollar amount reserved for current and future payment is usually 25% to 35% of the total financial liability cost to hospitals and healthcare systems. In a study of 8,151 claims against nurses, only 9.9% were related to obstetrical nursing care; however, the amount paid or severity of these claims ranked highest among other specialties, with assessment, monitoring, treatment, and care management making up the bulk of the allegations (Nurses Service Organization, 2009). Increasing patient safety decreases institutional and professional liability risk. All adverse outcomes cannot be prevented; however, defensibility is enhanced when care is consistent with current evidence and national standards and guidelines.

PERINATAL HIGH RELIABILITY

In 1999, the concept, theory, and attributes of high-reliability organizations (those that operate highly complex and hazardous technological systems essentially without mistakes over long periods of time) was applied to clinical perinatal practice (Knox, Simpson, & Garite, 1999). The description of high reliability perinatal units was based on observation differentiating units that produced more or less harm to patients using professional liability claims as a proxy for perinatal injury. The following attributes of low-risk, harm-free, highly reliable obstetric (OB) units were identified:

- Safety is declared as the hallmark of organizational culture and understood to be the responsibility and duty of every team member. Safety for mothers and babies is the number one priority and takes precedence over institution and provider convenience, production issues, and costs. Safety guides all unit operations and clinical actions. Decisions are made in the context of potential risks and benefits to patients. While institutional costs and financial resources are important and must be considered, patient safety is not at risk due to financial constraints. The administrative leadership team is committed to financially supporting the perinatal unit even if it is not one of the most profitable service lines. This commitment includes providing adequate personnel for leadership and clinical care and updated equipment as needed. Convenience is only a factor in decision making when there is no risk to patient safety. Patients are invited and encouraged to be actively involved in their care and are provided enough information to make decisions through a literacy-appropriate informed consent process.
- Patient safety is considered a team function rather than an individual function. All clinicians are considered competent, with an obligation to speak up if there is a question of safety. Team interaction is collegial rather than hierarchical. Hierarchy does not hinder any clinician from expressing concern in the face of potential risks. Any member of the team is able to offer opinions and speak up in the context of risk of patient harm. Those alerts and opinions are welcomed by the entire team regardless of discipline or rank.
- Respectful communication is highly valued and rewarded. Extensive, transparent communication is used to orient, plan, update, and adjust to the unexpected. Routine debriefing is practiced for critical, unusual, or unexpected events. Team members in high-reliability organizations do not wait until there is an adverse outcome to evaluate operations and practices. Evaluation is ongoing through use of established measurement processes.
- Emergencies are rehearsed and unexpected events anticipated. During board rounds and case conferences, possibilities for adverse events based on clinical situations are discussed and plans are developed and in place should they occur. Team-building exercises and simulation practices for obstetrical emergencies are conducted on a regular basis.
- Paradoxically, successful operations (absence of maternal, fetal, and neonatal injury) are viewed as potentially dangerous subject to risk of "normalization of deviance" (a degradation of professional, behavioral, and technical standards that occurs over time and increases probability of a major accident or harm). Because major accidents or patient harm occur only infrequently, clinical practice in the absence of professional standards and/or inaccurate processes (e.g., "work-arounds") may go undetected or deteriorate over long periods of time.

Perinatal units can be highly reliable in the care that is delivered by incorporating these basic principles into daily operations (Knox & Simpson, 2011; Knox, Simpson, & Townsend, 2003; Simpson & Knox, 2006). Other attributes of perinatal high reliability include effective leadership from the top down, professional behavior by all team members, and standardization of key clinical practices involving risk of adverse events that have a cumulative body of evidence and professional standards and guidelines to support development of clinical guidelines, algorithms, or protocols.

LEADERSHIP

Leadership structures and systems must be established to ensure that there is organization-wide awareness of patient safety performance gaps, direct accountability of leaders for those gaps, adequate investment in performance improvement abilities, and actions taken to ensure safe care of every patient served (National Quality Forum [NQF], 2010). Without effective leaders, staff members are challenged to implement essential criteria for safe care. The leadership team, composed of top hospital administrators, physician department chairs, department nurse leaders, unit nurse managers, clinical nurse specialists, educators, and charge nurses, must be enthusiastic participants actively engaged in promoting safe care as the number one priority. The fundamental goal of keeping patients safe from harm is worthy of sustained leadership attention and focus. Patient safety is a matter of integrity (Ryan, 2004). Leaders must be fully committed and have the will to do the right thing for mothers and babies, their families, their caregivers, and the institution, even when faced with the pressures of economics, productivity, and perceived provider convenience. This includes insisting on research-based, safe clinical practices and a professional environment where physicians and nurses are encouraged to work as a team, interact as colleagues, and collaborate on clinical solutions in a respectful manner. Our moral and ethical responsibility to do the right thing is discussed in detail in the *Code of Ethics for Nurses* (American Nurses Association [ANA], 2010). Adequate financial and personnel resource allocation and support for practices based on research findings that demonstrate safe and effective care are critical foundations of our moral and ethical responsibility to patients (ANA, 2010; Ryan, 2004).

A healthy work environment is critical to promoting patient safety. In 2005, the American Association of Critical-Care Nurses (AACN) published standards for establishing and sustaining healthy work environments. These standards have been endorsed by the Association of Women's Health, Obstetric and Neonatal Nurses (AWHONN). The role of nurses as integral members of the healthcare team and their contributions to patient outcomes are covered in detail. Support of the leadership team of the healthcare organization is essential for success. The AACN (2005) standards are summarized as follows:

- Skilled communication: Nurses must be as proficient in communication skills as they are in clinical skills.
- True collaboration: Nurses must be relentless in pursuing and fostering true collaboration.
- Effective decision making: Nurses must be valued and committed partners in making policy, directing and evaluating clinical care, and leading organizational operations.
- Appropriate staffing: Staffing must ensure the effective match between patient needs and nurse competence.
- Meaningful recognition: Nurses must be recognized and must recognize others for the value each brings to the work of the organization.
- Authentic leadership: Nurse leaders must fully embrace the imperative of a healthy work environment, authentically live it, and engage others in its achievement.

These standards offer a method of measuring performance of individual nursing units, healthcare organizations, and systems and reaffirm that safe and respectful environments are fundamental, requiring systems, structures, and cultures that support communication, collaboration, decision making, staffing recognition, and leadership (AACN, 2005). Implementation can lead to excellence when adoption and continued support occurs at every level of the healthcare organization from the bedside to the boardroom (AACN, 2005).

In 2011, the Society for Maternal–Fetal Medicine (SMFM) invited representatives from professional organizations involved in the care of mothers and babies to develop a call to action for quality care during labor and birth. Participating organizations included the American Academy of Family Physicians (AAFP), American Academy of Pediatrics (AAP), American College of Nurse Midwives (ACNM), ACOG, and AWHONN. Recommendations from *Quality Patient Care in Labor and Delivery: A Call to Action* (Lawrence et al., 2012) include:

- Ensure that patient-centered care and patient safety are organizational priorities that guide decisions for organizational policies and practices.
- Foster a just culture of openness by encouraging and promoting the active communication of good outcomes and opportunities for improvement.
- Develop forums to facilitate communication and tracking of issues of concern.
- Provide resources for clinicians to be educated in the principles of teamwork, safety, and shared decision making.
- Develop methods to systematically track and evaluate care processes and outcomes.
- Facilitate cross-departmental sharing of resources and expertise.
- Ensure that quality obstetric care is a priority that guides individual and team decisions.
- Identify and communicate the safety concerns and work together to mitigate potential safety risks.
- Disseminate and use the best available evidence, including individual and hospital-level data, to guide practice patterns.

These recommendations are based on the belief that mutual respect, patient-centered care, and shared decision making are essential for providing quality obstetric care (Lawrence et al., 2012). Improving safety requires teamwork and effective communication at multiple levels within the organization. With all professional disciplines working together, patient outcomes and satisfaction can be improved (Lawrence et al., 2012). Consensus on what needs to be accomplished for safe intrapartum care by these leading professional organizations is a powerful message to patients, healthcare providers, and administrators of shared goals for optimal outcomes. Leaders of the administrative and clinical teams in each hospital and healthcare team should support these recommendations and work to make them reality to promote the safest care possible for mothers and babies during labor and birth.

SHARED PHILOSOPHY OF CARE

In a high-reliability unit, there is an agreement that clinical practice will be based on the cumulative body of evidence and national professional standards and guidelines (Knox & Simpson, 2011). This shared philosophy should serve as a guide to develop unit policies and protocols and, ultimately, for how perinatal care is provided daily. An interdisciplinary practice committee, co-chaired by nurse and physician leaders, should be in place to guide unit operations and clinical care. This committee should include representatives from all disciplines (nurses, midwives, physicians) and specialty practice areas (obstetric, family medicine, pediatrics, neonatal, anesthesia), as well as leaders and direct care providers. The committee should be empowered to make policy changes as needed. There should be a standing agenda item each month to review the most recently published science and standards and guidelines from professional organizations and regulatory agencies such as ACOG, AAP, AWHONN, ACNM, the National Association of Neonatal Nurses (NANN), the Association of peri-Operative Registered Nurses (AORN), the American Society of PeriAnesthesia Nurses (ASPAN), the American Society of Anesthesiologists (ASA), TJC, the Centers for Disease Control and Prevention (CDC), the Institute for Safe Medication Practices (ISMP), the United States Department of Health and Human Services (HHS), the U.S. Preventative Services Task Force, and the U.S. Food and Drug Administration (FDA). Assigning committee members specific organizations to review each month and/or rotating responsibility among committee members for this review process will facilitate a comprehensive appraisal of recently published standards and guidelines and provide the committee with evidence upon which to promote practice changes. Discussion during the committee meetings should focus on how and when new standards and guidelines will be incorporated into unit operations and daily practice.

Patient safety must take priority over convenience, productivity, and costs. Standard unit polices and protocols should be in place for key clinical practices that are known to be associated with risk of adverse outcomes (Knox & Simpson, 2011). These include, but are not limited to, cervical ripening, labor induction, fetal assessment, perinatal group B streptococcus (GBS) prophylaxis, second-stage labor care, vaginal birth after cesarean birth (VBAC), operative vaginal birth, emergent cesarean birth, and neonatal resuscitation. All members of the interdisciplinary team must adhere to the unit policies. In rare cases where there may be a need to practice outside of unit policy, interdisciplinary discussion should occur, medical record documentation should be appropriately descriptive, and the case should be evaluated through the quality review process.

Patient safety is created through accountability based on standardization, simplification, and clarity, as supported by the principles of safety science (Kohn, Corrigan, & Donaldson, 1999). While standardization of unit practices and policies may be perceived as an inconvenience to some team members, it should be acknowledged that the collective good of mothers and babies is the primary concern. There is a growing body of evidence that establishing standardized clinical guidelines can lead to improved patient safety and clinical outcomes as well as a positive effect on malpractice litigation (Kirkpatrick & Burkman, 2010). Examples of standardized clinical guidelines include algorithms of care, templates for electronic medical records, standard provider order sets, surgical checklists, patient hand-off processes, and other protocols designed to improve patient care. Successful implementation has been shown to require more than just encouragement and educational efforts for the healthcare team members in some cases. Although voluntary participation is ideal, some healthcare systems have learned that "hard stops" and disciplinary or credentialing actions may be required to enforce clinical guidelines (Clark et al., 2010).

A conservative approach to perinatal practice based on cumulative evidence and published professional standards creates conditions that promote safer care and decrease the probability of preventable adverse outcomes. However, attempts to standardize basic aspects of care based on current evidence, standards, and guidelines can be met with resistance and may require much effort on the part of the leadership team. Barriers to changing practice include individual practice and clinician autonomy placed at a higher priority than patient safety ("No one is going to tell me how to practice"); a general aversion to change ("I like the status quo"), a false reassurance based on small numbers ("I've never had a problem doing it this way"), lack of accountability ("Peer review is nonexistent"), and hierarchical deference. Table 1–1 lists common barriers in promoting evidence-based care via quality improvement projects (Bingham & Main, 2010). Some hospitals and healthcare systems have implemented changes in practice through quality improvement projects. Strategies for successful implementation are listed in Table 1–2 (Bingham & Main, 2010). Each of these strategies requires sustained support and commitment from the administrative leadership team, the clinical leadership team, and front-line clinicians if it is to be successful. One key to success is putting patient safety and the needs of mothers and babies above all other priorities.

Maintaining a healthy work environment and supporting a quality workforce can be instrumental in providing quality care on a routine basis. When all team members have adequate education and support, feel part of the team, and get positive feedback on their efforts to provide optimal care, quality is enhanced. The Agency for Healthcare Research and Quality (AHRQ) (McHugh, Garman, McAlearney, Song, & Harrison, 2010) offers suggestions for workforce practices to

Table 1–1. COMMON BARRIERS TO IMPLEMENTATION OF EVIDENCE-BASED CLINICAL GUIDELINES AND PARTICIPATION IN QUALITY IMPROVEMENT PROJECTS

Leader barriers

Lack of leader knowledge to:	Design, plan, and implement quality improvement (QI)
	Perform QI data analysis
	Assess how to enhance their individual QI leadership abilities
Leader attitudes (beliefs and assumptions) that affect:	Topic selection
	QI topic goals
	Selection of QI implementation tactics
	Definitions of success
Leader practices	Lack of clarity of QI project goals
	Backing down or stop trying
	Lack of time and other resources
	Inadequate practices to ensure sustainability (e.g., new hires, staff returning from vacation, leaves of absences)

Clinician barriers

Lack of clinician knowledge:	About their own practices (lack adequate feedback)
	New or inexperienced
	Lack knowledge of the QI project
Clinician attitudes (beliefs and assumptions):	Not persuaded to change
	Want autonomy
Clinician practices:	Inertia—no motivation to change
	Forget
	Changes add more work or slow down usual work flow

Characteristics of the QI project

	Positive or negative effect(s) on clinician income or time
	Complexity of the QI project (e.g., how many groups work flow is affected by the QI project changes)

Implementation climate

	Type of hospital
	Amount of resources
	Type of community or population of patients

From Bingham, D., & Main, E. K. (2010). Effective implementation strategies and tactics for leading change on perinatal units. *Journal of Perinatal and Neonatal Nursing, 24*(1), 32–42.

Table 1–2. STRATEGIES FOR SUCCESSFUL IMPLEMENTATION OF EVIDENCE-BASED CLINICAL GUIDELINES

Education strategy

Examples of educational tactics	Definition
Grand rounds	*Physician educational sessions that are often held once a week.*
Classes or conferences	*Formal educational sessions developed on specific topics.*
Simulation training	*Simulation training is education that allows clinicians to practice skills and knowledge through a fabricated situation that mimics a complicated situation that they will face and need to practice how to respond.*
Competence fairs, tests, learning fairs, demonstrations	*Clinicians demonstrate their knowledge of a new concept or demonstrate their ability to perform a clinical skill.*
On-line learning	*The use of the internet for the transfer of information.*

Date strategy

Examples of data tactics	
Audit and feedback (group and individual)	*An examination of clinical records in order to gather specific pre-determined information. The information gathered is summarized and shared with the relevant group or individuals.*
Public release of data	*Details of care patterns and outcomes are reported openly to the community in such a way that anyone can access this information.*

Discourse strategy

Examples of discourse tactics	Definition
Meetings	*Group discussions (e.g., staff meetings).*
One-to-one discussions	*A discussion between a change leader and someone else whom they are seeking to influence to change.*
Academic detailing	*A review of relevant academic research by one leader meeting with one clinician at a time. A common tactic utilized by pharmaceutical representatives.*
Reminders	*A method for helping someone remember to perform specific tasks (e.g., checklists, order set).*
Newsletters	*A formal written update that is periodically distributed.*
Posters and bulletin boards	*A collection of data and information that is organized for display on poster board or a bulletin board.*
E-mails	*Electronic communications using either the Internet or Intranet that can be one-to-one or one-to-many.*
Rewards	*Something given in compensation for reaching a pre-determined goal (e.g., professional recognition, a bonus).*
Disciplinary discussions	*A discussion that is held by someone in the position to give employee feedback and a formal review of performance in order to outline how current behavior does not meet required expectations of job performance.*

From Bingham, D., & Main, E. K. (2010). Effective implementation strategies and tactics for leading change on perinatal units. *Journal of Perinatal and Neonatal Nursing, 24*(1), 32–42.

support high quality performance in their practical resource *Using Workforce Practices to Drive Quality Improvement: A Guide for Hospitals* (see Display 1–1).

Professional registered nurse staffing should be adequate to meet the needs of the service. The AWHONN (2010) staffing guidelines provide detailed recommendations for registered nurse staffing for perinatal units including various types of patients and clinical situations. These guidelines can be used as a basis for planning and implementing safe nurse staffing.

High Performance Work Practices

Organizational Engagement Practices
- Communicating mission, vision, and values
- Sharing performance information
- Involving employees in key decisions
- Tracking and rewarding performance

Staff Acquisition and Development Practices
- Rigorous recruiting
- Selective hiring
- Extensive education
- Career development

Frontline Empowerment Practices
- Employment security
- Reduced status distinctions
- Teams/decentralized decision making

Leadership Alignment and Development Practices
- Linking management training to organizational needs
- Planning succession
- Tracking and rewarding performance

Facilitators for Success
- Commit to an organizational culture that focuses on quality and safety
- Engage senior leadership support
- Involve the human resources department in strategic planning
- Identify opportunities for shared learning
- Hire human resources professionals with training and experience with high performance work practices
- Involve employee representatives
- Monitor progress

Adapted from McHugh, M., Garman, A., McAlearney, A., Song, P., & Harrison, M. (2010). *Using Workforce Practices to Drive Quality Improvement: A Guide for Hospitals* (AHRQ Publication No. 11-0003-EF). Rockville, MD: Agency for Healthcare Research and Quality.

PROFESSIONAL BEHAVIOR

Professionals should conduct themselves in a professional manner at all times. Expectations for professional behavior should be outlined explicitly in institutional policies for good citizenship and reaffirmed both by the leaders as well as each team member annually during contract renewal and performance reviews. Respectful, collegial interactions between nurses and physicians and with patients are the bedrock of the unit culture. The *different but equal* contribution of nurses to the care process and ultimate clinical outcomes should be recognized and valued. Poor behavior (e.g., throwing instruments or medical records, intimidation, having temper tantrums, making demeaning comments to team members and/or patients, or using

profanity) should not be defined or qualified by discipline. Exceptions should not be made because "he or she is a good clinician otherwise," "we need his patient volume," or "she's one of the few who is always willing to work overtime."

Disruptive behavior can be overt, such as yelling; using profanity; throwing instruments; slamming charts; physically threatening or abusing others; berating someone; displaying a rude, demeaning attitude; lying; not answering pages; and slow or no response when called for a bedside evaluation (Porto & Lauve, 2006). More subtle examples are disrespect, gossiping, nonverbal devaluation, eye rolling when a colleague makes a suggestion, not speaking to certain colleagues, gender discrimination, or sexual innuendo (Weber, 2004). Disruptive behavior is a significant threat to patient safety. After an experience with a disruptive clinician, many victims intentionally avoid additional interactions to minimize further opportunities for abuse (Rosenstein & O'Daniel, 2005). During labor, this can involve the nurse not calling the physician about an indeterminate or abnormal fetal heart rate (FHR) pattern because the last time they interacted, the nurse felt berated and demeaned (Simpson, James, & Knox, 2006; Simpson & Lyndon, 2009). Nurses may feel pressured to increase oxytocin rates during tachysystole and avoid speaking up to prevent another unpleasant encounter with the physician who believes more oxytocin will speed labor (Simpson et al., 2006). A nurse may be reluctant to seek advice from a nurse colleague concerning FHR interpretation because of past inferences of inadequacy during similar consultation. Because most (but not all) indeterminate FHR patterns are not the result of fetal acidemia and most (but not all) tachysystole will not cause maternal or fetal harm, these avoidance strategies will work for some time, until the inevitable adverse outcome occurs.

Respectful, collegial, professional behavior should be valued equally to competent clinical practice and patient volume. Processes for reporting disruptive behavior should be widely disseminated and their use actively encouraged and supported by the leadership team. There should be accountability for individual actions and meaningful follow-up with clear, actionable implications when disruptive behavior occurs. Each instance of disruptive behavior should be addressed in a timely manner, rather than delaying interventions until trends become apparent. Competent clinical practice is a basic expectation and cannot be substituted for irresponsible, inappropriate, dysfunctional, or abusive behavior. In the Joint Commission Sentinel Event Alert Number 40, *Behaviors that Undermine a Culture of Safety*, specific recommendations are listed for promoting professional behavior (TJC, 2008) (see Display 1–2). TJC has a leadership standard that addresses disruptive and inappropriate behaviors in

D I S P L A Y   1 – 2

Recommendations for Addressing Behaviors that Undermine a Culture of Safety

- Educate all team members—physicians, nurse midwives, nurses, and other personnel—on appropriate professional behavior defined by the organization's code of conduct. The code and education should emphasize respect. Include education in basic business etiquette (particularly phone skills) and people skills.
- Hold all team members accountable for modeling desirable behaviors, and enforce the code consistently and equitably among all staff regardless of seniority or clinical discipline in a positive fashion through reinforcement as well as punishment.
- Develop and implement policies and procedures/processes appropriate for the organization that address:
  - "Zero tolerance" for intimidating and/or disruptive behaviors, especially the most egregious instances of disruptive behavior such as assault and other criminal acts. Incorporate the zero-tolerance policy into medical staff bylaws and employment agreements as well as administrative policies.
  - Medical staff policies regarding intimidating and/or disruptive behaviors of physicians within a healthcare organization should be complementary and supportive of the policies that are present in the organization for other personnel.
  - Reducing fear of intimidation or retribution and protecting those who report or cooperate in the investigation of intimidating, disruptive, and other unprofessional behavior. Nonretaliation clauses should be included in all policy statements that address disruptive behaviors.
  - Responding to patients and/or their families who are involved in or witness intimidating and/or disruptive behaviors. The response should include hearing and empathizing with their concerns, thanking them for sharing those concerns, and apologizing.
  - How and when to begin disciplinary actions (e.g., suspension, termination, loss of clinical privileges, reports to professional licensure bodies).
- Develop an organizational process for addressing intimidating and disruptive behaviors that solicits and integrates substantial input from an interprofessional team including representation of medical and nursing staff, administrators, and other employees.
- Provide skills-based education and coaching for all leaders and managers in relationship-building and collaborative practice, including skills for giving feedback on unprofessional behavior and conflict resolution. Cultural assessment tools can also be used to measure whether or not attitudes change over time.
- Develop and implement a system for assessing staff perceptions of the seriousness and extent of instances of unprofessional behaviors and the risk of harm to patients.
- Develop and implement a reporting/surveillance system (possibly anonymous) for detecting unprofessional behavior. Include ombuds services and patient advocates, both of which provide important feedback from patients and families, who may experience intimidating or disruptive behavior from health professionals. Monitor system effectiveness through regular surveys, focus groups, peer and team member evaluations, or other methods. Have multiple and specific strategies to learn whether intimidating or disruptive behaviors exist or recur, such as through direct inquiries at routine intervals with staff, supervisors, and peers.
- Support surveillance with tiered, nonconfrontational interventional strategies, starting with informal "cup of coffee" conversations directly addressing the problem and moving toward detailed action plans and progressive discipline, if patterns persist. These interventions should initially be nonadversarial in nature, with the focus on building trust, placing accountability on and rehabilitating the offending individual, and protecting patient safety. Make use of mediators and conflict coaches when professional dispute resolution skills are needed.
- Conduct all interventions within the context of an organizational commitment to the health and well-being of all staff, with adequate resources to support individuals whose behavior is caused or influenced by physical or mental health pathologies.
- Encourage interprofessional dialogues across a variety of forums as a proactive way of addressing ongoing conflicts, overcoming them, and moving forward through improved collaboration and communication.
- Document all attempts to address intimidating and disruptive behaviors.

Adapted from Joint Commission. (2008). *Behaviors that undermine a culture of safety* (Sentinel Event Alert No. 40). Oakbrook Terrace, IL: Author.

two of its elements of performance: (1) the hospital/organization has a code of conduct that defines acceptable and disruptive and inappropriate behaviors; (2) leaders create and implement a process for managing disruptive and inappropriate behaviors (TJC, 2012). Further, standards in the medical staff chapter list core areas of competence that must be covered in the credentialing process, including interpersonal skills and professionalism (TJC, 2012). Similar expectations for ongoing competence validation are in effect for nurses (ANA, 2010; TJC, 2012).

COMMON AREAS OF LIABILITY AND PATIENT HARM IN CLINICAL PRACTICE

Following is a summary of the most common foci of professional perinatal liability claims, together with the most current applicable evidence and published standards and guidelines from professional associations and regulatory agencies (Simpson & Knox, 2003a, 2003b). The purpose of this discussion is to provide a framework for reviewing existing institutional protocols and developing future policies and guidelines that decrease professional liability exposure and minimize the risk of iatrogenic injury to mothers and babies.

Note that most publications about clinical practice from professional organizations include disclaimers that their recommendations are guidelines rather than standards of care. However, when clinical care results in litigation, both the plaintiff and defense teams frequently offer these professional publications as standards to support their case. Thus, while the intention is to offer guidelines based on the best evidence to date, publications from professional organizations such as ACOG, AAP, ASA, AWHONN, and ACNM do in fact become standards of care for all practical purposes in legal proceedings.

Allegations against nurses, nurse midwives, physicians, and/or institutions often result from a lack of knowledge of or commitment to practice based on current standards, guidelines, and evidence. In other cases, care is based on personal experience and history of practice over a long period during which the care provider has not experienced an adverse outcome. In obstetrics, complications leading to death are rare because mothers and babies are generally healthy. Even care that would be judged by expert peers to be substandard rarely results in injury or death. Without personal involvement in an adverse outcome, some practitioners tend to continue as they have in the past regardless of their true capabilities and limitations (Chauhan, Magann, McAninch, Gherman, & Morrison, 2003).

Although it is generally thought that practitioners with more experience have accumulated more knowledge and clinical skills and, therefore, provide higher quality care, researchers found the opposite to be true (Choudhry, Fletcher, & Soumerai, 2005). Physicians with more experience have less factual knowledge, are less likely to practice based on current science and standards from their professional associations, and are more likely to have a poor patient outcome when compared to physicians with fewer years of experience (Choudhry et al., 2005). While this study was about physicians, likely the same implications apply to nursing. Admittedly, some of the scientific evidence is counterintuitive and different from what we all learned years ago. For example, it seems likely that more oxytocin at higher rates will produce a more effective labor process and a clinically significant shorter labor. It also seems that pushing immediately at 10 cm and continuing to push despite an indeterminate or abnormal FHR pattern is the best and quickest way to deliver the baby. However, there is a growing body of evidence to the contrary. Given the odds of an adverse outcome for generally healthy patients and a practitioner's years of experience (with practice that may be no longer consistent with current standards, guidelines, and evidence),

practitioners are often surprised when the rare adverse outcome does occur (Chauhan et al., 2003). Moving toward a science-based clinical practice environment rather than "the way we've always done it" remains a significant challenge to promoting safe care. It should be noted that many times there is no cause-and-effect relationship between the allegations and an injury to a mother or baby. All adverse events are not preventable. There are times when patient are injured despite the best intentions of care providers based on multiple factors outside of their control. However, practices inconsistent with current standards, guidelines, and evidence offer opportunity for the plaintiff to demonstrate "breach of the standard of care," which can be challenging to overcome during a legal proceeding. There have been numerous discussions about strategies to decrease professional liability risk through liability reform legislation. These discussions have not led to significant changes in malpractice litigation processes or outcomes. One way to reduce liability exposure is to provide better care. In a study of 189 closed obstetric claims from a single liability insurance provider, 70% of claims were judged by expert reviewers to have involved substandard care (Clark et al., 2008). Similarly, in another study of 1,213 closed obstetric claims, 77% were found to involve substandard clinical judgment (Crico Strategies, 2010). Therefore, opportunities exist to improve care obstetric practices for mothers and babies to minimize risk of preventable harm and promote safe outcomes.

TELEPHONE TRIAGE

Common Allegations

- Failure to accurately assess maternal–fetal status over the telephone
- Failure to advise the woman to seek clinic, office, or inpatient evaluation and treatment
- Failure of the nurse to correctly communicate maternal–fetal status to the primary healthcare provider
- Failure of the physician/nurse midwife to come to the hospital to see the patient when requested by the nurse

Standards, Guidelines, and Recommendations

- Telephone advice to pregnant patients from labor and delivery nurses should be limited to two comments: "Call your primary healthcare provider" or "Come to the hospital to be evaluated." Ruling out labor and possible maternal–fetal complications cannot be done accurately over the phone. The liability for assessing and diagnosing conditions of pregnancy and labor should remain with the primary care providers rather than being assumed by the institution.

OBSTETRICAL TRIAGE

Common Allegations

- Failure to perform a medical screening exam for all pregnant women who present for care in the hospital
- Failure to include a timely assessment of fetal status as part of the maternal medical screening exam
- Delays in performing a medical screening exam (e.g., sending pregnant women who present for care to the waiting room before maternal–fetal status has been determined)
- Failure to have a policy in place delineating conditions that require bedside evaluation by a physician or midwife prior to discharge after medical screening exam by a labor nurse
- Failure of the provider to provide a bedside evaluation for pregnant women who present with high-risk medical or obstetric conditions
- Discharge of a pregnant woman without establishing fetal well-being (e.g., for women at 28 weeks or greater, a reactive nonstress test)
- Discharge of a pregnant woman who is unstable for discharge (e.g., in labor or with ongoing high-risk medical or obstetric conditions requiring inpatient care)
- Failure to meet all aspects of the Emergency Medical Treatment and Labor Act (EMTALA) regulations in assessing, treating, and discharging a pregnant women who presents for care

Standards, Guidelines, and Recommendations

- EMTALA imposes specific obligations on healthcare providers who offer triage care (a) to perform a medical screening examination to determine whether an emergency medical condition exists (including both the mother and the fetus), (b) to provide necessary stabilizing treatment when an emergency medical condition exists, and (c) to stabilize the patient, or, if the healthcare provider certifies that the benefits of transfer outweigh the risks, arrange for proper transfer to another hospital (The Consolidated Omnibus Budget Reconciliation Act [COBRA], 1985; United States Department of Health and Human Services, Centers for Medicare & Medicaid Services 2003, 2009). It is specifically prohibited to use the patient's insurance status and/or ability to pay for care as factors to determine whether a medical screening examination will be provided.
- Pregnant women may come to a hospital's labor and delivery area not only for obstetric care but also for evaluation and treatment of nonobstetric illness. Departments should agree on the conditions best treated in the labor and delivery area and those that should be treated in other hospital units. A pregnant woman who presents for care should be evaluated in a *timely* (not currently defined by AAP & ACOG, 2012) fashion. Minimally, the evaluation by an obstetric nurse should include assessment of maternal vital signs, FHR, and uterine contractions. Further evaluation includes assessment for vaginal bleeding, acute abdominal pain, temperature of 100.4°F or higher, preterm labor, preterm premature rupture of membranes, hypertension, and indeterminate or abnormal FHR pattern. If these findings are present or suspected, the responsible obstetric care provider should be promptly informed (AAP & ACOG, 2012).
- The initial triage process (10 to 20 minutes) requires one nurse to one woman presenting for care. This ratio may change to one nurse to two to three women as maternal–fetal status is determined to be stable, until patient disposition (AWHONN, 2010).
- Any patient suspected to be in labor or who has ruptured membranes or vaginal bleeding should be evaluated *promptly* (not currently defined by AAP & ACOG, 2012). Minimally, the following should be assessed: maternal vital signs; frequency and duration of uterine contractions; documentation of fetal well-being; urinary protein concentration; cervical dilatation and effacement, unless contraindicated (such as with placenta previa and preterm premature rupture of membranes), or cervical length as ascertained by transvaginal ultrasonography; fetal presentation and station of the presenting part; status of the membranes; estimated fetal weight; and assessment of maternal pelvis. Along with these assessment data, date and time of the patient's arrival and notification of the primary obstetric care provider should be included in the medical record (AAP & ACOG, 2012).
- If the woman has received prenatal care and a recent examination has confirmed the normal progress of pregnancy, her triage evaluation may be limited to an interval history and physical examination directed at the presenting condition. Previously identified risk factors should be considered and reassessed. If no new risk factors are found, attention may be focused on the following historical factors: time of onset and frequency of contractions; presence or absence of bleeding; fetal movement; history of allergies; time, content, and amount of the most recent food or liquid ingestion; and use of any medications (AAP & ACOG, 2012).

FETAL HEART RATE PATTERN INTERPRETATION, COMMUNICATION, AND DOCUMENTATION

Common Allegations

- Failure to accurately assess maternal–fetal status
- Failure to accurately distinguish, assess, and record FHR tracings of all fetuses in a multiple gestation pregnancy

- Failure to determine that the tracing being recorded is of maternal rather than fetal origin
- Failure to appreciate a deteriorating fetal condition
- Failure to appropriately treat an indeterminate or abnormal FHR in a timely manner (e.g., initiate intrauterine resuscitation measures based on the FHR pattern and/or plan for expeditious birth when appropriate)
- Failure to accurately communicate the maternal–fetal status to the physician/nurse midwife
- Failure to convey specific requests for bedside evaluation based on concern for fetal status to the physician/nurse midwife
- Failure of the physician/nurse midwife to respond appropriately when notified of indeterminate or abnormal fetal status
- Failure to institute the chain of consultation when there is a clinical disagreement between the nurse and responsible physician/nurse midwife regarding fetal status

Standards, Guidelines, and Recommendations

- Use the terminology recommended by the National Institute of Child Health and Human Development (NICHD) (Macones, Hankins, Spong, Hauth, & Moore, 2008), ACOG (2010a), and AWHONN (Lyndon & Ali, 2009) to describe FHR patterns in all professional communication and medical record documentation concerning fetal assessment via electronic fetal monitoring (EFM).
- Establish ongoing interdisciplinary fetal monitoring education (JCAHO, 2004). Knowledge and skills in fetal assessment are not discipline specific. Ensure and document that all care providers are competent to interpret EFM data (Minkoff & Berkowitz, 2009).
- All members of the team should participate in regularly scheduled case reviews that include the FHR tracing and offer suggestions for future care improvement.
- Include baseline rate, variability, presence or absence of accelerations and decelerations, clinical context, and pattern evolution in communication between team members about indeterminate or abnormal FHR patterns (Fox, Kilpatrick, King, & Parer, 2000).
- Establish a clear and agreed-upon definition of fetal well-being (e.g., accelerations 15 beats per minute above the baseline rate lasting for 15 seconds for the term fetus; a baseline rate within normal limits; no recurrent late, variable, or prolonged decelerations; and moderate variability) and document fetal well-being on admission prior to administration of pharmacologic agents for cervical ripening and labor induction, initiation of epidural analgesia, transfer to another unit, and discharge.
- Consider an initial assessment of fetal status via EFM on admission for women in labor when intermittent auscultation is planned for the primary method of fetal surveillance.
- Ensure ongoing, timely, and accurate assessment and determination of fetal well-being during labor.
- During absent or minimal baseline FHR variability, use stimulation to evaluate fetal well-being.
- Develop common expectations for intrauterine resuscitation based on the presumed etiology of the FHR pattern, including maternal repositioning, an intravenous fluid bolus of at least 500 mL of lactated Ringer's solution, oxygen administration at 10 L/min via nonrebreather facemask, reduction of uterine activity, correction of maternal hypotension, amnioinfusion, and modification of maternal pushing efforts during second stage labor (ACOG, 2010a; Simpson & James, 2005b).
- Establish agreement among team members concerning which type of FHR patterns require bedside evaluation by the primary care provider and the time frame involved (Fox et al., 2000).
- If continuous EFM is ordered, monitoring of FHR and uterine activity via EFM should continue until birth.
- Confirm maternal heart rate (HR) by palpation of maternal pulse during initiation of EFM and compare with FHR; repeat this confirmation periodically during labor. Be aware of abrupt changes in FHR that may indicate maternal HR is tracing. Recognize clinical situations that could result in maternal HR being recorded as FHR, including maternal tachycardia, contractions, maternal movement such as walking with the cordless transducer or telemetry, inaccurate transducer placement, extremes of maternal weight/size, and second stage labor pushing (e.g., accelerations with every contraction) (Simpson, 2011).
- Ensure that there are organizational resources and systems to support timely interventions (including emergent cesarean birth) when the FHR is indeterminate or abnormal.

ELECTIVE INDUCTION OF LABOR

Common Allegations

- Failure to fully inform the woman of the potential risks and benefits of elective induction
- Failure to accurately determine gestational age prior to elective induction
- Iatrogenic prematurity as the result of elective induction before 39 completed weeks of pregnancy
- Excessive doses of oxytocin resulting in uterine tachysystole (with or without the presence of an indeterminate or abnormal FHR pattern)
- Failure to accurately assess maternal–fetal status during labor induction

(See also FHR pattern interpretation, communication, and documentation; uterine tachysystole.)

Standards, Guidelines, and Recommendations

- Obtain informed consent and document it in the medical record (ACOG, 2009b; TJC, 2012). Ensure that the informed consent process is at the appropriate literacy level and in a language that the woman can understand (TJC, 2012).
- An established gestational age of at least 39 completed weeks by at least one of the following criteria should be documented prior to elective induction: (1) ultrasound measurement at less than 20 weeks of gestation supports gestational age of 39 weeks or greater; (2) fetal heart tones have been documented as present for 30 weeks by Doppler ultrasonography; (3) it has been 36 weeks since a positive serum or urine human chorionic gonadotropin pregnancy test result (ACOG, 2009b). Testing for fetal lung maturity should not be performed, and is contraindicated, when birth is mandated for fetal or maternal indications. Conversely, a mature fetal lung maturity test result before 39 weeks of gestation, in the absence of appropriate clinical circumstances, is not an indication for birth (ACOG, 2008a).
- Adhere to ACOG/AWHONN recommendations for dosages of pharmacologic agents (see misoprostol and oxytocin) (ACOG, 2009b; Simpson, 2013).
- Ensure adequate personnel are available to monitor maternal–fetal status (ACOG, 2009b) (e.g., one nurse to one woman receiving oxytocin for labor induction or augmentation) (AWHONN, 2010).
- Adhere to ACOG/AWHONN recommendations for maternal–fetal assessment: Assess characteristics of uterine activity and the FHR every 15 minutes during the active phase of the first stage of labor and every 5 minutes during the second stage of labor; assess maternal vital signs at least every 4 hours or more often if indicated (AAP & ACOG, 2012).

MISOPROSTOL (CYTOTEC) FOR CERVICAL RIPENING/LABOR INDUCTION

Common Allegations

- Excessive doses of misoprostol that resulted in uterine tachysystole (with or without an indeterminate or abnormal FHR pattern)
- Uterine rupture as a result of misoprostol administration
- Use of misoprostol for a woman with a history of a prior cesarean birth or uterine scar
- Failure to accurately assess maternal–fetal status during labor induction

(See also FHR pattern interpretation, communication, and documentation; uterine tachysystole.)

Standards, Guidelines, and Recommendations

- Obtain informed consent and document in the medical record. Ensure that the informed consent process is at the appropriate literacy level and in a language that the woman can understand (TJC, 2012).
- Have pharmacist prepare the tablets (100-microgram [mcg] tablets are not scored) (Simpson, 2013).
- Use the lowest possible dose to effect cervical change and labor progress (ACOG, 2009b).
- The initial dose should be 25 mcg (1/4 of 100-mcg tablet) inserted into the posterior vaginal fornix. The dose can be repeated every 3 to 6 hours, up to six doses in 24 hours as needed. There are lower rates of uterine tachysystole with lower dosages (25 mcg) and longer intervals between doses (q 6 hours rather than q 3 hours) (ACOG, 2009b).
- Re-dosing should be withheld if three or more contractions occur within 10 minutes, adequate cervical ripening is achieved with a Bishop score of 8 or more, the cervix is 80% effaced and 3 cm dilated, the patient enters active labor, or the FHR is indeterminate or abnormal (Simpson, 2013).
- If oxytocin is needed, it should not be given until at least 4 hours after the last dose (ACOG, 2009b).
- Misoprostol should be administered at or near the labor and birth suite, where uterine activity and FHR can be monitored continuously (Simpson, 2013).
- Misoprostol should not be administered to women with a history of prior cesarean birth or uterine scar (ACOG, 2009b, 2010b).

OXYTOCIN FOR LABOR INDUCTION/AUGMENTATION

Common Allegations

- Initiation of oxytocin in the absence of evidence of fetal well-being
- Failure to accurately assess maternal–fetal status during labor induction
- Excessive doses of oxytocin resulting in uterine tachysystole, with or without an indeterminate or abnormal FHR pattern

(See also FHR pattern interpretation, communication, and documentation; uterine tachysystole.)

Standards, Guidelines, and Recommendations

- Establish fetal well-being prior to initiation of oxytocin.
- Administer the lowest possible dose to achieve cervical change and labor progress (ACOG, 2009b).
- Starting at 1 to 2 mU and increasing by 1 to 2 mU/min no more frequently than every 30 to 40 minutes

will result in successful induction of labor for most women. Approximately 90% of women at term will have labor successfully induced with 6 mU/min or less (Arias, 2000).

- Based on physiologic and pharmacokinetic principles, a 30 to 40-minute interval between oxytocin dosage increases is optimal. The full effect of oxytocin on the uterine response to increases in dosage cannot be evaluated until steady-state concentration has been achieved. Increasing the infusion rate before steady-state concentration is achieved results in laboring women receiving higher than necessary doses of oxytocin, which increases risk of side effects such as uterine tachysystole and indeterminate or abnormal fetal status (Arias, 2000; Crane & Young, 1998; Phaneuf, Rodriguez-Linares, Tambyraja, MacKenzie, & Lopez Bernal, 2000).
- Titrate the dosage to the fetal response and uterine activity/labor progress (ACOG, 2009b; Simpson, 2013).
- Avoid uterine tachysystole and treat (decrease or discontinue oxytocin) in a timely manner if it occurs (ACOG, 2009b, 2010a; Simpson, 2013).
- If labor is progressing at 1 cm/hr cervical dilation, there is no need to increase the dosage rate (Crane & Young, 1998; Simpson, 2013).
- If using an active management of labor (AMOL) protocol, follow all aspects of the published protocol rather than just the oxytocin dosages and infusion frequencies. The protocol was designed to be used for nulliparous women in spontaneous active labor. The Dublin AMOL protocol is precisely described and, under these conditions, was found to be safe, although three subsequent studies in the United States (Frigoletto et al., 1995; Lopez-Zeno, Peaceman, Adashek, & Socol, 1992; Rogers, Gilson, Miller, Izquierdo, Curet, & Qualls, 1997) did not find that it led to a decrease in cesarean births: Candidates include only nulliparous women in spontaneous active labor with a singleton pregnancy, cephalic presentation, and no evidence of fetal compromise. To exclude false and prodromal labor, true labor is specifically defined as contractions with either bloody show, spontaneous rupture of membranes, or complete (100%) cervical effacement. Once labor is diagnosed, the woman receives continuous one-to-one labor support from a birth attendant (midwife). An amniotomy is performed if membranes are not spontaneously ruptured within 1 hour after labor has been diagnosed. If cervical dilation does not progress at least 1 cm/hr, oxytocin augmentation is initiated beginning at 6 mU/min, increasing by 6 mU/min every 15 minutes until adequate labor is established, to a maximum dose of 40 mU/min. "Hyperstimulation" of uterine activity is defined as more than seven contractions over 15 minutes (O'Driscoll, Jackson, & Gallagher, 1970).

- To enhance communication among members of the perinatal healthcare team and to avoid confusion, oxytocin administration rates should always be ordered by the physician or certified nurse midwife as mU/min and documented in the medical record as mU/min (Simpson, 2013).
- Ensure adequate personnel are available to monitor maternal–fetal status (ACOG, 2009b) (e.g., one nurse to one woman receiving oxytocin for labor induction or augmentation) (AWHONN, 2010).

UTERINE TACHYSYSTOLE

Common Allegations

- Failure to appropriately identify and treat uterine tachysystole (with and without an indeterminate or abnormal FHR pattern) in a timely manner
- Failure to decrease or discontinue the oxytocin infusion or delay the next dose of misoprostol during uterine tachysystole
- Physician/nurse midwife orders to continue oxytocin or administer misoprostol despite being notified of uterine tachysystole
- Failure to communicate with the physician/nurse midwife when uterine tachysystole occurs
- Failure to institute the chain of consultation when there is a clinical disagreement between the nurse and responsible physician/nurse midwife

(See also FHR pattern interpretation, communication, and documentation; elective induction of labor; misoprostol for cervical ripening/labor induction; oxytocin for labor induction/augmentation [Cytotec].)

Standards, Guidelines, and Recommendations

- A clear definition of tachysystole (e.g., a series of single contractions lasting 2 minutes or more, a contraction frequency of more than 5 in 10 minutes [averaged over 30 minutes], or contractions of normal duration occurring within 1 minute of each other [ACOG, 2003, 2009b; Macones et al., 2008; Simpson, 2013]) is essential in each institution because clinical management strategies, policies, and protocols should include expected actions when tachysystole is identified.
- All perinatal healthcare providers in each institution should be aware of clinical criteria established for tachysystole and the expected actions.
- While tachysystole can be the result of endogenous maternal oxytocin and prostaglandins, most excessive uterine activity is the result of administration of exogenous pharmacologic agents (Crane, Young, Butt, Bennett, & Hutchens, 2001).
- Treat tachysystole by decreasing or discontinuing oxytocin based on the individual clinical situation.

- Avoid prolonged periods of tachysystole that lead to progressive deterioration in fetal status (Bakker, Kurver, Kuik, & Van Geijn, 2007; Bakker & Van Geijn, 2008; Simpson & James, 2008) and subsequent indeterminate or abnormal FHR patterns (ACOG, 2010a; ACOG & AAP, 2003). Interventions for tachysystole should not be delayed until there is evidence of indeterminate or abnormal fetal status (Simpson, 2013).
- Empower and encourage all members of the perinatal team to be appropriately assertive in their actions and communications with colleagues to advocate for patient safety if they feel pressured to increase oxytocin rates during uterine tachysystole and/or indeterminate or abnormal FHR patterns (Clark, Simpson, Knox, & Garite, 2009; Simpson et al., 2006).

PAIN RELIEF DURING LABOR AND BIRTH

Common Allegations

- Failure to accurately identify and treat labor pain
- Use of "ability to pay" or insurance status as criteria for treatment of labor pain

Standards, Guidelines, and Recommendations

- Provide adequate pain relief for all women in labor as per their request regardless of ability to pay or whether they sought prenatal care (ACOG, 2006; TJC, 2012).
- Pain management is a moral imperative, a professional responsibility, and the duty of people in the healing professions (Institute of Medicine [IOM], 2011).
- Labor results in severe pain for many women. There is no other circumstance under which it is considered acceptable for a person to experience untreated severe pain, amendable to safe intervention, while under a physician's care. In the absence of a medical contraindication, maternal request is a sufficient medical indication for pain relief during labor and birth (ACOG, 2006). Maternal request represents sufficient justification for pain relief (ASA, 2007).
- The choice of technique, agent, and dosage should be based on patient preference, medical status, and contraindications. Decisions should be closely coordinated among the obstetrician, the anesthesia provider, the patient, and skilled support personnel (ACOG, 2006).
- There are conflicting data about the effect of epidural analgesia/anesthesia on the risk of cesarean birth; however, based on what is known at present, if the patient desires an epidural during the early stages of labor, there is no reason to deny that request if the denial is related to potential risk of cesarean birth (ACOG, 2006).

NURSES' ROLE DURING REGIONAL ANESTHESIA

Common Allegations

- Administration of bolus or change in medication rate of epidural anesthesia that resulted in subsequent maternal and/or fetal harm
- Nurses' actions beyond the scope of practice as defined by their professional association (AWHONN, 2012)

Standards, Guidelines, and Recommendations

- Adhere to the AWHONN clinical position statement that describes the role of the nurse during epidural anesthesia. Require that only qualified, credentialed anesthesia providers adjust the dosage for labor epidurals, including boluses, and increases or decreases in rate. Require that only qualified, credentialed anesthesia providers program the epidural pumps during regional anesthesia for labor (AWHONN, 2012).
- Acknowledge and support the responsibility of registered nurses to practice within the guidelines of their professional association. Expect that anesthesia providers will acknowledge this right and duty as well.

FUNDAL PRESSURE DURING THE SECOND STAGE OF LABOR

Common Allegations

- Application of fundal pressure during second stage of labor that resulted in shoulder dystocia and/or other maternal–fetal injuries
- Application of fundal pressure during shoulder dystocia that further affected the shoulder and delayed the birth, resulting in maternal–fetal injuries

  (See also shoulder dystocia.)

Standards, Guidelines, and Recommendations

- Fundal pressure applied during the second stage of labor is associated with risks of adverse outcomes to the mother and the baby (Simpson & Knox, 2001).
- Risks to the baby include inadvertent shoulder dystocia, which in turn places the baby at risk for brachial plexus injuries; fractures of the humerus and clavicles; hypoxemia, asphyxia, and death; an increase in fetal intracranial pressure, resulting in significant decreases in cerebral blood flow and indeterminate or abnormal FHR patterns; umbilical cord compression negatively affecting maternal–fetal exchange; functional alterations in the placental intervillous space, which increases the risk of fetal hypoxemia and

asphyxia; subgaleal hemorrhage; and spinal cord injuries (ACOG, 2002; Simpson & Knox, 2001).
- Risks to the mother include perineal injuries such as third- and fourth-degree lacerations, anal sphincter tears, uterine rupture and uterine inversion, pain, hypotension, respiratory distress, abdominal bruising, fractured ribs, and liver rupture (Simpson & Knox, 2001).
- Avoid fundal pressure to shorten an otherwise normal second stage of labor (Simpson & Knox, 2001).
- Avoid fundal pressure during shoulder dystocia (ACOG, 2002).
- Avoid clinical disagreements about fundal pressures at the bedside in front of the patient by having an agreed-upon policy.

SHOULDER DYSTOCIA

Common Allegations

- Failure to accurately predict risk of shoulder dystocia
- Failure to diagnose labor abnormalities
- Failure to appropriately initiate shoulder dystocia corrective maneuvers
- Failure to perform a cesarean birth
- Application of forceps or vacuum at high station or continued application without evidence of fetal descent, resulting in shoulder dystocia
- Application of fundal pressure during shoulder dystocia, further affecting the shoulder and delaying birth, thereby resulting in maternal–fetal injuries

(See also fundal pressure during the second stage of labor.)

Standards, Guidelines, and Recommendations

- Most cases of shoulder dystocia cannot be predicted or prevented (ACOG, 2002).
- There is no evidence that labor abnormalities are associated with risk of shoulder dystocia (ACOG, 2002).
- There is no evidence that any one maneuver is superior in releasing an impacted shoulder; however, the McRoberts maneuver and suprapubic pressure are easily implemented without an associated increase in risk of injury to the baby.
- Excess traction and fundal pressure should be avoided because of increased risk of injuries to the baby (ACOG, 2002).

SECOND-STAGE LABOR MANAGEMENT

Common Allegations

- Iatrogenic indeterminate or abnormal FHR patterns as a result of provider-coached maternal pushing efforts and/or uterine tachysystole
- Failure to appreciate deteriorating fetal status

D I S P L A Y   1 - 3

Suggestions for Medical Record Documentation (Simpson, 1999)

- Provide emergent nursing care to woman and newborn as a first priority.
- Avoid duplication in the documentation process. Ensure that documentation of the event by the provider and the nurse are in sync. The nurse may limit documentation to noting that a shoulder dystocia occurred and noting the nursing interventions, such as assisting the woman to McRoberts position and applying suprapubic pressure, while the provider may describe the head-to-body interval and maneuvers that were used.
- Provide a narrative note that summarizes the series of interventions and clinical events that have taken place, with a focus on a logical step-by-step approach to relieving the affected shoulder and resuscitating the newborn. Ideally, these data are entered by the birth attendant.
- Avoid documenting a minute-by-minute account of the emergency unless it is absolutely certain that the times included are accurate.
- Attempt to closely approximate the time interval between delivery of fetal head and body if possible.
- Review the EFM strip and talk with other providers in attendance to ensure the most accurate details of clinical circumstances are accurately recorded.
- Include fetal assessment data and/or attempts to obtain data about fetal status during the maneuvers.
- List the order of each maneuver used in clear and precise terms. Ideally, these data are entered by the birth attendant.
- Note that nursing assistance with these maneuvers was provided under the direction of the physician or nurse midwife.
- If suprapubic pressure was used, make sure it is noted as such to avoid later allegations of fundal pressure.
- If the baby appears depressed at birth, consider obtaining arterial cord blood gases.

- Failure to act on deteriorating fetal status by modifying maternal pushing efforts and initiating the usual intrauterine resuscitation measures
- Failure to anticipate resuscitation needs of baby after an indeterminate or abnormal FHR pattern during the second stage of labor
- Injuries to the perineum that resulted in perineal lacerations, loss of pelvic floor integrity, and sexual dysfunction

Standards, Guidelines, and Recommendations

- Follow ACOG (2000) and AWHONN (2008) recommendations for second-stage management.
- Develop common expectations among team members concerning when to begin pushing and how to encourage women to push.

- The active phase of second-stage labor is a period of stress for the fetus; thus, efforts should be made to minimize that stress by shortening the active pushing phase and using appropriate pushing techniques (AWHONN, 2008; Barnett & Humenick, 1982; Nordstrom, Achanna, Nuka, & Arulkumaran, 2001; Piquard, Schaefer, Hsiung, Dellenbach, & Haberey, 1989; Roberts, 2002).
- Women with epidural anesthesia who do not feel the urge to push at 10 cm cervical dilation should be allowed to rest until the fetus has descended enough to stimulate the urge to push (up to 2 hours for nulliparous women and up to 1 hour for multiparous women) (Fraser et al., 2000; Roberts, Torvaldsen, Cameron, & Olive, 2004). There is evidence to suggest that for women with epidurals, coached pushing does not significantly decrease the length of the second stage (Fraser et al., 2000; Hansen, Clark, & Foster, 2002; Mayberry, Hammer, Kelly, True-Driver, & De, 1999). Passive fetal descent will result in about the same length of the second stage for women with epidural analgesia/anesthesia as does the coached pushing approach.
- When the urge to push is noted, women should be encouraged to bear down as long as they can at the peak of the contraction, no more than three to four times per contraction (Mayberry, Gennaro, Strange, Williams, & De, 1999; Roberts, 2002).
- Women should not be told to take a deep breath and hold it while the care provider counts to 10 (AWHONN, 2008; Caldeyro-Barcia, 1979; Caldeyro-Barcia et al., 1981; Nordstrom et al., 2001; Sampselle & Hines, 1999; Simpson & James, 2005a). Discourage breath holding longer than 6 to 8 seconds per pushing effort (AWHONN, 2008; Barnett & Humenick, 1982; Roberts, 2002).
- Women should be assisted to appropriate positions for pushing, such as upright, semi-Fowlers, lateral, and squatting (AWHONN, 2008; Mayberry, Strange, Suplee, & Gennaro, 2003; Roberts, Algert, Cameron, & Torvaldsen, 2005). The supine lithotomy position and stirrups should not be used during pushing efforts (AWHONN, 2008; Tubridy & Redmond, 1996; Wong et al., 2003).
- The woman's knees should not be forcibly pushed back against her abdomen in positions that stretch the perineum or risk joint or nerve injury; rather, the woman should be allowed to position herself for comfort or keep her feet flat on the bed as desired (Simpson & James, 2005a; Tubridy & Redmond, 1996).
- Repetitive pushing efforts should not be encouraged if the FHR is indeterminate or abnormal. Instead, women should be coached to push with every other or every third contraction to maintain a stable baseline FHR and allow the fetus to recover between pushes (Simpson & James, 2005a). If the fetus is not responding well to coached pushing, stop pushing temporarily and let the fetus recover (AWHONN, 2008; Simpson & James, 2005a).
- Uterine tachysystole should be avoided during the second stage and the same intrauterine resuscitation techniques used during the first stage labor should be used during the second stage (Simpson & James, 2005a).
- As in the first stage of labor, the FHR pattern during the second stage should be used as an indicator of how well the fetus is responding. It is important to recognize indeterminate or abnormal FHR patterns and intervene appropriately. It is known that recurrent late and variable decelerations during the second stage are associated with respiratory acidemia at birth (Parer, King, Flanders, Fox, & Kilpatrick, 2006). Some fetuses may develop metabolic acidemia if this type of pattern continues over a long period (Parer et al., 2006). These babies are difficult to resuscitate and may not transition well to extrauterine life.

FORCEPS- AND VACUUM-ASSISTED BIRTH

Common Allegations

- Application of forceps/vacuum at high station that results in maternal–fetal injury
- Inappropriate timing or application of forceps, resulting in fetal injuries such as fractured skull, intracranial bleed, or facial paralysis
- Use of excessive force during a forceps- or vacuum-assisted birth
- Use of a vacuum for rotation of the fetal head
- Use of excessive pressures during a vacuum-assisted birth
- Excessive time of vacuum application

Standards, Guidelines, and Recommendations

- Adhere to ACOG (2000) indications for operative vaginal birth. No indication for operative vaginal birth is absolute; however, the following indications apply when the fetal head is engaged and the cervix is fully dilated: prolonged second stage for nulliparous women with lack of continuing progress for 3 hours with regional anesthesia or 2 hours without regional anesthesia, and prolonged second stage for multiparous women with lack of continued progress for 2 hours with regional anesthesia or 1 hour without regional anesthesia; suspicion of immediate or potential fetal compromise; and shortening of the second stage for maternal benefit.
- Operative vaginal birth should only be performed by individuals with privileges for such procedures and

in settings in which personnel are readily available to perform a cesarean birth in the event that operative vaginal birth is unsuccessful (ACOG, 2000).

Forceps–Assisted Vaginal Birth

- Adhere to ACOG (2000) criteria for types of forceps births:
  - *Outlet forceps:* The fetal scalp is visible at the introitus without separating the labia, the fetal skull has reached the pelvic floor, the sagittal suture is in anterior–posterior diameter or right or left occiput anterior or posterior position, the fetal head is at or on the perineum, and rotation does not exceed 45°.
  - *Low forceps:* The leading point of the fetal skull is at station ≥+2 cm and not on the pelvic floor, rotation is 45° or less (left or right occiput anterior to occiput anterior, or left or right occiput posterior to occiput posterior), and rotation is greater than 45°.
  - *Midforceps:* The station is above +2 cm but fetal head is engaged.
  - *High forceps:* This type is not included in classification and should not be permitted or attempted.

Vacuum–Assisted Vaginal Birth

- Follow the manufacturer's guidelines for the vacuum device being used. Generally, using no more than 600 mm Hg pressure and abandoning the procedure after three pop-offs and/or 20 minutes maximum total time of application is consistent with safe care and a decreased risk of fetal injuries (Bofill et al., 1996; Bofill, Martin, & Morrison, 1998).
- The vacuum pressure should not exceed 500 to 600 mm Hg, and the pressure should be released as soon as the contraction ends and the woman stops pushing (Brumfield, Gilstrap, O'Grady, Ross, & Schifrin, 1999).
- As a general guideline, progress in descent should accompany each traction attempt and no more than three pulls should be attempted (ACOG, 2000; Bofill et al., 1996; Bofill et al., 1998; Brumfield et al., 1999). Traction is only when the woman is actively pushing.
- The vacuum procedure should be timed from the moment of insertion of the cup into the vagina until birth and should not be on the fetal head for longer than 20 to 30 minutes (Bofill et al., 1998; Brumfield et al., 1999).
- When the cup has been applied at maximum pressure for more than 10 minutes, the rate of fetal injuries increases (Brumfield et al., 1999); thus, while total time of cup application can be between 20 and 30 minutes, the time of maximum pressure force should not exceed 10 minutes (Paluska, 1997).

- As with forceps, there should be a willingness to abandon attempts at a vacuum-assisted birth if satisfactory progress is not made. Three pop-offs, evidence of fetal scalp trauma, and/or no descent with appropriate application and traction should warrant abandoning the vacuum procedure (Bofill et al., 1998).
- The FDA (1998) recommendations for vacuum-assisted birth include rocking movements or torque should not be applied to the device; only steady traction in the line of the birth canal should be used and clinicians caring for the baby should be alerted that a vacuum device has been used so that they can adequately monitor the baby for the signs and symptoms of device-related injuries.
- Vacuum-assisted vaginal birth should not be performed before 34 weeks' gestation (ACOG, 2000).
- Persistent efforts to achieve a vaginal birth using different instruments may increase the potential for maternal and fetal injury. The incidence of injuries increase with combined methods (forceps and vacuum) of operative vaginal birth (ACOG, 2000).

VAGINAL BIRTH AFTER CESAREAN BIRTH (VBAC)

Common Allegations

- Failure to fully inform a woman with a history of a prior cesarean birth or uterine scar of risks and benefits of a trial of labor for VBAC
- Use of prostaglandin agents for cervical ripening or labor induction for a woman with a history of a prior cesarean birth or uterine scar that results in uterine rupture
- Use of excessive doses of oxytocin during labor induction or augmentation that results in uterine rupture
- Failure to have a heightened awareness of and identify signs and symptoms of uterine rupture such as indeterminate or abnormal changes in the FHR pattern
- Failure to treat uterine rupture in a timely manner
- Failure to have appropriate personnel and equipment in house during trial of labor for VBAC

Standards, Guidelines, and Recommendations

- Adhere to ACOG (2010b) recommendations for appropriate candidates (e.g., one or two prior low-transverse cesarean births, clinically adequate pelvis, no other uterine scars or previous rupture).
- Avoid use of prostaglandin agents for cervical ripening and labor induction (ACOG, 2010b).
- Avoid excessive use of oxytocin and tachysystole if labor induction is indicated (ACOG, 2010b).

- Ensure that a full surgical team (obstetrician/surgeon, surgical first assistant, anesthesia provider, scrub technician, circulating nurse, and personnel skilled in neonatal resuscitation) is in house during a trial of labor for patients attempting a VBAC (ACOG, 2010b).

MULTIPLE GESTATION

Common Allegations

- Failure to transfer care of high-risk pregnancy to appropriate healthcare provider or tertiary center
- Failure to diagnose multiple gestation
- Failure to determine chorionicity of multiple gestation
- Failure to accurately monitor all fetuses during labor and birth
- Failure to have in place appropriate personnel and equipment during birth of multiple gestation

Standards, Guidelines, and Recommendations

- Determine chorionicity during prenatal period using high-resolution ultrasound techniques by practitioners experienced with this technique.
- Anticipate vaginal birth if both twins are vertex; other presentations and higher-order multiples are usually delivered via cesarean birth.
- Attempt to continuously monitor all fetuses during the first and second stages of labor. This may be challenging with higher-order multiples.
- Have ultrasound equipment immediately available in the labor room to determine fetal presentation during the second stage of labor.
- Have personnel standing by in house for neonatal resuscitation and anesthesia during the second stage of labor.

IATROGENIC PREMATURITY

Common Allegations

- Failure to follow the ACOG (2009b) recommendations for gestational age for elective induction of labor or repeat cesarean section, resulting in iatrogenic prematurity and subsequent neonatal morbidity, neurological injury, or death
- Failure to accurately determine the gestational age prior to elective repeat cesarean birth or elective induction of labor

Standards, Guidelines, and Recommendations

- Avoid elective induction of labor and elective cesarean birth before 39 weeks of gestation (ACOG, 2009b). (See Elective Induction of Labor.)

PREVENTION OF PERINATAL GROUP B STREPTOCOCCAL DISEASE

Common Allegations

- Failure to adhere to the CDC guidelines for GBS prophylaxis, resulting in neonatal infection and subsequent neonatal neurological damage or death

Standards, Guidelines, and Recommendations

- Universal screening of all pregnant women at 35 to 37 weeks of gestation is the recommendation from the CDC (2010) for identifying those that would benefit from intrapartum GBS prophylaxis. These recommendations are supported by ACOG (2011b).
- All women in whom cultures are positive for GBS are to be given intrapartum antibiotic prophylaxis in labor unless a cesarean birth is performed before onset of labor in a woman with intact amniotic membranes.
- Cultures for GBS are not required in women who have group B streptococcal bacteriuria during the current pregnancy or who have previously given birth to a neonate with early-onset group B streptococcal disease because these women should receive intrapartum antibiotic prophylaxis.
- If at any time during pregnancy group B streptococcal bacteriuria is detected, antibiotics should be administered.
- Because women who had GBS colonization during a previous pregnancy are likely not to be colonized during subsequent pregnancies, they require culture evaluation for GBS with each pregnancy but not intrapartum antibiotic prophylaxis unless there is an indication for GBS prophylaxis during the current pregnancy.
- Refer to the entire recommendations from the CDC (2010) for specific details for identification of candidates for intrapartum prophylaxis and treatment of the newborn.

NEONATAL RESUSCITATION AT BIRTH

Common Allegations

- Failure to anticipate resuscitation needs of a baby whose mother experienced pregnancy complications and/or after an indeterminate or abnormal FHR pattern during labor
- Failure to have appropriate personnel and equipment available for neonatal resuscitation

Standards, Guidelines, and Recommendations

- All members of the perinatal team who are involved in labor and birth should have successfully completed the neonatal resuscitation course sponsored by AAP and the American Heart Association (AHA) (AAP & AHA, 2011).

- There should be one person at every birth whose primary responsibility is the baby and who is capable of initiating resuscitation (AAP & AHA, 2011).
- Either that professional or an alternate who is immediately available should have the skills required to perform a complete resuscitation, including endotracheal intubation and administration of medications (AAP & AHA, 2011).
- When resuscitation is needed, it must be initiated without delay. It is not sufficient to have someone on call (either at home or in a remote area of the hospital) for newborn resuscitation in the delivery room (AAP & AHA, 2011).
- If the birth is anticipated to be high risk, and thus may require more advanced resuscitation, at least two persons should be present solely to manage the baby: one with complete resuscitation skills and one or more to assist (AHA & AAP, 2011).

NURSE STAFFING

Common Allegations

- Failure to provide adequate registered nurse staffing to safely meet the needs of the perinatal unit, resulting in patient harm

Standards, Guidelines, and Recommendations

- *Guidelines for Professional Registered Nurse Staffing for Perinatal Units* (AWHONN, 2010) provide information for nurse staffing based on types of clinical situations and patients common in perinatal units (See Table 1–3). Refer to the *Guidelines* for specific details.
- Implement critical components of a well-designed nursing workforce that mutually reinforce patient safeguards, including the following: a nurse staffing plan with evidence that it is adequately resourced and actively managed and that its effectiveness is regularly evaluated with respect to patient safety (NQF, 2010; TJC, 2012). Senior administrative nursing leaders, such as a chief nursing officer, should be part of the hospital senior management team. Governance boards and senior administrative leaders should take accountability for reducing patient safety risks related to nurse staffing decisions and the provision of financial resources for nursing services. Provision of budgetary resources to support nursing staff in the ongoing acquisition and maintenance of professional knowledge and skills is required (NQF, 2010).

CONFLICT RESOLUTION

No group of individuals can work together in an organization and always share the same expectations, goals, and identical perspectives. Conflict is an inevitable result when reality does not meet with individual expectations. While individual expectations may differ, usually there exists among caregivers a basic commitment to quality and to the best possible outcomes for mothers and babies. Mutual trust and respect and the capacity to engage in agreeable disagreement are the hallmarks of a professional unit. When involved in a clinical or administrative situation that can potentially cause conflict, consider that both parties probably have the best interests of the patient in mind, although there may be different approaches proposed to achieve that goal. At times, clinical practice issues arise when the "way we've always done it" conflicts with a new or an alternate approach. Alternatively, all of the clinicians involved may not have the same perception of risk of patient harm; thus, they may have differing views of the next course of action (Lyndon et al., 2012).

If the conflict is not related to an emergent patient situation (e.g., there is at least some time for discussion), effective communication techniques can enhance the chances of conflict resolution to the satisfaction of both parties, or at least to reach a workable compromise. Taking time to really listen and understand the intent of the other person is a helpful starting point. While others express their concerns, give visual and verbal feedback to ensure that they know you take them seriously. For example, nod or say, "I see, please go on," or summarize what it is the other person is concerned about by saying, "Let me see if I understand you correctly." Then use phrases such as, "I have a different perspective." This usually works better in conflict resolution than, "You are wrong." Other successful strategies include a calm, collected attitude and careful consideration of the goal to be accomplished.

Communication in conflict resolution may not always be so rational and under one's control. This is especially true when dealing with difficult people, particularly those who are hostile or aggressive. These individuals manifest behavior that is abusive, abrupt, intimidating, and overwhelming. Being confronted by this behavior often catches the victim by surprise and generates feelings of helplessness. When being attacked, stand up for yourself and command respect. Calmly wait for the person to stop, then jump in. Use words that express your assertiveness. For example, say, "I am willing to discuss this with you when you are ready to speak to me with respect." This may help stop the verbal attack and allow time for more respectful discussion when the other person is rational.

Table 1–3. GUIDELINES FOR PROFESSIONAL REGISTERED NURSE STAFFING FOR PERINATAL UNITS[†]

Nurse-to-Woman or Nurse-to-Baby Ratio	Care Provided
Antepartum	
1:2–3	Women during nonstress testing
1:1	Woman presenting for initial obstetric triage
1:2–3	Women in obstetric triage after initial assessment and in stable condition
1:3	Women with antepartum complications in stable condition
1:1	Woman with antepartum complications who is unstable
1:1	Continuous bedside attendance for woman receiving IV magnesium sulfate for the first hour of administration for preterm labor prophylaxis and no more than 1 additional couplet or woman for a nurse caring for a woman receiving IV magnesium sulfate in a maintenance dose
1:2	Women receiving pharmacologic agents for cervical ripening
Intrapartum	
1:1	Woman with medical (such as diabetes, pulmonary or cardiac disease, or morbid obesity) or obstetric (such as preeclampsia, multiple gestation, fetal demise, indeterminate or abnormal FHR pattern, women having a trial of labor attempting vaginal birth after cesarean birth) complications during labor
1:1	Woman receiving oxytocin during labor
1:1	Woman laboring with minimal to no pain relief or medical interventions
1:1	Woman whose fetus is being monitored via intermittent auscultation
1:1	Continuous bedside nursing attendance to woman receiving IV magnesium sulfate for the first hour of administration; one nurse to one woman ratio during labor and until at least 2 hours postpartum and no more than one additional couplet or woman in the patient assignment for a nurse caring for a woman receiving IV magnesium sulfate during postpartum
1:1	Continuous bedside nursing attendance during initiation of regional anesthesia until condition is stable (at least for the first 30 minutes after initial dose)
1:1	Continuous bedside nursing attendance to woman during the active pushing phase of second-stage labor
1:2	Women in labor without complications
2:1	Birth; one nurse responsible for the mother and one nurse whose sole responsibility is the baby
Postpartum and Newborn Care	
1:1	Continuous bedside nursing attendance to woman in the immediate postoperative recovery period (for at least 2 hours)
1:3	Mother–baby couplets after the 2-hour recovery period (with consideration for assignments with mixed acuity rather than all recent post-cesarean cases)
1:2	Women on the immediate postoperative day who are recovering from cesarean birth as part of the nurse to patient ratio of one nurse to three mother–baby couplets
1:5–6	Women postpartum without complications (no more than two to three women on the immediate postoperative day who are recovering from cesarean birth as part of the nurse to patient ratio of one nurse to five to six women without complications)
1:3	Women postpartum with complications who are stable
1:5–6	Healthy newborns in the nursery requiring only routine care whose mothers cannot or do not desire to keep their baby in the postpartum room
1	At least one nurse physically present at all times in each occupied basic care nursery when babies are physically present in the nursery
1:1	Newborn boy undergoing circumcision or other surgical procedures during the immediate preoperative, intraoperative, and immediate postoperative periods
1:3–4	Newborns requiring continuing care
1:2–3	Newborns requiring intermediate care
1:1–2	Newborns requiring intensive care
1:1	Newborn requiring multisystem support
1:1 or greater	Unstable newborn requiring complex critical care
1	At least one nurse available at all times with skills to care for newborns who may develop complications and/or need resuscitation
Minimum Staffing	
2	A minimum of two nurses as minimum staffing even when there are no perinatal patients, in order to be able to safety care for a woman who presents with an obstetric emergency that may require cesarean birth (one nurse circulator; one baby nurse, one or both of whom should have obstetric triage, labor, and fetal assessment skills). A scrub nurse or surgical tech should be available in house or on call such that an emergent birth can be accomplished within 30 minutes of the decision to proceed. Another labor nurse should be called in to be available to care for any other pregnant woman who may present for care while the first two nurses are caring for the woman undergoing cesarean birth and during post-anesthesia recovery.

[†] It should be recognized that these staffing ratios represent minimal staffing, require further consideration based on acuity and needs of the service, and assume that there will be ancillary personnel to support the nurse.

From Association of Women's Health, Obstetric and Neonatal Nurses. (2010). *Guidelines for professional registered nurse staffing for perinatal units.* Washington, DC: Author.

Selecting the best time and place for interaction is also essential. Ideally, the setting will not allow opportunity for patients, family members, or other colleagues to overhear the discussion. The focus of the discussion should remain on the issue, preferably on the potential impact on patient care. If the conversation deteriorates beyond your personal capacity to handle it or the colleague becomes verbally abusive, end the discussion until a later time and inform a third party who has the ability to help or the responsibility to know about the interaction. An important strategy for promoting positive long-term professional collaboration is the development of interdisciplinary specialty practice opportunities where colleagues can come together to work toward a common goal. This can include developing unit guidelines, learning from a case review or grand rounds, examining quality of research findings, designing unit projects, or discussing conflict resolution. When colleagues come together to identify problems, define objectives, address alternatives, integrate changes, remain patient focused, disagree agreeably, negotiate, demonstrate mutual respect, and recognize and praise positive attributes and actions, it facilitates a professional culture for positive conflict resolution.

Some issues of conflict in the clinical setting cannot be solved at the lowest level and do not allow the luxury of time. If, after careful deliberation, the issue is determined to be a matter of maternal/fetal well-being or there is potential for the clinical situation to deteriorate rapidly, the nurse must initiate an appropriate course of action. One example is failure of the physician to respond to an abnormal FHR pattern or deteriorating maternal condition. Decisive, timely nursing intervention may be necessary to avoid a potentially adverse outcome. Knowledge and the use of the chain of consultation are ways to attempt to resolve differences of opinion in clinical practice settings. An example of chain of consultation is presented in Figure 1–1. If discussions with the physician or certified nurse midwife (CNM) do not result in care appropriate for the clinical practice situation, the nurse has the responsibility to use the perinatal unit institutional chain of consultation to avoid harm to the mother and/or baby. Frequently, this involves the staff nurse notifying the appropriate,

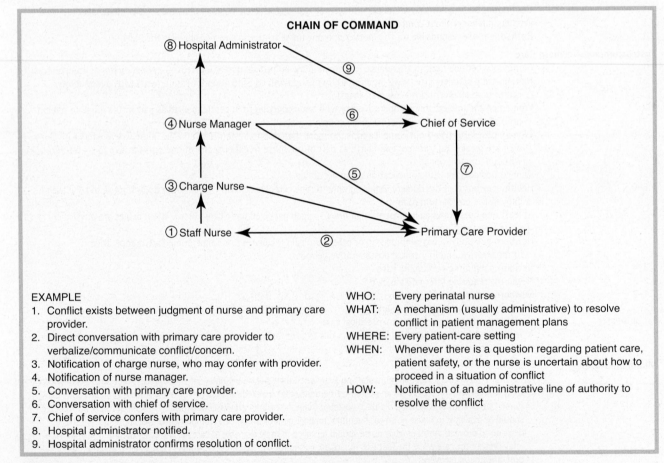

CHAIN OF COMMAND

⑧ Hospital Administrator

④ Nurse Manager   ⑥   Chief of Service

③ Charge Nurse

① Staff Nurse   ②   Primary Care Provider

EXAMPLE
1. Conflict exists between judgment of nurse and primary care provider.
2. Direct conversation with primary care provider to verbalize/communicate conflict/concern.
3. Notification of charge nurse, who may confer with provider.
4. Notification of nurse manager.
5. Conversation with primary care provider.
6. Conversation with chief of service.
7. Chief of service confers with primary care provider.
8. Hospital administrator notified.
9. Hospital administrator confirms resolution of conflict.

WHO: Every perinatal nurse
WHAT: A mechanism (usually administrative) to resolve conflict in patient management plans
WHERE: Every patient-care setting
WHEN: Whenever there is a question regarding patient care, patient safety, or the nurse is uncertain about how to proceed in a situation of conflict
HOW: Notification of an administrative line of authority to resolve the conflict

FIGURE 1–1. Each perinatal care setting should have its own administrative chain of consultation to assist in conflict resolution in the management of patients. Such a chain of command is illustrated here. Adapted from Chez, B. F., Harvey, C. J., & Murray, M. L. (1990). *Critical concepts in fetal heart rate monitoring.* (p. 32). Baltimore: Lippincott Williams & Wilkins.

immediately available supervisory nurse (e.g., charge nurse, nurse manager, or nursing supervisor) to provide assistance. In selected instances, it may be necessary to go further up the chain of consultation to resolve the situation. This process may require more time than the situation can accommodate. In other words, invoking the complete use of the chain of consultation is generally most successful when there is an urgent situation (e.g., progressively deteriorating FHR status) rather than an overt emergency (e.g., shoulder dystocia).

Institutions have a responsibility to support nurses who use the chain of consultation. Nurses may be reluctant to invoke this process due to intimidation, sense of personal or professional jeopardy, fear of retribution, or lack of confidence in the institutional lines of authority and responsibility. Medical hierarchy can be a powerful deterrent to speaking up when appropriate and following through on concerns about care that may not be in the best interests of the patient (Simpson & Lyndon, 2009). When all team members are not in agreement regarding potential risk of harm to the mother and/or baby, it can be a challenge to successfully advocate for a particular course of care. Speaking up in this context may be difficult, and successful resolution of the clinical conflict may not always occur (Lyndon et al., 2012). It is important that nurses and physicians know the institution's policy for chain of consultation, data about its use be collected and analyzed so that the process can be optimized, and personnel receive positive feedback for its appropriate use. Chain of consultation should not be the routine method of conflict resolution. Clinical disagreements that result in going up the chain are detrimental to nurse-physician relationships. Soon after a clinical disagreement that results in use of the chain of consultation, all those involved should meet and calmly discuss what happened and why. Having an objective third party such as the risk manager present during this discussion may facilitate the interaction. Prospective plans should then be developed to avoid this situation in the future. A positive corporate culture that includes selected use of the chain of consultation recognizes that when personnel are given the resources, support, and guidance that are necessary to carry out the responsibilities of their positions, everyone generally benefits: the institution, its employees, the medical staff, and the patients.

TEAM TRAINING AND DRILLS FOR OBSTETRIC EMERGENCIES

Positive long-term professional collaboration may also be enhanced by team-building exercises that focus on how clinicians work together to handle obstetric or neonatal emergencies. Interdisciplinary team training for obstetric and neonatal emergencies using in situ simulation is an effective learning method that reinforces the value of becoming an expert team member (Miller, Riley, Davis, & Hansen, 2008; Riley et al., 2008). Some hospitals and healthcare systems have found it valuable to provide interdisciplinary education on the principles of patient safety and communication skills. These educational sessions are often offered as a component of team training for obstetric and neonatal emergency drills. Crew resource training or Team STEPPS is one such curriculum and is available from AHRQ (2007); however, team training programs can be developed in house or arranged from private vendors. Team training involves the application of instructional strategies based on well-tested tools such as simulation, lectures, and videos to a specific set of skills (AHRQ, 2005). Effective team training reflects general learning theory principles, presents information about requisite team behaviors, affords team members the necessary skills practice, and provides them with remedial feedback (AHRQ, 2005). A team's utility and efficiency is tied directly to its team members and their ability to integrate various personal and situational characteristics. Each team member must understand the technical and tactical considerations of the required tasks for the specific clinical event, as well as the strengths and weaknesses of his or her teammates. In addition to carrying out his or her own responsibilities and altering them when necessary, each member must also monitor his or her teammates' activities and diffuse potential team conflicts. Effective teams exhibit these skills while maintaining a positive emotional attitude toward the team itself (AHRQ, 2005). Skills required for effective interdisciplinary team work are listed in Table 1–4.

Team training usually includes structured processes for communication such as team meetings, team huddles, care hand offs, and briefings and debriefings to facilitate information exchange and effective patient hand offs as well as working together efficiently during emergent events. Kaplan and Ballard (2012) summarized various types of structured communication processes used in healthcare. They include:

- SBAR (situation, background, assessment, recommendation), which provides a framework for communicating information that requires a clinician's immediate attention and action in a specific, structured format;
- DESC (describe, express, specify, consequences) as a method of conflict resolution;
- "Two-challenge rule" by which a patient safety concern must be raised a second time if it has gone unacknowledged and/or uncorrected;
- "Check backs" that require the receiver of an order or instruction to repeat it back to the sender to ensure it was clearly transmitted and understood;
- "Callouts" during an emergency when critical steps in a procedure are announced to team members so

Table 1–4. SKILLS REQUIRED FOR EFFECTIVE INTERDISCIPLINARY TEAM WORK

Competency	Definition	Behavioral Example
Situational awareness	Conscious, mindful observation of one's own environment or recognition of patient condition	Circulator entering the OR for Code CS becomes "task saturated" and "multitasks" for patient preparation. Situational awareness is maintained when he or she asks for help.
Closed-loop communication	Communication to a specific person that is acknowledged by the receiver and then affirmed by the sender (e.g., VORB)	Physician speaks to RN by name, requests 2 units of O-negative blood STAT. The RN replies, "I will order 2 units of O neg blood." Affirmed by physician.
SBAR-R	Technique of communication about a critical situation that involves clear specification of Situation–Background–Assessment–Recommendation–Response	S: The patient has intense supra pubic pain, bleeding. B: She is a VBAC. A: I think she may be rupturing. R: Do you want me to call the OR team for a Code CS? R: When can I expect you?
Shared mental model	A team trait characterized by an articulated common understanding of the problem and/or the plan. Everyone "being in the same movie."	Code Blue for a mother with amniotic fluid emboli—OB states: How long has she "been down"? "If there is no response, we need to get her into the OR within 5 minutes to save the baby." The Code team agrees.
Leadership and leadership transfer	Explicit handoff of responsibility or providing direction from one team member to another when team reforms or mission changes	The anesthesiologist calls out to the obstetrician: "Rx given, intubating now, you can 'cut'."
Team formation/ reformation	Assembly of a group of persons with special expertise to execute a specific task/addition or deletion of team members directly involved in the event.	Entering OR for a Code CS, the obstetrician speaks to the neonatal nurse practitioner: "This mother is a VBAC, term, may be rupturing, FHR has been 60 for 9 minutes."

FHR, fetal heart rate; OR, operation room; RN, registered nurse; STAT, immediate; VBAC, vaginal birth after cesarean; VORB, verbal order read back.
From Agency for Healthcare Research and Quality. (2007). *Team STEPPS curriculum.* Rockville, MD: Author; Riley, W., Hanson, H., Gurses, A., Davies, S., Miller, K., & Priester, R. (2008). The nature, characteristics, and patterns of perinatal critical events teams. In K. Henriksen, J. B. Battles, M. A. Keyes, & M. L. Grady (Eds.), *Advances in Patient Safety: New Directions and Alternative Approaches* (Vol. 3, pp. 131–144). Rockville, MD: Agency for Healthcare Research and Quality.

everyone is clear where they are in a given situation, and so the next step can be anticipated; and

- "Stop the line" in which a coded expression is chosen by the team to be used in front of a patient and understood by all team members to indicate a patient safety concern.

Healthcare organizations should establish a proactive, systematic, organization-wide approach to developing team-based care through teamwork training, skill building, and team-led performance improvement interventions that reduce preventable harm to patients (NQF, 2010). TJC (2004) recommends conducting team training in perinatal areas to teach staff to work together and communicate more effectively. For high-risk events, such as shoulder dystocia, emergency cesarean birth, maternal hemorrhage, and neonatal resuscitation, clinical drills should be conducted to help the team prepare for when such events actually occur along with debriefings to evaluate team performance and identify areas for improvement (JCAHO, 2004). These drills can be used to educate the clinical team regarding protocols, to refine local protocols, and to identify and fix systems problems that would prevent optimal care (TJC, 2010). In a study of team training for obstetrical emergencies, multiple institutional and unit policies and practices were identified during the

team training process that required revision to make care safer and more efficient (Andreatta, Frankel, Smith, Bullough, & Marzano, 2011). Hospitals and healthcare systems have reported success in reducing adverse events and professional liability by incorporating team training and obstetrical drills as a part of a comprehensive obstetrical patient safety program (Grunebaum, Chervenak, & Skupski, 2011; Pettker et al., 2009; Simpson, Kortz, & Knox, 2009; Wagner et al., 2012). As approximately 70% of adverse events in obstetrics can be linked to poor communication or miscommunication (JCAHO, 2004), team training and practice in handling obstetric and neonatal emergencies as an effective team have the potential to increase the likelihood that all caregivers know how to communicate and act on information shared in the clinical setting to decrease risk of patient harm (ACOG, 2011b).

PATIENT HANDOFFS

The "handoff" or transfer of patient care from one provider to another is a common procedure occurring multiple times each day in the healthcare setting, yet it is prone to errors and omissions that have the potential to negatively affect outcomes (Patterson, Roth, Woods, Chow, & Orlando, 2004). A report from AHRQ (2012) with results from 567,703 staff members from 1,128 U.S. hospitals found that 80% of hospital staff felt there was strong teamwork within units, but only 45% of hospital staff had positive perceptions of handoffs and transitions of care.

Care information should be transmitted and appropriately documented in a timely manner and in a clearly understandable form to patients and to all of the patient's healthcare providers/professionals, within and between care settings, who need that information to provide continued care (NQF, 2010). The healthcare organization should develop safe, effective communication strategies, structures, and systems to include the following: for verbal or telephone orders or for telephonic reporting of critical test results, verify the complete order or test result by having the person who is receiving the information record and "read back" the complete order or test result (NQF, 2010). A standardized list of "Do Not Use" abbreviations, acronyms, symbols, and dose designations that cannot be used throughout the organization should be developed and widely disseminated throughout the clinical areas to enhance safe communication among all members of the team (NQF, 2010; TJC, 2012). Ideally, the hand-off process occurs in a setting where the discussion is uninterrupted and free from distractions. However, in a busy unit, this is not often possible. Maintaining a focus on key aspects of care and treatment that need to be passed on can promote a concise discussion that can be accomplished within the time constraints of competing responsibilities and other required activities.

The associated risks related to hand offs are frequently unappreciated until there is an adverse event determined to be due to miscommunication between providers during a transition in patient care (Simpson, 2005b). Although the hand-off process is meant to promote continuity and efficiency, there are inherent vulnerabilities due to the human factors involved in the relay of critical information. Often, substantive portions of the communicated data are not transferred to the other professional as intended. A method to verify that the information has been received accurately via read back or by repeating key points of the assessment and plan should be included (ACOG, 2012). Ideally, the information transfer is uninterrupted and interactive (ACOG, 2012). Other industries have developed strategies to increase the likelihood that accurate and comprehensive information is transferred and that information is received and fully understood (Patterson et al., 2004). Some of these strategies are listed in Display 1–4 and others have been added and adapted to perinatal care.

Board rounds or huddles with as many members of the team in attendance as possible offer the opportunity to share perspectives on ongoing patient status with others and get updates on changes in the plan of care. The

---

DISPLAY 1 – 4

Strategies for Promoting Safe Handoffs

- Use face-to-face communication whenever possible with interactive questioning encouraged.
- Use "read backs" for verifying telephone communications and orders.
- Limit interruptions during updates and hand offs.
- Develop protocols for what type and amount of information must be included in a hand off for each clinical situation (i.e., labor, postpartum and newborn care).
- Solicit outgoing team's opinions about ongoing patient status and contingency plans for various potential variations in clinical condition.
- Assess patient status together (incoming and outgoing providers) at the bedside.
- Provide written summary of critical information.
- Ensure incoming providers have knowledge and access to the most up-to-date information.
- Ensure an unambiguous transfer of responsibility for key tasks that are left undone.
- Delay transfer of care responsibility when there is concern about status of the process or the ability of the incoming provider to safely handle the situation.
- During emergencies, remain involved until there is assurance and evidence that each piece of critical information has been accurately transferred and received by all members of the accepting team.
- Use role playing to teach new nurses how to effectively communicate during hand offs.
- Regularly observe hand offs in progress to evaluate the process and develop ideas for improvement.
- Use hand offs that are ideal and less than ideal as learning opportunities.

Adapted from Simpson, K. R. (2005). Handling handoffs safely. *MCN: The American Journal of Maternal Child Nursing, 30*(2), 76.

---

number and type of participants varies with the level of service offered and patient volume. For example, in a busy level III perinatal service, board rounds in the labor and birth unit can include the charge nurse, staff nurses, the clinical nurse specialist, resident physicians in training, the anesthesia provider, attending physicians, and representatives from the neonatal intensive care unit. Some labor and birth units conduct board rounds each day at 9 am and 9 pm while other units may choose times that meet their individual needs. Board rounds also work well for mother–baby units and neonatal units. Convening the team periodically each day to discuss clinical care may be beneficial in promoting teamwork and patient safety.

Handing off care at the bedside or bedside reporting has several benefits, including involving the patient and family members in the plan of care and providing the opportunity to see patients at the beginning of the shift (Griffin, 2010). With bedside reporting, patients and family members feel a part of the care transition and may appreciate the chance for input. Patients and family members may offer additional information from direct observation that is critical to the diagnosis, ongoing treatment plan, evaluation of patient status, and progress toward preparing for discharge (Griffin, 2010).

To ensure patient safety system robustness during hand offs, the perinatal team should develop and continually reevaluate effective communication and coordination strategies (Patterson et al., 2004). This is particularly important in emergent situations where the stress and stakes are high. The fresh perspective of the oncoming team can be helpful in reviewing the current plan. Open interaction about prior, ongoing, and expected maternal–fetal status should be encouraged. The hand-off process can be used to share experiences and expert knowledge of clinical situations and implications of patient assessment data with nurses new to the specialty (Simpson, 2005b). Critical thinking and professional nursing practice are enhanced when there is effective, efficient, and collegial communication during the shift report.

CHECKLISTS

Various types of checklists have been used prior to surgery for many years, usually individualized by each unit or institution. The preoperative checklist has been useful in making sure the history and physician examination and all of the patient's laboratory data is included in the medical record, consents have been signed, jewelry removed, and so forth. However, recently the surgical checklist process has been refined and standardized by the World Health Organization (World Alliance for Patient Safety, 2008) in an effort to promote patient safety and minimize risk of patient harm (Haynes et al., 2009). Use of a standardized surgical checklist has shown to be beneficial in reducing surgical complications and patient mortality (de Vries et al., 2010; Semel et al., 2010). The WHO (2008) surgical safety checklist can be adapted for cesarean birth (ACOG, 2011a). It includes verification of key issues prior to the surgery such as patient identification, allergies, airway assessment, and risk of blood loss. A time out confirms that all members of the team are introduced by name and role, reviews anticipated critical events, and confirms that prophylactic antibiotics have been given. The sign-out process includes a review of the procedure; sponge, instrument, and needle counts; and the key concerns regarding the immediate recovery period. One of the key aspects of the WHO's (2008) surgical safety checklist is communication among members of the team in a nonhierarchical style. Another important component is "sterile" communication, that is, no interruptions and all team members focused on the information that is being shared. Care providers are familiar with sterile technique as it applies to the instruments, equipment, and procedure but not necessarily with sterile communication. At times, the atmosphere in the surgical suite prior to the procedure can seem hurried, with each clinician focusing on his or her defined tasks. Sterile communication ensures that everyone is paying attention, has been provided essential information about the patient and the procedure, and has been allowed to voice any concerns that have the potential to affect the process and outcome. It is important to brief the patient and his or her support person about the surgical safety checklist process so they can be active participants and know what to expect. If this process is done well, the patient and her support person will have confidence that everything has been done to keep the mother and baby safe during the cesarean birth process.

Checklists can be developed for other aspects of perinatal care. For example, ACOG (2011d, 2011e) has published patient safety checklists for scheduling labor induction and scheduling cesarean birth. The purpose is to enhance patient safety by making sure all expected aspects of care are completed and verified prior to the procedure. A vital component of the scheduling process for elective births is establishing that the woman has reached 39 completed weeks of gestation. A more basic but equally important checklist is a universal protocol for preventing wrong site, wrong procedure, and wrong person surgery for all invasive procedures (NQF, 2010; TJC, 2012).

MEDICAL RECORD DOCUMENTATION

Medical record documentation is a vital nursing function. The purpose of the medical record is to communicate patient status to other members of the healthcare team and to provide an accurate, timely description of the course of care and the patient's response. The nurse providing care is in control of the information included in the nursing portions of the medical record; however, documentation has become one of the most time consuming of nursing activities and, therefore, one that is prone to omissions. Nurses often are concerned that medical record documentation forces them to focus on paperwork and/or the computer rather than patient care. Cumbersome documentation systems that require duplicate and triplicate entries of the same data contribute to this real problem. The ongoing challenge is to create a streamlined system for documentation that is cost effective, easy to use, an efficient use of nursing time, and sufficiently comprehensive for current or subsequent review. There are significant ramifications for inaccuracies and omissions in medical record documentation. Documentation deficiencies may result in decreased communication among team members, denied reimbursement by insurance carriers for care rendered, lost information for statistical or outcome data for quality purposes, and, in the case of litigation, increased difficulty for the defense to prove its case.

Of all strategies to decrease liability, accurate and thorough documentation may be the easiest to accomplish, yet it is the most common missing piece. The medical record is often the single most important document available in the defense of a negligent action. Frequently, in issues of litigation, the nurse cannot recall the specific patient or incident and, therefore, must rely on written or computerized nurses' notes completed at the time of patient contact. The time from event to formal legal inquiry may be several years, and the nurse may have limited independent recall without the documentation in the medical record. Without a complete and legible medical record, nurses may be unable to successfully defend themselves against allegations of improper care. Because lack of documentation equals a presumed lack of care, omissions are challenging to defend.

Litigation many times follows clinical events that result in significant adverse outcomes. Therefore, the most complete documentation should focus on the time period surrounding the adverse events. Obviously, during emergent situations, medical record documentation occurs retrospectively. The first priority during an emergency is to provide immediate patient care. Then, after the mother or fetus or newborn is stable, documentation is possible. Post-event documentation should focus on reconstructing a summary of all of the assessments, actions, and communication that transpired as accurately and timely as possible. For example, in the case of an abnormal FHR pattern of acute onset resulting in an emergent cesarean birth, summary documentation should include timely recognition of the problem, nursing actions initiated for maternal and/or fetal resuscitation, communication with team members and their responses, time to the surgical suite and incision, and chronologies of interventions performed (and by whom) for newborn resuscitation, followed by a note about the details of the discussion between the physician and the patient and her family. During emergent intrapartum situations, some nurses feel that documentation directly on the FHR strip can assist them in constructing notes after patient stabilization. If this approach is used, ensure that the narrative written or electronic notes written later coincide with the FHR strip annotations.

The medical record should provide a factual and objective account of care provided, including direct and indirect communication with other members of the healthcare team. Only clinically relevant information should be documented in the medical record. Address information not related to the patient's care, such as the filing of incident reports, short staffing, or conflicts between nurses and primary care providers, through the appropriate institutional channels rather than in the medical record.

Bedside use of a medical record as the single source of comprehensive data about the maternal–fetal status, nursing interventions, and the events of labor and birth documented in written or electronic flow sheets facilitate timely and accurate medical record data entry. Bedside documentation offers the opportunity for more direct patient observation and allows the patients to feel part of their care. Well-designed flow sheets are useful tools to prompt appropriate notations and practice consistency with unit guidelines, especially in the labor and birth setting. Ideally, this flow sheet is keyed to the NICHD terminology for FHR patterns to facilitate consistent medical record documentation concerning fetal status by all members of the team. Routine assessments and interventions can easily be documented in the flow sheet format. With the progressive use of electronic medical records, there has been a trend away from narrative notes; however, narrative notes offer the opportunity to include detailed information that is not included in the electronic flow sheet format. In the case of retrospective review, these additional details may be helpful in providing supplemental data that can assist in describing important aspects of care, communication with other members of the perinatal team, and the patient's response to interventions. Use narrative notes to document nonroutine care or events that are not included on the paper or electronic flow sheet. Also use narrative notes to document any nurse–physician communication, ongoing interventions for an indeterminate or abnormal FHR that does not resolve with the usual intrauterine resuscitation techniques, significant changes in maternal status, patient concerns or requests, and complete details of emergent situations and the outcome.

The practice of duplicate documentation of routine care on both the FHR strip and the medical record is outdated (Chez, 1997). Previously, perinatal nurses believed there should be enough documentation on the FHR strip so that the strip could stand alone for subsequent review. However, writing on the strip not only increases the amount of nursing time spent on inpatient care activities, but this practice also contributes to late entries on the medical record and can lead to errors in documentation. If the FHR strips are electronically archived, handwritten notes on the strip do not become part of the permanent medical record.

Retrospective charting is better than no documentation. However, late entries following an adverse outcome are often areas of controversy in litigation if they are written days after the event. Often, these types of late entries have a defensive tone. Ensure that the data entered are accurate and objective. Do not alter the medical record to include data that are not accurate, even if asked to do so by someone in a position of authority. Falsification of the medical record is not only dishonest and unethical, but it can lead to successful claims against the nurse and institution. Electronic medical records include an audit trail that can be used to determine the exact time data were entered and by whom.

One method to promote accurate and timely medical record documentation is to conduct routine medical record audits (see Display 1–5). Ideally, this process is coordinated by a committee of perinatal nursing peers who have volunteered to participate. An additional important by-product of medical record audits is the ability to evaluate unit and individual competence in various aspects of clinical care. When the fetal monitoring strip is used to compare FHR pattern interpretation and interventions documented in the medical record, valuable insight can be gained. Based on data collected, strategies can be developed for improvement for unit practice and/or individuals as appropriate.

INCIDENT MANAGEMENT

An incident may be defined as any happening that is not consistent with the routine care of a particular patient. Many adverse perinatal outcomes that result in litigation derive from perinatal incidents that are unexpected or are the result of an emergency

---

DISPLAY 1 – 5

Suggested Components of a Medical Record Audit

- Are the times noted on the Admission Assessment, Labor Flow Chart, and initial EFM strip consistent with each other within a reasonable time frame?
- If elective labor induction, is gestational age of at least 39 weeks confirmed?
- If elective (e.g., repeat or scheduled) cesarean birth, is gestational age of at least 39 weeks confirmed?
- Is it documented that the physician or midwife was notified of admission within the time frame outlined in the policies and procedures?
- Is fetal well-being established on admission?
- Is fetal well-being established prior to ambulation?
- Is fetal well-being established prior to medication administration?
- Does the EFM FHR baseline rate match the FHR baseline documented?
- Does the EFM FHR baseline variability match the FHR baseline variability documented?
- If there is evidence of absent or minimal FHR variability, is it documented?
- If there is evidence of absent or minimal FHR variability, are appropriate interventions documented?
- If there are FHR decelerations on the EFM strip, are they correctly documented?
- Are appropriate interventions documented during indeterminate or abnormal FHR patterns?
- Is there documentation of physician or midwife notification during indeterminate or abnormal FHR patterns?
- If FHR accelerations are documented, are they on the EFM strip?
- Are maternal assessments documented according to policy?
- If there is evidence of an indeterminate or abnormal FHR pattern, is oxytocin dosage increased?
- If there is evidence of an indeterminate or abnormal FHR pattern, is oxytocin dosage discontinued?
- If there is evidence of uterine tachysystole, are appropriate interventions documented?
- If there is evidence of adequate labor, is oxytocin dosage increased?

- If there is evidence of uterine tachysystole, is oxytocin dosage increased or decreased?
- Does the frequency of uterine contractions on the EFM strip match what is documented?
- Is the uterine activity monitor (external tocodynamometer or intrauterine pressure catheter [IUPC]) adjusted to maintain an accurate uterine activity baseline?
- Are oxytocin dosage increases charted when there is an inaccurate uterine baseline tracing or an uninterpretable FHR tracing?
- Is the physicians' and/or midwives' documentation of fetal status consistent with the nurses' documentation?
- Are automatically generated data from blood pressure devices and pulse oximeters accurate?
- Does documentation continue during the second stage of labor?
- Are patients in the second stage of labor encouraged to push before they feel the urge to push?
- Are patients in the second stage of labor encouraged to push with contractions when the FHR is indeterminate or abnormal (i.e., are there variable or late FHR decelerations occurring with each contraction)?
- When the FHR is indeterminate or abnormal during the second stage of labor, is pushing discontinued or encouraged with every other or every third contraction to maintain a stable baseline rate and minimize decelerations?
- If the FHR is indeterminate or abnormal during the second stage of labor, is oxytocin discontinued?
- Are uterine contractions continuously monitored during the second stage of labor via external tocodynamometer or IUPC?
- Does the time of birth on the medical record match the time of birth at end of the EFM strip?
- If the patient had regional analgesia/anesthesia, is a qualified anesthesia provider involved in the decision to discharge from postanesthesia care unit (PACU) care?
- If the patient had regional analgesia/anesthesia, is the discharge from PACU care scoring evaluation documented?
- Are maternal assessments documented during the immediate postpartum period every 15 minutes for at least 2 hours?
- Are newborn assessments documented during the transition to extrauterine life at least every 30 minutes until the newborn's condition has been stable for 2 hours?

occurrence. Emergency occurrences can be categorized as actual, evolving, or perceived. Actual emergencies may include maternal hemorrhage, prolapsed cord, amniotic fluid embolism, shoulder dystocia, or neonatal asphyxia. Evolving emergencies are those that develop gradually and go unrecognized until an acute situation occurs. Examples include progressive deterioration in fetal status evolving to terminal bradycardia, severe preeclampsia converting to overt eclampsia, or an unrecognized malpresentation progressing to precipitous birth without appropriate preparation. Finally, perceived emergencies are the near misses that have the potential to result in adverse outcomes. These may include insufficient resources, inadequate communication, professional knowledge deficits, or ineffective lines of authority and responsibility.

Incident management, therefore, plays an important role not only in reducing institutional liability but also in promoting a safer care environment. The goal is for members of the interdisciplinary perinatal team to objectively assess what happened (or what might have happened in the case of near misses) so that problem-prone systems or operations can be identified. After identification, there may be opportunities for improvement to prevent an adverse event or recurrence of the adverse event. This process requires time, extensive communication, and a systematic framework. Generally, incident management is a retrospective process that includes the examination of all of the events surrounding the incident. Key questions for the review include the following:

- What happened (or might have happened)?
- What were the contributing factors?
- Was it preventable?
- How was it handled?
- Were sufficient resources available?
- Was there an opportunity to handle it better?
- Is there a need for remedial action?
- What is the appropriate follow-up?
- What is the required documentation?

These questions can be addressed in a debriefing immediately following the event or as soon as possible. A post-event debriefing is a valuable tool to solicit feedback from all team members and may lead to discovery of important details that may be overlooked or forgotten in a more formal review that occurs days or weeks later. Ideally, someone is assigned to record the information that is produced through the debriefing process so it can be used to supplement the formal review process that may be necessary.

It is important to have a plan for disclosing events and their implications to the patient and family or support persons. Following serious unanticipated outcomes, including those that are clearly caused by systems failures, the patient and, as appropriate, the family should receive timely, transparent, and clear communication concerning what is known about the event (NQF, 2010). Care for the caregivers should not be overlooked in managing the aftermath of a serious event that results in patient harm. The caregivers involved in an adverse event may suffer psychological trauma as the second victims. At times, the caregivers have difficulties coming to terms with what happened and their role in the events and outcome even in cases when the event was deemed not to have been preventable. These problems may include questioning their judgment and clinical competence, negative feelings of self-worth, guilt, constantly reliving the events, fixating on "what ifs," and sleep difficulties similar to symptoms of post-traumatic stress. Following serious unintentional harm due to systems failures and/or errors that resulted from human performance failures, the involved caregivers (clinical providers, staff, and administrators) should receive timely and systematic care to include treatment that is just; respect; compassion; supportive medical care; and the opportunity to fully participate in event investigation, risk identification, and mitigation activities that will help to prevent future events (NQF, 2010).

SENTINEL EVENTS

Some incidents are of such serious nature that they are classified as sentinel events and require specific actions by Joint Commission–accredited institutions. A sentinel event is defined by TJC (2011a) as an unexpected occurrence involving death or serious physical or psychological injury, or the risk thereof. Serious injury specifically includes loss of limb or function. The phrase "or the risk thereof" includes any process variation for which a recurrence would carry a significant chance of a serious adverse outcome. Such events are called "sentinel" because they signal the need for immediate investigation and response (TJC, 2011a). The terms "sentinel event" and "error" are not synonymous as not all sentinel events occur because of an error, and not all errors result in sentinel events (TJC, 2011a). The goals of TJC sentinel event policy are (a) to have a positive impact in improving patient care, treatment, and services and on prevention; (b) to focus the attention of a hospital that has experienced a sentinel event on understanding the factors that contributed to the event (such as underlying causes, latent conditions and active failures in defense systems, or organizational culture), and on changing the hospital's culture, systems, and processes to reduce the probability of such an event in the future; (c) to increase the general knowledge about sentinel events, their contributing factors, and strategies for prevention; and (d) to maintain the confidence of the public and accredited hospitals in the accreditation process (TJC, 2011a).

Sentinel events in perinatal services that are subject to review by TJC include any occurrence that meets any of the following criteria (TJC, 2011a):

- The event has resulted in an unanticipated death or major permanent loss of function, not related to the natural course of the patient's illness or underlying condition.
- The event is one of the following (even if the outcome was not death or major permanent loss of function unrelated to the natural course of the patient's illness or underlying condition):
  - Suicide of any individual receiving care, treatment, or services in an around-the-clock care setting or within 72 hours of discharge
  - Unanticipated death of a full-term infant
  - Abduction of any patient receiving care, treatment, and services
  - Discharge of an infant to the wrong family
  - Rape (any staff-witnessed sexual contact as described by TJC [2011a] policy, including admission by the perpetrator that this sexual contact occurred on the premises and sufficient clinical evidence obtained by the hospital to support allegations of nonconsensual sexual contact)
  - Hemolytic transfusion reaction involving administration of blood or blood products having major blood group incompatibilities (ABO, Rh, other blood groups)
  - Surgery and nonsurgical invasive procedure on the wrong patient, wrong site, or wrong procedure
  - Unintended retention of a foreign object in an individual after surgery or other procedure
  - Severe neonatal hyperbilirubinemia (bilirubin >30 mg/dL)
  - Prolonged fluoroscopy with cumulative dose >1,500 rads to a single field or any delivery of radiotherapy to the wrong body region or >25% above the planned radiotherapy dose

Joint Commission–accredited organizations are expected to identify and respond appropriately to all sentinel events that occur in the organization or are associated with services that the organization provides or provides for (TJC, 2011a). Appropriate response includes conducting a timely, thorough, and credible root-cause analysis; developing an action plan to implement improvements to reduce risk of reoccurrence; implementing improvements; and monitoring the effectiveness of those improvements (TJC, 2011a). For a root-cause analysis to be considered credible, it is important to include members of the leadership team as well as those most closely involved in the processes and systems related to the event under review. Root-cause analysis is a process for identifying the basic or causal factors that are associated with variation in performance, including the occurrence or possible occurrence of a sentinel event (TJC, 2011a). A root-cause analysis focuses primarily on systems and processes, not individual performance. It begins with an analysis of special causes in clinical processes and progresses to common causes in organizational processes and identifies potential improvements in processes or systems that would tend to decrease the likelihood of such events in the future, or determines, after analysis, that no such improvement opportunities exist (TJC, 2011a).

In some cases, more than one root cause may be identified. There are often multiple factors that were involved in the adverse event, and each of these factors warrants thorough analysis. Critical to understanding the underlying potential causative factors is a review of the entire case rather than focusing on the immediate time frame surrounding the event. This more comprehensive analysis may reveal additional opportunities for improvement in systems and care practices. For example, in a case of delayed neonatal resuscitation resulting in the death of a term baby, review of the labor may reveal potential contributing factors such as a prolonged period of uterine tachysystole while oxytocin was infusing, an unrecognized indeterminate or abnormal FHR pattern, lack of initiation of timely and appropriate intrauterine resuscitation measures, and/or lack of modification of maternal pushing efforts when fetal status suggested evolving deterioration. In this example, neonatal resuscitation may not have been required had the care during labor been more consistent with expected interventions.

A root-cause analysis should produce an action plan that identifies the strategies that are intended to be implemented to reduce the risk of similar events occurring in the future. The plan should address responsibility for implementation, oversight, pilot testing as appropriate, time lines, and strategies for measuring the effectiveness of the actions (TJC, 2011a). Ideally, this process should be initiated and completed in a timely manner. TJC (2011a) recommends conducting the root-cause analysis and preparing an action plan within 45 days of the sentinel event.

Not all sentinel events are the result of errors. For example, a maternal death, while unexpected, may be unavoidable if the woman suddenly develops an amniotic fluid embolism or deteriorates as a result of consumptive coagulopathy. A term baby may not survive a complete placental abruption or prolapsed umbilical cord. The key issue is to carefully analyze the event through an interdisciplinary process with the goal of developing strategies to prevent future occurrences. The discussion should avoid blaming individuals and instead focus on systems that may have failed them. Some adverse outcomes in perinatal care are not predictable or avoidable, despite the best efforts of healthcare providers and the availability of sophisticated technology.

NEVER EVENTS

The term "never event" was introduced in 2002 by NQF. A never event is an adverse event that is unambiguous (clearly identifiable and measurable), serious (resulting in death or significant disability), should never occur, and is usually preventable (NQF, 2002). Twenty-seven never events were initially defined by NQF in 2002. The list was revised and expanded in 2006 (NQF, 2006). Never events are grouped into six categories of events: surgical, product or device, patient protection, care management, environmental, and criminal. Although most are focused on all patients in general, many apply or can be adapted to perinatal care (Simpson, 2006b). Display 1–6 lists examples of never events that can occur in the perinatal setting. Some of these events are consistent with sentinel events as classified by TJC (2011a).

METHODS OF MEASURING PATIENT SAFETY

Often, the first indication that there are significant gaps in the safety net is the occurrence of a near miss or an adverse outcome. Retrospective review of systems and routine clinical processes reveal areas for improvement, but in some cases they are too late for the patient and healthcare providers involved. Rather than a reactive approach based solely on review of errors and accidents, an ongoing prospective program that includes various measures of safety can be used to develop strategies to minimize the risk of patient harm (Simpson, 2006a).

Measuring things that do not occur (e.g., absence of patient harm as a result of the process of care) is a challenge. Nonetheless, various methods have been proposed as measures of patient safety, each with advantages and limitations. These include mainly structure, process, and outcomes measures. Structure measures cover the organizational context of care, for example, the fundamental infrastructure that is required to create conditions that promote patient safety, such as the existence of an interdisciplinary practice committee and key clinical protocols for areas of care known to be associated with patient risk, such as fetal assessment and neonatal resuscitation. Process measures evaluate how care is provided, for example, adherence to science- and standards-based clinical protocols or routinely beginning an emergent cesarean birth within 30 minutes of the decision to do so. Outcome measures for complication rates, morbidity, and mortality, such as the AHRQ (2011b) patient safety indicators (PSIs), TJC (2009a) *Perinatal Care Core*

DISPLAY 1–6

Obstetrical Never Events

- Infant abduction
- Infant discharged to the wrong person
- Infant death or serious disability (kernicterus) associated with failure to identify and treat hyperbilirubinemia
- Maternal or infant death or serious disability associated with a hemolytic reaction due to the administration of ABO-incompatible blood or blood products
- Maternal death or serious disability associated with labor and birth in a low-risk pregnancy while being cared for in a healthcare facility
- Maternal or infant death or serious disability associated with a medication error, for example, errors involving the wrong drug, wrong dose, wrong patient, wrong time, wrong rate, wrong preparation, or wrong route of administration (includes overdose of oxytocin, misoprostol, magnesium sulfate)
- Wrong surgical procedure performed on a mother or infant (e.g., circumcision, tubal ligation)
- Retention of a foreign object in a mother or infant after surgery or other procedure
- Maternal death after pulmonary embolism in untreated woman with known high-risk factors for DVT

- Infant breastfed by wrong mother or breast milk to wrong infant
- Death or serious disability of a fetus/infant with a normal FHR pattern on mother's admission for labor, barring any acute unpredictable event
- Prolapsed umbilical cord after elective rupture of membranes with the fetus at high station
- Prolonged periods of untreated uterine tachysystole during oxytocin or misoprostol administration
- Prolonged periods of an indeterminate/abnormal FHR pattern during labor unrecognized and/or untreated with the usual intrauterine resuscitation techniques or birth
- Ruptured uterus following prostaglandin administration for cervical ripening/labor induction to a woman with a known uterine surgical scar
- Missed administration of RhoGam to a mother who is an appropriate candidate
- Circumcision without pain relief measures
- Artificial insemination with the wrong donor sperm or wrong egg
- Neonatal group B streptococcus or HIV infection after missed intrapartum chemoprophylaxis
- Infant death or disability after multiple attempts with instruments to effect an operative vaginal birth
- Infant death or disability after prolonged periods of coached second stage labor pushing efforts during an indeterminate/abnormal FHR pattern

Adapted from National Quality Forum (2006). *Serious reportable events in healthcare.* Washington, DC: Author; and Simpson, K. R. (2006). Obstetrical "never events." *MCN: The American Journal of Maternal Child Nursing, 31*(2), 136.

DISPLAY 1-7

Joint Commission Perinatal Care Core Measure Set (2009)

Elective births before 39 completed weeks of gestation

Cesarean birth for low-risk first birth women

Administration of antenatal steroids to all appropriate candidates

Healthcare–associated bloodstream infections in newborns

Exclusive breast milk feeding in the inpatient setting

Measure Set (See Display 1–7), and the NQF (2009b) *National Voluntary Consensus Standards for Perinatal Care*, are the most widely used evaluation method in obstetrics. These measures are updated periodically as more data are available on gaps in quality and performance. Qualitative assessment methods also can provide rich actionable data. These include focus groups (Hesse-Biber & Leavy, 2006), storytelling (Beyea, Killen, & Knox, 2004), and executive walk rounds (Thomas, Sexton, Neilands, Frankel, & Helmreich, 2005). Other types of measurement tools include safety surveys such as the AHRQ (2011a) *Hospital Survey on Patient Safety Culture* and the *Safety Attitude Questionnaire* (Sexton et al., 2006).

STRUCTURE MEASURES

Structure measures are easy to analyze because they are based on concrete objective data. Most can be reported as a simple yes/no or in rates or percentages. Questions include the following: Is there an interdisciplinary practice committee? Are there standard unit policies for oxytocin, misoprostol, and magnesium sulfate administration? Is there a standard unit policy for avoiding elective births before 39 weeks gestation? Are there standard provider order sets? What percentage of the perinatal team holds certification in EFM? Is there an anonymous, nonpunitive error-reporting system? and so forth. Although it may be difficult to determine a direct cause-and-effect relationship between the existence of certain organizational structures and patient safety, it is generally assumed that they enhance the safe care environment (Leape & Berwick, 2005; Pronovost, Holzmueller, Ennen, & Fox, 2011; Pronovost, Nolan, Zeger, Miller, & Rubin, 2004; Simpson & Knox, 2011; Simpson, Knox, Martin, George, & Watson, 2011). (See Table 1–5 for examples of structure measures.)

PROCESS MEASURES

The degree to which institutions and healthcare providers adhere to processes that are supported by scientific evidence or recommended by professional organizations and regulatory agencies can be measured

(Pronovost et al., 2011; Pronovost et al., 2004). A process measure should have adequate specificity as defined by NQF (2002) (i.e., the process or manner of providing the service should be clearly defined and its essential components specified so that one could conduct an audit and readily determine whether the practice is in use). Many healthcare providers are accepting of process measures because they are more in control of and accountable for care processes than patient outcomes, which can be affected by many other variables (Pronovost et al., 2011; Pronovost et al., 2004; Simpson et al., 2011).

Process evaluation usually requires medical record review, which can be a time-consuming endeavor. Therefore, random samples of cases of each process under investigation are generally used rather than 100% of cases, particularly if the process is common (e.g., compliance with appropriate gestational age criteria for elective birth). If the process is rare (e.g., care during shoulder dystocia), review of all cases is feasible and should be considered. Although labor intensive, medical record review as a component of process measurement often uncovers important data concerning clinical care and documentation practices. Some process measures ideally should reveal nearly 100% adherence because there is a cumulative body of evidence or professional standards to support routine use in the absence of emergencies or patient refusal. For example, elective births should not occur before 39 completed weeks of gestation (ACOG, 2009b; NQF, 2009b; TJC, 2009a, 2009b), all baby boys should receive pain relief measures for circumcision (AAP, 1999 [reaffirmed 2005]; ACOG, 2001 [reaffirmed 2011]; AAP & ACOG, 2007, 2012), all pregnant women should be screened for perinatal GBS during their prenatal care and, if positive, treated with chemoprophylaxis during labor (ACOG, 2011c), and all mothers who are HIV positive should receive antiretroviral prophylaxis during labor (ACOG, 2008b). If the interdisciplinary perinatal practice committee has been empowered to enact policies and require routine adherence, other process measures can also be expected to have a 100% adherence rate. These include physician notification of specific indeterminate or abnormal FHR patterns and bedside evaluation of patients with certain maternal–fetal complications within designated time frames. (See Table 1–6 for examples of process measures.) A reliable and valid tool for measuring fetal safety during labor has been published: *Failure to Rescue, A Tool for Evaluating Team Response to Indeterminate or Abnormal Fetal Status During Labor* (Simpson, 2005a, 2006a). This tool can be used to evaluate the process of care during indeterminate or abnormal FHR patterns. Improvement in scores have shown to be possible with interdisciplinary education on fetal monitoring, attention to fetal well-being

Table 1–5. SELECTED STRUCTURE MEASURES FOR PERINATAL PATIENT SAFETY

Measure	Results
Interdisciplinary perinatal practice committee	Yes/No
Nurse and physician co-chairs of interdisciplinary practice committee	Yes/No
Regularly scheduled interdisciplinary case reviews	Yes/No
Interdisciplinary fetal monitoring education	Yes/No
Medical record documentation forms and electronic systems with cues for use of the NICHD terminology for FHR patterns	Yes/No
Weekly interdisciplinary fetal monitoring strip reviews	Yes/No
Routine medical record audits using fetal monitoring strips as part of the review	Yes/No
Uniform criteria for selecting cases for review	Yes/No
Standard policy for oxytocin administration (start at 1–2 mU/min and increase by 1–2 mU/min based on labor progress and fetal status, no more frequently than every 30–40 min; direct bedside physician evaluation required for increases beyond 20 mU/min; IV solution with 30 units in 500 mL for labor induction; IV solution with 20 units in 1,000 mL for immediate postpartum; IV solutions prepared by pharmacy)	Yes/No
Standard order set for oxytocin administration based on components of policy listed above	Yes/No
Standard policy for misoprostol administration (25 mcg as the initial dose; every 4–6 hours; oxytocin no sooner than 4 hours after last dose; continuous EFM for at least 4 hours after dose)	Yes/No
Standard order set for misoprostol administration based on components of policy listed above	Yes/No
Standard policy for magnesium sulfate administration (IV loading dose administered in 4 g [100 mL] or 6 g [150 mL] solution; maintenance solution 20 g in 500 mL; nurse double-checks for all dosage/pump changes; IV solutions prepared by the pharmacy)	Yes/No
Policy requiring full surgical team in house during labor of women attempting VBAC	Yes/No
Criteria for prioritizing labor inductions based on medical necessity	Yes/No
Requirement for 39 completed weeks of gestation before elective labor induction and elective cesarean birth	Yes/No
Agreed-upon definition of uterine tachysystole and expected interventions based on ACOG/AWHONN guidelines	Yes/No
Clinical algorithm for intrauterine resuscitation during indeterminate or abnormal FHR patterns	Yes/No
Protocol for second-stage labor care based on AWHONN guidelines	Yes/No
Policy for prevention of perinatal GBS based on AAP/ACOG/CDC recommendations	Yes/No
Policy for prevention of perinatal transmission of HIV based on ACOG/CDC recommendations	Yes/No
Policy for treatment of neonatal hyperbilirubinemia and kernicterus prevention based on AAP/TJC recommendations	Yes/No
Policy requiring analgesia and anesthesia for all circumcision	Yes/No
Criteria for transfer of high-risk mothers and babies	Yes/No
Nurse staffing based on AWHONN guidelines	Yes/No
Nurses' role in epidural anesthesia consistent with AWHONN guidelines (e.g., no programming epidural pumps, changing doses, or giving boluses)	Yes/No
Anonymous, nonpunitive error-reporting system	Yes/No
Good citizenship/professional behavior policy	Yes/No
All members of the perinatal leadership team are members of their professional association (ACOG, AAP, ASA, AWHONN, or NANN)	Yes/No
Percentage of physicians who are board-certified	
Percentage of nurses who hold certification in inpatient obstetrics	
Percentage of the perinatal team who hold certification in fetal monitoring	
Percentage of the perinatal team who have attended a fetal monitoring workshop within the past 2 years	
Percentage of the perinatal team who have completed the neonatal resuscitation program course within the past 2 years	

AAP, American Academy of Pediatrics; ACOG, American College of Obstetricians and Gynecologists; ASA, American Society of Anesthesiologists; AWHONN, Association of Women's Health, Obstetric and Neonatal Nurses; CDC, Centers for Disease Control and Prevention; EFM, electronic fetal monitoring; FHR, fetal heart rate; GBS, group B streptococcus; NANN, National Association of Neonatal Nurses; NICHD, National Institute of Child Health and Human Development; TJC, the Joint Commission; VBAC, vaginal birth after cesarean.

during labor, and appropriate and timely intrauterine resuscitation based on the FHR pattern (Simpson et al., 2011). Other tools for evaluating care during labor such as the *tachysystole tool* have shown similar improvements within this context (Simpson & Knox, 2009; Simpson et al., 2011) (See Display 1–8). Ongoing process evaluation can be a valuable tool for providing continuous feedback and educational reminders to clinicians and to identify gaps in routine care that can potentially be eliminated.

A successful clinical outcome does not mean that the process of care was appropriate or timely. There are not large numbers of maternal or infant deaths in individual hospitals or healthcare systems that allow statistically stable estimates of the death rates or statistical analyses that are usually used with outcome-based PSIs. When evaluating perinatal patient safety, process measurement is likely more useful to practicing clinicians and has more potential to identify errors, omissions, or miscommunication that can help the team develop strategies for improvement (Simpson, 2005a). Components of the care processes that are found to consistently work well can be shared with all members of the team and adopted as expectations for routine practice.

Table 1–6. SELECTED PROCESS MEASURES

Processes	Denominator	Numerator	Sample
Timely triage and disposition	Patients in sample who present to obstetric triage unit	All patients in denominator cohort who do not have documented decision for treatment or disposition within 2 hours of being seen in triage unit	30 medical records per month randomly selected from triage log who present to the obstetric triage unit
Adherence to unit policy for elective/repeat cesarean birth requiring 39 completed weeks of gestation	Patients in sample who have elective/repeat cesarean birth	All patients in denominator cohort who have cesarean birth before 39 completed weeks of gestation	30 medical records per month randomly selected from unit birth log of women who have elective/repeat cesarean birth
Adherence to unit policy for oxytocin administration for elective labor induction (appropriate gestational age of 39 completed weeks)	Patients in sample who have elective induction of labor	All patients in denominator cohort who are induced before 39 completed weeks of gestation	30 medical records per month randomly selected from unit birth log of women who had elective induction of labor
Adherence to unit policy for oxytocin administration for labor induction/augmentation (start at 1–2 mU/min and increase by 1–2 mU/min based on labor progress and fetal status no more frequently than every 30–40 min)	Patients in sample receiving oxytocin for labor induction/augmentation	All patients in denominator cohort who receive oxytocin outside the context of the policy dosage	30 medical records per month randomly selected from unit birth log of women who received oxytocin for labor induction/augmentation
Adherence to unit policy for oxytocin administration for labor induction/augmentation (physician evaluation for dose beyond 20 mU/min)	Patients in sample receiving oxytocin for labor induction/augmentation	All patients in denominator cohort who receive oxytocin dosage higher than 20 mU/min without documentation of bedside evaluation by an attending physician	30 medical records per month randomly selected from unit birth log of women who received oxytocin for labor induction/augmentation
Adherence to unit policy for oxytocin administration for labor induction/augmentation (tachysystole)	Patients in sample receiving oxytocin for labor induction/augmentation	All patients in denominator cohort with more than 20 min of unrecognized and untreated tachysystole	30 medical records per month randomly selected from unit birth log of women who received oxytocin for labor induction/augmentation (review includes EFM strip)
Adherence to unit policy for intra-uterine resuscitation	Patients in sample who have an indeterminate or abnormal FHR pattern during labor	All patients in denominator cohort with more than 10 min of unrecognized and untreated indeterminate or abnormal FHR pattern	30 medical records per month randomly selected from unit birth log of women who had an indeterminate or abnormal FHR pattern during labor (review includes EFM strip)
Pre-epidural IV fluid hydration	Patients in sample who have epidural anesthesia during labor	All patients in denominator cohort who do not receive at least 500 mL of lactated Ringer's solution IV prior to epidural anesthesia during labor	30 medical records per month randomly selected from unit birth log of women who had epidural anesthesia during labor
Promoting second-stage pushing fetal well-being	Patients in sample who have vaginal birth	All patients in denominator cohort who have unrecognized and untreated indeterminate or abnormal FHR during second-stage labor	30 medical records per month randomly selected from unit birth log of women who have vaginal birth
Prophylactic antibiotics prior to cesarean birth based on unit policy	Patients in sample who have cesarean birth	All patients in denominator cohort who do not receive antibiotics prior to cesarean birth	30 medical records per month randomly selected from unit birth log of women who have cesarean birth
Timely cesarean birth	Term patients in sample who have unscheduled cesarean birth after labor with an indication of maternal or fetal compromise	All patients in denominator cohort who do not have incision for cesarean birth within 30 min of the documented decision for cesarean birth	30 medical records per month randomly selected from unit birth log of women at term who had an unscheduled cesarean birth after labor with an indication of maternal or fetal compromise

EFM, electronic fetal monitoring; FHR, fetal heart rate.

DISPLAY 1-8

TACHYSYSTOLE TOOL

Tachysystole is defined as more than 5 contractions in 10 min (averaged over 30 min), contractions lasting 2 min or more, contractions of normal duration occurring within 1 min of each other (ACOG, 2003, 2009; AWHONN [Simpson], 2009; NICHD [Macones et al.] 2008).

Expected Care Process: Excessive uterine activity will be identified and interventions initiated within 20 min of its development. Interventions are based on whether or not the FHR pattern is normal.

CARE DATA	TIMES
Beginning	
Identification	
How many minutes before identification?	
Interventions initiated	Yes/No
Repositioning	Yes/No
IV fluid of lactated Ringer's solution	Yes/No
Decrease in oxytocin by ½ of current rate (normal FHR pattern)	Yes/No
Discontinuation of oxytocin (indeterminate or abnormal FHR pattern or if ½ dosage decrease does not correct excessive uterine activity)	Yes/No
Terbutaline 0.25 mg SQ	Yes/No
Resolution time	
Total length of excessive uterine activity period in minutes	

INDETERMINATE OR ABNORMAL FHR CHARACTERISTICS (IF APPLICABLE)

	Absent or Present	Accurately Interpreted
FHR (bradycardia or tachycardia)	Rate	Yes/No
Variability (absent or minimal)	Yes/No	Yes/No
Decelerations (late, variable, prolonged, recurrent, intermittent)	Yes/No	Yes/No

OVERALL EVALUATION OF CARE

EXPECTED CARE PROCESS MET	Yes	No

Adapted from Simpson, K. R., & Knox, G. E. (2009). Oxytocin as a high alert medication: Implications for perinatal patient safety. *MCN The American Journal of Maternal Child Nursing, 34*(1), 8–15.

OUTCOME MEASURES

The Agency for Healthcare Research and Quality (2011b) published a set of patient safety indicators (PSIs) that are intended to measure potentially preventable complications and iatrogenic events for patients treated in hospitals. The PSIs are for use with administrative data sets, particularly those found in hospital discharge abstract data. Many of the AHRQ PSIs exclude obstetric patients from their inclusion criteria. The indicators can be risk-adjusted using age, gender, and demographics (Johnson, Handberg, Dobalian, Gurol, & Pearson, 2005). The PSIs are designed to screen for adverse events that patients experience as a result of their exposure to the healthcare system; these events are likely amenable to prevention by changes at the system or provider level. The most useful PSIs measure conditions likely to reflect medical error, such as a foreign body accidentally left during a procedure or blood transfusion reaction. Those that measure conditions that conceivably, but not definitely, reflect medical error, such as death in low-mortality–diagnosis-related groups or postoperative infection, require more careful case analysis (AHRQ, 2011b).

Reliance on administrative data is both a strength and weakness of the AHRQ PSIs (Johnson et al., 2005). Administrative data sets allow the PSIs to be accessible and low-cost screening tools to help identify potential problems in quality of care and target promising areas for more in-depth review. Conversely, there are known limitations with using administrative data, including the difficulty in perfectly risk-adjusting outcomes and the lack of time relationships with events (Johnson et al., 2005). Reliability of administrative data is based on coding accuracy, timing of entries, and medical record documentation (Romano, Yasmeen, Schembri, Keyzer, & Gilbert, 2005). Errors in any of these areas can significantly obscure potential findings. Additionally, if the outcome is infrequent, it may take some time before providers can receive meaningful feedback in order to make practice changes (Pronovost et al., 2004). In cases of infrequent outcomes, process measures may be more valuable. For example, it may take 6 months to a year to see evidence of decreased rates of iatrogenic preterm birth using outcomes data, whereas improved adherence to 39 completed weeks of gestation as criteria for elective birth (ACOG, 2009b) may be seen within 1 month. Despite limitations, analysis of these inexpensive, readily available indicators may provide a screen for potential errors and a method of monitoring trends in care that put patients at risk.

In 2004, NQF identified National Voluntary Consensus Standards for Nursing-Sensitive Care. In 2009, (NQF, 2009a), these measures were updated. While some of the standards do not apply directly to perinatal care, several of the measures (falls prevalence, falls with injury, nursing skill mix, nursing care hours per patient day, practice environment scale—nursing work index, and nursing-sensitive care) are applicable. The nursing practice environment can be measured using the *Revised Nursing Work Index* (Aiken & Patrician, 2000; Lake, 2002). The value of this set of indicators is that they have been shown to reflect quality of nursing care (NQF, 2009a).

Often, clinical leaders desire a method that will allow more timely notification of clinical events that may warrant closer scrutiny, rather than waiting for information from administrative data sets. A set of clinical indicators can be developed with requirements for case review. For this process to be successful, all members of the perinatal team must be aware of the indicators and notification procedures. One method that works well is the creation of a form that can be affixed to the front matter of the paper portion of the medical record (but is not a permanent component) with a list of clinical indicators that require notification (see Display 1–9).

SAFETY ATTITUDE AND CLIMATE SURVEYS

Healthcare organizations should measure their culture, provide feedback to the leadership and staff, and undertake interventions that will reduce patient safety risk (NQF, 2010). Safety culture has been defined as the product of individual and group values, attitudes, perceptions, competence, and patterns of behavior that determine the commitment to and the style and proficiency of an organization's health and safety management (Nieva & Sorra, 2003). The term "safety culture" was first described after the Chernobyl nuclear power disaster that occurred in 1988 (Halligan & Zecevic, 2011). Over the years,

high-reliability organizations began to support the concept, and it eventually became integrated into the healthcare system as hospitals and clinicians worked to make care safer. Since the Institute of Medicine (Kohn et al., 1999) recommended changing healthcare organizational characteristics to create a culture of safety, surveys have been developed to measure safety attitudes and cultures. The most commonly known are the *Hospital Survey on Patient Safety Culture* (AHRQ, 2011a) and the *Safety Attitude Questionnaire* (SAQ) (Sexton et al., 2006). All use Likert scales to measure individual attitudes. Most cover the five common dimensions of the patient safety climate: leadership, policies and procedures, staffing, communication, and reporting. To date, there are limited data linking a better or improved safety climate score to meaningful patient outcomes. Only the SAQ (Sexton et al., 2006) has been tested to determine whether better scores are associated with improved outcomes; these studies demonstrated a relationship between higher SAQ scores and lower medication error and risk-adjusted mortality rates (Colla, Bracken, Kinney, & Weeks, 2005). The SAQ (Sexton et al., 2006) also specifically includes everyone practicing on the unit as participants rather than excluding nonemployees such as attending physicians. Healthcare organizations can use survey tools to better understand their

---

DISPLAY 1 – 9

Sample Form for Request for Review of Clinical Events

CONFIDENTIAL: NOT PART OF MEDICAL RECORD—DO NOT COPY OR RELEASE

This report is prepared for quality improvement and/or risk management purposes.   Patient Name
The report and the information contained herein are privileged under Peer Review Statute.

DATE: _____

_____ Fetal monitor strip review (e.g., abnormal FHR, tachysystole, second-stage management)
_____ APGAR score <7 at 5 minutes of life for a term (≥37 weeks) infant
_____ Umbilical artery cord blood <7.10
_____ Infant injury during birth: _____ Fracture _____ Laceration _____ Hematoma _____ Other: _____
_____ Transfer of term (≥37 weeks) infant
_____ Intrapartum fetal death ≥24 weeks (excludes fetal demise known prior to admission)
_____ Emergent "crash" cesarean birth: Time of decision: _____ Time of incision: _____
_____ Placental abruption
_____ Uterine rupture
_____ Shoulder dystocia (circle any maneuver used to disimpact the shoulders: suprapubic pressure, McRoberts maneuver,
         other: _____ .) Time elapsed from birth of fetal head to birth of body: _____ minutes.
_____ Other (e.g., amniotic fluid embolism, pulmonary embolism, etc.): _____
_____ Extensive episiotomy/perineal laceration tear and/or repair
_____ Maternal hemorrhage _____ Transfusion _____ Hysterectomy _____ Uterine _____ Artery ligation or embolization
_____ Unplanned maternal return to surgery
_____ Maternal transfer to intensive care unit
_____ Maternal death
_____ RN only present at birth (i.e., attending physician or CNM not present)

safety culture and identify areas for improvement. The safety culture assessment should be viewed as the starting point from which action planning begins and patient safety changes emerge (Nieva & Sorra, 2003).

QUALITATIVE METHODS

Focus groups, executive walk rounds, and storytelling are examples of qualitative methods to assess perinatal patient safety. These methods can provide rich data with detailed descriptions of system vulnerabilities that may not otherwise be noted using more traditional types of measurements (Hesse-Biber & Leavy, 2006). Participants often respond favorably to simple questions that ask their opinions and perceptions of safety. Bedside care providers have direct knowledge of how the system actually works and appreciate the opportunity to offer feedback. The potential value is acknowledging their wisdom and engaging them directly in improvement efforts (Thomas et al., 2005). Focus groups using open-ended questions such as "What could be done to improve patient safety on your unit?" or "Describe a common situation that you believe puts patients at risk for harm" work well to elicit responses that can be helpful in identifying gaps in the safety net. The facilitator can be a member of the leadership team or an external consultant. To be effective, however, participants must be confident that their comments will be confidential, and their suggestions for improvement should be acted on as appropriate within a reasonable time frame.

Executive walk rounds generally involve visits by hospital executives to patient units to discuss patient safety issues with direct care providers. Sample questions for executive walk rounds include "Have there been any near misses that almost caused patient harm but didn't?" "What aspects of the environment are likely to lead to the next patient harm?" "Is there anything we could do to prevent the next adverse event?" and "Can you think of a way in which the system or your environment fails you on a consistent basis?" The discussions should lead to action followed by feedback to participants (Thomas et al., 2005). Executive walk rounds are visible demonstrations of the executive and the organizational commitment to patient safety. Those who participate in the discussions may develop a more positive attitude about the safety climate in the organization (Thomas et al., 2005).

Patient safety can be enhanced by telling stories about clinical successes and events that did not go as planned. Detailed stories of how situations evolved into adverse events can be more helpful in teaching safety concepts than traditional methods such as lectures and assigned reading (Beyea et al., 2004). Stories help listeners remember facts and details that otherwise might be forgotten. Discussions concerning what worked and what could have been done differently in emergent situations are valuable in planning for future emergencies, particularly in avoiding similar types of errors or miscommunication that may have occurred (Simpson & Knox, 2003b). Storytelling opportunities may be provided during unit meetings, interdisciplinary case reviews, grand rounds, or informal teaching sessions.

EXTERNAL REVIEW AND RISK ASSESSMENT

Often, members of the leadership team desire external review to determine the state of perinatal patient safety in an individual hospital or entire healthcare system. Generally, this process includes a review of current clinical practices, policies, and protocols; selected medical records; recent sentinel events; and open and closed obstetric professional liability claims. Interviews with key members of the leadership team and individual care providers add qualitative data and confirmation of clinical practices identified during policy and medical record review. Ideally, the review team is interdisciplinary to enhance acceptance of the results and suggestions for improvement by all members of the perinatal team. Based on an objective review process, perinatal patient safety and professional liability risk can be determined. In some cases, external review is desired to confirm the leadership team's perceptions of quality care, while in other cases, the review follows an adverse outcome, series of adverse outcomes, or significant payout resulting from a successful malpractice claim. Whatever the reason, the process can be useful for identifying gaps in the safety net and planning for improvement.

PERINATAL PATIENT SAFETY NURSES

Some institutions have created a position for an advanced practice nurse whose primary responsibility is to promote safe care for mothers and babies by maintaining a focus on patient safety for all unit operations and clinical practices (Knox et al., 2003; Will, Hennicke, Jacobs, O'Neill, & Raab, 2006; Raab & Palmer-Byfield, 2011). Other responsibilities of the perinatal patient safety nurse include ensuring that all perinatal care providers and unit practices adhere to national professional standards as well as the principles of patient safety; coordinating professional communication education; maintaining professional collaboration and behavior; conducting ongoing objective analysis of practice based on structure, process, and outcome measures; and coordinating fetal monitoring education and certification (Knox et al., 2003; Will et al., 2006; Raab & Palmer-Byfield, 2011). Although the volumes in all hospitals may not support this position on a full-time basis, in some hospitals, a part-time position may be feasible.

SUMMARY

When the focus of care is putting safety of mothers and babies first, practice based on the cumulative body of science and national standards and guidelines is a natural and obvious conclusion. Keeping current is critically important for perinatal nurses to maximize safe care for mothers and babies and to minimize the risk of patient injuries and professional liability. Effective leadership and interdisciplinary collaboration are essential. When there is mutual respect and professional behavior among all members of the perinatal team, a safe care environment is enhanced. Practice in a perinatal setting where patient safety is the number one priority is professionally rewarding and personally fulfilling.

REFERENCES

Agency for Healthcare Research and Quality. (2005). *Medical Teamwork and Patient Safety: The Evidence-Based Relation*. Rockville, MD: Author.

Agency for Healthcare Research and Quality. (2007). *Team STEPPS Curriculum*. Rockville, MD: Author.

Agency for Healthcare Research and Quality. (2011a). *Hospital Survey on Patient Safety Culture*. Rockville, MD: Author.

Agency for Healthcare Research and Quality. (2011b). *Patient Safety Indicators*. Rockville, MD: Author.

Agency for Healthcare Research and Quality. (2012). *Hospital Survey on Patient Safety Culture: 2012 User Comparative Database Report* (6th ed.). Rockville, MD: Author.

Aiken, L. H., & Patrician, P. A. (2000). Measuring organizational traits of hospitals: The revised nursing work index. *Nursing Research, 49*(3), 146–153.

American Academy of Pediatrics. (1999). *Circumcision Policy Statement*. Reaffirmed in 2005. Washington, DC: Author.

American Academy of Pediatrics & American College of Obstetricians and Gynecologists. (2007). *Guidelines for Perinatal Care* (6th ed.). Elk Grove Village, IL: Authors.

American Academy of Pediatrics & American Heart Association. (2011). *Textbook of Neonatal Resuscitation* (6th ed.). Chicago, IL: Author.

American Association of Critical-Care Nurses. (2005). *AACN Standards for Establishing and Sustaining Healthy Work Environments*. Aliso Viejo, CA: Author.

American College of Obstetricians and Gynecologists. (2000). *Operative vaginal delivery* (Practice Bulletin No. 17). Washington, DC: Author.

American College of Obstetricians and Gynecologists. (2001). *Circumcision* (Committee Opinion No. 260; Reaffirmed 2011). Washington, DC: Author.

American College of Obstetricians and Gynecologists. (2002). *Shoulder dystocia* (Practice Bulletin No. 40; Reaffirmed 2010). Washington, DC: Author.

American College of Obstetricians and Gynecologists. (2003). *Dystocia and augmentation of labor* (Practice Bulletin No. 49; Reaffirmed 2011). Washington, DC: Author.

American College of Obstetricians and Gynecologists. (2006). *Analgesia and cesarean delivery rates* (Committee Opinion No. 339; Reaffirmed 2010). Washington, DC: Author.

American College of Obstetricians and Gynecologists. (2008a). *Fetal lung maturity* (Practice Bulletin No. 97). Washington, DC: Author. doi:10.1097/AOG.0b013e318188d1c2

American College of Obstetricians and Gynecologists. (2008b). *Prenatal and perinatal human immunodeficiency virus testing: Expanded recommendations* (Committee Opinion No. 418; Reaffirmed 2011). Washington, DC: Author. doi:10.1097/AOG.0b013e318188d29c

American College of Obstetricians and Gynecologists. (2009a). *2009 ACOG Survey on Professional Liability*. Washington, DC: Author.

American College of Obstetricians and Gynecologists. (2009b). *Induction of labor* (Practice Bulletin No. 107). Washington, DC: Author. doi:10.1097/AOG.0b013e3181b48ef5

American College of Obstetricians and Gynecologists. (2010a). *Management of intrapartum fetal heart rate tracings* (Practice Bulletin No. 116). Washington, DC: Author. doi:10.1097/AOG.0b013e3182004fa9

American College of Obstetricians and Gynecologists. (2010b). *Vaginal birth after previous cesarean delivery* (Practice Bulletin No. 115). Washington, DC: Author. doi:10.1097/AOG.0b013e3181eeb251

American College of Obstetricians and Gynecologists. (2011a). *Preoperative planned cesarean delivery* (Patient Safety Checklist No. 4). Washington, DC: Author. doi:10.1097/AOG.0b01.e31823ed223

American College of Obstetricians and Gynecologists. (2011b). *Preparing for clinical emergencies in obstetrics and gynecology* (Committee Opinion No. 487). Washington, DC: Author. doi:10.1097/AOG.0b013e31821922eb

American College of Obstetricians and Gynecologists. (2011c). *Prevention of early-onset group B streptococcal disease in newborns* (Committee Opinion No. 485). Washington, DC: Author. doi:10.1097/AOG.0b013e318219229b

American College of Obstetricians and Gynecologists. (2011d). *Scheduling induction of labor* (Patient Safety Checklist No. 5). Washington, DC: Author. doi:10.1097/AOG.0b013e318240d429

American College of Obstetricians and Gynecologists. (2011e). *Scheduling planned cesarean delivery* (Patient Safety Checklist No. 3). Washington, DC: Author. doi:10.1097/AOG.0b013e31823ed20d

American College of Obstetricians and Gynecologists. (2012). *Communication strategies for patient handoffs* (Committee Opinion No. 517). Washington, DC: Author. doi:10.1097/AOG.0b013e318249ff4f

American College of Obstetricians and Gynecologists & American Academy of Pediatrics. (2003). *Neonatal Encephalopathy and Cerebral Palsy: Defining the Pathogenesis and Pathophysiology*. Washington, DC: Author.

American Nurses Association. (2010). *Code of Ethics for Nurses*. Washington, DC: Author.

American Society of Anesthesiologists. (2007). Practice guidelines for obstetric anesthesia: An updated report by the American Society of Anesthesiologists task force on obstetric anesthesia. *Anesthesiology, 106*(4), 843–863.

Andreatta, P., Frankel, J., Smith, S. B., Bullough, A., & Marzano, D. (2011). Interdisciplinary team training identifies discrepancies in institutional policies and practices. *American Journal of Obstetrics and Gynecology, 205*(4), 298–301. doi:10.1016/j.ajog.2011.02.022

Arias, F. (2000). Pharmacology of oxytocin and prostaglandins. *Clinical Obstetrics and Gynecology, 43*(3), 455–468.

Association of Women's Health, Obstetric and Neonatal Nurses. (2008). *Nursing Management of the Second Stage of Labor* (Evidence-based clinical practice guideline). Washington, DC: Author.

Association of Women's Health, Obstetric and Neonatal Nurses. (2010). *Guidelines for Professional Registered Nurse Staffing for Perinatal Units*. Washington, DC: Author.

Association of Women's Health, Obstetric and Neonatal Nurses. (2012). *The Role of the Registered Nurse (RN) in the Care of Pregnant Women Receiving Analgesia/Anesthesia by Catheter Techniques (Epidural, Intrathecal, Spinal, PCEA Catheters)* (Clinical Position Statement). Washington, DC: Author.

Bakker, P. C., Kurver, P. H., Kuik, D. J., & Van Geijn, H. P. (2007). Elevated uterine activity increases the risk of fetal acidosis at birth. *American Journal of Obstetrics and Gynecology, 196,* 313.e1–313.e6. doi:10.1016/j.ajog.2006.11.035

Bakker, P. C., & Van Geijn, H. P. (2008). Uterine activity: Implications for the condition of the fetus. *Journal of Perinatal Medicine, 36*(1), 30–37.

Barnett, M. M., & Humenick, S. S. (1982). Infant outcome in second stage labor pushing method. *Birth and the Family Journal, 9,* 221–229.

Beyea, S. C., Killen, A., & Knox, G. E. (2004). Learning from stories: A pathway to patient safety. *AORN Journal, 79*(1), 224–226.

Bingham, D., & Main, E. K. (2010). Effective implementation strategies and tactics for leading change on perinatal units. *Journal of Perinatal and Neonatal Nursing, 24*(1), 32–42.

Bofill, J. A., Martin, J. N. Jr., & Morrison, J. C. (1998). The Mississippi operative vaginal delivery trial: Lessons learned. *Contemporary OB/GYN, 43*(10), 60–79.

Bofill, J. A., Rust, O. A., Schorr, S. J., Brown, R. C., Martin, R. W., Martin, J. N. Jr., & Morrison, J. C. (1996). A randomized prospective trial of the obstetric forceps versus the M-cup vacuum extractor. *American Journal of Obstetrics and Gynecology, 175*(5), 1325–1330.

Brumfield, C., Gilstrap, L. C., O'Grady, J. P., Ross, M. G., & Schifrin, B. S. (1999). Cutting your legal risks with vacuum-assisted deliveries. *OBG Management, 3,* 2–6.

Caldeyro-Barcia, R. (1979). The influence of maternal bearing-down efforts during second stage on fetal wellbeing. *Birth and the Family Journal, 6,* 17–21.

Caldeyro-Barcia, R., Giussi, G., Storch, E., Poseiro, J. J., Kettenhuber, K., & Ballejo, G. (1981). The bearing down efforts and their effects on fetal heart rate, oxygenation, and acid-base balance. *Journal of Perinatal Medicine, 9*(Suppl. 1), 63–67.

Centers for Disease Control and Prevention (2010). Prevention of perinatal group B streptococcal disease: Revised guidelines from CDC, 2010. *Morbidity and Mortality Weekly Report, 19*(RR-10), 1–36.

Chauhan, S. P., Magann, E. F., McAninch, C. B., Gherman, R. B., & Morrison, J. C. (2003). Application of learning theory to obstetric maloccurrence. *Journal of Maternal-Fetal and Neonatal Medicine, 13*(3), 203–207.

Chez, B. F. (1997). Electronic fetal monitoring: Then and now. *Journal of Perinatal and Neonatal Nursing, 10*(4), 1–4.

Choudhry, N. K., Fletcher, R. H., & Soumerai, S. B. (2005). Systematic review: The relationship between clinical experience and quality of health care. *Annals of Internal Medicine, 142*(4), 260–273.

Clark, S. L., Belfort, M. A., Dildy, G. A., & Meyers, J. A. (2008). Reducing obstetric litigation through alterations in practice patterns. *Obstetrics and Gynecology, 112*(6), 1279–1283. doi:10.1097/AOG.0b013e31818da2c7

Clark, S. L., Frye, D. R., Meyers, J. A, Belfort, B. A., Dildy, G. A., Kofford, S., . . . Perlin, J. A. (2010). Reduction in elective delivery <39 weeks of gestation: Comparative effectiveness of 3 approaches to change and the impact on neonatal intensive care admission and stillbirth. *American Journal of Obstetrics and Gynecology, 203*(5), 449.e1–e6. doi:10.1016/j.ajog.2010.05.036

Clark, S. L., Simpson, K. R., Knox, G. E., & Garite, T. J. (2009). Oxytocin: New perspectives on an old drug. *American Journal of Obstetrics and Gynecology, 200*(1), 35.e1–35.e6. doi:10.1016/j.ajog.2008.06.010

Colla, J. B., Bracken, A. C., Kinney, L. M., & Weeks, W. B. (2005). Measuring patient safety climate: A review of surveys. *Quality and Safety in Healthcare, 14*(5), 364–366.

The Consolidated Omnibus Budget Reconciliation Act (COBRA) of 1985, Pub. L. No. 9272, § 9121, 100 Stat. 82 (1986).

Crane, J. M., & Young, D. C. (1998). Meta-analysis of low-dose versus high-dose oxytocin for labour induction. *Journal of the Society of Obstetricians and Gynaecologists of Canada, 20,* 1215–1223.

Crane, J. M., Young, D. C., Butt, K. D., Bennett, K. A., & Hutchens, D. (2001). Excessive uterine activity accompanying induced labor. *American Journal of Obstetrics and Gynecology, 97*(6), 926–931.

Crico Strategies. (2010). *2010: Annual Benchmarking Report Malpractice Risks in Obstetrics.* Cambridge, MA: Author.

de Vries, E. N., Prins, H. A., Crolla, R. M., den Outer, A. J., van Andel, G., van Helden, S. H., . . . Boermeester, M. A. (2010). Effect of a comprehensive surgical safety system on patient outcomes. *New England Journal of Medicine, 363*(20), 1928–1937.

Food and Drug Administration. (1998). *Need for caution when using vacuum assisted delivery devices* (FDA Public Health Advisory). Washington, DC: Author.

Fox, M., Kilpatrick, S., King, T., & Parer, J. T. (2000). Fetal heart rate monitoring: Interpretation and collaborative management. *Journal of Midwifery and Women's Health, 45*(6), 498–507.

Fraser, W. D., Marcoux, S., Krauss, I., Douglas, J., Goulet, C., & Boulvain, M., for the PEOPLE (Pushing Early or Pushing Late with Epidurals) Study Group. (2000). Multicenter randomized trial of delayed pushing for nulliparous women in the second stage of labor with continuous epidural analgesia. *American Journal of Obstetrics and Gynecology, 182*(5), 1165–1172.

Frigoletto, F. D., Jr., Lieberman, E., Lang, J. M., Cohen, A., Barss, V., Ringer, S., et al. (1995). A clinical trial of active management of labor. *New England Journal of Medicine, 333*(12), 745–750.

Greenwald, L. M., & Mondor, M. (2003). Malpractice and the perinatal nurse. *Journal of Perinatal and Neonatal Nursing, 17*(2), 101–109.

Griffin, T. (2010). Bringing change-of-shift report to the bedside: A patient- and family-centered approach. *Journal of Perinatal and Neonatal Nursing, 24*(4), 348–353.

Grunebaum, A., Chervenak, F., & Skupski, D. (2011). Effect of a comprehensive obstetric patient safety program on compensation payments and sentinel events. *American Journal of Obstetrics and Gynecology, 204*(2), 97–105. doi:10.1016/j.ajog.2010.11.009

Halligan, M., & Zecevic, A. (2011). Safety culture in healthcare: A review of concepts, dimensions, measures and progress. *BMJ Quality and Safety, 20*(4), 338–343. doi:10.1136/bmjqs.2010.040964

Hansen, S. L., Clark, S. L., & Foster, J. C. (2002). Active pushing versus passive fetal descent in the second stage of labor: A randomized controlled trial. *Obstetrics and Gynecology, 99*(1), 29–34.

Haynes, A. B., Weiser, T. G., Berry, W. R., Lipsitz, S. R., Breizat, A. H., Dellinger, E. P., . . . Gawande, A. A. (2009). A surgical safety checklist to reduce global morbidity and mortality in a global population. *New England Journal of Medicine, 360*(5), 491–499.

Hesse-Biber, S. N., & Leavy P. (2006). *The Practice of Qualitative Research.* Thousand Oaks, CA: Sage.

Institute of Medicine. (2011). *Relieving Pain in America: A Blueprint for Transforming Prevention, Care, Education, and Research.* Washington, DC: The National Academies Press.

Johnson, C. E., Handberg, E., Dobalian, A., Gurol, N., & Pearson, V. (2005). Improving perinatal and neonatal patient safety: The AHRQ patient safety indicators. *Journal of Perinatal and Neonatal Nursing, 19*(1), 15–23.

Joint Commission. (2008). *Behaviors that Undermine a Culture of Safety* (Sentinel Event Alert No. 40). Oakbrook Terrace, IL: Author.

Joint Commission. (2009a). *Perinatal Care Core Measure Set.* Oakbrook Terrace, IL: Author.

Joint Commission. (2009b). *National Hospital Inpatient Quality Measures: Perinatal Care Core Measure Set.* Oakbrook Terrace, IL: Author.

Joint Commission. (2010). *Preventing Maternal Death* (Sentinel Event Alert No. 44). Oakbrook Terrace, IL: Author.

Joint Commission. (2011a). *Sentinel Event Policy and Procedures.* Oakbrook Terrance, IL: Author.

Joint Commission. (2011b). *Summary of Data of Sentinel Events Reviewed by the Joint Commission.* Oakbrook Terrace, IL: Author.

Joint Commission. (2012). *Comprehensive Accreditation Manual for Hospitals.* Oakbrook Terrance, IL: Author.

Joint Commission on Accreditation of Healthcare Organizations. (2004). *Preventing Infant Death and Injury During Delivery* (Sentinel Event Alert No. 30). Oak Brook, IL: Author.

Jury Verdict Research. (2009). *Current Award Trends in Personal Injury.* Horsham, PA: Author.

Kaplan, H. C., & Ballard, J. (2012). Changing practice to improve patient safety and quality of care in perinatal medicine. *American Journal of Perinatology, 29*(1), 35–42.

Kirkpatrick, D. H., & Burkman, R. T. (2010). Does standardization of care through clinical guidelines improve outcomes and reduce medical liability? *Obstetrics and Gynecology, 116*(5), 1022–1026. doi:10.1097/AOG.0b013e3181f97c62

Knox, G. E., & Simpson, K. R. (2011). Perinatal high reliability. *American Journal of Obstetrics and Gynecology, 204*(5), 373–377. doi: 10.1016/j.ajog.2010.10.900

Knox, G. E., Simpson, K. R., & Garite, T. J. (1999). High reliability perinatal units: An approach to the prevention of patient injury and medical malpractice claims. *Journal of Healthcare Risk Management, 19*(2), 24–32.

Knox, G. E., Simpson, K. R., & Townsend, K. E. (2003). High reliability perinatal units: Further observations and a suggested plan for action. *Journal of Healthcare Risk Management, 23*(4), 17–21.

Kohn, L. T., Corrigan, J. M., & Donaldson, M. S. (1999). *To Err is Human: Building a Safer Health System.* Washington, DC: National Academy Press.

Lake, E. T. (2002). Development of the practice environment scale of the nursing work index. *Research in Nursing and Health, 25*(3), 176–188.

Lawrence, H. C., Copel, J. A., O'Keeffe, D. F., Bradford, W. C., Scarrow, P. K., Kennedy, H. P., . . . Olden, C. R. (2012). Quality patient care in labor and delivery: A call to action. *American Journal of Obstetrics and Gynecology, 207*(3), 147–148. doi:10.1016/j.ajog.2012.07.018.

Leape, L. L., & Berwick, D. M. (2005). Five years after to err is human: What have we learned? *Journal of the American Medical Association, 293*(19), 2384–2390.

Lopez-Zeno, J. A., Peaceman, A. M., Adashek, J. A., & Socol, M. L. (1992). A controlled trial of a program for the active management of labor. *New England Journal of Medicine, 326*(7), 450–454.

Lyndon, A., & Ali, L. U. (Eds.). (2009). *AWHONN's Fetal Heart Monitoring* (4th ed.). Washington, DC: Kendall Hunt.

Lyndon, A., Sexton, B., Simpson, K. R., Rosenstein, A., Lee, K. A., & Wachter, R. M. (2012). Predictors of likelihood of speaking up about safety concerns in labour and delivery. *BMJ Quality and Safety, 21*(9), 791–799. doi:10.1136/bmjqs.2010.050211

Macones, G. A., Hankins, G. D. V., Spong, C. Y., Hauth, J., & Moore, T. (2008). The 2008 National Institute of Child Health and Human Development workshop report on electronic fetal monitoring. *Obstetrics and Gynecology, 112*(3), 661–666. doi:10.1097/AOG.0b013e3181841395

Mayberry, L. J., Gennaro, S., Strange, L., Williams, M., & De, A. (1999). Maternal fatigue: Implications of second stage nursing care. *Journal of Obstetric, Gynecologic and Neonatal Nursing, 28*(2), 175–181.

Mayberry, L. J., Hammer, R., Kelly, C., True-Driver, B., & De, A. (1999). Use of delayed pushing with epidural anesthesia: Findings from a randomized controlled trial. *Journal of Perinatology, 19*(1), 26–30.

Mayberry, L. J., Strange, L. B., Suplee, P. D., & Gennaro, S. (2003). Use of upright positioning with epidural analgesia: Findings from an observational study. *MCN: The American Journal of Maternal Child Nursing, 28*(3), 152–159.

McHugh, M., Garman, A., McAlearney, A., Song, P., & Harrison, M. (2010). *Using Workforce Practices to Drive Quality Improvement: A Guide for Hospitals* (AHRQ Publication No. 11-0003-EF). Rockville, MD: Agency for Healthcare Research and Quality.

Miller, K. K., Riley, W., Davis, S., & Hansen, H. E. (2008). In situ simulation: A method of experiential learning to promote safety and team behavior. *Journal of Perinatal and Neonatal Nursing, 22*(2), 105–113.

Minkoff, H., & Berkowitz, R. L. (2009). Fetal monitoring bundle. *Obstetrics and Gynecology, 114*(6), 1332–1335. doi:10.1097/AOG.0b013e3181bfb2bd

National Quality Forum. (2002). *Serious Reportable Events in Healthcare.* Washington, DC: Author.

National Quality Forum. (2006). *Serious Reportable Events in Healthcare.* Washington, DC: Author.

National Quality Forum. (2009a). *National Voluntary Consensus Standards for Nursing-Sensitive Care.* Washington, DC: Author.

National Quality Forum. (2009b). *National Voluntary Consensus Standards for Perinatal Care 2008: A Consensus Report.* Washington, DC: Author.

National Quality Forum. (2010). *Safe Practices for Better Healthcare.* Washington, DC: Author.

Nieva, V. F., & Sorra, J. (2003). Safety culture assessment: A tool for improving patient safety in healthcare organizations. *Quality and Safety in Health Care, 12*(Suppl. 2), 17–23.

Nordstrom, L., Achanna, S., Nuka, K., & Arulkumaran, S. (2001). Fetal and maternal lactate increase during active second stage labour. *British Journal of Obstetrics and Gynaecology, 108*(3), 263–268.

Nurses Service Organization. (2009). *CNA Healthpro Nurse Claims Study: An Analysis of Claims with Risk Management Recommendations 1997–2007.* Hatboro, PA: Author.

O'Driscoll, K., Jackson, R. J., & Gallagher, J. T. (1970). Active management of labor and cephalopelvic disproportion. *Journal of Obstetrics and Gynaecology of the British Commonwealth, 77*(5), 385–389.

Paluska, S. A. (1997). Vacuum-assisted vaginal delivery. *American Family Physician, 55*(6), 2197–2203.

Parer, J. T., King, T., Flanders, S., Fox, M., & Kilpatrick, S. J. (2006). Fetal acidemia and electronic fetal heart rate patterns: Is there evidence of an association? *Journal of Maternal-Fetal and Neonatal Medicine, 19*(5), 289–294.

Patterson, E. S., Roth, E. M., Woods, D. D., Chow, R., & Orlando, J. (2004). Handoff strategies in settings with high consequences for failure: Lessons for health care operations. *International Journal for Quality in Health Care, 16*(2), 125–132.

Pettker, C. M., Thung, S. F., Norwitz, E. R., Buhimschi, C. S., Raab, C. A., Copel, J. A., . . . Funai, E. F. (2009). Impact of a comprehensive patient safety strategy on obstetric adverse events. *American Journal of Obstetrics and Gynecology, 200*, 492.e1–492.e8. doi:10.1016/j.ajog.2009.01.022

Phaneuf, S., Rodriguez-Linares, B., Tambyraja, R. L., MacKenzie, I. Z., & Lopez Bernal, A. (2000). Loss of myometrial oxytocin receptors during oxytocin-induced and oxytocin-augmented labour. *Journal of Reproduction and Fertility, 120*, 91–97.

Piquard, F., Schaefer, A., Hsiung, R., Dellenbach, P., & Haberey, P. (1989). Are there two biological parts in the second stage of labor? *Acta Obstetricia et Gynecologica Scandinavica, 68*(8), 713–718.

Porto, G., & Lauve, R. (2006). Disruptive clinician behavior: A persistent threat to patient safety. *Patient Safety & Quality Healthcare* (July/August). Retrieved from http://www.psqh.com

Pronovost, P. J., Holzmueller, C. G., Ennen, C. S., & Foz, H. E. (2011). Overview of progress in patient safety. *American Journal of Obstetrics and Gynecology, 204*(1), 5–10.

Pronovost, P. J., Nolan, T., Zeger, S., Miller, M., & Rubin, H. (2004). How can clinicians measure safety and quality in acute care? *Lancet, 363*, 1061–1067.

Raab, C., & Palmer-Byfield, R. (2011). The perinatal patient safety nurse: Exemplar of transformational leadership. *MCN: The American Journal of Maternal Child Nursing, 36*(5), 280–287. doi:10.1097/NMC.0b013e31822631ec

Riley, W., Hanson, H., Gurses, A., Davies, S., Miller, K., & Priester, R. (2008). The nature, characteristics, and patterns of perinatal critical events teams. In K. Henriksen, J. B. Battles, M. A. Keyes, & M. L. Grady (Eds.), *Advances in Patient Safety: New Directions and Alternative Approaches* (Vol. 3, pp. 131–144). Rockville, MD: Agency for Healthcare Research and Quality.

Roberts, C. L., Algert, C. S., Cameron, C. A., & Torvaldsen, S. (2005). A meta-analysis of upright positions in the second stage to reduce instrumental deliveries in women with epidural analgesia. *Acta Obstetricia et Gynecologica Scandinavica, 84*(8), 794–798.

Roberts, C. L., Torvaldsen, S., Cameron, C. A., & Olive, E. (2004). Delayed versus early pushing in women with epidural analgesia: A systematic review and meta-analysis. *Journal of Obstetrics and Gynaecology, 111*(12), 1333–1340.

Roberts, J. E. (2002). The "push" for evidence: Management of the second stage. *Journal of Midwifery and Women's Health, 47*(1), 2–15.

Rogers, R., Gilson, G. J., Miller, A. C., Izquierdo, L. E., Curet, L. B., & Qualls, C. R. (1997). Active management of labor: Does it make a difference? *American Journal of Obstetrics and Gynecology, 177*(3), 599–605.

Romano, P. S., Yasmeen, S., Schembri, M. E., Keyzer, J. M., & Gilbert, W. M. (2005). Coding of perineal lacerations and other complications of obstetric care in hospital discharge data. *Obstetrics and Gynecology, 106*(4), 717–725.

Rosenstein, A. H., & O'Daniel, M. (2005). Disruptive behavior and clinical outcomes: Perceptions of nurses and physicians. *American Journal of Nursing, 105*(1), 54–64.

Ryan, M. J. (2004). Patient safety: A matter of integrity. *Journal of Innovative Management, 9*(1), 11–20.

Sampselle, C., & Hines, S. (1999). Spontaneous pushing during birth. Relationship to perineal outcomes. *Journal of Nurse Midwifery, 44*(1), 36–39.

Semel, M. E., Resch, S., Haynes, A. B., Funk, L. M., Bader, A., Berry, W. R., . . . Gawande, A. A. (2010). Adopting a surgical safety checklist could save money and improve the quality of care in U.S. hospitals. *Health Affairs Millwood, 29*(9), 1593–1599. doi:10.1377/hlthaff.2009.0709

Sexton, J. B., Helmreich, R. L., Neilands, T. B., Rowan, K., Vella, K., . . . Thomas, E. J. (2006). The Safety Attitudes Questionnaire: Psychometric properties, benchmarking data, and emerging research. *BMC Health Services Research, 3*(6), 44.

Simpson, K. R. (1999). Shoulder dystocia: Nursing interventions and risk management strategies. *MCN: The American Journal of Maternal Child Nursing, 24*(6), 305–311.

Simpson, K. R. (2005a). Failure to rescue: Implications for evaluating quality of care during labor and birth. *Journal of Perinatal and Neonatal Nursing, 19*(1), 23–33.

Simpson, K. R. (2005b). Handling handoffs safely. *MCN: The American Journal of Maternal Child Nursing, 30*(2), 76.

Simpson, K. R. (2006a). Measuring perinatal patient safety: Review of current methods. *Journal of Obstetric, Gynecologic and Neonatal Nursing, 35*(3), 432–442.

Simpson, K. R. (2006b). Obstetrical "never events." *MCN: The American Journal of Maternal Child Nursing, 31*(2), 136.

Simpson, K. R. (2013). *Cervical Ripening and Labor Induction and Augmentation* (Practice monograph). Washington, DC: Association of Women's Health, Obstetric and Neonatal Nurses.

Simpson, K. R. (2011). Avoiding confusion of maternal heart rate with fetal heart rate during labor. *MCN: The American Journal of Maternal Child Nursing, 36*(4), 272. doi:10.1097/NMC.0b013e318217a61a

Simpson, K. R., & James, D. C. (2005a). Effects of immediate versus delayed pushing during second-stage labor on fetal well-being: A randomized clinical trial. *Nursing Research, 54*(3), 149–157.

Simpson, K. R., & James, D. C. (2005b). Efficacy of intrauterine resuscitation techniques in improving fetal oxygen status during labor. *Obstetrics and Gynecology, 105*(6), 1362–1368.

Simpson, K. R., & James, D. C. (2008). Effects of oxytocin-induced uterine hyperstimulation during labor on fetal oxygen status and fetal heart rate patterns. *American Journal of Obstetrics and Gynecology, 199*, 34.e1–34.e5. doi:10.1016/j.ajog.2007.12.015

Simpson, K. R., James, D. C., & Knox, G. E. (2006). Nurse-physician communication during labor and birth: Implications for patient safety. *Journal of Obstetric, Gynecologic and Neonatal Nursing, 35*(4), 547–556.

Simpson, K. R., & Knox, G. E. (2001). Fundal pressure during the second stage of labor: Clinical perspectives and risk management issues. *MCN: The American Journal of Maternal Child Nursing, 26*(2), 64–71.

Simpson, K. R., & Knox, G. E. (2003a). Adverse perinatal outcomes: Recognition, understanding and prevention of common types of accidents. *AWHONN Lifelines, 17*(3), 225–236.

Simpson, K. R., & Knox, G. E. (2003b). Common areas of litigation related to care during labor and birth: Recommendations to promote patient safety and decrease risk exposure. *Journal of Perinatal and Neonatal Nursing, 17*(1), 94–109.

Simpson, K. R., & Knox, G. E. (2006). Essential criteria to promote safe care during labor and birth. *AWHONN Lifelines, 9*(6), 478–483.

Simpson, K. R., & Knox, G. E. (2009). Oxytocin as a high alert medication. *MCN: The American Journal of Maternal Child Nursing, 34*(1), 8–15. doi:10.1097/01.NMC.0000343859.62828.ee

Simpson, K. R., Knox, G. E., Martin, M., George, C., & Watson, S. R. (2011). MHA Keystone Obstetrics: A statewide collaborative for perinatal patient safety in Michigan. *Joint Commission Journal on Quality and Patient Safety, 37*(12), 544–552.

Simpson, K. R., Kortz, C. C., & Knox, G. E. (2009). A comprehensive perinatal patient safety program to reduce preventable adverse outcomes and costs of liability claims. *Joint Commission Journal on Quality and Patient Safety, 35*(11), 565–574.

Simpson, K. R., & Lyndon, A. (2009). Clinical disagreements during labor and birth: How does real life compare to best practice? *MCN: The American Journal of Maternal Child Nursing, 34*(1), 31–39. doi:10.1097/01.NMC.0000343863.72237.2b

Thomas, E. J., Sexton, J. B., Neilands, T. B., Frankel, A., & Helmreich, R. L. (2005). The effect of executive walk rounds on nurse safety climate attitudes: A randomized trial of clinical units. *BMC Health Services Research, 5*(1), 28–37.

Tubridy, N., & Redmond, J. M. (1996). Neurological symptoms attributed to epidural analgesia in labour: An observational study of seven cases. *Journal of Obstetrics and Gynaecology, 103*(8), 832–833.

United States Department of Health and Human Services, Centers for Medicare & Medicaid Services. (2003). *EMTALA: 42 CFR Parts 413, 482, and 489 [CMS-1063-F] RIN 0938-AM34 Medicare Program; Clarifying Policies Related to the Responsibilities of Medicare-Participating Hospitals in Treating Individuals with Emergency Medical Conditions* (Final Rule). Washington, DC: Author.

United States Department of Health and Human Services, Centers for Medicare & Medicaid Services. (2009). *Revisions to Appendix V, "Emergency Medical Treatment and Labor Act (EMTALA) Interpretive Guidelines"* (Publication 100-07). Washington, DC: Author.

Wagner, B., Meirowitz, N., Shah, J., Nanda, D., Reggio, L., Cohen, P., . . . Abrams, K. (2012). Comprehensive perinatal patient safety initiative to reduce adverse obstetric events. *Journal for Healthcare Quality, 34*(1), 6–15. doi:10.1111/j.1945-1474.2011.00134.x

Weber, D. O. (2004). Poll results: Doctors' disruptive behavior disturbs physician leaders. *The Physician Executive, 30*(5), 6–15.

White, A. A., Pichert, J. W., Bledsoe, S. H., Irwin, C., & Entman, S. S. (2005). Cause and effect analysis of closed claims in obstetrics and gynecology. *Obstetrics and Gynecology, 105*(5, Pt. 1), 1031–1038.

Will, S. B., Hennicke, K. P., Jacobs, L. S., O'Neill, L. M., & Raab, C. A. (2006). The perinatal patient nurse: A new role to promote safe care for mothers and babies. *Journal of Obstetric, Gynecologic and Neonatal Nursing, 35*(3), 417–423.

Wong, C. A., Scavone, B. M., Dugan, S., Smith, J. C., Prather, H., Ganchiff, J. N., . . . McCarthy, R. J. (2003). Incidence of postpartum lumbosacral spine and lower extremity nerve injuries. *Obstetrics and Gynecology, 101*, 279–288.

World Alliance for Patient Safety. (2008). *WHO Guidelines for Safe Surgery.* Geneva, Switzerland: World Health Organization.

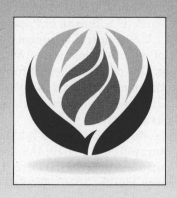

Lynn Clark Callister

CHAPTER 2

Integrating Cultural Beliefs and Practices When Caring for Childbearing Women and Families

Maria, a Mexican American woman having her first baby, attended a childbirth education class where the expectant fathers learned labor support techniques. She declined to lie on the floor surrounded by other men while her husband massaged her abdomen.

Hala, a Muslim Arabic woman experiencing her first labor, was attended by her mother and mother-in-law. As the labor slowly progressed and Hala began to be more uncomfortable, the two mothers alternated between offering her loving support, chastising her for acting like a child, and praying loudly that mother and baby will be safe from harm.

Nguyet, a primiparous Vietnamese immigrant, had been in the United States only a short time when she went into labor. She arrived at the birthing unit in active labor dilated to 5 cm. Nguyet and the father of the baby, Duc, spoke very limited English. Her labor was difficult, but she did not utter a sound. Duc entered the birthing room only when the nurses asked him to translate for Nguyet. After 20 hours of labor, a cesarean birth was performed. On the mother–baby unit, Nguyet cooperated with the instructions from the nurse to cough and deep breathe, but she became agitated when the nurse set up for a bed bath and began bathing her. When she was encouraged to walk, she shook her head and refused. She also refused the chilled apple juice the nurse brought to her. Because of abdominal distention and dehydration, a nasogastric tube was inserted, and intravenous fluids were restarted. No one could understand why she was so uncooperative.

Because of a nonreassuring fetal heart rate, Koua Khang needed an emergent cesarean birth. The nurse told her she would need to remove a nondescript white string bracelet from her wrist before surgery. Koua became hysterical, gesturing and trying to convey the message that the bracelet would protect her during the birth from evil spirits.

Michelle, a certified nurse midwife, cared for a Mexican immigrant mother who finally confided in her that during her postpartum hospitalization she went in the shower and turned on the water but was very careful not to get wet. She was following instructions from her nurse while trying to maintain her own cultural beliefs.

Mei Lin, a Chinese woman in graduate school in the United States, promised her mother she would follow traditional Asian practices after her son was born, including "doing the month" and subscribing to the hot/cold theory. Even though this woman was intellectually aware these practices had little scientific basis, she demonstrated her respect for her mother and her culture by honoring her mother's request.

Sameena was having a scheduled cesarean birth. Her family had a tradition that the newborn be placed immediately in a blanket that had been in the family for generations, but were concerned that since it was a surgical birth, the tradition would not be followed. The nurses accommodated this cultural tradition, and the blanket was placed inside the hospital receiving blanket when her child was born. The grandmother was pleased and grateful.

Childbirth is a time of transition and social celebration in all cultures. A Wintu child living in Africa, in deference to his mother, refers to her as, "She whom I made into mother." Culture also influences the experience of perinatal loss because the meaning of death and rituals surrounding death are culturally bound. Healthcare beliefs and health-seeking behaviors surrounding pregnancy, childbirth, and parenting are deeply rooted in cultural context. Culture is a set of behaviors, beliefs, and practices, a value system that is transmitted from one woman in a cultural group

41

to another (Lauderdale, 2007). It is more than skin color, language, or country of origin. Culture provides a framework within which women think, make decisions, and act. It is the essence of who a woman is. The extent to which a woman adheres to cultural practices, beliefs, and rituals is complex and depends on acculturation and assimilation into the dominant culture within the society, social support, length of time in the United States or Canada, generational ties, and linguistic preference. Even within individual cultural groups, there is tremendous heterogeneity. Although women may share a common birthplace or language, they do not always share the same cultural traditions (Moore, Moos, & Callister, 2010).

Diversity is a reality in the United States. Nurses provide care to immigrants, refugees, and women from almost everywhere in the world, many of whom are of childbearing age (Grewal, Bhagat, & Balneaves, 2008; McKeary & Newbold, 2010). More than 30% of the U.S. population now consists of individuals from culturally diverse groups other than non-Hispanic whites, whereas only 9% of registered nurses come from racial or ethnic minority backgrounds. It is projected that by the year 2050, minorities will account for more than 50% of the population of the United States. Each year, nearly 1 million immigrants come to the United States, half of whom are immigrant women of childbearing age.

Since 1980, more than 200,000 refugees have resettled in the United States (U.S. Bureau of Population, 2008). One in every 12 U.S. residents is foreign born. Twenty-seven percent of women living in the United States are women of color. One of the challenges for healthcare in this century is that members of racial and ethnic minorities make up a disproportionately high percentage of persons living in poverty.

Poverty brings many challenges in healthcare delivery (U.S. Census Bureau [USCB], 2010; U.S. Department of Health and Human Services [USDHHS], 2010; USDHHS Office of Minority Health, 2010). Women and families in poverty can be considered a culture associated with health disparities and increased vulnerability in childbearing women.

Clinical examples in this chapter represent only a fraction of the possible cultural beliefs, practices, and behaviors the perinatal nurse may see in practice (Display 2–1). It is beyond the scope of this chapter to thoroughly discuss in detail each cultural group. Although generalizations are made about cultural groups, a stereotypical approach to the provision of perinatal nursing care is not appropriate. Cultural beliefs and practices are dynamic and evolving, requiring ongoing exploration (Douglas & Pacquiao, 2010). In any given culture, each generation of childbearing families perceives pregnancy, childbirth, and parenting differently. Each individual

---

 D I S P L A Y   2 - 1

Culture and Birth Traditions

AFRICAN AMERICAN/BLACK
- Geophagia (ingestion of soil, chalk, or clay) may be present during pregnancy
- Strong extended family support
- Matriarchal society
- Present time orientation
- May engage in folk practices ("granny," "root doctor," voodoo priest, spiritualist) depending on background
- Tend to seek prenatal care after the first trimester

AMERICAN INDIAN AND NATIVE ALASKAN
- Healthcare decision making by families/tribal leaders
- Often stoic; don't make eye contact, limit touch
- Strong spiritual foundation
- May utilize a medicine man or shaman
- Present time orientation

ASIAN AMERICAN AND PACIFIC ISLANDER
- Culturally and linguistically heterogeneous
- Healthcare decision making by families
- "Hot/cold" theory of illness (pregnancy considered a "hot" condition, except among Chinese women, who consider it a "cold" condition)
- Asians are often stoic.

- Strong extended family support
- Asian fathers may choose not to attend the birth.
- Chinese postpartum focus on "doing the month"
- AAs have future orientation, PIs have present orientation
- Asians have high respect for others.
- Asians may utilize an acupuncturist/acupressurist, herbalist.

HISPANIC/LATINO
- Healthcare decision making by families
- Strong extended family support
- Prenatal care may not be valued because pregnancy is a healthy state.
- Enjoy strong extended family support
- Fathers may choose not to attend the birth.
- May use folk healers and Western medicine concurrently (curandero, espiritualista, yerbero)
- Present time orientation
- Believe in the "evil eye"
- Postpartum maternal/newborn dyad vulnerable or delicate

WHITE/CAUCASIAN
- Often considered a noncultural group
- Value autonomy and personal decision making
- Eastern European women avoid cutting or coloring hair during pregnancy.
- Future time orientation
- Focus on achievement

woman should be treated as an individual who may or may not espouse specific cultural beliefs, practices, and behaviors.

Cultures are not limited to the obvious traditional ethnic or racial groups. Examples of other "cultures" include refugees and immigrants, women living in poverty, women who have experienced ritual circumcision, adolescent childbearing women, women with disabilities, and deeply religious women such as those espousing the beliefs of Jehovah's Witnesses (Bircher, 2009; Braithwaite, Chichester, & Reid, 2010; Ogunleye, Shelton, Ireland, Glick, & Yeh, 2010; Wisdom et al., 2010). Perinatal nursing units may also be considered a culture, for some women a "foreign country" (Lewallen, 2011).

CULTURAL FRAMEWORKS AND CULTURAL ASSESSMENT TOOLS

Cultural frameworks and cultural assessment tools have been developed to guide perinatal nursing practice. The Sunrise Model is based on culture care theory (Fig. 2–1) (Leininger & McFarland, 2006). The Transcultural Assessment Model (Giger, 2008) includes variables such as communication, space, social organization, time, environmental control, and biologic variations (Fig. 2–2). Others have identified the dimensions of culture, including values, worldview, disease etiology, time orientation, personal space

orientation and touch, family organization, and power structure (Purnell & Paulanka, 2011). The Transcultural Nursing Model is illustrated in Figure 2–3 (Andrews & Boyle, 2007). Mattson (2011) has conceptualized specific ethnocultural considerations in caring for childbearing women (Fig. 2–4). Four assumptions define the influence culture has on pregnancy, childbirth, and parenting (Display 2–2). Models should focus on the person, the processes, the environment, and the outcomes.

CULTURAL COMPETENCE

The process of cultural competence in the delivery of healthcare includes cultural awareness, skills, encounters, and knowledge (Campinha-Bacote, 1994). Cultural competence is more than a nicety in healthcare. Cultural competence has become imperative because of increasing health disparities and population diversity; the competitive healthcare market; federal regulations on discrimination; complex legislative, regulatory, and accreditation requirements; and our litigious society (deChesnay, Wharton, & Pamp, 2005; Joint Commission for Accreditation of Healthcare Organizations, 2010; Rorie, 2008) (Fig. 2–5).

Acculturation is a complex variable that is challenging to measure, and current measures need to be refined (Beck, Froman, & Bernal, 2005). Acculturation can be at a cultural or group level and a psychological or individual level (Beck, 2006; Gorman, Madlensky,

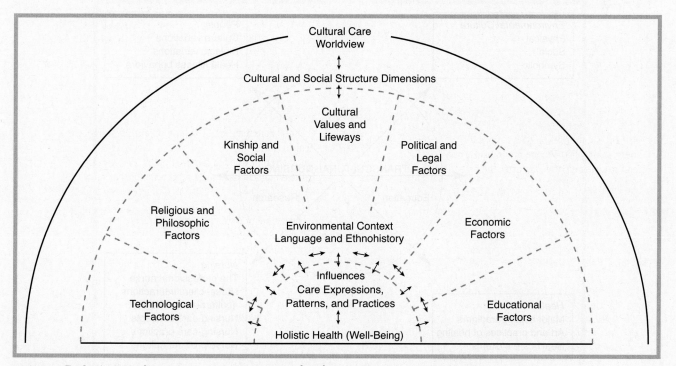

FIGURE 2-1. The Sunrise Model. (From Leininger, M., & McFarland, M. R. [2006]. *Cultural Care Diversity and Universality: A Worldwide Nursing Theory* [2nd ed.]. Sudbury, MA: Jones & Bartlett.)

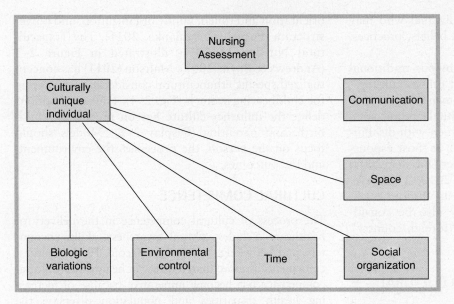

FIGURE 2-2. Transcultural model. (From Giger, J. N. [2007]. *Transcultural Nursing: Assessment and Intervention* [5th ed.] St. Louis, MO: Mosby–Year Book.)

Jackson, Ganiats, & Boles, 2007; Huang, Appel, & Ai, 2011). The General Acculturation Index scale can be used to assess level of acculturation, and it includes items such as written and spoken language, the country where the childhood was spent, the current circle of friends, and pride in cultural background (Balcazar, Peterson, & Krull, 1997). Other instruments include the Short Acculturation Scale, the Acculturation Rating Scale for Mexican Americans (ARSMA), the

ARSMA II, and the Bidimensional Acculturation Scale for Hispanics (Beck, 2006). A framework for acculturation has been identified by Berry (1980). Outcomes include assimilation, the establishment of relationships in the host society made at the expense of the patient's native culture; integration, in which cultural identity is retained and new relationships are established in the host society; rejection, in which one retains cultural identity and rejects the host society; and deculturation,

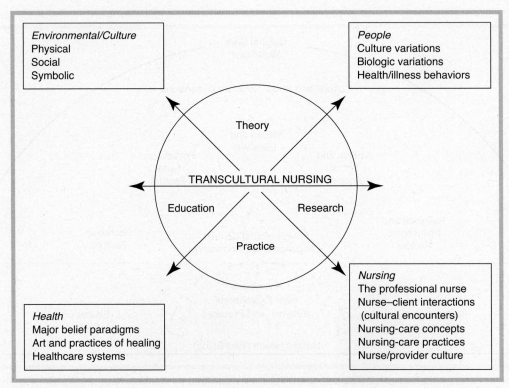

FIGURE 2-3. Transcultural nursing.

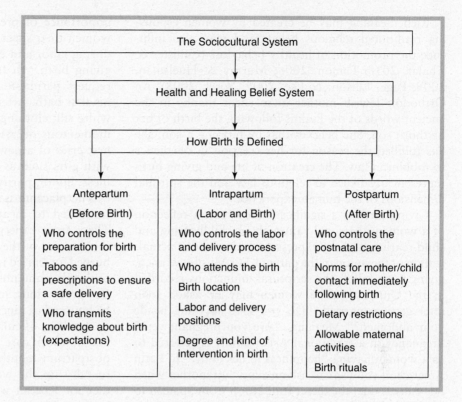

FIGURE 2-4. The sociocultural system, health and healing belief system, and how birth is defined. (From Mattson, S. [2011]. Ethnocultural considerations in the childbearing period. In S. Mattson & J. E. Smith [Eds.]. *Core curriculum for maternal-newborn nursing* [4th ed.] Philadelphia: Saunders.)

in which one values neither. Nurses will encounter immigrant women who fall into each of these categories of acculturation.

What constitutes a positive and satisfying birth experience varies from one culture to another (Amoros, Callister, & Sarkisyan, 2010; Callister, Holt, & Kuhre, 2010; Callister, Corbett, Reed, Tomao, & Thornton, 2010; Callister et al., 2007; Callister, Eads, Diehl, & See, 2011; Corbett & Callister, 2012; Johnson, Callister, Beckstrand, & Freeborn, 2007; Wilkinson & Callister,

2010). For example, within the Japanese culture, there is the belief in a process called "education of the unborn." A happy mother is thought to ensure joy and good fortune because the unborn child learns, communicates, and responds in utero. The individual personality is formed before birth. Such a belief about the fetus is reflected in many cultures, with concern during pregnancy about evil spirits and birthmarks. Other cultural considerations include fertility rites and beliefs about what determines the gender of the unborn child.

Influence of Culture on Pregnancy, Childbirth, and Parenting

- Within the framework of the *moral and value system*, cultural groups have specific *attitudes* toward childbearing and the meaning of the birth experience.
- Within the framework of the *ceremonial and ritual system*, cultural groups have specific *practices* associated with childbearing.
- Within the framework of the *kinship system*, cultural groups prescribe *gender-related roles* for childbearing.
- Within the framework of the *knowledge and belief system*, cultural groups influence *normative behavior* in childbearing and the *pain experience* of childbirth.

From Callister, L. C. (1995). Cultural meanings of childbirth. *Journal of Obstetric, Gynecologic, and Neonatal Nursing, 24*(4), 327–331.

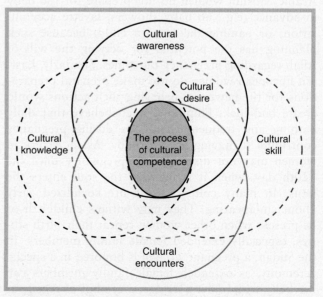

FIGURE 2-5. The process of cultural competence in the delivery of healthcare.

Rich meaning may be created by women espousing traditional religious beliefs and may also influence the promotion of healthy behaviors (Callister & Khalaf, 2010; Lemon, 2006; Murray & Huelsman, 2009; Page, Ellison, & Lee, 2009; Yosef, 2008). An Orthodox Jewish mother gives silent thanks in the ancient words of the Psalms following the birth of her firstborn son. She believes that by birthing a son, she has fulfilled the reason for her creation in obedience to rabbinical law. The creation of life and giving birth represent obedience to religious law and the spiritual dimensions of the human experience.

Giving birth is a significant life event, a reflection of a woman's personal values about childbearing and child rearing, and the expression and symbolic actualization of the union of the parents. For Muslim women, giving birth fulfills the scriptural injunctions recorded in the Quran. Muslim women may be asked soon after getting married, "Do you save anything inside your abdomen?" Meaning, "Are you pregnant yet?" Pregnancy in a traditional Asian family is referred to as a woman having "happiness in her body." In Latin America, if you were to ask an expectant mother when her baby is due, the direct translation from Spanish to English is, "When are you going to give light?"

PRACTICES ASSOCIATED WITH CHILDBEARING

There are many diverse cultural rituals, customs, and beliefs associated with childbearing. American Indian mothers believe tying knots or weaving will cause birth complications associated with cord accidents. Navajo expectant mothers do not choose a name or make a cradleboard because doing so may be detrimental to the well-being of the newborn. Arabic Muslim women do not prepare for the baby in advance (e.g., no baby showers, layette accumulation, or naming the unborn child) because such planning has the potential for defying the will of Allah regarding pregnancy outcomes. Similarly, Eastern European women do not make prenatal preparations for the newborn, believing such actions would create bad luck. Filipino women believe that daily bathing and frequent shampoos during pregnancy contribute to having a clean baby. Asian American women may not disclose their pregnancy until the 120th day, when it is believed the soul enters the fetus. In many cultures, girls are socialized early about childbearing. They may witness childbirth or be present when other women repeat their birth stories, especially extended female family members. In the Sudan, a pregnant woman is honored in a special ceremony, as extended female family members rub her belly with millet porridge, a symbol of regeneration, empowering her to give birth. Because of the

importance of preserving modesty, Southeast Asian women tie a sheet around their bodies like a sarong during labor and express a preference to squat while giving birth. An Italian maternal grandmother may request permission to give her newborn grandson his first bath. After the bath, she dresses him in fine, white silk clothing that she stitched by hand for this momentous occasion. When women in Bali hear the first cries of a newborn, they lavish the new mother with gifts such as dolls, fruit, flowers, or incense to bless, honor, purify, and protect the new child.

The placenta is called "el compañero" in Spanish, translated to mean, "the companion of the child." There are a variety of cultural rituals associated with the disposal of the placenta, including having it dried, burned, or buried in a specific way. Although disposing of the placenta must meet with standard infection control precautions, individual family preferences should be honored as much as possible.

A variety of cultural practices influence postpartum and newborn care. Laotian women stay home the first postpartum month near a fire or heater in an effort to "dry up the womb." The traditional postpartum diet for Korean women includes a soup made from beef broth and seaweed that is believed to cleanse the body of lochia and increase breast milk production. In Navajo tradition, a family banquet is prepared following the baby's first laugh because this touches the hearts of all those who surround the baby.

Care of the newborn's umbilical cord includes the use of a binder or belly band, the application of oil, or cord clamping, and then sterile excision. A Southeast Asian woman may fail to bring her newborn to the pediatrician during the first month after birth because this is considered to be a time for confinement and rest.

Postpartum cultural rituals are important for women of different cultures. Culturally diverse women experience postpartum depression, with an increased risk related to the gender of the child because in some societies male children are more highly valued (Callister, Beckstrand, & Corbett, 2010; Lau & Wong, 2008b).

GENDER ROLES

Many cultural groups show strong preference for a son. For example, according to Confucian tradition, only a son can perform the crucial rites of ancestor worship. A woman's status is closely tied to her ability to produce a son in many cultures.

A Mexican immigrant woman may prefer that her mother or sister be present during her childbirth, rather than the father of her child. In some cultures, fathers may prefer to remain in the waiting room until after the birth. Vietnamese fathers rarely participate in the birth of their children. Only after the newborn is bathed and dressed may the father see him or her. In cultures in which the husband's presence during birth is not thought to be appropriate, nurses should not assume this denotes lack of paternal involvement and support.

Modesty laws and the law of family purity found in the Torah prohibit the Orthodox Jewish husband from observing his wife when she is immodestly exposed and from touching her when there is vaginal bleeding. Depending on the specific religious sect, observance of the law varies from the onset of labor or bloody show to complete cervical dilation. Jewish husbands present at birth stand at the head of the birthing bed or behind a curtain in the room and do not observe the birth or touch their wives. Although cultural factors may limit a husband's ability to physically support or coach his wife during labor and birth, Jewish women still feel supported. Husbands praying, reading Psalms, and consulting with the rabbi represent significant and active support to these women (Noble, Engelhardt, Newsome-Wicks, & Woloski-Wruble, 2009; Noble, 2009; Zauderer, 2009).

CHILDBIRTH PAIN AND CULTURE

A major pain experience unique to women is that associated with giving birth. Many cultural differences related to the perception of childbirth pain have been identified (Callister, 2011). Some women feel that pain is a natural part of childbirth and that the pain experience provides opportunity for important and powerful growth. Others see childbirth pain as no different from the pain of an illness or injury; that it is inhumane and unnecessary to suffer.

Words used to describe the pain associated with childbirth vary. Labor pain has been described as horrible to excruciating, episiotomy pain described as discomforting and distressing, and postpartum pain described as mild to very uncomfortable. Korean women described pain with words such as "felt like dying" or the "the sky was turning yellow," or the sense of "tearing apart." Mexican American women view pain as a physical experience, composed of personal, social, and spiritual dimensions. Scandinavian women demonstrate a high level of resilience and hardiness when giving birth, as do Australian women. One Australian woman viewed birth as symbolic of the challenges of life: "[Giving birth] makes you more resilient. You know you are able to handle things that you didn't think you could. I think it gives you strength because you know if you can through that, you can cope with a lot of other things" (Callister, Holt, et al., 2010, p. 113). Women's perceptions of personal control have been found to positively influence their satisfaction with pain management during childbirth.

Pain behaviors also are culturally bound. Some Hispanic laboring women may moan in a rhythmic way and rub their thighs or abdomen to manage the pain.

During labor, Haitian women are reluctant to accept pain medication and instead use massage, movement, and position changes to increase comfort. Filipino women believe that noise and activity around them during labor increases labor pain. African American women are more vocally expressive of pain. American Indian women are often stoic, using meditation, self-control, and traditional herbs to manage pain. Puerto Rican women are often emotive in labor, expressing their pain vocally. There is disparity between the estimation of labor pain by caregivers and the pain the women reported they were experiencing. The Coping with Labor Algorithm is proving helpful in assessing pain in laboring women rather than use of the traditional pain scale (Roberts, Gulliver, Fisher, & Cloyes, 2010).

MAJOR CULTURAL GROUPS

The major cultural groups in the United States include African Americans/blacks (AA/B), American Indian/Alaska Native (AI/AN), Asian American/Pacific Islander (AA/PI), Hispanic/Latino (H/L), and white/Caucasian (W/C). Designation in one of these five categories is not equated with within-group homogeneity. The U.S. population by race and ethnic origin is shown in Figure 2–6 (USCB, 2010). The names used to identify these major U.S. cultural groups are those used by the USCB. The following two modifications were made in the year 2000 census data. The AA/PI category was separated into two categories, Asian American or Native Hawaiian/Pacific Islander; and Latino has been added to the Hispanic category (H/L).

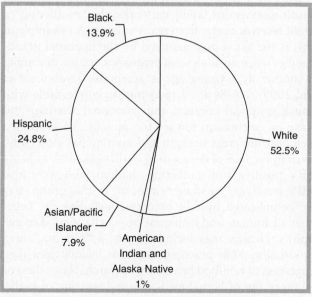

FIGURE 2-6. United States' predicted population by race and ethnic origin, 2050.

AFRICAN AMERICAN OR BLACK

According to 2010 census data, this group constitutes 12.6% of the population in the United States. This heterogeneous group has origins in black racial groups of Africa and the Caribbean Islands, including the West Indies, Dominican Republic, Haiti, and Jamaica. AA/B persons may speak French, Spanish, African dialects, and various forms of English. By 2050, the AA/B population is expected to nearly double its present size to 61 million. A disproportionate percentage of AA/Bs are disadvantaged because of poverty and low educational levels, and they are more likely to have only public insurance. Comparative lifetime pregnancy rates for U.S. women between the ages of 15 and 44 are 2.7 for W/Cs and 4.6 for AA/B and H/L women. Health disparities exist between W/C and AA/B women (Dominguez, 2011). Infant mortality rates for AA/Bs have consistently been twice those of the overall population (USDHHS, 2010). As a group, AA/Bs are at increased risk for diabetes, lupus, HIV/AIDS, sickle cell anemia, hypertension, and cancer of the esophagus and the stomach (Purnell & Paulanka, 2011; Spector, 2008).

Core Values

AA/B families display resilience and adaptive coping strategies in their struggles with racism and poverty. They have a strong religious commitment, as observed in Southern Baptist, fundamentalist, and black Muslim church communities, which helps to enhance their spiritual health and general well-being (Wehbe-Alamah, McFarland, Macklin, & Riggs, 2011). Fifty-one percent of AA/B families are headed by women, and more than 55% of all AA/B children younger than 3 years are born into single-parent families. AA/B families have extensive networks of extended families, friends, and neighbors who participate in child rearing with a high level of respect for elders. Children are highly valued, and as a result of extended family networks, the "mothering" a child receives comes from many sources. An example of this is the active role assumed by the maternal grandmother when an adolescent pregnancy occurs. Becoming a mother at a young age is acceptable (Nabukera et al., 2009). AA/Bs are demonstrative; comfortable with touch, physical contact, and emotional sharing; and have an orientation toward the present. AA/B women demonstrate great strength and matriarchal leadership, even in the face of devastating challenges, such as being HIV positive and mothering children who were also HIV positive. Providing healthcare to this group may be complicated by folk practices, including the belief that all animate and inanimate objects have good or evil spirits. Healers may include family, a "Granny," or a spiritualist. Folk practices may also include pica (i.e., ingestion of nonfood items such as starch, clay, ashes, or plaster); use of herbal medicine; and wearing of garlic, amulets, and copper or silver bracelets (Gunn & Davis, 2011; Spector, 2008).

Cultural Beliefs and Practices

Some American blacks may resent being called African Americans because this does not represent their origin (Moore et al., 2010). AA/Bs living in poverty may demonstrate a lack of respect for or fear of public clinics and hospitals. They tend to seek prenatal care later than other women, usually after the first trimester. The incidence of breastfeeding is related to the level of maternal education and social support. AA/B women are more expressive of pain and are usually accompanied during labor and birth by female relatives. Most male newborns are circumcised.

Haitian women are less likely than other groups to seek prenatal care. During pregnancy, they believe they should not swallow their saliva and instead carry a spit cup with them. Fathers are unlikely to be present during birth, believing it is an event only for women. Haitian women are encouraged by their community to breastfeed. However, some inaccurate beliefs, such as thick milk causing skin rashes and thin milk resulting in diarrhea, persist. During the postpartum period, women may believe that a series of three baths aids in their recovery. The first 3 days, women bathe in a special water infused with herbs. For the next 3 days, women bathe in water in which leaves have been soaked and warmed by the sun. After 4 weeks, a cold bath is taken that is believed to tighten muscles and bones loosened during the birth process. Women also believe that wearing a piece of linen or a belt tightly around the waist prevents the entry of gas into their body. Eating white foods such as milk, white lima beans, and lobster is avoided during the postpartum period because they are believed to increase vaginal discharge and hemorrhaging. Traditionally, Haitian women do not have their newborns circumcised because they believe circumcision decreases sexual satisfaction, but as acculturation occurs, this procedure is becoming more common. West Indian countries of origin are Trinidad, Jamaica, and Barbados. Traditionally, the father of the baby is not present during labor and birth.

Ghanian and other African childbearing women may believe in witchcraft and often access Western healthcare, ethnomedicine, and faith-based interventions simultaneously to ensure positive outcomes from pregnancy and childbirth (Farnes, Callister, & Beckstrand, 2011).

Ethiopian woman are considered to be in a delicate state after birth. To be protected from disease and harm, they remain secluded for at least 40 days. A special diet that includes milk and warm foods such as gruel made of oats and honey is thought to increase breast milk production.

Somali refugee women are resistive to and fearful of cesarean births and most technological perinatal interventions and are very afraid of dying in childbirth. As one woman said, "They got a C-section. . .They gonna die" (Brown, 2010, p. 220).

AMERICAN INDIAN AND ALASKAN NATIVE

Descendants of the original peoples of North America (i.e., American Indian, Eskimo, and Aleut) constitute 0.9% of the population. There are 500 federally recognized AI nations accessing healthcare from Indian Health Services and/or traditional healers.

AI/ANs have a higher unemployment and poverty rate than the general population. They average 9.6 years of formal education, the lowest rate of any major group in the United States. Urban AI/ANs have a much higher rate of low-birth-weight infants compared with urban W/Cs and rural AI/ANs and a higher rate of infant mortality than urban W/Cs. Urban AI/ANs have a high incidence of risk factors associated with poor birth outcomes, including delayed prenatal care, single marital status, adolescent motherhood, and use of tobacco and alcohol. These risk factors resemble the prevalence among AA/ABs except for the higher incidence of alcohol use among AI/ANs. Rural AI/ANs have lower rates of low-birth-weight infants and higher rates of timely prenatal care than their urban counterparts. As a group, AI/ANs have an increased risk for alcoholism, heart disease, cirrhosis of the liver, and diabetes mellitus (Purmell & Paulanka, 2011; Spector, 2008).

Core Values

In general, AI/ANs have a strong spiritual foundation in their lives with a holistic focus on the circular wheel of life. It is important to live in complete harmony with nature. Values include oral traditions passed from generation to generation. Elders play a dominant role in decision making and many AI/AN tribes are matrilineal, so involving maternal grandmothers in teaching young mothers is an important and culturally sensitive intervention. AI/ANs are present oriented, which may make it difficult to obtain an accurate health history because the past may be perceived as unrelated to current conditions. They believe in harmony. They may avoid eye contact and limit touch. Use of a formal interpreter increases the credibility of the healthcare provider because listening is highly valued.

Cultural Beliefs and Practices

During pregnancy, women avoid touching their hair. If an infant is born prematurely or expected to die, a family member may request to perform a ceremony that includes ritual washing of the hair. If hair is removed to initiate a scalp intravenous line on a newborn, some families want the hair returned to them. The mother and newborn remain indoors resting for 20 days or until the umbilical cord falls off. The umbilical cord may be saved, because some AI/ANs believe that it has spiritual significance. Patterns of infant care include group caregiving, living spiritually, merging the infant into Indian culture, using permissive discipline, and observing the child developing.

ASIAN AMERICAN AND PACIFIC ISLANDER

AA/PIs are people with origins in the Far East, Southeast Asia, the Indian subcontinent, or the Pacific Islands. AA/PIs constitute 3.6% of the population in the United States and are projected to make up 8.7% by 2050. There is great diversity in the 28 AA/PI groups designated in the census. Asians comprise 95% of this population and are divided into 17 groups, speaking 32 different primary languages plus multiple dialects. Major groups of AAs include Chinese, Japanese, Koreans, Filipinos, Vietnamese, Cambodians, and Laotians. The major groups, Chinese and Japanese, are the most long-standing groups of Asian immigrants.

PIs comprise 5% of AA/PIs, with specific groups including Hawaiian, Samoan, Guamanian, Tongan, Tahitian, North Marianas, and Fijian. There are more than 50 subgroups speaking at least 32 different languages. Approximately two thirds of Asians living in the United States are foreign-born. This group is culturally and linguistically heterogeneous. In the United States, AA/PIs are highly concentrated in the western states and in metropolitan areas.

There is a paucity of data regarding the health status of AA/PIs. Because they are a small minority, AA/PIs are often overlooked in healthcare services planning and research. In relation to healthcare, AA/PIs comprise the most misunderstood, underrepresented, underreported, and understudied ethnic population. They are often mistakenly referred to as the healthy minority (Kim & Keefe, 2010). Their educational attainment has a bimodal distribution, with 39% having college degrees and 5% assessed as functionally illiterate. They utilize primary and preventive care less often than non-Hispanic whites (Zhao, Esposito, & Wang, 2010). If they have limited English proficiency, barriers to healthcare include making an appointment, locating a health facility, communicating with healthcare providers, and acquiring health literacy (Kim & Keefe, 2010). Posttraumatic stress syndrome is of concern in AA/PI refugee women, especially Hmong women, who may have suffered atrocities while living in their country of origin. Infant mortality rates are highest in Native Hawaiians (11.4/1,000 live births). As a group, AA/PIs are at increased risk of hypertension, liver cancer, stomach cancer, and lactose intolerance (Purnell & Paulanka, 2011; Spector, 2008).

Core Values

Values embody the philosophical traditions of Buddhism, Hinduism, and Christianity. They believe events are predestined and strive for a degree of spirituality in their lives. Core values include cohesive families, filial piety and respect for the elderly, respect for authority, interdependence and reciprocity (group orientation), interpersonal harmony, and avoidance of disagreement and conflict. Pride, fatalism, education/achievement orientation, respect for tradition, and a strong work ethic are also core values. Asians seldom express strong reactions to emotionally arousing events and are taught to suppress feelings to maintain harmonious relationships with others. They avoid public displays of affection, except among family and close friends, and have clearly defined gender roles.

Traditional therapies are often employed concurrently with Western medicine, including acupuncture, herbs, nutrition, and meditation (Callister, Eads et al., 2011; Chuang et al., 2007; Chuang et al., 2009). Asian women may believe Western medicines are too strong and may halve the prescribed dosages. Chinese women avoid oral contraceptives because of a perception that hormones may be harmful. Screening exams such as cervical screening may be avoided because of modesty and discomfort with such intimate procedures.

Cultural Beliefs and Practices

Traditional Asian healthcare beliefs and practices are Chinese in origin, with the exception of Filipino beliefs and practices being based primarily on the Malaysian culture. The yin/yang polarity is a major life force and focuses on the importance of balance for the maintenance of health. Yin represents cold, darkness, and wetness; yang represents heat, brightness, and dryness. For those who subscribe to the hot/cold theory (including Asians and Hispanics), health requires harmony between heat and cold. Balance should be maintained for women to be in harmony with the environment. During pregnancy, women eat "cold" foods such as poultry, fish, fruits, and vegetables. Eating "hot" foods at this time, such as red peppers, spicy soups, red meat, garlic, ginger, onion, coffee, and sweets, is believed to cause abortion or premature labor (Le, Ngai, Lok, Yip, & Chung, 2009). A designation of "hot" or "cold" does not necessarily refer to physical temperature but the specific effects the food is believed to have on the body.

Because pregnancy is a "hot" condition, some expectant mothers may be reluctant to take prenatal vitamins, which are considered a "hot" medication. Encouraging the woman to take her prenatal vitamins with fruit juice may resolve the problem. Some pregnant Asian women believe that iron hardens bones and makes birth more difficult, and these women resist taking vitamin preparations containing iron. Many Southeast Asian women believe that exposure of the genital area is inappropriate because this is considered a sacred part of the body. They may be reluctant to have Pap smears, wait to seek prenatal care, and communicate poorly about physical changes of pregnancy. Sexual intercourse is avoided during the third trimester because it is thought to thicken amniotic fluid, causing respiratory distress in the newborn.

Vaginal exams and an open hospital gown may be deeply humiliating and unnerving to Southeast Asian women, who value humility and modesty. Giving birth is believed to deplete a woman's body of the "hot" element (blood) and inner energy. This places her in a "cold" state for about 40 days after birth, which is assumed to be the period for the womb to heal. Rice, eggs, beef, tea, and chicken soup with garlic and black pepper are foods high in "hotness" and are eaten by postpartum women. During postpartum, pericare and hygiene are considered important, but women are discouraged from showering for several days to 2 to 4 weeks. They believe that exposure to water cools the body and interrupts balance, which may cause premature aging. Differences between cultural traditions and the Western healthcare delivery system may cause cultural tension (Le et al., 2009). One woman said, "American hospital workers don't really understand Chinese traditional customs and what may be important to a Chinese mother" (Callister, Eads et al., 2011). Another Chinese woman noted,

> [The nurses] don't really know or understand. They just aren't aware. Right after birth, I told them I wanted to keep myself warm and I wanted more blankets but they said I didn't need blankets. As Chinese we are more afraid of the cold but the [nurses] didn't seem to think so. (Callister, Eads et al., 2011)

Most AA/PI women breastfeed for several years. Women in the Hmong community (originally from Laos) may choose to formula feed, inaccurately believing American women do not breastfeed because they do not see this practice in public like they did in their homelands (Riordan, 2005).

Korean mothers may believe that newborns need sleep and little stimulation. They are discouraged from touching the baby. Thus, they may not understand the amazing capabilities of the newborn to see, hear, and interact. Child rearing often occurs within the extended family. A newborn's head is considered sacred, the essence of his/her being. Touching the newborn's head is distressing to parents and should be avoided. Traditionally, newborns have not been circumcised, but as acculturation occurs, some AA/PIs have adopted this practice.

Cambodian women may avoid certain activities during pregnancy, such as standing in doorways, because they believe this will cause the baby to become stuck in the birth canal. Sexual intercourse is not permitted during the third trimester. It is thought that avoidance of sexual intercourse during pregnancy will produce a more attractive baby. Vernix caseosa is believed to be sperm. Cambodian woman will not be seen cuddling their newborns; instead, the newborn is held down and away from their body. Herbal medications are prepared during the third trimester to be eaten three to four times per day during the postpartum period to restore body heat. Along with eating special foods that are thought to restore lost heat, mothers wear heavy clothing during the postpartum period. Breastfeeding is delayed for several days because colostrum is thought to be harmful for the newborn.

Filipino women are discouraged from remaining in a dependent position late in pregnancy, because sitting or standing may cause retention of fluid. Sexual intercourse is discouraged for the last 2 months. The women eat eggs, believing that slippery foods help the baby move through the birth canal more easily. Filipino women are accompanied during labor by a woman who has experienced birth herself.

Korean women avoid certain animal foods during pregnancy because they believe these foods can harm the newborn's character or appearance. It is believed that eating duck can cause the newborn to be born with webs between his fingers and that eating eggs causes the child to be born without a spine. Dairy products are not traditionally part of the Korean diet, so care should be taken to ensure women are receiving adequate amounts of calcium during pregnancy. In the Korean culture, the new mother is perceived as being sick and needing care. Postpartum Korean women do not easily participate in self-care activities or care for their newborn. The husband's mother is responsible for caring for the newborn and the recovery of her daughter-in-law. The need to return the hot element to the body after childbirth is accomplished by eating a special seaweed soup made with beef broth and avoiding anything cold, such as ice. The soup is thought to increase breast milk production and rid the body of lochia. Korean women may refuse an ice pack or chemical cold pack for control of perineal edema because of the belief that coldness in any form may cause chronic illness such as arthritis. Women who breastfeed are reluctant to supplement with formula.

Samoan women do not eat octopus or raw fish during pregnancy. Women supporting the laboring woman often gently massage her abdomen to relieve discomfort and determine the position of the baby. Postpartum, the abdomen may be bound and massaged by the midwife. Women do not carry the newborn after dark or stand in front of windows with the newborn at night. Most women choose to breastfeed, and it is customary to abstain from sexual intercourse while breastfeeding. Generally, male infants are circumcised.

Vietnamese women must avoid sexual intercourse and be kept warm during their pregnancy. Special hygiene practices include using salt water to wash their teeth and gums.

Chinese women focus on "doing the month" (*zuo yue zi*), with elaborate and specific restrictions for the first month following giving birth designed to promote the health and well-being of both mother and newborn (Callister, Eads et al., 2011; Chin, Jaganthan, Hasmiza, & Wu, 2010; Tung, 2010; Wan et al., 2009). Sometimes nurses assume that with acculturation and education, childbearing women will be less likely to practice traditional beliefs, but many educated Chinese childbearing women do indeed "do the month" and value other cultural practices (Callister, Eads et al., 2011).

HISPANIC AND LATINO

H/L women have ethnic origins from countries where Spanish is the primary language, including Mexico, Puerto Rico, Cuba, Spain, and South or Central America. They constitute at least 13% of the population in the United States and are the fastest growing ethnic group (USCB, 2010). Immigration is estimated at one million people per year, and census data does not include the significant number of undocumented H/Ls living and working in the United States. Spanish is the most common second language spoken in the United States. Sixty-seven percent of Hispanics are of Mexican origin. Assimilation is minimal, with strongly held cultural beliefs and behaviors. Traditional beliefs, values, and customs govern decision-making behaviors.

Significant increases in the H/L population are related to a natural increase (births over deaths) of 1.8% and a fertility rate 50% higher than W/Cs. Women comprise the largest group among the H/L population in the United States, accounting for an estimated 11 million. Latino women are younger than non-H/L women at the age of first pregnancy. The fertility rate of H/L women is 84% higher than white women and 31% higher than black women. Although H/Ls are the most likely group of women to have children, they are the least likely to initiate early prenatal care (Ramos, Jurkowski, Gonzalez, & Lawrence, 2010).

Forty-three percent of H/L births were to unmarried mothers, with adolescents accounting for a large percentage of those births. Two thirds of H/L births are to Mexican American mothers. Unintended pregnancies are more common among H/Ls compared with other ethnic groups, especially among women of low socioeconomic status.

Compared with women born in the United States, foreign-born H/L women are more likely to be economically disadvantaged and uninsured, factors usually associated with poor outcomes and adjustments are made for maternal and healthcare factors (Ramos et al., 2010). H/Ls make up over 21% of the uninsured population. With larger families and inadequate sources of income, more than 30% of H/L live below the poverty level. Despite these factors, first-generation, or less acculturated, Mexican American women seem to have a perinatal advantage despite low levels of maternal education, low socioeconomic status, and less than adequate prenatal care. Aspects of their culture that seem to protect them include nutritional intake, lower prevalence of smoking and alcohol consumption, extended family support, and spirituality or a religious lifestyle.

Immigrants usually favor Depo-Provera or Norplant rather than oral contraceptives for family planning, and there is a shift toward less patriarchal control of family planning (Gonzalez, Sable, Campbell, & Dannerbeck, 2011). Use of the term "well woman visit" is more appropriate than "family planning visit" when scheduling an appointment. Because there may be much distress and embarrassment about touching and inserting fingers into the vagina, diaphragms are not a good choice as a family planning method. H/Ls may not perceive the need for routine checkups such as Pap smears.

As a group, H/Ls are at higher risk for diabetes (twice that of W/Cs—9.8% vs. 5%) (National Diabetes Information Clearinghouse, 2011), obesity (especially among adolescents), parasitic disease, and lactose intolerance (Mendelson, McNeese-Smith, Koniak-Griffin, Nyamathi, & Lu, 2008; Spector, 2008). H/Ls are not a homogenous group, and there are many significant variations between Puerto Rican, Mexican, Peruvian, Chilean, and other H/Ls.

Core Values

In the H/L community, there are strong family ties, large and cohesive kin groups, and a family decision-making process. It is believed that the family has a meditating effect on stress and depression (Sheng, Le, & Perry, 2010). Family values include pride and self-reliance, dignity, trust, intimacy, and respect for older family members and authority figures. H/L women usually consult their husbands, significant others, or other important family members such as godparents about major health decisions. "Curanderismo" or folk medicine is frequently used. Mexican Americans may seek the services of folk healers such as herbalists, bone and muscle therapists, and midwives. These practitioners are more prevalent in border towns and may be used there as an adjunct to the established healthcare systems. An emerging group of healthcare providers are bilingual nurse-curanderas. Culturally appropriate interventions such as the Hispanic Labor Friends Initiative and Familias Sanas are proving helpful for disadvantaged Hispanic childbearing women (Hazard,

Callister, Birkhead, & Nichols, 2009; Marsiglia, Bermudez-Parsai, & Coonrod, 2010).

Cultural Beliefs and Practices

Pregnancy is an important family event engendering extensive physical and emotional support from family members. Motherhood is seen as the most important role a woman can achieve. Most H/L babies are wanted, cherished, and pampered. They are thought to be untouched by sin and evil.

H/Ls have a present orientation. This orientation affects how prenatal care is accessed. Women are frequently late for or miss prenatal appointments and may not understand how high-risk behaviors affect maternal and fetal/neonatal well-being. H/Ls have a sense of fatalism, believing that their destiny is controlled by fate or by the will of God (Mann, Mannan, Quones, Palmer, & Torres, 2010). Hispanic women may consider early prenatal care to be unnecessary because pregnancy outcomes are beyond personal control. This sense of fatalism can also promote a sense of vulnerability and lack of control. They do expect personalism and respect from healthcare providers. During pregnancy, women maintain healthy diets and exercise, and they may take herbs and drink teas recommended by herbalists. Certain folk traditions are thought to prevent birth defects. A safety pin attached to an undergarment helps protect the fetus from a cleft lip or palate. If a pregnant Guatemalan woman sees an eclipse (i.e., a "bite" taken out of the moon), her unborn child may have a bite taken out of its mouth, resulting in a cleft lip or palate.

Some H/L women believe that unsatisfied cravings cause defects or injury to the fetus. For example, a strawberry nevus is believed to occur because the pregnant woman had an unsatisfied craving for strawberries during her pregnancy. Vitamins and iron are avoided by some women during pregnancy because they are thought to be harmful. Women believe that walking during labor makes birth occur more quickly and that inactivity decreases the amount of amniotic fluid and causes the fetus to stick to the uterus, delaying the birth. Many Hispanic women prefer not to have epidural analgesia/anesthesia. Cesarean birth may be feared and viewed as life threatening for the mother. Immigrant Hispanic women giving birth may exhibit "cultural passivity," demonstrating stoicism during labor and birth and deferring to healthcare providers for any decision making (Callister, Corbett, et al., 2010).

Postpartum women are discouraged from taking a shower for several days. Belief in the "evil eye" means that a fixed stare from a person believed to be envious may result in illness. "La manita de azabache," a black onyx hand, may be placed on or near the newborn to ward off the envious evil eye. An H/L mother may assume that a nurse who overly praises her new-born or is perceived as staring at the child can cause the child to cry excessively and be very restless. H/L women view colostrum as bad or old milk and may delay breastfeeding until several days after the birth (Riordan, 2005). Avoiding foods such as chilies and beans is thought to protect the newborn from illness. In the early postpartum period, the maternal/newborn dyad is considered "muy delicados" (vulnerable or delicate) and stays at home for 7 to 15 days; and for some, up to 40 days postpartum (Spector, 2008). H/L women experiencing symptoms of postpartum depression may not seek mental health services because of the stigma attached to doing so (Callister, Eads et al., 2011). Traditionally, circumcision has not been practiced, but as acculturation occurs, this practice is becoming more acceptable. Some H/L families may want to keep and bury the placenta. Whitaker, Kavanaugh, and Klima (2010) describe perinatal grief in H/L parents. Guidelines for providing culturally competent care for H/L families have been developed (USDHHS Health Resources and Services Administration, 2010).

WHITE OR CAUCASIAN

W/Cs have origins in Europe, North Africa, or the Middle East and constitute 83% of the population of the United States. There are 53 ethnic groups classified as W/C living in the United States. In many ways, W/Cs are perceived as being privileged. For example, there are substantial differences in sources of prenatal care, with 78% of W/C women receiving private care compared with 51% of Mexican American women, 44% of AA/B women, and 47% of Puerto Rican women.

W/C is generally acknowledged to be the dominant culture. This cultural group seems intent on achieving accomplishments quickly, contributing to a high-energy, high-stress lifestyle compared with other cultural groups that have more peaceful ways of life. Predominant belief systems accept the Western biotechnologic model of healthcare, including elective inductions, elective cesarean births, and assisted reproductive technology. Women in this group are more likely to embrace such practices, but paradoxically, like women in other cultural groups, most childbearing women want nurturing, supportive, and meaningful care (Callister, Holt, et al., 2010; Hidaka & Callister, 2011; Johnson et al., 2007; Matthews & Callister, 2004).

Core Values

Core values include individualism, self-reliance, personal achievement and independence, democratic ideals and egalitarianism, work and productivity, materialism, punctuality, and future time orientation, as well as openness, assertiveness, and directness in communication.

IMMIGRANT AND REFUGEE WOMEN

Increasingly, the United States is becoming a global village. Immigrant women are coping with tremendous cultural differences and issues related to making transitions that may be extremely stressful (Bircher, 2009; Birkhead, Kennedy, & Callister, 2010; Grewal et al., 2008; Ransford, Carrillo, & Rivera, 2010). In addition to multiple challenges, many demonstrate great resiliency and strength (deChesnay et al., 2005). Immigrant and refugee women may embrace distinct culture practices and are very heterogeneous.

Cultural beliefs and practices

As first-generation, less acculturated Americans, these women have stronger ties to cultural traditions and customs than second- or third-generation Americans. For instance, they may have given birth previously in their home attended by a traditional midwife and their mother or mother-in-law.

The biomedical and highly technological environment of birthing units in the United States may be foreign and frightening. There may be a deep sadness for these mothers as they give birth without the assistance of their own mothers. One Mexican immigrant mother explained her feelings: "When I had my baby, I felt like crying. I called for my mother but she could not come to help. My mother was here in my heart because she could not come" (Callister, Beckstrand, & Corbett, 2011). Many immigrants and refugees are migrant farm workers, living in unsanitary, unsafe, and crowded conditions. Language, illiteracy, and cultural barriers have a negative impact on access to healthcare.

Cultural beliefs, such as the belief among some African immigrants that condoms may lodge in the abdominal cavity and result in obstruction, infection, or cancer, also represent a significant challenge. Another cultural challenge is the resistance of Cambodian refugees to utilize contraception. Beliefs about gender inequalities and intimate partner violence compromise the health of immigrant childbearing women. Some may be at risk for perinatal depression (Callister, Beckstrand, et al., 2010), and immigrant status is a deterrent to seeking mental health services (Chen & Vargas-Bustamante, 2011; Callister, Beckstrand, et al., 2011; Lucero, Beckstrand, Callister, & Birkhead, 2012).

It is estimated that by 2025, there will be at least 15 million American Muslims, many of whom will be immigrants. Their beliefs include "shadadah" (monotheism), "salat" (prayer five times daily), "zakat" (purification), "sawm" (fasting during Ramadan), and "hajj" (a pilgrimage to Mecca). Islamic concepts include these five teachings, along with modesty, visiting the ill, and dietary and gender restrictions. The bride's status in the family is uncertain until she has proven fertility with the birth of her first child, and sons are highly valued. Seeking prenatal care is not considered important unless there are complications. Childbirth education classes are considered to be excessive planning that may negatively affect the outcomes of pregnancy (Moore et al., 2010).

As conservators of family health, the role of immigrant women in health promotion is critical. Refugees are eligible for special refugee medical assistance during their first 18 months in the United States. After this initial coverage, those who cannot afford private health insurance and are ineligible for Medicaid benefits may become medically indigent. Limitations in literacy and language make it difficult to enter the healthcare system. Feelings of fear and paranoia create circumstances where these women are unwilling to access care. Like other childbearing women, immigrant women appreciate supportive and respectful care.

It is interesting to note that foreign-born Chinese women have more positive perinatal outcomes, including fewer low-birth-weight or small-for-gestational-age newborns, or preterm birth (Li, Keith, & Kirby, 2010). Immigrant women may be more susceptible to helminthic diseases, including tapeworm, roundworm, and hookworm, because these are endemic in Asia. Eighty percent of the five million women of childbearing age who are HIV positive are from sub-Saharan Africa, with 90% of HIV cases in this area transmitted through heterosexual contact.

RITUALLY CIRCUMCISED WOMEN

It is estimated that at least 130 million women throughout the world have been ritually circumcised. Immigrants and refugee women from developing countries in Asia (e.g., Malaysia, India, Yemen, and Oman) and 28 African countries may have experienced female genital mutilation. Among Somali women, more than 98% of the women have experienced female circumcision/female genital mutilation. Egypt has the highest incidence worldwide (Dalal, Lawoko, & Jansson, 2010). Genital mutilation may occur at any point between the newborn period and the time a woman gives birth to her first child. These women experience severe pain and complications during childbirth because the inadequate vaginal opening and scarring may prevent cervical dilatation and fetal passage. After giving birth in their native countries, some women experience reinfibulation (i.e., suturing together of the labia). Because female circumcision is a culturally bound rite of passage, women may resent Western attitudes about this practice, which has strong social and cultural support. It is illegal in the United States, and professionals have position papers regarding the negative effects of this practice (American Academy of Pediatrics, 2010). Information is provided in the literature regarding management of women with female genital mutilation (Rashid & Rashid, 2007). Perinatal nurses need to create an environment of trust, establish rapport with male family members, ensure privacy, and be sensitive to the stoicism demonstrated toward childbirth pain. Cultural re-patterning may occur with the acceptance of alternatives such as flattening of the clitoris and symbolic cutting of the pubic hair.

DEEPLY RELIGIOUS WOMEN

Many religious and spiritual beliefs and practices influence childbearing (Callister & Khalaf, 2010). Orthodox Jews have a rich body of traditions associated with childbearing and great reverence for childbearing and child rearing. Some Jewish women feel a moral responsibility to bring at least two children into the world because of the destruction of their progenitors during the Holocaust. Circumcision is a Jewish ritual based on a Hebrew covenant in the Old Testament of the Bible (Genesis 17:10–14) performed on all male children by a mohel on the eighth day of life.

For Islamic women, creating an environment that honors traditional practices according to the precepts of Islam is important. Islamic women practice a cleansing process at the end of each menstrual period. Palestinian refugee women feel a strong obligation to bear a significant number of children, especially sons, to continue the generations of the Arabic bloodline. A woman espousing the beliefs of the Church of Jesus Christ of Latter-day Saints (Mormon) may request her husband to lay his hands on her head and give her a blessing for strength, comfort, and well-being as she labors and gives birth. Mexican American women often speak in terms of a person's soul or spirit (*alma* or *espíritu*) when referring to one's inner qualities.

The sacred day of worship varies. Sunday is the Sabbath for most Christians. The Muslim's holy day is sunset Thursday to sunset Friday. Jews and Seventh Day Adventists celebrate the Sabbath from sunset on Friday to sunset on Saturday. For an Orthodox Jewish woman, honoring the Sabbath may mean not raising the head of the bed to breastfeed and not turning on the call light to request assistance because, in the Orthodox culture, these acts would constitute work. Table 2–1 provides common religious dietary prohibitions.

There is a strong relationship between health status and spiritual well-being. Religiosity and a spiritual lifestyle have been found to be the source of powerful strength during childbearing, especially when complications such as fetal or neonatal demise occur (Marshall et al., 2011). For example, in a study of the lived experience of Jordanian Muslim women having a critically ill neonate, such experiences are considered a test of faith, qualified by the phrase "inshallah" or "as God wills" (Obeidat & Callister, 2011). Spiritual beliefs and religious affiliations may represent effective

Table 2-1. RELIGIOUS DIETARY PROHIBITIONS

Religion	Dietary Prohibitions
Hinduism	All meats are prohibited.
Islam	Pork and alcoholic beverages are prohibited.
Judaism	Pork, predatory fowl, shellfish, and blood by ingestion (e.g., blood sausage, raw meat) are prohibited. Foods should be kosher (i.e., properly prepared). All animals should be ritually slaughtered to be kosher. Mixing dairy and meat dishes at the same meal is prohibited.
Mormonism (Church of Jesus Christ of Latter-day Saints)	Alcohol, tobacco, coffee, and tea are prohibited.
Seventh-day Adventists	Pork, certain seafood (including shellfish), and fermented beverages are prohibited. A vegetarian diet is encouraged.

coping mechanisms and act as sources of support (Neu & Robinson, 2008).

HEALTH DIFFERENCES IN POPULATIONS OF CHILDBEARING WOMEN

There is a paucity of research identifying health differences among minority groups and the prevalence of illness among specific populations of childbearing women. As far as body structure is concerned, AA/PIs typically have small-for-gestational-age neonates. Birth weight is lower in AA/B newborns, but size for size, they are more mature for gestational age. AA/B newborns have a mean 9 days' shorter gestation period than other ethnic groups, and there is a slowing of intrauterine growth in black infants after 35 weeks' gestation. Infants born to AA/B women are 1.5 to 3 times more likely to die than other infants (CDC, 2011). Mongolian spots are commonly found in AA/B, AA/PI, AI/AN, and H/L infants.

In addition to physical differences, cultural practices may be misinterpreted during an initial examination. Dermal practices among Southeast Asian refugees may be noticed and assumed to be a sign of physical abuse. An example of a cultural practice that may be misinterpreted is "cupping." In this practice, a cup is heated and placed on the skin, leaving a circular ecchymotic area. Pinching and rubbing may produce bruises or welts. Rubbing the skin with a spoon or coin produces dermal changes. Touching a burning cigarette to the skin may also represent cultural self-care (Spector, 2008).

Chemical substances, including pharmaceuticals, are metabolized differently among groups. Ethnopharmacologic research is a growing and important specialty. It is essential that as part of a cultural assessment, specific questions are asked about the presence or absence of potentially adverse effects of medication. It may be possible in some instances to reduce dosages in culturally diverse women (Chuang et al., 2007; Chuang et al., 2009).

There is an increasing incidence of alcoholism among H/Ls and AA/Bs, while Asians have the lowest rates of alcoholism. Most Asians and AI/ANs experience a rapid onset but slow decrease in blood acetaldehyde levels, leaving long periods of exposure to substances that cause alcohol intoxication. Fetal alcohol syndrome, or its effect, is highest among AI/ANs. Caffeine is metabolized and excreted faster by W/Cs than Asians. The incidence of lactose intolerance is 94% in AA/PIs, 90% in AA/Bs, 79% in AI/ANs, 50% in H/Ls, and 17% in W/Cs. This can have a negative effect on breastfeeding because infants may be lactose intolerant as well.

The Rh negative factor, common in Caucasians, is rare in other groups (especially Asians) and essentially absent in Eskimos. There is a high incidence of diabetes in AI tribes, whereas the disease is rare in Alaskan Eskimos. The prevalence of insulin-dependent diabetes mellitus is highest among AA/Bs. Gestational diabetes mellitus occurs in 20% of pregnant women and is not attributed specifically to race or culture.

Communicable diseases that threaten foreign-born and new immigrants, particularly those from China, Korea, the Philippines, Southeast Asia, and the Pacific, are tuberculosis (TB) and hepatitis B. Half of the women who give birth to hepatitis B–carrier infants in the United States are foreign-born Asian women. There is a significantly higher incidence of TB in AI/ANs and foreign-born AA/PIs, and the incidence of TB is four times higher among Asians than the overall population. AA/PI and AI/AN women diagnosed with TB tend to be of childbearing age (CDC, 2011).

There is a higher incidence of hypertension in AA/Bs and H/Ls. The incidence of lupus is four times higher in AA/B women and is twice as prevalent in H/L women when compared to W/C women. Native Hawaiian and Samoan women are reported to have the highest obesity rates in the world, although maternal obesity is increasing at an alarming rate in the developed world in many populations.

Sickle cell anemia occurs predominately in AA/Bs. Tay-Sachs disease is predominately found in Hasidic Jews of Eastern European descent, particularly Ashkenazi and Sephardi women. Thalassemia is a genetic blood disorder found in women from the Mediterranean region, the Middle East, and Southeast Asia.

Researchers have also documented racial disparities in complications of pregnancy and childbirth. AA/B women were more likely to have 10 of 11 maternal perinatal complications than W/C women, including preterm labor, premature rupture of membranes (PROM), hypertensive disorders, diabetes, placenta previa (PP) and abruption, infection of the amniotic cavity (IAC), and cesarean birth. H/L women were at a higher risk than white women for diabetes, PP, PROM, IAC, and postpartum hemorrhage.

Access to care also differs depending on ethnicity and culture. Fifteen percent of the population of the United States as a whole does not have health insurance, compared to 33% of H/Ls, 19% of AA/Bs, and 18% of AA/PIs.

BARRIERS TO CULTURALLY COMPETENT CARE

Culturally competent care is more than a nicety: it is essential in the delivery of quality and safe care to childbearing women and their families (Ardoin & Wilson, 2010; U.S. Department of Health and Human Services Office of Minority Health, 2010). Barriers to culturally competent care include values, beliefs, and customs; communication challenges; and the biomedical healthcare environment.

DIFFERENCES IN VALUES, BELIEFS, AND CUSTOMS

"Ethnocentrism" is the belief that one's ways are the only way. "Cultural imposition" is the tendency to thrust one's beliefs, values, and patterns of behaviors on another culture. Characteristics of caregivers that influence their ability to be culturally competent include educational level, multicultural exposure, personal attitudes and values, and professional experiences. Identifying and understanding the childbearing woman's attitudes, behaviors, values, and needs assists the perinatal nurse in identifying interventions that are culturally appropriate; are acceptable to healthcare providers, the women, and their families; have the potential to increase adherence to therapeutic regimens; and will over time result in constructive changes in perinatal healthcare delivery.

Cross, Brazon, Dennis, and Isaacs (1989) originally developed the cultural competence continuum, which moves incrementally across six stages: destructiveness, incapacity, blindness, precompetence, competence, and proficiency. Nurses demonstrate various levels of

commitment when caring for culturally diverse women on a continuum from resistant care to generalist care to impassioned care (Kirkham, 1998). Nurses who are resistant judge behaviors, ignore client needs, and complain. Resistant nurses may ignore or resent culturally diverse women and their families. They may see culture as an inconvenience or problem. Nurses who provide generalist care are respectful and competent but do not differentiate cultural diversities. Culture, to them, is a nonissue. They may empathize with client experiences but don't feel empowered to bring about substantial change. Racist attitudes of colleagues are tolerated. Nurses who provide impassioned care have a high degree of personal commitment to provide culturally sensitive care. These nurses go beyond accommodation to an appreciation of cultural diversity. They are aware of the complexities of cultural competence and the variability of expressions within cultural groups. Creativity and flexibility are the hallmarks of the care they provide to culturally diverse clients. They feel empowered to make a difference through their clinical practice. Display 2–3 provides the characteristics of the culturally competent nurse. It is important

DISPLAY 2-3

Characteristics of the Culturally Competent Practitioner

- Move from cultural unawareness to an awareness and sensitivity to his/her own cultural heritage
- Recognize his/her own values and biases and are aware of how they may affect clients from other cultures
- Demonstrate comfort with cultural differences that exist between him/her and clients
- Know specifics about the particular cultural groups he/she works with
- Understand the significance of historic events and sociocultural context for specific cultural groups
- Respect and are aware of the unique needs of specific women
- Understand the diversity that exists within and between cultures
- Endeavor to learn more about cultural communities through interactions with diverse women, participation in cultural diversity workshops and community events, readings on cultural dynamics, and consultations with community experts
- Make a continuous effort to understand others' points of view
- Demonstrate flexibility and tolerance of ambiguity and be nonjudgmental
- Maintain a sense of humor
- Demonstrate willingness to relinquish control in clinical encounters, to risk failure, and to look within for sources of frustration, anger, and resistance
- Promote cultural practices that are potentially helpful, tolerate cultural practices that are harmless or neutral, and work to education women to avoid cultural practices that may be potentially harmful

for nurses to become more culturally aware. Cultural knowledge involves gaining knowledge of the world-views of others. Development of assessment skills to understand the values, beliefs, and practices of others means engaging in cross-cultural interactions rather than avoiding them.

It is essential that nurses examine their own cultural beliefs, biases, attitudes, stereotypes, and prejudices and ask, "Whose birth is it anyway?" The following story is told by Khazoyan and Anderson (1994, p. 226):

> Señor Rojas sat at the bedside of his laboring wife, held her hand, and spoke soft, encouraging words to her. This was the kind of support that she desired during her labor: his presence, his attention, and his affection. Following the birth of their child, Señora Rojas expressed contentment and proudly described the support that her husband had provided. He had met her expectations. The nurses, however, expected more. They had wanted Señor Rojas to participate more actively in his wife's labor by massaging her back and assisting her with breathing techniques.

COMMUNICATION

Communication barriers include lack of knowledge, fear and distrust, racism, bias and ethnocentrism, stereotyping, nursing rituals, and language barriers (Ebanks, McFarland, Mixer, Munox, Pacquiao, & Wenger, 2010). Communication (or lack of communication) between cultures occurs whenever a message produced in one culture must be processed into another culture. A significant barrier to culturally competent care is language and the lack of bilingual personnel and staff with culturally diverse backgrounds. Hospitals frequently enlist nonprofessional employees of the client's ethnic background to act as interpreters. These individuals are often unfamiliar with English medical terminology and may not be able to translate accurately. Interpreters who are members of the client's cultural group may be of a different social class than the client or may be more acculturated and anxious to appear part of the dominant culture. In some cases, interpreters may be disdainful or dismissive of the client's belief system. Using children or other family members to interpret may also lead to problems. Interpretation may be based on the perceptions of the interpreter as to what is best to communicate, and they often may omit important information. According to the USD-HHS Office of Minority Health's *National Standards for Culturally and Linguistically Appropriate Services in Health Care* (2001), using the woman's friends or family members is prohibited by the healthcare facility (Display 2–4). The standards for culturally and linguistically appropriate services are described in Display 2–5. Interpreters are visitors to the perinatal unit. They will need the help of the nursing staff

DISPLAY 2-4

Standards for Medical Interpreters

- Confidentiality
- Accuracy: conveying the content and spirit of what is said
- Completeness: conveying everything that is said
- Conveying cultural frameworks
- Nonjudgmental attitude about the content to be interpreted
- Client self-determination
- Attitude toward clients
- Acceptance of assignments
- Compensation
- Self-evaluation
- Ethical violations
- Professionalism

Adapted from National Council on Interpreting in Health Care. (2005). *National standards for medical interpreters.* Retrieved from http://www.ncihc.org/mc/page.do?sitePageId=57768&orgId=ncihc

to feel comfortable and effectively provide services to the non–English-speaking patient. Guidelines for perinatal nursing staff as they work with a medical interpreter are reviewed in Display 2–6.

HEALTHCARE ENVIRONMENT

This barrier includes bureaucracy (e.g., inability of the dietary department to provide culturally appropriate foods), unsupportive administration, lack of educational opportunities to promote cultural diversity, lack of translators, and rigid policies and protocols that do not support cultural diversity. Maternal child healthcare may be the first encounter immigrant women have with healthcare delivery systems in the United States. Consider how difficult it is for the woman who may be living in the United States without the support of extended family (especially female family members), speaking little or no English, having a limited understanding of the dominant culture, having little education, and working in a low-skills-level job without benefits. When this woman arrives at the birthing unit, the unfamiliar environment and procedures serve only to increase her stress. Being hospitalized means entering a new and foreign culture with a high level of technology, the necessity of conforming to unit policies and procedures and unfamiliar schedules, having one's privacy invaded, and behaving as a "patient." This may be very challenging for women.

Another issue is our birth language, which may not reflect how women feel about having a baby. For example, use of the term "delivery" versus "birth" diminishes what the woman's role really is, devaluing her accomplishment as a mother and de-emphasizing the important cultural and spiritual context of giving

DISPLAY   2 - 5

Standards for Culturally and Linguistically Appropriate Services (CLAS)

Standard 1. Healthcare organizations should ensure that the patients/consumers receive from all staff members effective, understandable, and respectful care that is provided in a manner compatible with their cultural health beliefs and practices and preferred language.

Standard 2. Healthcare organizations should implement strategies to recruit, retain, and promote at all levels of the organization a diverse staff and leadership that are representative of the demographic characteristics of the service area.

Standard 3. Healthcare organizations should ensure that staff at all levels and across all disciplines provide culturally competent care.

Standard 4. Healthcare organizations must offer and provide language assistance services, at no cost, to each patient/consumer with limited English proficiency at all points of contact in a timely manner during all hours of operation.

Standard 5. Healthcare organizations must provide to patients/consumers in their preferred language both verbal offers and written notices informing them of their right to receive language assistance services.

Standard 6. Healthcare organizations must ensure the competence of language assistance provided to limited English proficient patients/consumers by interpreters and bilingual staff. Family and friends should not be used to provide interpretation services (except at the request of the patient/consumer).

Standard 7. Healthcare organizations must make available easily understood patient-related materials and post signage in the language of the commonly encountered group or groups represented in the service area.

Standard 8. Healthcare organizations should develop, implement, and promote a written strategic plan that outlines clear goals, policies, and operational plans and management accountability/oversight mechanisms to provide culturally and linguistically appropriate services.

Standard 9. Healthcare organizations should conduct initial and ongoing organizational self-assessments of CLAS-related activities and are encouraged to integrate cultural and linguistic competence-related measures into their internal audits, performance improvement programs, patient satisfaction assessments, and outcome-based evaluations.

Standard 10. Healthcare organizations should ensure that data on the individual patient's/consumer's race, ethnicity, and spoken and written language are collected in health records, integrated into the organization's management information systems, and periodically updated.

Standard 11. Healthcare organizations should maintain a current demographic, cultural, and epidemiologic profile of the community as well as a needs assessment to accurately plan for and implement services that respond to the cultural and linguistic characteristics of the service area.

Standard 12. Healthcare should develop participatory, collaborative partnerships with communities and utilize a variety of formal and informal mechanisms to facilitate community and patient/consumer involvement in designing and implementing CLAS-related activities.

Standard 13. Healthcare organizations should ensure that conflict and grievance resolution processes are culturally and linguistically sensitive and capable of identifying, presenting, and resolving cross-cultural conflict or complaints by patients/consumers.

Standard 14. Healthcare organizations are encouraged to regularly make available to the public information about their progress and successful innovations in implementing the CLAS standards and to provide public notice in their communities about the availability of this information.

From United States Department of Health and Human Services Office of Minority Health. (2010). *Cultural competency.* Retrieved from http://minorityhealth.hhs.gov/templates/browse.aspx?lvl=1&lvlID=3

DISPLAY   2 - 6

Guidelines for Working with a Medical Interpreter

- Orient the interpreter.
- Request a female interpreter the approximate age of the woman.
- Be prepared prior to the interpreter coming, and try to communicate with the woman prior to the interpreter arriving.
- Ask the interpreter the best way to approach sensitive issues such as sexuality or perinatal loss.
- Face the woman and direct your questions to the woman rather than the interpreter.
- Ask about one problem at a time, using concise questions and phrases.
- Look for nonverbal cues.
- After the interaction, review the woman's answers with the interpreter.

Data from Ebanks, R. L., McFarland, M. R., Mixer, S. J., Munoz, C., Pacquiao, D. F., & Wenger, A. F. Z. (2010). Cross cultural communication. *Journal of Transcultural Nursing, 21*(4 Suppl.), 137S–150S. doi:10.1177/104365961037432

birth. The woman is not passively "delivered" by the omnipotent caregiver; she should be the central figure actively giving birth. Similarly, rather than "cesarean section," the focus should be on the woman giving birth rather than focusing on a surgical procedure, using the language "cesarean birth." These small but significant linguistic differences are important in the demonstration of respect.

TECHNIQUES TO INTEGRATE CULTURE INTO NURSING CARE

Understanding the cultural context in which patients live is important to fully appreciate their response to illness and is necessary for planning appropriate nursing and medical interventions. It is essential that culturally competent care be integrated into all standards of practice (Douglas et al., 2011). Becoming culturally competent is a developmental process.

DISPLAY 2–7

Changing Institutional Forces to Facilitate Culturally Competent Care

- Changing birthing room policies and unit protocols to promote individualized and family-centered care
- Lobbying for increased resources such as translation services and cultural mediators
- Designing continuing education opportunities to increase cultural competence
- Hiring a nursing staff reflecting the culture of the community
- Generating a pool of volunteer translators who meet women prenatally and follow them through their births and the postpartum period
- Increasing the availability of language line services
- Developing innovative programs addressing the unique needs of culturally diverse populations and integrating community and acute care services for childbearing women and their families

DISPLAY 2–8

Cultural Assessment of the Childbearing Woman

- How is childbearing valued?
- Is childbearing viewed as a normal physiologic process, a wellness experience, a time of vulnerability and risk, or a state of illness?
- Are there dietary, nutritional, pharmacologic, and activity prescribed practices?
- Is birth a private, intimate experience or a societal event?
- How is childbirth pain managed, and what maternal and paternal behaviors are appropriate?
- What support is given during pregnancy, childbirth, and beyond, and who appropriately gives that support?
- How is the newborn viewed, what are the patterns regarding care of the infant, and what are the relationships within the nuclear and extended families?
- What maternal precautions or restrictions are necessary during childbearing?
- What does the childbearing experience mean to the woman?

From Callister, L. C. (1995). Cultural meanings of childbirth. *Journal of Obstetric, Gynecologic, and Neonatal Nursing, 24*(4), 327–331.

As nurses become more sensitive to the issues surrounding healthcare and the traditional health beliefs of the women they care for, more culturally competent healthcare will be provided (Anderson et al., 2010). Examples of ways that perinatal nursing units might become more culturally competent are described in Display 2–7. Cooper, Grywalski, Lamp, Newhouse, and Studlien (2007) have described a program in their hospital to increase the cultural competence of nurses.

When the cultural expectations of the nurse and the woman conflict, both are left feeling frustrated and misunderstood. The woman's adherence to traditional practices may be seen as strange and backward to the nurse, who responds by trying to "fit" the woman into the biotechnologic Western system. For example, an AI/AN mother may avoid eye contact and fail to ask questions or breastfeed in the presence of the mother–baby nurse. For many women, including Southeast Asian women, there is "loss of face" because they feel responsible for any confusion or cultural conflict with the nurse, who is perceived as a social superior. This experience may discourage them from future contact with healthcare professionals. Moore and associates (2010) identified assessment information, including place of birth; how long the woman has lived in the United States; ethnic affiliation; and the strength of that affiliation, including ethnic communities, personal support systems, language and literacy, style of communication, religious practices, dietary practices, and socioeconomic status. Display 2–8 provides the components of a cultural assessment of the childbearing woman.

ENHANCING COMMUNICATION SKILLS

Display 2–9 contains suggestions for communicating effectively with childbearing women and their families. It is important to remember that effective communication requires a sincere desire to understand the other person's way of behaving and seeing the world. This allows for cultural reciprocity, when a woman feels that she has permission to share her cultural needs, concerns, and feelings. Respect and sensitivity

DISPLAY 2–9

Culturally Competent Communication

- Enhance communication skills (greet respectfully, establish rapport, demonstrate empathy, listen actively, provide appropriate feedback, demonstrate interest).
- Develop linguistic skills.
- Determine who the family decision makers are.
- Understand that agreement does not indicate comprehension.
- Use nonverbal communication.
- Use appropriate names and titles.
- Use culturally appropriate teaching techniques.
- Provide for sufficient time.

Data from Ebanks, R. L., McFarland, M. R., Mixer, S. J., Munoz, C., Pacquiao, D. F., & Wenger, A. F. Z. (2010). Cross cultural communication. *Journal of Transcultural Nursing, 21*(4 Suppl.), 137S–150S. doi:10.1177/104365961037432

characterize this kind of relationship. A perinatal nurse described the following experience:

> I cared for a Mexican-American woman in maternal/fetal testing. I was able to help her out by being her translator. Modesty was a big issue with her, and she was extremely uncomfortable with undoing her pants and showing her abdomen for the procedure. I felt that there was a unique bond and friendship that was created because of my understanding and sensitivity to her cultural values. It makes all the difference to the woman if she is able to communicate with you and you can convey that you really care.

Be considerate, be polite, and speak softly. Caring behaviors and personal attention from healthcare providers are important to individuals of all cultures. Spend a few minutes talking to the woman and her family as she is admitted to the birthing unit to build rapport. Just a greeting and knowing a few of the social words in the woman's language and use of culturally specific etiquette helps to establish rapport. It is essential to understand cultural communication patterns. For example, Native Americans may maintain silence and not interrupt others. Hispanics appreciate interactions that begin with personal conversation or small talk, which serves to promote trust.

DEVELOPING LINGUISTIC SKILLS

Learning a second language is an excellent way to lower cultural barriers. A labor and delivery nurse described her experience caring for a Mexican immigrant woman:

> When I stepped into the room and began to speak in my high-school-level Spanish, her face brightened and she quickly responded in a rapid flow of unintelligible (to me) foreign syllables. Soon, we were able to communicate quite well, and I became comfortable with her. I translated the physician's words and vice versa. I rubbed her leg and stroked her hair when she cried out or moaned. I'd then ask her about the pain and reassured her as much as I could.

Pay attention to changing trends in language and incorporate them into your spoken and written language. Avoid using complex words, medical terms, and jargon that are difficult to understand in any language. Keep instructions simple and repeat as necessary. Saying "I understand" may be patronizing. Speak slowly, speak distinctly, and try to appear unhurried. State your message slowly, sentence by sentence. Find creative ways to convey information. One mother–baby nurse described caring for a woman who spoke no English:

> I was left with hand gestures and body language for communication. It was very difficult for her to understand my actions. Her assessment was especially hard because I was unable to assess her pain, bleeding, and nipple tenderness adequately. I finally found an English to Spanish dictionary, but this was of limited help to me because I was so bad at pronouncing the words that she still had a very difficult time understanding me. Finally, I just let her read the words from the dictionary. This was the most effective way of communicating that I could come up with. I know that she felt somewhat isolated because she had a difficult time communicating her needs to me also.

DETERMINING WHO MAKES FAMILY DECISIONS

Ask women whom they wish to include in their birth experience and make sure those persons are present for all discussions and participate in decision making. Families fulfill several roles for women, including providers of security and support, caregivers, advocates, and liaisons. Families should be treated respectfully with the goal of establishing trust. For some cultural groups, conversation should be directed toward a specific family member. It is important to identify a spokesperson in the family, often the family member most proficient in English. Ask about family roles and respect the preferences of the woman and her family. When a Mexican immigrant woman was asked whether she wanted an epidural, the father of the baby answered, saying it was better for the baby to have an unmedicated labor and birth. The wife complied with this suggestion, and the nurse modeled support for the laboring woman and demonstrated respect for their decision as a couple. Many Mexican women may prefer not to have epidural analgesia/anesthesia.

Understanding the role of different family members in the Korean family system is important because a woman's mother-in-law traditionally cares for her and the newborn during the postpartum period. The nurse needs to recognize that any teaching she does must include the mother-in-law.

UNDERSTANDING THAT AGREEMENT MAY NOT INDICATE COMPREHENSION OR THE ABILITY TO ADHERE TO HEALTHCARE RECOMMENDATIONS

Maternal health literacy is an important consideration, since it has an effect on the health of the childbearing woman and her child. Screening tools that may be useful include REALM (Rapid Estimate of Adult Literacy in Medicine), TOFHLA (Test of Functional Health Literacy in Adults), and NVS (the Newest Vital Sign) (Ferguson, 2008).

The woman may pretend to understand in an effort to please the nurse and gain acceptance. The woman's smile may mask confusion, and her nod of assent or "uh-huh" may mean only that she hears, not that she understands or agrees. For example, a new mother who did not speak English was admitted to the mother–baby unit during the night shift. When asked if she was voiding sufficient amounts, she responded, "Yes." In the early morning hours, the mother began to complain of intense abdominal pain. She was catheterized and drained of more than 1,200 mL of urine. The nurse had incorrectly assumed that the woman had understood.

The story is told of a 14-year-old AN new mother who was instructed to return to the hospital lab within 24 hours to have her newborn's bilirubin level drawn. When the nurse inquired further, she learned that this young mother had only been in the city for 2 weeks and had never used public transportation and had no money. The nurse was able to assist with community resources to help this young mother, rather than judging her as neglectful for not following discharge instructions (Ebanks et al., 2010).

USING NONVERBAL COMMUNICATION

Use eye contact, friendly facial expressions, and face-to-face positions. Do not assume the woman dislikes you, does not trust you, or is not listening to you because she avoids eye contact. Koreans, Filipinos, and many other Asian groups, as well as AI/ANs, consider direct eye contact rude and confrontational. Islamic women are taught to lower their gaze with members of the opposite sex. Use touch to express caring and comfort. Nonverbal communication makes an important difference. A labor and delivery nurse said,

> I cared for a Korean first-time mother who came to the hospital fully dilated and gave birth to her son un-medicated. She did not speak any English, and her young husband was obviously uncomfortable and had little understanding about what was going on. As she gave birth, I could see the pain in her face, but she was stoic. I felt powerless because of her language and [other] cultural barriers, but I stayed with her and held her hand and encouraged her. Even though she could not understand my words, I hope she understood that I really cared.

Use universally understood language such as charades (acting out), drawings, and gestures, and repeat the message several times using different common words. Use of simple words that are easily translated serves to improve communication.

USING NAMES AND TITLES

Determine how the childbearing woman and her family wish to be addressed. Names and appropriate titles are often complex and confusing. Mexican American clients appreciate being addressed by their last name. In the Korean culture, family members are addressed in terms of their relationship to the youngest child in the family (e.g., "Sung's grandmother"). It is important to learn how the woman wants to be addressed and to record it in the patient record so she won't have to answer the question over and over again.

TEACHING TECHNIQUES

Use visual aids and demonstrations, and assist with return demonstrations. Do not assume that the woman

DISPLAY 2-10

Developing Culturally Appropriate Educational Material

- Be aware of your own assumptions and biases.
- Develop an understanding of the target culture, including core values.
- Work with a multicultural team.
- Develop materials in the native language rather than having materials translated.
- Have materials reviewed by members of the target cultural group.

can read or write. Ensure that teaching or educational materials can be understood by the client and are appropriate for the woman's cultural group and educational level. Display 2–10 contains suggestions for beginning the process of developing culturally appropriate patient education material. Appendix 2–A contains a sampling of culturally specific educational resources.

ACCOMMODATING CULTURAL PRACTICES

Stereotypical generalization involves two dynamics: stereotyping and generalizing. Stereotyping, or believing that something is the same for everyone in a group, should be avoided. Generalizing, however, must be done to understand potential cultural beliefs and practices. The goal of individualizing care is to achieve a balance between what is indigenous to the culture and what may be specific to an individual woman. An experience that made one nurse sensitive to differences among women within the same culture was when she assumed that birth in H/L culture was exclusively a woman's experience, with little involvement by the father of the baby. She said,

> When I helped a Hispanic couple having their first baby, much to my surprise the father was right in there coaching his wife. So I supported his efforts and tried to make the birth experience what they wanted it to be.

If in doubt, ask. A culturally competent labor and delivery nurse described the following experience with a Muslim family:

> I asked the father if there was anything I should know about their customs, and he told me that before anyone could handle the baby [besides the physician], the father had to hold the baby and whisper a prayer into the ear of the baby to protect the baby from evil. I told him that as long as there were no problems with the baby immediately after birth, I would hand him the baby, and if there were problems, he could 'do his thing' while the baby was under the warmer and stabilized. He agreed to that. There were no problems, and the father got his wishes and I had the opportunity to attend a wonderfully rich cultural birth.

One Muslim husband stayed with his wife 24 hours a day during her hospitalization. The husband observed the tradition of prayers five times each day, which is a religious duty specified in the Holy Quran. It was challenging for the nurse who walked into the room while he was praying on the floor on his prayer mat, but she did all she could to support these religious rituals.

In many cultures, there is a gender preference for male children. For example, a Korean mother gave birth to a healthy baby girl. Her husband was an active, supportive coach during the labor and birth. When he saw the baby girl, however, his demeanor changed, and he shouted at his wife and started to cry. The mother also cried and refused to hold or look at her newborn daughter. The father left the room, and the mother became subdued but still refused to hold the baby. Later, the nurse commented about the beautiful infant, referring to her not as a "baby girl," but as "the baby." The mother asked to hold her newborn. The father came back into the room, and the nurse told him his baby was perfect and beautiful. This reinforcement seemed to appease the father, who then held his infant.

It is important to respect the wisdom of other cultures. Healthcare beliefs and practices can be divided into three categories: potentially beneficial, harmless or neutral, and potentially harmful. Examples in each category are listed in Table 2–2. Preservation of potentially helpful beliefs or practices and harmless or neutral behaviors that respect the natural wisdom of the culture should be encouraged, valued, and celebrated. Beneficial as well as harmless or neutral practices and those of unknown efficacy may increase a woman's connection to her own historical and cultural roots. For example, an East Indian pregnant woman may softly sing songs passed from generation to generation, massaging her abdomen several times a day and continuing that practice with her infant through the first year of life.

Herbs commonly used in pregnancy include ginger, peppermint, chamomile, cinnamon, and red raspberry leaf for morning sickness; dandelion for constipation; field greens, dandelion, and red raspberry leaf for anemia; cranberry for urinary tract infections; and red raspberry leaf for prevention of preterm labor. Herbs should not be used in the first trimester of pregnancy, and some herbs, including blue or black cohosh, dong quai, ephedra chaste tree, and zinc, should never be used during pregnancy. Some nurse midwives recommend the use of black and blue cohosh for induction of labor in term women (Born & Barron, 2005).

Focus energy on changing harmful practices. For example, the motivator for a pregnant woman to discontinue a harmful practice, such as the use of certain herbs or smoking, is to appeal to her protective instincts toward her unborn child. It is essential to show genuine interest and appreciation. The culturally competent nurse seeks to understand the woman's unique way of experiencing birth and expressing what birth means. Failure of the nurse to demonstrate interest and caring toward cultural practices she does not understand causes women to lose confidence in the nurse and the larger healthcare system and may decrease adherence with suggested health promotion strategies.

Changes are needed in nursing education, healthcare delivery, and nursing research to increase cultural competence in perinatal nursing practice. The Institute of Medicine (2002, 2009) has called for healthcare providers and the healthcare delivery system to confront and overcome their racial and ethnic disparities.

NURSING EDUCATION

Most nursing students have little knowledge about any culture other than their own. Changes in basic nursing education programs should begin to increase cultural competence. National nursing education standards

Table 2-2. PERINATAL CULTURAL PRACTICES

Potentially Helpful	Harmless or Neutral	Potentially Harmful
Postpartum diet, hygiene practices	Avoidance of sexual activity during menstruation	Avoiding bathing during menstruation
Carrying the infant close in a sling	Yarn tied around the middle finger to give hope and signify spiritual wholeness	Avoiding iron supplements during pregnancy or lactation because of the belief that iron causes hardening of the bones and a hard labor
Breastfeeding on demand	Keeping the mother's head covered at all times with a scarf or wig	Belief that colostrum is "dirty" or "old" and unfit for the newborn
Spacing of children by long-term breastfeeding	Not allowing the newborn to see his/her image in a mirror	Prolonged bed rest after birth
Remaining active throughout labor	Garlic charm around the baby's neck to offer protection from the "evil eye"	Placing a raisin on the umbilical cord to prevent a hernia
Giving birth in nonrecumbent position	Eating garlic to prevent illness	Use of abdominal binders to prevent umbilical hernia

require that educational programs prepare nurses to understand the effect that cultural, racial, socioeconomic, religious, and lifestyle differences have on health status and responses to health and illness (American Association of Colleges of Nursing, 2010). Graduates should have the knowledge and skills to provide holistic care to culturally diverse women and their families (Maddalena, 2009). Nursing education should expose students to diversity in a variety of settings, include theoretical and factual information about cultural groups, identify strategies and skills useful in providing nursing care to culturally diverse clients, allow students the opportunity to examine their own personal values and attitudes, and encourage linguistic skills in a second language.

Cross-cultural health education materials are available on many Web sites, and sources are listed in Appendix 2–A.

HEALTHCARE DELIVERY

Most healthcare systems in the United States exhibit cultural blindness, ignoring differences as if they do not exist, but it is essential in moving toward a high-quality system of care for childbearing women that culture competence is a priority. Healthcare in the United States is a culture in itself, based on the dominant Western biomedical model of health beliefs and practices. In most hospitals, only American food is served, and there is a universal assumption that everyone seeking healthcare understands English. Nurses are in a position to challenge institutional forces that may inhibit culturally sensitive care. Display 2–11

DISPLAY 2-11

Strategies Fostering Culturally Competent Care on Perinatal Nursing Units

- Educational offerings on ethnic, religious, cultural, and family diversity
- Educational offerings about available community resources
- Literature searches focused on the predominant cultural groups cared for, followed by development of a resource binder available on the unit
- Generating a culture database
- Establishing a task force to create culturally sensitive birth plans for the predominant cultural groups cared for
- Establishing cultural competencies that are part of the yearly staff evaluation
- Making cultural competence part of the interview process
- Supporting each other in frustrating situations
- Nursing grand rounds focusing on cultural issues
- Celebrating successes by peers in providing culturally competent care
- Sharing resources such as books and professional journal articles
- Discouraging negativism and discrimination on the unit
- Creating connections between community and acute care settings

DISPLAY 2-12

Communication in a Multicultural Healthcare Team

- Assess the personal beliefs of members.
- Assess communication variables from a cultural perspective.
- Modify communication patterns to enhance communication.
- Identify mannerisms that may be threatening and avoid using them.
- Understand that respect for others and the needs they communicate is central to positive working relationships.
- Use validating techniques when communicating.
- Be considerate of a reluctance to talk when the subject might involve culturally taboo topics, such as sexual matters.
- Use team members from a different culture as resources but do not support a dependency by the team on those members.
- Support team efforts to plan and adapt care based on communicated needs and cultural backgrounds of individual patients.
- Identify potential interpreters for patients whenever necessary in order to improve communication.

provides examples of institutional changes and strategies that may facilitate culturally competent care. There are ethical issues related to caring for culturally diverse populations who do not speak English, including compromised quality of care, increased risk of adverse events, lack of access to healthcare, and lack of informed consent (Callister & Sudia-Robinson, 2011). In addition to diversity in women and their families receiving care, there is also growing diversity within the healthcare workforce. Display 2–12 describes how a multicultural healthcare team might improve communication between members.

NURSING RESEARCH

Culturally sensitive scholarship is essential in order for the delivery of culturally competent care to be evidence based (Engebretson, Mahoney & Carlson, 2008; Hulme, 2010). Many cultures are silent or invisible minorities because of the lack of research on their health needs, status, beliefs, behavior, and family roles. Cross-cultural comparative studies of childbirth demonstrate that much of the information available is medically oriented or narrowly anthropologic in focus. Much of the current literature on how culture influences childbirth is descriptive or focuses on a case study approach. There is a need for qualitative approaches to research, with women as participants or coinvestigators asking how sociocultural context and increasing technological approaches to childbirth influence childbearing in different cultures. Qualitative research approaches include focus groups with a bilingual discussion leader or participative research in which results are returned rapidly to participants to improve service. Such approaches are empowering and give legitimacy to healthcare issues of culturally diverse women. The ideal research team includes both members from within the culture being studied as well as nonmembers. Multidisciplinary research teams that include transcultural nurses, nurse anthropologists, sociologists, and others are effective. Cultural issues of specific interest to women have the potential to improve the quality of nursing care provided to women and their quality of life. One understudied area is the measurement of biologic and physiologic differences in cultural, ethnic, and racial groups of women. Studies on the sexual and emotional complications of genital mutilation also are needed. Another important research priority is intervention studies designed to measure the effectiveness of strategies for providing healthcare to vulnerable populations of culturally diverse women.

SUMMARY

The story is told of a Native American childbearing couple who seemed like a typical mainstream American family, but whose grandmother requested to take the placenta home. It would have been helpful if, on admission, the nurse had asked about their heritage and whether there were any cultural traditions that were important to them. The father would have perhaps responded that his mother was traditional and may want to take the placenta home. The nurse then would have had time to explain whether or not the request could be accommodated, demonstrating respect and providing culturally appropriate care (Leininger & McFarland, 2006). Nurses caring for childbearing women and their families should be respectful of women's cultural diversity and the societal context of their lives, balancing professional standards of care with attitudes, knowledge, and skills associated with cultural competence (Dean, 2010). Perinatal nurses should seek to create a healthcare encounter with childbearing women and their families that respects the sociocultural and spiritual context of life and moves beyond the superficial to understand the deeper meaning of childbearing. Perinatal nurses must never lose sight of the fact that a woman's childbirth experience is not only about making a baby but also about creating a mother—a mother who is strong and competent and who trusts her own capacities because she has been cared for by a culturally competent nurse. Giving birth has the potential to be a rich cultural and spiritual experience facilitated by such a nurse.

REFERENCES

American Academy of Pediatrics. (2010). Ritual genital cutting of female minors. *Pediatrics, 126*(1), 1088–1093. doi:10.1542/peds.2010-0187

American Association of Colleges of Nursing. (2010). *Cultural Competency in Baccalaureate Nursing Education.* Washington, DC: Author.

Amoros, Z. U., Callister, L. C., & Sarkisyan, K. (2010). Giving birth: The voices of Armenian women. *International Nursing Review, 57*(1), 135–141. doi:10.1111/j.1466-7657.2009.00775.x

Anderson, N. L. R., Boyle, J. S., Davidhizar, R. E., Giger, J. N., McFarland, M. R., Papadopoulos, I., . . . Wehbe-Alamah, H. (2010). Cultural health assessment. *Journal of Transcultural Nursing, 21*(4 Suppl.), 307S–336S. doi:10.1177/1043659610377208

Andrews, M. M., & Boyle, J. S. (2007). *Transcultural Concepts in Nursing* (5th ed). Philadelphia: Lippincott Williams & Wilkins.

Ardoin, K. B., & Wilson, K. B. (2010). Cultural diversity: What role does it play in patient safety? *Nursing for Women's Health, 14*(4), 322–326. doi:10.1111/j.1751-486X.2010.01563.x

Balcazar, H., Peterson, G. W., & Krull, J. L. (1997). Acculturation and family cohesiveness in Mexican American pregnant women: Social and health implications. *Family and Community Health, 20*(3), 16–31.

Beck, C. T. (2006). Acculturation: Implications for perinatal research. *MCN: The American Journal of Maternal Child Nursing, 31*(2), 114–120.

Beck, C. T., Froman, R. D., & Bernal, H. (2005). Acculturation level and postpartum depression in Hispanic mothers. *MCN: The American Journal of Maternal Child Nursing, 30*(5), 299–304. doi:10.1097/00005721-2005090000-00006

Berry, J. W. (1980). Acculturation as varieties of adaptation. In A. M. Padilla (Ed.), *Acculturation: Theories, Models and Some New Findings* (pp. 9–25). Boulder, CO: Westview Press.

Bircher, H. (2009). Perinatal care disparities and the migrant farm worker community. *MCN: The American Journal of Maternal Child Nursing, 34*(5), 303–307. doi:10.1097/01.NMC.60000366423.14110.96

Birkhead, A., Kennedy, H. P., & Callister, L. C. (2010). Navigating a new health care culture: Experiences of immigrant Hispanic women. *Journal of Immigrant and Migrant Health.* Advance online publication.

Born, D., & Barron, M. L. (2005). Herb use in pregnancy: What nurses should know. *MCN: The American Journal of Maternal Child Nursing, 30*(3), 201–206.

Braithwaite, P., Chichester, M., & Reid, A. (2010). When the pregnant Jehovah's Witness patient refuses blood. *Nursing for Women's Health, 14*(6), 464–470. doi:10.1111/j.1751-486X.2010.01593.x

Brown, E. (2010). "They get a C-section. . .They gonna die:" Somali women's fears of obstetrical interventions in the United States. *Journal of Transcultural Nursing, 21,* 220–227. doi:10.1177/1643659609358780

Callister, L. C. (1995). Cultural meanings of childbirth. *Journal of Obstetric, Gynecologic, and Neonatal Nursing, 24*(4), 327–331. doi:10.1111/j.1552-6909.1995.tb02484.x

Callister, L. C. (2011). The pain of childbirth: Its management among culturally diverse women. In K. H. Todd & M. Incayarwa (Eds). *Culture, genes, and analgesia: Understanding and managing pain in diverse populations.* New York, NY: Oxford University Press.

Callister, L. C., Beckstrand, R. L., & Corbett, C. (2010). Postpartum depression and culture: Pesado Corazon. *MCN: The American Journal of Maternal Child Nursing, 33*(5), 254–261. doi:10.1097/NMCb0Be3181e597bf

Callister, L. C., Beckstrand, R. L., & Corbett, C. (2011). Postpartum depression and help seeking behaviors in immigrant Hispanic women. *Journal of Obstetric, Gynecologic, and Neonatal Nursing, 40*(4), 440–449. doi:10.1111/j.1552-6909.2011.01254.x

Callister, L. C., Corbett, C., Reed, S., Tomao, C., & Thornton, K. (2010). Giving birth: The voices of Ecuadorian women. *Journal of Perinatal and Neonatal Nursing, 24*(2), 146–154. doi:10.1097/JPN.0b013e3181db2dda

Callister, L. C., Eads, M. C., Diehl, Y., & See, J. P. (2011). Perceptions of giving birth and adherence to cultural practices in Chinese women. *MCN: The American Journal of Maternal Child Nursing, 36*(6), 387–394. doi:10.1097/NMC.0b013e31822de397

Callister, L. C., Getmanenko, N., Garvrish, N., Marakova, O. E., Zotina, N.V., Lassetter, J., & Turkina, N. (2007). Giving birth: The voices of Russian women. *MCN: The American Journal of Maternal Child Nursing, 32*(1), 18–24. doi:10.1097/00005721-200701000-00005

Callister, L. C., Holt, S. F., & Kuhre, M. W. (2010). Giving birth: The voices of Australian women. *Journal of Perinatal and Neonatal Nursing, 24*(2), 128–136. doi:10.1097/JPN.0b013e3181cf0429

Callister, L. C., & Khalaf, I. (2010). Spirituality in childbearing women. *Journal of Perinatal Education, 19*(2), 16–24. doi:10.1624/105812410x495514

Callister, L. C., & Sudia-Robinson, T. (2011). An overview of ethics in maternal child nursing. *MCN: The American Journal of Maternal Child Nursing, 36*(3), 154–159. doi:10.1097/NMC.0b013e3182102175

Campinha-Bacote, J. (1994). *The process of cultural competence in healthcare: A culturally competent model of care.* Wyoming, OH: Transcultural CARE Associates. Retrieved from http://www.transcultural-care.net

Centers for Disease Control and Prevention. (2011). CDC health disparities and inequalities report: United States, 2011. *Morbidity and Mortality Weekly Report, 60*(Suppl.).

Centers for Disease Control and Prevention (2012). *Immigrant and refugee health.* Retrieved from http://www.cdc.gov/immigrantrefugeehealth/

Chen, J., & Vargas-Bustamante, A. (2011). Estimating the effects of immigration status on mental health care utilizations in the United States. *Journal of Immigrant and Minority Health.* Advance online publication. doi:10.1007/s10903-011-9445x

Chin, Y. M., Jaganthan, M., Hasmiza, A. M., & Wu, M. C. (2010). Zu yuezi practice among Malaysian Chinese women: Traditional versus modernity. *British Journal of Midwifery, 18*(3), 170–175.

Chuang, C. H., Chang, P., Hsieh, W. S., Tsai, Y. J., Lin, S. J., & Chen, P. C. (2009). Chinese herbal medicine use in Taiwan during pregnancy and the postpartum period. *International Journal of Nursing Studies, 46*, 787–795. doi:10.106/jinurstud.2008.12.015

Chuang, C. H., Hsieh, W. S., Guo, Y. L., Tsai, Y. J., Chang, P. J., Lin, S. J., & Chen, P. C. (2007). Chinese herbal medicines used in pregnancy. *Pharmacoepidemiology and Drug Safety, 16*, 446–448. doi:10.1002/peds.1382

Cooper, M., Grywalski, M., Lamp, J., Newhouse, L., & Studlien, R. (2007). Enhancing cultural competence: A model for nurses. *Nursing for Women's Health, 11*(2), 148–159.

Corbett, C., & Callister, L. C. (2012). Giving birth: The voices of women in Tamil, Nadu, India. *MCN: The American Journal of Maternal Child Nursing, 37*(5), 298–305. doi:10.1097/NMC.0b013e1826ba4d)

Cross, T. F., Brazon, B. J., Dennis, K. W., & Isaacs, M. R. (1989). *Toward a culturally competent system of care.* Washington, DC: Child and Adolescent Service System Program Technical Assistance Center.

Dalal, K., Lawoko, S., & Jansson, B. (2010). Women's attitudes toward discontinuation of female genital mutilation in Egypt. *Journal of Injury and Violence, 2*(1), 41–47. doi:10.5249/jvr.v2i1.33

D'Avanzo, C. E. (2008). *Pocket Guide to Cultural Health Assessment* (4th ed.). St Louis: Mosby.

Dean, R. A. K. (2010). Cultural competence: Nursing in a multicultural society. *Nursing for Women's Health, 14*(1), 50–59. doi:10.1111/j.1751-486X.2010.01507.x

deChesnay, M., Wharton, R., & Pamp, C. (2005). Cultural competence, resilience, and advocacy. In M. deChesnay (Ed.), *Caring for the Vulnerable* (pp. 31–41). Boston: Jones & Bartlett.

DeNavas-Walt, C., Proctor, B. D., & Smith, J. C. (2010). *Income, poverty, and health insurance coverage in the United States: 2009* (U.S. Census Bureau Current Population Report, P60-238). Washington, DC: U.S. Government Printing Office. Retrieved from http://www.census/gov/prod/2010pubs

Dominguez, T. P. (2011). Adverse birth outcomes in African American women: The social context of persistent reproductive disadvantage. *Social Work in Public Health, 26*, 4–16. doi:10.1080/10911350902986880

Douglas, M. K., & Pacquaio, D. F. (2010). Culturally based health and illness beliefs and practices across the lifespan. *Journal of Transcultural Nursing, 21*(Suppl. 1), 1525–1555. doi:10.1177/1043659610381094

Douglas, M., Pierce, J. U., Rosenkoetter, M., Pacquiao, D., Callister, L. C., . . . Purnell, L. (2011). Standards of practice for culturally competent nursing care: 2011 update. *Journal of Transcultural Nursing, 22*(4), 317–333. doi: 10.1177/1043659611412965

Ebanks, R. L., McFarland, M. R., Mixer, S. J., Munoz, C., Pacquiao, D. F., & Wenger, A. F. Z. (2010). Cross cultural communication. *Journal of Transcultural Nursing, 21*(4 Suppl.), 137S–150S. doi:10.1177/104365961037432

Engebretson, J., Mahoney, J., & Carlson, C. D. (2008). Cultural competence in the era of evidence-based practice. *Journal of Professional Nursing, 24*(3), 172–178. doi:10.1016/j.profnurs.2007.10.1012

Farnes, C., Callister, L. C., & Beckstrand, R. (2011). Help seeking behaviors among childbearing women in Ghana, West Africa. *International Nursing Review, 59*(4), 491–497. doi:10.1111/j.1466-7657.2011.00917.x

Ferguson, B. (2008). Health literacy and health disparities: The role they play in maternal and newborn nursing. *Nursing for Women's Health, 12*(4), 286–298. doi:10.1111/j.1751-486X.2008.00343.x

Giger, J. N. (2008). *Transcultural Nursing: Assessment and Intervention* (5th ed.). St. Louis, MO: Mosby-Year Book.

Gonzalez, E. U., Sable, M. R., Campbell, J. D., & Dannerbeck, A. (2011). The influence of patriarchal behavior on birth control access and use among recent Hispanic women. *Journal of Immigrant and Minority Health, 12*(4), 551–558. doi:10.1111/j.1523-536X.2007.0018.x

Gorman, J. R., Madlensky, I., Jackson, D. J., Ganiats, T. G., & Boles, E. (2007). Early postpartum breastfeeding and acculturation among Hispanic women. *Birth, 34*(4), 308–315. doi:10.1111/j.1523-536X.2007.00189.x

Grewal, S. K., Bhagat, R., & Balneaves, L. G. (2008). Perinatal beliefs and practices of immigrant Punjabi women living in Canada. *Journal of Obstetric, Gynecologic, and Neonatal Nursing, 37*(3), 290–300. doi:10.1111/j.1552-6909-2008.002.34.x

Gunn, J., & Davis, S. (2011). Beliefs, meanings, and practices of healing with botanicals recalled by elder African American women in the Mississippi Delta. *Online Journal of Cultural Competence in Nursing and Healthcare, 1*(1), 37–49.

Hazard, C. J., Callister, L. C., Birkhead, A., & Nichols, L. (2009). Hispanic Labor Friends Initiative: Supporting vulnerable women. *MCN: The American Journal of Maternal Child Nursing, 34*(3), 115–121. doi:10.1097/01.NMC.0000347306.15950.ae

Hidaka, R., & Callister, L. C. (2011). Giving birth with epidural analgesia: The experience of first-time mothers. *Journal of Perinatal Education, 21*(1), 24–35.

Huang, B., Appel, H., & Ai, A. L. (2011). The effects of discrimination and acculturation to service seeking satisfaction for Latina and Asian American women: Implications for mental health professionals. *Social Work in Public Health, 26*(1), 46–59. doi:10.1080/10911350093341077

Hulme, P. A. (2010). Cultural considerations in evidence-based practice. *Journal of Transcultural Nursing, 21,* 271–280. doi:10.1177/1043659609358782

Institute of Medicine. (2002). *Unequal Treatment: Confronting Racial and Ethnic Disparities in Health Care.* Washington, DC: Author.

Institute of Medicine. (2009). *Race, Ethnicity and Language Data: Standardization for Health Care Quality Improvement.* Washington, DC: Author

Johnson, T., Callister, L. C., Beckstrand, R., & Freeborn, D. (2007). Dutch women's perceptions of childbirth in the Netherlands. *MCN: The American Journal of Maternal Child Nursing, 32*(3), 170–177. doi:10.1097/01.NMC.0000269567.09809.65

Joint Commission for Accreditation of Healthcare Organizations. (2010). *Comprehensive Accreditation Manual for Hospitals.* Chicago: Author.

Khazoyan, C. M., & Anderson, N. L. R. (1994). Latina expectations of their partners during childbirth. *MCN: The American Journal of Maternal Child Nursing, 19*(4), 226–229.

Kim, W., & Keefe, R. H. (2010). Barriers to healthcare among Asian Americans. *Social Work in Public Health, 25,* 286–295. doi:10.1080/19371910903240704

Kirkham, S. R. (1998). Nurses' descriptions of caring for culturally diverse clients. *Clinical Nursing Research, 7*(2), 125–146. doi:10.1177/105477389800700204

Lau, Y., & Wong, D. F. K. (2008). The role of social support in helping Chinese women with perinatal depressive symptoms cope with family conflict. *Journal of Obstetric, Gynecologic, and Neonatal Nursing, 37*(5), 556–571. doi:10:1111/.1552-6909.2008.00273.x

Lauderdale, J. (2007). Transcultural perspectives in childbearing. In M. M. Andrews & J. S. Boyle (Eds.), *Transcultural Concepts in Nursing Care* (5th ed., pp. 85–115). St. Louis, MO: Mosby.

Le, D. T., Ngai, M. N., Lok, I. H., Yip, A. S., & Chung, T. K. (2009). Antenatal taboos among Chinese women in Hong Kong. *Midwifery, 25*(2), 104–113. doi:1016/j.midw.2007.01.008

Leininger, M., & McFarland, M. R. (2006). *Cultural Care Diversity and Universality: A Worldwide Nursing Theory.* Sudbury, MA: Jones and Bartlett.

Lemon, B. S. (2006). Amish health beliefs and practices in an obstetrical setting. *Journal of Multicultural Nursing and Health, 12*(3), 56–58.

Lewallen, L. P. (2011). The importance of culture in childbearing. *Journal of Obstetric, Gynecologic, and Neonatal Nursing, 40*(1), 4–8. doi:10.1111/j.1552-6909..2010.01209.x

Li, Q., Keith, L. G., & Kirby, R. S. (2010). Perinatal outcomes among foreign-born and US-born Chinese Americans. *Journal of Immigrant and Minority Health, 12*(3), 282–289. doi:10.1007/s10903-008-9191-x

Lucero, N. B., Beckstrand, R. L., Callister, L. C., & Birkhead, A. C. S. (2012). Prevalence of postpartum depression among Hispanic immigrant women. *Journal of the American Academy of Nurse Practitioners.* Early view. doi:10.111/j.1745-7599.2012.00744.x

Maddalena, V. (2009). Cultural competence and holistic practice. *Holistic Nursing Practice, 23*(3), 153–157. doi:10.1097/HNP.0b013e3181a056a0

Mann, J. R., Mannan, J., Quones, L. A., Palmer, A. A., & Torres, M. (2010). Religion, spirituality, social support, and perceived stress in pregnant and postpartum Hispanic women. *Journal of Obstetric, Gynecologic, and Neonatal Nurses, 39*(6), 645–657. doi:10.1111/j.1552-6909.2010.01188.x

Marshall, E. S., Carroll, L. S., Robinson, W. D., Callister, L. C., Olsen, S. F., Dyches, T. T., & Mandleco, B. (2011). Crucibles and healing: Illness and disability and perinatal loss, death, and bereavement. In D. C. Dollahite, A. J. Hawkins, & T. Draper (Eds.). *Successful Marriages and Families* (pp. 342–358). Salt Lake City, UT: Deseret Book.

Marsiglia, F. F., Bermudez-Parsai, M., & Coonrod, D. (2010). *Familias Sanas:* An intervention designed to increase rates of postpartum visits among Latinas. *Journal of Health Care for the Poor and Underserved, 21*(3), 119–131. doi:10.1353/hpu.0.0355

Matthews, R., & Callister, L. C. (2004). Childbearing women's perceptions of nursing care that promotes dignity. *Journal of Gynecologic, and Neonatal Nursing, 33*(4), 498–507. doi:10.1177/0884217504266896

Mattson, S. (2011). Ethnocultural considerations in the childbearing period. In S. Mattson & J. E. Smith (Eds). *Core Curriculum for Maternal Newborn Nursing* (4th ed, pp. 61–94). St. Louis: Elsevier & Saunders.

McKeary, M., & Newbold, B. (2010). Barriers to care: The challenges for Canadian refugees and their health care providers. *Journal of Refugee Studies, 23*(4), 524–545.

Mendelson, S. G., McNeese-Smith, D., Koniak-Griffin, D., Nyamathi, A., & Lu, M. C. (2008). A community based parish nurse intervention program for Mexican American women with gestational diabetes. *Journal of Obstetric, Gynecologic, and Neonatal Nursing, 37*(4), 415–425. doi:10.1111/j.1551-6909.2008.00262.x

Moore, M. L., Moos, M. K., & Callister, L. C. (2010). *Cultural Competence: An Essential Journey for Perinatal Nurses.* White Plains, NY: March of Dimes Foundation.

Murray, M. L., & Huelsman, C. M. (2009). Psyche, spirituality, and cultural dimensions of care. In M. Murray & G. Huelsmann (Eds.), *Labor and Delivery Nursing: A Guide to Evidence-Based Practice* (pp. 195–205). New York: Springer.

Nabukera, S. K., Wingate, M. S., Owen, J., Saliu, H. J., Swaminathan, S., Alexander, G. R., & Kirby, R. S. (2009). Racial disparities in perinatal outcomes and pregnancy spacing among women delaying initiation of childbearing. *Maternal Child Health Journal, 13*(1), 81–89. doi:10.1007/s10995-008-0330-8

National Diabetes Information Clearinghouse. (2011). *National diabetes statistics 2011.* Retrieved from http://diabetes.niddk.nih.gov/dm/pubs/statistics

Neu, M., & Robinson, J. (2008). Early weeks after premature birth as experienced by Latina adolescent mothers. *MCN: The American Journal of Maternal Child Nursing, 33*(3), 166–172. doi:10.1097/01.NMC.0000318352.1606.68

Noble, A. (2009). Jewish laws, customs and practice in labor, delivery and postpartum care. *Journal of Transcultural Nursing, 20*(3), 323–333. doi:10.1177/1043659609334930

Noble, A., Engelhardt, K., Newsome-Wicks, M., & Woloski-Wruble, A. C. (2009). Cultural competence and ethnic attitudes of midwives concerning Jewish couples. *Journal of Obstetric, Gynecologic, and Neonatal Nursing, 38*(5), 544–555. doi:10.1111/j.1551-69092009,0156.x

Obeidat, H., & Callister, L. C. (2011). The lived experience of Jordanian mothers with a preterm infant in the newborn intensive care unit. *Journal of Neonatal-Perinatal Medicine, 4*(2), 137–145. doi:10.3233/NPM-2011-2735

Ogunleye, O., Shelton, J. A., Ireland, A., Glick, M., & Yeh, J. (2010). Preferences for labor and delivery practices between pregnant immigrants and U.S.-born patients. *Journal of the National Medical Association, 102*(6), 481–484.

Page, R. L., Ellison, C. G., & Lee, J. (2009). Does religiosity affect health risk behaviors in pregnant and postpartum women? *Maternal Child Health Journal, 13*(5), 631–632. doi:10.1007/s10995-008-03945

Purnell, L. D., & Paulanka, B. J. (2011). *Transcultural Health Care: A Culturally Competent Approach* (3rd ed.). Philadelphia: F. A. Davis.

Ramos, B. M., Jurkowski, J., Gonzalez, B. A., & Lawrence, C. (2010). Latina women: Health and healthcare disparities. *Social Work in Public Health, 25*(3–4), 258–271. doi:10.1080/19379190903240605

Ransford, H. E., Carrillo, F. R., & Rivera, Y. (2010). Health-care seeking among Latino immigrants: Blocked access, use of traditional medicine, and the role of religion. *Journal of Health Care for the Poor and Underserved, 21*(3), 862–878. doi:10.1353/hpu0.0348

Rashid, M., & Rashid, M. H. (2007). Obstetric management of women with female genital mutilation. *The Obstetrician and Gynecologist, 9*(2), 95–101. doi:10.1576toag9.2.095

Riordan, J. (2005). The cultural context of breastfeeding. In J. Riordan (Ed.). *Breastfeeding and Human Lactation* (3rd ed., pp. 713–728). Boston: Jones & Bartlett.

Roberts, L., Gulliver, B., Fisher, J., & Cloyes, K. G. (2010). The Coping with Labor Algorithm: An alternate pain assessment tool for the laboring woman. *Journal of Midwifery and Women's Health, 55*(2), 107–116. doi:10.1016/j.jmwh.2009.11.002

Rorie, J. L. (2008). Cultural competence in midwifery practice. In H. Varney, J. M. Kriebs, & C. L. Gego (Eds.), *Varney's Midwifery* (6th ed.). Sudbury, MA: Jones & Bartlett.

Sheng, X., Le, H. N., & Perry, D. (2010). Perceived satisfaction with social support and depressive symptoms in perinatal Latinas. *Journal of Transcultural Nursing, 21,* 35–44. doi:10.1177/104365960348619

Spector, R. E. (2008). *Cultural Diversity in Health and Illness* (7th ed.). Upper Saddle River, NJ: Prentice Hall Health.

Tung, W. C. (2010). Doing the month and Asian culture: Implications for health care. *Home Health Management and Practice, 22*(5), 369–371. doi:10.1177/1084822310367473

U.S. Bureau of Population. (2008). *Refugee Admissions Program Fact Sheet.* Washington, DC: United States Department of State.

U.S. Department of Health and Human Services. (2010). *Healthy People 2020: Understanding and Improving Health* (3rd ed.). Rockville, MD: U.S. Government Printing Office.

U.S. Department of Health and Human Services, Health Resources and Services Administration. (2010). *Quality health services for Hispanics: The cultural competency component.* Retrieved from http://www.hrsa.gov/culturalcompetence/quality healthservices/basics.htm

U.S. Department of Health and Human Services, Office of Minority Health. (2001). *National Standards for Culturally and Linguistically Appropriate Services in Health Care.* Rockville, MD: Government Printing Office.

U.S. Department of Health and Human Services, Office of Minority Health. (2010). *Cultural competency.* Retrieved from http://minorityhealth.hhs.gov/templates/browse.aspx?lvl=1&lvlID=3

Wan, E. Y., Moyer, C. A., Harlow, S. D., Fan, Z., Jie, Y., & Yang, H. (2009). Postpartum depression and traditional postpartum care in China: Role of zuoyvei. *International Journal of Gynecology and Obstetrics, 104*(3), 209–213. doi:10.1016/j.ijgo.2008.10.1016

Wehbe-Alamah, H., McFarland, M., Macklin, J., & Riggs, N. (2011). The lived experiences of African American women receiving care from nurse practitioners in an urban nurse-managed clinic. *Online Journal in Cultural Competence in Nursing and Healthcare, 1*(1), 15–26.

Whitaker, C., Kavanaugh, K., & Klima, C. (2010). Perinatal grief in Latino parents. *MCN: The American Journal of Maternal Child Nursing, 35*(6), 341–345. doi:10.1097/NMC/)b04e181f2a111

Wilkinson, S. E., & Callister, L. C. (2010). Giving birth: The voices of Ghanian women. *Health Care for Women International, 31*(3), 201–220. doi:10.1080/073993343858

Wisdom, J. P., McGee, M. C., Horner-Johnson, W., Michael, Y. V., Adams, E., & Berlin, M. (2010). Health disparities between women with and without disabilities: A review of the research. *Social Work in Public Health, 25*(3–4), 368–386. doi:10.1080/19371910903240969

Yosef, A. R. O. (2008). Health beliefs, practice, and priorities for health care of Arab Muslims in the United States. *Journal of Transcultural Nursing, 19*(3), 284–291. doi:10.1177/043659608317450

Zauderer, C. (2009). Maternity care of Orthodox Jewish couples. *Nursing for Women's Health, 13*(2), 112–120. doi:10.1111/j.1751-486X.2009.01402.x

Zhao, M., Esposito, N., & Wang, K. (2010). Cultural beliefs and attitudes toward health and health care among Asian-born women in the United States. *Journal of Obstetric, Gynecologic, and Neonatal Nursing, 39*(4), 370–385. doi:10.1111/j.1552-6909.2010.01151.x

APPENDIX 2 – A

Culturally Competent Care Resources

AFRICAONLINE

http://www.africaonline.com/site/ (African topics such as health, women, and education and African countries)

AL-BAB.COM (ARAB TOPICS)

http://www.al-bab.com

ALLIANCE FOR HISPANIC HEALTH

http://www.hispanichealth.org

AMERICAN ACADEMY OF CHILD AND ADOLESCENT PSYCHIATRY

http://www.aacap.org/publications/factsfam/index.htm (Spanish, French, German, Malaysian, Polish, and Icelandic translations available with links from the site, although there is a disclaimer that they have not been reviewed for translation accuracy by the AACAP)

AMERICAN DIABETES ASSOCIATION

http://www.diabetes.org (English and Spanish)

AMERICAN IMMIGRATION RESOURCES ON THE INTERNET

http://www.theodora.com/resource.html (English, Chinese, Russian)

AMERISTAT

http://www.ameristat.org (graphics and text of U.S. population)

ASIAN AND PACIFIC ISLANDER AMERICAN HEALTH FORUM (NHPI AFFAIRS)

http://www.apiahf.org (focuses on health status of AA/PI communities)

AT&T LANGUAGE LINE

http://www.languageline.com (800) 752-0093

Translation into over 140 languages. Subscribed interpretation (organizations, frequent use); membership interpretation (organizations, predictable need); personal interpreter (individuals, occasional use)

BAYLOR UNIVERSITY REFUGEE HEALTH PAGE (SOUTHEAST ASIANS, CARVEL INSTITUTE)

http://www.bearingspace.baylor.edu/Charles_Kemp

CENTER FOR CROSS–CULTURAL HEALTH

http://www.crosshealth.com

CENTER FOR IMMIGRATION STUDIES

http://www.cis.org (immigration issues)

CENTER FOR REPRODUCTIVE LAW AND POLICY

http://www.crlp.org (global women's rights including reproductive rights)

CENTERS FOR DISEASE CONTROL AND PREVENTION

http://www.cdc.gov/epo/mmwr/international//world.html (Epidemiology International bulletins)
http://www.cdc.ogh (Office of Global Health)
http://www.cdc.gov/spanish (Spanish Web site)

CENTRAL INTELLIGENCE AGENCY (CIA) *WORLD FACTBOOK*

http://www.cia/gov/cia/publications/factbook

CROSS CULTURAL HEALTH CARE PROGRAM (CULTURAL COMPETENCE RESOURCE GUIDE)

http://www.xculture.org

CULTUREMED

http://www.suny.edu/library/culturemed/

DIVERSITY RX

http://www.diversityrx.org/

ETHNOMED

http://www.ethnomed.org/ (Amharic, Chinese, Hmong, Karen, Khmer, Oromo, Somali, Spanish, Tigrinya, Vietnamese)

GEORGETOWN UNIVERSITY CHILD DEVELOPMENT CENTER, NATIONAL CENTER FOR CULTURAL COMPETENCE

http://www.gucdc.georgetown.edu

HISPANIC HEALTH

http://www.hispanichealth.org

IMMIGRATION AND NATURALIZATION SERVICE (INS)

http://www.ins.gov

INDIAN HEALTH SERVICES

http://www.ihs.gov

MEDLINEplus HEALTH INFORMATION

http://www.nlm.nih.gov/medlineplus/populationgroups.html

MULTICULTURAL MENTAL HEALTH AUSTRALIA

http://www.atmhn.unimelb.edu.au (55 languages)

NATIONAL ASIAN WOMEN'S HEALTH ORGANIZATION

http://www.nawho.org

NATIONAL CENTER FOR CULTURAL COMPETENCE

http://nccc.georgetown.edu/

NATIONAL INSTITUTES OF HEALTH OFFICE OF ALTERNATIVE MEDICINE

http://altmed.od.nih.gov

NATIONAL INSTITUTES OF HEALTH OFFICE OF RESEARCH ON MINORITY HEALTH

http://www.od.nih.gov/ormh

NOAH: NEW YORK ONLINE ACCESS TO HEALTH

http://www.noah-health.org (English and Spanish)

OREGON HEALTH SCIENCES UNIVERSITY PATIENT EDUCATION RESOURCES FOR CLINICIANS

http://www.ohsu.edu/library/patiented/

PAN AMERICAN HEALTH ORGANIZATION (PAHO)

http://www.paho.org/

POPULATION REFERENCE BUREAU (PRB)

http://www.prb.org (U.S. and international population trends)

PRINCETON UNIVERSITY OFFICE OF POPULATION RESEARCH

http://www.opr.princeton.edu/archive

REPRODUCTIVE HEALTH OUTLOOK

http://www.rho.org (transcultural issues)

SAFE MOTHERHOOD INITIATIVE

http://www.safemotherhood.org

TRANSCULTURAL C.A.R.E. ASSOCIATES

http://www.transculturalcare.net

TRANSCULTURAL NURSING ASSESSMENT TOOL

http://www.culturaldiversity.org/assmtform.htm

TRANSCULTURAL NURSING SOCIETY

http://www.tcns.org/

UNICEF STATISTICAL DATA

http://www.unicef.org/statistics/

UNITED STATES CENSUS BUREAU, INTERNATIONAL STATISTICAL AGENCIES

http://www.census.gov/main/www/stat_int.html

UNITED STATES DEPARTMENT OF HEALTH AND HUMAN SERVICES

http://www.raceandhealth.hhs.gov

UNITED STATES DEPARTMENT OF HEALTH AND HUMAN SERVICES, OFFICE OF MINORITY HEALTH AND HEALTH DISPARITIES

http://minorityhealth.hhs.govwww.omhrc.gov

UTAH DEPARTMENT OF HEALTH, OFFICE OF ETHNIC HEALTH

http://minorityhealth.hhs.gov

WORLD HEALTH ORGANIZATION

http://www.who.int/

WORLD WIDE WEB VIRTUAL LIBRARY MIGRATION AND ETHNIC RELATIONS

http://www.ercomer.org/wwwvl/

JOURNALS

Cross Cultural Issues
Hispanic Health Care International (National Association of Hispanic Nurses)
http://springerpub.com/journal.aspx?jid=1540-4153

Hmong Studies Journal
Journal of Cultural Diversity
http://www.tuckerpub.com/jcd.htm

Journal of Multicultural Nursing and Health
http://findarticles.com/p/artixles/mi_qa3919/

Journal of Transcultural Nursing (Transcultural Nursing Society)
http://tcn.sagepub.com/

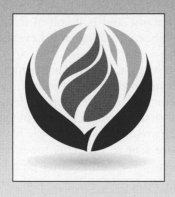

Susan Tucker Blackburn

CHAPTER 3

Physiologic Changes of Pregnancy

The pregnant woman experiences dramatic physiologic changes to meet the demands of the developing fetus, maintain homeostasis, and prepare for birth and lactation. Maternal adaptations during pregnancy result from the interplay of multiple factors, including the influences of reproductive and other hormones, growth factors, cytokines, and other signaling proteins, as well as mechanical pressures exerted by the growing fetus and enlarging uterus. An understanding of the normal physiologic changes of pregnancy is essential for discriminating between normal and abnormal states. Laboratory values and physical findings considered normal in the nonpregnant woman may not be normal for women during pregnancy. This chapter reviews physiologic changes during pregnancy to provide baseline information to guide the perinatal nurse in conducting an accurate and thorough assessment of the pregnant woman.

HORMONES AND OTHER MEDIATORS

Many of the physiologic changes during pregnancy are mediated by hormones. Hormones are responsible for maintaining homeostasis, regulation of growth, and development and cellular communication. They are transported by the blood from the site of production to their target cells throughout the pregnant woman's body and are responsible for many physiologic adaptations to pregnancy. During pregnancy, the placenta serves as an endocrine gland, secreting many hormones, growth factors, and other substances. The major hormones produced by the placenta are human chorionic gonadotropin (hCG), human placental lactogen (hPL), estrogen, and progesterone. However, the placenta also produces pituitary-like and gonad-like hormones (e.g., placental corticotropin, human chorionic thyrotropin, placental growth hormone), hypothalamus-like releasing hormones (e.g., human chorionic somatostatin, corticotropin-releasing hormone [CRH], gastrointestinal-like hormones (e.g., gastrin, vasoactive intestinal peptide), and parathyroid hormone–related protein (PTHrP) (Blackburn, 2012; Liu, 2009). The placental hormones are critical for many of the metabolic and endocrine changes during pregnancy. For example, PTHrP mediates placental calcium transport and fetal bone growth, and CRH release of prostaglandins (PGs) and has a major role in initiation of myometrial contractility and labor onset.

The placenta, membranes, and fetus also synthesize peptide growth factors such as epidermal growth factor, nerve growth factor, platelet-derived growth factor, transforming growth factor-β (TGF-β), skeletal growth factor, and insulin-like growth factor-I (IGF-I) and II (IGF-II) (Liu, 2009). These growth factors stimulate localized hormone release, regulate cell growth and differentiation, and enhance metabolic processes during pregnancy (Blackburn, 2012). For example, IGF-I and IGF-II enhance amino acid and glucose uptake and prevent protein breakdown, thus helping to regulate cell proliferation and differentiation to maintain fetal growth. TGF-β stimulates cell differentiation and is important in embryogenesis and neural migration and differentiation (Liu, 2009).

HUMAN CHORIONIC GONADOTROPIN

hCG is a glycoprotein with alpha and beta subunits. In early pregnancy, the beta subunits predominate, whereas the alpha units are more prevalent in late pregnancy (Cole, 2010). Assessment of free beta subunits is a component of first- and second-trimester maternal serum screening for fetal genetic disorders

(Nicolaides, 2011). hCG is secreted primarily by the placenta. The major function of hCG is to maintain progesterone and estrogen production by the corpus luteum until the placental function is adequate (about 10 weeks postconception). hCG may enhance uterine growth, maintenance of uterine quiescence, and immune function during pregnancy. hCG is also thought to have a role in fetal testosterone and corticosteroid production and angiogenesis (Cole, 2010). hCG is found in the blastocyst prior to implantation and is detected in maternal serum and urine around the time of implantation (7 to 8 days after ovulation) (Liu, 2009). Levels increase to peak about 60 to 90 days after conception, then decrease rapidly after 10 to 12 weeks (when the placenta becomes the main producer of estrogens and progesterone and the corpus luteum is no longer needed) to a nadir at 100 to 130 days (Liu, 2009). Maternal urine pregnancy testing assesses hCG levels and positive results are found by 3 weeks after conception (about 5 weeks after the last normal menstrual period) (Moore, Persaud, & Torchia, 2011). hCG levels are elevated in multiple and molar pregnancies and low with ectopic pregnancy or abnormal placentation (Liu, 2009).

HUMAN PLACENTAL LACTOGEN

hPL, also known as human chorionic somatomammotropin, is produced by the syncytiotrophoblast tissues of the placenta. Maternal serum hPL levels increase parallel to placental growth and peak near term. hPL is critical to fetal growth because it alters maternal protein, carbohydrate, and fat metabolism and acts as an insulin antagonist (Liu, 2009). This hormone increases free fatty acid availability for maternal metabolic needs and decreases maternal glucose uptake and use. Thus, glucose (the major fetal energy substrate) is reserved for fetal use, and free fatty acids are used preferentially by the mother (Blackburn, 2012). This preferred breakdown of free fatty acids increases levels of ketones and the risk of ketosis with significant decreased maternal food intake.

ESTROGENS

Estrogens (estrone, estradiol, and estriol) are steroid hormones secreted by the ovaries during early pregnancy and the placenta for most of pregnancy. Estrogen prevents further ovarian follicular development during pregnancy. Both luteinizing hormone (LH) and follicle-stimulating hormone (FSH) are inhibited by high concentrations of progesterone in the presence of estrogen. Estrogen affects the renin-angiotensin-aldosterone system and stimulates production of hormone-binding globulins in the liver during pregnancy. Estrogen also helps prepare the breasts for lactation, increases blood flow to the uterus, stimulates

the growth of the uterine muscle mass, enhances myometrial activity, and is involved in the timing of the onset of labor (Cunningham, Leveno, Bloom, & Hauth, 2009).

Estriol is the primary estrogen produced by the placenta during pregnancy. Production of estriol involves interaction of the mother, fetus, and placenta. The mother provides cholesterol and other precursors, which are metabolized by the placenta. These metabolites are sent to the fetus for further processing by the fetal liver and adrenal gland to produce dehydroepiandrosterone sulfate, which is sent back to the placenta to produce estriol. Maternal serum and urinary estriol levels increase throughout pregnancy, with a rapid rise during the last 6 weeks. This late increase in estriol alters the local (uteroplacental area) ratio of estrogens to progesterone, which is a factor in the onset of labor (Cunningham et al., 2009; Norwitz & Lye, 2009).

PROGESTERONE

Progesterone is initially produced by the corpus luteum in early pregnancy and later primarily by the placenta. Progesterone maintains decidual secretory activities required for implantation and helps to maintain myometrial relaxation by acting on uterine smooth muscle to inhibit PG production and down-regulating contraction-associated proteins such as gap junctions and PG and oxytocin receptors (Blackburn, 2012). Progesterone acts on smooth muscle in other areas of the body as well, especially in the gastrointestinal (GI) and renal system; relaxes venous walls to accommodate the increase in blood volume; alters respiratory center sensitivity to carbon dioxide; and aids in the development of acini and lobules of the breasts in preparation for lactation (Cunningham et al., 2009). Progesterone also mediates changes in immune function during pregnancy, which helps prevent rejection by the mother of the fetus and placenta as foreign antigens (Challis et al., 2009).

RELAXIN

Relaxin is secreted by the corpus luteum and later by the myometrium and placenta. Relaxin interacts with other mediators to inhibit uterine activity, thereby maintaining myometrial quiescence during pregnancy and diminishing the strength of uterine contractions. Relaxin also plays a role in cervical ripening and may help suppress oxytocin release during pregnancy (Goldsmith & Weiss, 2009).

PROSTAGLANDINS

PGs are found in high concentrations in the female reproductive tract and in the decidua and fetal membranes during pregnancy. PGs are part of a family of substances called eicosanoids that are synthesized from arachidonic acid, which is present in plasma membrane phospholipids. This family includes PGs, prostacyclins (PGI₂s), thromboxanes, and leukotrienes. Eicosanoids are released quickly with plasma membrane stimulation and act near the site of release. PGs affect smooth muscle contractility. The interplay between thromboxanes and PGI₂ is believed to contribute to hypertensive disorders in pregnancy. PGI₂ release is mediated by nitric oxide, which regulates vascular tone and is an important mediator of reduced vascular resistance and myometrial relaxation during pregnancy (Blackburn, 2012).

PGs mediate the onset of labor, myometrial contractility, and cervical ripening. Throughout most of pregnancy, myometrial PG receptors are down-regulated (Norwitz & Lye, 2009). Changes in receptor responsivity and increases in PG receptors and levels of stimulatory PG near the end of pregnancy are mediated by CRH, fetal cortisol, and uterine stretch (Romero & Lockwood, 2009). PGs play a critical role in labor onset via a variety of mechanisms, including formation of gap junctions (needed to transmit action potentials) and oxytocin receptors in the myometrium, increasing frequency of action potentials, stimulating myometrial contractility, and enhancing calcium availability (calcium is essential for smooth muscle contraction) (Norwitz & Lye, 2009; Romero & Lockwood, 2009). The physiologic roles of endogenous PGs have led to the use of various PGs for cervical ripening and induction of labor (Kelly, Malik, Smith, Kavanagh, & Thomas, 2009).

PROLACTIN

Prolactin is released from the anterior pituitary. This hormone is responsible for the increase in and maturation of ducts and alveoli in the breasts and for initiation of lactation after birth. During pregnancy, there is a marked increase of prolactin secondary to the effects of angiotensin II, gonadotropin-releasing hormone, and arginine vasopressin (AVP) on the pituitary. However, the high estrogen levels throughout pregnancy inhibit initiation of lactation. After birth, this inhibition quickly disappears with removal of the placenta, the major source of estrogen during pregnancy. The anterior pituitary begins to produce larger amounts of prolactin, which stimulate the breast to begin lactation. The serum prolactin concentration begins to rise in the first trimester and by term may reach 10 times the nonpregnant concentration (Liu, 2009). After birth, prolactin levels rise rapidly, returning to prepregnancy levels by 7 to 14 days in nonbreastfeeding mothers (Molitch, 2009). In lactating women, baseline prolactin levels are elevated further during sucking; the baseline decreases over the first months of lactation.

CARDIOVASCULAR SYSTEM

The cardiovascular system undergoes numerous and profound adaptations during pregnancy (Table 3–1). Cardiovascular anatomy, blood volume, cardiac output, and vascular resistance are altered to accommodate the additional maternal and fetal circulatory requirements. Increased ventricular wall muscle mass, an increased heart rate, cardiac murmurs, and dependent peripheral edema are evidence of these anatomic and functional changes. Physical symptoms may occur during pregnancy in response to normal cardiovascular changes. Some women report palpitations, light-headedness, or decreased tolerance for activity. Cardiovascular adaptations have a significant impact on all organ systems. Women with normal cardiovascular function are generally able to accommodate the dramatic cardiovascular changes associated with pregnancy. Women with cardiovascular disease are at increased risk for complications during pregnancy, labor, or the immediate postpartum period, in part because of alterations in blood and plasma volume and cardiac output (Curry, Swan, & Steer, 2009).

HEART

The position, appearance, and function of the heart change during pregnancy. As the growing uterus exerts pressure on the diaphragm, the heart is displaced upward, forward, and to the left, to lie in a more horizontal position. The first-trimester increase in ventricular muscle mass and the second- and early third-trimester increase in end-diastolic volume cause the heart to undergo a physiologic dilation (Monga, 2009). The point of maximal impulse is deviated to the left at the fourth intercostal space. During the first few days postpartum, the left atrium also appears to be enlarged because of the increased blood volume that occurs with removal of the placenta.

Table 3–1. CARDIOVASCULAR CHANGES DURING PREGNANCY

Parameter	Change
Heart rate	Increases 15%–20% (10–20 bpm)
Blood volume	Increases 30%–50% (1,450–1,750 mL)
Plasma volume	Increases 40%–60% (1,200–1,600 mL)
Red cell mass	Increases 20%–30% (250–450 mL)
Cardiac output	Increases 30%–50% (average 40%–45%)
Stroke volume	Increases 25%–30%
Systemic vascular resistance	Decreases 20%–30%
Colloid oncotic pressure	Decreases 20% (23 mm Hg)
Diastolic blood pressure	Decreases 10–15 mm Hg by 24–32 weeks

Maternal heart rate begins to increase at 4 to 5 weeks' gestation and peaks at about 32 weeks at 10 to 20 beats/min above baseline (Hegewald & Crapo, 2011; Monga, 2009). Heart rate and atrial size return to normal prepregnancy values in the first 10 days postpartum, whereas left ventricular size normalizes after 4 to 6 months (Cunningham et al., 2009; Monga, 2009).

Between 12 and 20 weeks, a change in heart sounds and a systolic murmur is heard in approximately 90% to 95% of pregnant women because of the increased cardiovascular load (Monga, 2009). Ninety percent of pregnant women have a wider split in the first heart sound (which also becomes louder) and an audible third heart sound. Around 30 weeks' gestation, the second heart sound also demonstrates an audible splitting. About 5% of pregnant women also have an audible fourth heart sound. Systolic murmurs are auscultated in more than 95% of pregnant women during the last two trimesters. However, systolic murmurs greater than grade 2/4 and any type of diastolic murmur are considered abnormal (Monga, 2009). Systolic murmurs can be best auscultated along the left sternal border and result from aortic and pulmonary artery blood flow (Blackburn, 2012).

BLOOD VOLUME

Blood volume increases approximately 30% to 50% beginning as early as 6 weeks and peaking at 28 to 34 weeks (Monga, 2009). Blood volume then plateaus or decreases slightly to term, returning to prepregnant values by 6 to 8 weeks postpartum or sooner (Monga, 2009). The increased blood volume is necessary to provide adequate blood flow to the uterus, fetus, and maternal tissues; to maintain blood pressure (BP); to assist with temperature regulation by increasing cutaneous blood flow; and to accommodate blood loss at birth (Blackburn, 2012). Failure of blood volume to increase is associated with altered fetal and placental growth. Blood volume is greater in multiple gestations and increases proportionally according to the number of fetuses (Monga, 2009).

Changes in blood volume are due to increases in both plasma volume and red blood cell (RBC) mass. Plasma volume increases approximately 50% (range, 40% to 60% or about 1,200 to 1,600 mL) by term, and red cell mass increases 20% to 30% (250 to 450 mL) (Monga, 2009). The rapid increase in plasma volume and later rise in RBC volume results in relative hemodilution. Even with increased RBC production, there is a decrease in both hemoglobin and hematocrit values during pregnancy.

One proposed mechanism for expansion of blood volume is hormonal stimulation of plasma renin activity and aldosterone levels. Increases in the renin-angiotensin-aldosterone system stimulate renal tubular reabsorption of sodium and a subsequent increase of 6 to 8 L in total body water (extracellular and plasma fluid volume) (Blackburn, 2012). Changes in systemic vascular resistance (SVR) decrease venous tone and increase the capacity of the blood vessels to accommodate the extra blood volume without overloading the maternal system.

The extra blood volume helps protect the woman from shock with the normal blood loss at birth. To prevent hemorrhage immediately after childbirth, the uterus contracts, shunting blood from uterine vessels into the systemic circulation and causing an autotransfusion of approximately 1,000 mL. Although up to 500 mL (10%) of blood may be lost with a vaginal birth and 1,000 mL (15% to 30%) with a cesarean birth, average loss is usually less. These changes are accompanied by a postpartum diuresis that further reduces the plasma volume during the first several days postpartum. Plasma volume returns to prepregnancy levels by 6 to 8 weeks and perhaps as early as 2 to 3 weeks postpartum (Blackburn, 2012).

CARDIAC OUTPUT

Cardiac output is the product of heart rate times stroke volume, both of which increase during pregnancy. Cardiac output is also influenced by blood volume, cardiac contractility, vascular resistance, and maternal position. Cardiac output increases 30% to 50% during pregnancy when measured in the left lateral recumbent position. This increase begins early, with approximately half of the increase occurring by 8 weeks' gestation; peaks in the second trimester; and then plateaus until term (Monga, 2009). In early pregnancy, the increase in cardiac output primarily results from an increase in stroke volume. Stroke volume increases by as early as 8 weeks, peaks at 16 to 24 weeks, and then declines to term. The increase in cardiac output results initially from the increase in both heart rate and stroke volume, but by late pregnancy is due primarily to the changes in heart rate, which continues increasing to term (Monga, 2009). Cardiac output increases are greater in multiple pregnancies, especially after 20 weeks' gestation (Blackburn, 2012).

Maternal position can greatly influence cardiac output, most dramatically during the third trimester. Cardiac output is optimized in the lateral position, somewhat decreased in the sitting position, and markedly decreased in the supine position (Tsen, 2005). In the supine position, pressure exerted on the inferior vena cava from the gravid uterus decreases venous return and results in decreased cardiac output. This position may lead to supine hypotension with diaphoresis and possible syncope.

Cardiac output rises progressively during labor (Harris, 2011; Monga, 2009). Changes in cardiac output during the intrapartum period depend on maternal position, type of anesthesia, and method of birth. During the first stage of labor, approximately 300 to 500 mL of blood are shunted from the uterus into the systemic circulation with each contraction. This results in a progressive and cumulative rise in cardiac output during the first and second stage of labor. Epidural anesthesia causes a sympathectomy and a marked decrease in peripheral vascular resistance that may cause a decrease in venous return, resulting in decreased cardiac output. An intravenous fluid bolus before epidural placement may mitigate these effects.

Immediately after birth, cardiac output is 60% to 80% higher than during prelabor levels, declining rapidly after 10 to 15 minutes to stabilize at prelabor values after 1 hour (Monga, 2009). As a result of these hemodynamic changes, the intrapartum and immediate postpartum periods are times of increased vulnerability in women with cardiovascular disease. Cardiac output remains high for 24 to 48 hours after birth and then progressively decreases and returns to nonpregnant levels by 6 to 12 weeks postpartum in most women (Blackburn, 2012).

DISTRIBUTION OF BLOOD FLOW

Most of the increase in blood volume during pregnancy is distributed to the uterus, kidneys, breasts, and skin. The uterus accommodates one third of the additional blood volume at term. The kidneys receive approximately 400 mL/min. Glandular growth, distended veins, and tissue engorgement reflect the increased blood flow to the breasts, which may lead to a sensation of heat and tingling. Hyperemia of the cervix and vagina is also evident. Blood flow to the maternal skin increases to compensate for the heat loss created by fetal and placental metabolism as well as increases in maternal metabolic rate. This increased blood flow can result in alterations in nail and hair growth, increased nasal congestion, rhinitis, increased risk of nosebleeds, and sensations of warm hands and feet (Blackburn, 2012; Kumar, Hayhurst, & Robson, 2011).

BLOOD PRESSURE

Maternal position during BP measurement significantly affects BP values. Sitting or standing BP measurement shows minimal change in systolic blood pressure (SBP) throughout pregnancy. Diastolic blood pressure (DBP), measured while in sitting or standing positions, gradually decreases by approximately 10 to 15 mm Hg over the first-trimester values, with lowest values seen at 24 to 32 weeks, followed by a gradual increase toward nonpregnant baseline values by term (Monga, 2009). Accurate comparison of BP values depends on consistent techniques of measurement and consistent maternal positioning. Changes in BP are thought to be related to the vasodilatory effects of nitric oxide, PGI_2, and relaxin that mediate a decrease in SVR (Monga, 2009).

SYSTEMIC VASCULAR RESISTANCE

SVR decreases by 20% to 30% (Hegewald & Crapo, 2011). Changes in SVR are related to the increased capacity of the uteroplacental blood vessels; the effects of progesterone, nitric oxide, and PGI_2 on vascular smooth muscle and vasodilation; and the softening of collagen fibers (Schrier, 2010). The uteroplacental vascular system is a low-resistance network that accommodates a large percentage of maternal cardiac output. Uterine vascular resistance also decreases during pregnancy and enhances uterine blood flow. SVR decreases by 5 weeks' gestation, is lowest at 16 to 34 weeks' gestation, and gradually increases by term, when the mean SVR may approximate nonpregnant values (Monga, 2009).

HEMATOLOGIC CHANGES

To meet additional oxygen requirements of pregnancy, RBC volume increases approximately 20% to 30% (Monga, 2009). However, because plasma volume increases to a greater degree than the erythrocyte volume, the hematocrit decreases approximately 3% to 5%. This decrease is most obvious during the second trimester, after blood volume peaks.

Hemoglobin levels during pregnancy are between 12 and 16 g/dL. With the increase in the number of RBCs, the need for iron for the production of hemoglobin also increases. Serum ferritin levels decrease, with the greatest decline seen at 12 to 25 weeks (Kilpatrick, 2009). Approximately 500 mg of iron is needed for the increases in maternal RBCs, 270 mg by the fetus and 90 mg by the placenta. Total iron needs during pregnancy, including replacement of losses, are estimated at 1 g. Iron needs increase from 0.8 g/day in early pregnancy to 7.5 mg/day by term (Kilpatrick, 2009; Monga, 2009).

The GI absorption of iron is increased during pregnancy, but additional iron supplementation is nonetheless necessary for most women to maintain maternal iron stores. If iron stores are initially low and supplemental iron is not added to enhance the diet, iron-deficiency anemia may result (Kilpatrick, 2009). There is controversy surrounding the efficacy and benefit of prophylactic oral iron supplementation during pregnancy (Peña-Rosas & Viteri, 2009; Sanghvi, Harvey, & Wainwright, 2010). Thus, supplementation may not be needed to prevent iron-deficiency anemia in a woman who has good iron stores prior to pregnancy and a diet during pregnancy that is high in bioavailable iron. However, many women of childbearing age have marginal iron stores (Monga, 2009). Iron supplementation does not prevent the normal fall in hemoglobin (due to hemodilution) but can prevent depletion of stores and onset of iron-deficiency anemia.

Leukocyte (especially neutrophil) production also increases in pregnancy. The average white blood cell (WBC) count in the third trimester is 5,000 to 12,000/mm^3 (Kilpatrick, 2009). Labor and early postpartum levels may reach 20,000 to 30,000/mm^3 without an infection. The increase in WBC count begins during the second month, and the level returns to the normal range for nonpregnant women by 6 days postpartum. Slight increases in eosinophil levels and slight decreases in basophil levels have also been reported (Kilpatrick, 2009). Platelet counts range between 150,000/mm^3 and 400,000/mm^3, with perhaps a slight decrease in the third trimester (McCrae, 2010).

Plasma proteins and other components are also altered during pregnancy. Serum electrolytes and osmolality decrease. Serum lipids, especially cholesterol (needed for steroid hormone synthesis) and phospholipids (needed for cell membranes), increase 40% to 60%. Total plasma protein decreases 10% to 14% due primarily to hemodilution, but with both absolute and relative decreases in serum albumin. This leads to decreased serum oncotic pressure that contributes to the dependent edema seen in many pregnant women. The decrease in albumin also results in less bound and increases in the free fraction of substances such as calcium and some drugs (Blackburn, 2012).

Coagulation and fibrinolytic systems undergo significant changes during pregnancy with alterations in coagulation (precoagulant) factors, coagulation inhibitors, and fibrinolysis. Pregnancy is considered a hypercoagulable state because of increased levels of many coagulation factors and a decrease in factors such as protein S that inhibit coagulation. The most marked increases occur in factors I (fibrinogen), VII, VIII, and X and von Willebrand factor (vWF) antigen (Montagnana, Franchi, Danese, Gotsch, & Guidi, 2010). These changes are partially balanced by alterations in the plasminogen system that enhances clot lysis. Prothrombin time (PT) and activated partial thromboplastin time (aPTT) decrease slightly as the pregnancy comes to term; however, bleeding time and clotting time remain unchanged despite the increase in clotting factors (Blackburn, 2012). The net effect of these alterations places pregnant women at increased risk for thrombus formation and consumptive coagulopathies. After birth, coagulation is initiated to prevent hemorrhage at the placental site. Fibrinogen and platelet counts decrease as platelet plugs and fibrin clots form to provide hemostasis.

RESPIRATORY SYSTEM

Changes in the respiratory system are essential to accommodate increased maternal–fetal requirements and to ensure adequate gas exchange to meet maternal and fetal metabolic needs. The respiratory system must provide an increased amount of oxygen and efficiently remove carbon dioxide. Changes in the respiratory system are due primarily to a combination of mechanical forces (e.g., the enlarging uterus) and biochemical effects, especially the effects of progesterone and PGs on the respiratory center and bronchial smooth muscle. Table 3–2 summarizes the changes in respiratory function during pregnancy.

STRUCTURAL CHANGES

Pressure from the uterus shifts the diaphragm upward approximately 4 cm, decreasing the length of the lungs. To adjust to this decreased length, the anteroposterior diameter of the chest enlarges by 2 cm. Increased pressure from the uterus widens the substernal angle 50%, from 68 to 103 degrees, and causes the ribs to flare out slightly (Bobrowski, 2010; Whitty & Dombrowski, 2009). The circumference of the thoracic cage may increase 5 to 7 cm, compensating for the decreased lung length (Bobrowski, 2010; Hegewald & Crapo, 2011). Many of these changes are probably caused by hormonal influence because they occur before pressure is exerted from the growing uterus. Despite the mechanical elevation of the diaphragm in pregnancy, most of the work of breathing remains diaphragmatic.

LUNG VOLUME

Lung volumes are altered during pregnancy. Total lung volume (i.e., the amount of air in lungs at maximal

Table 3–2. RESPIRATORY CHANGES DURING PREGNANCY

Parameter	Change
Tidal volume	Increases 30%–40% (500–700 mL)
Vital capacity	Unchanged
Inspiratory reserve volume	Unchanged
Expiratory reserve volume	Decreases 15%–20%
Respiratory rate	Unchanged
Functional residual capacity	Decreases 20%–30%
Total lung volume	Decreases 5%
Residual volume	Decreases 20%–30%
Minute ventilation	Increases 30%–50%
pH	Slight increase to 7.40–7.45
P$_a$O$_2$ (first trimester)	106–108 mm Hg
P$_a$O$_2$ (by term)	101–104 mm Hg
P$_a$CO$_2$	27–32 mm Hg
Bicarbonate	18–21 mEq/L (base deficit of –3 to –4 mEq/L)

inspiration) decreases slightly (5%). Residual volume (i.e., the amount of air in lungs after maximum expiration), expiratory reserve volume (i.e., the maximal amount of air that can be expired from the resting expiratory level), and functional residual capacity (i.e., the amount of air remaining in the lungs at resting expiratory level, permitting air for gas exchange between breaths) fall by about 18% to 20% (Hegewald & Crapo, 2011; Whitty & Dombrowski, 2009). Tidal volume (i.e., the amount of air inspired and expired with normal breath), increases 30% to 40% (500 to 700 mL/min) during pregnancy and compensates for decreases in expiratory reserve volume and residual volume. Vital capacity (i.e., the maximum amount of air that can be forcibly expired after maximum inspiration) and inspiratory reserve volume (i.e., the maximum amount of air that can be inspired at end of normal inspiration) remain unchanged. The net effect of these lung volume changes is that there is no change in maximum breathing capacity during pregnancy. Spirometric measurements used for the diagnosis of respiratory problems do not change and remain useful evaluation tools.

VENTILATION

Alveolar and minute ventilation increase. Minute ventilation (i.e., amount of air inspired in 1 minute) increases from the first trimester to values 30% to 50% higher by term. Minute ventilation is the product of the respiratory rate and the tidal volume. The increase in minute ventilation is caused by an increase in tidal volume because the respiratory rate remains unchanged or increases only slightly (Hegewald & Crapo, 2011). Progesterone stimulates ventilation by lowering the carbon dioxide threshold of the respiratory center and may also act as a primary stimulant to the respiratory center, independent of carbon dioxide sensitivity and threshold. For example, in the nonpregnant woman, an increase of 1 mm Hg in P_aCO_2 increases minute ventilation by 1.5 L/min, whereas in pregnancy this same change in P_aCO_2 results in a 6 L/min change in minute ventilation (Whitty & Dombrowski, 2009).

OXYGEN AND CARBON DIOXIDE EXCHANGE

Oxygen consumption increases to approximately 50 mL/min at term to meet increasing oxygen demand in maternal, placental, and fetal tissues. Further increases of 40% to 60% occur during labor (Whitty & Dombrowski, 2009). The increased oxygen demand during pregnancy is met by the increases in minute ventilation and cardiac output. Increased minute ventilation increases arterial partial pressures of oxygen (P_aO_2) and decreases alveolar carbon dioxide tension.

The P_aO_2 during pregnancy is mildly elevated to between 106 to 108 mm Hg during the first trimester and 101 to 104 mm Hg at term (Whitty & Dombrowski,

2009). P_aCO_2 is decreased to between 27 and 32 mm Hg (Bobrowski, 2010). The decrease in P_aCO_2 is accompanied by a fall in plasma bicarbonate concentration to 18 to 21 mEq/L (base deficit of -3 to -4 mEq/L). Decreased carbon dioxide levels in the blood lead to higher pH values that are compensated for by renal excretion of bicarbonate, and the woman maintains a normal pH in the range of 7.40 to 7.45. The result of these changes is mildly elevated P_aO_2 and decreased P_aCO_2 and serum bicarbonate levels compared with normal values for nonpregnant women (Blackburn, 2012). Thus, the acid-base status during pregnancy is that of a compensated respiratory alkalosis.

Up to 70% of pregnant women experience dyspnea (Whitty & Dombrowski, 2009). The exact cause of this dyspnea is unclear, but it may be due to the woman's sensation of hyperventilation, effects of progesterone, increased oxygen consumption, and decreased P_aCO_2 levels. Mechanical forces from pressure of the uterus on the diaphragm may increase the sensation of dyspnea, but these forces are not the primary cause because dyspnea usually begins during the first or second trimester. Symptoms of nasal stuffiness, rhinitis, and nosebleeds are also more common for pregnant women and are related to vascular congestion resulting from increased levels of estrogen (Hegewald & Crapo, 2011). The respiratory system rapidly returns to the prepregnant status within 1 to 3 weeks after birth.

RENAL SYSTEM

The renal system undergoes structural and functional changes during pregnancy. Changes in renal function accommodate the increased metabolic and circulatory requirements of pregnancy. The renal system excretes maternal and fetal waste products. Pressure placed on the renal system and the relaxant effects of progesterone on vascular tissue enhance the ability of the renal system to accommodate the cardiovascular changes of pregnancy.

STRUCTURAL CHANGES

Increased renal blood flow, interstitial volumes, and hormonal influences increase renal volume by 30% and lengthen the kidneys by approximately 1 cm (Monga, 2009). The relaxing effects of progesterone on smooth muscle are probably primarily responsible for the dilation of the renal calyces, pelvis, and ureters (Blackburn, 2012). This muscular relaxation, coupled with increased urine volume and stasis, is associated with an increased risk of urinary tract infection.

During late gestation, the growing uterus and the dilated ovarian vein plexus place pressure on and displace the ureters and bladder. The ureters become dilated, elongated, and more tortuous, primarily in portions above the pelvic rim. The urethra also lengthens. Dilation of the ureters on the right side is more pronounced than that on the left because of the cushioning that occurs on the left side and dextrarotation of the uterus by the sigmoid colon. The right ovarian vein crosses the pelvic brim and therefore experiences greater compression by the growing uterus than the left ovarian vein, which parallels the brim (Monga, 2009).

During the second trimester, hyperemia of pelvic organs, hyperplasia of all muscles and connective tissues, and the gravid uterus elevate the bladder trigone and cause thickening of the interuretic margin. The bladder is displaced forward and upward in late pregnancy. Mechanical pressure placed on the bladder by the gravid uterus changes it from a convex to a concave organ. Urine output is increased primarily due to changes in sodium excretion. Urinary frequency (>7 daytime voidings) is reported in about 60% of pregnant women, with an increased incidence of stress and urge incontinence (Fiadjoe, Kannan, & Rane, 2010). These changes regress after birth in most women. Nocturia is due to increased sodium and therefore water excretion, mediated by the effects of the lateral position, which decrease stasis and increase venous return renal blood flow and glomerular filtration rate (GFR) (Blackburn, 2012).

Pressure on the renal system can impair drainage of blood and lymph and impede urine flow, which increases risk of infection and trauma during pregnancy. Renal volumes normalize with the first week after birth. However, hydronephrosis and hydroureter may take 3 to 4 months to return to normal (Monga, 2009).

RENAL BLOOD FLOW, GLOMERULAR FILTRATION, AND TUBULAR FUNCTION

Renal plasma flow (RPF) increases 50% to 80% by the second trimester due to increased blood volume and cardiac output and the lowered SVR caused by progesterone. RPF then progressively decreases by term to a level 50% greater than nonpregnant values (Monga, 2009). Women lying in the supine position can have decreased RPF in late pregnancy, compared with values obtained while in lateral positions. An increase in the GFR is seen as early as 3 to 4 weeks after conception. GFR peaks by the end of the first trimester, at 40% to 60% greater than nonpregnant levels or at an average of 110 to 180 mL/min (Monga, 2009). This rise in GFR probably results from vasodilation of preglomerular and postglomerular resistance vessels without any alteration in glomerular capillary pressure.

The filtered load of many substances exceeds the tubular reabsorptive capacity. As a result, renal clearance of many substances is elevated during pregnancy, with increased excretion and a related decrease in serum levels of some substances. Amino acids, glucose, many electrolytes, and water-soluble vitamins are excreted in amounts higher than in nonpregnant women. Calcium excretion increases but is balanced by increased intestinal absorption. Serum potassium values are influenced by both elevated plasma aldosterone levels, which promote potassium excretion, and by progesterone, which promotes potassium retention (Monga, 2009). The net change favors potassium retention, with a net retention of 300 to 350 mEq/L. Because the extra potassium is used by maternal and fetal tissues, serum potassium is only slightly changed.

Serum urea, blood urea nitrogen, and creatinine levels decline because of increased GFR. Serum uric acid levels decrease in early pregnancy and rise after 24 weeks. As a result, normal lab values during pregnancy and critical values indicating abnormality may be altered. Examples of critical values indicative of abnormal renal function during pregnancy include plasma creatinine >0.8 mg/dL, blood urea nitrogen >14 mg/dL, and urinary protein >300 mg/dL (Blackburn, 2012; Podymow, August, & Akbari, 2010).

FLUID AND ELECTROLYTE BALANCE

The kidneys play a significant role in the regulation of body sodium and water content. Renal sodium is the primary determinant of volume homeostasis. The filtered load of sodium increases from nonpregnant levels of 20,000 mEq/day to approximately 30,000 mEq/day during pregnancy (Monga, 2009). Sodium balance is mediated by factors that promote sodium excretion versus those that promote sodium retention. Factors promoting sodium excretion during pregnancy include increased GFR, increased atrial natriuretic factor, decreased plasma albumin, elevated progesterone and PG levels, and decreased vascular resistance. The physiologic changes that cause excretion of sodium are accompanied by increases in tubular reabsorption of sodium to avoid sodium depletion. Increases in aldosterone, estrogen, and cortisol all contribute to sodium reabsorption (Blackburn, 2012). The end result favors sodium retention, with a net retention of 900 to 950 mg of sodium or an additional 2 to 6 mEq of sodium reabsorbed each day for fetal and maternal stores (Monga, 2009).

Sodium retention (and thus water retention, because as sodium is reabsorbed from the tubule back into the blood, it pulls water with it) is mediated by the changes in the renin-angiotensin-aldosterone system. Aldosterone acts on the distal tubule and cortical collecting ducts to enhance sodium reabsorption. Aldosterone release is controlled by a specialized region of the kidney that secretes the peptide hormone renin in response to decreases in BP or sodium contents of the renal tubules, and stimulation of the sympathetic nervous system. Renin converts angiotensinogen to angiotensin I. Angiotensin I is cleaved in the lungs by angiotensin-converting enzyme (ACE) to form angiotensin II. Angiotensin II is a potent stimulator of aldosterone secretion and a potent vasopressor. Angiotensinogen, plasma renin activity, plasma renin, angiotensin II, and aldosterone levels are all increased in pregnancy (Lindheimer & August, 2009).

During pregnancy, renin is produced by the uterus, placenta, and fetus as well as the kidney. Release is stimulated by estrogen, changes in BP, PGs, and progesterone (an aldosterone antagonist). Increased plasma levels of aldosterone promote water and sodium retention, which results in the natural volume-overload state of pregnancy. Despite the elevated levels of angiotensin II, BP is not elevated in normal pregnancy due to a 60% decrease in sensitivity of the blood vessels to the vasoconstrictor effects of angiotensin II. This decreased sensitivity is thought to be due to decreased responsiveness of angiotensin II receptors and the relaxant effects of vasodilatory PGs and endothelial factors such as nitric oxide. Women with preeclampsia do not maintain this reduced sensitivity to angiotensin II, and BP rises (Irani & Xia, 2011; Lindheimer & August, 2009). In healthy pregnant women, the net effect of these changes is the establishment of a new equilibrium that the women sense as normal. From this new baseline, she responds to changes in fluid and electrolytes in a manner similar to a nonpregnant woman (Blackburn, 2012).

GLYCOSURIA

During pregnancy, the amount of glucose that is filtered by the kidneys increases 10- to 100-fold due to the increased RPF and GFR. The renal tubules increase reabsorption of glucose from the tubules back into the blood but are unable to match the dramatic increase in filtered glucose. The glucose that cannot be absorbed is lost in the urine; therefore, glycosuria is common. The glucose tolerance test is normal with most pregnant women with glycosuria, suggesting that this glycosuria is secondary to altered renal function and not abnormal carbohydrate metabolism (Blackburn, 2012). Clinical management of the woman with diabetes requires serum glucose evaluation rather than urine glucose evaluation during pregnancy.

PROTEINURIA

Protein excretion is also increased during pregnancy because the increased filtered load of protein exceeds the tubular reabsorptive capacity. Thus, urinary protein measurements should not be considered abnormal until 24-hour urine values greater than 300 mg

are reached. Levels higher than 300 mg/24 hours may indicate renal disease, preeclampsia, or urinary tract infection (Hennessy & Makris, 2011; Podymow et al., 2010).

GASTROINTESTINAL SYSTEM

Nutritional requirements during pregnancy increase, and changes in the GI system meet these demands. The GI tract is altered physiologically and anatomically during pregnancy. Many of the common discomforts of pregnancy (e.g., heartburn, gingivitis, constipation, nausea, and vomiting) can be attributed to the GI system. Pregnancy is associated with increased appetite and consumption of food. Many women experience food cravings and avoidances, sometimes mediated by alterations in sensitivity to taste and smell.

MOUTH AND ESOPHAGUS

Pregnant women often experience gingival edema and hyperemia, which usually begins in the second month and peaks in the third trimester. Gingival changers are probably related to increased vascularity and blood flow, changes in connective tissue, and the release of inflammatory mediators. Tooth enamel is not altered, but increases in dental plaques and calculus have been reported (Blackburn, 2012). Existing periodontal disease may be exacerbated by pregnancy, and associations between periodontal disease and preterm birth and low birth weight have been reported in some studies (George et al., 2011; Polyzos et al., 2009; Uppal et al., 2010). Three percent to 5% of women develop an angiogranuloma (epulis) between their upper, anterior maxillary teeth. Epulis regresses postpartum but may recur with subsequent pregnancies (Blackburn, 2012).

Lower esophageal sphincter (LES) muscle tone and pressure decrease due to the effects of progesterone. LES function is further altered after the uterus is large enough to change the positioning of the stomach and intestines and to move the LES into the thorax (Cunningham et al., 2009; Kelly & Savides, 2009). These changes increase the risk of reflux and heartburn.

NAUSEA AND VOMITING

Nausea with or without vomiting affects 70% to 90% of pregnant women in Western cultures (Lee & Saha, 2011). The exact mechanism for nausea and vomiting of pregnancy (NVP) is unclear. Theories have focused on mechanical, endocrinologic, allergic, metabolic, genetic, and psychosomatic etiologies (Blackburn, 2012). The most frequent hormones linked with NVP are estrogens and especially hCG, whose secretion patterns parallel the appearance and disappearance of

NVP in most women. Many studies have examined this link; however, data are inconsistent and inconclusive (Lee & Saha, 2011). NVP usually begins between 4 and 6 weeks and peaks at 8 to 12 weeks but may begin earlier or last longer in some women (Blackburn, 2012). Treatment is supportive and involves suggesting that the woman avoid foods that trigger nausea and to eat frequent, small meals. Ginger has been reported to be effective in reducing nausea (Ebrahimi, Maltepe, & Einarson, 2010). Hyperemesis gravidarum is a more severe and persistent form of nausea and vomiting and is associated with weight loss, electrolyte imbalance, ketosis, and dehydration. Any underlying illness should be excluded; hospitalization for fluid and electrolyte replacement may be necessary.

STOMACH

Progesterone decreases stomach gastric smooth muscle tone and motility, while the gravid uterus displaces the stomach. Gastric emptying is probably unchanged in early pregnancy but may be delayed with a tendency toward reverse peristalsis later in gestation. Relaxation of the LES permits reflux of gastric contents into the esophagus, causing heartburn. Gastric reflux is more common later in pregnancy. Decreased gastric acidity may reduce symptoms in women with peptic ulcer (Kelly & Savides, 2009).

SMALL AND LARGE INTESTINES

The intestines are pushed upward and laterally. The appendix is displaced superiorly, reaching the right costal margin by term, which, along with milder guarding and rebound tenderness due to cushioning by the uterus, may delay diagnosis of appendicitis during pregnancy. Increased progesterone levels relax GI tract tone and decrease intestinal motility, allowing time for increased absorption from the colon. Increased height of the duodenal villi and activity of brush border enzymes also increase nutrient absorptive capacity (Kelly & Savides, 2009). As a result, absorption of substances such as calcium, amino acids, iron, glucose, sodium, chloride, and water are increased. Reduced motility, mechanical obstruction by the uterus, and increased water absorption from the colon increase the risk of constipation. Hemorrhoids may develop when there is straining during bowel movements related to constipation, and from the increased pressure exerted on the vessels below the level of the uterus.

LIVER

Liver size and morphology do not significantly change during pregnancy, but liver production of many proteins is altered due to the effects of estrogen. Hepatic blood flow increases during pregnancy, but the percentage of circulating blood volume reaching the liver remains unchanged. Some tests of liver function during pregnancy produce values that would suggest hepatic disease in nonpregnant women. For example, fibrinogen levels increase by 50% by the end of the second trimester. Plasma albumin concentration decreases, which in nonpregnant patients could indicate liver disease. Serum alkaline phosphatase activity and serum cholesterol concentration can be twice the normal range or even higher in multiple gestations (Blackburn, 2012). On the other hand, serum bilirubin, aspartate aminotransferase (AST), and alanine aminotransferase (ALT) are unchanged or slightly lower in normal pregnancy and therefore can be used to evaluate liver function during pregnancy.

GALLBLADDER

Gallbladder size and function are altered during pregnancy. Elevated progesterone levels cause the gallbladder to be hypotonic and distended. Gallbladder smooth muscle contraction is impaired and may lead to stasis. Emptying time is slow after 14 weeks' gestation. In the second and third trimesters, fasting and residual volumes are twice as large as in the nonpregnant woman. As a result of these changes, cholesterol may be sequestered in the gallbladder, increasing the risk of gall stones (Blackburn, 2012).

WEIGHT GAIN

Prenatal care, socioeconomic factors, and adequate nutrition influence pregnancy outcome. Women who are underweight before conception and women who have inadequate weight gain during pregnancy are at greater risk for having a low-birth-weight infant. The risk is greatest for women with both factors (Scotland, 2009). Maternal obesity and excessive weight gain during pregnancy have been associated with fetal macrosomia (Begum, Sachchithanantham, & De Somsubhra, 2011; Nelson, Matthews, & Poston, 2010). A nutritional assessment should be made at the initial prenatal visit, with referral to a registered dietitian as needed.

The woman's prepregnancy height and weight determine her actual caloric intake needs. On average, the increased demands of pregnancy require an additional 300 kcal each day. Women who are pregnant with twins or higher order multiples need an additional 300 kcal per fetus each day. There are differences in suggested weight gain based on prepregnancy weight and body mass index (BMI). The recently revised Institute of Medicine guidelines on weight gain during pregnancy assume a 1.1 to 4.0 lb weight gain during the first trimester. Recommended weight gain during the second and third trimester varies with BMI: 0.8 to 1.0 lb/week in women with a normal BMI; 1.0 to 1.3 lb/week in underweight women; 0.6 to 0.7 lb/week in overweight women and 0.4 to 0.6 lb/week in obese women (Rasmussen et al., 2010).

METABOLIC CHANGES

Profound metabolic changes occur throughout pregnancy to provide for the development and growth of the fetus. Adequate maternal weight gain and changes in maternal glucose, protein, and fat metabolism are important factors in normal fetal growth and development. During the course of pregnancy, approximately 3.5 kg of fat is deposited, approximately 30,000 kcal of energy is stored, and 900 g of new protein is synthesized to meet maternal and fetal needs (Blackburn, 2012). Estrogens, progesterone, and hPL influence metabolic processes during pregnancy by altering glucose utilization, fat metabolism and use, protein homeostasis, and insulin action. These changes meet fetal growth needs by increasing the availability of glucose and amino acid for transfer to the fetus while providing increased availability of fatty acids as an alternative energy substrate to meet maternal needs and maintain homeostasis (Blackburn, 2012). "The changes in carbohydrate and lipid metabolism parallel the energy needs of the mother and fetus, whereas the changes in maternal nitrogen and protein metabolism occur early in pregnancy, before fetal demand" (Blackburn, 2012).

Pregnancy can be divided into two metabolic phases: an initial anabolism dominant phase and a later catabolism predominant phase. During the first part of pregnancy, anabolism is prominent with nutrient uptake, energy stored as fat, and maternal weight gain. Estrogen stimulates pancreatic beta cell hypertrophy and hyperplasia with increased insulin production. During this phase, insulin sensitivity is not significantly affected, and insulin increases in response to the influx of glucose from the GI tract after a meal (Pridjian & Benjamin, 2010). The increased insulin promotes storage of glucose as glycogen, increased fat synthesis, storage of triglycerides and fat, fat cell hypertrophy, and inhibition of lipolysis. Both low-density and high-density lipoproteins increase (Herrera & Lasuncion, 2011). Maternal protein storage increases, with a net retention of 1.3 g/day of nitrogen for use both by the mother and the fetus (Blackburn, 2012).

As pregnancy progresses, the maternal metabolic status becomes more catabolic, and maternal weight gain is due primarily to fetal growth. Adipose tissue lipolytic activity is enhanced, and plasma, free fatty acids, glycerol, and ketones increase (Duttaroy, 2009;

Herrera & Lasuncion, 2011). These provide alternate energy sources for maternal needs, conserving glucose for transfer to the fetus. This is important since the fetus is an obligatory glucose user whose enzyme systems promote fat storage and who cannot readily break down fat to use for energy. During this phase, maternal urinary nitrogen excretion decreases, conserving protein for fetal transfer. Maternal insulin levels increase as insulin resistance in the peripheral tissues becomes prominent (Blackburn, 2012; Pridjian & Benjamin, 2010).

Insulin antagonism is caused by hPL and other placental hormones (e.g., progesterone, estrogen, cortisol, and prolactin) that oppose the action of insulin and promote maternal lipolysis (Moore & Catalano, 2009). Insulin normally helps to clear glucose from the blood and promotes glycogen and fat storage. Insulin resistance (mean insulin sensitivity decreases 50% to 70%) means that maternal glucose levels remain higher for a longer period of time after a meal to promote fetal transfer (Pridjian & Benjamin, 2010). Thus, decreased sensitivity to insulin in the liver and peripheral tissues leads to a persistent relative hyperglycemia after meals. This relative hyperinsulinemia and hyperglycemia of pregnancy has been referred to as a diabetogenic state.

Maternal metabolic responses alter responses on glucose tolerance tests so that these tests need to be interpreted using pregnancy-specific norms. These changes, in comparison to a nonpregnant individual, include (1) a lower initial fasting blood glucose value (due to decreased glucose utilization and increased fat utilization enhancing glucose availability for the fetus) and (2) elevated blood glucose for a longer period of time after ingestion of carbohydrates (due to insulin antagonism and decreased insulin sensitivity) (Moore & Catalano, 2009; Pridjian & Benjamin, 2010).

ENDOCRINE SYSTEM

THYROID GLAND

The production, circulation, and disposal of thyroid hormone are altered in pregnancy to support maternal metabolic changes and fetal growth and development. Increased vascularity and hyperplasia of the thyroid gland result in increased hormone production and an increase in thyroid size, although not in the form of a goiter in populations with adequate iodine intake (Alexander, 2009; Nader, 2009b). Most of the changes in the thyroid gland occur during the first half of pregnancy and lead to a state of "euthyroid hyperthyroxinemia," in which levels of thyroxine (T4) are elevated. These changes are due to estrogen (increasing thyroxine-binding globulin [TBG] production by the liver), hCG, and increased urinary iodide excretion (Alexander, 2009; Nader, 2009b). hCG, which has mild thyroid-stimulating–like activity, stimulates production of T4 and triiodo-thyronine (T3).

Total T4 and T3 increase and peak by 10 to 15 weeks and remain 40% to 100% higher to term (Galofre & Davies, 2009). Free T4 and T3 increase during the first trimester but decrease during the second and third trimesters as levels of TBG increase. Thus, more T3 and T4 are produced (increased total), but because much of the extra thyroid hormone is bound to TBG, the amount of free hormone is reduced. Serum protein-bound iodine increases. Increased production of thyroid hormone increases thyroid iodine uptake. At the same time, urinary iodide excretion increases and iodide is sent to the fetus, leading to a smaller iodine pool. These changes are partially compensated for by increased thyroid clearance and recycling of iodide; however, maternal iodide needs increase during pregnancy (Blackburn, 2012).

Maternal thyroid hormone is critical for fetal central nervous system (CNS) development, especially in early pregnancy, when the CNS undergoes critical development prior to the time the fetus is able to produce T4 (Melse-Boonstra & Jaiswal, 2010; Morreale de Escobar, Ares, Berbel, Obregón, & del Rey, 2008). Untreated maternal hypothyroidism increases the risk of pregnancy loss and altered fetal brain development and later mental retardation. Iodine supplementation has been found to decrease the incidence of these complications in populations with high endemic levels of hypothyroidism (Melse-Boonstra & Jaiswal, 2010).

Transient hyperthyroidism is seen during the first trimester in about 15% of healthy pregnant women (Galofre & Davies, 2009). Diagnosis of hyperthyroidism during pregnancy is challenging because normal signs of symptoms of pregnancy, including heat intolerance, tachycardia, wide pulse pressure, and vomiting, mimic hyperthyroidism (Fitzpatrick & Russell, 2010). Poor control during pregnancy can result in preterm labor, fetal loss, or thyroid crisis in these women. Diagnosis of abnormal thyroid function in the pregnant woman requires an understanding of the normal changes in thyroid function during pregnancy in order to appropriately interpret results of laboratory tests.

Transient postpartum thyroid disorder (PPTD) is seen in 6% to 9% of postpartum women and is thought to have an autoimmune basis. PPTD is usually characterized by a period (average, 2 to 4 months) of mild hyperthyroidism, followed by a period of hypothyroidism, with a return to normal thyroid function in most women by 12 months postpartum. Some women only experience one of these phases. Up to one fourth of these women develop permanent hypothyroidism within 5 to 15 years (Krassas, Poppe, & Glinoer, 2010).

PITUITARY GLAND

The anterior pituitary enlarges, with a 30% increase in weight and 2-fold increase in volume, and becomes more convex and dome shaped (Blackburn, 2012). These changes are primarily due to an increase in the group of cells that produce prolactin. Adrenocorticotropin (ACTH) secretion and serum levels increase, peaking during the intrapartum period (Vrekoussis et al., 2010). This increase is probably due primarily to stimulation by increased placental, rather than hypothalamic, CRH. Pituitary growth hormone secretion is suppressed by placental growth hormone, which increases from 15 to 20 weeks to term (Blackburn, 2012). FSH (stimulates ovum follicle growth) and LH (needed for ovulation) are both inhibited during pregnancy.

The posterior pituitary hormones are oxytocin and AVP. Oxytocin influences contractility of the uterus, and after birth, it stimulates milk ejection from the breasts. Secretion increases during the intrapartum and postpartum periods. AVP, also called antidiuretic hormone, causes vasoconstriction when released in large amounts, which increases BP. The major role of AVP is its antidiuretic action in the regulation of water balance. Secretion of AVP is controlled by changes in plasma osmolarity and blood volume. Plasma levels of AVP do not change during pregnancy, despite the changes in blood volume, indicating that AVP is secreted at a lower plasma osmolality in pregnancy (Blackburn, 2012).

ADRENAL GLANDS

The elevated ACTH stimulates increased cortisol production by the adrenal glands during pregnancy. The adrenal gland undergoes hypertrophy with increases in the zona fasciculata (the portion of the adrenal that produces glucocorticoids such as cortisol) (Nader, 2009a). Plasma levels of CRH progressively increase during the second and third trimesters of pregnancy. Circulating cortisol levels regulate carbohydrate and protein metabolism. Total and free cortisol increase 2- to 8-fold (Nader, 2009a). Thus, pregnancy is characterized by a transient hypercortisolemia (Mastorakos & Ilias, 2000). Normally increased cortisol would turn off ACTH release. Therefore, the increased ACTH with increased cortisol during pregnancy suggests changes in the set point for cortisol release. Thus, in spite of the elevated cortisol and ACTH, physiologic responses to stress (such as BP, heart rate, and cortisol reactivity) are maintained during pregnancy, although they may be somewhat blunted, with wide individual differences reported (Blackburn, 2012).

Other adrenal cortex hormones, aldosterone (see section on changes in the renal system), and steroid hormones also increase. Total testosterone levels also increase in pregnancy because of an increase in sex hormone–binding globulin. Free testosterone levels are low normal before 28 weeks' gestation.

PARATHYROID GLANDS

Parathyroid hormone (PTH) decreases during the first trimester, then increases to term. The early decrease is due to increased 1,25-dihydroxyvitamin D in response to PTHrP production by the fetus and placenta (Clarke & Khosla, 2010). Regulation of calcium is closely related to magnesium, phosphate, PTH, vitamin D, and calcitonin levels. Any alteration in one is likely to alter the others. Increases in serum-ionized calcium or magnesium suppress PTH levels, whereas decreases in serum-ionized calcium or magnesium stimulate the release of PTH.

Maternal calcium homeostasis changes during pregnancy. Total serum calcium falls, primarily related to the fall in albumin, reaching its lowest at 28 to 32 weeks, then plateaus or increases slightly to term (Blackburn, 2012). There is no significant change in mean serum-ionized calcium. Daily maternal intestinal calcium absorption increases and doubles by the third trimester due to increased calciferol (active form of vitamin D) and its binding proteins (Clarke & Khosla, 2010). This change begins in the first trimester, before fetal demand, so that maternal bone stores of calcium are increased during early pregnancy. These stores are used to meet the increased fetal demand in late pregnancy. Overall, significant maternal bone mass is not lost during pregnancy.

IMMUNE SYSTEM

One mystery in pregnancy is the process by which the mother's immune system remains tolerant of the foreign paternal antigens on fetal tissues and yet maintains adequate immune competence against microorganisms. Protection of the fetus from rejection is a multifactorial, complex process that seems to be predominately a localized uterine response, although there are also systemic responses mediated primarily by endocrine factors.

The mother initially has a weak immune response to the fetus/placenta that leads to an activation (facilitation) reaction rather than rejection. These initial responses, thought to help the mother recognize and protect the fetus, are mediated by Th2 cytokines (interleukins) and

growth factors. Trophoblast cells fail to express major histocompatibility complex class (MHC) I or II molecules, and this may be the major reason the fetus is not targeted by the maternal immune system. The absence of the usual MHC class I and II molecules prevents maternal T-cell activation and cytotoxic T-cell destruction (Petroff, 2011). Maternal tolerance of the fetus may be mediated by the presence of histocompatibility antigen, class 1, G (HLA-G), an MHC class I molecule found only on the trophoblast. This antigen is unique in that it may help the mother to recognize the fetus but does not elicit destructive responses from the T lymphocytes. Other factors that enhance maternal tolerance at the maternal–fetal interface include (1) progesterone, (2) blocking factors induced by progesterone, (3) altered natural killer (NK) cell function, (4) changes in the Th1–Th2 cytokine balance, (5) suppressor macrophages, and (6) toll-like receptors (Blackburn, 2012; Mor & Abrahams, 2009; Munoz-Suano, Hamilton, & Betz, 2011; Petroff, 2011). Cytokines, PGE$_2$, steroid hormones, estrogen, hCG, and various pregnancy-specific proteins exert immunosuppressive effects during pregnancy.

Immune responses include innate responses and adaptive responses. Both types of responses are altered during pregnancy with enhancement of innate and antibody-mediated responses in the systemic circulation of the pregnant woman. Innate responses include initial actions to the entry of pathogens and inflammatory reactions. Circulating WBCs (especially neutrophils and monocytes) are increased. However, decreased neutrophil chemotaxis (organized movement of neutrophils toward the site of pathogen entry) may delay initial responses to infection (Mor & Abrahams, 2009). Systemic NK cell cytotoxic activity is down-regulated by progesterone, especially in the second and third trimesters. Enhanced monocyte and neutrophil activity may enhance phagocytosis. Complement levels and activity are normal to increased but may be delayed (Blackburn, 2012).

Adaptive responses include antibody-mediated (B-lymphocyte) and cell-mediated (T-lymphocyte) responses. Pregnancy is characterized by a switch in the balance of Th1 to Th2 cytokines (Challis et al., 2009). Th1 and Th2 are subsets of T-lymphocyte helper cells that facilitate different components of the immune response. During pregnancy, Th2-type cytokines are increased, enhancing antibody-mediated immunity; while Th1 cytokines are decreased, reducing cell-mediated responses (associated with tissue rejection). B-lymphocyte function (antibody-mediated immunity) is not significantly altered and may be enhanced by the increase in Th2 cytokines. The slight decrease in immunoglobulin G (IgG) may increase the risk of bacterial colonization. Cell-mediated (T-lymphocyte) immunity is somewhat suppressed during pregnancy, which may help prevent maternal rejection of the fetus. This suppression is mediated by cortisol, hCG, progesterone, and alpha fetoprotein (Challis et al., 2009). T-cell total numbers are probably unchanged and systemic T-cell function maintained. However, selective localized (reproductive) immunosuppression may occur that may increase the risk of viral and mycotic infections.

NEUROMUSCULAR AND SENSORY SYSTEMS

In general, there are no major CNS changes during pregnancy, although several discomforts reported by pregnant women are associated with the nervous system. Mild frontal headaches may occur in the first and second trimesters and may be caused by tension or related to hormonal changes (Klein & Loder, 2010). Severe headache, especially after 20 weeks' gestation, may be associated with preeclampsia. This type of headache is a result of cerebral edema from vasoconstriction. Dizziness may result from vasomotor instability, postural hypotension, or hypoglycemia, especially after prolonged periods of sitting or standing. Paresthesia of the lower extremities can occur because of pressure from the gravid uterus, interfering with circulation. Excessive hyperventilation, resulting in lower P_aCO_2 levels, creates a tingling sensation in the hands (Blackburn, 2012).

Musculoskeletal alterations during pregnancy include changes in posture, gait, and ligament laxity. Early in pregnancy, the ligaments of the pregnant woman soften from the effects of progesterone and relaxin. This softening, especially evident in the sacroiliac, sacrococcygeal, and pubic joints of the pelvis, facilitates birth. The center of gravity changes with advancing pregnancy because of the increase in weight, fluid retention, lordosis, and mobilization of ligaments. To accommodate the increased weight of the uterus, the lumbodorsal spinal curve is accentuated, and the woman's posture changes. The rectus abdominis muscle may separate because of the pressure exerted by the growing uterus, producing diastasis recti. The risks of ligament injury, muscle cramps, back and joint pain, and falls are increased during pregnancy (Han, 2010; McCrory, Chambers, Daftary, & Redfern, 2010; Vermani, Mittal, & Weeks, 2010).

Sleep patterns change during pregnancy, mediated by hormonal changes and mechanical forces. Changes include an increase in total sleep time, insomnia, night awakenings, and daytime sleepiness and decreased stage 3 and 4 nonrapid eye movement sleep (Santiago, Nolledo, Kinzler, & Santiago, 2001). Night awakenings are often related to nocturia, fetal activity, backache, dyspnea, and heartburn. Sleep is also altered in the postpartum period, especially in the first 2 weeks.

The pregnant woman may experience ocular and otolaryngic changes. Intraocular pressure tends to drop during the second half of gestation. The cornea becomes thicker, and mild corneal edema may be present. These changes can slightly alter refractory power and may lead to mild discomforts in women who wear contact lenses. Otolaryngic changes are due to altered fluid dynamics, increased vascular permeability, vasomotor changes, increased vascularization, and the effects of estrogen. These changes can lead to an increase in ear and nasal stuffiness, hoarseness, and snoring (Blackburn, 2012; Kumar et al., 2011; Schmidt, Flores, Rossi, & Silveira, 2010).

INTEGUMENTARY SYSTEM

Skin changes induced by pregnancy include vascular alterations, variations in nail and hair growth, connective tissue changes, and altered pigmentation (Blackburn, 2012; Bremmer, Driscoll, & Colgan, 2010; Rapini, 2009). Blood flow to the skin increases three to four times above prepregnant levels. Vascular spider nevi appear on the face, neck, chest, arms, and legs. These are small, bright red elevations of the skin radiating from a central body. Spider nevi are related to increased subcutaneous blood flow and potentially to increased estrogen levels in the tissue. Palmar erythema is a normal vascular change during pregnancy, but it has also been associated with liver and collagen vascular diseases.

During early pregnancy, the number of hairs in the growth phase remains stable. In the later stages of pregnancy, however, hormonal levels apparently increase the number of hairs in the growth phase and decrease the number of hairs in the resting phase. After birth, the proportion of hairs that enters the resting phase doubles, and women may experience an increase in hair loss 2 to 4 months postpartum (Camacho-Martínez, 2009). Occasionally, nail growth may be affected, and nail changes include transverse grooving, softening, and increased brittleness.

Striae gravidarum (i.e., stretch marks) may occur on the skin of the breasts, hips, and upper thighs and are usually most pronounced on the abdomen. Striae, which result from the normal stretching of the skin and softening and relaxing of the dermal collagenous and elastic tissues during the last months of pregnancy, occur in about 50% of pregnant women (Blackburn, 2012).

Increases in estrogen and progesterone may cause an increase in melanocyte-stimulating hormone, causing hyperpigmentation in the integumentary system.

Darkening of the nipples, areolae, and perianal and genital areas occurs. The linea alba becomes the linea nigra and divides the abdomen longitudinally from the sternum to the symphysis. Melasma (i.e., the "mask of pregnancy," previously referred to as chloasma) appears as irregularly shaped brown blotches on the face, with a mask-like distribution on the cheekbones and forehead and around the eyes. Melasma is thought to result from elevated serum levels of estrogen and progesterone, which also stimulate melanin deposits. Melasma disappears after pregnancy but may reappear with excessive sun exposure or with oral contraceptive use (Jadotte & Schwartz, 2010; Rapini, 2009).

REPRODUCTIVE ORGANS

UTERUS

Before pregnancy, the uterus is a small, semisolid, pear-shaped organ that weighs 40 to 50 g. During pregnancy, the uterus becomes globular and increases in length. At term, the uterus weighs approximately 1,100 to 1,200 g, due to hypertrophy of the myometrial cells (Norwitz & Lye, 2009). Ten percent to 20% of the maternal cardiac output flows through the vascular system of the uterus (Monga, 2009). During the first few months of pregnancy, the wall of the uterus thickens due to myometrial hyperplasia and hypertrophy in response to elevated estrogen and progesterone levels. After this time, the muscle wall thins, allowing easier palpation of the fetus. The size and number of blood and lymphatic vessels increase.

The uterus remains relatively quiescent during most of pregnancy. Even in nonpregnant women, the myometrium has periodic low-frequency, low-amplitude activity. This baseline activity increases during pregnancy and becomes more apparent to the women as gestation progresses. Near the end of pregnancy, the myometrium goes through a preparatory stage for labor involving activation of uterine contractility, cervical ripening, and activation of fetal membranes. Activation is thought to be stimulated by uterotrophins such as estrogen and by increased formation of gap junctions (needed for transmission of the action potential between muscle cells), oxytocin receptors, PG receptor activation, and ion channels to enhance movement of calcium (essential for muscle contraction) into the myocytes (Norwitz & Lye, 2009).

Uteroplacental blood flow is essential for adequate fetal growth and survival. By term, the blood flow from the uterine and ovarian arteries to the uterus is approximately 500 to 600 mL/min, 80% of which is directed to the placental bed (Monga, 2009). Maternal position, maternal arterial pressure, and uterine contractility influence uterine blood flow. The uterine spiral arteries are altered by the fetal trophoblast cells, which migrate out of the placenta and remodel the elastic and muscle elements of the maternal spiral arteries underlying the site of placental implantation. As a result of these changes, the spiral arteries (often called uteroplacental arteries during pregnancy) are greatly increased in diameter and can accommodate the vast supply of blood needed to supply the placenta.

CERVIX

The cervix undergoes changes characterized by increased vascularity and water content, softening, and dilation (Timmons, Akins, & Mahendroo, 2010). Estrogen stimulates glandular tissue of the cervix, which increases the number of cells. Early in pregnancy, increased vascularity causes a softening and a bluish discoloration of the cervix known as Chadwick's sign. Endocervical glands, which occupy one half of the mass of the cervix at term, secrete a thick, tenacious mucus that forms the mucous plug and prevents bacteria and other substances from entering the uterus. This mucous plug is expelled before the onset of labor and may be associated with a bloody show. Hyperactive glandular tissue also causes an increase in the normal mucus production during pregnancy.

OVARIES

Ovulation ceases during pregnancy. Cells that line the follicles, known as thecal cells, become active in hormone production and serve as the interstitial glands of pregnancy. The corpus luteum persists and secretes progesterone until the 10th to 12th week, which maintains the endometrium until adequate progesterone is secreted by the placenta.

VAGINA

Vaginal epithelium and muscle layers undergo hypertrophy, increased vascularization, and hyperplasia during pregnancy in response to estrogen levels. Loosening of the connective tissue and thickening of the mucosa increase vaginal secretions. These secretions are thick, white, and acidic and play a role in preventing infection. By the end of pregnancy, the vaginal wall and perineal body become relaxed enough to permit stretching of the tissues to accommodate the birth of the infant.

BREASTS

Breasts increase in size and nodularity to prepare for lactation. Nipples become more easily erectile and veins are more prominent. Areolar pigmentation increases.

Montgomery's follicles, the sebaceous glands located in the areola, hypertrophy. Striae may develop as the breasts enlarge. Colostrum, a yellow secretion rich in antibodies, may leak from the nipples during the last trimester of pregnancy. Feelings of fullness, tingling, and increased sensitivity begin in the first few weeks of gestation.

SUMMARY

Significant physical, metabolic, and structural changes occur from conception until weeks into the postpartum period. A thorough understanding of these changes facilitates assessment of normal pregnancy progression. Recognition of variations from normal may result in early identification of risk factors and potential complications. Prompt management can be initiated to help ensure optimal outcomes for both mother and fetus.

REFERENCES

Alexander, E. K. (2009). Thyroid function: The complexity of maternal hypothyroidism during pregnancy. *Nature Reviews Endocrinology, 5*(9), 480–481. doi:10.1038/nrendo.2009.153

Begum, K. S., Sachchithanantham, K., & De Somsubhra, S. (2011). Maternal obesity and pregnancy outcome. *Clinical & Experimental Obstetrics & Gynecology, 38*(1), 14–20.

Blackburn, S. T. (2012). *Maternal, Fetal and Neonatal Physiology: A Clinical Perspective* (4th ed.). Philadelphia: Saunders Elsevier.

Bobrowski, R. A. (2010). Pulmonary physiology in pregnancy. *Clinical Obstetrics & Gynecology, 53*(2), 285–300. doi:10.1097/GRF.0b013e3181e04776

Bremmer, M., Driscoll, M. S., & Colgan, R. (2010). The skin disorders of pregnancy: A family physician's guide. *Journal of Family Practice, 59*(2), 89–96.

Camacho-Martínez, F. M. (2009). Hair loss in women. *Seminars in Cutaneous Medicine & Surgery, 28*(1), 19–32. doi:org/10.1016/j.sder.2009.01.001

Challis, J. R., Lockwood C. J., Myatt, L., Norman, J. E., Strauss, J. F. III, & Petraglia, F. (2009). Inflammation and pregnancy. *Reproductive Sciences, 16*(2), 206–215. doi:10.1177/1933719108329095

Clarke, B. L., & Khosla, S. (2010). Female reproductive system and bone. *Archives of Biochemistry & Biophysics, 503*(1), 118–128. doi:org/10.1016/j.abb.2010.07.006

Cole, L. A. (2010). Hyperglycosylated hCG, a review. *Placenta, 31*(8), 653–664. doi:10.1016/j.placenta.2010.06.005

Cunningham, G., Leveno, K., Bloom, S., & Hauth, J. (2009). *Williams Obstetrics* (23rd ed.). New York: McGraw-Hill.

Curry, R., Swan, L., & Steer, P. J. (2009). Cardiac disease in pregnancy. *Current Opinion in Obstetrics & Gynecology, 21*(6), 508–513. doi:10.1097/GCO.0b013e328332a762

Duttaroy, A. K. (2009). Transport of fatty acids across the human placenta: A review. *Progress in Lipid Research, 48*(1), 52–61. doi:10.1016/j.plipres.2008.11.001

Ebrahimi, N., Maltepe, C., & Einarson, A. (2010). Optimal management of nausea and vomiting of pregnancy. *International Journal of Women's Health, 4*(2), 241–248.

Fiadjoe, P., Kannan, K., & Rane, A. (2010). Maternal urological problems in pregnancy. *European Journal of Obstetrics, Gynecology, & Reproductive Biology, 152*(1), 13–17. doi:10.1016/j.ejogrb.2010.04.013

Fitzpatrick, D. L., & Russell, M. A. (2010). Diagnosis and management of thyroid disease in pregnancy. *Obstetrics & Gynecology Clinics of North America, 37*(2), 173–193. doi:10.1016/j.ogc.2010.02.007

Galofre, J. C., & Davies, T. F. (2009). Autoimmune thyroid disease in pregnancy: A review. *Journal of Women's Health, 18*(11), 1847–1856. doi:10.1089/jwh.2008.1234

George, A., Shamim, S., Johnson, M., Ajwani, S., Bhole, S., Blinkhorn, A., . . . Andrews, K. (2011). Periodontal treatment during pregnancy and birth outcomes: A meta-analysis of randomized trials. *International Journal of Evidence-Based Healthcare, 9*(2), 122–147. doi:10.1111/j.1744-1609.2011.00210.x

Goldsmith, L. T., & Weiss, G. (2009). Relaxin in human pregnancy. *Annals of the New York Academy of Sciences, 1160,* 130–135.

Han, I. H. (2010). Pregnancy and spinal problems. *Current Opinion in Obstetrics & Gynecology, 22*(6), 477–481. doi:10.1097/GCO.0b013e3283404ea1

Harris, I. S. (2011). Management of pregnancy in patients with congenital heart disease. *Progress in Cardiovascular Disease, 53*(4), 305–311. doi:10.1016/j.pcad.2010.08.001

Hegewald, M. J., & Crapo, R. O. (2011). Respiratory physiology in pregnancy. *Clinics of Chest Medicine, 32*(1), 1–13. doi:10.1016/j.ccm.2010.11.001

Hennessy, A., & Makris, A. (2011). Preeclamptic nephropathy. *Nephrology, 16*(2), 134–143. doi:10.1111/j.1440-1797.2010.01411.x

Herrera, E., & Lasuncion, M. A. (2011). Maternal-fetal transfer of lipid metabolites. In R. A. Polin, W. W. Fox, & S. H. Abman (Eds.), *Fetal and neonatal physiology* (4th ed.). Philadelphia: Saunders Elsevier.

Irani, R. A., & Xia, Y. (2011). Renin angiotensin signaling in normal pregnancy and preeclampsia. *Seminars in Nephrology, 31*(1), 47–58. doi:10.1016/j.semnephrol.2010.10.005

Jadotte, Y. T., & Schwartz, R. A. (2010). Melasma: Insights and perspectives. *Acta Dermatovenerol Croatica, 18*(2), 124–129.

Kelly, A. J., Malik, S., Smith, L., Kavanagh, J., & Thomas, J. (2009). Vaginal prostaglandin (PGE2 and PGF2a) for induction of labour at term. *Cochrane Database Systematic Review, 2009*(4), CD003101.

Kelly, T. F., & Savides, T. J. (2009). Gastrointestinal disease in pregnancy. In R. K. Creasy, R. Resnik, J. D. Iams, C. J. Lockwood, & T. Moore (Eds.). *Creasy & Resnik's Maternal-Fetal Medicine: Principles and Practice* (6th ed., pp. 1041–1058). Philadelphia: Saunders Elsevier.

Kilpatrick, S. J. (2009). Anemia and pregnancy. In R. K. Creasy, R. Resnik, J. D. Iams, C. J. Lockwood, & T. Moore (Eds.). *Creasy & Resnik's Maternal-Fetal Medicine: Principles and Practice* (6th ed., pp. 869–884). Philadelphia: Saunders Elsevier.

Klein, A. M., & Loder, E. (2010). Postpartum headache. *International Journal of Obstetric Anesthesia, 19*(4), 422–430. doi:10.1016/j.ijoa.2010.07.009

Krassas, G. E., Poppe, K., & Glinoer, D. (2010). Thyroid function and human reproductive health. *Endocrine Reviews, 31*(5), 702–755. doi:10.1210/er.2009-0041

Kumar, R., Hayhurst, K. L., & Robson, A. K. (2011). Ear, nose, and throat manifestations during pregnancy. *Otolaryngology Head & Neck Surgery, 145*(2), 188–198. doi:10.1177/0194599811407572

Lee, N. M., & Saha, S. (2011). Nausea and vomiting of pregnancy. *Gastroenterology Clinics of North America, 40*(2), 309–334. doi:10.1016/j.gtc.2011.03.009

Lindheimer, M. D., & August, P. (2009). Aldosterone, maternal volume status and healthy pregnancies: A cycle of differing views. *Nephrology Dialysis Transplantation, 24*(6), 1712–1714. doi:10.1093/ndt/gfp093

Liu, J. H. (2009). Endocrinology of pregnancy. In R. K. Creasy, R. Resnik, J. D. Iams, C. J. Lockwood, & T. Moore (Eds.). *Creasy & Resnik's Maternal-Fetal Medicine: Principles and Practice* (6th ed., pp. 111–124). Philadelphia: Saunders Elsevier.

Mastorakos, G., & Ilias, I. (2000). Maternal hypothalamic-adrenal axis in pregnancy and the postpartum period. Postpartum related disorders. *Annals of the New York Academy of Sciences, 900,* 95–106. doi10.1111/j1749-6632.2000.tb06220.x

McCrae, K. R. (2010). Thrombocytopenia in pregnancy. *Hematology American Society of Hematology Education Program Book, 2010, 397–402.* doi:10.1182/asheducation-2010.1.397

McCrory, J. L., Chambers, A. J., Daftary, A., & Redfern, M. S. (2010). Dynamic postural stability in pregnant fallers and nonfallers. *British Journal of Obstetrics & Gynecology, 117(8),* 954–962. doi: 10.1111/j.1471-0528.2010.02589.x

Melse-Boonstra, A., & Jaiswal, N. (2010). Iodine deficiency in pregnancy, infancy and childhood and its consequences for brain development. *Best Practice & Research Clinical Endocrinology & Metabolism, 24(1),* 29–38. doi:10.1016/j.beem.2009.09.002

Molitch, M. E. (2009). Prolactin in human reproduction. In J. F. Strauss & R. L. Barbieri (Eds.), *Yen & Jaffe's Reproductive Endocrinology* (6th ed., pp. 57–78). Philadelphia: Saunders Elsevier.

Monga, M. (2009). Maternal cardiovascular, respiratory and renal adaptation to pregnancy. In R. K. Creasy, R. Resnik, J. D. Iams, C. J. Lockwood, & T. Moore (Eds.). *Creasy & Resnik's Maternal-Fetal Medicine: Principles and Practice* (6th ed., pp. 101–110). Philadelphia: Saunders Elsevier.

Montagnana, M., Franchi, M., Danese, E., Gotsch, F., & Guidi, G. C. (2010). Disseminated intravascular coagulation in obstetric and gynecologic disorders. *Seminars in Thrombosis & Hemostasis, 36(4),* 404–418.

Moore, K. L., Persaud, T. V. N., & Torchia, M. G. (2011). *The Developing Human: Clinically Oriented Embryology* (9th ed.). Philadelphia: Saunders Elsevier.

Moore, T. R., & Catalano, P. (2009). Diabetes and pregnancy. In R. K. Creasy, R. Resnik, J. D. Iams, C. J. Lockwood, & T. Moore (Eds.). *Creasy & Resnik's Maternal-Fetal Medicine: Principles and Practice* (6th ed., pp. 953–994). Philadelphia: Saunders.

Mor, G., & Abrahams, V. M. (2009). The immunology of pregnancy. In R. K. Creasy, R. Resnik, J. D. Iams, C. J. Lockwood, & T. Moore (Eds.), *Creasy & Resnik's Maternal-Fetal Medicine: Principles and Practice* (6th ed., pp. 87–100). Philadelphia: Saunders.

Morreale de Escobar, G., Ares, S., Berbel, P., Obregón, M. J., & del Rey, F. E. (2008). The changing role of maternal thyroid hormone in fetal brain development. *Seminars in Perinatology, 32(6),* 380–386. doi:10.1053/j.semperi.2008.09.002

Munoz-Suano, A., Hamilton, A. B., & Betz, A. G. (2011). Gimme shelter: The immune system during pregnancy. *Immunological Reviews, 241(1),* 20–38. doi: 10.1111/j.1600-065X.2011.01002.x

Nader, S. (2009a). Other endocrine disorders of pregnancy. In R. K. Creasy, R. Resnik, J. D. Iams, C. J. Lockwood, & T. Moore (Eds.), *Maternal-Fetal Medicine: Principles and Practice* (6th ed., pp. 1015–1040). Philadelphia: Saunders.

Nader, S. (2009b). Thyroid disease and pregnancy. In R. K. Creasy, R. Resnik, J. D. Iams, C. J. Lockwood, & T. Moore (Eds.), *Maternal-Fetal Medicine: Principles and Practice* (6th ed., pp. 995–1014). Philadelphia: Saunders.

Nelson, S. M., Matthews, P., & Poston, L. (2010). Maternal metabolism and obesity: Modifiable determinants of pregnancy outcome. *Human Reproduction Update, 16(3),* 255–275. doi:10.1093/humupd/dmp050

Nicolaides, K. H. (2011). Screening for fetal aneuploidies at 11 to 13 weeks. *Prenatal Diagnosis, 31(1),* 7–15. doi:10.1002/pd.2637

Norwitz, E. R., & Lye, S. J. (2009). Biology of parturition. In R. K. Creasy, R. Resnik, J. D. Iams, C. J. Lockwood, & T. Moore (Eds.). *Creasy & Resnik's Maternal-Fetal Medicine: Principles and Practice* (6th ed., pp. 69–86). Philadelphia: Saunders Elsevier.

Peña-Rosas, J. P., & Viteri, F. E. (2009). Effects and safety of preventive oral iron or iron+folic acid supplementation for women during pregnancy. *Cochrane Database Syst Rev, 4,* CD004736.

Petroff, M. G. (2011). Review: Fetal antigens—identity, origins, and influences on the maternal immune system. *Placenta, 32,* S176–S181. doi:10.1016/j.placenta.2010.12.014

Podymow, T., August, P., & Akbari, A. (2010). Management of renal disease in pregnancy. *Obstetrics & Gynecology Clinics of North America, 37(2),* 195–210. doi:10.1016/j.ogc.2010.02.012

Polyzos, N. P., Polyzos, I. P., Mauri, D., Tzioras, S., Tsappi, M., Cortinovis, I., & Casazza, G. (2009). Effect of periodontal disease treatment during pregnancy on preterm birth incidence: A metaanalysis of randomized trials. *American Journal of Obstetrics & Gynecology, 200(3),* 225–232. doi:10.1016/j.ajog.2008.09.020

Pridjian, G., & Benjamin, T. D. (2010). Update on gestational diabetes. *Obstetrics & Gynecology Clinics of North America, 37(2),* 255–267. doi:10.1016/j.ogc.2010.02.017

Rapini, R. P. (2009). The skin and pregnancy. In R. K. Creasy, R. Resnik, J. D. Iams, C. J. Lockwood, & T. Moore (Eds.). *Creasy & Resnik's Maternal-Fetal Medicine: Principles and Practice* (6th ed., pp. 1123–1134). Philadelphia: Saunders.

Rasmussen, K. M., Abrams, B., Bodnar, L. M., Butte, N. F., Catalano, P. M., & Maria Siega-Riz, A. (2010). Recommendations for weight gain during pregnancy in the context of the obesity epidemic. *Obstetrics & Gynecology, 116(5),* 1191–1195. doi:10.1097/AOG.0b013e3181f60da7

Romero, R., & Lockwood, C. J. (2009). Pathogenesis of spontaneous preterm labor. In R. K. Creasy, R. Resnik, J. D. Iams, C. J. Lockwood, & T. Moore (Eds.). *Creasy & Resnik's Maternal-Fetal Medicine: Principles and Practice* (6th ed., pp. 521–544). Philadelphia: Saunders Elsevier.

Sanghvi, T. G., Harvey, P. W., & Wainwright, E. (2010). Maternal iron-folic acid supplementation programs: Evidence of impact and implementation. *Food & Nutrition Bulletin, 31(2 Suppl.),* S100–S107.

Santiago, J. R., Nolledo, M. S., Kinzler, W., & Santiago, T. V. (2001). Sleep and sleep disorders in pregnancy. *Annals of Internal Medicine, 134(5),* 396–408.

Schmidt, P. M., Flores, F. T., Rossi, A. G., & Silveira, A. F. (2010). Hearing and vestibular complaints during pregnancy. *Revista Brasileira de Otorrinolaringologia, 76(1),* 29–33.

Schrier, R. W. (2010). Systemic arterial vasodilation, vasopressin, and vasopressinase in pregnancy. *Journal of the American Society of Nephrology, 21(4),* 570–572. doi:10.1681/ASN.2009060653

Scotland, N. E. (2009). Maternal nutrition. In R. K. Creasy, R. Resnik, J. D. Iams, C. J. Lockwood, & T. Moore (Eds.). *Creasy & Resnik's Maternal-Fetal Medicine: Principles and Practice* (6th ed., pp. 143–150). Philadelphia: Saunders Elsevier.

Timmons, B., Akins, M., & Mahendroo, M. (2010). Cervical remodeling during pregnancy and parturition. *Trends in Endocrinology & Metabolism, 21(6),* 353–361. doi:10.1016/j.tem.2010.01.011

Tsen, L. C. (2005). Gerald W. Ostheimer "What's New in Obstetric Anesthesia" Lecture. *Anesthesiology, 102(3),* 672–679.

Uppal, A., Uppal, S., Pinto, A., Dutta, M., Shrivatsa, S., Dandolu, V., & Mupparapu, M. (2010). The effectiveness of periodontal disease treatment during pregnancy in reducing the risk of experiencing preterm birth and low birth weight: A meta-analysis. *Journal of the American Dental Association, 141*(12), 1423–1434.

Vermani, E., Mittal, R., & Weeks, A. (2010). Pelvic girdle pain and low back pain in pregnancy: A review. *Pain Practice, 10*(1), 60–71. doi:10.1111/j.1533-2500.2009.00327.x

Vrekoussis, T., Kalantaridou, S. N., Mastorakos, G., Zoumakis, E., Makrigiannakis, A., Syrrou, M., . . . Chrousos, G. P. (2010). The role of stress in female reproduction and pregnancy: An update. *Annals of the New York Academy of Science, 1205,* 69–75. doi:10.1111/j.1749-6632.2010.05686.x

Whitty, J. E., & Dombrowski, M. P. (2009). Respiratory diseases in pregnancy. In R. K. Creasy, R. Resnik, J. D. Iams, C. J. Lockwood, & T. Moore (Eds.), *Creasy & Resnik's Maternal-Fetal Medicine: Principles and Practice* (6th ed., pp. 927–952). Philadelphia: Saunders Elsevier.

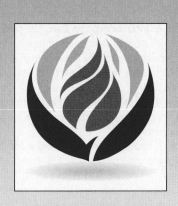

Mary Lee Barron

CHAPTER 4

Antenatal Care

Care of the pregnant woman in the antenatal setting is multifaceted, requiring knowledge of the normal and abnormal pregnancy, risk factors affecting pregnancy outcome, screening tests, common pregnancy discomforts and treatments, and psychosocial tasks and issues surrounding the childbearing continuum and appropriate nursing interventions. The purpose of this chapter is to present an overview of essential aspects of preconception and prenatal care for perinatal nurses caring for women during the childbearing process. Complications which may result in a high-risk pregnancy and require additional medical and nursing intervention are discussed in detail in Chapters 5 through 12.

PRECONCEPTION CARE

Prenatal care begins with preconception healthcare. The purpose of preconception care is to deliver risk screening, health promotion, and effective interventions as a part of routine healthcare (Centers for Disease Control and Prevention [CDC], 2006a). Preconception healthcare is critical because the behaviors and exposures that occur before prenatal care is initiated may affect fetal development and subsequent maternal and perinatal outcomes. The CDC (2006a) developed 10 recommendations for improving preconception and interconception care as part of a strategic plan to improve the health of women, their children, and their families (Display 4–1). These recommendations, based on existing knowledge and evidence-based practice, were developed for improving preconception health through changes in consumer knowledge, clinical practice, public health programs, healthcare financing, and data and research activities. Each recommendation has specific action steps toward the continuing

goal of achieving the *Healthy People 2020* objectives to improve maternal and child health outcomes. The recommendations are aimed at achieving four goals, based on personal health outcomes:

Goal 1. Improve the knowledge and attitudes and behaviors of men and women related to preconception health.

Goal 2. Ensure that all women of childbearing age in the United States receive preconception care services (i.e., evidence-based risk screening, health promotion, and interventions) that will enable them to enter pregnancy in optimal health.

Goal 3. Reduce risks indicated by a previous adverse pregnancy outcome through interventions during the interconception period.

Goal 4. Reduce the disparities in adverse pregnancy outcomes.

Preconception care should be tailored to meet the needs of the individual woman. Because preconception care needs to be provided across the life span and not during only one visit, certain recommendations will be more relevant to women at different life stages and with varying levels of risk. Intuitively, it makes sense to deliver preconception care in the context of primary care. All women attempting a pregnancy should follow the same behavioral recommendations, such as avoiding smoking and alcohol use and using only medications known to be safe in pregnancy. All women of childbearing age should take a daily folic acid supplement. Beginning pregnancy with nondepleted iron stores is beneficial for the maternal iron status during pregnancy and infant birth weight (Ribot et al., 2012). The importance of preconception advice to ensure that women have adequate iron stores prior to, or early in, pregnancy when supplemented

89

DISPLAY 4-1

Recommendations to Improve Preconception Health

Recommendation 1. Individual Responsibility across the Life Span. Each woman, man, and couple should be encouraged to have a reproductive life plan.

Recommendation 2. Consumer Awareness. Increase public awareness of the importance of preconception health behaviors and preconception care services by using information and tools appropriate across various ages; literacy, including health literacy; and cultural/linguistic contexts.

Recommendation 3. Preventive Visits. As a part of primary care visits, provide risk assessment and educational and health promotion counseling to all women of childbearing age to reduce reproductive risks and improve pregnancy outcomes.

Recommendation 4. Interventions for Identified Risks. Increase the proportion of women who receive interventions as follow-up to preconception risk screening, focusing on high-priority interventions (i.e., those with evidence of effectiveness and greatest potential impact).

Recommendation 5. Interconception Care. Use the interconception period to provide additional intensive interventions to women who have had a previous pregnancy that ended in an adverse outcome (e.g., infant death, fetal loss, birth defects, low birth weight, or preterm birth).

Recommendation 6. Prepregnancy Checkup. Offer, as a component of maternity care, one prepregnancy visit for couples and persons planning pregnancy.

Recommendation 7. Health Insurance Coverage for Women with Low Incomes. Increase public and private health insurance coverage for women with low incomes to improve access to preventive women's health and preconception and interconception care.

Recommendation 8. Public Health Programs and Strategies. Integrate components of preconception health into existing local public health and related programs, including emphasis on interconception interventions for women with previous adverse outcomes.

Recommendation 9. Research. Increase the evidence base and promote the use of the evidence to improve preconception health.

Recommendation 10. Monitoring Improvements. Maximize public health surveillance and related research mechanisms to monitor preconception health.

Centers for Disease Control and Prevention. (2006a). Recommendations to improve preconception health and health care—United States: A report of the CDC/ATSDR preconception care work group and the select panel on preconception care. *Morbidity and Mortality Weekly Report Recommendations and Reports, 55*(RR 06), 1–23.

with moderate daily iron doses should not be underestimated. Health promotion, risk screening, and interventions are different for a young woman who has never experienced pregnancy than for a woman aged 35 years who has had three children. Women who present with chronic diseases, previous pregnancy complications, or behavioral risk factors might need more intensive interventions. Social determinants of women's health also play a role in birth outcome. Low socioeconomic status is a long-known risk factor for preterm birth. Identified modifiable risk factors include isotretinoin (Accutane) use, alcohol misuse, antiepileptic drug use, diabetes (preconception), folic acid deficiency, hepatitis B, HIV/AIDS, hypothyroidism, maternal phenylketonuria, rubella seronegativity, obesity, oral anticoagulant use, sexually transmitted disease (STD), and smoking (CDC, 2006a). The American College of Obstetricians and Gynecologists (ACOG, 2005a) identified the following as core preconception care factors:

- Undiagnosed, untreated, or poorly controlled medical conditions
- Immunization history
- Medication and radiation exposure in early pregnancy
- Nutritional issues
- Family history and genetic risk
- Tobacco and substance abuse and other high-risk behaviors
- Occupational and environmental exposures
- Social issues
- Mental health issues

Implementation of the CDC recommendations is targeted toward (1) women and men of childbearing age having high reproductive awareness (i.e., they understand risk factors related to childbearing), (2) women and men having a reproductive life plan, (3) pregnancies being intended and planned, (4) women and men of childbearing age having healthcare coverage, (5) women of childbearing age being screened before pregnancy for risks that could affect the pregnancy, and (6) women with previous adverse pregnancy outcomes (e.g., infant death, very low birth weight, or preterm birth) having access to interconception care aimed at reducing their risks. The reader is referred to http://www.cdc.gov/mmwr/preview/mmwrhtml/rr5506a1.htm for complete recommendations.

PRENATAL CARE

The American Academy of Pediatrics (AAP) and ACOG (2007a) describe prenatal care thusly: "A comprehensive antepartum care program involves a coordinated approach to medical care and psychosocial support that optimally begins before conception and extends throughout the antepartum period." This comprehensive program includes (1) preconceptional care, (2) prompt diagnosis of pregnancy, (3) initial prenatal evaluation, and (4) follow-up prenatal visits. Quality prenatal care includes education and support for the pregnant woman, ongoing maternal–fetal assessment, preparation for parenting, and promotion of a positive physical and emotional family experience. Comprehensive services include health education; nutrition education; the Women, Infants, and Children's (WIC) program; social services assessment; assessment for intimate partner violence, depression screening; medical risk assessment; and referral as appropriate. To provide optimal, individualized care, nurses must recognize the effect of pregnancy on a woman's life span. Although a woman's preconceptional health has an impact on pregnancy, it is also true that childbearing is an event that may affect her long-term health. It is important to consider pregnancy within the larger context of women's health and primary care.

Continued contact with the pregnant woman through comprehensive prenatal care provides an ideal opportunity for the healthcare provider to assess for and identify potential problems that may place the woman and fetus at risk. The question of the necessary number of visits has been explored by researchers for several decades. The U.S. Department of Health and Human Services (USDHHS) Expert Panel on the Content of Prenatal Care (1989) recommended that healthy, pregnant women who are at low risk for pregnancy complications could attend fewer visits without negative consequences. For nulliparous women, nine visits were recommended; for multiparous women, seven visits were recommended. However, these recommendations have been slow to be adopted. Dowswell and colleagues (2010) reported that in settings with limited resources, reduced visit programs are associated with higher perinatal mortality when compared to standard prenatal care. Women in all settings were less satisfied with the reduced visits schedule and perceived the gap between visits as too long. Although reduced visits may be associated with lower costs, visits should not be reduced without close monitoring on fetal and neonatal outcomes. See Display 4–2 for guidelines for routine prenatal care visits.

Another model of prenatal care, Centering Pregnancy, was developed in 1998 and integrates group support with prenatal care. Centering Pregnancy uses the essential components of prenatal care: risk assessment, health promotion, medical and psychosocial interventions, and follow-up. Group prenatal care intuitively seems to be an efficient method of simultaneously communicating the same message to multiple patients as well as promoting the development of an instant support group for women and families. This model involves 10 90- to 120-minute sessions that begin at 16 weeks' gestation and conclude with a postpartum meeting (Rising, 1998; Rising, Kennedy, & Klima, 2004). The initial prenatal visit is an individual appointment. Each woman is invited to join a group of 8 to 12 other women with similar estimated dates of birth. Sessions allow for individual time with the care provider and group sharing and education. Groups are led by advanced practice nurses or other healthcare professionals with expertise in group process. Group prenatal care results in equal or improved perinatal outcomes without added cost (Ickovics et al., 2007; Kennedy et al., 2011). See https://www.center-inghealthcare.org/index.php for more information. Nurses must be aware of these prenatal care models in order to offer the highest quality evidence-based care to pregnant women.

Regardless of the approach to delivery of prenatal care, evidence-based recommendations for prenatal care have been established (National Guideline Clearinghouse [NGC] and the Institute for Clinical Systems Improvement [ICSI] are readily located at http://guidelines.gov). Display 4–2 is a summary of the content, timing, counseling and education that should be delivered in prenatal care.

Because early initiation of prenatal care is important to the health of the mother and to the optimization of pregnancy outcomes, a goal of increasing the proportion of pregnant women who initiate prenatal care in the first trimester to 90% was established as one of the *Healthy People 2000* objectives and retained as a *Healthy People 2010* objective (*Objective 16–6a*). Between 1980 and 1991, three of every four (76%) pregnant women in the United States who had a live birth began prenatal care in the first trimester (Lewis, Matthews, & Heuser, 1996). Although this proportion increased to 84% in 2002, it remains below the *Healthy People 2010* goal of 90% (USDHHS, 2000). In the most recent objectives, Healthy People 2020, the target is 77.9%, a 10% improvement from the baseline of 70.8% of women delivering a live birth who received prenatal care in the first trimester in 2007 (USDHHS, 2010). Therefore, little progress has been made on early initiation of prenatal care.

Promotion of early pregnancy recognition could be a means of improving birth outcomes as early pregnancy recognition is associated with improved timing and number of prenatal care visits (Ayoola, Nettleman, Stommel, & Canady, 2010). Nurses can encourage and empower women to access prenatal care at a critical point in fetal development.

PRENATAL RISK ASSESSMENT

The goal of risk assessment is to identify women and fetuses at risk for developing antepartum, intrapartum, postpartum, or neonatal complications to promote risk-appropriate care that will enhance the perinatal outcome. The underlying causes of preterm labor and intrauterine growth restriction (IUGR) are not fully understood. However, a large

D I S P L A Y   4 – 2

Guidelines for Prenatal Care
National Guideline Clearinghouse (NGC) and the Institute for Clinical Systems Improvement (ICSI) 2010

EVENT	PRECONCEPTION VISIT	VISIT 1[b] 6–8 WEEKS	VISIT 2 10–12 WEEKS	VISIT 3 16–18 WEEKS	VISIT 4 22 WEEKS	VISIT 5 28 WEEKS	VISIT 6 32 WEEKS	VISIT 7 36 WEEKS	VISIT 8–11 38–41 WEEKS
Screening Maneuvers	Risk profiles	Risk profiles	Weight	Weight	Weight	Preterm labor risk	Weight	Weight	Weight
	Height and weight/BMI	GC/Chlamydia	Blood pressure	Blood pressure	Blood pressure	Weight	Blood pressure	Blood pressure	Blood pressure
	Blood pressure	Height and weight/BMI	Fetal aneuploidy screening	Depression	Fetal heart tones	Blood pressure	Fetal heart tones	Fetal heart tones	Fetal heart tones
	History and physical	Blood pressure	Fetal heart tones	Fetal aneuploidy screening		Depression	Fundal height	Fundal height	Fundal height
	Cholesterol and HDL	History and physical[a]		Fetal heart tones		Fetal heart tones		Cervix exam	Cervix exam
	Cervical cancer screening	Rubella		OB ultrasound (optional)		Fundal height		Confirm fetal position	
	Rubella/rubeola	Varicella		Fundal height		GDM		Culture for group B streptococcus	
	Varicella	Intimate partner violence				Domestic abuse			
	Intimate partner violence	Depression				[Rh antibody status]			
	Depression	CBC				[Hepatitis B surface Ag]			
		ABO/Rh/Ab				[GC/Chlamydia]			
		Syphilis							
		Urine culture							
		HIV							
		[Blood lead screening]							
		[VBAC]							
		Viral hepatitis							

	Visit 1	Visit 2	Visit 3	Visit 4	Visit 5	Visit 6	Visit 7	Visit 8	Visit 9
Counseling Education Intervention	Preterm labor education and prevention Substance use Nutrition and weight Intimate partner violence List of medications, herbal supplements, vitamins Accurate recording of menstrual dates	Preterm labor education and prevention Prenatal and life-style education • Physical activity • Nutrition • Follow-up on modifiable risk factors • Nausea and vomiting • Warning signs • Course of care • Physiology of pregnancy Discuss fetal aneuploidy screening	Preterm labor education and prevention Prenatal and life-style education • Fetal growth • Review lab results from visit 1 • Breastfeeding • Nausea and vomiting • Physiology of pregnancy • Follow-up on modifiable risk factors	Preterm labor education and prevention Prenatal and life-style education • Follow-up on modifiable risk factors • Physiology of pregnancy • Second trimester growth • Quickening	Preterm labor education and prevention Prenatal and lifestyle education • Follow-up on modifiable risk factors • Classes • Family issues • Length of stay • GDM • [RhoGAM]	Psychosocial risk factors Preterm labor education and prevention Prenatal and life-style education • Follow-up on modifiable risk factors • Work • Physiology of pregnancy • Preregistration • Fetal growth • Awareness of fetal movement	Preterm labor education and prevention Prenatal and life-style education • Follow-up on modifiable risk factors • Travel • Contraception • Sexuality • Pediatric care • Episiotomy Labor and delivery issues Warning signs/pregnancy-induced hypertension [VBAC]	Prenatal and life-style education • Follow-up on modifiable risk factors • Postpartum care • Management of late pregnancy symptoms • Contraception • When to call provider • Discussion of postpartum depression	Prenatal and life-style education • Follow-up on modifiable risk factors • Postpartum vaccinations • Infant CPR • Post-term management Labor and delivery update
Immunization and Chemoprophylaxis	Tetanus booster Rubella/MMR [Varicella/VZIG] Hepatitis B vaccine Folic acid supplement [ABO/Rh/Ab] [RhoGAM]	Tetanus booster Nutritional supplements Influenza [Varicella/VZIG][c] Pertussis		[Progesterone]					

[Bracketed] items refer to high risk groups only.

[a] It is acceptable for the history and physical and laboratory tests listed under Visit 1 to be deferred to Visit 2 with the agreement of both the patient and the provider.

[b] Should also include all subjects listed for the preconception visit if none occurred.

[c] Administration of the varicella vaccine during pregnancy is contraindicated.

Ab, antibody; ABO, blood group system; Ag, antigen; BMI, body mass index; CBC, complete blood count; CPR, cardiopulmonary resuscitation; GC, gonococci; GDM, gestational diabetes mellitus; HDL, high density lipoprotein; MMR, measles/mumps/rubella; OB, obstetrics; RhoGAM, Rho(D) immune globulin; VBAC, vaginal birth after cesarean; VZIG, varicella zoster immune globulin. Institute for Clinical Systems Improvement. (2010). *Routine Prenatal Care*. Bloomington, MN: Author. Retrieved from http://guidelines.gov/content.aspx?id=24138&search=prenatal+care

body of knowledge regarding risk factors associated with prematurity and low birth weight has developed. These factors include demographic, medical, obstetric, sociocultural, lifestyle, and environmental risks. It is important to note that many risk factors have been identified in studies of women who develop complications of pregnancy or deliver preterm; however, no firm cause-and-effect relationship between some of the commonly associated risk factors and poor outcome has been established. Risk-assessment tools may be helpful in distinguishing between women at high and low risk (Display 4–3). Unfortunately, the predictive value of these tools is limited. Enthusiasm for risk assessment must be tempered with reality. Identification of real or potential problems should be a shared process in which the nurse assesses the woman's individual perception of risk. Risk presented as a calculation of odds may not resonate with the pregnant woman; most women use a set of values that is rooted in their lives, personal philosophies, and family and health histories to make sense of risk (Carolan, 2009). Approximately one third of the potential complications of pregnancy occur during the intrapartum period and are not predictable by current risk-assessment systems (AAP & ACOG, 2007). However, risk assessment directs the

---

DISPLAY 4 – 3

Risk Assessment

OBSTETRIC HISTORY

History of infertility

Grand multiparity

Previous stillborn/neonatal death

Incompetent cervix

Previous multiple gestation

Uterine or cervical anomaly

Previous prolonged labor

Previous preterm labor or preterm birth

Previous low-birth-weight infant

Previous cesarean birth

Previous midforceps delivery

Previous macrosomic infant

Previous pregnancy loss (spontaneous or induced)

Last delivery <1 year before present conception

Previous hydatidiform mole or choriocarcinoma

Previous infant with neurologic deficit, birth injury, or congenital anomaly

MEDICAL HISTORY

Cardiac disease	History of abnormal Pap smear
Metabolic disease	Previous surgeries, particularly
Gastrointestinal disorders	involving the reproductive
Seizure disorders	organs
Malignancy	Pulmonary disease
Reproductive tract anomalies	Chronic hypertension
Renal disease, repeat urinary	Endocrine disorders
tract infections, bacteriuria	Hemoglobinopathies
Emotional disorders, mental	Sexually transmitted diseases
retardation	Surgery during pregnancy
Family history of severe	
inherited disorders	

CURRENT OBSTETRIC STATUS

Inadequate prenatal care	Large-for-gestational-age
Intrauterine growth–restricted	fetus
fetus	Placenta previa
Polyhydramnios	Abnormal presentation

Maternal anemia

Weight gain <10 lb

Weight loss >5 lb

Sexually transmitted diseases

Pregnancy-induced hypertension, preeclampsia

Premature rupture of membranes

Rh sensitizations

Preterm labor

Overweight or underweight

Immunization status

Fetal or placental malformations

Abnormal fetal surveillance tests

Abruptio placentae

Multiple gestation

Postdatism

Fibroids

Fetal manipulation

Cervical cerclage

Maternal infection

PSYCHOSOCIAL FACTORS

Inadequate finances

Poor housing

Social problems

Unwed, father of baby uninvolved or unsupportive

Adolescent

Minority status

Poor nutrition

Parental occupation

More than two children at home, no help

Inadequate support systems

Unacceptance of pregnancy

Dysfunctional grieving

Psychiatric history

Attempt or ideation of suicide

Intimate partner violence

Demographic Factors

    Maternal age <16 or >35 years

    Education <11 years

Lifestyle

    Smokes >10 cigarettes/day

    Alcohol intake

    Substance abuse

    Heavy lifting, long periods of standing

    Long commute

    Unusual stress

provider toward areas in which intervention can have a positive impact on perinatal outcomes. The nurse's knowledge of prenatal risk assessment allows for anticipatory planning, individualized education, and appropriate referral. Outcomes of risk assessment provide guidelines by which the effectiveness of the care can be evaluated. The nurse's role in prenatal care is discussed within these parameters.

INITIAL PRENATAL VISIT

Antepartum assessment begins with the first prenatal visit. Generally, a woman with an uncomplicated pregnancy is examined approximately every 4 weeks for the first 28 weeks of pregnancy, every 2 to 3 weeks until 36 weeks' gestation, and weekly thereafter. Women with medical or obstetric problems may require closer surveillance. Intervals between visits are determined by the nature and severity of the problem (AAP & ACOG, 2007).

The initial prenatal visit is of vital importance and requires careful attention to detail. The nurse is obligated to practice within the framework of professional standards, such as the Association of Women's Health, Obstetric and Neonatal Nurses' (AWHONN) *Standards and Guidelines* (2009) and *Guidelines for Perinatal Care* (AAP & ACOG, 2007), which provide guidelines for practice in the ambulatory care setting. During the first prenatal visit, baseline health data are obtained and assessed, a patient-centered relationship is established, and the plan of care is initiated. Risk assessment during the initial prenatal visit should include the following:

- A careful family medical history, individual medical history, reproductive health history, psychosocial history, and genetic history
- A comprehensive physical examination designed to evaluate potential risk factors
- Appropriate prenatal laboratory screening
- Individualized, risk-appropriate laboratory evaluation
- Fetal assessment, as developmentally appropriate (e.g., fetal heart rate [FHR], fetal activity, kick counts) and individualized fetal surveillance, as indicated (e.g., ultrasonography, biophysical profile [BPP])

Maternal Age

The association between Down syndrome and advanced maternal age has been long documented (Hook, 1981). Maternal age of 35 years and older is associated with an increased risk of fetal death (Huang, Sauve, Birkett, Fergusson, & van Walraven, 2008; Silver, 2007) and obstetrical complications, perinatal morbidity, and mortality. Children born to mothers younger than 19 or older than 35 years of age have an increased risk of prematurity, congenital anomalies, and risks from other complications of pregnancy (March of Dimes,

2011a). However, researchers report that pregnancy outcomes previously linked to maternal age are mitigated by poverty (Cunningham et al., 2010; Markovitz, Cook, Flick, & Leet, 2005). With poor socioeconomic status, the risk of perinatal morbidity increases after the age of 35, but with adequate income and healthcare, women in that age group experienced only a slight increase in gestational diabetes (GDM), pregnancy-induced hypertension, placenta previa or placental abruption, and cesarean birth (Markovitz et al., 2005).

Complications common in pregnant adolescents include low birth weight, preeclampsia and pregnancy-induced hypertension, IUGR, and preterm labor. In younger mothers, socioeconomic factors largely explain increased neonatal mortality risk (Markovitz et al., 2005). Although much of the literature links advanced maternal age to adverse perinatal outcomes, there is a paucity of data linking advanced maternal age with outcomes of preterm newborns. Recently, Kanungo and colleagues (2011) reported that among preterm newborns, the odds of survival without major morbidity improved by 5% and mortality (8%), necrotizing enterocolitis (11%), and sepsis (9%) reduced as maternal age group increased by 5 years. Knowledge of these risks and outcomes serves as a guide for counseling women for whom age is a risk factor.

Medical and Obstetric History

Assessment of health factors that may influence pregnancy outcome includes careful evaluation of the woman's individual medical, gynecologic, obstetric, psychosocial, and environmental history. Pertinent family history of the woman and her partner is necessary for complete evaluation. Maternal–family reproductive health history (e.g., preeclampsia, hypertension, diabetes, preterm birth) may be particularly significant. The additional physiologic stress of pregnancy affects chronic conditions (e.g., diabetes, hypertension, cardiac disease). Likewise, factors such as a recent history of STDs or chemical dependency may be indicative of lifestyle behaviors that threaten maternal–fetal well-being.

Obstetric history, such as length of previous labors, cesarean birth, birth weight, gestational age, history of preterm labor or preterm birth, grand multiparity, elective or spontaneous abortion, instrument-assisted birth, previous stillbirth, or uterine or cervical anomaly may indicate potential risks for the current pregnancy. Apply these risk factors within the context of the gestational age. For example, a history of preterm birth would be a pertinent risk to a woman who is presently at 20 weeks' gestation but is not relevant when the woman is at 37 weeks' gestation. Note familial history, including cardiac disease, diabetes, and bleeding disorders. The woman may also be affected by her mother's obstetric history. There is a familial predisposition to develop preeclampsia. The medical and genetic history of the birth parents serves to guide counseling and testing for predisposed genetic complications. The family history is the most important source of genetic information. The ideal time for genetic screening is before attempting pregnancy. Although general population screening is not considered appropriate, Williams and Lea (2003) recommend that persons with the following conditions be offered genetic screening:

- Developmental disability of unknown etiology, including women with developmental disabilities who present for preconception or prenatal care
- Autism
- Unexplained mental retardation or developmental delay, particularly if the member of the family is related to the patient through females
- Family history of fragile X syndrome
- Family history that suggests increased risk for specific autosomal recessive disease

Probably the most common indications for genetic counseling and prenatal diagnosis are maternal age and abnormal maternal serum screening. If the initial prenatal risk assessment reveals factors that carry risk for the baby (e.g., Tay-Sachs, sickle cell disease/trait, thalassemia, cystic fibrosis), the woman (and her partner) should be offered genetic counseling and additional testing if the woman so desires.

Genetic counseling has grown into a well-recognized specialty. Our understanding of genetics and genomics in healthcare has changed in recent years, however. Genetic conditions inherited in families are caused by gene mutations present on one or both chromosomes of a pair. The three main patterns of Mendelian inheritance are autosomal dominant, autosomal recessive, and X-linked (Fig. 4–1). The term "genomics" refers to the study of all the genes in the human genome together, including their interactions with each other and the environment (Feetham, Thomson, & Hinshaw, 2005). Genes can cause diseases, and they also may affect disease susceptibility and resistance, prognosis and progression, and responses to illnesses and their treatments. This range of responsiveness results in variable testing sensitivity, specificity, and predictive value of the genetic test (Feetham et al., 2005).

As knowledge of the behavioral, environmental, and genetic mechanisms of disease increases, individuals and families will need to reframe their concepts and experiences with diagnosis, treatment, and prevention (Feetham et al., 2005). Therefore, individualized education, planning, and support are vital to the process of genetic counseling. Genetic counseling and fetal surveillance techniques force a woman (and her partner) to consider the amount and kind of information desired, subsequent decisions related to that information, and what those decisions may reflect about their self-image and personal values. Nurses are knowledgeable, nonthreatening confidants as the woman and her partner sort through the information and decision making. Nurses, therefore, need to be cognizant of the benefits, limitations, and social implications of the counseling and testing process.

Lifestyle Factors

Lifestyle or behavioral factors significantly affect women's health in general and perinatal health specifically. Living conditions, marital status, occupation, nutrition, and use of tobacco, alcohol, and illicit substances can all affect pregnancy outcome. Socioeconomic factors may influence gestational age at entry to prenatal care, nutritional status, and availability of support systems. Number of years of

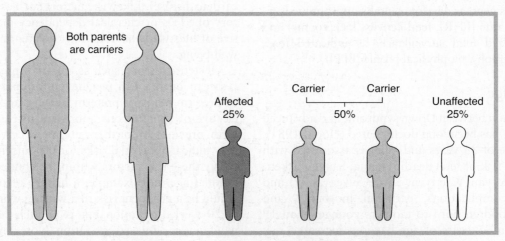

FIGURE 4–1. The inheritance pattern of offspring when both parents are carriers of an autosomal recessive gene.

completed maternal education has been correlated with birth weight, perinatal mortality and morbidity, and neonatal neurologic sequelae. In general, as years of maternal education increase, incidence of perinatal mortality and morbidity decreases. Not surprisingly, adolescents are more likely to begin prenatal care later than adults (March of Dimes, 2011b). Pregnant women who have more education are more likely to start prenatal care early and have more visits. Between 1989 and 1997 (the last data analysis that was performed), the percentage of women with delayed prenatal care or no prenatal care decreased from 25% to 18%, with improvement in both delayed prenatal care (from 22% to 16%) and in no prenatal care (from 2% to 1%). Groups more likely to have delayed or no prenatal care between 1989 and 1997 included non-Hispanic blacks, Hispanics, women aged <20 years, women with <12 years of education, and multiparous women (CDC, 2000). This association may be a reflection of education as an indicator of socioeconomic status. Women in lower socioeconomic groups tend to initiate prenatal care later than their middle socioeconomic group counterparts. The three most common reasons for late entry into care are (1) no knowledge that she was pregnant, (2) financial barriers, and (3) inability to get an appointment (CDC, 2000).

The marital status of the mother and the presence of the father as related to perinatal outcome are complex social phenomena. Marital status may be a marker for the presence or absence of social, emotional, and financial resources. Infants of mothers who are not married have been shown to be at higher risk for poor outcomes. In 2006, infants of unmarried mothers had an infant mortality rate of 9.19 per 1,000, 80% higher than the rate for infants of married mothers (Mathews & MacDorman, 2010).

Findings of older studies demonstrated an increase in perinatal morbidity and mortality associated with single motherhood (Bennett, Braveman, Egerter, & Kiely, 1994; Cooperstock, Bakewell, Herman, & Schramm, 1998; Hein, Burmeister, & Papke, 1990; Luo, Wilkins, & Kramer, 2004; Mathews, MacDorman, & Menacker, 2002). That unmarried mothers often are younger, are less well educated, and have a lower socioeconomic status than married mothers was controlled for in the older studies. More recently, births to women who live in an intimate relationship with a partner but without legal marriage have become increasingly common and widely accepted in many Western societies. However, pregnancy outcomes are worse among mothers in common-law unions versus traditional marriage relationships. One study found an overall 20% increase of adverse outcomes in unmarried, cohabiting mothers, and that free maternity care did not overcome the difference (Raatikainen, Heiskanen, & Heinonen,

2005. The highest incidence of perinatal morbidity and loss occurs in families where the father is not present (Luo et al., 2004).

When employment status of the Finnish parents in 24,939 pregnancies was examined, unemployment was associated with adolescent maternal age, unmarried status, overweight, anemia, smoking, alcohol consumption, and prior pregnancy terminations. Although antenatal care is free in Finland, this was unable to fully overcome the adverse pregnancy outcomes associated with unemployment, and small-for-gestational-age risk is highest when both parents are unemployed (Raatikainen, Heiskanen, Verkasalo, & Heinonen, 2006).

Teratogen Exposure

The cause of congenital malformations can be divided into three categories: unknown, genetic, and environmental. The cause of a majority of human malformations is unknown. Both maternal and paternal environmental exposures can produce human developmental disease including preterm birth, growth restriction, functional or structural abnormalities, or death.

More than 50 teratogenic environmental drugs, chemicals, and physical agents have been described using modern epidemiologic tools and clinical dysmorphology. Severe congenital malformations occur in 3% of births. According to the CDC (Martin et al., 2006), severe congenital malformations include birth defects that cause death, hospitalization, or mental retardation; necessitate significant or repeated surgical procedures; are disfiguring; or interfere with physical performance. Each year in the United States, 120,000 newborns are born with severe birth defects (CDC, 2008). Our understanding of this process is evolving:

> Whereas single genes and individual chemical exposures are responsible for some instances of adverse pregnancy outcome or developmental disease, gene–environment interactions are responsible for the majority. These gene–environment interactions may occur in the father, mother, placenta or fetus, suggesting that critical attention be given to maternal and paternal exposures and gene expression as they relate to the mode of action of the putative developmental toxicant both prior to and during pregnancy (Mattison, 2010, p. 208).

Counseling regarding possible teratogenic influences should be performed in a factual yet sympathetic and supportive way so the woman is not unduly alarmed or burdened with guilt (ACOG, 1997). Nurses should also be cognizant of the common potential teratogens in the population for which they provide care. For example, if the majority of the women come from an urban setting in which it is known that lead exposure is problematic, the history should include special attention to the risk. Maternal blood lead levels of approximately 10 mcg/dL have been linked to increased risks of pregnancy hypertension, spontaneous abortion, and reduced neurobehavioral development in the child (Bellinger, 2005).

Teratogen exposure may be associated with an occupation (e.g., X-rays, chemicals, viruses) or a lifestyle. The most common substances used by pregnant women include tobacco, alcohol, and marijuana. Alcohol is a potent teratogen in humans, and prenatal alcohol exposure is a leading preventable cause of birth defects and developmental disabilities. The harm from substance use and abuse is well known and may have disastrous effects in pregnancy, affecting all body systems and causing cardiac, pulmonary, gastrointestinal, and psychiatric complications. "Although the prevalence of substance abuse is significantly lower in pregnant women compared to nonpregnant women, some groups remain vulnerable to continued use, including those who did not intend to get pregnant and those who are less educated, unemployed, unmarried, and exposed to violence" (Massey et al., 2011, p. 143). The effects of tobacco use in pregnancy are well documented. No amount of alcohol is safe in pregnancy. Marijuana is the most commonly used illicit substance taken during pregnancy. The impact on the child is not clear. While prenatal marijuana use does not increase the risk of preterm birth, birth defects, or mortality in the first 2 years of life in exposed infants, emerging evidence indicates effects on later functioning. These effects include cognitive deficits, especially in visuospatial function, impulsivity, inattention and hyperactivity, depressive symptoms and substance use disorders, and cancer (Gray, Day, Leech, & Richardson, 2005; Huizink & Mulder, 2006). Methamphetamine abuse is becoming more common among women of reproductive age. "Meth," also known as speed or chalk, or as ice, crystal, and glass when smoked, is a powerfully addictive stimulant and a known neurotoxic agent that damages the endings of brain cells containing dopamine. Definitive information on the impact of exposure to methamphetamine in utero is lacking. There is fair to good evidence that amphetamines do not cause congenital anomalies. Studies consistently show amphetamine exposure during pregnancy is associated with an increased risk of preterm birth, low birth weight, and birth of small-for-gestational-age infants, but most of these studies have not adjusted for confounding factors, such as tobacco use, polydrug exposure, nutrition, and access to prenatal care (UpToDate, 2012). Screening for alcohol and substance use and abuse is discussed in more detail later in this chapter.

Assessing the use of prescription or over-the-counter medications and use of complementary and alternative therapies such as herbs, homeopathy, and folk remedies is crucial. This provides nurses with a more complete picture of the woman's approach to healthcare and allows them to identify potentially harmful practices. Commonly, pregnant women are counseled that using acetaminophen is safe whereas using a nonsteroidal anti-inflammatory drug (NSAID) such as ibuprofen is not. If there is a potential substance or practice about which there is a question of teratogenicity, nurses can contact the Organization of Teratology Information Services at its toll-free number ([866] 626-OTIS or [866] 626-6847) or visit http://www.otispregnancy.org for more information. This organization is a national service that can answers questions or refer pregnant women or nurses to local resources.

Over the last three decades, first trimester use of prescription medications increased by more than 60% and the use of four or more medications more than tripled; approximately half of childbearing-aged women use at least one medication (Mitchell et al., 2011). As more women delay childbearing and as the population has grown more obese, there are more likely to be women of childbearing age using medications for chronic diseases such as diabetes, hypertension, and hyperlipidemia. Medications to treat the later disorders include angiotensin-converting enzyme inhibitor (ACE inhibitor), angiotensin receptor blocker (ARB), or HMG-coenzyme A reductase inhibitor (statin). Use of ACE inhibitors and ARBs are associated with well-established risks: oligohydramnios, fetal renal dysplasia, IUGR, and fetal death (Morrical-Kline, Walton, & Guildenbacher, 2011). Statin use during pregnancy is contraindicated with case reports demonstrating vertebral, anal, cardiac, tracheal, esophageal, renal, and limb anomalies (Patel, Edgerton, & Flake, 2006). Consequently, it is important for the primary care provider as well in women's health to be cognizant of this growing shift in the population of childbearing women with regard to medication use and to counsel women appropriately.

Nutrition

The impact of nutrition on maternal and fetal well-being cannot be underestimated. The special physiology of a woman creates variable nutrient requirements during different stages of the life cycle. Nutritional practices influence every pregnancy, as well as a woman's risk for anemia, diabetes mellitus, cardiovascular disease, osteoporosis, and several types of cancer. Specific complications of pregnancy, such as preeclampsia, preterm birth, IUGR, and low-birth-weight infants with associated detrimental outcomes, can be correlated to nutritional status. A healthy, well-nourished woman has a surplus of all nutrients. The key components of a health-promoting lifestyle during pregnancy include appropriate weight gain; appropriate physical activity; consumption of a variety of foods in accordance with the Dietary Guidelines for Americans 2005; appropriate and timely vitamin and mineral supplementation; avoidance of alcohol, tobacco, and other harmful substances; and safe food handling.

Approximately 60% of American women do not gain the appropriate amount of weight during pregnancy, with more gaining too much, especially those with a high prepregnancy BMI (Olson, 2008). Current weight gain guidelines are described in Table 4–1. In 2005, the U.S. Department of Agriculture created an interactive Web-based MyPyramid, now ChooseMyPlate. The Web site provides food intake and physical activity recommendations for persons aged 2 and older, replacing healthy foods for unhealthful and offering diet tracking, menu planning, nutrition information, and personalized advice. The strategies are easy to understand for the lay public. The information should be used to complement and not substitute for prenatal education (Shieh & Carter, 2011). The nurse is encouraged to explore the Web site for use with preconception, prenatal, and lactating women: http://www.choosemyplate.gov.

The nutrition assessment includes diet intake information (3-day recall), monitoring weight gain, and hematologic assessment. Assessment of usual dietary patterns provides a basis for understanding nutritional health. Variations from the normal dietary routine, such as eating disorders, food avoidance, or special diets; food resources; and metabolic disorders such as diabetes, warrant additional interventions. Women who have eating disorders may be reticent to reveal this information. This assessment may require a number of prenatal visits and a building of a trusting relationship between the nurse and the woman. After an eating disorder is revealed, the nurse should ask the woman how she manages eating food and meals, as well as what her attitude is toward eating (e.g., preoccupation with food, feeling guilty after eating, engaging in dieting, enjoyment of food).

Most nutritional advice for pregnant women is based on the 1990 Institute of Medicine (IOM) Pregnancy Report, the 2005 Dietary Guidelines for Americans by the USDHHS and U.S. Department of Agriculture, and the 2006 IOM publication, *Dietary Reference Intakes: The Essential Guide to Nutrient Requirements*. The current dietary recommendations developed by the IOM include (1) increased intake of protein from 60 to 80 g/day (1.1 g/kg/day); (2) 340 additional calories per day in the second trimester and 452 calories per day in the third trimester; (3) increased iron intake from 15 to 30 g/day; and (4) increased folate consumption from 400 to 800 mcg/day. The recommended amount of calcium for women aged 19 to 50, pregnant or not, is 1,000 mg/day; for adolescents up to age 18, it is 1,300 mg daily. There are certain special circumstances that may affect these recommendations. For example, if there is a history of a child with a neural tube defect (NTD), the folic acid recommendation is increased to 4 mg rather than 0.4 to 0.8 mg/day. Nurses should encourage women to consume a variety of foods, eat at regular intervals (three meals a day and healthy snacks), drink milk two to three times per day, reduce caffeine, and avoid alcohol. Common discomforts (e.g., nausea and vomiting of pregnancy, heartburn, and varied reactions to taste or smell of food) can prove challenging to the woman who is trying to follow pregnancy dietary recommendations. Knowledge of safe remedies is the basis for advice when helping women with these discomforts. For example, acupressure wristbands and small, frequent feedings can be of help to some women to decrease nausea.

Another aspect of the nutritional assessment is the use of vitamins and herbs. Because herbs and vitamins are considered dietary supplements, these products are not regulated in the same manner that prescription and over-the-counter medications are. Often the products are labeled as "natural," and the woman may conclude that the product is therefore not harmful. Excesses of one nutrient can alter the need for, absorption of, or use of other nutrients. Supernutrient regimens or megadoses of vitamins (especially those that are fat soluble) may be harmful and cannot ensure a healthy pregnancy.

Vitamin D deficiency is the most common nutritional deficiency worldwide in both children and adults. It has also been observed that vitamin D deficiency is linked to preeclampsia during pregnancy and an increased risk of having a cesarean section (Bodnar et al., 2007; Merewood, Mehta, Chen, Bauchner, & Holick, 2009).

Table 4–1. RECOMMENDATIONS FOR WEIGHT GAIN DURING PREGNANCY

Prepregnant Status	BMI	Weight Gain (Pounds/ Kilograms)
Singleton pregnancy		
Underweight	<18.5	28–40 lb (12.7–18.2 kg)
Normal weight	18.5–24.9	25–35 lb (11.4–15.9 kg)
Overweight	25.0–29.9	15–25 lb (7.0–11.5 kg)
Obese	>30	11–20 lb (5.0–9.0 kg)
Twin pregnancy		
Underweight	<18.5	No recommendation due to insufficient data
Normal weight	18.5–24.9	37–54 lb (16.8–24.5 kg)
Overweight	25.0–29.9	31–50 lb (14.1–22.7 kg)
Obese	>30	11–20 lb (11.4–19.1 kg)

From Institute of Medicine (2009). *Weight Gain During Pregnancy: Reexamining the Guidelines*. http://www.iom.edu/Reports/2009/Weight-Gain-During-Pregnancy-Reexamining-the-Guidelines.aspx

However, it is not necessary to screen vitamin D levels in the general population of pregnant women. Instead, a dietary supplement of 400 IU (10 mcg) daily is recommended and can be found in most prenatal vitamins. There is insufficient evidence to recommend more than what is contained in prenatal vitamins. Women at risk of vitamin D deficiency (low dietary intake as in vegetarians, inadequate sunlight exposure, and ethnic minorities, especially those with darker skin) can be screened and treated (1,000 to 2,000 IU/day) if low levels are found (ACOG, 2011).

Fish are an excellent source of protein, are low in saturated fats, and contain omega-3 fatty acids. Nearly all fish and shellfish contain trace amounts of mercury; therefore, pregnant and lactating women are advised to avoid fish with potentially high methylmercury levels: shark, swordfish, king mackerel, and tile fish. Pregnant women ingest no more than 12 oz or two servings of canned tuna per week and no more than 6 oz of albacore or "white" tuna (U.S. Environmental Protection Agency, 2011). If the mercury content of locally caught fish is unknown, then overall fish consumption should be limited to 6 oz per week.

Avoidance of foodborne illnesses (e.g., norovirus causing acute gastroenteritis, *Salmonella*, listeriosis, *Escherichia coli*, or hepatitis A), which cause maternal disease, congenital defects, preterm labor, miscarriage, and fetal death, is also important for the nurse to assess and to teach the woman. To reduce the risk of foodborne illness, it is important for the woman to:

- Practice good personal hygiene (hand washing and care of kitchen utensils, cookware, and surfaces).
- Consume meats, fish, poultry, and eggs that are fully cooked.
- Avoid unpasteurized dairy and fruit/vegetable products.
- Wash fresh fruits and vegetables prior to eating.
- Avoid raw sprouts (alfalfa, clover, radish, and mung bean).
- Avoid listeriosis by refraining from processed/deli meats, hot dogs, soft cheeses, smoked seafood, meat spreads, and pate.

The FDA provides advice on food safety for women at http://www.fda.gove/food/resourcesforyou/health educators/ucm081785.htm.

Many pregnant women experience pica (eating non-food substances) during pregnancy. Some women are embarrassed to tell the nurse about these cravings, yet they may significantly interfere with dietary intake of proper nutrients during pregnancy. Pica cravings are not limited to any one group, educational level, race, ethnic group, income level, or religious belief but rather are universal; however, the type of substance ingested does seem to be culturally influenced (Young, 2010). In the United States, the practice of pica during pregnancy is linked to lower income women, African American heritage, family or personal history of pica during childhood or before pregnancy, strong cravings during pregnancy, and cultural groups that endorse pica during pregnancy as important for fertility and femininity (Corbett, Ryan, & Weinrich, 2003). As a part of nutrition assessment, nurses should question (in a nonjudgmental style) patients at each prenatal visit regarding pica practice. Pica may be practiced for cultural or other reasons unknown to nurses. Working with patients to discover what they are eating and helping them to substitute foods with nutritional value can be a part of a nursing care plan that results in a positive pregnancy outcome (Corbett et al., 2003).

Occupation

Women in low-income positions or employed as unskilled laborers are at increased risk for preterm labor. A meta-analysis of working conditions and pregnancy outcome showed a significant positive association between preterm birth and physically demanding work, shift work, standing for longer than 3 hours/day or standing as the predominant occupational posture, and a high cumulative work fatigue score. Additionally, physically demanding work is positively associated with small-for-gestational-age babies, hypertension, and/or preeclampsia. Working long hours was not associated with an adverse pregnancy outcome (Mozurkewich, Luke, Avni, & Wolf, 2000). However, decreasing or eliminating work during pregnancy may place the woman at greater socioeconomic risk by threatening her livelihood. Activities that cause excessive fatigue such as heavy work, job-related stress, and psychosocial stress may stimulate uterine contractions and increase the risk of perinatal complication (Mozurkewich et al., 2000; Papiernik, 1993). Areas to ask about in the nature of the woman's job include whether she sits or stands continuously, lifts heavy objects, perceives problems with ventilation, and is exposed to toxic chemicals or radiation. Hobbies and the home environment should be assessed also. Household tasks may be a source of fatigue equal to or greater than job-related fatigue.

Psychosocial Screening

Psychosocial screening of every woman presenting for prenatal care is an important step toward improving the woman's health and the birth outcome. In this way, the nurse can identify areas of concern, validate major issues, and make suggestions for possible changes. Depending on the nature of the identified problem, a referral may be made to an appropriate member of the healthcare team. A woman may be reluctant to share information until a trusting relationship has been formed. Questions asked at the first prenatal visit bear repeating with ongoing prenatal care. The woman may need reassurance as to the confidentiality of the information. For example, if she reveals she uses cocaine, would she be turned over to the judicial system and possibly jailed? Nurses are obligated to know how to answer the woman when these issues arise.

Pregnancy affects the entire family, and, therefore, assessment and intervention must be considered in a family-centered perspective. Stress has been suggested as a potential contributor to preterm birth and physical complications during pregnancy and birth, including prolonged labor, increased use of intrapartum analgesics and barbiturates, and other complications. Unusual stressful events, such as the death of a significant family member or friend, job loss, or a problematic relationship with the baby's father may increase risk of poor pregnancy outcome. Home conditions (e.g., private or government housing), quality of comfort (e.g., heat, water), housekeeping burden, and number and age of previous children influence stress levels. Nurses should be aware that many women continue to work under hazardous or stressful conditions out of economic necessity, but that they will attempt to minimize any known risk factors as much as possible. Additionally, nurses should assess how the woman appraises her situation (e.g., what one woman finds stressful, another may not). Nurses should identify resources available to the pregnant woman (e.g., support groups, social worker, counselor, etc.).

Symptoms of dysfunctional family relationships, such as violence toward the pregnant woman, child abuse, or psychosomatic illnesses, are also indicative of risk and warrant investigation. Intimate partner violence is a serious problem in the United States. Victims are found among women of all ages, socioeconomic classes, and ethnicities. Intimate partner violence against women covers a broad spectrum of behaviors, including actual or threatened physical, sexual, or psychological abuse between family members or intimate partners. The CDC reports that approximately 4.8 million episodes of intimate partner violence occur every year in the United States in women 18 years and older (CDC, 2006b). Exposure to intimate partner violence is associated with a range of negative psychobehavioral risks and health outcomes including increased risk of poor physical health, physical disability, psychological distress, mental illness, and heightened substance use including alcohol and illicit drugs. Additionally, abuse during pregnancy is linked to significantly higher rates of depression and suicide attempts as well as use of tobacco, alcohol, and illicit drugs (Kiely, El-Mohandes, El-Khorazaty, & Gantz, 2010).

Separated and divorced women are at greater risk for intimate partner violence (Coker, Smith, McKeown, &

King, 2000). The National Violence Against Women Survey report demonstrated that women had an increased risk of injury if the perpetrator was an intimate partner (vs. a non-intimate partner) (Tjaden & Thoennes, 2000). There is an increased risk of intimate partner violence if the couple was cohabitating rather than married. Married women living apart from their husbands were more likely to be victims of rape, physical assault, and/or stalking (Tjaden & Thoennes, 2000).

AWHONN (2004) has long urged nurses to routinely assess all pregnant women for intimate partner violence. There is no evidence that one screening tool is better than another at present and there are a variety of tools available (see http://www.nnvawi.org/assessment.htm). The nurse should ask the woman whether she is safe in her home, particularly if she presents with injuries. Integrating a standardized screening protocol into routine history-taking procedures increases identification, documentation, and referral for intimate partner violence. There is no single profile of the woman who suffers abuse, and the abuse is likely to continue or escalate during pregnancy (AAP & ACOG, 2007).

Yost, Bloom, McIntire, and Leveno (2005) surveyed 16,041 women presenting to a labor and delivery unit. They found that when compared with women denying intimate partner violence, women (n = 949) reporting verbal abuse had an increased rate of low-birth-weight infants, and neonatal deaths were significantly increased in women experiencing physical abuse. Second, women who declined to participate (n = 94) in their survey were found to have significantly increased rates of a variety of pregnancy complications that adversely affected their infants' outcomes (Yost et al., 2005).

Assessing for abuse carries the responsibility of intervention if abuse is identified or suspected. At minimum, nurses should have referral sources readily available. Nurses should document the frequency and severity of present and past abuse (using patient quotes as much as possible), location and extent of injuries, treatments, interventions, escape plan, and educational materials (including phone numbers to a shelter and the police). Discuss a plan of escape and document whether shelter assistance was declined or accepted by the woman. Counseling and intervention can reduce intimate partner violence and improve pregnancy outcome (Kiely et al., 2010). For more information on this important topic and an Abuse Assessment Screening tool (Nursing Network on Violence Against Women, International [NNVAWI], 2003), the reader is directed to http://www.nnvawi.org/assessment.htm.

Addressing psychosocial issues during pregnancy has the potential to reduce costs to the individual and to society (ACOG, 2006; AWHONN, 2004). A simple screening tool to open a discussion with the patient about perinatal psychosocial risk factors was developed by the Healthy Start Program of the Florida Department of Health and has been refined and in use since 1992 (Florida Department of Health, 1997). The patient should be asked whether she:

- Has any problems (job, transportation, etc.) that prevent her from keeping healthcare appointments
- Feels unsafe where she lives
- Has used any form of tobacco in the past 2 months
- Has used drugs or consumed alcohol (including beer, wine, or mixed drinks) in the past 2 months
- Has been threatened, hit, slapped, or kicked by anyone she knows
- Has been forced by anyone to perform a sexual act she did not want to do
- Can rate her stress level on a scale of 1 to 5
- Has moved in the past 12 months, and if so, how many times
- Would change the timing of this pregnancy if she could

Major depression is one of the most frequently encountered medical complications in pregnancy, and the risk for depression increases even more during the postpartum period (Gaynes et al., 2005). Prevalence estimates suggest that as many as 18.4% of all pregnant women are depressed during their pregnancy (i.e., from conception to birth), with as many as 12.7% having a major depressive episode. Lower figures were found in a very recent study, in which 7.4% women were diagnosed as having a depressive disorder at least once during pregnancy. The prevalence of major depression was 5.2% at 12 to 16 weeks, 2.6% at 22 to 26 weeks, and 3.5% at 32 to 36 weeks of pregnancy (Bunevicius et al., 2009).

Depression in pregnancy is associated with greater maternal lifestyle risks, increased incidence of postpartum depression, suicide, and adverse birth outcomes (Beck, 2008; Pereira et al., 2011). The impact of depression during pregnancy is significant for the mother and her baby. Researchers during the past decade have identified that untreated maternal depression that extends into the postpartum period has a negative effect on the emotional, cognitive, and developmental growth of young infants (Rahman, Bunn, Lovel, & Creed, 2007; Van den Bergh, Mulder, Mennes, & Glover, 2005). While it is unclear as to why pregnancy and childbirth represent a time of increased vulnerability for the onset or exacerbation of depression, it may be that it is the combination of hormonal shifts, neuroendocrine changes, and psychosocial adjustments (Pereira et al., 2011).

Recognition, diagnosis, and treatment of depression in pregnancy are vital. Brief screenings for symptoms of depression in pregnancy during the initial interview assist clinicians in identifying pregnant women who have symptoms of depression. Effective identification of depression in obstetrical practice meets Healthy People 2020's (USDHHS, 2010) recommendation for additional research to discover health indicators that place women at risk in pregnancy. The U.S. Preventive Task Force (Pignone et al., 2002) recommended that the following two questions be part of the basic repertoire of every adult patient visit:

- "Over the past 2 weeks have you felt down, depressed, or hopeless?"
- "Over the past 2 weeks, have you felt little interest in doing things?"

Jesse and Graham (2005) validated the use of these two questions in pregnancy; sensitivity was 91%, and specificity was 52%. If the responses are positive, nurses must assess the patient's safety (i.e., risk of suicide). These questions can be the first step in determining which women should be referred for a clinical diagnostic evaluation by a psychiatric nurse practitioner, social worker, psychologist, or a psychiatrist. For some women, a pregnancy support group may be helpful. Women who are diagnosed with depression during pregnancy should be followed carefully for postpartum depression. Predisposing risk factors for the development of postpartum depression have been identified (Display 4–4).

DISPLAY 4 – 4

Predisposing Factors for Postpartum Depression

Anxiety or depression during pregnancy

History of depression

Not being married or cohabiting with partner; poor marital relationship

Poor social support

Low socioeconomic status; Medicaid insurance

Intimate partner violence

Unintended pregnancy

Smoking

Stressful life event during pregnancy and/or puerperium
- Loss of loved one (fetus, newborn, partner, or other child)
- Illness of partner, parent, or child
- Financial difficulties
- Job loss
- Move of household

Adapted from Beck, C. T. (2008). State of the science on postpartum depression—What nurse researchers have contributed: Part 1. *MCN: The American Journal of Maternal/Child Nursing, 3,* 121–126; Lancaster, C., Gold, K., Flynn, H., Yoo, H., Marcus, S., & Davis, M. (2010). Risk factors for depressive symptoms during pregnancy: A systematic review. *American Journal of Obstetrics & Gynecology, 202,* 5–14.

It is possible to identify prenatally women who are at risk for experiencing parenting difficulties. Asking the woman how she thinks her pregnancy is progressing and questions about her preparations for the care of the baby opens up areas of discussion that may provide insight into positive or negative reactions to the experience of pregnancy and preparation for parenthood. The woman is given the opportunity to verbalize thoughts about the changes she is experiencing, fantasies about the baby, and acceptance of pregnancy and the child by the family.

Substance Abuse

Alcohol use has long been identified as a preventable cause of birth defects. Drinking while pregnant is still a problem; one in eight pregnant women drink alcohol (Denny, Tsai, Floyd, & Green, 2009). Fetal alcohol syndrome (FAS) has four criteria: maternal drinking during pregnancy, a characteristic pattern of facial abnormalities, growth retardation, and brain damage (often manifested by intellectual difficulties or behavioral problems). As surveillance and research have progressed, it has become clear that FAS is a rare example of a wide array of defects that can occur from fetal exposure to alcohol (Krulewitch, 2005).

Substance abuse or chemical dependency affects all body systems and can cause cardiac, pulmonary, gastrointestinal, and psychiatric complications. The relationships between substance abuse, stress, psychiatric comorbidities, intimate partner violence, and the lack of healthcare are striking. Simmons, Havens, Whiting, Holz, and Bada (2009) note the connections:

- General health status declines with use of illicit drugs, including cocaine, opiates, and amphetamines, even after controlling for other psychosocial and biological covariates.
- Stress is strongly associated with substance use. Stress has been associated with abnormal functioning of the hypothalamic-pituitary-adrenal axis.
- Psychiatric comorbidity is also common in individuals with substance use disorders. Individuals with mental and substance use comorbidities are less likely to receive mental health treatment.
- Research demonstrates women who use drugs or drink alcohol are more likely to be battered and injured.
- Women who experience interpersonal violence (IPV) are more likely to be frequent substance users and have a greater number of substance disorder symptoms than women who do not experience IPV.
- Previous research has demonstrated a link between receipt of welfare benefits and increased risk of illicit drug use, but Medicaid policies make it difficult for clients to obtain substance abuse treatment services.

Chasnoff, Wells, McGourty, and Bailey (2007) validated a five-item brief screening instrument, 4Ps Plus©, to identify pregnant women at highest risk for substance use receiving prenatal care. The questions are easily integrated into prenatal care. The four screening questions are aimed at the following:

1. Parents: Did either of your parents ever have a problem with alcohol or drugs?
2. Partner: Does your partner have a problem with alcohol or drugs?
3. Past: Have you ever drunk beer, wine, or liquor?
4. Pregnancy: In the month before you knew you were pregnant, how many cigarettes did you smoke? In the month before you knew you were pregnant, how many beers/how much wine/how much liquor did you drink?

The women fall into low-, average-, and high-risk categories based on these questions. High risk are those women who used any alcohol or smoked three or more cigarettes in the month before pregnancy. Because substance abuse or chemical dependency can adversely affect the health of the woman and the fetus, it is essential to include drug use assessment and education strategies in prenatal and women's healthcare encounters.

Cigarette Smoking

Cigarette smoking has been linked to an increased incidence of low birth weight and prematurity (ACOG, 2005b) and remains a problem. In the United States, combined data for 2000 to 2005 indicated that 22.5% of those reported smoking before or during pregnancy or after delivery. Compared with nonsmokers, women who smoked were significantly more likely to be younger (aged <25 years), non-Hispanic white, have <12 years of education, be unmarried, have an annual income of <$15,000, be underweight, have an unintended pregnancy, be first-time mothers, have initiated prenatal care later, be Medicaid enrolled, and be enrolled in WIC during pregnancy. This indicates that the problem is pretty much unchanged from previous studies (Tong, Jones, Dietz, D'Angelo, & Bombard, 2009).

From a preventive perspective, it is not enough to discourage smoking in pregnant women. The focus must be on discouraging smoking in any woman of childbearing age who may potentially become pregnant. Smoking during pregnancy presents major, avoidable health risks to the fetus. Smoking has been linked to increased risk of miscarriage, IUGR, low birth weight and very low birth weight, preterm labor and premature birth, placenta previa, placental abruption, perinatal loss, and sudden infant death syndrome (SIDS). Infants and young children are affected by environmental tobacco smoke, which has been linked with an increased risk of lower respiratory infections in children, fluid in the middle ear, symptoms of upper respiratory tract irritation, reduced lung function, and additional episodes and increased severity of asthma in children (AWHONN, 2000).

The risk of fetal death is typically 1.5-fold over nonsmokers; the risk decreases to that of nonsmokers in women who stop smoking after the first trimester (Silver, 2007). Infants who live with a smoker face an increased risk of SIDS. During pregnancy, many women are more highly motivated to stop or decrease their smoking; however, simply providing information may not be enough for the pregnant woman with a long history of smoking. The U.S. Preventive Services Task Force (USPSTF; 2009) recommends that clinicians ask all pregnant women about tobacco use and provide augmented, pregnancy-tailored counseling for those who smoke. In pregnant women, the USPSTF found convincing evidence that smoking cessation counseling sessions, augmented with messages and self-help materials tailored for pregnant smokers, increases abstinence rates during pregnancy compared with brief, generic counseling interventions alone. Tobacco cessation at any point during pregnancy yields substantial health benefits for the expectant mother and baby.

Counseling interventions of at least 10 minutes have been shown to increase quit rates (AWHONN, 2000). One evidence-based approach is the "5 A's." In practices that have used the 5 A's approach, quit rates among pregnant women have risen by 30% or more (Martin et al., 2006). This approach to smoking cessation is easily integrated into prenatal care:

- *Ask:* Ask the patient to choose a statement that best describes her smoking status.
- *Advise:* Ask permission to share the health message about smoking during pregnancy.
- *Assess:* Readiness to change
- *Assist:* Briefly explore problem-solving methods and skills for smoking cessation.
- *Arrange:* Let the woman know that you will be following up on each visit; assess smoking status at subsequent prenatal visits; affirm efforts to quit. (USPSTF, 2009)

Physical Activity

Despite the fact that pregnancy is associated with profound anatomic and physiologic changes, exercise has confirmed benefits and minimal risks for most women. A woman's overall health, including obstetric and medical risks, should be assessed before initiating an exercise program (Display 4–5). Generally, participation in a wide range of recreational activities appears to be safe during pregnancy; however, each sport should be reviewed individually for its potential risk, and activities with a high risk of falling or those with a high risk of abdominal trauma should be avoided during pregnancy. Scuba diving also should be avoided throughout pregnancy because the fetus is at an increased risk for decompression sickness during this activity. In the absence of either medical or obstetric complications, 30 minutes or more of moderate exercise a day on

---

DISPLAY 4 – 5

Exercise during Pregnancy

ABSOLUTE CONTRAINDICATIONS TO AEROBIC EXERCISE DURING PREGNANCY

- Hemodynamically significant heart disease
- Restrictive lung disease
- Incompetent cervix/cerclage
- Multiple gestation at risk for premature labor
- Persistent second- or third-trimester bleeding
- Placenta previa after 26 weeks' gestation
- Premature labor during the current pregnancy
- Ruptured membranes
- Preeclampsia/pregnancy-induced hypertension

RELATIVE CONTRAINDICATIONS TO AEROBIC EXERCISE DURING PREGNANCY

- Severe anemia
- Unevaluated maternal cardiac arrhythmia
- Chronic bronchitis
- Poorly controlled type 1 diabetes
- Extreme morbid obesity
- Extreme underweight (BMI <12)
- History of extremely sedentary lifestyle
- Intrauterine growth restriction in current pregnancy
- Poorly controlled hypertension
- Orthopedic limitations
- Poorly controlled seizure disorder
- Poorly controlled hyperthyroidism
- Heavy smoker

WARNING SIGNS TO TERMINATE EXERCISE WHILE PREGNANT

- Vaginal bleeding
- Dyspnea prior to exertion
- Dizziness
- Headache
- Chest pain
- Muscle weakness
- Calf pain or swelling (need to rule out thrombophlebitis)
- Preterm labor
- Decreased fetal movement
- Amniotic fluid leakage

From American College of Obstetricians and Gynecologists. (2002b). *Exercise during Pregnancy and the Postpartum Period* (Committee Opinion No. 267). Washington, DC: Author.

most, if not all, days of the week is recommended for pregnant women (ACOG, 2002b).

Many women are committed to exercising regularly and wish to continue throughout the pregnancy. Pregnant women who have been sedentary before pregnancy should gradually progress up to 30 minutes a day (Artal & O'Toole, 2003). Overall exercise benefits the woman psychologically and physically. Recreational and competitive athletes with uncomplicated pregnancies may remain active during pregnancy and modify their usual exercise routines to refrain from contact sports or other activities that might possibly cause abdominal distress. Particular attention should be paid to maintaining proper hydration during these exercise sessions. Pregnant women with diabetes, morbid obesity, or chronic hypertension should have individualized exercise prescription. Women with medical or obstetric complications should be carefully evaluated before recommendations on physical activity participation during pregnancy are made. Because of increased relaxation of ligaments during pregnancy, flexibility exercise should be individualized. A typical exercise prescription should promote musculoskeletal fitness and address type, intensity and progression, quantity and duration, and frequency. A typical session includes:

- Warm-ups and stretching (5 to 10 minutes)
- Exercise program (30 to 45 minutes)
- Cool down (5 to 10 minutes)

Maternal Infections

Maternal infections have long been recognized as risk factors for adverse pregnancy outcomes. Infections have been reported to account for 10% to 25% of fetal deaths in developed countries (Cunningham et al., 2010; Silver, 2007). Factors such as maternal serologic status, timing of infection during pregnancy, mode of acquisition, and immunologic status influence disease course and pregnancy outcomes (Cunningham et al., 2010). The mechanism likely involves both maternal and fetal inflammatory responses but is unknown. There is epidemiologic, microbiologic, and clinical evidence of an association between infection and preterm birth. Spontaneous preterm birth epidemiologic studies reveal that births at less than 34 weeks' gestation are much more frequently accompanied by clinical or subclinical infection than those at more than 34 weeks. Both maternal and neonatal infections are more common after preterm than term birth. The earlier the birth, the more risk there is of an associated infection (Boggess, 2005).

The proportion of fetal deaths due to viral infections is uncertain because there is no way to systematically evaluate by cultures. Prevention is key (see Appendix 4–A for information regarding vaccination in pregnancy).

Parvovirus B19 (B19V) is perhaps the most common viral infection to cause pregnancy loss (Dijkmans et al., 2012; Silver, 2007). Erythema infectiosum, also known as Fifth's disease, is a relatively benign disease affecting mainly children and young adults. Infection with B19V usually occurs through respiratory droplets and can be transmitted vertically from mother to fetus (Dijkmans et al., 2012). Maternal infection can occur without symptoms. The mechanism causing pregnancy loss is thought to be fetal anemia leading to fetal hydrops. The prevalence of IgG antibodies to B19V, evidence of a status after infection, in the population ranges from 2% to 15% in children 1 to 5 years old, 15% to 60% in children 16 to 19 years old, and 30% to 60% in adults (Heegaard & Brown, 2002). No vertical transmission has been described if the mother has IGG antibodies against B19V at the time of exposure. When maternal infection occurs, maternal viremia peaks at approximately 1 week and the risk of vertical transmission has been estimated to be around 25% (de Jong, Walther, Kroes, & Oepkes, 2011).

The most common viral infection is cytomegalovirus, found in 2.3% of U.S. pregnant women (Hyde, Schmid, & Cannon, 2010). Day care providers have an annual rate of 8.5% (Hyde et al., 2010). Transmission usually occurs by contact with infected nasopharyngeal secretions or other body fluids. Maternal transmission to the fetus or newborn is most common following primary maternal infection. Routine screening is not recommended because:

- No vaccine is available.
- In seropositive pregnant women, it is difficult to distinguish between primary and nonprimary infection.
- There is no evidence that antiviral drug treatment of primary infection in pregnant women changes the outcome in the neonate.
- When fetal infection occurs, there is no way to accurately predict whether or not the fetus will develop significant sequelae.

Coxsackie virus has also been reported to cause fetal death as well as other sporadically occurring viruses (e.g., echoviruses, enteroviruses, chickenpox, measles, mumps, and rubella).

Genital herpes simplex virus (HSV) is rarely transmitted in utero; however, this infection is one of the most common STDs. The latest HSV data indicates that overall national HSV-2 prevalence remains high (16.2%) and that the disease continues to disproportionately burden African Americans (39.2% prevalence), particularly black women (48.0% prevalence), who face a number of factors putting them at greater risk, including higher community prevalence and biologic factors that put women of all races at greater risk for HSV-2 than men. Most persons with HSV-2 have not received a diagnosis.

Currently, ACOG (2007) does not recommend routine HSV screening of pregnant women. There is controversy over the cost/benefit ratio of universal screening and the number of neonatal deaths prevented from doing such screening. Most primary and first-episode infections in early pregnancy are not associated with spontaneous abortion or stillbirth, but a late pregnancy primary infection may be associated with preterm labor. Neonatal transmission is by three routes: (1) intrauterine in 5%, (2) peripartum in 85%, or (3) postnatal in 10% (Cunningham et al., 2010). The fetus becomes infected by virus shed from the cervix and/or lower genital tract. The virus either invades the uterus following membrane rupture or is transmitted by contact with the fetus at delivery. The rate of transmission is 1 in 3,200 to 1 in 30,000 births depending on the population studied (Cunningham et al., 2010). Antiviral therapy with acyclovir has been used for treatment and will decrease the duration of symptoms and viral shedding in women with a primary outbreak in pregnancy. Acyclovir appears safe for pregnant women. ACOG (2007) recommends viral therapy at or beyond 36 weeks for women who have any recurrence during pregnancy. Whether suppression is needed for women with outbreaks before but not during pregnancy has not been determined (Cunningham et al., 2010).

HIV attacks the CD4 cells of the immune system. Infection with HIV occurs primarily through sexual contact, contaminated blood or blood products through exposure to contaminated needles and syringes, and mother-to-child transmission. High-risk factors include injection drug use, prostitution, a suspected or known HIV-infected sexual partner, multiple sexual partners, or a diagnosis of another STD. HIV is transmitted during pregnancy in utero, during vaginal delivery, and through breast milk of an HIV-infected woman.

According to the CDC (2009) HIV surveillance report, women comprised 24% of all diagnoses of HIV infection in the United States among adults and adolescents. Most HIV-infected women are of reproductive age. Minority women are disproportionately affected: black and Hispanic women are at increased risk of HIV infection (1 in 32 black women and 1 in 106 Hispanic/Latina women compared with 1 in 526 white or Asian women). The estimated number of perinatally acquired AIDS cases had decreased dramatically over the last two decades. The Perinatal HIV Guidelines Workgroup (2008) suggests that this is predominantly due to the implementation of prenatal HIV testing with antiviral therapy given to the pregnant woman and then to her neonate. The CDC (2009), the ACOG (2008), and the U.S. Preventive Services Task Force (2005) recommend prenatal screening using an "opt-out approach." This means that the woman is notified that HIV testing is included in a comprehensive panel of prenatal tests, but testing may be declined. Women are given information regarding HIV but are not required to sign a specific consent. Through the use of such opt-out strategies, HIV testing rates have increased.

In addition to the standard prenatal assessment for all pregnant women, the initial lab evaluation of an HIV-infected woman should include:

- History of use (prior and current) of antiretroviral medications
- Renal and liver function
- HIV-1 RNA viral level
- CD4+ lymphocyte count, CD4+ percentage
- Complete blood count (CBC) with differential
- Platelet count
- Screen for STD
- Screen for hepatitis B and C
- Screen for cytomegalic virus (CMV) and toxoplasmosis
- Pap smear
- Purified protein derivative (PPD) for tuberculosis
- Assessment of supportive care needs

During pregnancy, most women with HIV are advised to take combination antiretroviral regimens to reduce perinatal transmission treatment and treatment of maternal HIV disease. This regimen may need adjustment in the woman who was already taking a regimen of medications. When possible, zidovudine (ZDV) is included because it has been shown to significantly reduce the risk of passing HIV to the infant and is thought to be safe to take during pregnancy. A combination regimen is more effective in reducing HIV transmission than a single-drug regimen (Sweet & Gibbs, 2009)

Medical and nursing care of HIV-infected pregnant women requires coordination and communication between HIV specialists and obstetrical healthcare providers. General counseling should include current knowledge about risk factors for perinatal transmission. Risk of perinatal transmission of HIV has been associated with potentially modifiable factors including cigarette smoking, illicit drug use, genital tract infections, and unprotected sexual intercourse with multiple partners during pregnancy. Besides improving maternal health, cessation of cigarette smoking and drug use, treatment of genital tract infections, and use of condoms with sexual intercourse during pregnancy may reduce risk of perinatal transmission (National Institute of Health, 2011). A resource available to nurses is the National Perinatal HIV Hotline (1-888-448-8765), a federally funded service providing free clinical consultation to providers caring for HIV-infected women and their infants.

Maternal genitourinary and reproductive tract infections have been implicated as a main risk factor in 15% to 25% of preterm deliveries (Denney & Culhane, 2009). Bacterial vaginosis is a maldistribution of normal vaginal flora occurring in up to 20% of all pregnancies (Boggess, 2005). Numbers of lactobacilli are decreased, and overrepresented species are anaerobic bacteria, including *Gardnerella vaginalis*, *Mobiluncus*, and some *Bacteroides* species. Treatment is reserved for symptomatic women, who usually complain of a fishy-smelling discharge. However, treatment does not reduce preterm birth, and routine screening is not recommended (ACOG, 2001b).

As a routine part of prenatal practice, nurses can assess maternal dentition and advise on proper brushing and flossing techniques and encourage women to seek dental care. Continuing or acquiring dental care during pregnancy should be a routine recommendation to pregnant women, as there has been evidence to support an association between gingivitis and preterm birth, low birth weight, and preeclampsia (Xiong, Buekens, Fraser, Beck, & Offenbacher, 2006). Gingivitis occurs in 60% to 75% of pregnant women, and it surfaces most frequently during the second trimester (Barak et al., 2003; Khader & Ta'ani, 2005). Symptoms include swollen red gums and bleeding with brushing the teeth. Elevated levels of estrogen and progesterone cause the gums to react differently to the bacteria found in plaque. Gums infected with periodontal disease become toxic reservoirs of bacteria resulting in increased prostaglandin production (Barak et al., 2003).

Although multiple studies have shown an association between periodontal infection and adverse pregnancy outcomes, treatment of periodontal disease during pregnancy has not been shown to improve birth outcomes. Recently, Jeffcoat and colleagues (2010) did demonstrate that successful routine periodontal treatment (scaling and root planing plus oral hygiene instruction) is associated with a decreased incidence of spontaneous preterm birth.

Culture

Cultural assessment is an important part of prenatal care. A comprehensive discussion of culture as it relates to pregnancy and childbirth practices is presented in Chapter 2. Cultural beliefs and practices can affect the health status of the woman by influencing her use of healthcare services, confidence in and acceptance of recommended prevention and treatment strategies, and global beliefs regarding her body, illness, religion, and so forth (Seidel et al., 2010). Principal beliefs, values, and behaviors that relate to pregnancy and childbirth should be identified, taking care to avoid sweeping generalizations about cultural characteristics or cultural values. Not every individual in a culture may display certain characteristics, as there are variations among cultures and within cultures. Planning culturally specific care requires information about ethnicity, degree of affiliation with the ethnic group, religion, patterns of decision making, language, style of communication, norms of etiquette, and expectations about the healthcare system (Seidel et al., 2010). Nutritional practices and beliefs about medication are particularly significant during pregnancy. Certain behavioral differences can be expected if a culture views pregnancy as an illness, as opposed to a natural occurrence; for example, seeking prenatal care may or may not be important if pregnancy is viewed as a natural occurrence. Healthcare practices during pregnancy are influenced by numerous factors, such as the prevalence of folk remedies, the prevalence of indigenous healers, and the influence of professional healthcare workers. Socioeconomic status and living in an urban or rural setting affect patterns of use of home remedies and use of the healthcare system.

Without cultural awareness, nurses and other healthcare providers tend to project their own cultural responses onto women and families from different socioeconomic, religious, or educational groups. This leads caregivers to assume patients are demonstrating a certain type of behavior for the same reason that they themselves would. Additionally, some nurses may fail to recognize that healthcare has its own culture, which has been dominated historically by traditional middle-class values and beliefs. In an ethnocentric approach, caregivers sometimes believe that if members of other cultures do not share Western values, they should adopt them. An example of this is a nurse who values equality of the sexes dealing with an Asian woman who defers to the husband to make the decisions. Pressuring the woman to defy cultural values and beliefs can prove stressful for the woman and significantly interfere with a therapeutic relationship.

When a language barrier exists, the woman may be reluctant to provide information if the interpreter is male, a relative, or a child of the pregnant woman. Reviewing the goals and purposes of the interview with the interpreter in advance generally enhances the interaction with the woman. Gender is an important factor in health beliefs. In many cultures, a male physician would not be allowed to examine a woman, much less deliver her baby.

Nurses cannot expect to be culturally competent for every woman they care for. However, culturally responsive behaviors can enhance prenatal care. If a particular ethnic group dominates the local population, it is a professional responsibility to learn as much about that culture so as to provide optimal care.

Current Pregnancy Status

Assessment of current pregnancy status includes analysis of current pregnancy history, psychosocial factors, nutritional status, and laboratory data; a review of symptoms guided by the gestational age that may reflect medical or pregnancy complications; assessment of the pregnant woman's concerns; and a complete physical examination. Symptom review includes questions about nausea and vomiting, headache, abdominal or epigastric pain, visual changes, fever, viral illness, vaginal bleeding, dysuria, cramping, and other concerns. This screening process incorporates assessment of historical and social factors with current health status. Evaluation of current pregnancy status provides baseline data that guides planning for future evaluation and health promotion activities.

The physical examination is comprehensive and covers a review of the cardiovascular, respiratory, neurologic, endocrine, gastrointestinal, reproductive, and genitourinary systems. Particular attention should be directed to the anthropometric assessment, including the woman's height, weight, and pelvimetry data, because these physical characteristics can influence the pregnancy course and birth (Cunningham et al., 2010). Pelvic examination includes measurement of cervical length, a Pap smear, and assessment for STDs. The abdominal examination compares data from the woman's report of her last menstrual period with physical findings. Depending on weeks of gestation, the FHR may be auscultated.

Selected laboratory data are valuable to the assessment process. Biochemical information provides information about current prenatal health as well as general wellness status. Evaluation of specific laboratory data is discussed later in this chapter.

ONGOING PRENATAL CARE

Nurses who interact with the childbearing family in the prenatal period assess the well-being of the woman and the growth and well-being of the fetus. Nursing intervention is directed by the data obtained from ongoing comprehensive maternal–fetal assessments. Evaluation of the growth and development of the fetus can be shared with the parents to promote prenatal parent–infant attachment.

Risk status in pregnancy is a dynamic process that affects clinical and nonclinical parameters. Psychosocial factors, socioeconomic factors, and lifestyle patterns also require ongoing evaluation. Employment status, family economic status, and relationship status could change from visit to visit. These changes affect the woman's psychosocial stress level, potentiating existing risk factors. In general, factors with potential to affect the pregnancy are in a constant state of fluctuation and require continued surveillance.

Subsequent prenatal visits should be structured to promote continuous, rather than episodic, risk assessment. Each prenatal visit should include a maternal–fetal

physical assessment, including vital signs, weight, fundal height, FHR, and fetal movement, as well as a review of pertinent laboratory data, dating data, the problem list, and the woman's response to recommended interventions (e.g., smoking cessation). At return prenatal visits, risk factors must be analyzed to evaluate their relevance to the gestational age. For example, if a woman has a history of preterm labor and is at 37 weeks' gestation in the current pregnancy, this risk factor would no longer be relevant. Conversely, new risk factors may develop during the pregnancy, such as preeclampsia or GDM. Ongoing prenatal care is a dynamic process in which risk factors may change from month to month. Achieving healthy pregnancy outcomes is a multifaceted and sometimes complex process. Nurses can be credible sources of information, offering support as the woman and her partner or family sort through information and decision making during pregnancy.

Particular attention should be given to evaluation of blood pressure trends (see Chapter 5 for a complete discussion of hypertensive disease during pregnancy). During pregnancy, blood pressure values decrease slightly during the second trimester but return to early pregnancy values by the third trimester. Ideally, during preconception care or early prenatal care, a baseline blood pressure is noted. It is important to evaluate and document blood pressure measurements in the same arm with the woman in the same position (e.g., sitting or semi-Fowler's) with the blood pressure cuff at the level of the heart. Use of the same device for assessing blood pressure is also critical to accuracy. Consistency in blood pressure monitoring allows for more accurate assessment and comparison across prenatal visits.

A blood pressure reading of >140/90 mm Hg is considered elevated (ACOG, 2002b). Other clinical data are important to assess as blood pressure change is not usually a lone sign of complications. When there is a change in blood pressure, the woman should be assessed for the concurrent development of proteinuria, headaches, dizziness, visual disturbances, epigastric pain, or edema. Gestational hypertension is defined as systolic blood pressure ≥140 mm Hg and/or diastolic blood pressure ≥90 mm Hg in a previously normotensive pregnant woman who is ≥20 weeks of gestation and has no proteinuria (ACOG, 2002b; Sibai, 2005). The blood pressure readings should be documented on at least two occasions at least 6 hours apart. It is considered severe when sustained elevations in systolic blood pressure ≥160 mm Hg and/or diastolic blood pressure ≥110 mm Hg are present for at least 6 hours (ACOG, 2002b). Gestational hypertension is a temporary diagnosis for hypertensive pregnant women who do not meet criteria for preeclampsia (both hypertension and proteinuria) or chronic hypertension (hypertension first detected before the 20th week of pregnancy). The diagnosis is changed to:

- Preeclampsia, if proteinuria develops
- Chronic hypertension, if blood pressure elevation persists ≥12 weeks postpartum
- Transient hypertension of pregnancy, if blood pressure returns to normal by 12 weeks postpartum

Basic fetal surveillance includes assessment of fundal height, FHR, and fetal activity. Fundal height is the measurement of the uterus from the symphysis pubis to the top of the fundus. The measurement of the fundal height in centimeters (±2 cm) should correlate with gestational age between 22 and 34 weeks. Fundal height less than gestational age may be indicative of IUGR. Fundal height greater than gestational age may indicate multiple gestation, polyhydramnios, macrosomia, fibroids, or other conditions that cause uterine distension. Fetal activity is an indirect measure of central nervous system function and is predictive of fetal well-being. Fetal movement counting (i.e., "kick counts") is discussed later in this chapter.

PRETERM LABOR AND BIRTH

Following a long period of fairly steady increase, the U.S. preterm birth rate declined in 2007 (from 12.8% to 12.7%), and then again in 2008 (to 12.3%), marking the first 2-year downturn in this rate in nearly three decades. Declines in preterm birth rates from 2006 to 2008 were observed for mothers of all age groups under age 40, for the three largest race and Hispanic origin groups, for the majority of all states, and for all types of deliveries. Nationally, the preterm birth rate declined 4% between 2006 and 2008 from 12.8% to 12.3% of live births (Martin, Osterman, & Sutton, 2010). Preterm and low-birth-weight births are considered by many to be the most urgent problem in the care of pregnant women. Because this is such an important issue in prenatal care, the reader is referred to Chapter 7 for an in-depth discussion of this topic.

BIOCHEMICAL SCREENING AND LABORATORY ASSESSMENT

Selected biochemical screenings may be repeated at specific intervals during pregnancy. Subsequent prenatal visits usually include urinalysis by dipstick for evidence of proteinuria, glucosuria, and ketonuria. Although it is common practice, there is little evidence to suggest routine urinalysis by means of dipstick provides useful clinical information or is predictive of women who will develop complications of pregnancy. The practice is currently questioned in the national guidelines for prenatal care (Agency for Healthcare Quality, 2010). Dipstick urinalysis does not detect proteinuria reliably in patients with early preeclampsia; measurement of

24-hour urinary protein excretion is the gold standard but is not always practical. Trace glycosuria also is unreliable, although higher concentrations may be useful (Kirkham, Harris, & Grzybowski, 2005).

After a baseline CBC is obtained, periodic assessment of hematocrit and hemoglobin values may be indicated for certain at-risk populations. Additionally, laboratory data such as urinalysis, urine culture, blood type and Rhesus factor (Rh), antibody screen, rubella titer, rapid plasma reagin test, hepatitis B surface antigen, gonorrhea and chlamydia testing, and cervical cytology should be obtained from all pregnant women. Additional laboratory tests (e.g., sexually transmitted infection [STI] screenings; group B streptococci; fetal fibronectin [fFN]; toxoplasmosis, rubella, cytomegalovirus, herpes simplex, and HIV [TORCH] titers; tuberculin testing; toxicology screenings; and genetic screenings) should be performed as indicated, based on historical indicators or clinical findings (AAP & ACOG, 2007).

Chlamydia testing is recommended for all pregnant women (AAP & ACOG, 2007). A nucleic acid amplification test (NAAT) of the cervix is the most sensitive test available with excellent specificity (CDC, 2002). ACOG (2008) supports universal HIV testing of pregnant women early in the pregnancy using an opt-out approach; that is, the test is offered to all and the woman may opt-out if she desires to decline testing. In this way, appropriate medical management can be initiated early to reduce the possibility of perinatal transmission. Appropriate counseling and referral services should be available for women with positive test results.

Screening for GDM is generally carried out at 24 to 28 weeks' gestation using a 1-hour, 50-g glucose challenge test (ACOG, 2001a; World Health Organization, 2006). Serum glucose evaluation before 24 to 28 weeks' gestation (i.e., at the first visit) may be indicated based on family history or maternal factors such as glucosuria, advanced maternal age, marked obesity, family history of diabetes mellitus, personal history of GDM, previous macrosomic infant, or previous unexplained fetal loss. The woman does not need to be fasting for the screening test. One hour after ingesting a glucose load (Glucola), the serum glucose level should be less than 140 mg/dL. The American Diabetes Association (ADA) recommends a cutoff value after 1 hour of either 140 mg/dL (7.8 mmol/L), which is said to identify 80% of women with GDM, or 130 mg/dL (7.2 mmol/L), which should identify 90%. Problems have also been reported for the glucose challenge test: there are many false-positives and sensitivity is only 86% at best (Menato et al., 2008). Nonfasting plasma glucose over 200 mg/dL on screening or a fasting greater than 105 mg/dL is indicative of diabetes mellitus and no oral glucose tolerance test (OGTT) is necessary for diagnosis.

If the screening result is greater than or equal to 140 mg/dL, a diagnostic test using a 3-hour 100-g OGTT is recommended. The diagnostic test for GDM is administered after a fast of at least 8 hours, but with the patient consuming her usual unrestricted daily diet in the days preceding the test. On the day of the test, only water may be consumed, and cigarette smoking should be avoided. Diagnosis of GDM is based on two or more abnormally elevated venous plasma glucose values (ADA, 2008). Women diagnosed with GDM require education about appropriate nutrition, self-management, and self-glucose monitoring and referral for appropriate medical care and counseling. The diagnosis of GDM is made when two or more of the values at the 3-hour OGTT are elevated above the following values (in plasma mg/dL):

Fasting: 105
1 hour: 190
2 hour: 165
3 hour: 145

If only one level is elevated, repeat testing at a later gestation may be ordered or dietary restriction recommended. Approximately 15% to 20% of those with GDM will develop overt diabetes mellitus.

Maternal serum alpha-fetoprotein (MSAFP) screening (including PAPPA) should be offered to all pregnant women between 15 and 20 weeks' gestation (AAP & ACOG, 2007; ACOG, 2007a). The goal of MSAFP is to identify women who have an increased risk of NTDs, Down syndrome, or trisomy 21. Screening should be voluntary, and the woman should be counseled about its limitations and benefits (ACOG, 2007a).

Alpha-fetoprotein (AFP) is a protein that is produced in the fetal yolk sac during the first trimester and in the fetal liver during later gestation. The concentration of AFP in maternal serum is altered by factors that include inaccurate dating of gestational age, maternal weight and race, multiple gestation, and maternal diabetes. Most screening programs establish a cutoff of 2.0 to 2.5 times the median values (2.0 to 2.5 MoM) to be designated as a positive result for NTD (AAP & ACOG, 2007). In contrast to the absolute cutoff of 2.0 to 2.5 MoM used in NTD screening, Down syndrome screening uses a series of age-specific cutoff levels for each MSAFP level. There is a direct relationship between the age of the patient and the chance of her result being designated as positive.

Abnormally elevated MSAFP levels have been associated with birth defects and chromosomal anomalies, such as open NTDs, open abdominal defects, and congenital nephrosis (AAP & ACOG, 2007). High MSAFP levels also may result from multiple gestations. Low MSAFP levels have been associated with Down syndrome and other chromosomal anomalies (AAP & ACOG, 2007). Double-marker (i.e., AFP and human chorionic gonadotropin [hCG]), triple-marker (i.e., AFP, hCG, and estriol), and quadruple-marker (AFP, hCG, estriol, and inhibin A) screening is also available to screen for trisomy 18, trisomy 21, and NTDs. Average hCG levels are higher and unconjugated estriol levels are lower in Down syndrome pregnancies. The hCG and estriol levels are lower in trisomy 18 pregnancies. When more parameters are evaluated, there is an increased accuracy in diagnosis. Although maternal serum screening with the use of double and triple markers is superior to the use of MSAFP alone when screening for fetal Down syndrome, this method still fails to detect Down syndrome in women less than 35 years of age (AAP & ACOG, 2007). The quadruple is the most effective multiple-marker screening test for Down syndrome in the second trimester. This approach yields an 81% detection rate and a false-positive rate of 5% (Dugoff et al., 2005).

Women should be counseled that maternal serum screening tests are optional, about the limited sensitivity and specificity of maternal screening tests, and the psychological implications of a positive test prior to the performance of the tests. Any abnormal finding warrants additional testing; however, screening protocols vary. If the initial ultrasound examination does not provide an explanation for the MSAFP elevation (such as inaccurate dating, multiple gestation, or fetal demise), a comprehensive (level II) ultrasound examination is performed to evaluate the fetus for malformations. Genetic counseling and amniocentesis may be offered in some centers as a follow-up to abnormal findings as well. Hemoglobin electrophoresis is used to detect genetic hemoglobin disorders, including sickle cell anemia, sickle cell disease, and thalassemia. These recessive inherited conditions occur in the United States, primarily in families of African descent, but can also be found in families of Asian, Middle Eastern, or Mediterranean descent (Larrabee & Cowan, 1995). Women of African descent are routinely screened for these disorders. Although prevalence of sickle cell trait is common among African Americans (8% to 12%), information related to inheritance patterns is not well known to those at risk. Figure 4–1 and Display 4–6 provide teaching tools that may be helpful in explaining the genetic transfer of sickle cell trait and sickle cell disease to women and their partners.

Nuchal Translucency

An ultrasound scan is carried out to assess the amount of fluid behind the neck of the fetus, known as nuchal translucency (NT). Fetuses at risk of Down syndrome tend to have a higher amount of fluid around the neck. The nuchal scan is most accurate between 11 and 14 weeks. The scan is obtained with the fetus in sagittal section and a neutral position of the fetal head

DISPLAY 4-6

Patient Teaching Tool for Genetic Transfer of Sickle Cell Disease/Trait

1. Two parents affected with sickle cell trait:
   SA+SA = 25% of children will have sickle cell disease
   50% of children will have sickle cell trait
   25% of children will not be affected by the trait or disease
2. One parent affected with sickle cell trait, one parent affected with sickle cell disease:
   SA+SS = 50% of children will have sickle cell disease
   50% of children will have sickle cell trait
   0 children will not be affected by the trait or disease
3. Two parents affected by sickle cell disease:
   SS+SS = 100% of children will have sickle cell disease
   0 children will have sickle cell trait
   0 children will not be affected by the disease
4. One parent affected by sickle cell disease, one parent unaffected:
   SS+AA = 100% of children will have sickle cell trait
   0 children will have sickle cell disease
   0 children will not be affected by trait
5. One parent affected by sickle cell trait, one parent unaffected:
   SA+AA = 50% of children will have sickle cell trait
   50% of children will not be affected by the trait
   0 children will be affected by sickle cell disease

AA, unaffected; SA, sickle cell trait; SS, sickle cell disease.
From Larrabee, K., & Cowan, M. (1995). Clinical nursing management of sickle cell disease and trait during pregnancy. *Journal of Perinatal and Neonatal Nursing, 9*(2), 29–41.

(neither hyperflexed nor extended, either of which can influence the NT thickness). The fetal image is enlarged to fill 75% of the screen, and the maximum thickness is measured, from leading edge to leading edge. When combined with serum markers, NT measurement detects 79% to 87% of Down fetuses (ACOG, 2007a).

PRENATAL DIAGNOSIS

Prenatal diagnostic evaluation should be offered to families with any of the following: maternal age of 35 years or more, maternal age of 32 or more and pregnant with twins, women carrying a fetus with an ultrasonographically identified structural anomaly, women with ultrasound markers of aneuploidy (including increased nuchal thickness), women with a known positive serum screen, a family history of chromosomal anomalies, parental balanced translocation carrier, the mother a known or at-risk carrier for X-linked disorder, parents who are carriers of an autosomal recessive disorder detectable in utero, a parent affected with an autosomal dominant disorder detectable in utero, a family history of NTDs (Kirkham et al., 2005).

Chorionic Villus Sampling

Chorionic villus sampling (CVS) involves the removal of a small sample of chorionic (placental) tissue through a catheter inserted through the cervix. The villi are harvested and cultured for chromosomal analysis and processed for DNA and enzymatic analysis as indicated. Results are available in 4 days. CVS is ideally performed between 10.0 and 11.5 weeks' gestation. The risk of fetal loss is approximately 1%. As with amniocentesis, information about benefits and risks must be provided before the procedure (Cunningham et al., 2010).

Ultrasonography

Ultrasonography (i.e., fetal imaging by intermittent, high-frequency sound waves) is the most commonly used prenatal diagnostic procedure. Indications vary widely and depend on gestational age and type of diagnostic information sought. During early pregnancy, ultrasound is frequently used to determine presence of an intrauterine gestational sac, fetal number, and cardiac activity and to measure crown-rump length. Early ultrasonography (i.e., before 14 weeks' gestation) accurately determines gestational age (±1 week), decreases the need for labor induction after 41 weeks' gestation, and detects multiple pregnancies (ACOG, 2001b). Components of the basic ultrasound examination include the following:

- Presence of gestational sac and an evaluation of uterus and adnexa when performed during the first trimester
- Estimated gestational age
- Number of fetuses
- Viability
- Location of placenta
- Volume of amniotic fluid
- Fetal presentation and anatomical survey when performed during the second and third trimesters

Ultrasound during the second and third trimesters can be useful when there is a discrepancy between the woman's last menstrual period and uterine size, to detect fetal anatomic defects, abnormal fetal growth, and for placental localization and amniotic fluid volume estimates. When maternal or fetal complications are suspected or identified, ultrasonography serves as a valuable tool to confirm the diagnosis and follow-up on fetal status. Ultrasonography is also used to guide the obstetrician during other diagnostic procedures, such as CVS, amniocentesis, and fetal blood sampling. In women for whom preterm birth is a concern, cervical length can be measured via ultrasound. However, the value of doing this test lies in its negative predictive value. That is, the test is more useful for those women who are not likely to experience preterm labor than for predicting preterm labor (ACOG, 2001b).

Controversy exists over the benefits of routine ultrasound examination for all pregnant women. Advocates suggest routine screening can decrease incidence of labor induction for suspected postdate pregnancies and avoid undiagnosed fetal anomalies and twin gestations. However, no evidence directly links improved fetal outcomes with routine ultrasound screening (Kirkham et al., 2005).

Amniocentesis

Amniocentesis is the collection of a sample of amniotic fluid from the amniotic sac for identification of genetic diseases, selected birth defects, and fetal lung maturity; therapy for polyhydramnios; and progressive evaluation of isoimmunized pregnancies. Amniocentesis for genetic evaluation may be performed between 15 and 20 weeks' gestation. Genetic amniocentesis allows for detection of chromosomal anomalies, biochemical disorders, NTDs, some ventral wall defects, and DNA analysis for a number of single-gene disorders. Early amniocentesis, between 11 and 14 weeks' gestation, is offered at some centers with outcomes similar to midtrimester amniocentesis (Cunningham et al., 2010). Before testing, families should be given information about indications for amniocentesis, how the procedure is done, risks involved, and ramifications of findings.

Fetal Blood Sampling

Fetal blood sampling, also known as percutaneous umbilical blood sampling (PUBS) or cordocentesis, allows direct evaluation of fetal blood obtained from the umbilical cord. The procedure is not often performed and is only done in centers that have the expertise. Using ultrasonography to guide placement, a needle is inserted into one of the umbilical vessels (usually the vein), and a small amount of blood is withdrawn. Valuable information can be gained from analysis of fetal blood, including prenatal diagnosis of fetal blood disorders, isoimmunization, metabolic disorders, infections, and karyotyping (Cunningham et al., 2010). Cordocentesis can also be used for fetal therapies such as red blood cell and platelet transfusions.

Biochemical Markers

Fetal fibronectin (fFN), a protein secreted by the trophoblast, can be detected by use of a monoclonal antibody: FDC-6. The exact function is unknown, but this protein is thought to play a role in mediating placental–uterine attachment. fFN is normally present in the cervical or vaginal fluid before 20 weeks' gestation. However, after 20 weeks, the presence of fFN may indicate a disruption of the attachment of the fetal membranes, and therefore it has been investigated as an early marker for preterm birth.

Predicting women truly at risk for preterm birth and those destined to deliver at term may result in the ability to initiate interventions to prolong pregnancy and avoid preterm birth (see Chapter 7). fFN is a glycoprotein found in high concentrations in the amniotic fluid. It is normally found in the cervical and vaginal secretions before 16 to 20 weeks' gestation, but its presence in the cervicovaginal secretion after 20 weeks' gestation is abnormal, except as a marker of the imminent onset of labor at term (Cunningham et al., 2010). Elevation of fFN levels is hypothesized to reflect mechanical or inflammatory damage to the membranes or placenta. The fFN cutoff for a positive test is ≥ 50 ng/mL (Cunningham et al., 2010). The cervicovaginal fFN assay has limited accuracy in predicting preterm within 7 days of sampling in symptomatic pregnant women (Sanchez-Ramos, Delke, Zamora, & Kaunitz, 2009).

The fFN test is best used in the evaluation of women with preterm contractions in whom the diagnosis of preterm labor is uncertain. A negative test together with other reassuring factors (e.g., no signs of intrauterine infection or active abruption, no progressive cervical change or increase in uterine contraction intensity) can be used to avoid interventions (e.g., admission to the hospital, tocolysis, glucocorticoid administration). The high negative predictive value has proved most useful. In a large seminal study, 99.5% of pregnant women presenting to their physicians with signs and symptoms of preterm labor, and who subsequently had a negative cervicovaginal fFN test, failed to deliver within 7 days (Peaceman et al., 1997)

To collect a specimen for fFN testing, a Dacron swab is placed in the posterior fornix of the vagina and rotated for 10 seconds. Sexual activity within 24 hours of sample collection, recent cervical examination, and vaginal bleeding may result in false-positive tests (Adeza Biomedical, 2005). For this reason, a specimen should not be collected if the patient has had intercourse within 24 hours, and the specimen should be collected before performance of a digital cervical exam, measurement of transvaginal cervical length, or performance of Pap smear or cervical cultures. fFN testing should be limited to women with intact amniotic membranes and cervical dilatation <3 cm. This provides the nurse with the opportunity to review signs and symptoms of preterm labor and to address any fears or anxieties the woman or family may have regarding preterm birth.

FETAL SURVEILLANCE

Fetal assessment is an integral component of prenatal care. Careful assessment of fetal well-being enhances perinatal outcome through early identification and intervention for fetal compromise. The goal of antepartum

Indications for Antepartum Fetal Surveillance

MATERNAL CONDITIONS

- Antiphospholipid syndrome
- Hyperthyroidism (poorly controlled)
- Hemoglobinopathies (hemoglobin SS, SC, or S-thalassemia)
- Cyanotic heart disease
- Systemic lupus erythematosus
- Chronic renal disease
- Type 1 diabetes mellitus
- Hypertensive disorders

PREGNANCY-RELATED CONDITIONS

- Pregnancy-related hypertension
- Decreased fetal movement
- Oligohydramnios
- Polyhydramnios
- Intrauterine growth restriction
- Postterm pregnancy
- Isoimmunization
- Previous fetal demise (unexplained or recurrent risk)
- Multiple gestation (with significant growth discrepancy)

From American College of Obstetricians and Gynecologists. (1999). *Antepartum Fetal Surveillance* (Practice Bulletin No. 9). Washington, DC: Author.

fetal surveillance is to prevent fetal death. Display 4–7 provides the indications for antepartum fetal surveillance. Techniques based on FHR patterns have been in use since the 1970s (ACOG, 1999). Ultrasonography may be used as indicated throughout the pregnancy to assess fetal growth and development.

ASSESSMENT OF FETAL ACTIVITY

Fetal movement counting (i.e., "kick counts") has been proposed as a primary method of fetal surveillance for all pregnancies. Cessation of fetal movement is correlated with fetal death. The mother's observation of fetal movement has been validated through an 80% to 90% correlation of maternal perception of movement with movement detected on real-time ultrasonography (Moore & Piacquadio, 1989).

Several methods of fetal movement counting have been proposed; however, neither the ideal number of kicks nor the ideal duration for movement counting has been defined (ACOG, 1999). Perception of 10 distinct movements in a period of up to 2 hours is considered reassuring. After 10 movements have been perceived, the count may be discontinued. Another approach is to instruct women to count fetal movements for 1 hour three times per week. The count is considered reassuring if it equals or exceeds the woman's established baseline count (ACOG, 1999). Monitoring of fetal movement is recommended for pregnant women at

high risk for antepartum fetal death beginning as early as 26 to 28 weeks' gestation. For most at-risk patients, however, initiating testing at 32 to 34 weeks is appropriate (ACOG, 1999). Because fetal movement counting is inexpensive, reassuring, and a relatively easily taught skill, all women could benefit from instruction on fetal activity assessment.

Although fetal activity is a reassuring sign, decreased fetal movement is not necessarily ominous. A healthy fetus usually has perceivable movements within 10 to 60 minutes (Cunningham et al., 2010). However, perception of fetal movement can be influenced by many factors, including time of day, gestational age, placental location, glucose loading, maternal smoking, maternal medications, and decreased uterine space as gestation increases. Decreased fetal movement may also reflect the fetal sleep state. Early identification of conditions that can affect pregnancy outcome can minimize perinatal morbidity by allowing for the establishment of an appropriate treatment plan and referrals (AAP & ACOG, 2007). Report of decreased fetal movement is an indication for further assessment. The woman should be instructed to have something to eat and drink, rest, and focus on fetal movement for 1 hour. Four movements in 1 hour are considered reassuring. If fewer than four movements are perceived in 2 hours, the woman should call her primary healthcare provider immediately.

NONSTRESS TEST

The nonstress test (NST) is one of the most common methods of prenatal screening and involves electronic FHR monitoring for approximately 20 minutes. The NST is based on the premise that the normal fetus moves at various intervals and that the central nervous system and myocardium responds to movement with acceleration of the FHR. Acceleration of the FHR during fetal activity is a sign of fetal well-being (ACOG, 1999). Various definitions of reactivity have been used. Using the most common definition, the NST is considered to be reactive when two or more FHR accelerations of 15 beats per minute above baseline and lasting at least 15 seconds occur within a 20-minute time frame with or without perception of fetal movement by the woman (ACOG, 1999). These accelerations should occur within 40 minutes of testing. An NST that does not meet these criteria is nonreactive. A reactive NST is reassuring, indicating less than a 1% chance of fetal death within 1 week of a reactive NST. Most deaths within 1 week of a reactive NST fall into nonpreventable categories, such as abruptio placentae, sepsis, and cord accidents. However, a nonreactive NST is not necessarily an ominous sign. Rather, the nonreactive NST indicates a need for further testing and should be followed by a contraction stress test or BPP (Cunningham et al., 2010). The NST of the noncompromised preterm fetus (24 to 28 weeks' gestation) is frequently nonreactive, and up to 50% of NSTs may not be reactive from 28 to 32 weeks' gestation (ACOG, 1999). Prior to 32 weeks, some practitioners consider that the test is reactive if FHR increases 10 beats for 10 seconds twice in a 20-minute period.

BIOPHYSICAL PROFILE

The BPP combines electronic FHR monitoring with ultrasonography to evaluate fetal well-being based on multiple biophysical variables. Five parameters are assessed: fetal muscle tone, fetal movement, fetal breathing movements, amniotic fluid volume, and FHR reactivity as demonstrated by NST. Each item has a maximum score of 2, with a summed score of 8 to 10 indicating fetal well-being (i.e., reassuring). A score of 6 is considered "equivocal," and the test should be repeated the next day in a preterm fetus. A term fetus should be delivered. A score of 4 usually indicates that birth is warranted, although for extremely premature pregnancies, management is individualized. Scores of 0 to 3 are "abnormal," with expeditious birth considered (ACOG, 1999). Indications for BPP are those listed for antepartum fetal surveillance, with weekly testing usually recommended.

MODIFIED BIOPHYSICAL PROFILE

The modified BPP combines the use of an NST as a short-term indicator of fetal well-being, with the assessment of amniotic fluid index (AFI) as an indicator of long-term placental function. The AFI is the sum of the measurements of the deepest cord-free amniotic fluid pocket in each of the four abdominal quadrants. An AFI value greater than 5 cm generally is considered to represent an adequate volume of fluid. A modified BPP is considered reassuring if the NST is reactive and the AFI is greater than 5 but abnormal if the NST is nonreactive or the AFI is 5 or less (ACOG, 1999). The modified BPP is less cumbersome and appears to be as predictive of fetal status as other approaches of biophysical fetal surveillance (AAP & ACOG, 2007).

NURSING ASSESSMENT AND INTERVENTIONS

Nursing interventions are based on a collaborative approach to the identification of strengths and conditions with potential to increase risk of complications. Together, the nurse and woman set goals and strategize ways to implement a plan of care to meet these goals. During the antepartum period, nursing care typically includes comfort promotion (i.e., measures to relieve discomforts caused by the physiologic changes of pregnancy), counseling for family adaptation in planning the addition of a new member, and encouraging behaviors to enhance maternal and fetal well-being. Providing education, especially for the woman experiencing a first-time pregnancy, is an important aspect of antepartum care. The nurse has the opportunity and the responsibility to teach the woman and her family about beneficial and detrimental lifestyle practices, potential risks, and care required to promote maternal and fetal well-being. The nurse in ambulatory care provides anticipatory planning, assesses all available data, and structures education and nursing interventions accordingly. Inherent in competent antenatal nursing practice are the ability to differentiate between normal pregnancy variations and high-risk complications and the initiation of appropriate nursing interventions.

Total care management of the childbearing family requires cooperation, collaboration, and communication across disciplines. Risk factors must be evaluated in terms of individual risk versus benefit to be effective. Healthcare providers are charged with the task of finding the goodness of fit between the recommended healthcare regimen and the individual's reality to optimize outcome. Case management allows for a single healthcare professional to coordinate healthcare management in collaboration with the pregnant woman.

CASE MANAGEMENT

The childbearing woman and her family are the core of the perinatal healthcare team. Family-centered perinatal care is a model of care based on the philosophy that the physical, social, spiritual, and economic needs of the total family unit should be integrated and considered collectively (AWHONN, 2009). The nurse's role as case manager, advocate, and educator is of primary importance in facilitating a family-friendly system that validates the woman's own knowledge and promotes empowered healthcare decision making.

Nutrition

Nutrition assessment and counseling is a vital component of prenatal care. The woman may benefit from regularly scheduled appointments with the nutritionist during an early prenatal visit and again at 28 weeks' gestation. Additional visits with the nutritionist should be scheduled as indicated (e.g., for inadequate or excessive weight gain, anemia, metabolic disorders such as GDM). Weight-gain charts; 24-hour diet recall; or simple, self-report dietary assessment tools are valuable education resources.

Nutritional status may change because of availability of appropriate foods and financial resources for groceries. The most significant food shortages for low-income women occur at the end of the month, when federal and local resources are depleted or when food is shared among a disproportionate number of household members. Likewise, religious practices may dictate fasting during specific times of the year (e.g., Lent or

Ramadan), limiting the woman's food intake. Awareness and ongoing assessment of these factors allows for timely interventions and appropriate referral to nutrition counseling, social work, and community support services. Referrals to food and nutrition supplement programs may be warranted. Women in the United States should be referred to the Special Supplemental Feeding Program for WIC. Other supplemental food and nutrition programs are available to childbearing families on a regional or local basis. The prenatal healthcare team must be knowledgeable about such resources in their area.

Social Services

The emphasis on individualized, holistic prenatal care, encompassing physiologic and psychosocial needs, promotes a prevention-oriented model of care. Today's families may face unemployment, homelessness, chemical dependency, increased family and neighborhood violence, and lack of support systems that may precipitate crises and affect perinatal outcome. Early recognition of potential risk allows for prompt intervention and referral. The role of the perinatal social worker is critical in providing interventions that relieve stress, providing for woman's basic needs, following crisis situations, and facilitating healthcare decision making. Social work referrals are appropriate for pregnant women experiencing medical, psychological, or socioeconomic crises. Psychosocial and socioeconomic factors are evaluated on a continuing basis, with referral to social services as needed.

From a practical point of view, pregnant women have much to benefit from a team approach. The woman has access to health professionals offering expertise in a specific area, and the perinatal team may be more likely to thoroughly assess and plan for a woman's individual needs. A pregnant woman may communicate about some concern to a nutritionist or social worker regarding a problem area that she did not reveal to the physician or nurse. With professional collaboration and communication among team members, problems can be better identified and addressed.

Education and Counseling

Educational and health promotional activities that include the father (depending on his relationship with the pregnant woman) can be integrated into prenatal care. Prenatal education should focus not only on a positive labor and birth experience but, more importantly, on laying the groundwork for a successful pregnancy outcome and family experience (AWHONN, 2009). Education regarding nutrition, sexuality, stress reduction, lifestyle behaviors, and hazards in the workplace is appropriate to include in prenatal education (Display 4–8). Chapter 17 provides a comprehensive review of childbirth education.

Early identification of conditions that can affect pregnancy outcome can minimize perinatal morbidity by allowing for the establishment of an appropriate treatment plan and referrals (AAP & ACOG, 2007). Women must receive information regarding risk factors, warning signs, and criteria for provider notification. Routine prenatal care should include education to enhance recognition of warning signs of preterm labor and preeclampsia, fever, rupture of membranes or leaking of fluid, decreased fetal movement, vaginal bleeding, persistent nausea and vomiting, and signs and symptoms of viral or bacterial infection.

With current postpartum lengths of stay, it is increasingly difficult to teach the woman and family all they need to know about maternal–newborn care during hospitalization. The last trimester of pregnancy may be a potentially effective time to introduce maternal–newborn care content, including parenting issues and family planning information. Because there is no accurate way to predict which women will develop postpartum emotional disorders, all childbearing women and family members should be provided with information about postpartum depression and where to seek help.

Confidence-building strategies that promote breastfeeding are an important component of prenatal nutrition education. Providing information about breastfeeding convenience, infant benefits, and potential formula cost savings can enhance maternal motivation. Acknowledging that some women may feel embarrassed or uncomfortable about breastfeeding and providing tips for discreet breastfeeding techniques are also helpful approaches.

Maternal breastfeeding self-efficacy is a significant predictor of breastfeeding duration and level. Breastfeeding duration is significantly associated with psychological factors including dispositional optimism, breastfeeding self-efficacy, faith in breast milk, breastfeeding expectations, anxiety, planned duration of breastfeeding, and the time of the infant feeding decision (O'Brien, Buikstra, & Hegney, 2008). Self-efficacy enhancing strategies to increase a new mother's confidence in her ability to breastfeed can easily be integrated into prenatal nursing care. Chezem, Friesen, and Boettcher (2003) studied infant feeding plans and breastfeeding confidence to explore their effect on actual practices. Breastfeeding knowledge was strongly correlated with breastfeeding confidence and actual lactation duration. Expectations and the actual breastfeeding experience differed among women planning to combination feed and those planning to exclusively breastfeed. Whether as a cause or consequence, daily human milk substitute feeding was associated with negative breastfeeding outcomes (Chezem et al., 2003). Breastfeeding promotion interventions increase duration of breastfeeding (Chung, Raman, Trikalinos, Lau, & Ip, 2008). However, combining both prenatal

DISPLAY 4 – 8

Prenatal Education Topics

FIRST TRIMESTER

What to expect during prenatal care; scope of services offered in the practice which the patient is attending; anticipated schedule of visits

Healthy lifestyle

Nutrition

Dental care

Smoking cessation

Teratogen avoidance including medication use, hot tub exposure

Alcohol avoidance

Illicit drug avoidance

Seat belt use

Sexuality

Work and rest patterns

Physiologic changes of pregnancy

Emotional changes of pregnancy

Discomforts of pregnancy

Screening, diagnostic tests

Nipple assessment, breastfeeding promotion

Warning signs of pregnancy complications

Criteria and mechanism for notification of healthcare provider

(Information may be given at individual prenatal care visit or early pregnancy class)

SECOND TRIMESTER

Nutrition

Smoking cessation

Teratogen avoidance

Alcohol avoidance

Illicit drug avoidance

Prenatal laboratory tests

Physiologic changes of pregnancy

Emotional changes of pregnancy

Healthy lifestyle

Discomforts of pregnancy

Sexuality

Family roles

Fetal growth and development

Breastfeeding promotion

Childbirth education

Travel

Perineal exercises

Clothing choices/shoes

Body mechanics

Preterm birth prevention

Preeclampsia precautions/warning signs of pregnancy complications

THIRD TRIMESTER

Reproductive health; family planning

Discomforts of pregnancy

When to stop working

Where to go/who to call; physician coverage in labor and delivery

Warning signs of pregnancy complications

Fetal growth and development

Cord blood banking

Newborn care

Infant car seat use

Discussion of planned infant feeding

Childbirth education

Postpartum self-care choices

Postpartum emotional changes

Preparation for childbirth

Adapted from American Academy of Pediatrics & American College of Obstetricians and Gynecologists. (2007). *Guidelines for Perinatal Care* (6th ed.). Elk Grove, IL: Author; U.S. Department of Health and Human Services Expert Panel on the Content of Prenatal Care. (1989). *Caring for Our Future: The Content of Prenatal Care.* Washington, DC: U.S. Public Health Service.

and postnatal interventions are more effective than either prenatal or postnatal alone. Group education (peer support) is a more effective strategy to extend the duration of breastfeeding than usual prenatal care. Class information commonly given to pregnant mothers includes benefits of breastfeeding, early initiation, how breast milk is produced, hazards of bottle feeding, breastfeeding on demand, prolonged breastfeeding, family planning, and the lactational amenorrhea method. A session with the nutritionist focusing on nutrition during lactation may be helpful in encouraging initiation of breastfeeding and a successful breastfeeding experience. Chapter 20 provides an in-depth discussion about breastfeeding.

The childbearing continuum is a transition involving each family member. Childbirth education provides the opportunity for enhancement of family systems and facilitation of empowered behaviors that may last a lifetime. Over 40 years ago, the first childbirth education classes began as a means to provide information for women wishing to be awake, active participants in the birth of their child. Since then, childbirth education focusing on coping strategies for labor has been shown to decrease use of anesthesia in labor and enhance maternal confidence and satisfaction. Today, childbirth education goes well beyond basics to include information about birth as a natural process; environments that enhance the woman's ability to give birth;

care options; and, most important, the tools necessary to make informed healthcare decisions that are appropriate for individual families. Childbirth education has expanded in some centers to meet consumers' need for information concerning preconception wellness, care provider and birthing options, and maternal–newborn care during the postpartum period. Current, accurate information; effective coping skills; and intact support systems fostered by childbirth education provide families with the skills to explore alternatives and make informed decisions that are congruent with their personal goals. It is important that childbirth education is available to all women. Perinatal nurses are challenged to move childbirth education from traditional services to time frames and locations that meet consumer needs.

HEALTH PROMOTION

Preconception health promotion is increasingly recognized as an important factor influencing perinatal outcome. The addition of a prepregnancy visit and the recommended prenatal and postpartum visits has been identified as an essential step toward improving pregnancy outcomes, particularly for those planning pregnancy (CDC, 2006a). If women have not been exposed to this information before pregnancy, healthcare professionals should seize the opportunity to provide information and experiences that promote these activities during prenatal care. Awareness of reproductive risk, healthy lifestyle behaviors, and reproductive options is essential in improving pregnancy outcome. Additionally, use the interconception period to provide additional intensive interventions to women who have had a previous pregnancy that ended in an adverse outcome (e.g., infant death, fetal loss, birth defects, low birth weight, or preterm birth). Experiencing an adverse outcome in a previous pregnancy is an important predictor of future reproductive risk. However, many women with adverse pregnancy outcomes do not receive targeted interventions to reduce risks during future pregnancies (CDC, 2006a). Whereas a preterm birth is identified on birth certificates and a woman's primary care provider typically knows this information, professional guidelines do not include systematic follow-up and intervention for women with this critical predictor of risk.

SUMMARY

Prenatal care provides numerous opportunities for increasing reproductive awareness from a woman's health perspective. Aside from providing valuable information regarding the current pregnancy, laboratory evaluation also provides indicators of general health status and opportunities for health promotion. Screening tests that allow for health promotion are also offered during pregnancy. Nursing care during the prenatal period is multifaceted, requiring knowledge of the psychosocial tasks and issues surrounding the childbearing continuum, as well as knowledge of normal physiologic processes and potential risks. Anticipatory guidance during the prenatal period can have a significant impact on perinatal outcome. Education based on individual assessment empowers women and underscores their partnership in healthcare decision making. The goal of prenatal care must go a step farther than targeting a positive physical outcome. Rather, we must work toward providing care and education that facilitates holistic family wellness and the best possible outcomes for mothers and babies.

REFERENCES

Adeza Biomedical. (2005). *Fetal Fibronectin Enzyme Immunoassay and Rapid fFN for the TLi™ System: Information for Health Care Providers*. Sunnyvale, CA: Author.

Agency for Healthcare Quality. (2010). *National guideline clearinghouse: Prenatal care*. Retrieved from http://www.guidelines.gov/content.aspx?id=24138&search=prenatal+care

American Academy of Pediatrics & American College of Obstetricians and Gynecologists. (2007). *Guidelines for Perinatal Care* (6th ed.). Elk Grove Village, IL: Author.

American College of Obstetricians and Gynecologists. (1997). *Teratology* (Educational Bulletin No. 236). Washington, DC: Author.

American College of Obstetricians and Gynecologists. (1999). *Antepartum Fetal Surveillance* (Practice Bulletin No. 9). Washington, DC: Author.

American College of Obstetricians and Gynecologists. (2001a). *Gestational Diabetes* (Practice Bulletin No. 30). Washington, DC: Author.

American College of Obstetricians and Gynecologists (2001b). *Assessment of Risk Factors for Preterm Birth* (Practice Bulletin No. 31). Washington, DC: Author.

American College of Obstetricians and Gynecologists. (2002a). *Diagnosis and Management of Preeclampsia and Eclampsia* (Practice Bulletin No. 33). Washington, DC: Author.

American College of Obstetricians and Gynecologists. (2002b). *Exercise during Pregnancy and the Postpartum Period* (Committee Opinion No. 267; Reaffirmed 2009). Washington, DC: Author.

American College of Obstetricians and Gynecologists. (2005a) The importance of preconception care in the continuum of women's health care (ACOG Committee Opinion #313, September 2005; Reaffirmed 2012). *Obstetrics & Gynecology, 106*(3), 665-666.

American College of Obstetricians and Gynecologists. (2005b). *Smoking Cessation During Pregnancy* (Committee Opinion No. 316). Washington, DC: Author.

American College of Obstetricians and Gynecologists. (2006). *Psychosocial Risk Factors: Perinatal Screening and Intervention* (Committee Opinion No. 343). Washington, DC: Author.

American College of Obstetricians and Gynecologists. (2007). *Management of Herpes in Pregnancy* (Practice Bulletin No. 31). *Obstetrics & Gynecology, 109*(6), 1489–1498.

American College of Obstetricians and Gynecologists. (2008). *Prenatal and Perinatal Human Immunodeficiency Virus Testing: Expanded Recommendations for Fetal Chromosomal Abnormalities* (Committee Opinion No. 418; Reaffirmed 2011). Washington, DC: Author.

American College of Obstetricians and Gynecologists. (2011). *Vitamin D: Screening and Supplementation During Pregnancy* (Committee Opinion No. 495). Washington, DC: Author.

American Dietetic Association. (2008). Position of the American Dietetic Association: Nutrition and lifestyle for a healthy pregnancy outcome. *Journal of the American Dietetic Association, 108*, 553–561.

Artal, R., & O'Toole, M. (2003). Guidelines of the American College of Obstetricians and Gynecologists for exercise during pregnancy and the postpartum period. *British Journal of Sports Medicine, 37*(1), 6–12. doi:10.1136/bjsm.37.1.6

Association of Women's Health, Obstetric and Neonatal Nurses. (2000). *Smoking and Childbearing* (Clinical Position Statement). Washington, DC: Author.

Association of Women's Health, Obstetric and Neonatal Nurses. (2004). *Response to the U.S. Preventive Services Task Force Report on Screening for Family and Intimate Partner Violence Published in the March 2 Annals of Internal Medicine*. Washington, DC: Author.

Association of Women's Health, Obstetric and Neonatal Nurses. (2009). *Standards and Guidelines for Professional Nursing Practice in the Care of Women and Newborns* (7th ed.). Washington, DC: Author.

Ayoola, A. B., Nettleman, M., Stommel, M., & Canady, R. B. (2010). Time of pregnancy recognition and prenatal care use: A population-based study in the United States. *Birth, 37*(1), 37–43. doi:10.1111/j.1523-536X.2009.00376.x

Ayoola, A. B., Stommel, M., & Nettleman, M. (2009). Late recognition of pregnancy as a predictor of adverse birth outcomes. *American Journal of Obstetrics & Gynecology, 201*, 156e1–156e6.

Barak, S., Oettinger-Barak, O., Oettinger, M., Machtei, E. E., Peled, M., & Ohel, G. (2003). Common oral manifestations during pregnancy: A review. *Obstetrical and Gynecological Survey, 58*(9), 624–628.

Beck, C. T. (2008). State of the science on postpartum depression—What nurse researchers have contributed: Part 1. *MCN: The American Journal of Maternal/Child Nursing, 33*(2), 121–126. doi:10.1097/01.NMC.0000313421.97236.cf

Bellinger, D. C. (2005). Teratogen update: Lead and pregnancy. *Birth Defects Research, 73*(6), 409–420. doi:10.1002/bdra.20127

Bennett, T., Braveman, P., Egerter, S., & Kiely, J. L. (1994). Maternal marital status as a risk factor for infant mortality. *Family Planning Perspectives, 26*(6), 252–256, 271.

Bodnar, L. M., Catov, J. M., Simhan, H. N., Holick, M. F., Powers, R. W., & Roberts, J. M. (2007). Maternal vitamin D deficiency increases risk of pre-eclampsia. *Journal of Clinical Endocrinology & Metabolism, 92*(9), 3517–3522. doi:10.1210/jc.2007-0718

Boggess, K. A. (2005). Pathophysiology of preterm birth: Emerging concepts of maternal infection. *Clinics in Perinatology, 32*(3), 561–569. doi:10.1016/j.clp.2005.05.002

Bunevicius, R., Kusminskas, L., Bunevicius, A., Nadisauskiene, R. J., Jureniene, K., & Pop, V. J. (2009). Psychosocial risk factors for depression during pregnancy. *Acta Obstetricia et Gynecologica Scandinavica, 88*(5), 599–605. doi:10.1002/da.20276

Carolan, M. (2009). Towards understanding the concept of risk for pregnant women: Some nursing and midwifery implications. *Journal of Clinical Nursing, 18*(5), 652–658. doi:10.1111/j.1365-2702.2008.02480.x

Centers for Disease Control and Prevention. (2000). Entry into prenatal care—United States, 1989–1997. *Morbidity and Mortality Weekly Report, 49*(18), 393–398.

Centers for Disease Control and Prevention. (2002). Screening tests to detect chlamydia trachomatis and Neisseria gonorrhoeae infections—2002. *Morbidity and Mortality Weekly Report, 51*(RR-15), 1.

Centers for Disease Control and Prevention. (2006a). Recommendations to improve preconception health and health care—United States: A report of the CDC/ATSDR preconception care work group and the select panel on preconception care. *Morbidity and Mortality Weekly Report Recommendations and Reports, 55*(RR 06), 1–23.

Centers for Disease Control and Prevention. (2006b). *Intimate partner violence: Fact sheet*. Retrieved from http://www.cdc.gov/violenceprevention/pdf/ipv-factsheet-a.pdf

Centers for Disease Control and Prevention. (2008). Update on overall prevalence of major birth defects—Atlanta, Georgia, 1978–2005. *Morbidity and Mortality Weekly Report Recommendations and Reports, 57*(1), 1–6

Centers for Disease Control and Prevention. (2009). *HIV in women*. Retrieved from http://www.cdc.gov/hiv/topics/women/

Chasnoff, I. J., Wells, A. M., McGourty, R. F., & Bailey, L. K. (2007). Validation of the 4P's Plus screen for substance use in pregnancy validation of the 4P's Plus. *Journal of Perinatology, 27*(12), 744–748. doi:10.1038/sj.jp.7211823

Chezem, J., Friesen, C., & Boettcher, J. (2003). Breastfeeding knowledge, breastfeeding confidence, and infant feeding plans: Effects on actual feeding practices. *Journal of Obstetric, Gynecologic, and Neonatal Nursing, 32*(1), 40–47. doi:10.1177/0884217502239799

Chung, M., Raman, G., Trikalinos, T., Lau, J., & Ip, S. (2008). Interventions in primary care to promote breastfeeding: An evidence review for the U.S. Preventive Services Task Force. *Annals of Internal Medicine, 149*, 565–582.

Coker, A., Smith, P., McKeown, R., & King, M. (2000). Frequency and correlates of intimate partner violence by type: Physical, sexual, and psychological battering. *American Journal Public Health, 90*(4), 553–559. doi:10.2105/AJPH.90.4.533

Cooperstock, M. S., Bakewell, J., Herman, A., & Schramm, W. F. (1998). Effects of fetal sex and race on risk of very preterm birth in twins. *American Journal of Obstetrics & Gynecology, 179*(3, Pt. 1), 762–765.

Corbett, R. W., Ryan, C., & Weinrich, S. P. (2003). Pica in pregnancy: Does it affect pregnancy outcomes? *MCN: The American Journal of Maternal Child Nursing, 28*(3), 183–191.

Cunningham, F. G., Leveno, K. J., Bloom, S. L., Hauth, J. C., Rouse, D. J., & Spong, C. Y. (2010). *William's Obstetrics* (23rd ed.). New York: McGraw-Hill. Retrieved from http://www.accessmedicine.com/content.aspx?aID=6052072

de Jong, E. P., Walther, F. J., Kroes, A. C., & Oepkes, D. (2011). Parvovirus B19 infection in pregnancy: New insights and management. *Prenatal Diagnosis, 31*(5), 419–425. doi:10.1002/pd.2714

Denney, J. M. & Culhane, J. (2009). Bacterial vaginosis: A problematic infection from both a perinatal and neonatal perspective. *Seminars In Fetal & Neonatal Medicine, 14*(4), 200–203. doi:10.1016/j.siny.2009.01.008

Denny, C. H., Tsai, J., Floyd, R. L., & Green, P. P. (2009). Alcohol use among pregnant and nonpregnant women of childbearing age—United States, 1991–2005. *Morbidity and Mortality Weekly Report Recommendations and Reports, 58*, 529–532.

Dijkmans, A. C., de Jong, E. P., Lopriore, E., Vossen, A., Walther, F. J., & Oepkes, D. (2012). Parvovirus B19 in pregnancy: Prenatal diagnosis and management of fetal complications. *Current Opinion in Obstetrics & Gynecology, 24*(2), 95–101. doi:10.1097/GCO.0b013e3283505a9d

Dowswell, T., Carroli, G., Duley, L., Gates, S., Gülmezoglu, A. M., Khan-Neelofur, D., & Piaggio, G. G. (2010). Alternative versus standard packages of antenatal care for low-risk pregnancy. *Cochrane Database Systematic Reviews, 10*, CD000934.

Dugoff, L., Hobbins, J. C., Malone, F. D., Vidaver, J., Sullivan, L., Canick, J. A., . . . D'Aton M. E. (2005). FASTER Trial Research Consortium. Quad screen as a predictor of adverse pregnancy outcome. *Obstetrics and Gynecology, 106*(2), 260–267. doi:10.1097/01.AOG.0000172419.37410.eb

Feetham, S., Thomson, E. J., & Hinshaw, A. S. (2005). Nursing leadership in genomics for health and society. *Journal of Nursing Scholarship, 37*(2), 102–110. doi:10.1111/j.1547-5069.2005.00021.x

Florida Department of Health. (1997). Florida's Healthy Start Prenatal Risk Screening Instrument. Tallahassee, FL: Florida Department of Health.

Gaynes, B. N., Gavin, N., Meltzer-Brody, S., Lohr, K. N., Swinson, T., Gartlehner, G., . . . Miller, W. C. (2005). *Perinatal depression: Prevalence, screening accuracy, and screening outcomes* (Summary, Evidence Report/Technology Assessment No. 119; AHRQ Publication No. 05-E006–1). Rockville, MD: Agency for Healthcare Research and Quality. Retrieved from http://www.ahrq.gov/clinic/epcsums/peridepsum.htm#Contents

Gray, K. A., Day, N. L., Leech, S., & Richardson, G. A. (2005). Prenatal marijuana exposure: Effect on child depressive symptoms at ten years of age. *Neurotoxicology Teratology, 27*(3), 439–448. doi:org/10.1016/j.ntt.2005.03.010

Heegaard, E. D., & Brown, K. E. (2002). Human parvovirus B19. *Clinical Microbiology Review, 15*(3), 485–505. doi:10.1128/CMR.15.3.485-505.2002

Hein, H. A., Burmeister, L. F., & Papke, K. R. (1990). The relationship of unwed status to infant mortality. *Obstetrics & Gynecology, 76*(5, Pt. l)., 763–768.

Hook, E. B. (1981). Rates of chromosome abnormalities at different maternal ages. *Obstetrics and Gynecology, 58*, 282–285.

Huang, L., Sauve, R., Birkett, N., Fergusson, D., & van Walraven, C. (2008). Maternal age and risk of stillbirth: A systematic review. *Canadian Medical Association Journal, 178*(2), 165–172. doi:10.1503/cmaj.070150

Huizink, A. C., & Mulder, E. J. (2006). Maternal smoking, drinking or cannabis use during pregnancy and neurobehavioral and cognitive functioning in human offspring. *Neuroscience Biobehavioral Review, 30*(1), 24–41, doi:10.1016/j.neubiorev.2005.04.005

Hyde, T. B., Schmid, D. S., & Cannon, M. J. (2010). Cytomegalovirus seroconversion rates and risk factors: Implications for congenital CMV. *Reviews in Medical Virology, 20*(5), 311–326. doi:10.1002/rmv.659

Ickovics, J. R., Kershaw, T. S., Westdahl, C., Magriples, U., Massey, Z., Reynolds, H., & Rising, S. S. (2007). Group prenatal care and perinatal outcomes. *Obstetrics and Gynecology, 110*(1, Pt. 2), 330–339. doi:10.1097/01.AOG.0000270153.59102.40

Institute for Clinical Systems Improvement. (2010). Routine prenatal care. *Institute for Clinical Systems Improvement (ICSI)*.

Institute of Medicine. (2009). *Weight Gain During Pregnancy: Reexamining the Guidelines*. Washington, DC: National Academy Press. Retrieved from http://www.iom.edu/Reports/2009/Weight-Gain-During-Pregnancy-Reexamining-the-Guidelines.aspx

Jeffcoat, M., Parry, S., Sammel, M., Clothier, B., Catlin, A., & Macones, G. (2010). Periodontal infection and preterm birth: Successful periodontal therapy reduces the risk of preterm birth. *British Journal of Obstetrics & Gynecology, 118*, 250–256. doi:10.1111/j.1471-0528.2010.02713.x. Advance online publication.

Jesse, D. E., & Graham, M. (2005). Are you often sad and depressed? Brief measures to identify women at risk for depression in pregnancy. *MCN: The American Journal of Maternal Child Nursing, 30*(1), 40–45.

Kanungo, J., James, A., McMillan, D., Lodha, A., Faucher, D., Lee, S., & Shah, P. (2011). Advanced maternal age and the outcomes of preterm neonates: A social paradox? *Obstetrics & Gynecology, 118*(4), 872–877. doi:10.1097/AOG.0b013e31822add60

Kennedy, H., Farrell, T., Paden, R., Hill, S., Jolivet, R., Cooper, B., & Rising, S. (2011). A randomized clinical trial of group prenatal care in two military settings. *Military Medicine, 176*, 1169–1177.

Khader, Y. S., & Ta'ani, Q. (2005). Periodontal diseases and the risk of preterm birth and low birth weight: A meta-analysis. *Journal of Periodontology, 76*(1), 161–165. doi:10.1902/jop.2005.76.2.161

Kiely, M., El-Mohandes, A. A., El-Khorazaty, M. N., & Gantz, M. G. (2010). An integrated intervention to reduce intimate partner violence in pregnancy: A randomized controlled trial. *Obstetrics & Gynecology, 115*(2, Pt. 1), 273–283. doi:10.1097/AOG.0b013e3181cbd482

Kirkham, C., Harris, S., & Grzybowski, J. (2005). Evidence based prenatal care: Part I. General prenatal care and counseling issues. *American Family Physician, 71*(7), 1307–1316.

Krulewitch, C. J. (2005). Alcohol consumption during pregnancy. *Annual Review of Nursing Research, 23*(1), 101–134.

Lancaster, C., Gold, K., Flynn, H., Yoo, H., Marcus, S., & Davis, M. (2010). Risk factors for depressive symptoms during pregnancy: A systematic review. *American Journal of Obstetrics and Gynecology, 202*(1), 5–14. doi:10.1016/j.ajog.2009.09.007

Larrabee, K., & Cowan, M. (1995). Clinical nursing management of sickle cell disease and trait during pregnancy. *Journal of Perinatal and Neonatal Nursing, 9*(2), 29–41.

Lewis, C. T., Matthews, T. J., & Heuser, R. L. (1996). Prenatal care in the United States, 1980–94. *Vital and Health Statistics, 21*, 117.

Luo, Z. C., Wilkins, R., & Kramer, M. S. (2004). Disparities in pregnancy outcomes according to marital and cohabitation status. *Obstetrics and Gynecology, 103*(6), 1300–1307.

March of Dimes. (2011a). *Toward Improving the Outcome of Pregnancy III*. White Plains, NY: March of Dimes Birth Defects Foundation.

March of Dimes. (2011b). *Peristats*. White Plains, NY: March of Dimes Birth Defects Foundation.

Markovitz, B. P., Cook, R., Flick, L. H., & Leet, T. L. (2005). Socioeconomic factors and adolescent pregnancy outcomes: Distinctions between neonatal and post-neonatal deaths? *BMC Public Health, 5*, 79. doi:10.1186/1471-2458-5-79

Martin, J. A., Hamilton, B. E., Sutton, P. D., Ventura, S. J., Menacker, F., & Kirmeyer, S. (2006). Births: Final data for 2004. *National Vital Statistics Reports, 55*(1), 1–102.

Martin, J. A., Osterman, M., & Sutton, P. D. (2010). *Are preterm births on the decline in the United States?* (NCHS Data Brief 39). Hyattsville, MD: National Center for Health Statistics. Retrieved from http://www.cdc.gov/nchs/data/databriefs/db39.htm

Massey, S. H., Lieberman, D. Z., Reiss, D., Leve, L. D., Shaw, D. S., & Neiderhiser, J. M. (2011). Association of clinical characteristics and cessation of tobacco, alcohol, and illicit drug use during pregnancy. *The American Journal on Addictions, 20*, 143–150. doi:10.1111/j.1521-0391.2010.00110.x

Mathews, T. J., & MacDorman, M. F. (2010). Infant mortality statistics from the 2006 period linked birth/infant death data set. *National Vital Statistics Reports: From The Centers of Disease Control and Prevention, National Center For Health Statistics, National Vital Statistics System, 58*(17), 1–31.

Mathews, T. J., MacDorman, M. F., & Menacker, F. (2002). Infant mortality statistics from the 1999 period linked birth/infant death data set. *National Vital Statistics Reports, 50*, 1–28.

Mattison, D. R. (2010). Environmental exposures and development. *Current Opinion in Pediatrics, 22*(2), 208–218. doi:10.1097/MOP.0b013e32833779bf

Menato, G., Bo, S., Signorile, A., Gallo, M., Cotrino, I., Poala, C. B., . . . Massobrio, M. (2008). Current management of gestational diabetes mellitus. *Expert Review of Obstetrics & Gynecology, 3*(1), 73–91. doi:10.1586/17474108.3.1.73

Merewood, A., Mehta, S. D., Chen, T. C., Bauchner, H., & Holick, M. F. (2009). Association between vitamin D deficiency and primary cesarean section. *Journal of Clinical Endocrinology and Metabolism, 94*(3), 940–945. doi:10.1210/jc.2008-1217

Mitchell, A. A., Gilboa, S. M., Werler, M. M., Kelley, K. E., Louik, C., & Hernandez-Diaz, S. (2011). Medication use during pregnancy, with particular focus on prescription drugs: 1976–2008. *American Journal of Obstetrics and Gynecology, 205*(1), 51.e1–51.e8. doi:10.1016/j.ajog.2011.02.029

Moore, T. R., & Piacquadio, K. (1989). A prospective evaluation of fetal movement screening to reduce the incidence of antepartum fetal death. *American Journal of Obstetrics and Gynecology, 160*(5, Pt. 1), 1075–1080. doi:10.1016/0002-9378(89)90164-6

Morrical-Kline, K. A., Walton, A. M., & Guildenbacher, T. M. (2011). Teratogen use in women of childbearing potential: An intervention study. *The Journal of the American Board of Family Medicine, 24*(3), 262–271. doi:10.3122/jabfm.2011.03.100198

Mozurkewich, E. L., Luke, B., Avni, M., & Wolf, F. M. (2000). Working conditions and adverse pregnancy outcome: A meta-analysis. *Obstetrics and Gynecology, 95*(4), 623–635.

National Institute of Health. (2011, September). *Panel on treatment of HIV-infected pregnant women and prevention of perinatal transmission. Recommendations for use of antiretroviral drugs in pregnant HIV-1-infected women for maternal health and interventions to reduce perinatal HIV transmission in the United States.* Retrieved from http://aidsinfo.nih.gov/contentfiles/PerinatalGL.pdf

Nursing Network on Violence Against Women, International. (2003). *Abuse assessment screen.* Retrieved from http://www.nnvawi.org/assessment.htm

O'Brien, M., Buikstra, E., & Hegney, D. (2008). The influence of psychological factors on breastfeeding duration. *Journal of Advanced Nursing, 63*(4), 397–408. doi:10.1111/j.1365-2648.2008.04775.x

Olson, C. M. (2008). Achieving a healthy weight gain during pregnancy. *Annual Review of Nutrition, 28,* 411–423.

Papiernik, E. (1993). Prevention of preterm labor and delivery. *Balliere's Clinical Obstetrics and Gynecology, 7*(3), 499–521. doi:10.1016/S0950-3552(05)80446-8

Patel, C., Edgerton, L., & Flake, D. (2006). What precautions should we use with statins for women of childbearing age? *Journal of Family Practice, 55*(1), 75–77.

Peaceman, A. M., Andrews, W. W., Thorp, J. M., Cliver, S. P., Lukes, A., Iams, J. D., . . . Pietrantoni, M. (1997). Fetal fibronectin as a predictor of preterm birth in patients with symptoms: A multicenter trial. *American Journal of Obstetrics and Gynecology, 177*(1), 13–18.

Pereira, A., Bos, S., Marques, M., Maia, B., Soares, M., Valente, J., . . . Azevedo, M. (2011). The postpartum depression screening scale: Is it valid to screen for antenatal depression? *Archives of Women's Mental Health, 14,* 227–238.

Perinatal HIV Guidelines Workgroup. (2008). *Public Health Service Task Force recommendations for use of antiretroviral drugs in pregnant HIV infected women for maternal health and interventions to reduce perinatal HIV transmission in the United States.* Retrieved from http://aidsinfo,nih.gov/ContentFiles/PerinatalGL.pdf

Pignone, M. P., Gaynes, B. N., Rushton, J. L., Burchell, C. M., Orleans, C. T., Mulrow, C. D., . . . Lohr, K. N. (2002). Screening for depression in adults: A summary of the evidence for the U.S. Preventive Services Task Force. *Annals of Internal Medicine, 136*(10), 765–776.

Raatikainen, K., Heiskanen, N., & Heinonen, S. (2005). Marriage still protects pregnancy. *British Journal of Obstetrics and Gynaecology, 112*(10), 1411–1416. doi:10.1111/j.1471-0528.2005.00667.x

Raatikainen, K., Heiskanen, N., Verkasalo, P., & Heinonen, S. (2006). Good outcome of teenage pregnancies in high-quality maternity care. *European Journal of Public Health, 16*(2), 157–161. doi:10.1093/eurpub/cki158

Rahman, A., Bunn, J., Lovel, H., & Creed, F. (2007). Association between antenatal depression and low birthweight in a developing country. *Acta Psychiatria Scandinavia, 115,* 481–486. doi:10.1111/j.1600-0447.2006.00950.x

Ribot, B., Aranda, F., Viteri, F., Hernandez-Martinez, C., Canals, J., & Arija, V. (2012). Depleted iron stores without anemia early in pregnancy carries increased risk of lower birthweight even when supplemented daily with moderate iron. *Human Reproduction, 27*(5), 1260–1266. doi:10.1093/humrep/des026

Rising, S. S. (1998). Centering pregnancy. An interdisciplinary model of empowerment. *Journal of Nurse Midwifery, 43*(1), 46–54. doi:10.1016/S0091-2182(97)00117-1

Rising, S., Kennedy, H., & Klima, C. (2004). Redesigning prenatal care through Centering Pregnancy. *Journal of Midwifery & Women's Health, 49*(5), 398–404. doi:10.1111/j.1542-2011.2004.tb04433.x

Sanchez-Ramos, L., Delke, I., Zamora, J., Kaunitz, A. M. (2009). Fetal fibronectin as a short-term predictor of preterm birth in symptomatic patients: A meta-analysis. *Obstetrics & Gynecology, 114*(3), 631–640. doi:10.1097/AOG.0b013e3181b47217

Seidel, H. M., Ball, J. W., Dains, J. E., Flynn, J. A., Solomon, B. S., & Stewart, R. W. (2010). *Mosby's Guide to Physical Examination* (6th ed.). Philadelphia: CV Mosby.

Shieh, C., & Carter, A. (2011). Online prenatal nutrition education. *Nursing for Women's Health, 15*(1), 27–35. doi:10.1111/j.1751-486X.2011.01608.x

Sibai, B. M. (2005). Diagnosis, prevention, and management of pre-eclampsia. *Obstetrics & Gynecology, 105*(2), 402–410. doi:10.1097/01.AOG.0000152351.13671.99

Silver, R. M. (2007). Fetal death. *Obstetrics and Gynecology, 109*(1), 153–167. doi:10.1097/01.AOG.0000248537.89739.96

Simmons, L. A., Havens, J. R., Whiting, J. B., Holz, J. L., & Bada, H. (2009). Illicit drug use among women with children in the United States: 2002–2003. *Annals of Epidemiology, 19,* 187–193. doi:10.1016/j.annepidem.2008.12.007

Sweet, R., & Gibbs, R. (2009). *Infectious Diseases of the Female Genital Tract.* Philadelphia: Lippincott Williams & Wilkins.

Tjaden, P., &. Thoennes, T. (2000). *Extent, Nature, and Consequences of Intimate Partner Violence.* Washington, DC: National Institute of Justice. Retrieved from http://www.ncjrs.gov/txtfiles1/nij/181867.txt

Tong, V. T., Jones, J. R., Dietz, P. M., D'Angelo, D., & Bombard, J. M. (2009). Trends in smoking before, during, and after pregnancy—Pregnancy Risk Assessment Monitoring System (PRAMS), United States, 31 sites, 2000–2005. *Morbidity and Mortality Weekly Report Recommendations and Reports, 29*(58), 1–29.

UpToDate. (2012). *Substance use in pregnancy.* Retrieved from http://www.uptodate.com/contents/substance-use-in-pregnancy?source=search_result&search=substance+use+in+pregnancy&selectedTitle=1~150

U.S. Department of Health and Human Services. (2010). *Healthy People 2020: Understanding and Improving Health* (2nd ed.). Washington, DC: U.S. Government Printing Office.

U.S. Department of Health and Human Services Expert Panel on the Content of Prenatal Care. (1989). *Caring for our Future: The Content of Prenatal Care.* Washington, DC: United States Public Health Service.

U.S. Environmental Protection Agency. (2004). *What you need to know about mercury in fish and shellfish.* Retrieved from www.epa.gov/waterscience/fish/advice/

U.S. Preventive Services Task Force. (2005). *Screening for HIV.* Available at: http://www.uspreventiveservicestaskforce.org/uspstf05/hiv/hivrs.htm

U.S. Preventive Services Task Force. (2009). Counseling and interventions to prevent tobacco use and tobacco-caused disease in adults and pregnant women: U.S. Preventive Services Task Force reaffirmation recommendation statement. *Annals of Internal Medicine, 150,* 551–555.

Van den Bergh, B. R., Mulder, E. J., Mennes, M., & Glover, V. (2005). Antenatal maternal anxiety and stress and the neurobehavioral development of the fetus and child: Links and possible mechanisms. A review. *Neuroscience Biobehavioral Review, 29*(2), 237–258. doi:10.1016/j.neubiorev.2004.10.007

Williams, J. K., & Lea, D. H. (2003). *Genetic Issues for Perinatal Nurses* (Nursing Module; 2nd ed.). White Plains, NY: March of Dimes Birth Defects Foundation.

World Health Organization. (2006). *Definition and Diagnosis of Diabetes Mellitus and Intermediate Hyperglycemia.* Author. Geneva, Switzerland

Xiong, X., Buekens, P., Fraser, W. D., Beck, J., & Offenbacher, S. (2006). Periodontal disease and adverse pregnancy outcomes: A systematic review. *BJOG: An International Journal of Obstetrics and Gynaecology, 113*(2), 135–143. doi:10.1111/j.1471-0528.2005.00827.x

Yost, N. P., Bloom, S. L., McIntire, D. D., & Leveno, K. J. (2005). A prospective observational study of domestic violence during pregnancy. *Obstetrics and Gynecology, 106*(1), 61–65. doi: 10.1097/01.AOG.0000164468.06070.2a

Young, S. L. (2010). Pica in pregnancy: New ideas about an old condition. *Annual Review of Nutrition, 30,* 403–422. doi:10.1146/annurev.nutr.012809.104713

APPENDIX 4 – A

Vaccines and Immune Globulin During Pregnancy

RECOMMENDED VACCINES DURING PREGNANCY

Influenza

Recommended for all women regardless of stage of pregnancy.

CONTRAINDICATED/NOT RECOMMENDED VACCINES IN PREGNANCY

Anthrax	BCG measles	Mumps
Rubella	Varicella	Yellow fever
Zoster		

RISK VS. BENEFIT: NOT ROUTINELY RECOMMENDED EXCEPT IN PERSONS AT INCREASED RISK OF EXPOSURE

Polio	Plague	Typhoid

CONTRAINDICATED BUT NO ADVERSE OUTCOMES REPORTED IF GIVEN IN PREGNANCY

Varicella

INDICATIONS FOR VACCINE THAT ARE NOT ALTERED BY PREGNANCY

Cholera	Pneumococcus
Hepatitis A	Rabies
Hepatitis B	Tetanus-diphtheria
Meningococcus	

INDICATED FOR IMMUNOGLOBULINS AS POSTEXPOSURE PROPHYLAXIS

Hepatitis A	Rabies
Hepatitis B	Tetanus
Measles	Varicella

Adapted from American College of Obstetricians and Gynecologists. (2009). *Update on Immunization and Pregnancy: Tetanus, Diptheria, and Pertussis Vaccination* (Committee Opinion No. 438). Washington, DC: Author; American College of Obstetrician and Gynecologists. (2010). *Influenza Vaccination During Pregnancy* (Committee Opinion No. 468). Washington, DC: Author; Centers for Disease Control and Prevention. (2007). *Guidelines for vaccinating pregnant women.* Retrieved from http://www.cdc.gov/vaccines/pubs/preg-guide.htm

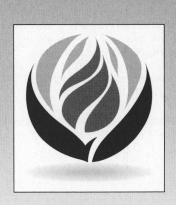

Judith H. Poole

CHAPTER 5

Hypertensive Disorders of Pregnancy

Hypertension is a common medical complication of pregnancy and a leading cause of maternal morbidity and mortality. The woman may present with hypertension that predates her pregnancy or be diagnosed for the first time after the pregnancy is established. Regardless of when the diagnosis is made, it is important for the healthcare provider to recognize that the hypertensive disorders of pregnancy are part of a spectrum of diagnoses. This spectrum of diagnoses is categorized by the gestational age at the onset of hypertension and the presence of proteinuria. This chapter will discuss the current terminology for the diagnosis of hypertension during pregnancy, common risk factors, pathophysiology, and management. Assessment of maternal–fetal status and implications for the perinatal nurse are included.

CLASSIFICATION AND DEFINITIONS

Terminology used to describe the hypertensive disorders of pregnancy has suffered from imprecise usage, causing confusion for healthcare providers caring for women with hypertensive complications during pregnancy, childbirth, and postpartum. *The National High Blood Pressure Education Program Working Group Report on High Blood Pressure in Pregnancy*, published through the National Institutes of Health and the National Heart, Lung, and Blood Institute, outlines current accepted terminology for the hypertensive disorders of pregnancy (National High Blood Pressure Education Program [NHBPEP], 2000; NHBPEP Working Group, 2000). See Table 5–1 for the current classification of hypertension in pregnancy. The American College of Obstetricians and Gynecologists (ACOG) published a practice bulletin in 2002, reaffirmed in 2008, on the diagnosis and management of preeclampsia endorsing the new classification scheme. Clinically, there are two basic types of hypertension during pregnancy: chronic hypertension and gestational hypertension. The distinction is based on the gestational age at onset of the disease and the presence of proteinuria.

CHRONIC HYPERTENSION

Chronic hypertension is hypertension present and observable before the pregnancy, diagnosed before 20 weeks' gestation, or hypertension continuing beyond the 12th week postpartum (ACOG, 2012; NHBPEP, 2000; NHBPEP Working Group, 2000). Hypertension is defined as a systolic blood pressure equal to or greater than 140 mm Hg or a diastolic blood pressure equal to or greater than 90 mm Hg (ACOG, 2012; NHBPEP, 2000; NHBPEP Working Group, 2000). Hypertension is diagnosed when either value is above the defined values; elevation of both systolic and diastolic pressures is not necessary for the diagnosis. The severity of hypertension is determined by the higher value, even if the other value is within normal parameters.

GESTATIONAL HYPERTENSION

Gestational hypertension is the onset of hypertension, generally after the 20th week of gestation, in a previously normotensive woman, appearing as a marker of a pregnancy-specific vasospastic condition (Roberts & Funai, 2008). Gestational hypertension in clinical practice is a retrospective diagnosis. If hypertension is first diagnosed during pregnancy, is transient, does not progress into preeclampsia, and the woman is normotensive by 12 weeks postpartum, the diagnosis is gestational hypertension; if the blood pressure elevation persists, then the

Table 5-1. CLASSIFICATION OF HYPERTENSIVE DISORDERS OF PREGNANCY

Type of Hypertension	Diagnostic Criteria	Significance

Gestational hypertension	• New onset of hypertension, generally after 20 weeks of gestation
	• Hypertension defined as:
	  ○ SBP ≥140 mm Hg, *OR*
	  ○ DBP ≥90 mm Hg
	• Absence of proteinuria
		• Replaces pregnancy-induced hypertension
		• A retrospective diagnosis
		• BP normalizes to prepregnancy values by 12 weeks' postpartum
		• Think oxygenation and perfusion

Preeclampsia	• Gestational hypertension plus gestational proteinuria in a previously normotensive woman before 20 weeks of gestation
	• Gestational proteinuria defined as
	  ○ >300 mg on random specimen
	  ○ ≥1+ on dipstick
		• In absence of proteinuria, suspect if any of the following are present:
		  ○ Headache
		  ○ Blurred vision
		  ○ Abdominal pain
		  ○ Abnormal laboratory tests

Severe preeclampsia	• Diagnosis of preeclampsia plus at least one of the following:
	  ○ SBP ≥160 mm Hg
	  ○ DBP ≥110 mm Hg
	  ○ Proteinuria >2 g/24 hr
	  ○ Serum creatinine >1.2 mg/dL
	  ○ Platelets <100,000
	  ○ ↑ LD (hemolysis)
	  ○ ↑ ALT or AST
	  ○ Persistent headache or cerebral/visual disturbances
	  ○ Persistent epigastric pain
		• One of sickest patients on unit
		• At increased risk for complications
		• Additional criteria for diagnosis may include:
		  ○ Oliguria defined as <500 mL/24 hr
		  ○ Pulmonary edema
		  ○ Impaired liver function of unclear etiology
		  ○ IUGR
		  ○ Oligohydramnios
		  ○ Grand mal seizures (eclampsia)

HELLP syndrome	• Diagnosis based on presence of:
	  ○ Hemolysis
	  ○ Elevated liver enzymes
	  ○ Low platelets
	• Hemolysis
	  ○ Abnormal peripheral smear
	  ○ LD >600 U/L
	  ○ Total bilirubin ≥1.2 mg/dL
	• Elevated liver enzymes
	  ○ Serum aspartate aminotransferase >70 U/L
	  ○ LD >600 U/L
	• Low platelets <150,000
		• Form of severe preeclampsia
		• Laboratory diagnosis
		• Impairs oxygenation and perfusion
		• Severity of disease, morbidity/mortality, and recovery related to platelet levels
		  ○ <150,000 but >100,000
		  ○ <100,000 but >50,000
		  ○ <50,000

Eclampsia	• Diagnosis of preeclampsia
	• Occurrence of seizures
	• No other possible etiology for seizure
		• Critically ill patient
		• At risk for cerebral hemorrhage, aspiration, or death
		• Foley's Rule of 13:
		  ○ 13% mortality
		  ○ 13% abruption
		  ○ 13% seize after MgSO4 therapy
		  ○ 13% seize >48 hr postpartum

Chronic hypertension	• Hypertension defined as:
	  ○ SBP ≥140 mm Hg, *OR*
	  ○ DBP ≥90 mm Hg
	• Hypertension
	  ○ Present and observable before pregnancy
	  ○ Diagnosed before 20 weeks' gestation
	  ○ Persists beyond 12 weeks' postpartum
		• Diagnosis may not be known prior to pregnancy
		• Places pregnancy at increased risk for abruption

Superimposed preeclampsia	• Diagnosis based on presence of one or more of the following in the woman with chronic hypertension:
	  ○ New onset of proteinuria
	  ○ Hypertension and proteinuria before 20th week of gestation
	  ○ Sudden ↑ in proteinuria
	  ○ Sudden ↑ BP (previously well controlled)
	  ○ ↑ ALT or AST to abnormal levels
	  ○ Thrombocytopenia
		• Prognosis worse for woman and fetus
		• Mandates close observation
		• Timing of birth indicated by overall assessment of maternal–fetal well-being rather than fixed end point

ALT, alanine aminotransferase; AST, aspartate aminotransferase; DBP, diastolic blood pressure; IUGR, intrauterine growth restriction; LD, lactate dehydrogenase; SBP, systolic blood pressure; U/L, Units per liter.

Adapted from American College of Obstetricians and Gynecologists. (2002). *Diagnosis and Management of Preeclampsia and Eclampsia* (Practice Bulletin No. 33; Reaffirmed 2008). Washington, DC: Author. Retrieved from http://mail.ny.acog.org/website/SMIPodcast/DiagnosisMgt.pdf; National High Blood Pressure Education Program. (2000). *National High Blood Pressure Education Program Working Group Report on High Blood Pressure in Pregnancy* (NIH Publication No. 00-3029). Bethesda, MD: National Institute of Health; National Heart, Lung, and Blood Institute; and National High Blood Pressure Education Program; National High Blood Pressure Education Program Working Group. (2000). Report of the National High Blood Pressure Education Program Working Group on high blood pressure in pregnancy. *American Journal of Obstetrics and Gynecology, 183*(1), S1–S22. doi:10.1067/mob.2000.107928

diagnosis is chronic hypertension (NHBPEP, 2000; NHBPEP Working Group, 2000). These two types of hypertension (chronic hypertension and gestational hypertension) may occur independently or simultaneously.

Once gestational hypertension is present, hypertension is further classified according to the maternal organ systems affected. The practitioner must keep in mind that hypertension during pregnancy represents a continuum of disease processes. Hypertension may be the first sign, but the underlying pathophysiology can involve all major organ systems.

PREECLAMPSIA

Preeclampsia is characterized by renal involvement, as evidenced by the onset of proteinuria. It must be remembered that preeclampsia is a pregnancy-specific syndrome of reduced organ perfusion, including the utero–placental–fetal unit, secondary to cyclic vasospasms and activation of the coagulation cascade (NHBPEP, 2000; NHBPEP Working Group, 2000). The disease process is said to be mild or severe on the basis of maternal or fetal findings. If signs and symptoms of preeclampsia or eclampsia occur in women with chronic hypertension, the diagnosis of superimposed preeclampsia or eclampsia is made.

HELLP SYNDROME

HELLP syndrome is a clinical and laboratory diagnosis characterized by hepatic involvement as evidenced by Hemolysis, Elevated Liver enzymes, and Low Platelet count. HELLP syndrome is not part of the current classification system but is a reflection of disease progression to severe preeclampsia.

ECLAMPSIA

Eclampsia is characterized by the onset of seizure activity or coma in the woman diagnosed with preeclampsia with no history of preexisting neurologic pathology or other identifiable cause (NHBPEP, 2000; NHBPEP Working Group, 2000).

SIGNIFICANCE AND INCIDENCE

Hypertensive disorders of pregnancy are one of the most common medical complications during pregnancy, labor, birth, and the postpartum period. Between 2000 and 2009, the rate of chronic hypertension complicating pregnancy increased 67% from a rate of 7.6 per 1,000 births to a rate of 12.7. In contrast, the rate for gestational hypertension has increased slightly from 39.4 per 1,000 births in 2008 to a rate of 41.2 in 2009 (Martin et al., 2011). A diagnosis of hypertension complicating pregnancy challenges the care provider, who must weigh the risk, benefits, and alternatives of treatment related to maternal, fetal, and neonatal well-being. Everyone caring for the woman during her pregnancy must be aware of the significance of the disease process, current diagnostic criteria, and management recommendations. Prompt recognition of the disease process and monitoring for potential complications decreases the risk of significant morbidity for the woman and her baby.

Preeclampsia is a significant contributor to maternal and perinatal morbidity and mortality, complicating approximately 5% to 8% of all pregnancies not terminating in first-trimester abortions (Han & Norwitz, 2011). In 2009, hypertension, both chronic and pregnancy related, complicated 221,403 (5.36%) of the 4.13 million pregnancies in the United States (Martin et al., 2011).

Maternal race influences the rate of gestational hypertension complicating pregnancy, with the highest rates seen for non-Hispanic black women (50.2/1,000 live births). The rate for non-Hispanic white women is 46.1 per 1,000 live births, and for Hispanic women the rate is 28.9 per 1,000 live births. Non-Hispanic black women also have higher rates for chronic hypertension (25.7/1,000) when compared to non-Hispanic white (12.3/1,000) and Hispanic (6.8/1,000) women. Maternal age distributions demonstrate women older than 30 years of age have the highest rates of hypertension for all reported races (Martin et al., 2011).

MORBIDITY AND MORTALITY

In the United States, pregnancy-associated hypertension is a leading cause of maternal death. Final mortality data for 2007 reported a total of 548 maternal deaths, producing a rate of 12.7 deaths per 100,000 live births (Xu, Kochanek, Murphy, & Tejada-Vera, 2010). The overall rate of maternal death from preeclampsia or eclampsia was 8.4 per 100,000 live births, which was one of the leading specific causes of death identified. There is a large disparity among rates of maternal death by race. African American women are more likely to die of preeclampsia. The overall maternal death rate for African American women was 26.5 per 100,000 live births in 2007, compared with 10.0 for white women and 21.7 for all other races. Of those maternal deaths from preeclampsia or eclampsia, the maternal mortality rate was 6.6 for whites, 17.3 for African Americans, and 14.6 for all other races (Xu et al., 2010).

In 2003, the Department of Health and Human Services and the Centers for Disease Control and Prevention (CDC) published data from the Pregnancy Mortality Surveillance System reporting pregnancy-related mortality from 1991 to 1999 (Chang et al., 2003). This publication examined the pregnancy-related mortality by pregnancy outcome. Hypertension remained a leading cause of maternal death, accounting for 15.7% of all maternal deaths from 1991 to 1999. For women who had hypertension as the cause of death, 19.3% gave birth to a living infant and 20% had a stillbirth; for 11.8%, the pregnancy outcome was unknown (Chang et al., 2003). The cause-specific, pregnancy-related mortality ratio was three to four times higher for African American women diagnosed with a hypertensive disorder (Chang et al., 2003).

The significance of preeclampsia as a contributor to maternal morbidity and mortality has recently been addressed in the Sentinel Event Alert *Preventing Maternal Death* published by The Joint Commission (TJC, 2010). In the alert, TJC identified the leading causes of maternal death: hemorrhage, hypertensive disorders, pulmonary embolism, amniotic fluid embolism, infection, and preexisting chronic conditions. Of those maternal deaths related to hypertension, TJC identified two commonly preventable errors. The failure to adequately control blood pressure in the hypertensive woman and the failure to adequately diagnose and treat pulmonary edema in women with preeclampsia contribute to preventable maternal mortality (TJC, 2010).

Hypertension during pregnancy predisposes the woman to potentially lethal complications such as abruptio placentae, disseminated intravascular coagulation (DIC), cerebral hemorrhage, cerebral vascular accident, hepatic failure, and acute renal failure. Leading causes of maternal death from hypertension complicating pregnancy include complications from abruptio placentae, hepatic rupture, and eclampsia (Roberts & Funai, 2008). The risk of stroke is disproportionately high among women diagnosed with either preeclampsia or eclampsia. While rare, there is a fourfold increased risk of stroke in this population either during the pregnancy or later in life (Bushnell & Chireau, 2011).

Maternal hypertension contributes to intrauterine fetal death and perinatal mortality. The main causes of neonatal death are placental insufficiency and abruptio placentae (Roberts & Funai, 2008). Intrauterine growth restriction (IUGR) is common in babies of women with preeclampsia. The exact cause is unknown, but fetal and neonatal consequences of preeclampsia may be related to the changes in the uteroplacental unit. Histologic findings of placentas from pregnancies complicated by preeclampsia are consistent with poor uteroplacental perfusion, which can lead to chronic hypoxemia in the fetus (Roberts, 2004).

RISK FACTORS

Preeclampsia is a subtle and insidious disease process unique to human pregnancy. The signs and symptoms of preeclampsia become apparent relatively late in the course of the disease, usually during the third trimester of pregnancy. However, the underlying pathophysiology may be present as early as 8 weeks of gestation.

Historically, several well-defined risk factors have been identified for the development of preeclampsia (Display 5–1). Although risk factors are identified, the individual predictive values of the risk factors for screening and risk identification purposes have not been verified. Women should not be arbitrarily labeled as low- or high-risk patients based solely on historical risk factors.

Of interest today is the identification of physiologic or biochemical markers that would allow early identification of the woman at risk for the development of preeclampsia. Such markers would permit healthcare providers the opportunity to target close surveillance and timely interventions to the subpopulation of hypertensive women that would best benefit from the interventions. Biomarkers currently being investigated include soluble fms-like tyrosine kinase I (sflt-I), soluble endoglin (sEng), placental growth factor (PlGF), placental protein 13 (PP-13), a disintegrin and metalloprotease 12 (ADAM12), Pentraxin 3 (PTX3), pregnancy-associated plasma protein A (PAPP-A), Visfatin, and adrenomedullin (Grill et al., 2009). Of interest, the identified biomarkers may be more predictive in combination than as an isolated finding.

DISPLAY 5-1

Historical Risk Factors for the Development of Preeclampsia

- First pregnancy or pregnancy of a new genetic makeup
- Multiple gestations
- Preexisting diabetes, collagen vascular disease, hypertension, or renal disease
- Hydatidiform mole
- Fetal hydrops
- Maternal age
- African American race
- Family history of pregnancy-induced hypertension
- Antiphospholipid antibody syndrome
- Angiotensin gene T235
- Socioeconomic status
- Failure to demonstrate hemodilution
- Failure to demonstrate a decrease in systemic vascular resistance and second-trimester mean arterial pressures
- Use of contraceptives that prevent exposure to sperm
- Pregnancy achieved through artificial donor insemination
- Obesity or insulin resistance
- Thrombophilic disorders, including hyperhomocysteinemia
- Regular physical activity
- Gestational diabetes

PREVENTION STRATEGIES

EXERCISE

Regular physical activity may provide a protective effect against the development of preeclampsia (Sorensen et al., 2003; Weissgerber, Wolfe, & Davies, 2004). Sorensen and colleagues (2003) examined the relationship of regular exercise and physical activity in the year preceding pregnancy and for the first 20 weeks of gestation to the risk of developing preeclampsia. Compared to inactive women, women who participated in physical activity and regular exercise during the first 20 weeks of gestation experienced a 35% reduced risk for developing preeclampsia (OR, 0.65; 95% CI, 0.43–0.99). As the level of physical activity or exercise increased, the risk for preeclampsia decreased. Participation in light to moderate activity reduced the risk for preeclampsia by 24% (95% CI, 0.48–1.20); participation in vigorous activities reduced the risk by 54% (95% CI, 0.27–0.79; Sorensen et al., 2003). Similar results were seen in women who participated in regular exercise or physical activity for the year before becoming pregnant.

ANTIPLATELET THERAPY

Early studies examining the use of antiplatelet therapy to prevent preeclampsia failed to demonstrate a significant difference in outcomes between treatment and control groups for most women, including nulliparas. However, a recent review of 59 trials by The Cochrane Collaboration did demonstrate a 17% reduction in the risk of preeclampsia with the use of antiplatelet agents (Duley, Henderson-Smart, Meher, & King, 2007). When stratified for risk level, there was no statistical difference in the relative risk based on maternal risk factors, but there was a significant increase in the absolute risk reduction of preeclampsia for high-risk women. Antiplatelet use was also associated with a reduction in the relative risk for preterm birth (8%), fetal/neonatal deaths (14%), and small-for-gestational-age babies (10%).

DIETARY SUPPLEMENTATION

Dietary supplementation to reduce the risk or development of preeclampsia includes vitamin, mineral, and antioxidant supplementation. Calcium supplementation has demonstrated a reduction in hypertension; the greatest effect was seen in women with low calcium intake (Hofmeyr, Lawrie, Atallah, & Duley, 2010). Currently, there are no data to support the use of antioxidants (e.g., vitamin C, vitamin E, selenium, lycopene) to reduce the risk of preeclampsia or other complications of pregnancy (Rumbold, Duley, Crowther, & Haslam, 2008). Fish/marine oil supplementation, like other dietary supplementation, has failed to reduce the incidence of preeclampsia in low- and high-risk populations (Makrides, Duley, & Olsen, 2006).

The use of nitric oxide donors (glyceryl trinitrate) or precursors (L-arginine) has also been investigated as a means for reducing the risk of or preventing preeclampsia. While investigations continue, to date there is insufficient evidence to draw reliable conclusions related to effectiveness (Meher & Duley, 2007).

PATHOPHYSIOLOGY OF PREECLAMPSIA

Preeclampsia has been called the "disease of theories." There is not one established cause. Research is ongoing to identify the pathophysiology. Although the exact mechanism is unknown, preeclampsia is thought to occur because of changes within the maternal cardiovascular, hematologic, and renal systems.

Normal physiologic adaptations to pregnancy include an increase in plasma volume, vasodilation of the vascular bed, decreased systemic vascular resistance, elevation of cardiac output, and increased prostacyclin production. Physical assessment findings consistent with these changes are dilutional anemia, lower systemic blood pressures and mean arterial pressure (MAP), a slight increase in heart rate, and peripheral edema. In preeclampsia, these normal adaptations are altered. Instead of plasma volume expansion and hemodilution, there is a decrease in circulating plasma volume resulting in hemoconcentration. Women with preeclampsia have inadequate plasma volume expansion, with an average plasma volume 9% below expected values for mild disease and up to 40% below normal with severe disease. Further intravascular volume depletion may occur from endothelial injury and increased capillary permeability. The volume depletion may result in increased blood viscosity, leading to a decrease in maternal organ perfusion, including the uteroplacental unit.

Maternal intravascular volume depletion has been associated with fetal morbidity. The reduction in plasma volume may be more closely related to IUGR than hypertension. The vascular bed demonstrates increased sensitivity to vasoactive substances, resulting in vasoconstriction and increased vascular tone. Vasoconstriction results in increased systemic vascular resistance and hypertension. The hypertension is further aggravated by vasospasms of the arterial bed, the underlying mechanism for observed signs and symptoms of the disease process. The cumulative effect of decreased intravascular volume and vasoconstriction leads to a decreased organ perfusion. As the process worsens, hemolysis may also compromise tissue oxygen delivery.

Vasoconstriction and a further increase in cardiac output above the normal pregnancy elevation result in arterial vasospasms, endothelial damage, and an imbalance in endothelial prostacyclin and thromboxane ratios. Tables 5–2 and 5–3 provide highlights of the pathophysiology of disease progression and multiple organ system involvement.

Of interest is ongoing research examining the relationship of endothelial dysfunction and alterations in the immune response with the development of preeclampsia (Chaiworapongsa et al., 2004; Dechend et al., 2005; González-Quintero et al., 2004; Lévesque, Moutquin, Lindsay, Roy, & Rousseau, 2004; Magnini et al., 2005; NHBPEP Working Group, 2000; Waite, Louie, & Taylor, 2005; Wang, Gu, Zhang, & Lewis, 2004; Yamamoto, Suzuki, Kojima, & Suzumori, 2005). Vascular endothelial cells play a role in the modulation of vascular smooth muscle contractile activity and the coagulation and regulation of blood flow. Receptors within the endothelial

cells respond to vasodilators and vasoconstrictors while producing vasoactive substances such as hormones, autacoids, and mitogenic cytokines, including PGI_2, nitric oxide, and endothelin. The underlying processes are not fully understood, but women diagnosed with preeclampsia exhibit histologic evidence of increased circulating markers of endothelial activation. Endothelial dysfunction and subsequent increased capillary permeability in turn leads to the pathway of reduced organ perfusion.

The "two stage model of preeclampsia" is the most recent area of investigation related to the pathophysiology of preeclampsia (Redman & Sargent, 2005; Roberts & Hubel, 2009). This model proposes that the processes that eventually lead to preeclampsia originate within the placenta. Stage 1 results from reduced placental perfusion, secondary to failed remodeling of the maternal vessels supplying the intervillus space, and leads to the clinical manifestations of preeclampsia. The

Table 5-2. PHYSIOLOGIC AND PATHOPHYSIOLOGIC CHANGES ASSOCIATED WITH PREECLAMPSIA

Feature	Normal Pregnancy	Preeclampsia Alterations
Blood volume	50%↑	Smaller ↑
Plasma volume	50%↑	Little or no change
Red cell mass	20%↑	Hemoconcentration
Cardiac output	40%–50%↑	Variable
	Widening pulse pressure	↓ Vascular compliance
Blood pressure	↓ Initially with return to prepregnant values by 3rd trimester	Hypertension
Peripheral vascular resistance	↓ Total peripheral resistance	↑ Resistance
		↑ Vascular reactivity
Renal function	↑ Venous capacitance	Vasospasms
RPF	↑	↓
GFR	75%↑	↓
BUN	50%↑	↓
Creatinine clearance	↓	↑
Serum creatinine	↑	↓
Uric acid	↓	↑
Renin–angiotensin–aldosterone system	Markedly activated and responds appropriately to posture and salt intake	Plasma renin concentration and activity suppressed
		Loss of antagonists (vasodilators) to AII
		Increased sensitivity to vasoactive substances
Coagulation system		
Fibrinogen	↑	Normal with mild disease
Factors VII, VIII, IX, X	All ↑	Normal initially, then ↓
		Increase in ratio of von Willebrand factor to factor VII, coagulant activity increased leading to consumption of factor VI
Fibrinolytic activity	↓	↑
Platelet count	Normal	↓
Bleeding time	Normal	Prolonged

AII, angiotensin II; BUN, blood urea nitrogen; GFR, glomerular filtration rate; RPF, renal plasma blood flow.
Adapted from Roberts, J. (1994). Current perspectives on preeclampsia. *Journal of Nurse-Midwifery, 39*(2), 70–90. doi:10.1016/0091-2182(94)90015-9

Table 5-3. PREECLAMPSIA PATHOPHYSIOLOGY AS A MULTIORGAN SYSTEM DISEASE

System	Effect of Preeclampsia	Clinical Implications
Vascular bed 1. Endothelial dysfunction 2. Altered coagulation 3. Altered response to vasoactive substances	• Increased release of cellular fibronectin, growth factors, VCAM-1, factor VIII antigen, and peptides • Endothelial cell injury initiates coagulation either by intrinsic pathway (contact adhesion) or extrinsic pathway (tissue factor) • Decreased production of prostacyclin and alteration in prostacyclin/thromboxane ratio	Endothelial dysfunction presents before clinical signs of disease Increased thrombus formation, including pulmonary and cerebral emboli Vasoconstriction and vasospasm Increased sensitivity to vasoactive substance Capillary permeability, which contributes to edema formation
Cardiovascular and pulmonary 1. ↑ Vascular resistance 2. ↑ Cardiac output and stroke volume 3. ↓ Colloid osmotic pressure	• Arteriolar narrowing • ↑ Sympathetic activity • ↑ Levels of endothelin-1, a vasoconstrictor • ↑ Sensitivity to endogenous pressors, including vasopressin, epinephrine, and norepinephrine • ↑ Capillary permeability • Further depletion of intravascular colloids through capillary permeability and renal excretion of proteins	Increased blood pressure Hyperdynamic cardiac activity Epidurals can be used safely, but must be cautious if ephedrine is used to correct hypotension Subendocardial hemorrhages are present in >50% of women who die of eclampsia At risk for pulmonary edema, myocardial ischemia, left ventricular dysfunction
Renal 1. Proteinuria 2. Altered function	• Slight decrease in glomerular size • Diameter of glomerular capillary lumen decreased • Glomerular endothelial cells are greatly enlarged and may occlude the capillary lumen • Glomerular capillary endotheliosis • Thickening of renal arterioles	Proteinuria plus hypertension is the most reliable indicator of fetal jeopardy; indicative of glomerular dysfunction ↑ Serum uric acid secondary to a ↓ urate clearance (uric acid better predictor of outcome than blood pressure) ↓ Creatinine clearance with an elevation of serum creatinine levels ↑ BUN mirrors changes in creatine clearance and also a function of protein intake and liver function Urine sediment analysis may not be beneficial At risk for oliguria, acute tubular necrosis (ATN), renal failure
Hepatic 1. Hepatic dysfunction 2. Hepatic rupture	• Changes consistent with hemorrhage into hepatic tissue • Later changes consistent with hepatic infarction • ↑ Hepatic artery resistance • Fibrin deposition • Hepatocellular necrosis	Elevations of liver function tests; the association of microangiopathic anemia and elevations of AST/ALT carries ominous prognosis for mother and fetus HELLP syndrome Possible elevations in bilirubin Signs of liver failure: malaise, nausea, epigastric pain, hypoglycemia, hemolysis, anemia
Hematologic 1. Thrombocytopenia 2. Altered platelet function 3. Hemolysis	• ↑ Platelet destruction • ↑ Platelet aggregation • ↓ Platelet life span • Hemolytic anemia • Destruction of red blood cells (RBCs) in microvasculature	Platelets <100,000 increased risk of coagulopathy Platelets <50,000 increased risk of hemorrhage Platelets <20,000 increased risk for spontaneous bleeding Decreased oxygen-carrying capacity and organ oxygenation
Central nervous system (CNS) 1. Hyperreflexia	• May indicate increasing CNS involvement, but not diagnostic of disease • Alteration of cerebral autoregulation with seizures • ↑ Intracranial pressures	Cerebral edema with severe disease Signs of CNS alterations: headache, dizziness, changes in vital signs, diplopia, scotomata, blurred vision, amaurosis, tachycardia, alteration in level of consciousness
Fetal/neonatal 1. Fetal intolerance to labor 2. Preterm birth 3. Oligohydramnios 4. IUGR 5. IUFD 6. Abruptio placentae	• Alteration in placental function • At risk for indicated preterm birth secondary to maternal disease process	Must monitor for signs of fetal compromise Monitoring for IUGR and IUFD At risk for abruptio placentae, oligohydramnios, indeterminate or abnormal fetal heart rate patterns
Uteroplacental 1. Spiral arteries 2. Changes consistent with hypoxia	• Abnormal invasion • Retain nonpregnant characteristics • Limited vasodilatation • Vessel necrosis	Decreases in uteroplacental perfusion Increased risk for fetal compromise and IUGR

ALT, alanine aminotransferase; AST, aspartate aminotransferase; BUN, blood urea nitrogen; IUFD, intrauterine fetal demise; IUGR, intrauterine growth restriction; VCAM-1; vascular cell adhesion molecule 1.

pathophysiologic abnormalities associated with Stage 1 include inadequate maternal vascular response to placentation, endothelial dysfunction, abnormal angiogenesis, and an exaggerated inflammatory response with resultant generalized vasospasm, activation of platelets, and abnormal hemostasis (Roberts & Hubel, 2009). Once there are clinical signs and symptoms of the disease, the woman enters Stage 2 of the disease process.

CLINICAL MANIFESTATIONS OF PREECLAMPSIA–ECLAMPSIA

Historically, the classic triad for preeclampsia has included hypertension, proteinuria, and edema. However, not all of these parameters must be present for the diagnosis of preeclampsia. The NHBPEP has published recommendations that clarified the differences in diagnostic criteria previously published by ACOG, the Australasian Society for the Study of Hypertension in Pregnancy, and the Canadian Hypertension Society. These recommendations include eliminating edema from the diagnostic criteria, eliminating the use of blood pressure changes in defining hypertension, using both systolic and diastolic pressures to define hypertension, and adding systemic changes to the diagnostic criteria (NHBPEP, 2000; NHBPEP Working Group, 2000). Hypertension and proteinuria are the most significant indicators. Edema is significant only if hypertension, proteinuria, or signs of multisystem organ involvement are present.

The clinical manifestations of preeclampsia are directly related to the presence of vascular vasospasms. These vasospasms result in endothelial injury, red blood cell destruction, platelet aggregation, increased capillary permeability, increased systemic vascular resistance, renal and hepatic dysfunction, and other systemic changes.

HYPERTENSION

Although controversy exists about the most appropriate definition of hypertension, ACOG (2002), the NHBPEP (2000), and the NHBPEP Working Group (2000) define hypertension as a sustained blood pressure elevation of 140 mm Hg or more systolic or 90 mm Hg or more diastolic after the 20th week of gestation that is recorded on two or more measurements. The use of elevations above baseline values, specifically a 30 mm Hg increase in the systolic blood pressure or a 15 mm Hg increase in diastolic blood pressure above baseline values, to define hypertension is of questionable value for the diagnosis of preeclampsia and is no longer part of the diagnostic criteria for identifying hypertension (ACOG, 2002; NHBPEP, 2000; NHBPEP Working Group, 2000). Women who demonstrate an elevation in baseline blood pressure

but fail to reach an absolute blood pressure of 140 mm Hg systolic or 90 mm Hg diastolic or higher are not likely to suffer adverse perinatal outcomes without other risk factors. However, it is prudent to carefully observe women who have a rise of 30 mm Hg systolic or 15 mm Hg diastolic blood pressure if this change is accompanied by proteinuria or hyperuricemia (uric acid [UA] $\geq$6 mg/dL; NHBPEP, 2000; NHBPEP Working Group, 2000).

Measurement of blood pressure is important in the evaluation, diagnosis, and management of hypertension. In the past, Korotkoff 4 (K4, muffling of sound) has been used to identify the diastolic pressure. However, current recommendations are to use Korotkoff 5 (K5, disappearance of sound) (NHBPEP, 2000; NHBPEP Working Group, 2000). It is also important to keep in mind that the diagnosis of hypertension is not made based on one blood pressure evaluation. In an ambulatory setting, the diagnosis of hypertension is based on two determinations, generally within a week. The degree of suspected hypertension will determine the interval between blood pressure determinations.

In addition to the recommendation of using K5, patient position will also influence blood pressure readings. Historically, blood pressure determinations were obtained in a left lateral position with the blood pressure cuff placed on the right arm. However, this position will falsely lower systolic, diastolic, and mean pressures. Current recommendations are to evaluate the blood pressure with the woman in a sitting position, with placement of the cuff on the left arm with the arm positioned at heart level. If reevaluation is required, the patient should be in the same position as the initial evaluation. If the left lateral position is being maintained by the patient, the blood pressure will still be taken in the left arm; the arm should not be under the patient or lower than heart level.

Earlier research suggests that an increase in mean arterial pressure in the second trimester (MAP-2) of more than 85 mm Hg is useful in identifying the women at risk for developing hypertension during pregnancy. Several investigators have correlated an elevation of MAP-2 with an increased risk for maternal hypertension and for fetal and neonatal risks; however, more definitive research is needed.

PROTEINURIA

Proteinuria is defined as the urinary excretion of 0.3 g of protein/L (300 mg/L) in a 24-hour urine specimen (NHBPEP, 2000). Random determinations for urine protein excretion are often monitored with dipstick analysis. The stated threshold of 0.3 g/L correlates with 30 mg/dL or "1+" or greater on dipstick analysis (NHBPEP, 2000). However, urine dipstick evaluation is a poor quantifier of protein excretion. Studies comparing traditional urine dipstick analysis to 24-hour urine protein quantitation to determine proteinuria found that in routine clinical practice, a finding of "negative" or "trace" proteinuria misses significant proteinuria in up to 40% of hypertensive women. When feasible, evaluation of total protein excretion should be done by 24-hour urine protein quantitation rather than by urinalysis or dipstick analysis (NHBPEP, 2000; NHBPEP Working Group, 2000). If a 24-hour urine for protein quantitation is not possible or feasible, a timed collection corrected for creatinine excretion can be performed (NHBPEP, 2000; NHBPEP Working Group, 2000).

Proteinuria, which should occur for the first time during the pregnancy, may indicate a worsening of the disease process and increased risk of adverse outcome for the woman and fetus. There is a positive correlation between the degree of proteinuria and perinatal mortality and fetal growth restriction. The concentration of urine protein is extremely variable. Urinary protein concentration is influenced by factors such as contamination of the specimen with vaginal secretions, blood, or bacteria; urine specific gravity and pH; exercise; and posture.

EDEMA

Edema is a common finding of pregnancy and is not necessary for the diagnosis of preeclampsia (NHBPEP, 2000; NHBPEP Working Group, 2000). Dependent edema in the absence of hypertension or proteinuria is generally related to changes in interstitial and intravascular hydrostatic and osmotic pressures that facilitate movement of intravascular fluid into the tissues. Compression of the iliac vein increases venous hydrostatic pressure; this promotes fluid shifting into the interstitial space. Plasma volume expansion results in a decreased serum albumin levels; this lowers the colloid osmotic pressure promoting fluid leaving the intravascular space. Together, these two physiologic adaptations of pregnancy result in benign dependent edema.

With preeclampsia, edema becomes pathologic when accompanied by hypertension, proteinuria, or signs of organ dysfunction. Intracellular and extracellular edema represents a generalized and excessive accumulation of fluid in tissue. As vasospasms worsen, capillary endothelial damage results in increased systemic capillary permeability (i.e., leakage), which leads to hemoconcentration and increases the risk of pulmonary edema.

HYPERREFLEXIA

Hyperreflexia is not considered diagnostic for preeclampsia or a risk factor for eclampsia. In healthy young women, hyperreflexia can be a common finding. Deep tendon reflexes (DTRs) are evaluated once magnesium sulfate therapy is begun to assess for early signs of magnesium toxicity.

PREECLAMPSIA VERSUS SEVERE PREECLAMPSIA

The diagnosis of preeclampsia has significant implications for both maternal and fetal/neonatal well-being. Because other conditions can mimic preeclampsia, it is important to look for systemic manifestations of disease progression such as ascites, hydrothorax, increased neck vein distention, gallop rhythm, pulmonary rales, or generalized bruising or petechiae. To identify the progression of preeclampsia to severe disease or to increase the certainty of the diagnosis, nursing management requires accurate and thorough observation and assessments as well as possible preparation for birth of the baby. Display 5–2 lists criteria for confirming the diagnosis of preeclampsia and progression to severe preeclampsia. Display 5–3 lists the potential maternal and fetal complications of severe preeclampsia.

D I S P L A Y　5 - 2

Criteria for Diagnosis of Preeclampsia

- Blood pressure of 140 mm Hg or more systolic, **OR** 90 mm Hg or more diastolic on two occasions at least 6 hours or more apart. For severe preeclampsia, blood pressure of 160 mm Hg or more systolic, **OR** 110 mm Hg or more diastolic on two occasions at least 6 hours or more apart. If severe hypertension is present, the caregiver must treat and not wait for follow-up blood pressure to establish diagnosis.
- Proteinuria of 2.0 g or more in 24 hours (2+ or 3+ on qualitative examination). For severe preeclampsia, proteinuria of 5.0 g or more in 24 hours (3+ on qualitative examination). Proteinuria should occur for the first time in pregnancy, and the condition resolves postpartum.
- Increased serum creatinine (>1.2 mg/dL, unless known to be previously elevated)
- Platelet count <100,000 cells/mm³ and/or evidence of microangiopathic hemolytic anemia (with increased lactic acid dehydrogenase [LDH])
- Elevated liver enzymes (alanine aminotransferase [ALT] or aspartate aminotransferase [AST])
- Persistent headache or other cerebral or visual disturbances
- Persistent epigastric pain
- Oliguria, 24-hour urinary output of <500 mL
- Pulmonary edema or cyanosis
- Intrauterine growth restriction (IUGR)

Data from National High Blood Pressure Education Program. (2000). *National High Blood Pressure Education Program Working Group Report on High Blood Pressure in Pregnancy* (NIH Publication No. 00-3029). Bethesda, MD: National Institute of Health; National Heart, Lung, and Blood Institute; and National High Blood Pressure Education Program; Walfisch, A., & Hallak, M. (2006). Hypertension in pregnancy. In D. K. James, P. J. Steer, C. P. Weiner, & B. Gonik (Eds.), *High Risk Pregnancy: Management Options* (3rd ed., pp. 772–789). Philadelphia, PA: Saunders Elsevier.

Potential Maternal and Fetal Complications of Severe Preeclampsia

Cardiovascular:
- Hypoperfusion
- Severe hypertension
- Hypertensive crisis
- Pulmonary edema
- Congestive heart failure
- Future cardiac dysfunction

Pulmonary:
- Pulmonary edema
- Hypoxemia/acidemia

Renal:
- Oliguria
- Acute renal failure
- Impaired drug metabolism and excretion

Hematologic:
- Hemolysis
- Decreased oxygen-carrying capacity
- Thrombocytopenia
- Coagulation defects, including disseminated intravascular coagulation (DIC)
- Anemia

Neurologic:
- Eclampsia
- Cerebral edema
- Intracerebral hemorrhage
- Stroke
- Amaurosis (cortical blindness)

Hepatic:
- Hepatocellular dysfunction
- Hepatic rupture
- Hypoglycemia
- Coagulation defects
- Impaired drug metabolism and excretion

Uteroplacental:
- Abruptio placentae
- Decreased uteroplacental perfusion

Fetal:
- Intrauterine growth restriction (IUGR)
- Intrauterine fetal demise (IUFD)
- Fetal intolerance to labor
- Preterm birth
- Low birth weight
- Decreased oxygenation

While caring for women with hypertensive disorders of pregnancy, nursing assessments focus on identification of the disease progression. Preeclampsia is a systemic disease in which one or more organ systems are involved. The wide range of symptoms and multiple organ system involvement can sometimes result in misdiagnosis and delay in treatment. Cocaine intoxication, lupus nephritis, chronic renal failure, and acute fatty liver of pregnancy are examples of conditions that may mimic preeclampsia and eclampsia. Women with chronic hypertension or any preexisting medical condition that predisposes to the development of hypertension are at increased risk for superimposed preeclampsia and eclampsia. Care of the woman with severe preeclampsia or HELLP syndrome is best referred to a tertiary perinatal center.

NURSING ASSESSMENT AND INTERVENTIONS FOR PREECLAMPSIA

Basic to the management of preeclampsia is a philosophic understanding of the disease process in that (1) birth is always the appropriate therapy for the woman but not always for the fetus; (2) the signs and symptoms of preeclampsia are not of pathogenetic importance; and (3) the pathogenetic changes of preeclampsia are present for an extended time before clinical signs and symptoms are present. Once clinical signs and symptoms are observed (e.g., headaches, epigastric pain, visual disturbances), underlying pathophysiologic changes within all major organ systems are present; the degree of organ system dysfunction parallels disease progression. The only definitive therapy for preeclampsia is birth. The decision to initiate birth versus expectant management must be individualized. Decisions for management are determined by maternal and fetal status and gestational age.

HOME CARE MANAGEMENT

Mild preeclampsia may be managed at home with frequent follow-up care, including telephone contact between the woman and a high-risk perinatal nurse and periodic nurse home visits. Criteria for home management vary among primary perinatal healthcare providers and home care agencies. The woman must be in a stable condition with no evidence of worsening maternal or fetal status.

INPATIENT MANAGEMENT

Women with mild preeclampsia may be evaluated in the inpatient setting and remain hospitalized. Women with severe preeclampsia or eclampsia are managed in the hospital. A woman with a fetus at an early gestational age, usually less than 34 weeks, is generally managed in a tertiary center because of the ability to provide advanced neonatal care if birth is indicated. Nursing care involves accurate and astute observations and assessments. Comprehensive knowledge regarding pharmacologic therapies, management regimens, and possible complications is also required.

The most important aspect of care for women with hypertension in pregnancy is recognition of the abilities of the facility and the obstetric and neonatal staff to handle potential emergencies. The decision to transfer a patient to a perinatal center should be based on the level of care required for the woman or should be made because the fetus is preterm and neonatal support will be required. It is best not to attempt expectant management of patients with severe preeclampsia (antepartum or postpartum) unless in a tertiary care center. However, providers of obstetric care, regardless of level of care provided, must be able to stabilize the woman before transport.

CONTROVERSIAL MANAGEMENT PROTOCOLS: USE OF COLLOIDS AND DIURETICS

Some management protocols are considered to be inappropriate in the care of women with preeclampsia. Diuretics and administration of high concentrations of colloid solutions (e.g., albumin, Hespan) should not be used to decrease peripheral edema or increase urine output. Preeclampsia is associated with a decrease in plasma volume expansion leading to hemoconcentration and a relative hypovolemia. The administration of diuretics further decreases intravascular volume, leading to further compromise of renal perfusion and urine output. Administration of high concentrations of colloid solutions, in theory, would increase intravascular osmotic pressure, causing interstitial fluid to be drawn back into the intravascular compartment; this would decrease peripheral edema. However, preeclampsia is a disease of endothelial dysfunction and capillary permeability. The increase in intravascular colloid osmotic pressure is only transient and the colloids "leak" into the interstitial space, further depleting intravascular volume. The combination of diuretics and administration of high concentrations of colloid solutions further depletes intravascular volume and increases the risk of pulmonary edema and uteroplacental insufficiency.

Intravenous fluid therapy is not without risk in the management of a woman with preeclampsia. Administration of intravenous fluids decreases intravascular colloid osmotic pressure, but the administration of colloid solutions, such as Hespan or albumin, is not indicated. The administration of colloid solutions theoretically increases intravascular colloid osmotic pressure, but the proteins in these solutions leak into the tissues as a result of capillary injury and increased capillary permeability. There is a resulting alteration in the hydrostatic and osmotic forces that potentiate the development of pulmonary edema and further depletion of intravascular volume. The administration of colloids in any clinical situation in which endothelial injury and capillary permeability complicate the disease process is contraindicated.

Valium is no longer the first-line agent to stop seizure activity because of the depressant effect on the fetus and depression of the maternal gag reflex. Seizure precautions should be followed according to institution protocol. It is important to avoid insertion of a padded tongue blade to the back of the throat; a nasopharyngeal airway may be appropriate, if available. Heparin should not be administered as prophylaxis against coagulopathies because it increases the risk for intracranial bleeding.

ANTEPARTUM MANAGEMENT

Antepartum management of the woman diagnosed with mild preeclampsia remains controversial. Key to the debate is whether the woman should be hospitalized or whether ambulatory management would be appropriate. In the face of severe disease, the woman should be hospitalized with the timing of birth dictated by maternal and fetal status.

Historically, women diagnosed with mild preeclampsia were admitted to the hospital for two reasons: to prevent eclampsia and to improve perinatal outcome. However, researchers have questioned the practice of routine hospitalization of women diagnosed with mild preeclampsia. Outpatient management for women with mild preeclampsia is a viable option for those who agree to follow established protocols, can have frequent office or home visits, and can perform blood pressure monitoring.

The role of antihypertensive medication in the expected management of women with mild preeclampsia is controversial. Antihypertensive regimens reported in prospective and retrospective studies include hydralazine, methyldopa, nifedipine, prazosin, diuretics, and beta-blockers. Although these studies examined the effect of different antihypertensive agents, none reported a better perinatal outcome compared with management without antihypertensives. There are insufficient data to support prophylactic use of antihypertensive therapy in the management of mild preeclampsia.

Traditionally, women diagnosed with severe preeclampsia remote from term are delivered expeditiously. Although this approach may allow recovery from the disease process for the woman, it may not improve fetal and neonatal outcomes. The use of conservative management for severe preeclampsia remote from term has suggested that pregnancy may be prolonged to gain fetal maturity without increased risk to the woman (Coppage & Sibai, 2004; Haddad et al., 2004). With strict criteria for patient selection and intensive maternal and fetal surveillance, pregnancy may be prolonged. Assessments are aimed at early identification of worsening in maternal or fetal status or evidence of end-organ dysfunction. Table 5–4 provides the selection criteria for expectant management of severe preeclampsia remote from term.

Table 5-4. EXPECTANT MANAGEMENT SELECTION CRITERIA FOR PATIENT WITH SEVERE PREECLAMPSIA REMOTE FROM TERM

Management Approach (if one or more of the clinical findings present)	Clinical Findings
Expeditious birth (within 72 hr)	Maternal: • Uncontrolled hypertension (defined as blood pressure persistently >160/110 despite maximum recommended doses of two antihypertensive medications) • Eclampsia • Platelet count <100,000 mm^3 • AST or ALT >2x upper limit of normal with epigastric pain or RUQ tenderness • Pulmonary edema • Compromised renal function (rise in serum creatinine of at least 1 mg/dL over baseline values) • Abruptio placentae • Persistent severe headache or visual changes Fetal: • Recurrent late or variable decelerations • BPP <4 on two occasions, 4 hr apart • AFI <2 cm • Ultrasound estimated fetal weight <5th percentile • Reverse umbilical artery diastolic flow
Consider expectant management	Maternal: • Controlled hypertension • Urinary protein of any amount • Oliguria (<0.5 mL/kg/hr), which resolves with hydration • AST/ALT >2x upper limit of normal without epigastric pain or RUQ tenderness Fetal: • BPP >6 • AFI >2 cm • Ultrasound estimated fetal weight >5th percentile

AFI, amniotic fluid index; ALT, alanine aminotransferase; AST, aspartate aminotransferase; BPP, biophysical profile; RUQ, right upper quadrant.
Data from Coppage, K. H., & Sibai, B. M. (2004). Hypertensive emergencies. In M. R. Foley, T. H. Strong, Jr., & T. J. Garite (Eds.), *Obstetric Intensive Care Manual* (2nd ed., pp. 51–65). New York, NY: McGraw-Hill; Haddad, B., Deis, S., Goffinet, F., Paniel, B. J., Cabrol, D., & Sibai, B. M. (2004). Maternal and perinatal outcomes during expectant management of 239 severe preeclamptic women between 24 and 33 weeks' gestation. *American Journal of Obstetrics and Gynecology, 190*(6), 1590–1595; Sibai, B. M. (2002). High-risk pregnancy series: An expert's view. Chronic hypertension in pregnancy. *Obstetrics and Gynecology, 100*(2), 369–377. doi:10.1016/S0029-7844(02)02128-2; Sibai, B. M., & Hnat, M. (2002). Delayed delivery in severe preeclampsia remote from term. *OBG Management, 14*(5), 92–108.

ACTIVITY RESTRICTION

Activity restriction, varying from frequent rest periods with legs elevated to complete bed rest in the full lateral position, is frequently prescribed for women with preeclampsia (ACOG, 2002). While on bed rest, blood pressure decreases, and interstitial fluid is mobilized into the intravascular space, enhancing flow to the uterus and kidneys. Controversy exists about whether the reduction of systolic blood pressure associated with bed rest improves maternal or fetal outcomes. For pregnancies complicated with nonproteinuric hypertension, bed rest does not appear to significantly improve outcome; however, for women with proteinuric preeclampsia, bed rest does seem to have some benefit. It is unclear whether bed rest in a hospital setting improves outcomes because of concurrent intensive inpatient maternal–fetal assessments and appropriate medical intervention or is beneficial when considered as an independent factor.

ONGOING ASSESSMENT

Preeclampsia can appear to occur without warning or be recognized with the gradual development of symptoms. A key goal is early identification of women at risk for development of preeclampsia. A review of the major organ systems adds to the database for detecting changes from baseline in blood pressure, weight gain and patterns of weight gain, increasing edema, and presence of proteinuria. The nurse should note whether the woman complains of unusual, frequent, or severe headaches; visual disturbances; or epigastric pain.

Accurate and consistent blood pressure assessment is important for establishing a baseline and monitoring subtle changes throughout the pregnancy. Blood pressure readings are affected by maternal position and measurement techniques. Consistency must be ensured with the use of proper equipment and cuff size, correct maternal positioning, a rest period before recording the pressure, and recording of Korotkoff 5 (i.e., disappearance of sound) (NHBPEP, 2000;

NHBPEP Working Group, 2000). K4 is typically 5 to 10 mm Hg higher than K5. Ideally, blood pressure measurements should be recorded with the woman in a semi-Fowler's position, with the arm at heart level. If the initial measurement indicates an elevation, the woman should be allowed to relax and have a repeat measurement performed, again in a semi-Fowler's position (Beevers, Lip, & O'Brien, 2001). Use of electronic blood pressure devices produces different values than those obtained with a manual cuff and stethoscope. Electronic blood pressure devices systematically underestimate diastolic pressure values by approximately 10 mm Hg and overestimate systolic pressure values by approximately 4 to 6 mm Hg. These differences are related to the normal hemodynamic changes that occur during pregnancy and the subsequent changes in Korotkoff sounds able to be heard with the human ear compared with the electronic device. There is a widening of pulse pressure when using electronic blood pressure devices compared with manual readings; however, MAP is unchanged (Marx, Schwalbe, Cho, & Whitty, 1993). The main points to remember are that blood pressure measurements should be taken in a consistent manner and that assessment focuses on trends, rather than on a single reading. This may support use of MAP for the diagnosis of hypertension. Since outpatient settings may use a combination of auscultation and automated technology and inpatient settings typically rely on automated technology, a common reference point allows for more consistency when comparing trends.

Presence of edema, in addition to hypertension, warrants additional investigation. Edema, assessed by distribution and degree, is described as dependent or pitting. If periorbital or facial edema is not obvious, the pregnant woman is asked if it was present when she awoke.

DTRs are evaluated if preeclampsia is suspected. The biceps and patellar reflexes and ankle clonus are assessed and the findings recorded. The evaluation of DTRs is especially important if the woman is being treated with magnesium sulfate; absence of DTR is an early indication of impending magnesium toxicity.

Proteinuria is determined from dipstick testing of a clean-catch or catheter urine specimen. A reading greater than +1 on two or more occasions at least 4 hours apart should be followed by a 24-hour urine collection. A 24-hour collection for protein and creatinine clearance is more reflective of true renal status because proteinuria is a later sign in the course of preeclampsia. Urine output is assessed for volume of at least 25 to 30 mL/hr or 100 mL/4 hours. Placement of an indwelling Foley catheter with a urometer facilitates accurate assessment of urine output and may assist with the detection of early signs of renal compromise.

An important ongoing assessment is determination of fetal status. Uteroplacental perfusion decreases in women with preeclampsia, thereby placing the fetus in jeopardy. The uterine spiral arteries of the placental bed are subject to vasospasm. When this occurs, perfusion between maternal circulation and intervillous space is compromised, decreasing blood flow and oxygenation to the fetus. Oligohydramnios, IUGR, fetal compromise, and intrauterine fetal death are all associated with preeclampsia. The fetal heart rate (FHR) should be assessed for baseline rate, variability, and normal versus indeterminant or abnormal patterns. The presence of abnormal baseline rate, minimal or absent variability, or late decelerations may indicate fetal intolerance to the intrauterine environment. Because of the poor positive predictive value of indeterminate or abnormal fetal findings to detect fetal acidemia at birth, maternal and fetal status is evaluated to determine when birth should occur. The presence of variable decelerations, antepartum or intrapartum, may suggest decreased amniotic fluid volume (i.e., oligohydramnios), increasing the risk of umbilical cord compression, and possible fetal compromise. Biophysical or biometric monitoring for fetal well-being may be ordered. These tests include fetal movement counting, nonstress testing (NST), contraction stress test (CST), biophysical profile (BPP), and serial ultrasonography. As long as the fetus continues to grow in an appropriate manner and biophysical findings are reassuring, it can be inferred that the placenta and uterine blood flow are appropriate.

If labor is suspected, a vaginal examination for cervical changes is indicated. Uterine tonicity is evaluated for signs of labor and abruptio placentae. Preterm contractions or a tense, tender uterus may be early indications of an abruptio placentae.

Assessments target signs of deterioration from mild preeclampsia to severe preeclampsia or eclampsia. Signs of liver involvement (e.g., epigastric pain, elevated liver function test, thrombocytopenia), renal failure, worsening hypertension, cerebral involvement, and developing coagulopathies must be assessed and documented. Lung sounds are assessed for rales (i.e., crackles) or diminished breath sounds, which may indicate pulmonary edema. Noninvasive assessment parameters to assess maternal status include level of consciousness, blood pressure, hemoglobin oxygen saturation (i.e., pulse oximetry), electrocardiogram (ECG) findings, and urine output. Invasive hemodynamic monitoring with a flow-directed pulmonary artery catheter (Swan-Ganz) may be indicated in selected patients.

LABORATORY TESTS

The nurse assists in obtaining a number of blood and urine specimens to aid in the diagnosis of preeclampsia, HELLP syndrome, or chronic hypertension. No known laboratory tests predict the development of preeclampsia. Laboratory abnormalities are nonspecific in preeclampsia, but changes can reflect underlying multiorgan system dysfunctions. Thrombocytopenia is the most common hematologic abnormality, but routine assessment of the other coagulation factors is not recommended until the platelet concentration is less than 100,000/mm^3. Unless a preexisting coagulopathy is present, the woman is not at an increased risk for developing a coagulopathy until the platelet level falls below 100,000/mm^3. Baseline laboratory test information is useful in the early diagnosis of preeclampsia and for comparison with results obtained to evaluate progression and severity of disease. Display 5–4 provides the common laboratory assessments for a woman with hypertension during pregnancy.

PHARMACOLOGIC THERAPIES

Pharmacologic therapies are instituted for two purposes: seizure prophylaxis and antihypertensive management.

DISPLAY 5 - 4

Laboratory Values Assessed for Women with Hypertension during Pregnancy

Complete blood count:
- Hemoglobin
- Hematocrit
- Platelet count

Chemistry:
- Electrolytes
- Blood urea nitrogen (BUN)
- Serum creatinine
- Serum albumin

Uric acid:
- Serum calcium
- Serum sodium
- Serum magnesium
- Serum glucose
- Liver function tests: lactate dehydrogenase (LDH), aspartate aminotransferase, alanine aminotransferase
- May consider serum amylase and lipase
- May consider cardiac enzymes

Urine:
- Urinalysis for protein
- 24-hour creatinine clearance may be measured in patients with chronic hypertension or renal disease
- 24-hour urine for sodium excretion
- Specific gravity

Coagulation profile:
- Platelet count and function
- Prothrombin and partial thromboplastin times
- Fibrinogen
- Fibrin split or fibrin degradation products
- Bleeding time
- D-dimer

Magnesium Sulfate

Magnesium sulfate is the drug of choice in the management of preeclampsia to prevent seizure activity (ACOG, 2002; NHBPEP, 2000; NHBPEP Working Group, 2000). (Magnesium sulfate safety is presented in the "Ongoing Assessment" section under "Nursing Assessment and Interventions for Preeclampsia.") For seizure prophylaxis, magnesium sulfate is administered as a secondary infusion by an infusion-controlled device to achieve serum levels of approximately 5 to 8 mg/dL (4 to 7 mEq/dL). The loading dose is a 4- to 6-g intravenous bolus over 15 to 30 minutes, followed by a maintenance infusion of 2 to 3 g/hour.

The action of magnesium sulfate as an anticonvulsant is controversial, but it is thought to block neuromuscular transmission and decrease acetylcholine excretion at the end plate, depressing the vasomotor center and thereby depressing central nervous system (CNS) irritability. Magnesium circulates largely unbound to protein and is almost exclusively excreted in the urine. In patients with normal renal function, the half-time for excretion of magnesium is approximately 4 hours. In women with decreased glomerular filtration and renal hypoperfusion, such as seen in preeclampsia, the half-time for excretion is delayed, increasing the risk for toxicity.

Signs and symptoms of hypermagnesemia are assessed for the duration of the infusion. Clinically significant findings of hypermagnesemia are related primarily to magnesium's cellular effects. Intravenous magnesium, more so than oral, slows or blocks neuromuscular and cardiac conducting system transmission, decreases smooth muscle contractility, and depresses CNS irritability. Although the desired anticonvulsant effect can be achieved easily with current dosing regimes, the nurse must be aware of the potential for untoward effects, including decreased uterine and myocardial contractility, depressed respirations, and interference with cardiac conduction that places the woman at risk for cardiac dysrhythmias or cardiac arrest. Contrary to popular belief, magnesium sulfate has little effect on maternal blood pressure when administered appropriately.

The effect of magnesium sulfate on fetal heart baseline variability is controversial. Fetal serum levels for magnesium will approximate maternal levels, so fetal sedation is possible. However, minimal to absent baseline variability should not be seen as a side effect of maternal magnesium sulfate therapy until fetal hypoxemia has been ruled out.

Nursing responsibilities and assessments for women receiving magnesium sulfate include:

- Obtain patient history, including drug history and any known allergies; note renal function or history of heart block, myocardial damage, or concurrent use of CNS depressants, digoxin, or neuromuscular blocking agents. (Make sure anesthesia personnel are aware of infusion.)

- Assess maternal baseline vital signs, DTRs, neurologic status, and urinary output before initiation of therapy and reassess per institution protocol.
- Administer magnesium sulfate according to protocol; all infusions should be prepared by the facility pharmacy, or the facility should use commercially prepared solutions.
- Establish the primary intravenous line and intravenously administer magnesium sulfate piggyback by means of a controlled-infusion device; infuse via a separate line and do not mix with other intravenous drugs unless compatibility has been established.
- Avoid administration of any solution of magnesium sulfate if particulate matter, cloudiness, or discoloration is noted.
- Document magnesium sulfate infusion in grams per hour.
- Continue fetal assessment.
- Keep calcium gluconate (1 g of a 10% solution) immediately available in a secure medication area on the unit (e.g., drug dispenser system or locked emergency medication area).
- Be cautious with concurrent administration of narcotics, CNS depressants, calcium channel blockers, and beta-blockers; discontinue magnesium sulfate and notify the physician if signs of toxicity occur.
- Monitor for signs of magnesium toxicity (e.g., hypotension, loss of DTRs, respiratory depression, respiratory arrest, oliguria, shortness of breath, chest pains, electrocardiographic changes [increased PR interval, widened QRS complex, prolonged QT interval, heart block]); if toxicity is suspected, discontinue infusion and notify provider.
- Monitor serum magnesium levels as indicated based on maternal status or if toxicity suspected; routine serum magnesium levels are not required in the absence of comorbidities. (Depression of DTRs occurs at serum concentrations lower than those associated with adverse cardiopulmonary effects, and the presence of DTRs indicates magnesium levels that are not too high.) See Table 5-5 for effects associated with various serum magnesium levels.
- Maintain strict intake and output and keep patient hydrated; urine output should be at least 25 mL/hr while administering parenteral magnesium; magnesium sulfate may cause a transient osmotic diuresis.
- Maintain seizure precautions and neurologic evaluations.
- Prepare for neonatal resuscitation.
- Follow the Guidelines for Professional Registered Nurse Staffing for Perinatal Units (Association of Women's Health, Obstetric and Neonatal Nurses [AWHONN], 2010) regarding nurse-to-patient ratios during magnesium sulfate administration. These include 1 nurse to 1 woman in continuous bedside attendance for the woman receiving IV

Table 5-5. SERUM MAGNESIUM LEVELS AND ASSOCIATED EFFECTS

Effect	Serum Level (mg/dL)
Anticonvulsant prophylaxis	5–8
Electrocardiographic changes	5–10
Loss of deep tendon reflexes	8–12
Somnolence	10–12
Slurred speech	10–12
Muscular paralysis	15–17
Respiratory difficulty	15–17
Cardiac arrest	20–35

Data from Coppage, K. H., & Sibai, B. M. (2004). Hypertensive emergencies. In M. R. Foley, T. H. Strong, Jr., & T. J. Garite (Eds.), *Obstetric Intensive Care Manual* (2nd ed., pp. 51–65). New York: McGraw-Hill; Roberts, J. M., & Funai, E. F. (2008). Pregnancy-related hypertension. In R. K. Creasy, R. Resnik, & J. D. Iams (Eds.), *Maternal-Fetal Medicine: Principles & Practice* (6th ed., pp. 651–690). Philadelphia: Saunders.

magnesium sulfate during the first hour of administration; a 1 nurse to 1 woman ratio during labor and until at least 2 hours postpartum and no more than 1 additional couplet or woman in the patient assignment for a nurse caring for a woman receiving IV magnesium sulfate during postpartum (AWHONN, 2010).

Phenytoin

Phenytoin (Dilantin) has also been proposed for eclampsia prophylaxis; however, it is not a first-line therapy in the United States. Clinical studies have not demonstrated better results with phenytoin compared with magnesium sulfate. Because of a lack of experience with phenytoin and the significant maternal side effects, magnesium sulfate remains the first-line drug in the United States. However, phenytoin may be considered when the use of magnesium sulfate is associated with increased risk of maternal complications, such as with myasthenia gravis or markedly reduced renal function. However, if phenytoin is used, extreme care must be taken and caregivers must be familiar with the expected side effects and potential complications, and resuscitation equipment must be immediately available.

Antihypertensive Therapy

Pharmacologic therapies directed at the control of significant hypertension include a variety of agents. Several general precautions should be considered when antihypertensive agents are ordered: antihypertensive therapy is initiated when diastolic blood pressure is sustained at greater than 110 mm Hg **or** systolic blood pressure is sustained at greater than 160 mm Hg to prevent maternal cerebral vascular accident (ACOG, 2011). The effect of the antihypertensive agent may

Indications for Antihypertensive Therapy

Antepartum and Intrapartum

Persistent elevations for at least 1 hour:
- Systolic blood pressure (SBP) ≥160 mm Hg, or
- Diastolic blood pressure (DBP) ≥110 mm Hg, or
- Mean arterial pressure (MAP) ≥130 mm Hg

Persistent elevations for at least 30 minutes:
- SBP ≥200 mm Hg, or
- DBP ≥120 mm Hg, or
- MAP ≥140 mm Hg

Thrombocytopenia or congestive heart failure with persistent elevations for at least 30 minutes:
- SBP ≥160 mm Hg
- DBP ≥105 mm Hg
- MAP ≥125 mm Hg

Postpartum (persistent elevations for at least 1 hour):
- SBP ≥160 mm Hg
- DBP ≥105 mm Hg
- MAP ≥125 mm Hg

DBP, diastolic blood pressure; MAP, mean arterial pressure; SBP, systolic blood pressure.

Data from American College of Obstetricians and Gynecologists. (2011). *Emergent Therapy for Acute-Onset, Severe Hypertension with Preeclampsia or Eclampsia.* (ACOG Committee Opinion No. 514). Washington, DC: Author; Coppage, K. H., & Sibai, B. M. (2004). Hypertensive emergencies. In M. R. Foley, T. H. Strong, Jr., & T. J. Garite (Eds.), *Obstetric Intensive Care Manual* (2nd ed., pp. 51–65). New York, NY: McGraw-Hill.

depend on intravascular volume status and hypovolemia resulting from increased capillary permeability, and hemoconcentration may need correction before the initiation of therapy. Diastolic blood pressure should be maintained between 90 and 100 mm Hg to maintain uteroplacental perfusion (NHBPEP, 2000; NHBPEP Working Group, 2000). See Display 5–5 for indications for antihypertensive therapy. See Table 5–6 for dosing, mechanism of action, and considerations for commonly used antihypertensive agents.

Hydralazine Hydrochloride

Hydralazine hydrochloride (Apresoline) is considered by many to be the first-line agent to decrease hypertension. Dosage regimens vary (see Table 5–6), but intermittent intravenous boluses generally work equally as well as continuous infusions; there is also less chance of rebound hypotension with intermittent boluses. Side effects of hydralazine include flushing, headache, maternal and fetal tachycardia, palpitations, and uteroplacental insufficiency with subsequent fetal tachycardia and late decelerations. Because hydralazine increases maternal cardiac output and heart rate,

if hypertension is more a force issue (i.e., elevated cardiac output, hypervolemia, or tachycardia), the clinical state may worsen with blood pressure either not lowering or possibly increasing.

Labetalol Hydrochloride

Labetalol hydrochloride (Normodyne or Trandate) has been used in place of hydralazine for the management of hypertension. Dosage regimens vary based on physician experience and preference; however, stacked dosing generally provides better results (see Table 5–6). Labetalol hydrochloride is contraindicated in women with asthma and those with greater than first-degree heart block. Because of labetalol's alpha- and beta-adrenergic blockage, transient fetal and neonatal hypotension, bradycardia, and hypoglycemia are possible. The combined alpha- and beta-adrenergic blockades decrease the incidence of rebound maternal tachycardia, making it an attractive alternative to Apresoline, especially in women with cardiac disease who cannot tolerate tachycardia.

POSTPARTUM MANAGEMENT

Immediate postpartum curettage has been associated with a more rapid recovery for women with severe preeclampsia, although more research is needed in this area. Most women are clinically stable within 48 hours after birth. However, because of the risk of eclampsia during the first 24 to 48 hours postpartum, careful monitoring is essential and should include frequent assessments of vital signs, level of consciousness, DTRs, urinary output, and laboratory data. Intravenous magnesium sulfate is usually continued for 24 hours postpartum. It is important to be alert for early signs and symptoms of complications of preeclampsia such as postpartum hemorrhage, DIC, pulmonary edema, HELLP syndrome, increased intracranial pressure, and intracranial hemorrhage. Intensity of monitoring and progression of activity are based on the patient's condition. After vital signs and mental status are stable, laboratory data indicate that condition is improving, urinary output is reassuring, and intravenous magnesium sulfate is discontinued, the frequency of maternal assessments can be decreased from 1 to 2 hours to 4 to 8 hours, the Foley catheter can be removed, and the patient can be encouraged to ambulate. It is important to provide assistance and assess stability during initial ambulation, after bed rest, and after intravenous administration of magnesium sulfate during the intrapartum and postpartum period. Efforts should be made to initiate maternal–newborn attachment by bringing the newborn, if stable, to visit the mother. Photographs of the newborn can be taken and provided to the woman if the maternal or newborn condition prevents visitation.

Table 5-6. ANTIHYPERTENSIVE THERAPY FOR PREECLAMPSIA AND ECLAMPSIA

Generic Name	Trade Name	Mechanism of Action	Dosage	Considerations
Hydralazine	Apresoline	• Direct-acting dilator of smooth muscle • Primary effect is arterial dilation, with minor venodilator effects • ↓ Systemic, pulmonary, and renal resistance • Systemic vasodilation results in ↓ systemic vascular resistance, ↓ arterial pressure, ↑ SV, ↑ rate of ventricular pressure rise • Reflex tachycardia may occur secondary to vasodilation • Onset of action is 15–20 min • Duration of effect is approximately 2–6 hr • Metabolized by liver	• 5 mg or 10 mg IV over 2 min • If either threshold is still exceeded, administer 10 mg IV over 2 min • If either threshold is still exceeded, administer labetalol	• Must wait 20 min for response between IV doses • After dosing, if either threshold is exceeded, repeat dose and continue to monitor BP closely • After second dose, if either threshold is exceeded, change to labetalol • Rebound hypotension • Reflex ↑ in CO and HR (Hyperdynamic circulatory changes also include ↑ LV pressure rise, and SV may be dangerous in patients with certain cardiovascular disorders) • Monitor BP and HR • Maximal BP ↓ within 10 min • ↓ Dose with hepatic dysfunction, low cardiac output, and severe renal dysfunction • Use with caution in patients with coronary artery disease (reflex tachycardia can produce anginal attacks or AMI) • Contraindicated in patients with rheumatic mitral valve disease (↑ PAP) • Not recommended for BP control in patients with dissecting aortic aneurysm (↑ rate of LV pressure rise stresses dissecting aortic segment, worsens aortic injury, and propagates dissection) • Because of postural hypotension, give with caution in patients with cerebrovascular disease • Excessive dosing may result in too rapid and too profound reduction in BP causing ↓ uteroplacental blood flow and ↓ oxygen delivery to the fetus • May ↓ hemoglobin, neutrophil, WBC, granulocyte, platelet, and RBC counts
Labetalol	Normodyne Trandate	• Selective (α-adrenergic and nonselective β-adrenergic) blocking agent • Induces a controlled rapid decrease in BP • ↓ in catecholamine–induced cardiac stimulation and direct vasodilation • ↓ SVR and arterial pressure without reflex tachycardia • β-Blocking effects also blunt rate of LV pressure rise usually associated with vasodilator drugs, ↓ stress on aortic wall • Hypotensive effect usually seen within 2–5 min, peaks at 10 min, and persists for 2–6 hr after IV administration • Metabolized by liver and excreted in urine and bile	Initial dose 20 mg IV over 2 min; if either threshold is exceeded after 10 min, repeat with stacked dosing every 10 min of 40 mg–80 mg–80 mg–80 mg IV for a maximum dose of 300 mg	• Monitor HR and BP • Consider ECG monitoring for bradydysrhythmias and heart block • Monitor blood glucose levels • ↓ Amplitude and frequency of FHR accelerations; may ↓ FHR baseline • Monitor newborn for hypoglycemia, hypotension, and bradycardia • Not a titratable drug; effect of increases in IV infusion rate may not be noted for approximately 10 min; diminution of the drug effect may not be noted for several hours following reduction of dose or discontinuation of drug • Valuable in managing hypertensive crisis as a result of dissecting aortic aneurysm or traumatic dissection of aorta • Effectively ↓ cerebral perfusion pressures without ↓ cerebral perfusion • ↓ Dose with hepatic dysfunction or hepatic hypoperfusion

Drug	Action	Dosage	Comments
			• ↓ Dosage necessary in patients with creatinine clearances <10 mL/min • Adverse reactions related to α-blockade include orthostatic hypotension • Potential β-blockade reactions include bronchospasm, ↓ myocardial contractility and SV, and bradycardia (dose related) • Patient should not be quickly raised to a sitting position during therapy and for at least 2 hr after last dose • ↑ Uteroplacental perfusion and ↓ uterine vascular resistance • May exert a positive effect on early fetal lung maturation in patients remote from term • May ↑ transaminase and urea levels
Nifedipine Procardia Adalat	• Calcium channel blocker • Thought to inhibit calcium ion influx across cardiac and smooth-muscle cells decreasing contractility and smooth-muscle oxygen demand • May dilate coronary arteries and arterioles • Effect seen within 20 min, with peak action within 30–60 min with duration of 4–8 hr	10 mg PO, may be repeated × 1 after 30 min	• Oral route only; sublingual dosing can result in excessive hypotension, acute myocardial ischemia, and death • Possible exaggerated effect if used with MgSO$_4$, including severe hypotension with resulting ↓ uteroplacental perfusion and maternal neuromuscular blockade (muscle weakness, jerky movements of extremities, difficulty in swallowing, paradoxical respirations, and inability to lift head from pillow) • Principal side effects include headache and cutaneous flushing • May ↑ ALT, AST, alkaline phosphatase, and LD levels
Nitroglycerin Nitrostat IV Tridil Nitro–Bid IV	• Relaxation of venous vascular smooth muscle and, to a lesser degree, arterial smooth muscle • Venodilatation associated with *marked* ↓ in preload; slight arterial dilator effect produces a *slight* ↓ in SVR (afterload reduction) that, in turn, is associated with an ↑ SV • Reflex tachycardia may occur in response to vasodilation • Also dilates the epicardial and collateral coronary arteries while preserving coronary autoregulation so that coronary blood flow is not shunted away from ischemic myocardium (coronary steal) • Onset of hypotensive effect approximately 1–5 min, duration of effect is 5–10 min • Very short hemodynamic half-life • Undergoes hepatic metabolism	Continuous IV infusion beginning at 5 mcg/min; increase by 5–10 mcg every 5 min until BP, wedge pressure response, or relief of pain is obtained	• Requires critical care consultation or comanagement • There is no maximal dose, but most believe that if 200 mcg/min do not provide relief of hypertension or ischemic pain, higher doses are unlikely to provide additional benefit • Monitor BP, HR, and ECG for worsening or resolution of ischemic changes • PAP and PACP should be monitored in hemodynamically unstable patients • Latent or overt hypovolemia may be associated with a marked ↓ in BP • Hypotension may worsen myocardial ischemia • Restoring circulatory volume by fluid loading generally stabilizes the patient's response to nitroglycerin • Larger doses of nitroglycerin were required following volume expansion; the ability to effect a smoother and more controlled drop in BP required prevasodilator hydration • Occasionally, bradycardia and severe hypotension occur during IV infusion (Bezold-Jarisch reflex)

(continued)

Table 5–6. ANTIHYPERTENSIVE THERAPY FOR PREECLAMPSIA AND ECLAMPSIA *(Continued)*

Generic Name	Trade Name	Mechanism of Action	Dosage	Considerations
Sodium Nitroprusside	Nipride Nitropress	• Extremely potent direct-acting dilator of both veins and arteries of systemic, coronary, pulmonary, and renal circulations • ↓ Preload, mediated by vasodilation, associated with ↓ right and left ventricular filling volume and pressure, ↓ size and wall stress of both ventricles, and ↓ pulmonary vascular congestion and therefore pulmonary pressures • ↓ Afterload (mediated by arteriolar dilation) results in ↓ systemic and pulmonary vascular resistance and an ↑ SV • Both preload and afterload reduction ↓ myocardial oxygen consumption • Reflex tachycardia may result from ↓ BP • Titrate dosing to desired response • 10 mcg/kg/min considered usual maximal dose • Onset of effects within 30–60 sec; BP begins to rise almost immediately after discontinuation and reaches pretreatment levels within 1–10 min • Rapidly metabolized in presence of RBCs	0.25 mcg/kg/min infusion; increase by 0.25 mcg/kg/min q5 min	• May cause headache because of direct cerebral vasodilation • Methemoglobin may result from higher doses (7 mcg/kg/min) • Patients with normal arterial oxygen saturation who appear cyanotic should be evaluated for toxicity, defined as a methemoglobin level >3% • May ↓ FHR baseline variability • Critical care drug requiring critical care management • Invasive hemodynamic monitoring required • Ferrous ion in the nitroprusside molecule reacts rapidly with the sulfhydryl compounds in RBCs, resulting in release of cyanide; cyanide further metabolized in the liver to thiocyanate • Drug is photosensitive and degrades rapidly in light; IV bag should always be covered with metal foil or another opaque material; do not need to cover tubing or drip chamber • Should be observed for signs of thiocyanate and cyanide toxicity • Signs of thiocyanate toxicity include weakness, rashes, tinnitus, lactic acidosis, blurred vision, seizures, psychotic behavior, and mental confusion • Metabolic acidosis one of the earliest signs of plasma accumulation of cyanide radical • Therapy should not exceed 48 hr • Does cross placenta with fetal cyanide concentrations higher than maternal levels • Transient fetal bradycardia possible • Monitor maternal serum pH, plasma cyanide, red-cell cyanide, and methemoglobin levels • Correction of hypovolemia prior to initiation of nitroprusside infusion is essential in order to avoid abrupt and often profound drops in BP

ALT, alanine aminotransferase; AMI, acute myocardial infarction; AST, aspartate aminotransferase; BP, blood pressure; CO, cardiac output; ECG, electrocardiogram; FHR, fetal heart rate; HR, heart rate; IV, intravenous; LD, lactate dehydrogenase; LV, left ventricular; PACP, pulmonary artery capillary pressure; PAP, pulmonary artery pressure; RBC, red blood cell; SV, stroke volume; SVR, systemic vascular resistance; WBC, white blood cell count.

Data from American College of Obstetricians and Gynecologists. (2011). Emergent Therapy for Acute-Onset, Severe Hypertension with Preeclampsia or Eclampsia. (ACOG Committee Opinion No. 514). Washington, DC: Author. doi:10.1097/AOG.0b013e31823ed1ef

HELLP SYNDROME

HELLP syndrome, a multisystem disease, is a form of severe preeclampsia in which the woman presents with a variety of complaints and exhibits common laboratory markers for a syndrome of hemolysis (H), elevated liver enzymes (EL), and low platelets (LP). This subset of women progresses from preeclampsia to the development of multiple organ involvement and damage. The complaints range from malaise, epigastric pain, nausea, and vomiting to nonspecific viral syndrome–like symptoms. On presentation, these patients are generally in the second or early third trimester and initially may show few signs of preeclampsia. Because of the presenting symptoms, these patients may receive a nonobstetric diagnosis, delaying treatment and increasing maternal and perinatal morbidity and mortality. Assessments and management of the woman diagnosed with HELLP syndrome are the same as those for the woman with severe preeclampsia.

ECLAMPSIA

Eclampsia is the development of seizures, coma, or both in a woman with signs and symptoms of preeclampsia. Other causes of seizures must be excluded. Eclampsia can occur antepartum, intrapartum, or postpartum; approximately 50% of cases occur antepartum. The immediate care during a seizure is to ensure a patent airway. Once this has been attained, adequate oxygenation must be maintained by use of supplemental oxygen. Magnesium sulfate (and amobarbital sodium for recurrent convulsions) is given according to the institutional protocol. Aspiration is a leading cause of maternal morbidity after an eclamptic seizure. After initial stabilization and airway management, the nurse should anticipate orders for a chest radiograph and possible arterial blood gas determination to exclude the possibility of aspiration. Rapid assessments of uterine activity, cervical status, and fetal status are performed. During the seizure, membranes may rupture, and the cervix may dilate because the uterus becomes hypercontractile and hypertonic. If birth is not imminent, the timing and route of delivery and the induction of labor versus cesarean birth depend on maternal and fetal status. All medications and therapy are merely temporary measures.

SUMMARY

Perinatal nurses may be challenged by the complications of pregnancy, especially when they occur unexpectedly in the low-risk setting. A thorough knowledge of the nursing care for common perinatal complications, including timely identification and appropriate interventions, is required to ensure optimal outcomes for mothers and babies.

REFERENCES

American College of Obstetricians and Gynecologists. (2002). *Diagnosis and Management of Preeclampsia and Eclampsia* (Practice Bulletin No. 33; Reaffirmed 2008). Washington, DC: Author. Retrieved from http://mail.ny.acog.org/website/SMIPodcast/DiagnosisMgt.pdf

American College of Obstetricians and Gynecologists. (2011). *Emergent Therapy for Acute-Onset, Severe Hypertension with Preeclampsia or Eclampsia*. Washington, DC: Author. doi:10.1097/AOG.0b013e31823ed1ef

American College of Obstetricans and Gynecologists. (2012). *Chronic Hypertension in Pregnancy* (Practice Bulletin No. 125). Washington, DC: Author. doi:10.1097/AOG.0b013e318249ff06

Association of Women's Health, Obstetric and Neonatal Nurses. (2010). *Guidelines for Professional Registered Nurse Staffing for Perinatal Units*. Washington, DC: Author.

Beevers, G., Lip, G. Y. H., & O'Brien, E. (2001). ABC of hypertension. Blood pressure measurement. Part I—Sphygmomanometry: Factors common to all techniques. *British Medical Journal, 322,* 981–985. doi:10.1136/bmj.322.7292.981

Bushnell, C., & Chireau, M. (2011). Preeclampsia and stroke: Risks during and after pregnancy. *Stroke Research and Treatment.* Retrieved from http://www.hindawi.com/journals/srt/2011/858134/

Chaiworapongsa, T., Romero, R., Espinoza, J., Bujold, E., Mee Kim, Y., Conçalves, L. F., & Edwin, S. (2004). Evidence supporting a role for blockade of the vascular endothelial growth factor system in the pathophysiology of preeclampsia. *American Journal of Obstetrics and Gynecology, 190*(6), 1541–1550. doi:10.1016/j.ajog.2004.03.043

Chang, J., Elam-Evans, L. D., Berg, C. J., Herndon, J., Flowers, L., Seed, K. A., & Syverson, C. J. (2003). Pregnancy-related mortality surveillance—United States, 1991–1999. *Morbidity and Mortality Weekly Report: Surveillance Summaries, 52*(SS02), 1–8.

Coppage, K. H., & Sibai, B. M. (2004). Hypertensive emergencies. In M. R. Foley, T. H. Strong, Jr., & T. J. Garite (Eds.), *Obstetric Intensive Care Manual* (2nd ed., pp. 51–65). New York: McGraw-Hill.

Dechend, R., Gratze, P., Wallukat, G., Shagdarsuren, E., Plehm, R., Bräsen, J. H., . . . Müller, D. N. (2005). Agonistic autoantibodies to the AT1 receptor in a transgenic rat model of preeclampsia. *Hypertension, 45*(4), 742–746. doi:10.1161/01.HYP.0000154785.50570.63

Duley, L., Henderson-Smart, D. J., Meher, S., & King, J. F. (2007). Antiplatelet agents for preventing pre-eclampsia and its complications. *Cochrane Database of Systematic Reviews,* (2), CD004659. doi:10.1002/14651858.CD004659.pub2

González-Quintero, V. H., Smarkusky, L. P., Jiménez, J. J., Mauro, L. M., Jy, W., Hortsman, L. L., . . . Ahn, Y. S. (2004). Elevated plasma endothelial microparticles: Preeclampsia versus gestational hypertension. *American Journal of Obstetrics and Gynecology, 191*(4), 1418–1424. doi:10.1016/j.ajog.2004.06.044

Grill, S., Rusterholz, C., Zanetti-Dällenbach, R., Tercanli, S., Holzgreve, W., Hahn, S., & Lapaire, O. (2009). Potential markers of preeclampsia—A review. *Reproductive Biology and Endocrinology, 7,* 70. Retrieved from http://www.rbej.com/content/7/1/70

Haddad, B., Deis, S., Goffinet, F., Paniel, B. J., Cabrol, D., & Sibai, B. M. (2004). Maternal and perinatal outcomes during expectant management of 239 severe preeclamptic women between 24 and 33 weeks' gestation. *American Journal of Obstetrics and Gynecology, 190*(6), 1590–1595. doi:10.1016/j.ajog.2004.03.050

Han, C. S., & Norwitz, E. R. (2011). Expectant management of severe preeclampsia remote from term: Not for everyone. *Contemporary OB GYN, 56*(2), 50–55.

Hofmeyr, G. J., Lawrie, T. A., Atallah, A. N., & Duley, L. (2010). Calcium supplementation during pregnancy for preventing hypertensive disorders and related problems. *Cochrane Database of Systematic Reviews*, (8), CD001059. doi:10.1002/14651858.CD001059.pub3

Lévesque, S., Moutquin, J. M., Lindsay, C., Roy, M. C., & Rousseau, F. (2004). Implication of an AGT haplotype in a multigene association study with pregnancy hypertension. *Hypertension, 43*(1), 71–78. doi:10.1161/01.HYP.0000104525.76016.77

Magnini, L. E., Latthe, P. M., Villar, J., Kilby, M. D., Carroli, G., & Khan, K. S. (2005). Mapping the theories of preeclampsia: The role of homocysteine. *Obstetrics and Gynecology, 105*(2), 411–425. doi:10.1097/01.AOG.0000151117.52952

Makrides, M., Duley, L., & Olsen, S. F. (2006). Marine oil, and other prostaglandin precursor, supplementation for pregnancy uncomplicated by pre-eclampsia or intrauterine growth restriction. *Cochrane Database of Systematic Reviews*, (3), CD003402. doi:10.1002/14651858.CD003402.pub2

Martin, J. A., Hamilton, B. E., Ventura, S. J., Osterman, M. J. K., Kirmeyer, S., Mathews, T. J., & Wilson, E. C. (2011). Births: Final data for 2009. *National Vital Statistics Reports, 60*(1). Retrieved from http://www.cdc.gov/nchs/data/nvsr/nvsr60/nvsr60_01.pdf

Marx, G. F., Schwalbe, S. S., Cho, E., & Whitty, J. E. (1993). Automated blood pressure measurements in laboring women: Are they reliable? *American Journal of Obstetrics and Gynecology, 168*(3, Pt. 1), 796–798. doi:10.1016/S0002-9378(12)90822-4

Meher, S., & Duley, L. (2007). Nitric oxide for preventing preeclampsia and its complications. *Cochrane Database of Systematic Reviews*, (2), CD006490. doi:10.1002/14651858.CD006490

National High Blood Pressure Education Program. (2000). *National High Blood Pressure Education Program Working Group Report on High Blood Pressure in Pregnancy* (NIH Publication No. 00-3029). Bethesda, MD: National Institutes of Health; National Heart, Lung, and Blood Institute; and National High Blood Pressure Education Program.

National High Blood Pressure Education Program Working Group. (2000). Report of the National High Blood Pressure Education Program Working Group on high blood pressure in pregnancy. *American Journal of Obstetrics and Gynecology, 183*(1), S1–S22. doi:10.1067/mob.2000.107928

Redman, C. W., & Sargent, I. L. (2005). Latest advances in understanding preeclampsia. *Science, 308*(5728), 1592–1594. doi:10.1126/science.1111726

Roberts, J. (1994). Current perspectives on preeclampsia. *Journal of Nurse-Midwifery, 39*(2), 70–90. doi:10.1016/0091-2182(94)90015-9

Roberts, J. M., & Funai, E. F. (2008). Pregnancy-related hypertension. In R. K. Creasy, R. Resnik, & J. D. Iams (Eds.), *Maternal-Fetal Medicine: Principles & Practice* (6th ed., pp. 651–690). Philadelphia: Saunders.

Roberts, J. M., & Hubel, C. A. (2009). The two stage model of preeclampsia: Variations on the theme. *Placenta, 30*(Suppl. A), S32–S37. doi:10.1016/j.placenta.2008.11.009

Rumbold, A., Duley, L., Crowther, C. A., & Haslam, R. R. (2008). Antioxidants for preventing pre-eclampsia. *Cochrane Database of Systematic Reviews*, (1), CD004227. doi:10.1002/14651858.CD004227.pub3

Sibai, B. M. (2002). High-risk pregnancy series: An expert's view. Chronic hypertension in pregnancy. *Obstetrics and Gynecology, 100*(2), 369–377. doi:10.1016/S0029-7844(02)02128-2

Sibai, B. M., & Hnat, M. (2002). Delayed delivery in severe preeclampsia remote from term. *OBG Management, 14*(5), 92–108.

Sorensen, T. K., Williams, M. A., Lee, I. M., Dashow, E. E., Thompson, M. L., & Luthy, D. A. (2003). Recreational physical activity during pregnancy and risk of preeclampsia. *Hypertension, 41*(6), 1273–1280. doi:10.1161/01.HYP.0000072270.82815.91

The Joint Commission. (2010). *Preventing Maternal Death* (Sentinel Event Alert No. 44). Oakbrook Terrace, IL; Author. Retrieved from http://www.jointcommission.org/assets/1/18/sea_44.pdf

Waite, L. L., Louie, R. E., & Taylor, R. N. (2005). Circulating activators of peroxisome proliferator-activated receptors are reduced in preeclamptic pregnancy. *Journal of Clinical Endocrinology and Metabolism, 90*(2), 620–626. doi:10.1210/jc.2004-0849

Walfisch, A., & Hallak, M. (2006). Hypertension in pregnancy. In D. K. James, P. J. Steer, C. P. Weiner, & B. Gonik (Eds.), *High Risk Pregnancy: Management Options* (3rd ed., pp. 772–789). Philadelphia: Saunders Elsevier.

Wang, Y., Gu, Y., Zhang, Y., & Lewis, D. F. (2004). Evidence of endothelial dysfunction in preeclampsia: Decreased endothelial nitric oxide synthase expression is associated with increased cell permeability in endothelial cells from preeclampsia. *American Journal of Obstetrics and Gynecology, 190*(3), 817–824. doi:10.1016/j.ajog.2003.09.049

Weissgerber, T. L., Wolfe, L. A., & Davies, G. A. (2004). The role of regular physical activity in preeclampsia prevention. *Medicine and Science in Sports and Exercise, 36*(12), 2024–2031.

Xu, J. Q., Kochanek, K. D., Murphy, S. L., & Tejada-Vera, B. (2010). Deaths: Final data for 2007. *National Vital Statistics Reports, 58*(19). Retrieved from http://www.cdc.gov/nchs/data/nvsr/nvsr58/nvsr58_19.pdf

Yamamoto, T., Suzuki, Y., Kojima, K., & Suzumori, K. (2005). Reduced flow-mediated vasodilation is not due to a decrease in production of nitric oxide in preeclampsia. *American Journal of Obstetrics and Gynecology, 192*(2), 558–563. doi:10.1016/j.ajog.2004.08.031

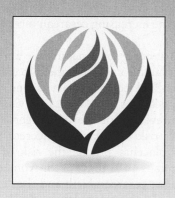

Mary Ellen Burke Sosa

CHAPTER 6

Bleeding in Pregnancy

SIGNIFICANCE AND INCIDENCE

Hemorrhagic complications during pregnancy are a significant causative factor of adverse maternal–fetal outcomes. Major blood loss predisposes the woman to an increased risk of hypovolemia, anemia, infection, preterm labor/birth, and maternal death. Although bleeding can cause considerable problems for the mother, the fetus is especially in jeopardy because significant maternal blood loss can result in negative alterations in maternal hemodynamic status and decreased oxygen-carrying capacity. When bleeding decreases blood flow to the placenta, maternal–fetal gas exchange is reduced and the fetus is at risk for progressive physiologic deterioration (e.g., hypoxemia, hypoxia, asphyxia, and death). This risk is directly related to the amount and duration of blood loss.

Hemorrhage during pregnancy is one of the leading causes of maternal death in the United States, along with embolism and hypertensive disorders (Berg, Callaghan, Syverson, & Henderson, 2010; Paxton & Wardlaw, 2011; The Joint Commission [TJC], 2010). According to the most recent data available from the Centers for Disease Control and Prevention (Berg et al., 2010), the aggregate pregnancy-related mortality ratio for the 8-year period from 1998 to 2005 was 14.5 per 100,000 live births, which is higher than any period in the previous 20 years of the Pregnancy Mortality Surveillance System. African American women continued to have a threefold to fourfold higher risk of pregnancy-related death (Berg et al., 2010), which may reflect social, economic, and cultural barriers to healthcare (Mahlmeister, 2010). The proportion of deaths attributable to hemorrhage and hypertensive disorders declined from previous years, whereas the proportion from medical conditions,

particularly cardiovascular, increased (Berg et al., 2010). Nevertheless, hemorrhage related to pregnancy remains a significant issue in the United States as seven causes of death, including hemorrhage, thrombotic pulmonary embolism, infection, hypertensive disorders of pregnancy, cardiomyopathy, cardiovascular conditions, and noncardiovascular medical conditions, each contributed 10% to 13% of maternal deaths (Berg et al., 2010). It is estimated that 70% to 92% of maternal deaths from hemorrhage are preventable (Berg et al., 2005). When considering all maternal deaths, the outcome of pregnancy was helpful in identifying specific risks. For example, no maternal deaths were reported as a result of a molar pregnancy, while 93% of deaths of women with ectopic pregnancy were hemorrhage related (Berg et al., 2010). When the outcome of pregnancy was live birth, maternal deaths were caused by a number of factors, including uterine rupture, placental abruption, placenta previa, placenta accreta, retained placental fragments, coagulopathies, and uterine atony (Berg et al., 2010). Significant causes of death in women whose pregnancy ends in stillbirth are hemorrhage from placental abruption and uterine rupture (Berg et al., 2010; Chang et al., 2003). Placental abruption and uterine rupture also are significant causes of fetal death (Silver, 2007).

As noted in The Joint Commission's (2010) Sentinel Event Alert *Preventing Maternal Death,* the nurse must be alert to the symptoms of hemorrhage and shock and be prepared to act quickly to minimize blood loss and hasten maternal and fetal stabilization. Up to 15% of maternal cardiac output (750 mL to 1,000 mL/min) flows through the placental bed at term; unresolved bleeding can result in maternal exsanguination in 8 to 10 minutes (Rajan & Wing, 2010). In addition to the physiologic implications of bleeding during pregnancy, the mother experiences emotional stress as she worries about the outcome for herself and her baby. Although maternal mortality decreased approximately 99% during the 20th century, hemorrhage remains a major cause of maternal death in all parts of the world. According to the most recent data, maternal mortality rates in the United States increased from 7.6 per 100,000 live births in 1996, 9.8 per 100,000 live births in 2000, and 12.1 per 100,000 live births in 2003 to approximately 15.4 per 100,000 live births in 2005 (Berg et al., 2010; Hoyert, 2007). The increase is significant as these rates had remained constant for the previous two decades (Clark et al., 2008) after many years of decreasing (e.g., 607.9 per 100,000 live births in 1915; 83.3 per 100,000 live births in 1950) (Hoyert, 2007). It is unclear whether the increase represents more women actually dying or improved coding and data collection methods (Berg et al., 2010).

Bleeding complicates approximately one in five pregnancies; the incidence and cause of bleeding vary by trimester (MacMullen, Dulski, & Meagher, 2005). Most bleeding occurring in the first trimester of pregnancy is related to spontaneous abortion and is generally not life threatening. Ectopic pregnancy is the leading cause of life-threatening hemorrhage during the first trimester, although the maternal mortality rate declined from 13.0% of all maternal deaths from 1970 to 1989 and to 6.0% from 1991 to 1999 (Creanga et al., 2011). Hemorrhage during the antepartum period usually results from disruption of the placental implantation site (involving a normally implanted placenta or placenta previa) (Hull & Resnik, 2009). Most serious obstetric hemorrhage occurs in the postpartum period as a result of uterine atony after placental separation (American College of Obstetricians and Gynecologists [ACOG], 2006; Driessen et al., 2011). Other causes of postpartum hemorrhage include retained placenta, uterine rupture, abnormal placental implantation, uterine inversion, genital tract trauma, and coagulopathy (ACOG, 2006; Oyelese & Ananth, 2010).

Symptomatic placenta previa is identified in approximately 0.3% to 0.5% of pregnancies (Harper, Obido, Macones, Crane, & Cahill, 2010; Oyelese & Smulian, 2006). Low implantation of the placenta is much more common during early pregnancy; however, most of these cases resolve or are not found to be clinically significant as pregnancy progresses (Harper et al., 2010; Oyelese & Smulian, 2006). Placentas may be classified as low lying during the second trimester by routine abdominal ultrasonography because it is difficult to determine which placentas cross the cervical os during ultrasonographic examination in early pregnancy. Transvaginal ultrasound remains a more accurate way to diagnose placenta previa and to measure the distance from the placental edge to the cervical os (Oyelese & Smulian, 2006; Vergani et al., 2009). The incidence of placenta previa is increasing, most likely secondary to the increasing cesarean birth rate (Hull & Resnik, 2009).

Placenta accreta is an uncommon abnormality of placental implantation where the placenta is abnormally adherent. Placenta accreta is one of the most serious complications of placenta previa. In addition to placenta previa, prior uterine surgery significantly increases the risk of placenta accreta (Comstock, 2011). With placenta previa, the risk of developing placenta accreta is 10% to 25% for women with a history of one prior cesarean birth and rises to more than 38% for women with two or more cesarean births or second-trimester pregnancy terminations (Comstock, 2011; Snegovskikh, Clebone, & Norwitz, 2011). The incidence of placenta accreta is rising secondary to an increase in the cesarean birth rate (Eller et al., 2011; Mahlmeister, 2010).

The incidence of abruptio placentae varies in the literature according to the population studied and diagnostic criteria. In the United States, the reported incidence of abruptio placentae is approximately 1% of all pregnancies (Hull & Resnik, 2009). Risk of recurrence in subsequent pregnancies has been reported to be as high as 5.5% to 16.6%. This rate is approximately 30 times higher than the rate for pregnant women without a history of prior abruptio placentae. The strongest risk factor for abruption is a history of placental abruption in a previous pregnancy (Hull & Resnik, 2009). The risk of recurrence for women with a history of two placental abruptions increases to approximately 25% (Hull & Resnik, 2009).

Vasa previa is a condition in which umbilical arteries and veins abnormally implanted throughout the amnion traverse the cervical os in front of the presenting part of the fetus. Vasa previa is a rare but life-threatening complication for the fetus at the time of rupture of membranes (Oyelese & Smulian, 2006; Robinson & Grobman, 2011). The reported incidence of vasa previa is approximately 1 in 2,500 births (Robinson & Grobman, 2011). Rupture of the vessels during spontaneous or artificial rupture of membranes usually leads to fetal exsanguination or severe neurologic fetal injury secondary to fetal hemorrhage before the cause of bleeding is recognized and before an emergent cesarean birth can be accomplished (Silver, 2007). Fetal death occurs in 60% to 75% of cases of ruptured vasa previa (Oyelese & Smulian, 2006).

Uterine rupture is another significant cause of maternal hemorrhage. The risk of uterine rupture for women attempting vaginal birth after cesarean birth (VBAC) is less than 1%; however, the consequences can be catastrophic for the mother and baby (ACOG, 2010; Spong & Queenan, 2011; Tillett, 2010). The risk of uterine rupture depends on the number, type, and location of the previous incisions (ACOG, 2010; Lang &

Landon, 2010). Although risk of uterine rupture has been reported as nearly five times greater for women with a history of two prior low transverse cesarean births when compared to women with one prior cesarean birth (ACOG, 2010), a large multicenter study did not find a difference in rupture rates in these two groups (Cahill & Macones, 2007; Landon et al., 2006; Lang & Landon, 2010). Women with a previous low-vertical uterine incision have a similar success rate for having a VBAC as those women with a previous low transverse incision (ACOG, 2010; Cahill & Macones, 2007). The risk of uterine rupture is increased for women with a T-shaped incision (ACOG, 2010).

Waiting for spontaneous labor, thus avoiding pharmacologic cervical ripening agents and oxytocin, appears to significantly decrease the risk of uterine rupture for women attempting VBAC (ACOG, 2010; Landon et al., 2005; Lang & Landon, 2010). There are enough data to suggest that prostaglandins and high rates of oxytocin infusion increase the risk for rupture (ACOG, 2010; Lang & Landon, 2010). Uterine ruptures at the scar site and remote from the previous scar site have been reported with high doses of oxytocin (Lang & Landon, 2010). It has been theorized that prostaglandins induce local biochemical modifications that weaken the prior uterine scar, thus predisposing it to rupture (Lang & Landon, 2010). Due to the risk of uterine rupture with the use of misoprostol or any prostaglandin agent for cervical ripening or induction, ACOG (2010) does not recommend prostaglandins for women attempting VBAC. If labor needs to be induced in a patient with a previous scar for a clear and compelling clinical indication, the potential increased risk of uterine rupture with the use of prostaglandins should be discussed with the patient and documented in the medical record (ACOG, 2010).

The incidence of uterine inversion is approximately 1 case in 2,500 births, although the range varies among studies (You & Zahn, 2006). It is difficult to ascertain the true incidence because uterine inversion is not often reported in the literature. Improper management of the third stage of labor increases the likelihood of iatrogenic uterine inversion (Oyelese & Ananth, 2010).

Postpartum hemorrhage remains one of the leading causes of maternal death worldwide (Burke, 2010; Callaghan, Kuklina, & Berg, 2010; Oyelese & Ananth, 2010). Early or primary postpartum hemorrhage (within 24 hours after birth) is most frequently caused by uterine atony, retained placental fragments, lower genital tract lacerations, uterine rupture, uterine inversion, placenta accreta, and coagulopathies. Late or secondary postpartum hemorrhage (>24 hours to 6 weeks after birth) is more likely to be caused by infection, placental site subinvolution, retained placental fragments, and coagulopathy (Rajan & Wing, 2010).

DEFINITIONS AND CLINICAL MANIFESTATIONS

The definitions, cause, pathophysiology, and clinical manifestations of the most frequently occurring causes of bleeding and bleeding disorders in pregnancy are described in the following sections. A diagnosis-specific summary of expected management is included. A more detailed summary of nursing interventions for bleeding during pregnancy concludes this section.

PLACENTA PREVIA

Placenta previa is the abnormal implantation of the placenta in the lower uterine segment. The reported incidence of placenta previa at birth varies widely. This variation results from differences in the time of diagnosis. Asymptomatic placenta previa is often diagnosed during routine ultrasound performed in the second trimester; most cases of placenta previa are detected before the third trimester (Oyelese & Smulian, 2006). These women are at increased risk for other obstetric complications such as placental abruption, intrauterine growth restriction (IUGR), and hemorrhage. It has been theorized that the placental tissue that surrounds the cervical os does not develop as well as the placental tissue that is in the myometrium (Hull & Resnik, 2009; Oyelese & Smulian, 2006). By the end of 40 weeks of pregnancy, the incidence of placenta previa is approximately 0.05% (Harper et al., 2010). The most significant risk factors include prior uterine surgery resulting in uterine scarring and history of a prior placenta previa (Hull & Resnik, 2009; Oyelese & Smulian, 2006). Late development and implantation of the ovum, more frequently occurring in older women, may also play a role in placenta previa. Display 6–1 lists the risk factors associated with placenta previa.

DISPLAY 6 – 1

Risk Factors Associated with Placenta Previa

- Previous placenta previa
- Previous cesarean birth
- Induced or spontaneous abortions involving suction curettage
- Multiparity
- Advanced maternal age (>35 years)
- Cigarette smoking
- Multiple gestation
- Fetal hydrops fetalis
- Large placenta
- Uterine anomalies
- Fibroid tumors
- Endometritis
- African American or Asian ethnicity

Placental implantation has traditionally been classified as normal, low-lying, partial placenta previa, and total placenta previa (Fig. 6–1). Clark (1999) proposed a new classification system: placenta previa, in which the placenta covers the internal os in the third trimester, and marginal placenta previa, in which the placenta is within 2 to 3 cm of the internal os but does not cover the os. The rationale for this classification system is the ambiguity and lack of clinical utility of the term *low-lying placenta*. Until Clark's (1999) classification, there had been no accepted definition of how close the placenta must be to mandate cesarean birth or double setup examination. It is now known that there is no increased risk of intrapartum hemorrhage if the distance from the lower margin of the placenta to the internal os is at least 2 to 3 cm (Vergani et al., 2009). As the ability to more accurately visualize placental location increases because of advancements in ultrasound technologies, this classification system has been adopted in clinical practice. The term *placental migration* (a misnomer) has been used to describe the apparent movement of the placenta away from the cervical os. The placenta does not move; it remains in place as the uterus expands away from the os.

Clinical Manifestations

Painless uterine bleeding during the second or third trimester characterizes placenta previa. The first significant bleeding episode may occur before 30 weeks' gestation; some women never exhibit bleeding as a symptom until labor develops (Hull & Resnik, 2009). Rarely is the first bleeding episode life threatening or a cause of hypovolemic shock. The bright red bleeding may be intermittent or continuous. After the bleeding episode, women may demonstrate "spotting" of bright red or dark brown blood on the peripad.

Diagnosis

The standard for the diagnosis of placenta previa is an ultrasound examination. It may be a transabdominal, transvaginal, or translabial ultrasound. Transvaginal ultrasound provides precise information regarding the placement of the placenta in relation to the cervical os (Hull & Resnik, 2009; Oyelese & Smulian, 2006). If ultrasound reveals a normally implanted placenta, a speculum examination is performed to exclude local causes of bleeding (e.g., cervicitis, polyps, carcinoma of the cervix) and a coagulation profile is obtained

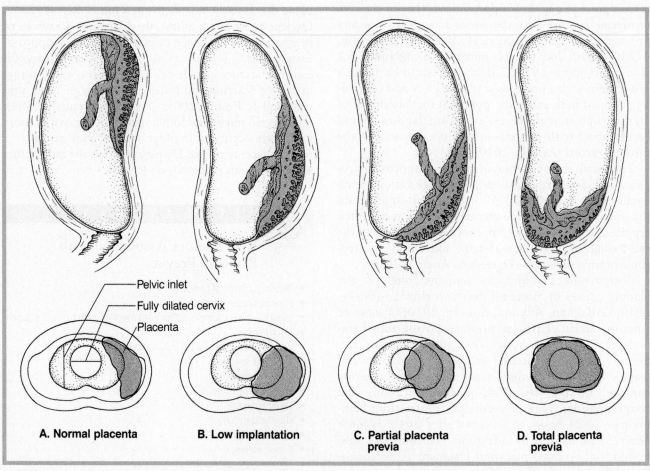

Pelvic inlet
Fully dilated cervix
Placenta

A. Normal placenta   **B. Low implantation**   **C. Partial placenta previa**   **D. Total placenta previa**

FIGURE 6-1. Placenta previa.

to exclude other causes of bleeding. Diagnosis of placenta previa increased dramatically with the advent of transabdominal ultrasound; the rate has decreased with the use of transvaginal or translabial ultrasound (Oyelese & Smulian, 2006). Placenta previa is most often diagnosed before the onset of bleeding when an ultrasound examination is performed for other indications.

Management

Conservative management is usually possible when the fetus is not mature and maternal status is stable. When survival is likely and fetal lung maturity is achieved, birth can be accomplished. Most births are by cesarean section, although vaginal birth may be achieved if the placental edge does not completely cover the cervical os. This type of vaginal birth occurs in the operating room with personnel and equipment available for a cesarean birth if needed (i.e., a double setup).

Patients are frequently hospitalized with the initial bleeding episode. Those with recurrent bleeding episodes, recurrent uterine activity associated with bleeding, or evidence of fetal or maternal compromise usually remain hospitalized until the birth. Some women will have a life-threatening bleeding event. For women who are unstable, blood can be cross-matched at all times and intravenous (IV) access maintained. For stable patients with occasional spotting, a saline lock may be used to maintain an IV access site. In the event of sudden-onset hemorrhage, a second IV line should be initiated with a large bore catheter because it is very difficult to obtain IV access when the woman is in shock. Women who experience an initial bleeding episode that resolves, are hemodynamically stable, demonstrate fetal well-being, and have emergency services readily available to them are candidates for expectant management as outpatients (Hull & Resnik, 2009; Oyelese & Smulian, 2006).

ABRUPTIO PLACENTAE

Abruptio placentae, or premature separation of the placenta, is the detachment of part or all of the placenta from its implantation site, typically occurring after the 20th week of pregnancy (Fig. 6–2). Premature separation of the placenta is a serious event and accounts for about 15% of all neonatal deaths (Witlin, Saade, Mattar, & Sibai, 1999). More than 50% of these deaths are the result of preterm birth. Other causes of fetal death include hypoxia and asphyxia. Risk factors associated with abruptio placentae are listed in Display 6–2. Despite these reported risk factors, the exact cause of abruptio placentae is unknown. There may be some type of disease or damage to the blood vessels; this may be of long duration. The risk of recurrence in subsequent pregnancies has been reported as high as 5% to 16% (Hull & Resnik, 2009). Women with two previous placental abruptions have a risk of recurrence of 25% (Hull & Resnik, 2009). Women with severe preeclampsia and eclampsia are at high risk for abruptio placentae. This high-risk status includes women with mild pregnancy-induced or chronic hypertension. A placental abruption significant enough to cause fetal death is less common (1 in 420 births), but as use of cocaine has increased, fetal death associated with abruptio placentae has risen in selected populations (Hull & Resnik, 2009).

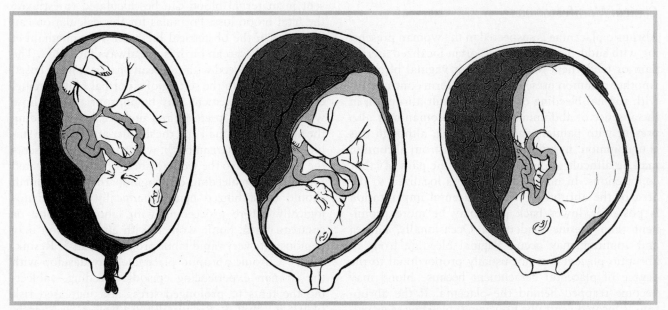

FIGURE 6–2. Abruptio placentae at various separation sites. (*Left*) External hemorrhage. (*Center*) Internal or concealed hemorrhage. (*Right*) Complete separation.

Risk Factors Associated with Abruptio Placentae

- Partial abruption of current pregnancy
- Prior abruptio placentae
- Rapid decompression of the uterus, such as birth of the first of multiple fetuses and amniotic reduction therapy in polyhydramnios
- Hypertension
- Preterm premature rupture of membranes <34 weeks' gestation
- Prior cesarean birth
- Blunt abdominal trauma
- Thrombophilias
- Multiparity
- Cocaine use
- Cigarette smoking
- Extremely short length of the umbilical cord
- Uterine anomalies
- Uterine fibroids at the placental implantation site
- Use of intrauterine pressure catheters during labor

Quantitative proteinuria and the degree of blood pressure elevation are not predictive of an abruption (Witlin et al., 1999). Investigators concluded that the greatest morbidity occurred in preeclamptic women with preterm gestations not receiving prenatal care (Witlin et al., 1999). Thrombophilias, such as factor V Leiden or the antiphospholipid antibody syndrome, were thought to be associated with an increased risk of abruption (Sibai, 2005); however, studies have shown that there is no increased risk of abruption with factor V Leiden mutation (Hull & Resnik, 2009).

Clinical Manifestations

Abruptio placentae is suspected in the woman presenting with sudden-onset, intense, often localized uterine pain or tenderness with or without vaginal bleeding. Another common presentation is preterm contractions with vaginal bleeding or with an occult abruption in the absence of abdominal pain. The woman may also present with painless vaginal bleeding, although this is uncommon. In mild cases, the pain from abruption may be difficult to distinguish from the pain of labor contractions. In many cases, pain is localized to the area of the abruption. When placental implantation is posterior, lower back pain may be more prominent than uterine tenderness. Occasionally, nausea and vomiting may occur. Vaginal bleeding from an abruptio placentae is not usually proportional to the degree of placental detachment because blood may become trapped behind the placenta. If the abruption is located centrally, no vaginal bleeding is visualized initially. Approximately 10% of women present

with concealed hemorrhage (Hull & Resnik, 2009). Marginal separations and large abruptions are associated with bright red bleeding and are almost always accompanied by contractions that are usually of low amplitude and high frequency (Hull & Resnik, 2009; Oyelese & Ananth, 2010; Oyelese & Smulian, 2006).

Contractions may be difficult to record if there is an increase in uterine resting tone and for women at earlier gestations. Palpation for uterine contractions or hypertonus is necessary. The contraction pattern of women with an evolving placental abruption often will show frequent contractions of short duration. Fetal assessment by electronic fetal monitoring (EFM) should be accomplished before obtaining a full uterine ultrasound because most placental abruptions cannot be accurately identified with ultrasonography. More than 50% of placental abruptions are not visible on ultrasound (Hull & Resnik, 2009; Oyelese & Ananth, 2010).

The fetal response to abruptio placentae depends on the volume of blood loss and the extent of uteroplacental insufficiency. Anticipatory nursing care includes being alert to the possibility of an abruption in the presence of any or all of the following: fetal tachycardia; bradycardia; loss of variability; presence of late decelerations; decreasing baseline (especially from tachycardia to a normal or near normal baseline with minimal or absent variability); a sinusoidal fetal heart rate (FHR) pattern; low-amplitude, high-frequency contractions; uterine hypertonus; and abdominal pain.

The Kleihauer–Betke (KB) test may be performed on the mother's serum or vaginal blood to test for the presence of fetal red blood cells (RBCs). Fetal-to-maternal transfer of blood is documented by the presence of fetal cells in maternal serum (Silver, 2007). Depending on fetal age and size, the number of fetal RBCs present in maternal blood can be calculated to estimate the fetal blood loss. Formulas for this calculation can be found in the obstetrical literature (Cunningham et al., 2010). Cesarean birth is not always indicated. The decision to proceed with cesarean birth is usually based on fetal status. In the setting of a normal FHR tracing, expectant management may be appropriate for those women who are preterm and not in labor, providing the abruption is small and the mother and fetus are stable. Labor or cesarean birth, whichever mode presents the fewest risks to the woman and/or fetus, is indicated for significant bleeding or coagulopathy. The woman should be stabilized hemodynamically and hematologically before proceeding with labor initiation or cesarean birth. Some women with an abruption may demonstrate very rapid labor progress (Hull & Resnik, 2009). Chronic abruptio placentae may develop with the woman experiencing episodic bleeding, subjecting the fetus to prolonged stress and increased risk of IUGR (Hull & Resnik, 2009; Oyelese & Ananth, 2010). Risk of developing disseminated intravascular coagulation (DIC) exists during placental abruption because of release of thromboplastin from the site into the maternal bloodstream.

Diagnosis

The diagnosis of abruptio placentae is based on the woman's history, physical examination, and laboratory studies. Examination of the placenta at birth or by a pathologist confirms the diagnosis. Ultrasonography is used to exclude placenta previa; however, it is not diagnostic for abruption (Hull & Resnik, 2009). Abruptions are classified as partial, marginal (i.e., only the margin of the placenta is involved), or total (i.e., complete).

Management

Treatment depends on maternal and fetal status. In the presence of fetal compromise, severe hemorrhage, coagulopathy, poor labor progress, or increasing uterine resting tone, an emergent cesarean birth is performed once efforts to stabilize the woman have been initiated. In an older but reliable study, 22% of all perinatal deaths from abruption occurred after the patient was hospitalized, with 30% occurring in the first 2 hours (Knab, 1978). If the mother is hemodynamically stable, the fetus is alive with a normal FHR tracing (or an indeterminate FHR tracing with imminent birth), or if the fetus is dead, a vaginal birth may be attempted. If the mother is hemodynamically unstable, attempts are first directed at maternal stabilization.

IV access is established; if possible, two lines are placed. Blood replacement products and lactated Ringer's solution are infused in quantities necessary to maintain urine output of 30 to 60 mL/hr and a hematocrit of approximately 30%. Some experts suggest 1 Unit of blood replacement for every 4 L of IV fluid or 3 mL of crystalloid solution for every milliliter of blood loss (Clark, 2004). Blood loss is almost always underestimated (Oyelese & Smulian, 2006). Fluid resuscitation is aggressive in the presence of hemorrhage. With rapid volume IV infusions, the nurse anticipates the possibility of pulmonary edema due to lower colloid osmotic pressure in pregnancy. DIC may develop, placing the mother at significant risk for maternal morbidity and mortality.

ABNORMAL PLACENTAL IMPLANTATION

Abnormal adherence of the placenta occurs for unknown reasons but is thought to be the result of zygote implantation in an area of defective decidua basalis (Comstock, 2011). The risk has greatly increased in the last 10 years with the rapidly rising rate of cesarean births (Eller et al., 2011; You & Zahn, 2006). The risk of placenta accreta increases with the number of previous cesarean births; the odds ratio increases from 1.3 for a second cesarean birth to 29.8 for the sixth or greater cesarean births (ACOG, 2006; Comstock, 2011; Wright et al., 2011). When pregnancy is complicated by placenta previa, the risk of accreta is much greater, increasing to 67% for women with four or more cesarean births presenting with anterior or central placenta previa (Lyndon et al., 2010; Wright et al., 2011). Patients with one prior cesarean birth who present with anterior or central placenta previa in the subsequent pregnancy have a 24% risk of placenta accreta (ACOG, 2002). Placenta accreta and uterine atony are the two most common causes of postpartum hysterectomy (ACOG, 2006; Eller et al., 2011). Other risk factors include advanced maternal age, smoking, and a short interconceptual period.

Clinical Manifestations

Placenta accreta occurs when there is a lack of decidua basalis, so that the placenta is implanted directly into the myometrium. Complete accreta occurs when the entire placenta is adherent; partial accreta occurs with one or more cotyledons adherent; and focal accreta occurs with one piece of a cotyledon adherent. Placenta increta is the abnormal invasion of the trophoblastic cells into the uterine myometrium. Placenta percreta occurs when the trophoblast cells penetrate the uterine musculature and the placenta develops on organs in the vicinity of the percreta. Placenta percreta can adhere to the bladder and other pelvic organs and vessels. Placenta percreta accounts for only 5% to 7% of cases of abnormal adherence. Placenta increta occurs in 15% to 18% of cases, and placenta accreta is the most common form, accounting for 75% to 80% of cases (Comstock, 2011; You & Zahn, 2006). Figure 6–3 demonstrates abnormal adherence of the placenta.

Diagnosis

Placental attachment disorders in women who have a placenta implanted over a uterine scar can be accurately diagnosed prior to 20 weeks' gestation by ultrasound,

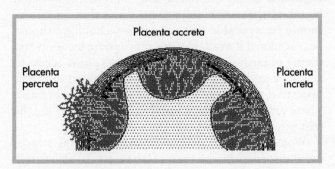

FIGURE 6-3. Abnormal adherence of the placenta.

and placenta increta and percreta can be accurately diagnosed in the second trimester by ultrasound or MRI (Comstock, 2011; Yang et al., 2006). Second trimester maternal serum alpha-fetoprotein (MSAFP) levels were noted in recent studies to be elevated in women with placenta previa and accreta (Lyndon et al., 2010). The diagnosis of an abnormally adherent placenta was made historically when manual separation of a retained placenta was attempted. If the placenta does not separate readily, rapid surgical intervention may be indicated. The woman with an abnormally attached placenta is at increased risk for hemorrhage; 90% of women lose more than 3,000 mL of blood intraoperatively, and the maternal mortality rate has been reported as high as 7% to 10% (Wright et al., 2011; You & Zahn, 2006).

Management

Maternal morbidity due to placental attachment disorders is decreased in women who are diagnosed before birth and treated by a multidisciplinary team. The goal is to prevent shock, thrombosis, infection, ureteral injury, and adult respiratory distress syndrome (ARDS). Patients may receive erythropoietin before the surgery and thrombosis prevention, antibiotics, and fluid resuscitation during the surgery. Invasive hemodynamic monitoring is continuous. It is recommended that 8 to 10 units of packed RBCs be available in the operating room, with the blood bank maintaining the same amount (Eller et al., 2011). Anesthesia, surgery, and urology services may be involved in the cesarean hysterectomy. An interventional radiologist may be needed if selective embolization of the hypogastric arteries with an absorbable gel is performed to reduce blood loss (Eller et al., 2011; You & Zahn, 2006).

It is recommended that women with a history of prior cesarean birth have an ultrasound to determine if there is a placenta previa. If so, further screening for an accreta via ultrasound and/or MRI is recommended (Lyndon et al., 2010). Planning for the potential of significant maternal blood loss and its sequelae is critical. If there is a diagnosis or strong suspicion of placenta accreta prior to birth, ACOG (2006) recommends the following measures: the woman should be counseled about the likelihood of hysterectomy and blood transfusion, blood products and clotting factors should be available and cell savor technology should be considered if available, the appropriate location and timing of birth should be considered to allow access to adequate surgical personnel and equipment, and preoperative anesthesia assessment should be obtained. These anticipatory steps improve the potential for the best possible outcome.

Women who are diagnosed with placental attachment disorders at the time of birth are at higher risk for developing the previously described complications, as well as for an increased risk of death. Mobilization of nursing and medical staff, anesthesia, blood bank, surgery, and radiology is necessary immediately to perform the cesarean hysterectomy (Snegovskikh et al., 2011). In hospitals where specialized services may not be immediately available, the nurse can anticipate the need for calling in extra staff, alerting on-call physicians, obtaining uncrossed O-negative blood, and proceeding to hysterectomy.

VASA PREVIA

Clinical Manifestations/Diagnosis

Vasa previa is the result of a velamentous insertion of the umbilical cord. With vasa previa, the umbilical cord is implanted into the membranes rather than into the placenta. The vessels then traverse within the membrane, crossing the cervical os before reaching the placenta. The umbilical vein and arteries are not surrounded by Wharton's jelly, so they have no supportive tissue, which predisposes the umbilical blood vessels to laceration; this condition occurs most often during either spontaneous or artificial rupture of the membranes (Oyelese & Smulian, 2006; Robinson & Grobman, 2011). The sudden appearance of bright red blood at the time of spontaneous or artificial rupture of the membranes, coupled with the sudden onset of an indeterminate or abnormal FHR pattern, should immediately alert the nurse to the possibility of vasa previa. Bleeding that is fetal in origin is always significant because of the small volume of fetal blood. Total blood volume in the fetus is approximately 80 to 100 mL/kg, and rapid exsanguination can result in severe neurologic injury or fetal death (Silver, 2007).

Management

Immediate cesarean birth is indicated in the presence of vasa previa. Vasa previa rupture may also occur before or after rupture of the membranes; the diagnosis is considered for women with limited antenatal bleeding and indeterminate or abnormal FHR patterns. Risk factors associated with vasa previa are listed in Display 6–3.

DISPLAY 6 - 3

Risk Factors Associated with Vasa Previa

- Succenturiate-lobed placenta
- Bilobed placenta
- Placenta previa
- In vitro fertilization
- Multiple gestation
- Fetal anomaly

Although it rarely occurs (approximately 1 in 2,500 births or 1 in 50 cases in which there is a velamentous insertion of the cord), vasa previa is associated with high incidence of fetal morbidity and mortality because fetal bleeding rapidly leads to shock and exsanguination (Oyelese et al., 2004; Robinson & Grobman, 2011). Vasa previa is occasionally diagnosed before rupture of the membranes by examiners performing an ultrasound for other indications, palpating a pulsing vessel, directly visualizing a vessel, or identifying fetal blood cells in vaginal blood. Diagnosis before birth may be made with transvaginal color Doppler ultrasound. It has been suggested that an increased rate of diagnosis may occur if routine ultrasound examinations include an evaluation of placental cord insertion. Transvaginal ultrasound is indicated if placental cord insertion cannot be determined transabdominally (Hull & Resnik, 2009; Oyelese & Smulian, 2006). If noted, planned cesarean birth is accomplished at 34 to 35 weeks' gestation (Robinson & Grobman, 2011). The survival rate in one retrospective study was 56% without a prenatal diagnosis versus 97% with a prenatal diagnosis (Oyelese et al., 2004).

In the case of an antenatal bleeding event, some practitioners suggest obtaining a KB or Apt test to determine if the blood is fetal in origin. These tests have limited clinical utility during labor because of the short time required from rupture to birth to save the fetus; complete exsanguination can occur in less than 10 minutes as all of the fetal cardiac output moves the umbilical cord (Hull & Resnik, 2009).

UTERINE RUPTURE

Uterine rupture may be a catastrophic event for the woman and fetus, whether related to rupture of a uterine scar from prior uterine surgery, tachysystole, trauma, or, rarely, spontaneous rupture of the uterus. The terms "uterine rupture" and "uterine dehiscence" are sometimes used interchangeably in the literature. Uterine rupture refers to the actual separation of the uterine myometrium or previous uterine scar, with rupture of the membranes and possible extrusion of the fetus or fetal parts into the peritoneal cavity. Dehiscence refers to a separation of the old scar with the uterine serosa remaining intact; the fetus remains inside the uterus (Lang & Landon, 2010). Excessive bleeding usually occurs with uterine rupture, whereas bleeding is generally minimal with dehiscence.

Uterine rupture occurs most frequently in women with a previous uterine incision through the myometrium and usually occurs during labor, although it can occur in the antepartum period. Tachysystole or hypertonus of the uterus caused by oxytocin or prostaglandin administration can cause uterine rupture even in the unscarred uterus (Catanzarite, Cousins, Dowling,

DISPLAY 6-4

Risk Factors Associated with Uterine Rupture

- Previous uterine surgery
- High dosages of oxytocin
- Prostaglandin preparations (e.g., misoprostol, dinoprostone)
- Tachysystole
- Hypertonus
- Grand multiparity
- Blunt or penetrating abdominal trauma
- Midforceps rotation
- Maneuvers within the uterus
- Obstructed labor
- Abnormal fetal lie
- Previous termination(s) of pregnancy
- Vigorous pressure on the uterus at birth

& Daneshmand, 2006; Lang & Landon, 2010; Mazzone & Woolever, 2006). The use of misoprostol is contraindicated for third trimester use (ACOG, 2010; Scott, 2011). Invasive or blunt trauma, seen in women after a motor vehicle accident, battery, fall, or with knife or gunshot wound, is an additional cause of uterine rupture. Uterine rupture may also occur spontaneously with no history of uterine surgery or terminations of pregnancy. Display 6–4 describes the risk factors associated with uterine rupture.

Clinical Manifestations

The clinical presentation of the woman experiencing a uterine rupture depends on the specific type of rupture and may develop over several hours or several minutes. Impending rupture may be preceded by increasing uterine hypertonus or tachysystole (Lang & Landon, 2010; Sheiner et al., 2004). Contrary to earlier reports, *usually* there is no decrease in uterine tone or cessation of contractions prior to or during uterine rupture (ACOG, 2010; Lang & Landon, 2010), although this finding has been reported by some researchers (Sheiner et al., 2004). Indeterminate or abnormal changes in the FHR pattern are early signs of impending or evolving uterine rupture and are seen in up to 70% of cases of uterine rupture (ACOG, 2010; Cahill & Macones, 2007; Lang & Landon, 2010; Sheiner et al., 2004). The FHR pattern prior to rupture or as the rupture is evolving may be characterized by a decrease in variability; recurrent variable, prolonged, or late decelerations followed by bradycardia; or sudden onset of fetal bradycardia (Ayres, Johnson, & Hayashi, 2001; Lang & Landon, 2010; Menihan, 1999; Ridgeway, Weyrich, & Benedetti, 2004). The most consistent indeterminate or abnormal FHR patterns noted with uterine rupture are recurrent variable or late decelerations and fetal bradycardia (ACOG, 2010; Ayres et al., 2001; Lang & Landon, 2010; Ridgeway et al., 2004). If the uterine rupture is preceded by late decelerations, the fetus will tolerate a shorter period of prolonged decelerations. Significant neonatal morbidity has been reported when the time between onset of prolonged decelerations and birth is equal to or greater than 17 minutes (Scott, 2011). Jauregui, Kirkendall, Ahn, and Phelan (2000) reported a significant risk of brain damage, intrapartum death, and death within 1 year of life for infants who were partially or completely extruded into the maternal abdomen during uterine rupture.

The woman with a uterine rupture may complain of abdominal pain and tenderness and/or have vomiting, syncope, vaginal bleeding, tachycardia, or pallor. If unrecognized, bleeding can quickly cause maternal hypotension and shock. A traumatic rupture may be apparent almost immediately in the woman who complains of sharp, tearing pain, "like something has given way or popped open." There may be an inability on the part of the practitioner to reach the presenting part on vaginal examination, demonstrating loss of fetal station. Uterine contractions may decrease in frequency and intensity or demonstrate tachysystole (Lang & Landon, 2010; Scott, 2011). The fetus may be palpated through the abdominal wall. Bleeding may be vaginal or into the abdominal cavity or both. Intraabdominal bleeding is suspected if the woman has a tense, acute abdomen with shoulder pain. Signs of shock appear soon after a catastrophic rupture, and complete cardiovascular collapse rapidly follows without prompt intervention.

Dehiscence of a prior lower segment cesarean scar is usually asymptomatic initially. The woman may continue to have contractions without further dilation of the cervix; if an intrauterine pressure catheter is in place for labor assessments, there may be little or no change in intrauterine pressure or resting tone pressures. If the dehiscence extends past the scar tissue, the woman may begin to complain of pain in the lower abdomen that is unrelieved with analgesia or epidural anesthesia.

Common sequelae associated with uterine rupture include excessive hemorrhage requiring surgical exploration; need for hysterectomy; need for blood product transfusion; hypovolemia; hypovolemic shock; injury to the bladder or ureters; bowel laceration; extrusion of any part of the fetus, umbilical cord, or placenta through the disruption; emergent cesarean birth for suspected rupture; emergent cesarean birth for indeterminate or abnormal fetal status; and general anesthesia (ACOG, 2010; Landon et al., 2004; Paré, Quiñones, & Macones, 2006; Scott, 2011). Many women with uterine rupture experience more than one of these complications (Landon et al., 2004). Maternal death due to uterine rupture is a rare complication (Chauhan, Martin, Henrichs, Morrison, & Magann, 2003; Landon et al., 2004).

Diagnosis

The key to diagnosis is suspicion that uterine rupture has occurred. The nurse immediately should inform the primary healthcare provider at the first suspicion of a uterine rupture based on characteristics of the FHR pattern and maternal condition. Diagnosis is confirmed at birth.

Management

Treatment includes maternal hemodynamic stabilization and immediate cesarean birth. If possible, the uterine defect is repaired or hysterectomy is performed. Uterine rupture is discussed further in Chapter 14.

INVERSION OF THE UTERUS

Inversion of the uterus (i.e., turning inside out) after birth is a potentially life-threatening complication. The incidence of uterine inversion is approximately 1 in 2,500 births (You & Zahn, 2006). Fundal pressure and traction applied to the cord may result in inversion (Oyelese & Ananth, 2010). Fundal implantation occurs in approximately 10% of pregnancies but is the recorded site in the majority of reported inversions (Thorp, 2009). Other risk factors associated with inversion of the uterus are listed in Display 6–5. Partial inversion occurs when only the fundus inverts. A complete inversion occurs when the fundus passes through the opening of the cervix (Thorp, 2009; You & Zahn, 2006). Although proper management of the third stage of labor prevents most uterine inversions, some uterine inversions are spontaneous and otherwise unavoidable. Regardless of the precipitating factor, once an inversion occurs, prompt recognition and correction is necessary to reduce maternal morbidity and mortality.

Clinical Manifestations/Diagnosis

In addition to possible visualization of the inversion, the primary presenting symptoms of uterine inversion are hemorrhage and hypotension. The woman may

DISPLAY   6 - 5

Risk Factors Associated with Uterine Inversion

- Uterine atony
- Abnormally adherent placental tissue
- Fetal macrosomia
- Fundal placentation
- Uterine anomalies
- Use of oxytocin
- Use of fundal pressure
- Traction on the umbilical cord
- Abnormally short umbilical cord

experience sudden, acute pelvic pain. Attempts to massage the fundus are unsuccessful because the fundus has inverted into the uterus or vaginal vault, or it is visible at or through the introitus. On bimanual examination, there will be a firm mass below or near the cervix along with the absence of an identification of the uterine corpus on abdominal examination (Thorp, 2009).

Management

Uterine inversion is an emergent situation associated with severe hemorrhage and requiring immediate attempts to replace the uterus. If the inversion occurs before placental separation, removal of the placenta will result in additional hemorrhage (ACOG, 2006), although some providers believe it is easy to replace the uterus if the placenta has been removed (Thorp, 2009). The largest amounts of blood loss are those reported with delivery of the placenta prior to attempting to reposition the uterus (You & Zahn, 2006). Replacement of the uterus involves the birth attendant placing the palm of the hand against the fundus (now inverted and lowermost at or through the cervix) as if holding a tennis ball, with the fingertips exerting upward pressure circumferentially (ACOG, 2006). If attempts to replace the uterus are not quickly successful, administration of tocolytics (e.g., terbutaline, magnesium sulfate, nitroglycerin) or general anesthesia may be necessary (ACOG, 2006; Thorp, 2009; You & Zahn, 2006). Manual replacement with or without uterine relaxants is usually successful (ACOG, 2006; Thorp, 2009). Laparotomy may be required in unusual cases. Oxytocin is withheld until the uterus has been repositioned.

Monitoring of maternal vital signs is extremely important because the pharmacologic agents directed at relaxing the uterine myometrium may exacerbate maternal hypotension. Automatic blood pressure cuffs, in use in the majority of hospitals, overestimate systolic values by 4 to 6 mm Hg and underestimate diastolic values by 10 mm Hg. Fluid resuscitation should be initiated to prevent shock. Blood replacement therapy is administered as indicated by maternal hematologic status. Broad-spectrum antibiotic therapy and placement of a nasogastric tube may be initiated as indicated. Uterine inversion may occasionally recur during a subsequent birth.

POSTPARTUM HEMORRHAGE

Postpartum hemorrhage is defined as a 10% decrease in hematocrit from admission assessment to postpartum data collection and the need to administer a transfusion of RBCs or hemodynamic instability (Oyelese & Ananth, 2010; Rajan & Wing, 2010). Blood loss is traditionally underestimated (Callaghan et al., 2010; Lyndon et al., 2010) and is therefore an unreliable determinant of hemorrhage or excessive blood loss. Treatment is based on clinical signs and symptoms. Postpartum hemorrhage is the leading cause of maternal morbidity and mortality worldwide (Callaghan et al., 2010; Driessen et al., 2011; You & Zahn, 2006). Complications of postpartum hemorrhage depend on the severity of the hemorrhage and range from anemia to maternal death.

Postpartum hemorrhage can result from abnormal implantation of the placenta; lacerations of the cervix, vagina, or perineum; uterine inversion; and DIC. However, the most common cause of postpartum hemorrhage worldwide is uterine atony, occurring in over 70% of cases (Driessen et al., 2011; Oyelese & Ananth, 2010). Early postpartum hemorrhage occurs after the delivery of the placenta, up to 24 hours after birth; late postpartum hemorrhage occurs 24 hours to 6 weeks after birth. Late postpartum hemorrhage is associated with subinvolution of the uterus and with retained placental tissue that may be the result of abnormal placental implantation. Display 6–6 lists the risk factors for postpartum hemorrhage. A thorough discussion of postpartum hemorrhage is presented in Chapter 17.

DISPLAY 6-6

Risk Factors Associated with Postpartum Hemorrhage

- Uterine atony
- Precipitous labor
- Intraamniotic infection (IAI)
- Macrosomia
- Multifetal gestation
- History of uterine atony
- Retained products of conception
- Clotted blood in uterus
- Polyhydramnios
- Prolonged labor
- High parity
- Prostaglandin ripening or induction
- Oxytocin induction or augmentation
- Anesthesia effects
- Trauma to genital tract
  ○ Large episiotomy, including extensions; lacerations of the perineum, vagina, or cervix; ruptured uterus
- Genital tract lacerations
- Genital tract hematoma
- Compound presentation
- Precipitous birth
- Forceps birth
- Vacuum extraction
- Episiotomy extension
- Coagulation defects
- Sepsis
- Poorly perfused myometrium because of hypotension, hemorrhage, or conduction anesthesia

Uterine Atony

Uterine atony is marked hypotonia of the uterus. Because of the increased blood flow to the placenta in late pregnancy (approximately 750 to 1,000 mL/min), failure of the uterus to contract after placental separation can result in very rapid and significant blood loss. The usual methods to prevent postpartum hemorrhage are uterine massage and administration of oxytocin (10 to 40 Units/liter [U/L] titrated to control atony).

Uterine atony is more likely to occur when the uterus is overdistended (e.g., multiple gestations, macrosomia, polyhydramnios). In such conditions, the uterus is "overstretched" and contracts poorly. Other causes of atony include induction or augmentation of labor, traumatic birth, halogenated anesthesia, tocolytics, rapid or prolonged labor, intraamniotic infection, and multiparity.

Lacerations of the Birth Canal

Birth canal lacerations may include injuries to the labia, perineum, vagina, and cervix. Lacerations secondary to birth trauma occur more commonly with operative vaginal birth (i.e., forceps or vacuum assisted) (Burke, 2010). Other risk factors include fetal macrosomia, precipitous labor and birth, and episiotomy. Prevention, recognition, and prompt, effective treatment of birth canal lacerations are vital. Lacerations may be anticipated if the uterus is well contracted but bleeding remains brisk. Some birth canal lacerations may result in a hematoma, which may not always be immediately recognized. Severe pelvic pain may be the first reported symptom, although maternal vital signs may deteriorate as the amount of blood loss in the hematoma increases. Because hematoma formation may conceal the blood loss, the woman may develop shock in the absence of other signs of hemorrhage. Pain unrelieved by the usual oral analgesic agents administered postpartum should be investigated.

Severe pelvic pain and continued bleeding despite efficient postpartum uterine contractions with a firm uterus warrants reexamination of the birth canal by the physician or midwife. Continuous bleeding from minor sources may be just as dangerous over time as a sudden loss of a large amount of blood.

Prevention

Active management of the third stage of labor has been found to decrease risk of postpartum hemorrhage by 60% to 70%. Active management occurs by administering oxytocin with delivery of the anterior shoulder, clamping/cutting the umbilical cord within 2 to 3 minutes of birth, controlling traction of the umbilical cord with the provider's hand supporting the uterus to prevent uterine inversion, and performing vigorous fundal massage for at least 15 seconds (Burke, 2010; Lyndon et al., 2010; Rajan & Wing, 2010).

Management

The first step in the treatment of postpartum bleeding is to evaluate the uterus to determine if it is firmly contracted and, if not, to continue uterine massage. IV access with two 16- to 18-gauge catheters may be obtained if not already established. Generally, 20 to 40 units of oxytocin in 1 L of crystalloid solution is given intravenously initially at a rate of 10 to 15 mL/min and then continued for at least 3 or 4 hours following stabilization at a slower rate, as determined by the provider. If the uterus initially fails to respond to oxytocin, 0.2 mg of methylergonovine may be given intramuscularly to correct uterine atony via tetanic uterine contractions. If methylergonovine fails to resolve uterine atony or is contraindicated (e.g., hypertension), 15-methyl-prostaglandin $F_{2\alpha}$ may be administered intramuscularly or intrauterine as long as the woman does not have asthma or systemic lupus. Most hemorrhage is controlled with one or two injections of 0.25 mg of 15-methyl-prostaglandin $F_{2\alpha}$ by intramuscular or intramyometrial routes, depending on the type of birth (Hoffman, 2009). Various dosages of misoprostol (800 to 1,000 mcg) per rectum have been reported in the literature as a successful alternative to the traditional drugs used for postpartum hemorrhage related to uterine atony (Hoffman, 2009; Rajan & Wing, 2010). Misoprostol may be used in the woman who has asthma. Table 6–1 lists the uterotonic agents used for postpartum hemorrhage.

In the event that uterotonic agents are unable to decrease bleeding, the provider may apply uterine tamponade via packing the uterus with gauze or inflating a balloon device that can hold 400 to 500 cc of saline and has a port that allows for assessment of continued bleeding. Assessment of fundal height is very important prior to packing the uterus or placing a balloon device; continued rising of fundal height is indicative of ongoing bleeding (Rajan & Wing, 2010).

Blood transfusion and treatment of shock may be urgently needed during postpartum hemorrhage. The use of autologous transfusion and cell-saver technology, in which the patient's blood is collected during surgery, washed, filtered, and transfused back to the patient, has been used since the early 1970s. Autologous transfusion is considered safe for pregnant women with severe hemorrhage (ACOG, 2006; Fuller & Bucklin, 2010; Porreco & Stettler, 2010); however, autologous transfusion requires anticipation of a need for transfusion, clinicians who are educated in using the technique, and minimum hematocrit concentrations that are often above those of a pregnant woman.

The interior of the uterus is explored so that retained products of conception can be removed and possible rupture of the uterus diagnosed. If the blood fails to

Table 6-1. UTEROTONIC AGENTS USED FOR POSTPARTUM HEMORRHAGE

		Medical Management of Postpartum Hemorrhage		
Medication	Route/Dose	Frequency	Side Effects	Comments/Contraindications
Oxytocin (Pitocin)	IV: 10–40 units in 1 L normal saline or lactated Ringer's solution IM: 10 units	Continuous	Usually none, but N&V and water intoxication have been reported	Avoid undiluted rapid IV infusion, which can cause hypotension
Methylergonovine (Methergine)	IM 0.2 mg	Every 2–4 hr	Hypertension, hypotension, N&V	Avoid if patient is hypertensive
15-methyl-prostaglandin $F_{2\alpha}$ (Carboprost, Hemobate)	IM: 0.25 mg	Every 15–90 min, 8 doses maximum	N&V, diarrhea, flushing or hot flashes, chills or shivering	Avoid in asthmatic patients; relative contraindication if hepatic, renal, and cardiac disease Diarrhea, fever, and tachycardia can occur
Dinoprostone (Prostin E_2)	Suppository; vaginal or rectal 20 mg	Every 2 hr	N&V, diarrhea, fever, headache, chills or shivering	Avoid if patient is hypotensive. If available, 15-methyl-prostaglandin $F_{2\alpha}$ is preferred. Fever is common. Stored frozen, it must be thawed to room temperature.
Misoprostol (Cytotec, PGE_1)	800–1,000 mcg rectally 600 mcg sublingually	1 dose	Fever, chills or shivering	Usually used when other medications have not resulted in resolution of hemorrhage

IM, intramuscularly; IV, intravenously; N&V, nausea and vomiting; PG, prostaglandin.
Adapted from American College of Obstetricians and Gynecologists. (2006). *Postpartum Hemorrhage* (Practice Bulletin No. 76). Washington, DC: Author; Rajan, P. V., & Wing, D. A. (2010). Postpartum hemorrhage: Evidence-based medical interventions for prevention and treatment. *Clinical Obstetrics and Gynecology, 53*(1), 165–181. doi:10.1097/GRF.0b013e3181ce0965

clot, DIC may be developing, and prompt, appropriate treatment may be life saving. The treatment for DIC is to cure the underlying problem. Figure 6–4 provides a management plan for postpartum hemorrhage.

NURSING ASSESSMENT

A medical and obstetric history is usually available in the prenatal record and can be assessed for previous bleeding or bleeding disorders in order to assist the nurse in identifying risk factors for obstetrical precursors to hemorrhage. Assessment of the woman who is bleeding begins with careful evaluation of the amount and color of blood loss, character of uterine activity, presence of abdominal pain, stability of maternal vital signs, and fetal status. Bright red vaginal bleeding suggests active bleeding, and dark or brown blood may indicate past blood loss. Display 6–7 presents nursing assessments and interventions for abnormal bleeding and/or hemorrhage.

Maternal or fetal tachycardia and maternal hypotension suggest hypovolemia; however, hypotension is a late sign. Historically, the frequency of vital signs depends on patient stability. Vital signs are usually repeated every 15 minutes until the bleeding is controlled and the vital signs remain or return to normal. Vital signs are performed more frequently (every 1 to 5 minutes) when there is evidence of instability including systolic blood pressure less than 90 mm Hg, maternal tachycardia, decreasing level of consciousness, and oliguria.

When using an automatic blood pressure cuff, ensure that the Doppler is placed directly over the brachial artery for a more accurate recording. However, in severe hypotensive states, the automatic blood pressure device is less accurate. Many automatic blood pressure monitors calculate mean arterial pressure (MAP = systolic blood pressure +2 × diastolic blood pressure ÷ 3), which provides a quick number for reference and is a more stable parameter of hemodynamic function. The normal value for mean arterial pressure in the second trimester of pregnancy is approximately 80 mm Hg (Page & Christianson, 1976) and is 90 mm Hg at term. When the blood pressure cannot be assessed with a blood pressure cuff, systolic blood pressure may be estimated by the presence of a radial, femoral, or brachial pulse. The presence of a radial pulse is associated with a systolic blood pressure of approximately 80 mm Hg, a femoral pulse with a blood pressure of 70 mm Hg, and a carotid pulse with a blood pressure of 60 mm Hg (Ruth & Miller, 2012). Placement of an arterial line in the woman who is hemorrhaging allows for continuous, accurate blood pressure monitoring and provides a means for drawing blood for arterial blood gas analysis and other laboratory values. Invasive

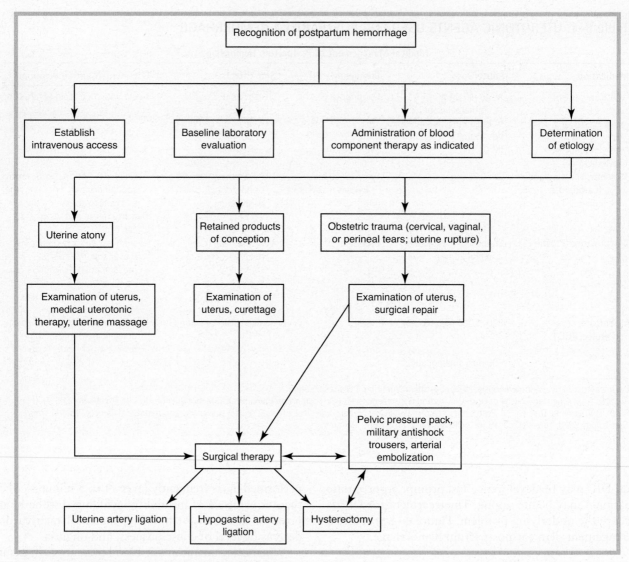

FIGURE 6-4. Management plan for postpartum hemorrhage.

DISPLAY 6-7

Nursing Assessments and Interventions for Abnormal Bleeding/Hemorrhage

INITIAL NURSING INTERVENTIONS
- Notify physician and/or nurse midwife and anesthesia providers.
- Secure airway and start oxygen via nonrebreather mask at 10 L/min.
- Establish intravenous (IV) access if there is not an existing IV line: infuse lactated Ringer's solution (or normal saline) wide open, start another IV with a 16-gauge catheter. (Do not infuse IV solutions containing glucose.)
- Perform uterine massage.
- Obtain complete blood count (CBC), fibrinogen, prothrombin time (PT), partial thromboplastin time (PTT), and other laboratory tests.
- Draw 5 mL of the patient's blood in a clean red-top tube and observe frequently. If no clot forms within 8 to 10 minutes, suspect coagulopathy.

- Type and cross match 4 units of packed red blood cells (PRBCs).
- Administer oxytocin, Methergine, prostaglandin $F_{2\alpha}$, and Cytotec as ordered.
- Administer blood products as ordered.

SECONDARY NURSING INTERVENTIONS
- Insert Foley catheter with urimeter; assess for output of at least 30 mL/hr.
- Apply oxygen saturation monitor.
- Assess maternal vital signs per hospital policy.
- Call for additional nursing help so that one nurse can be responsible for patient care and another nurse can be available for obtaining necessary medications, administering IV fluids, and monitoring intake and output if possible.
- Obtain CBC, PT, PTT, fibrinogen, ionized Ca, K after 5 to 7 units of PRBCs.
- Anticipate surgical intervention such as exploratory laparotomy, Bakri balloon, uterine artery embolization, bilateral uterine artery ligation, B-lynch suture, hypogastric artery ligation, and hysterectomy. Notify members of the surgical team and ensure that a surgical suite is readied.

hemodynamic monitoring with a flow-directed pulmonary artery catheter (Swan-Ganz) may be indicated in selected patients, especially in patients who remain oliguric after fluid resuscitation (Clark, Greenspoon, Aldahl, & Phelan, 1986) or who have other complications such as sepsis, cardiac or pulmonary disease, or severe hypertension related to preeclampsia. Skin and mucous membrane color is noted. Inspection also includes looking for oozing at the sites of incisions or injections and detecting petechiae or ecchymosis in areas not associated with surgery or trauma.

Antenatally, FHR is continuously assessed and the uterus is palpated for contractions, especially in early gestations. In an emergent situation, use of electronic FHR and uterine monitoring provides continuous data about the fetus and uterus, allowing the nurse time to simultaneously initiate other needed treatments. The pregnant woman is positioned in the lateral or modified Trendelenburg position, if possible. If the patient is in Trendelenburg or supine position, a wedge is placed under one hip to alleviate compression of the vena cava and aorta by the gravid uterus. Caution must be used in placing a pregnant woman in Trendelenburg because the pressure of the gravid uterus may interfere with optimal cardiopulmonary functioning. If the mother is hemodynamically unstable, oxygen is administered by nonrebreather facemask at 10 L/min to maintain maternal–fetal oxygen saturation. Mentation is assessed frequently and provides additional indication of maternal blood volume and oxygen saturation.

Blood is drawn to assess maternal hemoglobin, hematocrit, platelet count, and coagulation profile. Display 6–8 lists the blood tests commonly ordered for the woman who is bleeding. In an emergent situation, blood may be drawn into a plain additive-free red-top (clot) tube, the tube taped to a wall and then visually evaluated

DISPLAY 6-8

Laboratory Values Assessed in Pregnant Women Who Are Bleeding

- Complete blood count
- Fibrinogen concentration
- Prothrombin time
- Activated partial thromboplastin time
- Fibrin degradation products or fibrin split products
- Platelet count
- Blood type, Rh, and antibody screen
- Clot retraction

POSSIBLY INDICATED
- Kleihauer–Betke test
- Apt test
- Ivy bleeding time
- D-dimer
- Serum creatinine
  - Blood urea nitrogen (BUN)
- Urine creatinine clearance
- Urine sodium excretion
- Liver function test, including serum glucose
- Antithrombin III
- Arterial blood gases
- Urine or serum drug screen

for clot formation. Treatment for a significant coagulopathy should be initiated if no sign of clotting is evident within 5 to 10 minutes (Lyndon et al., 2010; Rajan & Wing, 2010). Massive hemorrhage protocols offer guidance for volume replacement. The California Maternal Quality Care Collaborative (CMQCC) recommends a ratio of 6 units packed red blood cells (PRBCs); 4 units fresh frozen plasma (FFP); and 1 unit pheresis platelets

Table 6-2. BLOOD REPLACEMENT PRODUCTS

Blood Component Therapy			
Product	Volume (mL)[a]	Contents	Effect (per unit)
Fresh whole blood	500	Red blood cells, all procoagulants	Increase hematocrit by 3 percentage points, hemoglobin by 1 g/dL
Packed red blood cells	240	Red blood cells, white blood cells, plasma	Increase hematocrit by 3 percentage points, hemoglobin by 1 g/dL
Platelets	50	Platelets, red blood cells, plasma; small amounts of fibrinogen, factors V and VIII	Increase platelet count 5,000–10,000/mm³ per unit
Fresh frozen plasma	250	Fibrinogen, antithrombin III, factors V and VIII	Increase fibrinogen by 10 to 25 mg/dL
Cryoprecipitate	40	Fibrinogen, factors VIII and XIII, von Willebrand factor	Increase fibrinogen by 10 to 25 mg/dL

[a]Volume depends on individual blood bank.
Adapted from American College of Obstetricians and Gynecologists. (2006). *Postpartum hemorrhage* (Practice Bulletin No. 76). Washington, DC: Author; Rajan, P. V., & Wing, D. A. (2010). Postpartum hemorrhage: Evidence-based medical interventions for prevention and treatment. *Clinical Obstetrics and Gynecology, 53*(1), 165–181. doi:10.1097/GRF.0b013e3181ce0965

(Lyndon et al., 2010). Table 6–2 lists blood replacement products, factors present, and the expected effect per unit administered.

Circulating volume is usually restored with IV crystalloid solution administration. Two large-bore IV lines are needed for fluid replacement and administration of drug therapies. Blood and blood products are administered as needed or as soon as they are available. Breath sounds are auscultated before fluid volume replacement, if possible, to provide a baseline for future assessment. Massive fluid replacement during pregnancy or the immediate postpartum period for the woman who is hemorrhaging increases the potential for development of pulmonary edema. However, fluid replacement is necessary to restore circulatory volume, and the nurse anticipates and assesses for the development of peripheral or pulmonary edema and treatment with furosemide as ordered. Hemoglobin arterial oxygen saturation is monitored with a pulse oximeter. Pulse oximeters are an adjunct to assessment; they are not always accurate, especially in a patient in hypovolemic shock. In the hemorrhagic patient, blood flow to the extremities is decreased, and the oxygen saturation displayed may not accurately reflect tissue oxygenation status or the pulse oximeter may not be able to display a value at all. Arterial blood gas analysis may therefore be necessary to determine oxygen status. A maternal oxygen saturation level of at least 95% and a PaO_2 of at least 65 mm Hg as determined by blood gas analysis are necessary for the fetus to maintain adequate oxygenation.

Continuous electrocardiogram (ECG) monitoring is indicated for the woman who is hypotensive or tachycardic, continuing to bleed profusely, or in shock. Maternal hypovolemia leading to hypoxia and acidosis may result in maternal heart rate dysrhythmias, including premature ventricular contractions, sinus or atrial tachycardia, and atrial or ventricular fibrillation.

A Foley catheter with a urometer is inserted to allow for hourly assessment of urine output. The most objective and least invasive assessment of adequate organ perfusion and oxygenation is urinary output of at least 30 mL/hr (Ruth & Kennedy, 2011). Attempts should be made to maintain urine output of at least 30 mL/hr because this is an objective and noninvasive means of evaluating adequate end-organ perfusion. In addition to volume, urine is assessed for the presence of blood and protein and for specific gravity.

NURSING INTERVENTIONS

Evaluation and management of acute episodes of bleeding during pregnancy usually occur in the inpatient setting. An exception is spotting during early gestation. After stabilization and a period of hospitalization, selected women may be managed at home.

HOME CARE MANAGEMENT

Controversy exists concerning home care management of women with placenta previa and marginal separation of the placenta; however, women in stable condition increasingly are being cared for in the home, with visits by perinatal nurses or daily provider-initiated phone contact. Criteria for home care management vary with the primary perinatal provider and home care agency. The woman must be in stable condition with no evidence of active bleeding and have resources to be able to return to the hospital immediately if active bleeding resumes. Bed rest at home remains a controversial topic; there are few data to determine how much time a women should be in bed or whether bed rest affects outcome in a positive manner. Complete or partial bed rest has long-term deleterious effects on the woman, physically and psychologically (Maloni, 2011).

INPATIENT MANAGEMENT

When the woman is admitted to the hospital, the nurse begins assessment of the bleeding. The woman with acute bleeding requires continuous, ongoing nursing assessments and interventions. Maternal vital signs are assessed frequently, according to individual clinical situations. Careful assessments are mandatory. Vital signs and noninvasive assessments of cardiac output (e.g., skin color, skin temperature, pulse oximetry, mentation, urinary output) are obtained frequently to observe for signs of declining hemodynamic status.

Because an indeterminate or abnormal FHR pattern may be the first sign of maternal or fetal hemodynamic compromise, electronic FHR and uterine activity monitoring should be continuous. It is important to appreciate how rapidly maternal–fetal status can deteriorate as a result of maternal hemorrhage. Blood is shunted away from the uterus when the mother experiences hypotension or hypovolemic shock. Because of the potential for maternal–fetal mortality, it is essential to be prepared for an emergent birth at all times when caring for a pregnant woman who is bleeding. Supportive staff necessary for an emergency cesarean birth (i.e., anesthesia personnel, surgical team, and neonatal resuscitation team) should be notified and on standby (if possible, in the hospital). Hemorrhage from placenta previa, abruptio placentae, or uterine rupture requires expeditious birth. Two large-bore IV catheters (at least 18-gauge) are placed if the woman is experiencing heavy bleeding. If consistent with institution policy, a 14- or 16-gauge IV catheter may be considered. The need to replace fluids and blood is determined by a number of parameters, including vital signs, amount of blood loss, mental status, laboratory values, and fetal condition.

Fluid replacement consists of administering lactated Ringer's or normal saline solution, PRBCs, FFP, and possibly platelets. Fluid is replaced in a ratio of 3 cc:1 cc lost blood. Blood product replacement therapy is anticipated, and communication with the blood bank is essential. Significant hemorrhage resulting in syncope or hypovolemic shock generally necessitates transfusion.

Blood type, Rh, and antibody screen should be obtained on admission; crossmatching is ordered as necessary. The use of blood components in conjunction with crystalloid solutions, rather than with whole blood, is usually a better treatment option because it provides only the specific components needed (Fuller & Bucklin, 2010; Ruth & Kennedy, 2011). By using only the specific products required for the emergency, blood resources are conserved, and there is a decreased risk of blood replacement complications. Transfusion reactions may be demonstrated by chills, fever, tachycardia, hypotension, shortness of breath, muscle cramps, itching, convulsions, and ultimately cardiac arrest. The woman is assessed throughout the procedure. In the event of a reaction, the transfusion is immediately discontinued, and the IV line is flushed with normal saline. Treatment is then based on clinical symptoms. The development of anaphylaxis should be considered and appropriate treatment made available.

Careful fetal surveillance is critical to ensure fetal well-being during transfusion of multiple blood products. The increased incidence of uteroplacental insufficiency is related to complications of coagulation factor replacement therapy and the amount and duration of blood loss. Administration of multiple replacement blood products leads to increased intravascular fibrin formation. Deposition of fibrin in the decidual vasculature of the chorionic villi may cause fetal compromise.

Because of the normal hemodynamic changes that occur, pregnant women may lose more than one fourth of their fluid volume before displaying signs of shock (Clark, 2004). Women who are bleeding should be monitored carefully for the actual amount of blood loss, although this is sometimes difficult to assess in an emergent situation and is usually underestimated (Ruth & Kennedy, 2011). Sheets or pads can be inspected and weighed. Accurate intake and output measurement and documentation are critical. Ideally, one nurse is assigned to monitor intake and output during a period of massive fluid and blood replacement. In an emergent situation in which the obstetrician and anesthesiologist may be ordering or adding replacement fluid to multiple IV lines, it becomes essential that one of the nurses records and maintains a running total of intake and output in addition to signing for blood products and overseeing administration.

The woman may develop a coagulopathy. Display 6–9 lists the risk factors for DIC. Pulmonary edema and renal failure, as evidenced by oliguria proceeding to anuria, must be anticipated. Systolic blood pressures of less than 60 mm Hg are associated with acute renal failure. The woman is at risk for development of acute tubular necrosis from lack of perfusion to the kidneys (i.e., prerenal failure). Prolonged periods of severe hypotension may result in renal cortical necrosis. Urine output of less than 30 mL/hr should be reported to the primary care provider immediately.

In the case of severe hemorrhage, control of abdominal bleeding may be achieved by the placement of medical antishock trousers (MAST suit), which are used in prehospital settings and in emergency and trauma units to control bleeding. Consensus does not exist about the benefits of using MAST suits; however, MAST suits are used in many institutions. Care must be taken not to put any pressure on the pregnant abdomen past midgestation, but MAST suits can be used for postpartum hemorrhage (Brown, 2009). A nonpneumatic antishock garment (NASG) is also available, and there is some data to support its use during a hemorrhagic situation (Lyndon et al., 2010).

HEMORRHAGIC AND HYPOVOLEMIC SHOCK

Hemorrhagic and hypovolemic shock is an emergent situation in which the perfusion of body organs may become severely compromised and death may ensue. Aggressive treatment is necessary to prevent adverse sequelae (e.g., cellular death, fluid overload, ARDS, oxygen toxicity). Common clinical symptoms of inadequate intravascular volume (i.e., hypovolemia) that necessitate blood replacement include evidence of hemorrhage (i.e., loss of a large amount of blood externally or internally in a short period of time), evidence of hypovolemic shock (e.g., increasing pulse, cool clammy skin,

---

DISPLAY 6 - 9

Obstetric Risk Factors Associated with Disseminated Intravascular Coagulation

- Abruptio placentae
- Hemorrhage
- Preeclampsia or eclampsia
- Amniotic fluid embolism
- Saline termination of pregnancy
- Sepsis
- Dead fetus syndrome
- Cardiopulmonary arrest
- Massive transfusion therapy

rapid breathing, restlessness, reduced urine output), or a decrease in hemoglobin and hematocrit below acceptable levels for trimester of pregnancy or the nonpregnant state.

Aggressive fluid and blood replacement is not without risk. The 24 hours after the shock period are critical. Observe for fluid overload, ARDS, and oxygen toxicity. Transfusion reactions may follow administration of blood or blood components. Even in an emergency, each unit should be checked per hospital protocol. Rapid transfusion with cold blood can chill the woman and cause vasoconstriction, arrhythmia, or cardiac arrest. Banked blood may be calcium deficient, increasing the risk for arrhythmias and further bleeding. Potassium levels may increase to dangerous levels. Laboratory values for other parameters are usually checked at least every 4 to 6 hours or as indicated by the woman's condition. Display 6–10 suggests a management plan for hypovolemic shock (Fuller & Bucklin, 2010; Ruth & Kennedy, 2011). In keeping with TJC's (2010) call for maternal safety, most hospitals have developed massive transfusion guidelines or policies for patients who are anticipated to or who actually need greater than 10 units of PRBCs. Infection is another complication of hemorrhage. Causes of infection may include surgical procedures, multiple pelvic examinations, anemia, and loss of the white blood cell component of the blood. It is anticipated that the patient may receive prophylactic antibiotics or treatment for signs of infection.

Hemorrhage is a nursing and medical emergency requiring rapid and efficient teamwork from all members of the healthcare team. Perinatal nurses play an important role in the initial assessments, early interventions, and stabilization of the woman. Recognition that blood loss is out of proportion to the patient's clinical presentation is important because initial vital signs may remain within normal range in the presence of a significant hemorrhage. Anticipating that a woman who is bleeding may rapidly proceed to hypovolemic shock can prevent complications and decrease maternal and fetal morbidity and mortality.

THROMBOPHILIAS IN PREGNANCY

Acquired and/or inherited thrombophilias in pregnancy are associated with a myriad of maternal and fetal complications, including maternal thrombosis/embolism, although it remains controversial as to if and how strong an association there is with early onset severe preeclampsia, abruption, IUGR, intrauterine fetal death (IUFD), indeterminate or abnormal FHR patterns, preterm birth, and recurrent miscarriage (ACOG, 2011b; Silver, 2007). The most common acquired thrombophilia during pregnancy is antiphospholipid antibody syndrome (APLA syndrome) (ACOG, 2011a; Sibai, 2005). Of the antiphospholipid antibodies, lupus anticoagulant (a misnomer because it causes thrombosis), anticardiolipin antibody, and anti-β_2–glycoprotein have the highest association with pregnancy complications. The antibodies are the result of antigenic changes in endothelial and platelet cell membranes, which promote thrombosis.

Inherited thrombophilias vary in prevalence and ability to cause thrombosis. The most common inherited thrombophilias most likely to cause thrombosis in pregnancy are mutations in Factor V Leiden, antithrombin deficiency, prothrombin gene G20210A mutation, tetrahydrofolate reductase, deficiencies in proteins C and S, and platelet collagen receptor alpha-2-beta-1 (ACOG, 2011b; Sibai, 2005). Other factors that contribute to thrombosis formation in pregnancy include the normal hypercoagulable state and venous stasis.

Management

Women who have been identified as having a thrombophilia need to be counseled as to current recommendations regarding anticoagulation during pregnancy. Surveillance alone versus prophylaxis/anticoagulation therapy is individualized by history and current clinical indicators. Anticoagulation is not

---

DISPLAY 6 - 10

Management Plan for Obstetric Hypovolemic Shock

GOALS
- Maintain systolic blood pressure ≥90 mm Hg, urine output ≥30 mL/hr, and normal mental status.
- Identify and eliminate source of hemorrhage.
- Avoid overzealous volume replacement that may contribute to pulmonary edema.

MANAGEMENT
- Establish two large-bore intravenous lines.
- Place woman in Trendelenburg position (wedge under hip if undelivered).
- Rapidly infuse 5% dextrose in lactated Ringer's solution while blood products are obtained.
- Infuse fresh whole blood or packed red blood cells, as available.
- Infuse platelets and fresh frozen plasma only as indicated by documented deficiencies in platelets (<30,000/mL) or clotting parameters (fibrinogen, prothrombin time [PT], partial thromboplastin time [PTT]).
- Search for and eliminate the source of hemorrhage.
- Use invasive hemodynamic monitoring if the woman fails to respond to clinically adequate volume replacement.
- Critical laboratory tests include complete blood count, platelet count, fibrinogen, PT, PTT, and arterial blood gas determinations.

recommended if the woman has no history of venous thromboembolism (VTE) or poor pregnancy outcome. Full- or adjusted-dose anticoagulation with low-molecular-weight heparin (LMWH) is recommended antenatally and 6 weeks postpartum for women who have antithrombin deficiency, homozygosity for the factor V Leiden mutation, the prothrombin gene G20210A mutation, compound heterozygosity for both mutations, or a current VTE. The same is recommended antenatally and long term for women receiving vitamin K antagonist therapy (ACOG, 2011b; James, Abel, & Brancazio, 2006). Women with a history of antiphospholipid antibody syndrome with a previous thrombosis (history of two or more early pregnancy losses, one or more late loss, IUGR, abruption, or preeclampsia) are offered antepartum a low dose of aspirin, an intermediate dose of unfractionated heparin (UFH), or prophylactic LMWH. Women who have a history of a single episode of VTE and thrombophilia or a strong family history of thrombosis may receive intermediate dose LMWH or UFH antepartum followed with postpartum anticoagulants.

LMWH has fewer side effects and a longer half-life than UFH. Because of the longer half-life of LMWH, women may not be able to receive regional anesthesia; many women are switched to UFH during the latter part of the third trimester. Controversy exists regarding which women should be screened for thrombophilias. Individual screening is done based on the woman's history and current pregnancy status. Screening for thrombophilias is considered for women with a history of a VTE with nonrecurrent condition or women with a first-degree relative with a history of high risk for VTE or a VTE prior to the age of 50 years with no known risk factors. Thrombophilia screening is no longer recommended for women with a history of recurrent fetal loss, IUGR, preeclampsia, or abruption (ACOG, 2011b). As the current pregnancy progresses, the woman can be tested for thrombophilias if she develops signs and symptoms of VTE.

UFH is associated with the development of osteoporosis and a 2% risk of vertebral fracture, as well as heparin-induced thrombocytopenia (HIT). LMWHs are actually fragments of UFHs, which have more activity against factor Xa. There is a lower risk of developing osteoporosis and HIT (James et al., 2006). However, LMWH is more costly, and the longer half-life increases the risk of bleeding in the intrapartum period. Neither UFH nor LMWH crosses the placenta.

Fetal surveillance may be beneficial. Serial ultrasounds for growth, and twice-weekly nonstress tests or biophysical profiles can be instituted at 24 to 25 weeks' gestation. The mother can be monitored closely for the development of preeclampsia.

MATERNAL TRAUMA

The perinatal nurse may encounter pregnant women who have experienced trauma as they may be admitted to the labor and delivery unit or to an obstetric triage unit. In most institutions, women with major trauma are stabilized in the emergency department with the assistance of perinatal healthcare providers who are called to the department for consultation and assessment of fetal well-being, whereas women with minor trauma may be sent directly to the labor and delivery unit. The focus of this discussion is women who present with seemingly minor or non–life-threatening trauma. A thorough knowledge of the normal physiologic changes during pregnancy, complications of bleeding and preterm labor, and maternal–fetal assessment is necessary to provide optimum care for pregnant women after trauma.

Approximately 5% to 8% of women experience trauma during pregnancy (Barraco et al., 2010; Brown, 2010). Of women that present to the hospital for treatment, approximately 6% of maternal trauma patients have significant orthopedic injuries, which often are associated with additional adverse outcomes such as increased risk of preterm birth, placental abruption, and perinatal mortality when compared to pregnant women with trauma excluding orthopedic injuries (Cannada et al., 2010). Therefore, traumatized pregnant women with orthopedic injuries are high-risk obstetrical patients and may benefit from referral to a medical center capable of handling both the primary injury and the potential preterm birth associated with the injury (Cannada et al., 2010). Approximately two thirds of all trauma events during pregnancy are the result of motor vehicle accidents (which may or may not include an orthopedic injury). Motor vehicle accidents are the most significant cause of fetal death due to trauma (Barraco et al., 2010; Brown, 2010). The incidence and severity of injuries can be reduced by appropriate use of automobile safety restraints, but many pregnant women do not use safety restraints while driving or riding as a passenger in a car.

Other significant causes of trauma during pregnancy are falls and direct assaults to the abdomen. During pregnancy, falls are the most common cause of minor injury and are estimated to cause 17% to 39% of trauma that results in emergency department visits and hospital admissions, second only to motor vehicle accidents (Dunning, LeMasters, & Bhattacharya, 2010). In a study of 3,997 women who had given birth within the previous 2-month period, 27% reported falling at least once during their pregnancy and 10% indicated they fell at least twice (Dunning et al., 2010). Of those who fell, 20% sought medical care and 21% had 2 or more days of restricted activity. Women aged 20 to

24 years had an almost twofold risk of falling more than those over 35 years. Approximately 56% of falls occurred indoors, 39% on stairs, and 9% reported falling from a height greater than 3 ft (Dunning et al., 2010). Injuries associated with falls during pregnancy include fractures, sprains/strains, head injury, rupture of internal organs, placental abruption, uterine rupture, rupture of membranes, and occasionally maternal or fetal death (Dunning et al., 2010).

Intimate partner violence is becoming an increasing source of trauma during pregnancy. Data about incidence of intimate partner violence have been difficult to accumulate because of reporting issues and the frequency of inaccurate description of the causative factors for injury given by the woman. It is estimated that up to one out of every four women in the United States are victims of intimate partner violence each year (Shay-Zapien & Bullock, 2010). Fetal loss resulting from abdominal trauma may occur because of abruptio placentae or other placental injury, direct fetal injury, uterine rupture, maternal shock, maternal death, or a combination of these events (Barraco et al., 2010; Oxford & Ludmir, 2009).

Nursing assessment and interventions for the pregnant woman who has experienced trauma are based on the clinical situation and maternal–fetal status. A thorough history is essential and should include the nature of the trauma event, condition and symptoms at time of injury, and current clinical symptoms. The principles of management of preterm labor and complications of bleeding are applied based on the clinical situation. Ongoing maternal–fetal assessments and accurate reporting of findings to the primary healthcare provider are important.

Fortunately, most women who experience trauma suffer only minor injuries that do not require inpatient evaluation for the nonpregnant population. However, approximately 5% to 25% of women who experience minor trauma have an adverse maternal or fetal outcome (Curet, Shermer, Demarest, Bieneik, & Curet, 2000; El Kady, Gilbert, Anderson, Danielsen, & Smith, 2004). Up to 50% of fetal losses and other adverse fetal outcomes related to trauma occur in women with seemingly minor or nonsignificant injuries (El Kady, et al., 2004) Careful evaluation of maternal–fetal status is warranted when pregnant women present with reports of any type of trauma (Cannada et al., 2010). Reliability of methods to predict which women are at risk for adverse outcomes remains low. Retrospective data demonstrate that a positive KB test (the presence of fetal RBCs in the maternal circulation, indicating that a fetomaternal or transplacental hemorrhage has occurred) predicts preterm labor and adverse outcomes better than clinical assessment (Muench et al., 2004). The usual signs of complications, including bleeding, uterine tenderness, contractions, and loss of amniotic fluid, are valuable, but they may not be present in all cases (Curet et al., 2000; Muench et al., 2004). Use of ultrasound to exclude abruptio placentae has the potential to miss 50% of cases (Reis, Sander, & Pearlman, 2000). Continuous EFM is useful for ongoing evaluation of fetal status and uterine activity. Recommended duration of continuous EFM after trauma ranges from 6 to 24 hours based on clinical signs and symptoms and the mechanism of injury (Curet et al., 2000; Mattox & Goetzl, 2005). Monitoring should be continued, and further evaluation is warranted if uterine contractions, an indeterminate or abnormal FHR pattern, vaginal bleeding, significant uterine tenderness or irritability, serious maternal injury, or rupture of the membranes occurs (Mattox & Goetzl, 2005). Women with a positive KB test may benefit greatly from continuous EFM and assessment of serial KB testing every 6 to 12 hours to determine if the KB value is falling. If the KB value decreases and EFM is normal, the woman may be evaluated for discharge. Rh immune globulin may need to be administered dependent on the results of the KB test in an Rh-negative woman. If the KB test is negative, extended EFM is not necessary (Muench et al., 2004). The decision to continue inpatient evaluation, discharge to home, or transfer to another facility is made in collaboration with the primary healthcare provider, consistent with maternal–fetal status, and as outlined in the federal Emergency Medical Treatment and Labor Act (EMTALA). See Chapter 13 for maternal transport.

SUMMARY

When bleeding complicates pregnancy, there is significant risk for adverse outcomes. A thorough knowledge of nursing care for bleeding complications, including timely identification and appropriate interventions, is required to ensure optimal outcomes for mothers and babies.

REFERENCES

American College of Obstetricians and Gynecologists. (2002). *Placenta Accreta* (Committee Opinion No. 266). Washington, DC: Author.

American College of Obstetricians and Gynecologists. (2006). *Postpartum Hemorrhage* (Practice Bulletin No. 76). Washington, DC: Author.

American College of Obstetricians and Gynecologists. (2010). *Vaginal Birth After Previous Cesarean Delivery* (Practice Bulletin No. 115). Washington, DC: Author. doi:10.1097/AOG.0b013e3181eeb251

American College of Obstetricians and Gynecologists. (2011a). *Antiphospholipid Syndrome* (Practice Bulletin No. 118). Washington, DC: Author. doi:10.1097/AOG.0b013e31820a61f9

American College of Obstetricians and Gynecologists. (2011b). *Inherited Thrombophilias in Pregnancy.* (Practice Bulletin No. 124). Washington, DC: Author. doi:10.1097/AOG.0b013e3182310c6f

Ayres, A. W., Johnson, T. R., & Hayashi, R. (2001). Characteristics of fetal heart rate tracings prior to uterine rupture. *International Journal of Gynaecology and Obstetrics, 74*(3), 235–240.

Barraco, R. D., Chiu, W. C., Clancy, T. V., Como, J. J., Ebert, J. B., Hess, H. L., . . . Weiss, P. M. (2010). Practice management guidelines for the diagnosis and management of injury in the pregnant patient: The EAST Practice Management Guidelines Work Group. *The Journal of Trauma: Injury, Infection, and Critical Care, 69*(1), 211–214. doi:10.1097/TA.0b013e3181dbe1ea

Berg, C. J., Callaghan, W. M., Syverson, C., & Henderson, Z. (2010). Pregnancy-related mortality in the United States, 1998 to 2005. *Obstetrics and Gynecology, 116*(6), 1302–1309. doi: 10.1097/AOG.0b013e3181fdfb11

Berg, C. J., Harper, M. A., Atkinson, S. M., Bell, E. A., Brown, H. L., Hage, M. L., . . . Callaghan, W. M. (2005). Preventability of pregnancy-related deaths: Results of a state-wide review. *Obstetrics and Gynecology, 106*(6), 1228–1234. doi:10.1097/01.AOG.0000187894.71913.e8

Brown, H. L. (2009). Trauma in pregnancy. *Obstetrics and Gynecology, 114*(1), 147–160. doi:10.1097/AOG.0b013e3181ab6014

Brown, H. L. (2010). Trauma in pregnancy. *Obstetric Anesthesia Digest, 30*(3), 144–145. doi:10.1097/01.aoa.0000386814.84816.cd

Burke, C. (2010). Active versus expectant management of the third stage of labor and implementation of a protocol. *Journal of Perinatal and Neonatal Nursing, 24*(3), 215–228. doi:10.1097/JPN.0b013e3181e8ce90

Cahill, A. G., & Macones, G. A. (2007). Vaginal birth after cesarean delivery: Evidence-based practice. *Clinical Obstetrics and Gynecology, 50*(2), 518–525. doi:10.1097/GRF.0b013e31804bde7b

Callaghan, W. M., Kuklina, E. V., & Berg, C. J. (2010). Trends in postpartum hemorrhage: United States, 1994–2006. *American Journal of Obstetrics and Gynecology, 202*(4), 353e1–353e6. doi:10.1016/j.ajog.2010.01.011

Cannada, L. K., Pan, P., Casey, B. M., McIntire, D. D., Shafi, S., & Leveno, K. J. (2010). Pregnancy outcomes after orthopedic trauma. *The Journal of Trama: Injury, Infection, and Critical Care, 69*(3), 694–698. doi:10.1097/TA.0b013e3181e97ed8

Catanzarite, V., Cousins, L., Dowling, D., & Daneshmand, S. (2006). Oxytocin-associated rupture of an unscarred uterus in a primagravida. *Obstetrics and Gynecology, 108*(3, Pt. 2), 723–725. doi:10.1097/01.AOG.0000215559.21051.dc

Chang, J., Elam-Evans, L. D., Berg, C. J., Herndon, J., Flowers, L., Seed, K., & Syversen, C. J. (2003). Pregnancy-related mortality surveillance, United States, 1991–1999. *Morbidity and Mortality Weekly Report, 52*(2), 1–8.

Chauhan, S. P., Martin, J. N. Jr., Henrichs, C. E., Morrison, J. C., & Magann, E. F. (2003). Maternal and perinatal complications with uterine rupture in 142,075 patients who attempted vaginal birth after cesarean delivery: A review of the literature. *American Journal of Obstetrics and Gynecology, 189*(2), 408–417. doi:10.1067/S0002-9378(03)00675-6

Clark, S. L. (1999). Placenta previa and abruptio placenta. In R. K. Creasy, R. Resnik, & J. Iams (Eds.), *Maternal-Fetal Medicine* (4th ed., pp. 616–631). Philadelphia: Saunders.

Clark, S. L. (2004). Placenta previa and abruptio placenta. In R. K. Creasy, R. Resnik, & J. Iams (Eds.), *Maternal-Fetal Medicine* (5th ed., pp. 707–722). Philadelphia: Saunders.

Clark, S. L., Belfort, M. A., Dildy, G. A., Herbst, M. A., Meyers, J. A., & Hankins, G. D. (2008). Maternal death in the 21st century: Causes, prevention, and relationship to cesarean delivery. *American Journal of Obstetrics and Gynecology, 199*(1), 36.e1-36.e5; discussion 91–92. doi:10.1016/j.ajog.2008.03.007

Clark, S. L., Greenspoon, J. S., Aldahl, D., & Phelan, J. P. (1986). Severe preeclampsia with persistent oliguria: Management of hemodynamic subsets. *American Journal of Obstetrics and Gynecology, 154*(3), 490–494.

Comstock, C. (2011). The antenatal diagnosis of placental attachment disorders. *Current Opinion in Obstetrics and Gynecology, 23*(2), 117–122. doi:10.1097/GCO.0b013e328342b730

Creanga, A., Shapiro-Mendoza, C. K., Bish, C. L., Zane, S., Berg, C. J., & Callaghan, W. M. (2011). Trends in ectopic pregnancy mortality in the United States: 1980–2007. *Obstetrics and Gynecology, 117*(4), 837–843. doi:10.1097/AOG.0b013e3182113c10

Cunningham, F. G., Leveno, K. J., Bloom, S. L., Hauth, J. C., Rouse, D. J., & Spong, C. Y. (Eds.). (2010). Obstetrical hemorrhage. In *Williams Obstetrics* (23rd ed., pp. 757–803). New York: McGraw Hill.

Curet, M. J., Shermer, C. R., Demarest, G. B., Bieneik, E. J. III, & Curet, L. B. (2000). Predictors of outcome in trauma during pregnancy: Identification of patients who can be monitored for less than 6 hours. *Journal of Trauma, 49*(1), 18–25.

Driessen, M., Bouvier-Colle, M. H., Dupont, C., Khoshnood, B., Rudigoz, R. C., & Deneux-Tharaux, C. (2011). Postpartum hemorrhage resulting from uterine atony after vaginal delivery: Factors associated with severity. *Obstetrics and Gynecology, 117*(1), 21–31. doi:10.1097/AOG.0b013e318202c845

Dunning, K., LeMasters, G., & Bhattacharya, A. (2010). A major public health issue: The high incidence of falls during pregnancy. *Maternal Child Health Journal, 14*(5), 720–725. doi:10.1007/s10995-009-0511-0

El Kady, D., Gilbert, W. M., Anderson, J., Danielsen, B., & Smith, L. H. (2004). Trauma during pregnancy: An analysis of maternal and fetal outcomes in a large population. *American Journal of Obstetrics and Gynecology, 190*(6), 1661–1668. doi:10.1016/j.ajog.2004.02.051

Eller, A. G., Bennett, M. A., Sharshiner, M., Masheter, C., Soisson, A. P., Dodson, M., & Silver, R. M. (2011). Maternal morbidity in cases of placenta accreta managed by a multidisciplinary care team compared with standard obstetric care. *Obstetrics and Gynecology, 117*(2, Pt. 1), 331–337. doi:10.1097/AOG.0b013e3182051db2

Fuller, A. J., & Bucklin, B. A. (2010). Blood product replacement for postpartum hemorrhage. *Clinical Obstetrics and Gynecology, 53*(1), 196–208. doi:10.1097/GRF.0b013e3181cc42a0

Harper, L. M., Obido, A. O., Macones, G. A., Crane, J. P., & Cahill, A. G. (2010). Effect of placenta previa on fetal growth. *American Journal of Obstetrics and Gynecology, 203*(4), 330e1–330e5. doi:10.1016/j.ajog.2010.05.014

Hoffman, C. (2009). Postpartum hemorrhage. *Postgraduate Obstetrics & Gynecology, 29*(2), 1–6. doi:10.1097/01.PGO.0000342884.77973.30

Hoyert, D. L. (2007). Maternal mortality and related concepts. *Vital and Health Statistics, 3*(33), 1–20.

Hull, A. D., & Resnik, R. (2009). Placenta previa, placenta accreta, abruptio placentae, and vasa previa. In R. K. Creasy, R. Resnik, J. D. Iams, C. J. Lockwood, & T. R. Moore (Eds.), *Creasy and Resnik's Maternal–Fetal Medicine: Principles and Practice* (6th ed., pp. 725–737). Philadelphia, PA: Saunders Elsevier.

James, A. H., Abel, D. E., & Brancazio, L. R. (2006). Anticoagulants in pregnancy. *Obstetrical and Gynecological Survey, 61*(1), 59–69.

Jauregui, I., Kirkendall, C., Ahn, M. O., & Phelan, J. (2000). Uterine rupture: A placentally mediated event? *Obstetrics and Gynecology, 95*(4, Suppl. 1), S75. doi:10.1016/S0029-7844(00)00754-7

The Joint Commission. (2010). *Preventing Maternal Death* (Sentinel Event Alert No. 44). Oak Brook Terrace, IL: Author. Retrieved from http://www.jointcommission.org/assets/1/18/sea_44.PDF

Knab, D. R. (1978). Abruptio placenta: An assessment of the time and method of delivery. *Obstetrics and Gynecology, 52*(5), 625–629.

Landon, M. B., Hauth, J. C., Leveno, K. J., Spong, C. Y., Leindecker, S., Varner, M. W., . . . Gabbe, S. G. (2004). Maternal and perinatal outcomes associated with a trial of labor after prior cesarean delivery. *New England Journal of Medicine, 351*(25), 2581–2589. doi:10.1056/NEJMoa040405

Landon, M. B., Leindecker, S., Spong, C. Y., Hauth, J. C., Bloom, S., Varner, M. W., . . . Gabbe, S. G. (2005). The MFMU Cesarean Registry: Factors affecting the success of a trial of labor after previous cesarean delivery. *American Journal of Obstetrics and Gynecology, 193*(3, Pt. 2), 1016–1023. doi:10.1016/j.ajog.2005.05.066

Landon, M. B., Spong, C. Y., Thom, E., Hauth, J. C., Bloom, S. L., Varner, M. W., . . . Gabbe, S. G. (2006). Risk of uterine rupture with a trial of labor in women with multiple and single prior cesarean delivery. *Obstetrics and Gynecology, 108*(1), 12–20. doi:10.1097/01.AOG.0000224694.32531.f3

Lang, C., & Landon, M. (2010). Uterine rupture as a source of obstetrical hemorrhage. *Clinical Obstetrics and Gynecology, 53*(1), 237–251. doi:10.1097/GRF.0b013e3181cc4538

Lyndon, A., Lagrew, D., Shields, L., Melsop, K., Bingham, D., & Main, E. (Eds.). (2010). *Improving Health Care Response to Obstetric Hemorrhage.* (California Maternal Quality Care Collaborative Toolkit to Transform Maternity Care). Developed under contract ##08-85012 with the California Department of Public Health: Maternal, Child and Adolescent Health Division; Published by the California Maternal Quality Care Collaborative. Retrieved from http://www.cmqcc.org/ob_hemorrhage

MacMullen, N. J., Dulski, L. A., & Meagher, B. (2005). Red alert: Perinatal hemorrhage. *MCN: The American Journal of Maternal Child Nursing, 30*(1), 46–51.

Mahlmeister, L. R. (2010). Best practices in perinatal care: Strategies for reducing maternal death rate in the United States. *The Journal of Perinatal & Neonatal Nursing, 24*(4), 297–301. doi:10.1097/JPN.0b013e3181f918bb

Maloni, J. A. (2011). Lack of evidence for prescription of antepartum bed rest. *Expert Review of Obstetrics & Gynecology, 6*(4), 385–393. doi:10.1586/eog.11.28

Mattox, K. L., & Goetzl, L. (2005). Trauma in pregnancy. *Critical Care Medicine, 33*(10), S385–S389.

Mazzone, M. E., & Woolever, J. (2006). Uterine rupture in a patient with an unscarred uterus: A case study. *Wisconsin Medical Journal, 105*(2), 64–66.

Menihan, C. A. (1999). The effect of uterine rupture on fetal heart rate patterns. *Journal of Nurse-Midwifery, 44*(1), 40–46. doi:10.1016/S0091-2182(98)00076-7

Muench, M. V., Baschat, A. A., Reddy, U. M., Mighty, H. E., Weiner, C. P., Scalea, T. M., & Harman, C. R. (2004). Kleihauer-Betke testing is important in all cases of maternal trauma. *Journal of Trauma: Injury, Infection & Critical Care, 57*(5), 1094–1098.

Oxford, C. M., & Ludmir, J. (2009). Trauma in pregnancy. *Clinical Obstetrics and Gynecology, 52*(4), 611–629. doi:10.1097/GRF.0b013e3181c11edf

Oyelese, Y., & Ananth, C. V. (2010). Postpartum hemorrhage: Epidemiology, risk factors, and causes. *Clinical Obstetrics and Gynecology, 53*(1), 147–156. doi:10.1097/GRF.0b013e3181cc406d

Oyelese, Y., Catanzarite, V., Prefumo, F., Lashley, S., Schachter, M., Tovbin, Y., . . . Smulian, J. C. (2004). Vasa previa: The impact of prenatal diagnosis on outcomes. *Obstetrics and Gynecology, 103*(5, Pt. 1), 937–942. doi:10.1097/01.AOG.0000123245.48645.98

Oyelese, Y., & Smulian, J. C. (2006). Placenta previa, placenta accreta, and vasa previa. *Obstetrics and Gynecology, 107*(4), 927–941. doi:10.1097/01.AOG.0000207559.15715.98

Page, E. W., & Christianson, R. (1976). The impact of mean arterial pressure in the middle trimester upon the outcome of pregnancy. *American Journal of Obstetrics and Gynecology, 125*(6), 740–746.

Paré, E., Quiñones, J. N., & Macones, G. A. (2006). Vaginal birth after caesarean section versus elective repeat caesarean section: Assessment of maternal downstream health outcomes. *BJOG: An International Journal of Obstetrics and Gynaecology, 113*(1), 75–85. doi:10.1111/j.1471-0528.2005.00793.x

Paxton, A., & Wardlaw, T. (2011). Are we making progress in maternal mortality? *New England Journal of Medicine, 364*(21), 1990–1993. doi:10.1056/NEJMp1012860

Porreco, R. P., & Stettler, R. W. (2010). Surgical remedies for postpartum hemorrhage. *Clinical Obstetrics and Gynecology, 53*(1), 182–195. doi:10.1097/GRF.0b013e3181cc4139

Rajan, P. V., & Wing, D. A. (2010). Postpartum hemorrhage: Evidence-based medical interventions for prevention and treatment. *Clinical Obstetrics and Gynecology, 53*(1), 165–181. doi:10.1097/GRF.0b013e3181ce0965

Reis, P. M., Sander, C. M., & Pearlman, M. D. (2000). Abruptio placentae after auto accidents: A case control study. *Journal of Reproductive Medicine, 45*(1), 6–10.

Ridgeway, J. J., Weyrich, D. L., & Benedetti, T. J. (2004). Fetal heart rate changes associated with uterine rupture. *Obstetrics and Gynecology, 103*(3), 506–512.

Robinson, B. K., & Grobman, W. A. (2011). Effectiveness of timing strategies for delivery of individuals with vasa previa. *Obstetrics and Gynecology, 117*(3), 542–549. doi:10.1097/AOG.0b013e31820b0ace

Ruth, D., & Kennedy, B. B. (2011). Acute volume resuscitation following obstetric hemorrhage. *Journal of Perinatal & Neonatal Nursing, 25*(3), 253–260. doi:10.1097/JPN.0b013e31822539e3

Ruth, D., & Miller, R. S. (2012). Trauma in pregnancy. In N. H. Troiano, C. J. Harvey, & B. F. Chez (Eds.), *High-Risk and Critical Care Obstetrics* (3rd ed., pp. 343–356). Philadelphia: Lippincott Williams & Wilkins.

Scott, J. R. (2011). Vaginal birth after cesarean delivery: A common-sense approach. *Obstetrics and Gynecology, 118*(2, Pt. 1), 342–350. doi:10.1097/AOG.0b013e3182245b39

Shay-Zapien, G., & Bullock, L. (2010). Impact of intimate partner violence on maternal child health. *MCN: The American Journal of Maternal Child Nursing, 35*(4), 206–212. doi:10.1097/NMC.0b013e3181dd9d6e

Sheiner, E., Levy, A., Ofir, K., Hadar, A., Shoham-Vardi, I., Hallak, M., . . . Mazor, M. (2004). Changes in fetal heart rate and uterine patterns associated with uterine rupture. *Journal of Reproductive Medicine, 49*(5), 373–378.

Sibai, B. M. (2005). Thrombophilia and severe preeclampsia: Time to screen and treat in future pregnancies? *Hypertension, 46*(6), 1252–1253. doi:10.1161/01.HYP.0000188904.47575.7e

Silver, R. M. (2007). Fetal death. *Obstetrics and Gynecology, 109*(1), 153–167. doi:10.1097/01.AOG.0000248537.89739.96

Snegovskikh, D., Clebone, A., & Norwitz, E. (2011). Anesthetic management of patients with placenta accreta and resuscitation strategies for associated massive hemorrhage. *Current Opinion in Anaesthesiology, 24*(3), 274–281. doi:10.1097/ACO.0b013e328345d8b7

Spong, C. Y., & Queenan, J. T. (2011). Uterine scar assessment: How should it be done before trial of labor after cesarean delivery? *Obstetrics and Gynecology, 117*(3), 521–522. doi:10.1097/AOG.0b013e31820ce593

Thorp, J. M. Jr. (2009). Clinical aspects of normal and abnormal labor. In R. K. Creasy, R. Resnik, J. D. Iams, C. J. Lockwood, & T. R. Moore (Eds.). *In Creasy and Resnik's Maternal–Fetal Medicine: Principles and Practice* (6th ed., pp. 691–724). Philadelphia: Saunders Elsevier.

Tillett, J. (2010). Understanding and explaining risk. *Journal of Perinatal & Neonatal Nursing, 24*(3), 196–198. doi:10.1097/JPN.0b013e3181e7c6f9

Vergani, P., Ornaghi, S., Pozzi, I., Beretta, P., Russo, F. M., Follesa, I., & Ghidini, A. (2009). Placenta previa: Distance to internal os and mode of delivery. *American Journal of Obstetrics and Gynecology, 201*(3), 266e1–266e5. doi:10.1016/j.ajog.2009.06.009

Witlin, A. G., Saade, G. R., Mattar, F., & Sibai, B. M. (1999). Risk factors for abruptio placentae and eclampsia: Analysis of 445 consecutively managed women with severe preeclampsia and eclampsia. *American Journal of Obstetrics and Gynecology, 180*(6, Pt. 1), 1322–1329. doi:10.1016/S0002-9378(99)70014-1

Wright, J. D., Pri-Paz, S., Herzog, T. J., Shah, M., Bonanno, C., Lewin, S. N., . . . Devine, P. (2011). Predictors of massive blood loss in women with placenta accreta. *American Journal of Obstetrics and Gynecology, 205*(1), 38.e1–38.e6. doi:10.1016/j.ajog.2011.01.040

Yang, J. I., Lim, Y. K., Kim, H. S., Chang, K. H., Lee, J. P., & Ryu, H. S. (2006). Sonographic findings of placental lacunae and the prediction of adherent placenta in women with pla-

centa previa totalis and prior cesarean section. *Ultrasound in Obstetrics and Gynecology, 28*(2), 178–182. doi:10.1002/uog.2797

You, W. B., & Zahn, C. M. (2006). Postpartum hemorrhage: Abnormally adherent placenta, uterine inversion, and puerperal hematomas. *Clinical Obstetrics and Gynecology, 49*(1), 184–197.

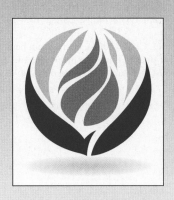

Nancy Jo Reedy

CHAPTER 7

Preterm Labor and Birth

SIGNIFICANCE AND INCIDENCE

Preterm birth (PTB) is birth occurring before 37 completed weeks of gestation. Based on the most recent data available, in 2010, the PTB rate in the United States was approximately 12% (Hamilton, Martin, & Ventura, 2011). This rate reflects an increase of 30% between 1981 and 2006. Although there was a slight decline in the PTB rate between 2007 and 2010, it remains higher than any year in the period between 1981 and 2006 (Martin, 2011; Martin, Osterman, & Sutton, 2010). For the last two decades, the largest contribution to the increase in PTBs was late PTBs between 34 and 36 completed weeks of gestation (Raju, Higgins, Stark, & Leveno, 2006). From 1992 to 2002, two thirds of the increase in the rate of PTBs in the United States was in this subset of preterm babies (Davidoff et al., 2006). The small drop in the PTB rate for 2010 was primarily among babies born late preterm, which decreased 2% from 8.66% in 2009 to 8.49%. The 2010 late preterm rate was 7%, lower than the 2006 high (9.14%). The 2010 rate for early preterm births (less than 34 weeks of gestation) was essentially stable at 3.50%, with 1.53% between 32 and 33 weeks and 1.97% less than 32 weeks (Hamilton et al., 2011). In 2010, late PTBs continued to comprise two thirds of the total PTBs, with 8.5% late preterm and 12% total preterm (Hamilton et al., 2011).

The Institute of Medicine (IOM; 2007) report on PTB cited "troubling and persistent disparities in PTB rates among different ethnic and racial groups" (p. 1). The highest rates of PTB are among non-Hispanic blacks (17.15% in 2010). Although this is the lowest PTB rate for non-Hispanic blacks in over three decades,

it is still 46% higher than Hispanic infants and 59% higher than non-Hispanic white infants (Hamilton et al., 2011; Martin et al., 2011). Other racial and ethnic groups have lower rates, but all are still unacceptably high. The rate of PTB for American Indians is 13.9%; for Hispanics, 11.97%; for non-Hispanic whites, 10.9%; and for Asians, 10.9%. PTB is the leading source of neonatal mortality and morbidity in the United States (IOM, 2007); thus, PTB is a problem that has attracted decades of research in an attempt to discover possible causes and cures.

The rising rates of PTB in the United States contrast with the drop in rates of infant mortality since the 1950s. In 2007, the rate of infant mortality for the United States was 6.75%; in 1950, by comparison, it was 29.2% (MacDorman & Mathews, 2011; March of Dimes, 2012a). This dramatic change occurred because of the emergence of the science of neonatal care, with more babies now living past their first birthday despite being born at earlier gestational ages. Sophisticated neonatal care has also allowed more preterm babies to survive, although for many of the smallest preterm babies, that survival is liable to come with significant morbidity, which could last throughout their lives.

It is important when discussing PTB that everyone uses the same definitions. Although they are different entities, often with separate etiologies, the terms *preterm birth* and *low birth weight* (LBW) are commonly used interchangeably. In fact, most of the long-term follow-up studies of children and adults quoted in the literature are of very-low-birth weight (VLBW) or extremely-low-birth weight (ELBW) children because assessment of gestational age was not common in perinatal care until recent decades. Birth weight has been, and continues to be, a simple and definitive assessment, thus easier to access. PTB refers only to gestational age at birth, no matter the birth weight. Although the term *preterm birth* (<37 weeks) is commonly used, other classifications in the literature of babies born preterm include moderately preterm (32 to 34 weeks), late preterm (34 to 36 weeks), and very PTB (<32 weeks). Preterm babies may be, but do not have to be, low birth weight. A preterm baby born to a mother with gestational diabetes, for instance, might be of normal birth weight and yet be born preterm. The prematurity would then dictate the health problems of the baby, as lung, central nervous system, or gastrointestinal immaturity would pose health risks.

LBW refers only to weight at birth, no matter the gestational age. A baby is considered LBW if it is born <2,500 g (5.5 lb). VLBW is defined as birth <1,500 g (3.5 lb), and ELBW is <1,000 g (<2.2 lb). LBW babies may be born before 37 weeks but can also be born at term (e.g., a baby at 41 weeks gestational age could weigh 1,800 g because of intrauterine growth restriction [IUGR]). Risk factors, causes, and outcomes for LBW, growth restriction, and PTB are interrelated but can cause some confusion when reviewing the literature.

The rates of LBW and PTB in the United States are different. The LBW rate increased more than 20% from the mid-1980s through 2006 but has trended slightly downward since. In 2010, the LBW rate was 8.15%. The rate of VLBW was 1.45% in 2010, unchanged from 2009. The VLBW rate increased during the 1980s and 1990s, peaking at 1.49% in 2007, but declined to 1.45% to 1.46% for 2008 to 2010 (Hamilton et al., 2011).

Much research has been conducted on the sequelae of LBW, VLBW, and ELBW. Babies with the most mortality and morbidity are the VLBW and ELBW babies. A baby born at VLBW (<1,500 g) is at high risk for neonatal mortality (De Jesus et al., 2012; Morales et al., 2005) and, when compared with normal birth weight children, is at higher risk for learning disabilities and cognitive deficiencies during childhood (Litt, Taylor, Klein, & Hack, 2005; Orchinik et al., 2011). Low gestational age is a corresponding risk factor for neonatal morbidity. Although the majority of babies with gestational ages of greater than or equal to 24 weeks survive, there are high rates of morbidity among survivors. In a study of 9,575 babies of extremely low gestational age (22 to 28 weeks) and VLBW or ELBW (401 to 1,500 g), babies at the lowest gestational ages were at greatest risk for morbidities (Stoll et al., 2010). Overall, 93% had respiratory distress syndrome, 46% had patent ductus arteriosus, 16% had severe intraventricular hemorrhage, 11% had necrotizing enterocolitis, 36% had late-onset sepsis, and 68% had bronchopulmonary dysplasia with

greater than 50% undetermined retinopathy status at the time of discharge from the neonatal intensive care unit (NICU).

VLBW children followed through adulthood have been found to have poorer educational achievement, higher blood pressures, poorer respiratory function, and generally poorer physical abilities than their peers who were born at normal birth weight (Hack, 2006). ELBW babies demonstrate restricted growth patterns during their NICU stays and into their childhoods (Carroll, Slobodzian, & Steward, 2005). A meta-analysis of studies of overall brain growth demonstrated reduction in size of all major brain structures in 818 children and adolescents born at <32 weeks or <1,500 g when compared with 450 peers born at term (de Kieviet, Zoetebier, van Elburg, Vermeulen, & Oosterlaan, 2012). It has also been shown that there are gender differences in the viability of ELBW infants, with females having a 1-year survival advantage (Morse et al., 2006). The outcomes for children followed to 8 years of age who had been ELBW infants (<1,000 g) are even worse. These children have been shown to have significantly more chronic health conditions and need for special services than normal birth weight babies; their health problems include more instances of cerebral palsy, asthma, poor vision, low IQ (<85), poor academic skills, and poor motor skills (Hack et al., 2011; Hack et al., 2005; IOM, 2007; Mikkola et al., 2005). Predictors of cognitive impairment for ELBW babies include thrombosis of fetal vessels in the placenta, severe fetal growth restriction, male gender, and maternal obesity (Helderman et al., 2012; Kent, Wright, & Abdel-Latif, 2012; Morsing, Asard, Ley, Stjerngvist, & Marsál, 2011). Predictors of mortality within 2 years after NICU discharge for ELBW babies include African American race, male gender, and prolonged NICU stay (De Jesus et al., 2012; Kent et al., 2012).

Consequences of PTB continue to devastate families, communities, and healthcare in general. Unfortunately, there is no cure in sight. PTB is a serious and costly health problem, affecting approximately one in eight births in the United States. It is estimated that PTBs are responsible for approximately 70% of neonatal deaths and 36% of infant deaths as well as 25% to 50% of cases of long-term neurologic impairment in children in the United States (American College of Obstetricians and Gynecologists [ACOG], 2012c). The healthcare community is concerned about all PTBs, but the most costly births of all are those <32 weeks. Although they make up only about 2% of all births, they result in the most devastating consequences for babies and families (Green et al., 2005). The costs to society in the United States alone for prematurity complications were estimated to be $26.2 billion in 2005 (IOM, 2007). The March of Dimes commissioned a study of the cost of prematurity to employers (Thomson Reuters, 2008). The study found that babies with a diagnosis of prematurity/LBW cost $64,713 for mother and baby compared with $15,047 for an uncomplicated birth and healthy newborn. Costs for a preterm/LBW baby were more than 10 times the cost of a normal newborn. Preterm infants are twice as likely to die by their first birthday and are more likely to suffer morbidity such as respiratory distress syndrome, intraventricular hemorrhage, and necrotizing enterocolitis than infants born at term (March of Dimes, 2012b). Clearly, there is great need for more research about this costly public health problem to find successful methods of prevention.

LATE PRETERM BIRTHS

Most PTBs are between 34 and 36 completed weeks of gestation (Martin et al., 2011) and do not represent infants with the most severe morbidities. However, these infants have their own set of physiologic and developmental problems, which until recently have been poorly recognized because of concentration on the dramatically severe difficulties encountered by the <32-week infants. Late preterm infants are now the focus of much research and intervention. In July 2005, the National Institute of Child Health and Human Development (NICHD, 2005) convened a panel of experts to discuss the definition and terminology, epidemiology, etiology, biology or maturation, clinical care, surveillance, and public health aspects of "near term" PTB and "near term" infants (Raju et al., 2006). However, the panel came to the consensus that "late preterm birth" and "late preterm infants" were better descriptors because they highlight the physiologic vulnerability of this group of preterm infants. Along with the March of Dimes, ACOG, and the American Academy of Pediatrics (AAP), the Association of Women's Health, Obstetric and Neonatal Nurses (AWHONN) was an invited participant and has been one of the professional organizations leading the way to increase awareness among healthcare providers and the public and to promote better outcomes. Before the NICHD expert panel meeting, AWHONN established its "Late Preterm Infant Initiative," a conceptual framework for optimizing the health of these babies (Medoff-Cooper, Bakewell-Sachs, Buus-Frank, & Santa-Donato, 2005; Santa-Donato, 2005). This ongoing program is focused on developing evidence-based practices for caring for the subset of preterm babies born between 34 weeks and 0/7 days and 36 weeks and 6/7 days (Raju et al., 2006).

Evaluation of the issue of late preterm infants by AWHONN (Medoff-Cooper et al., 2005) found that these infants are often overlooked in research because they may not seem dramatically sick; they are, however, immature at birth, and have missed 4 to 6 weeks of the third trimester of gestation, putting them at risk for many health problems. There is a growing body of evidence that, compared to term babies, late preterm babies have more problems with temperature stability, feeding, hypoglycemia, respiratory distress, apnea/bradycardia, symptoms suggesting the need for sepsis evaluation, and clinical jaundice (Medoff-Cooper et al., 2005; Raju et al., 2006). They also are at greater risk for kernicterus, apnea, seizures, and rehospitalization (Mally, Bailey, & Hendricks-Muñoz, 2010). It is estimated that the brain size of a fetus or a baby born at 34 to 35 weeks of gestation is only 60% of that of a baby born at term (Raju et al., 2006), and these infants are at risk for neurologic compromise if born late preterm (Kinney, 2006). Late preterm infants, once thought to be just lighter than full-term infants, are now known to be at higher risk for multiple morbidities, as well as infant mortality risk (Mally et al., 2010). Display 7–1 lists the adverse outcomes that are significantly increased in late preterm infants. Because late preterm babies reflect such a large proportion of all preterm babies, even a modest increase in the PTB rate of this group can have a significant impact on human and healthcare costs. Possible causes for the increase in late PTBs include increasing proportions of pregnant women over 35 years of age, multiple births, medically indicated births secondary to better surveillance of the mother and fetus, attempts to reduce stillbirths, stress from a variety of sources, and early elective births for convenience (Raju et al.,

DISPLAY 7 - 1

Adverse Outcomes Significantly Increased in Late Preterm Infants

- Respiratory distress syndrome
- Transient tachypnea of the newborn
- Pulmonary infection
- Unspecified respiratory failure
- Recurrent apnea
- Temperature instability
- Jaundice as a cause for discharge delay
- Bilirubin-induced brain injury
- Clinical problems with one or more diagnoses
- Rehospitalization for all causes
- Rehospitalization for neonatal dehydration
- Feeding difficulties
- Long-term neurodevelopmental delay
- Periventricular leukomalacia

2006). Late preterm infants are discussed in detail in Chapter 21.

EARLY TERM BIRTHS

Elective births comprise a significant proportion of babies born at 37 and 38 weeks of gestation. In 2010, the March of Dimes suggested using *early term* to define the subset of babies born between 37 0/7 and 38 6/7 weeks of gestation, often electively (Fleischman, Oinuma, & Clark, 2010). The rate of early term induction rose from 2% to 8% from 1991 to 2006 in the United States, representing a 300% increase (Murthy, Grobman, Lee, & Holl, 2011). Although it is well known that significant excess costs are associated with elective births before 37 completed weeks of gestation (Gilbert, Nesbitt, & Danielsen, 2003), electively born early term babies also generate appreciable costs including admission to the NICU due to iatrogenic morbidity related to being born too soon (Clark et al., 2010). When compared to babies born at 39 weeks or greater, babies born electively via cesarean at 37 or 38 weeks are at higher risk for neonatal morbidity such as adverse respiratory outcomes, mechanical ventilation, newborn sepsis, hypoglycemia, admission to the NICU, and hospitalization for 5 days or more (Tita et al., 2009). Clark and colleagues (2009) found similar neonatal outcomes when comparing babies electively born at 39 weeks or greater with babies electively born between 37 0/7 and 38 6/7 weeks.

There has been an emphasis on lung maturity as a determining factor in predicting risks of neonatal morbidity and mortality; however, the role of maturation of other organ systems is getting more attention (March of Dimes, 2011). For example, the brain continues to develop throughout pregnancy, including rapid growth in the last month (Noble, Fifer, Rauh, Nomura, & Andrews, 2012). Being born at term, but earlier than 39 weeks' gestation, can have significant negative neurologic effects as children develop. In a study of 128,050 children who were born at term (≥37 weeks' gestation), researchers linked birth data to children's school records 8 years later and found that, even among the "normal term" range, gestational age was an important independent predictor of academic achievement (Noble et al., 2012). Gestational age within the normal term range was significantly and positively related to reading and math scores in third grade, with achievement scores for children born at 37 and 38 weeks significantly lower than those for children born at 39, 40, or 41 weeks; this effect was independent of birth weight as well as a number of other obstetric, social, and economic factors (Noble et al., 2012).

Elective labor inductions and elective cesarean births are preventable factors contributing to the increase in late preterm and early term births and associated costs (March of Dimes & California Maternal Quality Care Collaborative, 2010). Evidence supports induction of labor for postterm gestation, premature rupture of membranes at term, and premature rupture of membranes near term with documented fetal lung maturity as well as significant maternal compromise such as HELLP syndrome or nonremedial fetal compromise such as fetal hydrops (ACOG, 2009; Mozurkewich, Chilimigras, Koepke, Keeton, & King, 2009). Other medical indications for induction before 39 completed weeks of gestation suggested by ACOG (2009) include abruptio placentae, chorioamnionitis, fetal demise, gestational hypertension, preeclampsia, eclampsia, maternal medical conditions (e.g., diabetes mellitus, renal disease, chronic pulmonary disease, chronic hypertension, antiphospholipid syndrome), and fetal compromise (e.g., severe fetal growth restriction, isoimmunization, oligohydramnios). In 2011, further recommendations for timing of medically indicated births before 39 completed weeks of gestation were published by the NICHD based on a review of the evidence by an expert panel of perinatal clinicians and scientists (Spong et al., 2011). See Table 7–1 for the NICHD recommendations.

Because late preterm and early term births without medical indications have potential to result in a preventable neonatal morbidity, professional organizations have promulgated recommendations to avoid their occurrence. Estimations of the "due date" can often be miscalculated by up to 2 weeks; therefore, ACOG, AAP, and the National Institutes of Health (NIH) recommend that gestational age of 39 completed weeks of gestation be confirmed by at least one method before elective labor induction, repeat cesarean birth, or nonmedically indicated cesarean birth to avoid iatrogenic PTB (AAP & ACOG, 2012; ACOG, 2009; NIH, 2006). These methods include an ultrasound measurement at less than 20 weeks of gestation that supports gestational age of 39 weeks or greater, fetal heart tones have been documented as present for 30 weeks by Doppler ultrasonography, or it has been 36 weeks since a positive serum or urine human chorionic gonadotropin pregnancy test result (ACOG, 2009). Testing for fetal lung maturity should not be performed, and is contraindicated, when birth is required for fetal or maternal indications. Conversely, a mature fetal lung maturity test result before 39 weeks of gestation, in the absence of appropriate clinical circumstances, is not an indication for birth (ACOG, 2008a). Adoption and consistent use of the ACOG (2009) and NICHD (Spong et al., 2011) guidelines for medically indicated births before 39 weeks

Table 7-1. GUIDANCE REGARDING TIMING OF DELIVERY WHEN CONDITIONS COMPLICATE PREGNANCY AT OR AFTER 34 WEEKS OF GESTATION

Condition	Gestational Age* at Delivery	Grade of Recommendation[†]
Placental and uterine issues		
Placenta previa[†]	**36–37 wk**	B
Suspected placenta accreta, increta, or percreta with placenta previa[†]	**34–35 wk**	B
Prior classical cesarean (upper segment uterine incision)[†]	**36–37 wk**	B
Prior myomectomy necessitating cesarean delivery[†]	37–38 wk (may require earlier delivery, similar to prior classical cesarean, in situations with more extensive or complicated myomectomy)	B
Fetal issues		
Fetal growth restriction-singleton	**38–39 wk:**	
	• Otherwise uncomplicated, no concurrent findings	B
	34–37 wk:	
	• Concurrent conditions (oligohydramnios, abnormal Doppler studies, maternal risk factors, comorbidity)	B
	Expeditious delivery regardless of gestational age:	
	• Persistent abnormal fetal surveillance suggesting imminent fetal jeopardy	
Fetal growth restriction-twin gestation	**36–37 wk:**	
	• Dichorionic-diamniotic twins with isolated fetal growth restriction	B
	32–34 wk:	
	• Monochorionic-diamniotic twins with isolated fetal growth restriction	B
		B
	• Concurrent conditions (oligohydramnios, abnormal Doppler studies, maternal risk factors, comorbidity	
	Expeditious delivery regardless of gestational age:	
	• Persistent abnormal fetal surveillance suggesting imminent fetal jeopardy	
Fetal congenital malformations[†]	**34–39 wk:**	B
	• Suspected worsening of fetal organ damage	
	• Potential for fetal intracranial hemorrhage (e.g., vein of Galen aneurysm, neonatal alloimmune thrombocytopenia)	
	• When delivery prior to labor is preferred (e.g., EXIT procedure)	
	• Previous fetal intervention	
	• Concurrent maternal disease (e.g., preeclampsia, chronic hypertension)	
	• Potential for adverse maternal effect from fetal condition	
	Expeditious delivery regardless of gestational age:	B
	• When intervention is expected to be beneficial	
	• Fetal complications develop (abnormal fetal surveillance, new-onset hydrops fetalis, progressive or new-onset organ injury)	
	• Maternal complications develop (mirror syndrome)	
Multiple gestations: dichorionic-diamniotic[†]	**38 wk**	B
Multiple gestations: monochorionic-diamniotic[†]	**34–37 wk**	B
Multiple gestations: dichorionic-diamniotic or monochorionic-diamniotic with single fetal death[†]	If occurs at or after 34 wk, consider delivery (recommendation limited to pregnancies at or after 34 wk; if occurs before 34 wk, individualize based on concurrent maternal or fetal conditions)	B
Multiple gestations: monochorionic-monoamniotic[†]	**32–34 wk**	B
Multiple gestations: Monochorionic-monoamniotic with single fetal death[†]	Consider delivery; individualized according to gestational age and concurrent complications	B
Oligohydramnios—isolated and persistent[†]	**36–37 wk**	B
Maternal issues		
Chronic hypertension—no medications[†]	**38–39 wk**	B
Chronic hypertension—controlled on medications[†]	**37–39 wk**	B
Chronic hypertension—difficult to control (requiring frequent medication adjustments)[†]	**36–37 wk**	B

Table 7-1. GUIDANCE REGARDING TIMING OF DELIVERY WHEN CONDITIONS COMPLICATE PREGNANCY AT OR AFTER 34 WEEKS OF GESTATION (*Continued*)

Condition	Gestational Age* at Delivery	Grade of Recommendation[†]
Gestational hypertension[§]	37–38 wk	B
Preeclampsia—severe[†]	At diagnosis (recommendation limited to pregnancies at or after 34 wk)	C
Preeclampsia—mild[†]	37 wk	B
Diabetes—pregestational well controlled[†]	LPTB or ETB not recommended	B
Diabetes—pregestational with vascular disease[†]	37–39 wk	B
Diabetes—pregestational, poorly controlled[†]	34–39 wk (individualized to situation)	B
Diabetes—gestational well controlled on diet[†]	LPTB or ETB not recommended	B
Diabetes—gestational well controlled on medication[†]	LPTB or ETB not recommended	B
Diabetes—gestational poorly controlled on medication[†]	34–39 wk (individualized to situation)	B
Obstetric issues		
Prior stillbirth-unexplained[†]	LPTB or ETB not recommended	B
	Consider amniocentesis for fetal pulmonary maturity if delivery planned at less than 39 wk	C
Spontaneous preterm birth: preterm premature rupture of membranes[†]	34 wk (recommendation limited to pregnancies at or after 34 wk)	B
Spontaneous preterm birth: active preterm labor[†]	Delivery if progressive labor or additional maternal or fetal indication	B

ETB, early term birth as 37 0/7 weeks through 38 6/7 weeks; LPTB, late preterm birth at 34 0/7 weeks through 36 6/7 weeks.

*Gestational age is in completed weeks; thus, 34 weeks includes 34 0/7 weeks through 34 6/7 weeks.

[†]Grade of recommendations are based on the following: recommendations or conclusions or both are based on good and consistent scientific evidence (A); limited or inconsistent scientific evidence (B); primarily consensus and expert opinion (C). The recommendations regarding expeditious delivery for imminent fetal jeopardy were not given a grade. The recommendation regarding severe preeclampsia is based largely on expert opinion; however, higher-level evidence is not likely to be forthcoming because this condition is believed to carry significant maternal risk with limited potential fetal benefit from expectant management after 34 weeks.

[†]Uncomplicated, thus no fetal growth restriction, superimposed preeclampsia, and so forth. If these are present, then the complicating conditions take precedence and earlier delivery may be indicated.

[§]Maintenance antihypertensive therapy should not be used to treat gestational hypertension.

From Spong, C. Y., Mercer, B. M., D'Alton, M., Kilpatrick, S., Blackwell, S., & Saade, G. (2011). Timing of indicated late-preterm and early-term birth. *Obstetrics and Gynecology, 118*(2, Pt. 1), 323–333. doi:10.1097/AOG.0b013e3182255999

should have a positive influence on avoidance of preventable adverse neonatal morbidity related to elective early term births.

The American College of Nurse-Midwives (ACNM, 2010, 2012) and AWHONN (2012) recommend awaiting spontaneous onset of labor unless there are evidence-based medical indications that outweigh the risks of induction. Awaiting spontaneous labor in the absence of medical indications for birth not only will reduce elective early term births but can also decrease the cesarean birth rate (Fisch, English, Pedaline, Brooks, & Simhan, 2009; Reisner, Wallin, Zingheim, & Luthy, 2009).

WHY HAS THE RATE OF PRETERM BIRTHS INCREASED?

Contributing factors to the increase in PTBs over the last three decades include increasing use of infertility treatments producing twins and higher order multiples, more births to women at older ages (>35 years of age), more medically induced prematurity (including early labor inductions), early repeat cesarean births, primary cesarean births without a medical indication, advances in maternal and fetal medicine and neonatal care (which lead both providers and patients to believe that birth at earlier gestations is not an insurmountable health hazard), more pregnancies in very-high-risk women who then require early birth, and an increase in fetal complications leading to early birth, such as IUGR (Green et al., 2005; Murthy et al., 2011). As some of these issues (e.g., morbidities related to late PTB, elective early labor inductions, early cesarean births) have gained more attention, the PTB rate appears to have stabilized and even decreased slightly (Hamilton et al., 2011). It is too early to know whether this trend will continue and represent actual and sustainable improvement for this serious public health problem.

The issue of PTB of multiples and higher order multiples is particularly problematic. The twin birth rate in 2009 was 32.2 twins per 1,000 live births, a record high (Martin et al., 2011). Of the more than 4 million U.S. live births in 2009, there were 137,217 twin births, 5,905 triplet births, 355 quadruplet births, and 80 quintuplet and higher multiples births (Martin et al., 2011). The rate of triplet and other higher order multiple births in 2009 was 153.5 per 100,000 births. The twin birth rate increased by 76% since 1980 and by 47% since 1990 but has now stabilized, rising about 1% annually (Martin et al., 2011). During that same time, the rate of higher order multiples rose more than 500% but has declined slightly since 2004 (Martin et al., 2011). About 58.8% of twins are born preterm (Martin et al., 2011). The PTB rate is 94.4% for triplets, 98.3% for quadruplets, and 97% for higher order multiples (Martin et al., 2011). In 2006, 1% of singletons died in infancy compared with 3% of twins and 7% of triplets (Luke & Brown, 2007). It must be remembered, however, that the high rates of PTB in the United States cannot be attributed solely to the rates of multiple births, since the preterm rate for singletons also rose 23.7% from 9.7% in 1990 to 12% in 2010 (Hamilton et al., 2011).

WHAT IS PRETERM LABOR?

The diagnosis of preterm labor generally is based on clinical criteria of regular uterine contractions accompanied by a change in cervical dilation, effacement, or both, or initial presentation with regular contractions and cervical dilation of at least 2 cm (ACOG, 2012c). Display 7–2 lists the diagnostic criteria for preterm labor. Less than 10% of women with the clinical diagnosis of

preterm labor actually give birth within 7 days of presentation (ACOG, 2012c). It is estimated that approximately 30% of preterm labor resolves spontaneously and 50% of women hospitalized for preterm labor actually give birth at term (ACOG, 2012c). Although it is important to recognize that women who present with irregular contractions might not be in actual preterm labor at that time since they do not meet diagnostic criteria (ACOG, 2012c), women who report these symptoms need careful assessment and follow-up to decrease the risk of progressing to active preterm labor.

PATHOPHYSIOLOGY OF PRETERM LABOR AND BIRTH

In nearly 40% of PTBs, the cause is unknown (March of Dimes, 2011). Based on what has been learned from the research over the past few decades, it is doubtful that one causative factor for preterm labor will be discovered. All indications are that preterm labor has multiple causes, including social factors, physiologic factors, medical history factors, and illness factors (Green et al., 2005). The March of Dimes has characterized preterm labor as a series of complex interactions of factors and pathways (Green et al., 2005). Figure 7–1 illustrates the determinants of preterm labor conceptualized by Green and colleagues (2005). This conceptualization suggests that genetics, environment, stress, and psychosocial factors all play a role in the development of preterm labor leading to PTB. No single factor is thought to act alone; rather, factors interact in as yet unknown ways to initiate the cascade of events that result in preterm labor and birth. The external environment, including personal behaviors (e.g., smoking and drug use), psychosocial factors, nutrition, immune status, medical conditions, and medical interventions, interacts with genetics and family history through pathways that include inflammation and infection, maternal/fetal stress, abnormal uterine distention, bleeding/thrombophilia, and other possible pathways such as hormones and toxins. These factors and pathways, combined with racial and ethnic disparities, fetal growth, and preterm premature rupture of membranes, finally result in preterm labor/birth (Muglia & Katz, 2010). When thought of in this manner, it is clear that there is no one "cause" of preterm labor and birth, and therefore, no one single "cure." Multiple causes require research into multiple cures and preventive measures. One of the significant barriers in studying the causative factors of preterm labor and birth is the lack of knowledge regarding the exact physiologic mechanism responsible for initiation of term labor and birth. As with preterm labor, multiple theories have been proposed concerning what factors are responsible for spontaneous term labor, but none has proven conclusive.

D I S P L A Y   7 – 2

Clinical Criteria for Diagnosis of Preterm Labor

- 20 and 0/7 to 36 and 6/7 weeks' gestation
  And
- Regular uterine contractions
  And
- Change in cervical dilation
  And/Or
- Change in cervical effacement by digital examination or transvaginal assessment of cervical length
  Or
- Initial presentation with regular contractions and cervical dilation ≥2 cm

Adapted from American College of Obstetricians and Gynecologists. (2012c). *Management of Preterm Labor* (Practice Bulletin No 127). Washington, DC: Author. doi:10.1097/AOG.0b013e31825af2f0

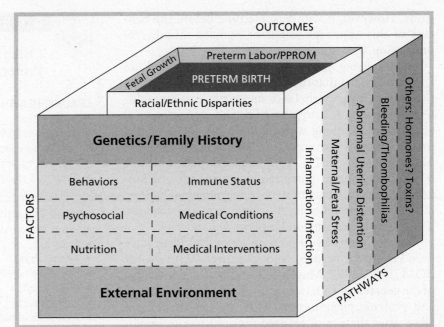

FIGURE 7-1. Determinants of preterm labor.

Although research has not found the cause or causes of preterm labor, some evidence suggests avenues for further research. According to the March of Dimes (2011), there may be four main routes leading to spontaneous premature labor:

1. *Infections/Inflammation.* Preterm labor is often triggered by the body's natural immune response to certain bacterial infections, such as those involving the genital and urinary tracts and fetal membranes. Even infections far away from the reproductive organs, such as periodontal disease, may contribute to PTB.

2. *Maternal or fetal stress.* Chronic psychosocial stress in the mother or physical stress (e.g., insufficient blood flow from the placenta) in the fetus appears to result in production of a stress-related hormone called corticotropin-releasing hormone. Corticotropin-releasing hormone may stimulate production of a cascade of other hormones that trigger uterine contractions and premature birth.

3. *Bleeding.* Placental abruption triggers the release of various proteins involved in blood clotting, which also appear to stimulate uterine contractions.

4. *Uterine stretching.* Overdistension of the uterus due to multiple gestation, polyhydramnios, or uterine or placental abnormalities can lead to the release of chemicals that stimulate uterine contractions.

Knowledge about these four routes may help scientists develop more effective interventions that can halt the various chemical cascades that lead to PTB (March of Dimes, 2011).

Not all PTBs can or should be prevented. About 25% of PTBs are intentional and occur because of health problems of the mother or the fetus (e.g., IUGR, preeclampsia, abruptio placentae, pulmonary or cardiac disease); another 25% of PTBs follow rupture of membranes (a cause not currently known to be preventable). Recently, researchers have proposed reconceptualizing how we think about PTB in order to more clearly differentiate the various pathways to PTB (Goldenberg et al., 2012; Kramer et al., 2012; Villar et al., 2012).

RISK FACTORS FOR PRETERM LABOR AND BIRTH

Risk factors for preterm labor and birth have been published and refined since the early 1980s (IOM, 1985). Historically, risk factors and gestational age have defined the conversation about preterm labor and birth. However, recent international discussions suggest moving away from a gestational age–focused conceptualization of PTB to a more complex model that considers all births (including stillbirths) between 16 and 38 6/7 weeks' gestation to be preterm and considers five components in assigning a PTB phenotype: maternal conditions, fetal conditions, placental conditions or pathology, signs of labor, and the pathway to birth (clinician initiated vs. spontaneous) (Villar et al., 2012). This model considers only the index pregnancy and not risk factors in assigning a phenotype for PTB. It is hoped that the proposed phenotypic classification system may improve future understanding of PTB by teasing out the heterogenous causes of PTB for more focused study. However, it will be some time before the benefits of this approach might be realized in concrete prevention strategies.

In addressing prevention of PTB, the March of Dimes suggested that there are three important known risk factors for preterm labor and birth (current multifetal pregnancy, history of a PTB, and uterine/cervical abnormalities), along with multiple categories of risk for subgroups of women (Freda & Patterson, 2004; March of Dimes, 2011). Additional risk factors include medical conditions predating the pregnancy, demographic factors, behavioral and environmental factors, illnesses occurring during the pregnancy, and genetics. These factors are listed in Displays 7–3 and 7–4.

Some of the risks of preterm labor and birth have been known for decades, and some are new to the list (IOM, 1985, 2007; Muglia & Katz, 2010). Knowledge of the genetics of PTB (see next section) is clearly a new and evolving phenomenon, as is the risk of preterm labor after the use of assisted reproductive technologies (ARTs), proposed in a study by Jackson, Gibson, Wu, and Croughan (2004). They performed a meta-analysis of 15 studies, examining the outcomes of singletons conceived through in vitro fertilization (n = 12,282) compared to 1.9 million spontaneously conceived singletons. Controlling for maternal age and parity, they found significantly higher odds ratios for PTB and other adverse perinatal outcomes in the singletons conceived through ART. Further risks of ART include multiple gestation, which carries a greater risk of PTB. Of live births from pregnancies conceived in ART cycles using fresh nondonor eggs or embryos in 2009, 28.9% were twins and 1.6% were higher order multiples (Centers for Disease Control and Prevention [CDC], American Society for Reproductive Medicine, & Society for Assisted Reproductive Technology, 2011). Among ART births in 2009, 60% of twins and 97.5% of higher order multiples were born preterm, and 56.1% of twins and 92.1% of higher order multiples were LBW (CDC et al., 2011).

Another risk that has received recent attention in the literature is periodontal disease (Offenbacher et al., 2006). Follow-up studies of interventions in periodontal disease have attempted to identify specific interventions that are effective. A French study failed to

DISPLAY 7-4

Other Possible Risk Factors for Preterm Labor

CHRONIC HEALTH PROBLEMS
- Hypertension
- Diabetes mellitus
- Clotting disorders/thrombophilia
- Low prepregnancy weight
- Obesity (as related to comorbidities such as hypertension and diabetes; not a risk factor for spontaneous preterm labor)

BEHAVIORAL AND ENVIRONMENTAL RISKS
- Late or no prenatal care
- Smoking
- Alcohol abuse
- Use of illicit drugs
- DES exposure
- Intimate partner violence
- Lack of social support
- High levels of stress
- Long working hours
- Long periods of standing

DEMOGRAPHIC RISKS
- Non-Hispanic black race
- Age <17 years
- Age >35 years
- Low socioeconomic status

GENETICS–ASSISTED REPRODUCTIVE TECHNOLOGIES MEDICAL RISKS IN CURRENT PREGNANCY
- Infection (especially genitourinary infections)
- Short interpregnancy interval
- Fetal anomalies
- Preterm premature rupture of membranes
- Vaginal bleeding (especially in the second trimester or in more than one trimester)
- Periodontal disease
- Being underweight prior to the pregnancy

demonstrate improved outcome with improved dental care (Vergnes et al., 2011). A South African study identified specific periodontopathogens that, when treated together, showed improved outcome (Africa, Kayitenkore, & Bayingana, 2010). More research is needed to further define the role and intervention in periodontal risk.

Clearly, the list of PTB risk factors is lengthy (Goldenberg et al., 2012). A number of these risk factors are not modifiable, but some are. Some of the current thinking in this field proposes that preconception care, or care begun before a pregnancy has been conceived, could ameliorate some of these preexisting factors, such as smoking cessation, tight control of preexisting diabetes or hypertension, obesity, or low prepregnancy weight (ACOG, 2005; Freda, Moos, & Curtis, 2006; Moos, 2003). The CDC held a major

DISPLAY 7-3

Risk Factors for Preterm Birth

The three most common risk factors for preterm birth are:
- Current multifetal pregnancy
- History of a preterm birth
- Uterine/cervical abnormalities

conference dedicated to this topic in 2005 and has published recommendations for preconception care, all of which are aimed at reducing PTB and other poor pregnancy outcomes (Johnson et al., 2006).

GENETIC INFLUENCES

In the late 1970s, when the topic of preterm labor and birth became prominent as an important entity for research and prevention, no thought was given to the possibility that preterm labor could have a genetic component. For decades, diligent researchers in medicine, epidemiology, public health, and nursing focused on physical symptoms, biologic pathways, and social interventions in their efforts to prevent this costly and dangerous complication of pregnancy. It was not until 2003 that the director of the National Human Genome Research Institute at the NIH announced that the sequencing of the human genome had been completed (Lewis, 2006). This event ushered in the genomic era of health research and has impacted the study of PTB in extraordinary ways. What we once thought of as strictly a social phenomenon or a biologic accident might actually have a genetic component that could hold promise for exciting new interventions unheard of previously in history.

The possibility that preterm labor and birth has a genetic component provides us with new targets for prevention. For instance, Wang and colleagues (2002) found that infant birth weight is particularly vulnerable in women who smoke and possess a certain gene polymorphism. This could be the answer for why some women smoke during pregnancy and give birth to normal weight babies at term, and others who smoke have preterm, small babies who are at risk for more health problems. The clinical implication is that smoking cessation could be strongly targeted toward women who smoke and have the polymorphism. This sort of tailored intervention is an example of how advances in our understanding of genetics and biomarkers could transform the way we look at PTB prevention.

It has been known for some time that women who were themselves born preterm have a higher chance of having preterm labors and births themselves (Plunkett et al., 2009; Ward, 2003; Ward, Argyle, Meade, & Nelson, 2005). Is it possible that these women and their sisters and mothers have a genetic predisposition toward PTB? If so, can it be altered? More genetic research on this topic may answer these questions.

Genetic polymorphisms have been implicated in PTB (Kalish, Vardhana, Normand, Gupta, & Witkin, 2006). Giarratano (2006) described the effect of genetics on PTB and provided information about the genes that could possibly be implicated in preterm labor and birth. These data are reproduced here as Tables 7–2 through 7–4. These genes control pro-inflammatory cytokines (involved in possible infection and preterm premature rupture of membranes), the labor cascade genes (being studied for their role in the initiation of labor), and the vasculopathic genes (involved in vascular problems such as preeclampsia and thrombophilias). None of these lines of genetic inquiry has reached maturity, but they have given researchers entirely new areas in which to discover more information about how preterm labor begins, and how, possibly, to avoid it.

Table 7-2. PRO-INFLAMMATORY CYTOKINES

Candidate Genes	Symbol	Polymorphisms	Role of Candidate Gene in Preterm Labor and Birth	Speculated Impact of the Polymorphism
Interleukin 6	IL-6	G-174C Other SNPs: C/C G/G G/C	Critical in the cascade of host response; activates the acute phase response, stimulates T lymphocytes, induces differentiation of B lymphocytes; increases seen in gestational tissues in PTL.	Women with C/C variation produce less IL-6 and are less likely to manifest the inflammatory cascade leading to PTL. C/C variation lacking in African American women in PTB cases <34 weeks.
Interleukin 1 beta	IL-1β	IL-1β+3953*1 IL 1RN*2	A key pro-inflammatory cytokine correlated to prostaglandin production and increased uterine activity. Found in membranes in PTL.	Fetal carriage of these variations possibly increases the IL-1β cytokine production and risk for PTB.
Tumor necrosis factor-α promotor gene	TNF-α	G-308A (TNFA2 or Allele 2)	Pro-inflammatory cytokine. Elevated in the amniotic fluid of women experiencing preterm labor, PPROM, and positive amniotic fluid cultures.	TNFA2 allele causes elevated levels of TNF-α protein, leading to immune hyperresponsiveness to environmental factors, such as bacterial vaginosis, causing chorioamnionitis.

PPROM, preterm premature rupture of membranes; PTB, preterm birth; PTL, preterm labor; SNPs, single nucleotide polymorphisms.
From Giarratano, G. (2006). Genetic influences on preterm birth. *MCN: The American Journal of Maternal Child Nursing, 31*(3), 169–175.

Table 7-3. LABOR CASCADE PATHWAYS

Candidate Genes	Symbol	Polymorphisms	Role of Candidate Gene in Preterm Labor and Birth	Speculated Impact of the Polymorphism
Oxytocin receptors	OTRs	OTR Allele 1; OTR Allele 2 (Allele 2 has a 30 base pair C-A repeat)	In normal labor onset, OTRs are thought to increase myometrial sensitivity to oxytocin before labor onset. The binding of oxytocin to the myometrial receptor promotes the influx of calcium from the intracellular stores, as one pathway to activate contractions.	No published studies regarding this specific polymorphism. Continued study occurs to explore how the "normal" pathways of labor probably differ in cases of PTL and PPROM, with subsequent labor.
Corticotropin-releasing hormone	CRH	T255G Other SNPs: T/T T/G G/G	CRH is synthesized in the hypothalamus in response to stress, and in the placenta and membranes in pregnancy. CRH metabolic pathway promotes production of prostaglandins and PTL onset.	Research related to PTB in progress; in an obesity study, T/G variation in combination with a glucocorticoid polymorphism increased cortisol levels.

PPROM, preterm premature rupture of membranes; PTB, preterm birth; PTL, preterm labor; SNPs, single nucleotide polymorphisms.
From Giarratano, G. (2006). Genetic influences on preterm birth. *MCN: The American Journal of Maternal Child Nursing, 31*(3), 169–175.

PRETERM BIRTH RISK IN THE CONTEXT OF THE LIFE COURSE

Several investigators have observed that PTB is characterized by complex interactions between genes, environment, and socioeconomic factors. It is presently believed that preconception stress and/or cumulative activation of stressors, such as racism and economic stress, across the life course may contribute to the observed racial disparity in PTB in the United States, although the exact mechanisms of this effect are unclear (Kramer, Hogue, Dunlop, & Menon, 2011). Better understanding of social inequities, including local environmental exposures, in conjunction with genetic responses and gene–environment interaction may ultimately explain disparities in U.S. birth outcomes and contribute to the development of more effective prevention strategies (Culhane & Goldenberg, 2011; Dunlop, Kramer, Hogue, Menon, & Ramakrishan, 2011; Menon, Dunlop, Kramer, Fortunato, & Hogue, 2011).

Table 7-4. VASCULOPATHIC PATHWAYS

Candidate Genes	Symbol	Polymorphisms	Role of Candidate Gene in Preterm Labor and Birth	Speculated Impact of the Polymorphism
Vascular endothelial growth factor	VEGF	C936T Other SNPs: T/T	VEGF is a major angiogenic factor and regulates endothelial cell proliferation. Threshold levels are required for fetal and placental vascular development and inhibition of cell death in the placenta.	C936T is associated with lower VEGF production; an association was found between this variation and an increased risk of spontaneous PTB.
		C677T A1298C	An abnormal vascular network is hypothesized to predispose to spontaneous abortion or to early labor and birth.	
Methylenetrahydrofolate reductase (enzyme)	MTHFR	Risks results from a Vitamin B$_{12}$ deficiency, plus mutation	Elevates homocysteine, a risk factor associated with many vascular disorders in adults. In pregnancy, associated with uteroplacental vasculopathy, such as thrombosis and placental infarcts, seen with PTB.	Both mutations associated with decreased MTHFR activity, which increases homocysteine concentrations, particularly with low folate. Association of this mutation with PTB is unknown.

PTB, preterm birth; SNPs, single nucleotide polymorphisms.
From Giarratano, G. (2006). Genetic influences on preterm birth. *MCN: The American Journal of Maternal Child Nursing, 31*(3), 169–175.

RISK FACTORS AS SCREENING METHODS TO PREDICT PRETERM LABOR AND BIRTH

Because there is as yet no known single causative factor for preterm labor and about 50% of all PTBs occur in women with no known risk factors (Goldenberg & Rouse, 1998), it must be concluded that all pregnant women are at some risk for preterm labor and birth. Many studies in the 1980s and 1990s attempted to use risk-screening tools to determine which women were at risk for PTB and then, based on their risk status, initiate preventative interventions; disappointingly, none of those studies produced a drop in the rate of PTB (Collaborative Group on Preterm Birth Prevention, 1993; Herron, Katz, & Creasy, 1982).

Risk screening for PTB (as well as other obstetric or medical complications of pregnancy) is still conducted during the prenatal period; however, risk screening should be considered as part of a comprehensive assessment process rather than an efficacious method to accurately identify women who will give birth preterm and to allow opportunities to intervene using approaches that have proven successful. A problem as pervasive as preterm labor and birth must be explained to all pregnant women during routine prenatal care (i.e., education about signs and symptoms of preterm labor and what to do should they occur) in order to make sure that women who have any symptoms of early labor tell their healthcare providers immediately.

CAN PRETERM LABOR AND BIRTH BE PREVENTED?

The search for prevention of PTB has been ongoing for decades. It would be comforting to think that simple strategies such as prenatal care could prevent PTB, but studies have not shown that to be true (Krans & Davis, 2012; Lu, Tache, Alexander, Kotelchuck, & Halfon, 2003). However, preconception, interconception, and prenatal care do provide opportunities for reducing or eliminating modifiable risk factors for PTB (Johnson et al., 2006). Substance abuse, interpersonal violence, and smoking are all risk factors that clinicians may be able to help women modify or eliminate during prenatal care. Likewise, clinicians can also address internutritional status and optimal interpregnancy intervals during preconception and interconception care, in addition to partnering with women to obtain optimal control of chronic diseases prior to and during pregnancy (Berghella, Iams, Reedy, Oshiro, & Wachtel, 2010; Moos, Badura, Posner, & Lu, 2011). Mental health is an important factor in predicting a healthy pregnancy outcome. In a study of 14,175 women who completed the Edinburgh Postnatal Depression Scale between 24 and 28 weeks of pregnancy, women with depressive symptoms were more likely to give birth preterm, including birth at <37, <34, <32, and <28 weeks of gestation (Straub, Adams, Kim, & Silver, 2012).

Psychosocial assessment and nursing intervention have shown promise in preventing PTB in specific at-risk situations such as military families, lack of partner involvement, and other family system disruptions (Lederman, 2011). Research is needed to confirm the effectiveness of specific interventions. Although prenatal care is important as a healthcare strategy for all pregnant women, it is not a prevention method for PTB. At this point in time, no prevention strategy for all women has been discovered. In lieu of that, many studies have examined smaller scale prevention efforts aimed at specific subgroups of at-risk women. Other interventions, which previously had been thought to be preventive and evolving strategies, follow.

HOME UTERINE ACTIVITY MONITORING

Home uterine activity monitoring (HUAM) was a system of care to detect preterm labor using a combination of recording uterine activity with a tocodynamometer, transmitting it by phone or the Internet to the healthcare provider, and providing daily telephone calls from a healthcare provider (usually a perinatal nurse) to offer the woman support and advice. For several decades, it was thought that HUAM would be able to identify increased uterine activity before the woman was aware and, thus, provide opportunity to prevent PTB. Prospective studies were never able to confirm that premise (ACOG, 2001; Brown et al., 1999; Dyson et al., 1998). One randomized study found that women who were helped by HUAM received more benefit from the nursing telephone support they received than from the machine (Iams, Johnson, O'Shaughnessy, & West, 1987). Based on published research about efficacy and the significant cost of the system, ACOG (2001, 2012b) has not recommended the use of HUAM for singleton or multiple pregnancies for more than a decade. HUAM rarely is used today and is essentially "obstetric history." It should be remembered, however, that the contact with the nurse was found to be effective and is beneficial without a home monitor.

BIOCHEMICAL FETAL MARKERS

The search for early predictive factors for preterm labor and birth has included the use of biochemical markers, most notably fetal fibronectin. The U.S. Food and Drug Administration (FDA) approved fetal fibronectin testing for preterm labor in 1995. Fetal fibronectin is an extracellular matrix glycoprotein produced in the decidual cells of the uterus. Fetal fibronectin is thought to be the trophoblastic "glue" in the formation of the uteroplacental junction. It is normally absent from vaginal secretions from 24 to 36 weeks of pregnancy. Lockwood and colleagues (1991) first published a study suggesting that fetal fibronectin found in vaginal secretions between 24 and 34 weeks at a level greater than 50 ng/mL is a predictor of preterm labor.

It has been theorized that preterm labor breaks the bonds between the placenta and the amniotic membranes, causing a release of fetal fibronectin into the vaginal secretions. Several factors may affect the accuracy of the results of fetal fibronectin testing, including sexual activity within 24 hours of sample collection, cervical examination within 24 hours of sample collection, vaginal probe ultrasound, vaginal bleeding, intraamniotic and vaginal infections, and use of douches or vaginal lubricants. When a woman who is a potential candidate for fetal fibronectin testing presents with signs and symptoms of preterm labor, it is important to delay digital examination of the cervix until the test has been completed.

The potential value of the test is in deciding who is at immediate risk of preterm labor and who is not. The negative predictive value of the fetal fibronectin test is high (up to 95%), whereas the positive predictive value is low (25% to 40%). Therefore, the test is most effective in predicting who will not experience preterm labor rather than who will experience it. Fetal fibronectin testing is useful in determining which women will not go into preterm labor within a few days and, therefore, do not need to be considered for immediate steroid administration, tocolysis, or transport to tertiary care. Women between 24 and 34 weeks of gestation who have a negative fetal fibronectin test have a 0.5% to 5% chance of giving birth within 7 to 14 days (March of Dimes, 2012c). Women with a positive fetal fibronectin test signal the need for further evaluation, education, and possible interventions such as steroid administration and tocolysis. There may be potential value of contingent or combined assessment for preterm labor using both cervical length and fetal fibronectin testing (Audibert et al., 2010; Bolt et al., 2011); however, more data are needed before routine practice can be recommended (ACOG, 2012c).

CERVICAL LENGTH MEASUREMENTS

Measuring cervical length has been thought to be predictive of PTB because, in some populations, it has been shown that a short cervical length can be a precursor to preterm labor. Various definitions of short cervical length as identifying risk for PTB exist, ranging from <30 to <15 mm. The shorter the cervical length, the higher the risk. In a meta-analysis of five studies of asymptomatic women at risk for PTB, Romero and colleagues (2012) used ≤25 mm as the definition of short cervix as measured by ultrasound. Others have used ≤20 mm as a predictor of high risk for PTB (Moroz & Simhan, 2012; Society for Maternal–Fetal Medicine [SMFM], 2012).

Transvaginal ultrasound is the gold standard for cervical length measurement (SMFM, 2012) and is valid between 15 and 28 weeks' gestation, but this technology requires significant skill and resources. Nonsonographic cervical length measurement using a measuring probe (Cervilenz) may be useful as a screening tool when ultrasound is not available or easily accessible and as a cost-saving method to identify women who truly need sonographic evaluation (Ross & Beall, 2009). Nonsonographic measurement of cervical length using a measuring probe has shown to be more accurate than digital examination and may be comparable to fetal fibronectin as a screening tool (Burwick, Lee, Benedict, Ross, & Kjos, 2009; Burwick, Zork, Lee, Ross, & Kjos, 2011); however, more research is needed in the form of randomized clinical trials to rigorously evaluate its efficacy before routine clinical use.

Research on the administration of vaginal progesterone to women with a short cervix (Hassan et al., 2011; Romero et al., 2012) suggests that an effective intervention is available and therefore provides a reason to measure the cervix in at-risk women (e.g., women with a positive fetal fibronectin test). The value of measuring the cervix in *all* pregnant women requires further research. According to ACOG (2012b), although results of observational studies have suggested knowledge of fetal fibronectin status or cervical length may assist in reducing use of unnecessary resources, these findings have not been confirmed by randomized clinical trials. Furthermore, the positive predictive value of a positive fetal fibronectin test result or a short cervix alone is poor and should not be used exclusively to direct management in the setting of acute symptoms (ACOG, 2012c). As with so much about PTB prevention, more data are needed before universal clinical recommendations can be offered.

BED REST

According to Maloni (2010), from 700,000 to 1 million women each year are placed on antepartum bed rest for risk of pregnancy complications, including PTB. Bed rest is the most commonly ordered intervention, despite the fact that no evidence supports its effectiveness in actually preventing PTB (Goldenberg & Rouse, 1998; Maloni et al., 1993; Sciscione, 2010). Bigelow and Stone (2011) noted that approximately 70% of maternal–fetal medicine specialists include bed rest in their treatment of preterm labor, and 95% of obstetricians prescribe bed rest for pregnancy complications in general. Maloni, Alexander, Schluchter,

Shah, and Park (2004) found that after only 3 days of bed rest, muscle tone decreases, calcium is lost, and glucose intolerance develops. One study measured loss of gastrocnemius muscle tone in women on antepartum bed rest, the symptoms of which continued into the postpartum period (Maloni & Schneider, 2002). After longer periods of bed rest, women experience bone demineralization, constipation, fatigue, anxiety, and depression (Maloni et al., 2004). Dysphoria, or negative affect, also has been described in women placed on bed rest (Maloni & Park, 2005).

Bed rest may cause more harm than therapeutic benefit. Maloni (2010) presented a comprehensive model for the complex physiologic effects of bed rest, including alterations in fluid and electrolyte balance and alterations in cardiovascular, cardiopulmonary, endocrine, gastrointestinal, renal, musculoskeletal, sensory, and behavioral function. Maloni and colleagues (2004) also showed significant maternal weight loss in mothers on antepartum bed rest, as well as lower infant birth weights across all gestational ages. Two decades ago, Goldenberg and colleagues (1994) found that bed rest had a major financial impact for families and for society in lost wages, household help expenses, and hospital costs. In addition, women who have been on bed rest suffer substantial physical and emotional symptoms during the bed rest period and after the infant's birth, including fatigue, mood changes, difficulty concentrating, back soreness, dry skin, and headaches (Maloni & Park, 2005). According to the latest review in the *Cochrane Database of Systematic Reviews*, due to the potential adverse effects of bed rest for women and their families and the increased healthcare costs, clinicians should not routinely advise women at risk of PTB to rest in bed (Sosa, Althabe, Belizán, & Bergel, 2004). Despite all the literature describing the harmful effects of bed rest and recommendations from ACOG (2012c) to avoid its routine use, bed rest is still ordered frequently for women at risk for PTB. Display 7–5 describes nursing care measures for women who are prescribed bed rest during pregnancy. Some form of activity restriction, rather than strict bed rest, is another option that physicians may order for women at risk for preterm labor and birth. Activity restriction for this population is similarly lacking evidence of efficacy, as is bed rest.

INTRAVENOUS HYDRATION

One common strategy used in the inpatient setting to reduce preterm contractions is IV hydration. Significant amounts of IV fluids are usually administered to increase vascular volume and because, anecdotally, it is thought that uterine contractions are quieted by hydration. There has been no evidence found that hydration indeed can avert a PTB (Freda & DeVore, 1996; Lu et al., 2003). Similar to bed rest therapy, however, intravenous (IV) fluid therapy is a traditional treatment that continues to be used despite recommendations to the contrary (ACOG, 2012c). This therapy is not without side effects. Nurses should be cautious when administering IV fluids for this purpose because if uterine activity continues, the next treatment could be IV administration of tocolytic agents, which carry a possible side effect of pulmonary edema. Careful attention to intake and output and auscultation of the lungs are essential to monitor for the development of pulmonary edema.

According to the latest review in the *Cochrane Database of Systematic Reviews*, available data do not support any advantage of hydration as a treatment for women who present in preterm labor, although hydration may be beneficial for women with evidence of

---

DISPLAY 7-5

Nursing Care for Women Prescribed Bed Rest as Therapy

- Assist the family in becoming involved in the nursing care plan.
- Assist the woman and healthcare team in clarifying what is meant by "bed rest" (e.g., Allowed to sit up? Shower? Make dinner? Use the stairs __ times per day?).
- If the family is not available, suggest that the woman ask friends for help during this time.
- Maintaining hydration while on bed rest is important; suggest that a cooler be kept beside the bed.
- Bed rest can lead to muscle wasting; teach passive limb exercises.
- Anxiety and depression are common during bed rest; teach the family to expect this and talk about their feelings.
- The woman should be in a place where she can interact with her family rather than in a bedroom alone.
- Instruct the woman not to do any nipple preparation for breastfeeding; nipple stimulation can cause uterine contractions.
- Some women find that keeping a journal helps them deal with the isolation and boredom of bed rest.
- Household jobs that can be done while in bed (e.g., paying bills, mending, folding laundry) help the woman feel more a part of the family.
- This is a good time to provide short educational videos about all aspects of pregnancy, labor, birth, and parenting.
- A laptop computer, smart phone, or tablet with Internet access can help the woman keep in touch with friends and access support and information.
- Provide referral information for online support groups to women with computer and Internet access.
- Encourage the woman to develop a support system of people with whom she can talk and vent her feelings.
- Educate the family about the emotional and behavioral responses they can expect from other children, according to the ages and developmental stages of other children in the family.

dehydration (Stan, Boulvain, Pfister, & Hirsbrunner-Almagbaly, 2002). Based on the preponderance of the evidence, therefore, according to ACOG (2012b), bed rest, hydration, and pelvic rest do not appear to improve the rate of PTB and should not be routinely recommended.

PROPHYLACTIC ANTIBIOTICS

Prophylactic antibiotics to prevent PTB have been studied, and no evidence exists that they can prevent PTB (ACOG, 2012c; Lu et al., 2003). ACOG (2011b) supports following protocols for prevention of early onset perinatal group B streptococcus (GBS) recommended by the CDC (Verani, McGee, & Schrag, 2010) as the best use of antibiotic therapy in women with preterm labor because it can prevent infection in the newborn. ACOG (2011c) also recommends antibiotics to prolong latency (the period between rupture of membranes and onset of labor) in women with preterm premature rupture of membranes. Figure 7–2 presents the CDC (Verani et al., 2010) algorithm for screening for GBS colonization and use of intrapartum prophylaxis for women with preterm labor. Table 7–5 presents the CDC (Verani et al., 2010) recommended regimens for intrapartum antimicrobial prophylaxis for perinatal GBS disease prevention. Figure 7–3 presents the CDC (Verani et al., 2010) algorithm for screening for GBS colonization and use of intrapartum prophylaxis for women with preterm premature rupture of membranes. Figure 7–4 presents the CDC (Verani et al., 2010) recommended regimens for intrapartum antibiotic prophylaxis for prevention of early-onset GBS disease. Care of the baby exposed to GBS is presented in Chapter 21.

CERVICAL CERCLAGE

Recent studies on implications and management of women with a short cervix have resulted in a resurgence of the study of cerclage in relation to PTB. However, all of the researchers did not use the same definition of "short cervix," so comparing findings across studies is challenging. The general consensus is that a cervix less than 30 mm long is a concern and less than 15 mm is greatest concern. A study of cerclage in women with a cervix less than 25 mm did not show a reduction in PTB (Owen et al., 2009). A meta-analysis of four randomized trials comparing cervical length–indicated cerclage versus history-indicated cerclage found that women with a singleton pregnancy and history of PTB can be followed with measurement of cervical length and cerclage placed only if short cervix (<25 mm) is identified (Berghella & Mackeen, 2011). The SMFM issued an evidence-based guideline (see Fig. 7–5) recommending cerclage (in addition to progesterone therapy) for women with a prior history

of preterm birth and a cervical length <25 mm on transvaginal ultrasound (SMFM, 2012). Cerclage without consideration of cervical length is reserved for women with multiple midtrimester losses who fit the diagnosis of cervical insufficiency (Berghella & Mackeen, 2011).

PROGESTERONE

The use of progesterone has been studied as a preventive measure for women at risk of PTB. Meis and colleagues (2003) published the first randomized clinical trial of weekly injections of 250 mg of 17-alpha-hydroxyprogesterone (generally referred to in the literature as "17P"), starting at 16 to 20 weeks of gestation for prevention of PTB, and found that the group receiving 17P had significantly fewer PTBs. The women who benefitted from treatment in these studies had experienced spontaneous singleton PTB, with or without premature rupture of membranes, prior to 28 weeks. Benefit was noted for women who gave birth up to 37 weeks, although less dramatic reduction in recurrence of PTB than the earlier gestation. Spong and colleagues (2005) found that progesterone given to women who had previously given birth at <34 weeks was associated with a prolonged gestation in a subsequent pregnancy. Although the results from Spong and colleagues (2005) and Meis and colleagues were favorable for this specific high-risk population, further research with multiple gestation, women undergoing cerclage, and other pregnancies at high risk for preterm labor have not benefited from 17P.

As more studies with progesterone have been conducted, there has been renewed interest in its use as a potential preventative agent for PTB. A multicenter, randomized, double-blind, placebo-controlled study demonstrated benefit of vaginal progesterone in reducing PTB in women with a short cervix (Hassan et al., 2011). These researchers found that women with a short cervix (10 to 20 mm) on sonogram who were given midtrimester vaginal progesterone had a 45% reduction in births prior to 33 weeks and improved neonatal outcomes compared to placebo (Hassan et al., 2011). In a later meta-analysis of five studies that included asymptomatic women with a short cervix (≤25 mm), vaginal progesterone administration was found to reduce the risk of PTB prior to 33 weeks and neonatal morbidity and mortality such as respiratory distress syndrome, birth weight <1,500 g, admission to the NICU, and requirements for mechanical ventilation (Romero et al., 2012).

Success of vaginal progesterone in reducing PTB in a number of studies has now compelled serious reconsideration of the role of progesterone. The SMFM (2012) and ACOG (2008b) have recommended that women with a history of spontaneous PTB should be offered antenatal progesterone. The SMFM (2012) also recommends vaginal progesterone for women

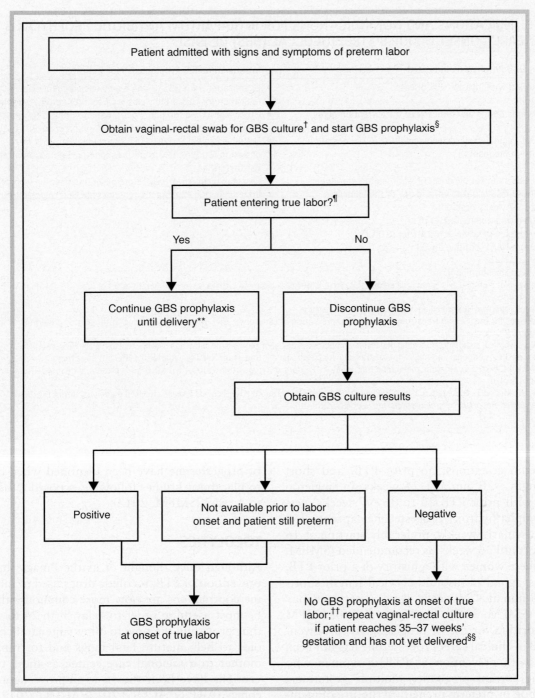

FIGURE 7–2. Algorithm for screening for group B streptococcal (GBS) colonization and use of intrapartum prophylaxis for women with preterm* labor (PTL). *t <37 weeks and 0 days' gestation. [a]If patient has undergone vaginal–rectal GBS culture within the preceding 5 weeks, the results of that culture should guide management. GBS-colonized women should receive intrapartum antibiotic prophylaxis. No antibiotics are indicated for GBS prophylaxis if a vaginal–rectal screen within 5 weeks was negative. [b]See Figure 7–4 for recommended antibiotic regimens. [c]Patient should be regularly assessed for progression to true labor; if the patient is considered not to be in true labor, discontinue GBS prophylaxis. [d]If GBS culture results become available prior to birth and are negative, then discontinue GBS prophylaxis. [e]Unless subsequent GBS culture prior to birth is positive. [f]A negative GBS screen is considered valid for 5 weeks. If a patient with a history of PTL is readmitted with signs and symptoms of PTL and had a negative GBS screen more than 5 weeks prior, she should be rescreened and managed according to this algorithm at that time. (From Verani, J. R., McGee, L., & Schrag, S. J. [2010]. Prevention of perinatal group B streptococcal disease—Revised guidelines from CDC, 2010. *Morbidity and Mortality Weekly Report, Recommendations and Reports, 59*[RR-10], 1–32.)

Table 7-5. INDICATIONS AND NONINDICATIONS FOR INTRAPARTUM ANTIBIOTIC PROPHYLAXIS TO PREVENT EARLY-ONSET GROUP B STREPTOCOCCAL (GBS) DISEASE

Intrapartum GBS Prophylaxis Indicated	Intrapartum GBS Prophylaxis Not Indicated
• Previous infant with invasive GBS disease	• Colonization with GBS during a previous pregnancy (unless an indication for GBS prophylaxis is present for current pregnancy)
• GBS bacteriuria during any trimester of the current pregnancy[a]	• GBS bacteriuria during previous pregnancy (unless an indication for GBS prophylaxis is present for current pregnancy)
• Positive GBS vaginal–rectal screening culture in late gestation[b] during current pregnancy[a]	• Negative vaginal and rectal GBS screening culture in late gestation[†] during the current pregnancy, regardless of intrapartum risk factors
• Unknown GBS status at the onset of labor (culture not done, incomplete, or results unknown) and any of the following: — Birth at <37 weeks' gestation[c] — Amniotic membrane rupture ≥18 hr — Intrapartum temperature ≥100.4°F (≥38.0°C)[d] — Intrapartum NAAT[e] positive for GBS	• Cesarean birth performed before onset of labor on a woman with intact amniotic membranes, regardless of GBS colonization status or gestational age

NAAT, nucleic acid amplification tests.
[a]Intrapartum antibiotic prophylaxis is not indicated in this circumstance if a cesarean birth is performed before onset of labor on a woman with intact amniotic membranes.
[b]Optimal timing for prenatal GBS screening is at 35 to 37 weeks' gestation.
[c]Recommendations for the use of intrapartum antibiotics for prevention of early-onset GBS disease in the setting of threatened preterm birth are presented in Figures 7–2 and 7–3.
[d]If amnionitis is suspected, broad-spectrum antibiotic therapy that includes an agent known to be active against GBS should replace GBS prophylaxis.
[e]NAAT testing for GBS is optional and might not be available in all settings. If intrapartum NAAT is negative for GBS but any other intrapartum risk factor (birth at <37 weeks' gestation, amniotic membrane rupture at ≥18 hours, or temperature ≥100.4°F [≥38.0°C]) is present, then intrapartum antibiotic prophylaxis is indicated.
From Verani, J. R., McGee, L., & Schrag, S. J. (2010). Prevention of perinatal group B streptococcal disease—Revised guidelines from CDC, 2010. *Morbidity and Mortality Weekly Report, Recommendations and Reports, 59*(RR-10), 1–32.

with singleton gestations, no prior PTB, and short cervical length ≤20 mm at ≤24 weeks. In singleton gestations with prior PTB 20 to 36 6/7 weeks' gestation, 17-alpha-hydroxy-progesterone caproate 250 mg intramuscularly weekly, preferably starting at 16 to 20 weeks until 36 weeks, is recommended (SMFM, 2012). In these women with a history of a prior PTB, if the transvaginal ultrasound cervical length shortens to <25 mm at <24 weeks, cervical cerclage may be offered (SMFM, 2012). See Figure 7–5 for SMFM (2012) algorithm for use of progestogens in prevention of PTB in clinical care. Progesterone has not been associated with prevention of PTB in women who have in the current pregnancy multiple gestations, preterm labor, or preterm premature rupture of membranes; therefore, there is insufficient evidence to recommend the use of progesterone in women with any of these risk factors, with or without a short cervical length (SMFM, 2012). Routine cervical length screening remains controversial; however, it is not unreasonable for individual providers to use this strategy (SMFM, 2012).

Further study about the safety and long-term effects of progesterone on both the mother and the baby and its usefulness in preventing PTB in other populations such as women with multiple gestations are needed before this therapy can be used routinely for *all* women at risk for PTB. To date, no negative long-term effects

of progesterone have been identified when compared to placebo in studies following exposed fetuses for up to 4 years (SMFM, 2012).

TOCOLYTICS

Although once thought of as the "magic bullet" for prevention of PTB, tocolytic drugs used to inhibit uterine contractions are now more commonly thought to be most useful in order to delay birth 24 to 48 hours, thus providing the time to allow antenatal corticosteroids to help mature fetal lungs and to transport the mother to a regional care center, as these two interventions have been shown to improve neonatal outcomes (AAP & ACOG, 2012; ACOG, 2012c; Bieber, Barfield, Dowling-Quarles, Sparkman, & Blouin, 2010; Goldenberg & Rouse, 1998). Evidence does not support the use of tocolytic maintenance therapy, nor is there sufficient evidence to support a clear choice for the first-line agent to use for short-term therapy (ACOG, 2012b; Conde-Agudelo, Romero, & Kusanovic, 2011). Given the potential for serious adverse effects from all tocolytic agents, neither maintenance treatment with tocolytic drugs nor repeated acute tocolysis should be undertaken as a general practice (AAP & ACOG, 2012; ACOG, 2012c).

Several classes of drugs have been used in an effort to stop preterm labor, although none has been shown to be

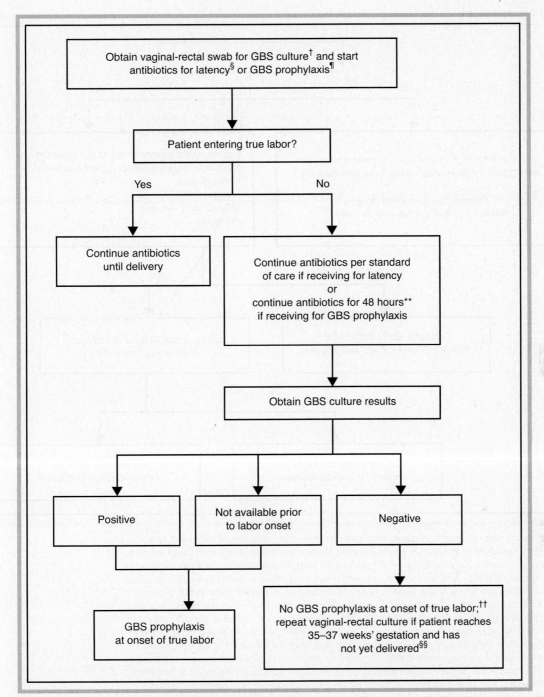

FIGURE 7–3. Algorithm for screening for group B streptococcal (GBS) colonization and use of intrapartum prophylaxis for women with preterm* premature rupture of membranes (pPROM). *At <37 weeks and 0 days' gestation. [†]If patient has undergone vaginal–rectal GBS culture within the preceding 5 weeks, the results of that culture should guide management. GBS-colonized women should receive intrapartum antibiotic prophylaxis. No antibiotics are indicated for GBS prophylaxis if a vaginal–rectal screen within 5 weeks was negative. [§]Antibiotics given for latency in the setting of pPROM that include ampicillin 2 g intravenously (IV) once, followed by 1 g IV every 6 hours for at least 48 hours, are adequate for GBS prophylaxis. If other regimens are used, GBS prophylaxis should be initiated in addition. [¶]See Figure 7–4 for recommended antibiotic regimens. [**]GBS prophylaxis should be discontinued at 48 hours for women with pPROM who are not in labor. If results from a GBS screen performed on admission become available during the 48-hour period and are negative, GBS prophylaxis should be discontinued at that time. [††]Unless subsequent GBS culture prior to birth is positive. [§§]A negative GBS screen is considered valid for 5 weeks. If a patient with pPROM is entering labor and had a negative GBS screen more than 5 weeks prior, she should be rescreened and managed according to this algorithm at that time. (From Verani, J. R., McGee, L., & Schrag, S. J. [2010]. Prevention of perinatal group B streptococcal disease—Revised guidelines from CDC, 2010. *Morbidity and Mortality Weekly Report, Recommendations and Reports, 59*[RR-10], 1–32.)

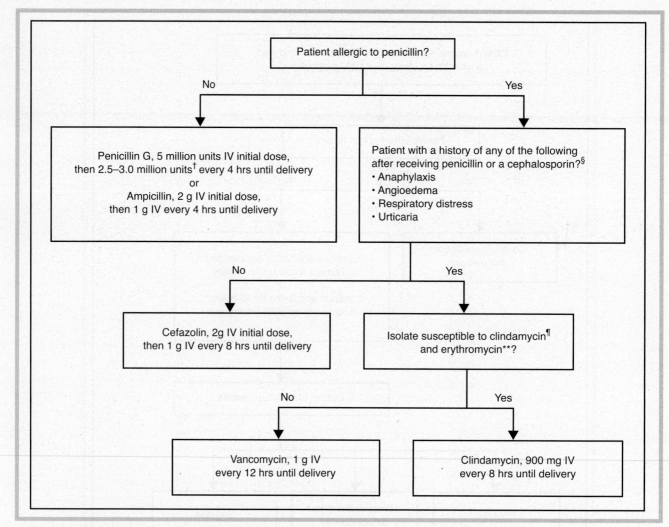

FIGURE 7-4. Recommended regimens for intrapartum antibiotic prophylaxis for prevention of early-onset group B streptococcal (GBS) disease. *Broader-spectrum agents, including an agent active against GBS, might be necessary for treatment of chorioamnionitis. [a]Doses ranging from 2.5 to 3.0 million units are acceptable for the doses administered every 4 hours following the initial dose. The choice of dose within that range should be guided by which formulations of penicillin G are readily available to reduce the need for pharmacies to specially prepare doses. [b]Penicillin-allergic patients with a history of anaphylaxis, angioedema, respiratory distress, or urticaria following administration of penicillin or a cephalosporin are considered to be at high risk for anaphylaxis and should not receive penicillin, ampicillin, or cefazolin for GBS intrapartum prophylaxis. For penicillin-allergic patients who do not have a history of those reactions, cefazolin is the preferred agent because pharmacologic data suggest it achieves effective intraamniotic concentrations. Vancomycin and clindamycin should be reserved for penicillin-allergic women at high risk for anaphylaxis. [c]If laboratory facilities are adequate, clindamycin and erythromycin susceptibility testing should be performed on prenatal GBS isolates from penicillin-allergic women at high risk for anaphylaxis. If no susceptibility testing is performed or the results are not available at the time of labor, vancomycin is the preferred agent for GBS intrapartum prophylaxis for penicillin-allergic women at high risk for anaphylaxis. [d]Resistance to erythromycin is often but not always associated with clindamycin resistance. If an isolate is resistant to erythromycin, it might have inducible resistance to clindamycin, even if it appears susceptible to clindamycin. If a GBS isolate is susceptible to clindamycin, resistant to erythromycin, and testing for inducible clindamycin resistance has been performed and is negative (no inducible resistance), then clindamycin can be used for GBS intrapartum prophylaxis instead of vancomycin. IV, intravenously. (From Verani, J. R., McGee, L., & Schrag, S. J. [2010]. Prevention of perinatal group B streptococcal disease: Revised guidelines from CDC, 2010. *Morbidity and Mortality Weekly Report, Recommendations and Reports, 59*[RR-10], 1–32. Reprinted with permission.)

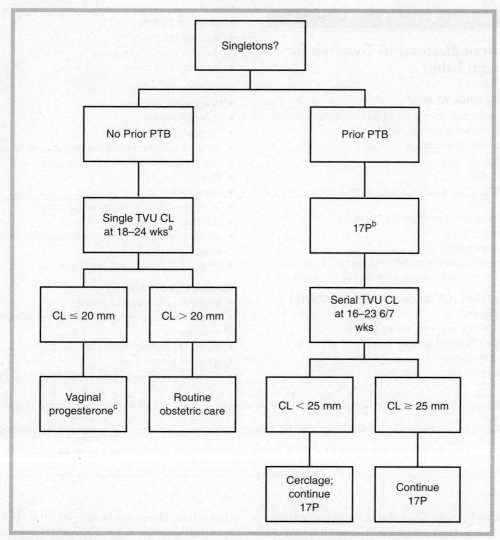

FIGURE 7-5. Algorithm for use of progestogens in prevention of preterm birth (PTB) in clinical care. [a]If transvaginal ultrasound (TVU) screening is perfomed. [b]117-alpha-hydroxy-progesterone caproate (17P) 250 mg intramuscularly every week from 16 to 20 weeks until 36 weeks. [c]For example, daily 200-mg suppository or 90-kg gel from time of diagnosis of short cervical length (CL) to 36 weeks. (From Society for Maternal–Fetal Medicine. [2012]. Progesterone and preterm birth prevention: Translating clinical trials data into clinical practice. *American Journal of Obstetrics and Gynecology, 206*[5], 376–386. doi:10.1016/j.ajog.2012.03.010. Reprinted with permission.)

effective for more than 24 to 48 hours (ACOG, 2012c; Goldenberg & Rouse, 1998; Sciscione et al., 1998). There are conflicting results among beta-mimetics, magnesium sulfate, calcium channel blockers, and non-steroidal anti-inflammatory drugs (NSAIDs); all have demonstrated only limited benefit (Berghella et al., 2009; Conde-Agudelo et al., 2011; King, Flenady, Cole, & Thornton, 2005; Loe, Sanchez-Ramos, & Kaunitz, 2005). If a tocolytic drug is used to stop preterm contractions, the choice of that drug can only be made based on the individual woman and her health status at the time. All of the drugs used for tocolysis have major side effects for the mother or the fetus and should only be used with extreme care. Displays 7–6, 7–7, and 7–8 describe contraindications to tocolytic

therapy, complications that can arise when tocolytics are used, and nursing care for women undergoing tocolytic therapy.

Serious Safety Concerns Related to Tocolytics

Careful, expert nursing care is essential for all women who receive tocolytic therapy. In 1997 and 1998, the FDA issued warnings to healthcare providers about the potential risks of using terbutaline pumps to prevent PTB (Nightingale, 1998). In April 2011, the FDA issued a warning to the public and healthcare providers that injectable terbutaline should not be used in pregnant women. The FDA (2011) cited data on serious side effects of injectable terbutaline, including maternal

DISPLAY 7-6

Contraindications to Tocolysis for Preterm Labor

GENERAL CONTRAINDICATIONS[a]

- Acute fetal compromise (except for intrauterine resuscitation)
- Intraamniotic infection/chorioamnionitis
- Eclampsia or severe preeclampsia
- Intrauterine fetal demise
- Lethal fetal anomaly
- Fetal maturity
- Placental abruption
- Maternal bleeding with hemodynamic instability
- Intolerance to tocolytics
- Pulmonary hypertension
- Preterm premature rupture of membranes (except for the purpose of maternal transport, steroid administration, or both)

CONTRAINDICATIONS FOR SPECIFIC TOCOLYTIC AGENTS

Beta-mimetic Agents

- Tachycardia-sensitive maternal cardiac disease
- Poorly controlled maternal diabetes mellitus
- Maternal hyperthyroidism
- Maternal seizure disorders

Magnesium Sulfate

- Maternal hypocalcemia
- Maternal myasthenia gravis
- Maternal renal failure

Indomethacin

- Gestation ≥32 weeks
- Maternal asthma
- Coronary artery disease
- Maternal gastrointestinal bleeding (current or past)
- Platelet dysfunction or bleeding disorder
- Oligohydramnios
- Renal failure
- Suspected fetal cardiac or renal anomaly
- Maternal liver disease
- Allergy to aspirin or other nonsteroidal anti-inflammatory drug
- Presence of fetal growth restriction

Calcium Channel Blockers

- Maternal cardiovascular disease
- Maternal preload-dependent cardiac lesions such as aortic insufficiency
- Maternal hemodynamic instability
- Maternal hypotension
- Avoid combining with beta-sympathomimetic drugs

---

[a]Relative and absolute contraindications to tocolysis are based on the clinical circumstances and should take into account the risks of continuing the pregnancy versus those of birth.

Adapted from American College of Obstetricians and Gynecologists. (2012b). *Management of Preterm Labor* (Practice Bulletin No. 127). Washington, DC: Author. doi:10.1097/AOG.0b013e31825af2f0

Lowe, N. K., & King, T. L. (2011). Labor. In T. King & M. C. Brucker (Eds.), *Pharmacology for Women's Health* (pp. 1086–1116). Sudbury, MA: Jones and Bartlett.

---

cardiac effects and death. They did acknowledge usage for 48 to 72 hours but condemned usage beyond 72 hours and outpatient/home usage. The FDA (2011) also warned against using oral terbutaline in pregnancy, citing the same dangers and no evidence of efficacy.

In October 2005 and June 2006, the Institute for Safe Medication Practices (ISMP) issued the Medication Safety Alert *Preventing Magnesium Toxicity in Obstetrics*. Numerous cases of magnesium overdoses that resulted in maternal respiratory arrest have been reported to ISMP in the past 9 years. Maternal deaths have been reported with use of magnesium sulfate (Simpson & Knox, 2004). Available data do not support the role of tocolytic agents in reducing the incidence of preterm labor, increasing the interval from onset to birth, or reducing the incidence of PTB (ACOG, 2012c), but they are still frequently used as a secondary intervention in the United States.

Beta-Mimetics

Ritodrine hydrochloride (Yutopar) was the only agent approved by the FDA for use as a tocolytic in the United States; however, the manufacturer discontinued the drug in September 2003. All drugs used for tocolysis are used "off label" (i.e., used for a purpose other than that approved by the FDA). Terbutaline (Brethine) is a beta-agonist commonly used for asthma, as was ritodrine, and is sometimes used off label for tocolysis. With recent FDA warnings, terbutaline may be used by injection in an inpatient setting for 24 to 72 hours only. Terbutaline pumps and oral terbutaline for tocolysis are strongly cautioned against and not recommended. Beta-mimetics (also called beta-adrenergic receptor agonists) stimulate beta-receptor cells located in smooth muscle. Theoretically, beta-agonist agents work by relaxing the smooth muscle, which decreases or stops uterine contractions. The beta-receptors are also located in smooth muscle in the cardiovascular, pulmonary, and gastrointestinal systems. Effects of beta-mimetic agents are related directly to dosage and route of administration. Maternal side effects are common and uncomfortable. Fetal side effects are thought to be the same as those in the mother because beta-mimetics rapidly cross the placenta. Beta-mimetic agents are contraindicated in patients with known cardiac disease.

Conscientious nursing care for the woman receiving beta-mimetic therapy is essential and includes ongoing assessment and monitoring of side effects. Maternal pulse rate must be monitored for any patient who

DISPLAY 7-7

Potential Complications and/or Side Effects of Tocolytic Agents

BETA–ADRENERGIC AGENTS
Maternal
- Hyperglycemia
- Hypokalemia
- Hypotension
- Flushing
- Pulmonary edema
- Cardiac insufficiency
- Tachycardia
- Arrhythmias
- Palpitations
- Nausea and vomiting
- Shortness of breath
- Chest discomfort
- Maternal death

Fetal/Neonatal
- Fetal cardiac effects such as tachycardia
- Alterations in fetal glucose metabolism/hyperglycemia/hyperinsulinemia
- Neonatal hypoglycemia, hypocalcemia, hypotension

MAGNESIUM SULFATE
Maternal
- Maternal lethargy
- Flushing
- Drowsiness
- Double vision
- Nausea
- Vomiting
- Diaphoresis
- Headache
- Pulmonary edema
- Loss of deep tendon reflexes
- Respiratory depression*
- Cardiac arrest*
- Maternal tetany*

- Profound muscular paralysis*
- Profound hypotension*
- When used with calcium channel blockers: suppresses heart rate, contractility, and left ventricular systolic pressure; produces neuromuscular blockade

Fetal/Neonatal
- Hypotonia
- Lethargy
- Bone demineralization
- Neonatal depression

INDOMETHACIN
Maternal
- Nausea and vomiting
- Esophageal reflux
- Gastritis
- Hepatitis[†]
- Renal failure[†]
- Gastrointestinal bleeding[†]

Fetal/Neonatal
- Oligohydramnios
- Transient hypotension
- Premature closure of fetal ductus arteriosus
- Necrotizing enterocolitis in preterm newborn
- Intraventricular hemorrhage in newborn

CALCIUM CHANNEL BLOCKERS
Maternal
- Dizziness
- Flushing
- Transient hypotension
- Headache
- Nausea
- Palpitations
- Edema
- Elevation of hepatic transaminases
- When used with magnesium sulfate: suppression of heart rate, contractility, and left ventricular systolic pressure

Fetal/Neonatal
- No known adverse effects

*Effect is rare and seen with toxic levels.
[†]Effect is rare and associated with chronic use.

Adapted from American College of Obstetricians and Gynecologists. (2012b). *Management of Preterm Labor* (Practice Bulletin No. 127). Washington, DC: Author. doi:10.1097/AOG.0b013e31825af2f0
Lowe, N. K., & King, T. L. (2011). Labor. In T. King & M. C. (Eds.), *Pharmacology for Women's Health* (pp. 1086–1116). Sudbury, MA: Jones and Bartlett.

is administered a beta-mimetic agent. A heart rate of 120 beats per minute or greater may warrant continuous electrocardiogram monitoring and discontinuation of tocolytic therapy. A heart rate greater than 120 beats per minute is associated with a decreased ventricular filling time and, therefore, with decreased cardiac output. Over time, if the left ventricular filling time is decreased, less blood is pumped to the myocardium, resulting in decreased myocardial perfusion. This is reflected by the patient's complaints of chest heaviness, shortness of breath, or chest pain.

Myocardial infarction may result if the agent is not discontinued. Mothers may also experience hypotension, cardiac arrhythmias, pulmonary edema, and alterations in metabolism. Fetal effects can include tachycardia and ischemia, hyperglycemia, and hyperinsulinemia (ACOG, 2012c; Lowe & King, 2011).

Oxytocin Receptor Antagonists

Atosiban, an oxytocin receptor antagonist, was tested in the United States as a tocolytic during the 1990s. It was felt that this tocolytic could be effective in

Nursing Care for Women Receiving Tocolytic Therapy

- Know the contraindications and potential complications of tocolytic therapy.
- Encourage the woman to assume a side-lying position to enhance placental perfusion.
- Explain the purpose and common side effects of the medication.
- Assess maternal vital signs according to institutional protocol.
- Notify the provider if the maternal vital signs fall outside the designated parameters.
- Assess for signs and symptoms of pulmonary edema.
- Assess intake and output at least every hour (unless on low-dose maintenance therapy).
- May limit intake to 2,500 mL/day (90 mL/hr) for some tocolytics.
- Provide psychosocial support.

stopping preterm labor and also have few side effects for the mother or the baby. Six clinical trials were conducted, but atosiban did not reduce PTB significantly (Papatsonis, Flenady, Cole, & Liley, 2005) and was not approved for use in the United States. Atosiban continues to be used in countries other than the United States for tocolysis.

Magnesium Sulfate

IV magnesium sulfate is a commonly used pharmacologic agent in intrapartum settings in the United States to stop preterm contractions. Despite widespread use in the United States, the effectiveness of magnesium sulfate therapy for tocolysis remains controversial because studies and meta-analyses have shown conflicting results. A Cochrane review concluded that magnesium was ineffective as a tocolytic agent and potentially increased risk of neonatal death (Crowther, Hiller, & Doyle, 2002; Grimes & Nanda, 2006). A later Cochrane review evaluated magnesium sulfate for tocolytic maintenance therapy and found insufficient evidence of therapeutic benefit (Han, Crowther, & Moore, 2010). Other meta-analyses found magnesium sulfate to be as effective as other tocolytic agents in delaying birth (Conde-Agudelo et al., 2011; Haas et al., 2009). Unfortunately, placebo-controlled trials have not been done for several agents, including magnesium, terbutaline, and nifedipine, which makes it much more difficult to determine their efficacy.

Magnesium sulfate use for preterm labor tocolysis is considered off label. The exact mechanism of action is unknown. Theoretically, magnesium interferes with calcium uptake in the cells of the myometrium. Because myometrial cells are thought to need calcium to contract, decreasing the amount of calcium decreases or stops contractions. Magnesium sulfate relaxes smooth muscle throughout the body, and a decrease in blood pressure may be observed with the administration of a loading dose or at high infusion rates. Maternal side effects include flushing, headache, nausea and vomiting, shortness of breath, chest pain, and pulmonary edema. Many practitioners feel comfortable using this agent because they have experience in its administration for the prevention of eclamptic seizures. Institutional protocols differ widely for how this drug is used in women with preterm labor.

Often, women in preterm labor receive magnesium sulfate after significant amounts of IV fluids have been infused in an effort to inhibit contractions. This practice increases the risk for pulmonary edema. Therefore, careful assessment of respiratory status, including rate and clarity of breath sounds, is required as well as accurate recording of fluid intake and output (Simpson & Knox, 2004). Signs and symptoms of pulmonary edema include shortness of breath, chest tightening or discomfort, cough, oxygen saturation below 95%, increased respiratory and heart rates, and adventitious breath sounds. Changes in behavior such as apprehension, anxiety, or restlessness may be additional signs of pulmonary edema or hypoxemia and should be closely monitored, documented, and reported (Simpson & Knox, 2004). The provider should be notified if a woman experiences any of the following symptoms (Simpson & Knox, 2004):

- Significant changes in blood pressure from baseline values
- Double (or blurring of) vision
- Tachycardia or bradycardia
- Respiratory rate below 14 or above 24
- Oxygen saturation below 95%
- Changes in breath sounds suggestive of pulmonary edema
- Changes in level of consciousness or neurologic status
- Absent deep tendon reflexes
- Urinary output less than 30 mL/hr
- Indeterminate or abnormal fetal heart rate pattern

Maternal respiratory rate, oxygen saturation, deep tendon reflexes, and state of consciousness should be monitored closely to detect progressive magnesium toxicity (Display 7–9). Magnesium toxicity results in loss of deep tendon reflexes and progressive muscle weakness, including the diaphragm and other respiratory muscles, leading to acute respiratory failure. In addition, an overdose of magnesium sulfate depresses the respiratory center in the brain, further inhibiting respirations. Hypotension, complete heart block, and cardiac arrest can occur. One ampule of calcium gluconate, 1 g (10 mL of a 10% solution), should be clearly labeled with directions for administration and kept in the nearest locked drug cabinet (Simpson & Knox, 2004).

DISPLAY 7-9

Safe Care Practices for the Use of Intravenous Magnesium Sulfate in Obstetrics

Intravenous (IV) magnesium sulfate may be administered to pregnant women for preterm labor prophylaxis, neuroprotection of the preterm fetus, or seizure prophylaxis for women with preeclampsia.

- The pharmacy should supply high-risk IV medications such as magnesium sulfate in prepackaged-premixed solutions.
- Magnesium sulfate only should be administered via controlled infusion pump.
- The infusion pump should not be preprogrammed to change the dose in the absence of direct bedside attendance of the nurse.
- A second nurse should double check all doses and pump settings.
- Use a 100 mL (4 g)/150 mL (6 g) IV piggyback solution for the initial bolus instead of bolusing from the main bag with a rate change on the pump.
- Use 500-mL IV bags with 20 g of magnesium sulfate versus 1,000-mL IV bags with 40 g of magnesium sulfate for the maintenance fluids.
- Use color-coded tags on the lines as they go into the pumps and into the IV ports.
- Maternal–fetal status should be assessed and documented before the medication is administered. Assessments include maternal vital signs, oxygen saturation, level of consciousness, characteristics of the fetal heart rate, and uterine activity.
- All maternal–fetal status parameters, including how the woman is tolerating magnesium sulfate, should be documented in the medical record every 15 minutes during the first hour, every 30 minutes during the second hour, and at least every hour while the maintenance dose is infusing (even for those patients who are considered to be stable).

- Signs and symptoms of magnesium toxicity should be evaluated and ruled out during each assessment. Deep tendon reflexes should be assessed prior to administration of the medication, at least every 2 hours thereafter, and as needed based on maternal signs and symptoms. Oxygen saturation should be assessed once per hour. Continuous pulse oximetry is not recommended. Breath sounds should be auscultated before the initial administration of magnesium sulfate, then every 2 hours thereafter.
- Provide one nurse to one woman continuous nursing care at the bedside during the first hour of administration.
- Provide one nurse to one woman ratio during labor and until at least 2 hours postpartum.
- Patient assignment should be no more than one additional couplet or woman for a nurse caring for a woman receiving IV magnesium sulfate in a maintenance dose.
- Provide nursing care during the maintenance dose in a clinical setting where the patient is close to the nurses' station rather than on the general antepartum or postpartum nursing unit where there is less intensive nursing care.
- Consider that a woman receiving magnesium sulfate remains high risk even when symptoms of preeclampsia or preterm labor are stable.
- When care is transferred to another nurse, have both nurses together at the bedside assess patient status, review dosage and pump settings, and review written physician medication orders.
- After the medication therapy is completed, discontinue the medication by removing the line from the IV port to prevent accidental infusion and potential magnesium sulfate overdose.
- Conduct periodic magnesium overdose drills with airway management and calcium administration with physician and nurse team members participating together.
- Maintain calcium antidote in an easily accessible locked medication kit with the dosage and administration (1 g of calcium gluconate should be given intravenously over 3 minutes) clearly printed on the kit.

Adapted from Simpson, K. R. (2006). Minimizing risk of magnesium sulfate overdose in obstetrics. *MCN: The American Journal of Maternal Child Nursing, 31*(5), 340; Simpson, K. R., & Knox, G. E. (2004). Obstetrical accidents involving intravenous magnesium sulfate: Recommendations to promote patient safety. *MCN: The American Journal of Maternal Child Nursing, 29*(3), 161–171.

If respiratory depression occurs, 1 g calcium gluconate should be given intravenously over 3 minutes (Sibai, 2002). If respiratory arrest occurs, ventilation should be supported until the antidote takes effect (Sibai, 2002). IV fluids administered at a rapid infusion rate can assist excretion of magnesium sulfate. Although significantly high values (30 to 35 mg/dL) are frequently reported as being necessary to cause cardiac arrest, it is important to remember that an untreated respiratory arrest will lead to cardiac arrest as the cardiac muscle becomes hypoxic and ischemic. Thus, cardiac arrest can occur at magnesium levels consistent with respiratory failure if the respiratory failure is not identified and treated immediately. Magnesium levels causing cardiotoxicity are not required to cause cardiac arrest.

Magnesium sulfate is on the *ISMP List of High-Alert Medications* because there is serious risk of causing significant patient harm when used in error (Simpson, 2006). Although errors with these drugs may not be more common than those with other medications, consequences of errors are more devastating (ISMP, 2006). Essential components of safe nursing care for women receiving IV magnesium sulfate have been described (ISMP, 2005, 2006; Simpson & Knox, 2004). See Display 7–9 for safe care practices when using magnesium sulfate in obstetrics. Because accidents and adverse outcomes continue to occur with magnesium sulfate in obstetrics, it is important to review important safety procedures that can minimize risk.

Magnesium Sulfate for Neuroprotection

In a multicenter randomized trial conducted in the United States, Rouse and colleagues (2008) found that magnesium sulfate, when given to the mother before PTB, may be beneficial to the preterm newborn in preventing cerebral palsy. Babies who survive PTB whose mothers were given magnesium sulfate prior to the birth were shown to have a decreased incidence of cerebral palsy when followed up to 2 years of life. A previous randomized controlled trial in Australia found similar results (Crowther, Hiller, Doyle, & Haslam, 2003). A review by the Cochrane Collaboration (Doyle, Crowther, Middleton, Marret, & Rouse, 2009) concluded that magnesium sulfate given to the mother prior to PTB is effective for neuroprotection of the preterm newborn. At least one subsequent analysis (Huusom et al., 2011) has questioned whether or not there is enough evidence to support or refute neuroprotective effectiveness. Huusom and colleagues (2011) expressed concern about the methodologic problems inherent in studying a condition that is rare, such as cerebral palsy, and drawing conclusions based on small samples of the five studies evaluated in the Doyle and colleagues (2009) Cochrane Review.

In a 2010 committee opinion, ACOG and SMFM supported use of magnesium sulfate as a potential benefit to the preterm newborn when given to women at high risk for birth before 32 weeks' gestation. However, the potential neuroprotective effects of magnesium sulfate should not be the basis for decision making about which agent to use for tocolysis (ACOG & SMFM, 2010). Hospitals that elect to use magnesium sulfate for fetal neuroprotection should develop uniform and specific guidelines for their departments regarding inclusion criteria, treatment regimens, concurrent tocolysis, and monitoring in accordance with one of the larger clinical trials that showed effectiveness (ACOG & SMFM, 2010). In 2012, ACOG offered more specific suggestions when using magnesium sulfate for neuroprotection. Criteria for use included gestational age less than or equal to 31 6/7 weeks *and* singleton or multiple pregnancy at risk for birth within the next 30 minutes to 24 hours *and either* active preterm labor with cervix 4 to 8 cm dilated or preterm premature rupture of membranes if rupture occurred later than 22 weeks *or* indicated PTB within the next 24 hours (ACOG, 2012b). Clarification about dosing was added: if the woman's condition leading to the planned PTB is for severe preeclampsia or hemolysis, elevated liver enzymes, and low platelet count (HELLP) syndrome, the full antiseizure magnesium sulfate regimen should be administered as minimal therapy (ACOG, 2012b). Suggestions for dosing of IV magnesium sulfate for neuroprotection were based on one of three previous clinical trials (Crowther et al., 2003; Marret et al., 2007; Rouse et al., 2008). Therefore, three different dosing regimens are listed as appropriate (ACOG, 2012b). The clinical leadership team at each site can determine which regimen will work best for their perinatal service. For medication safety reasons, ideally one regimen should be chosen for each perinatal service. There remain many unanswered questions about the use of magnesium sulfate for neuroprotection, including which women and fetuses are the best candidates and the optimal dosing regimen. More research is needed for answers on safety and benefit for the preterm newborn.

Calcium Channel Blockers

Calcium channel blockers are another class of drugs that have been used to suppress contractions. They cause the myometrial muscle to relax by interfering with the movement of extracellular calcium into the calcium channels of the cells. This prevents the electrical system from passing the current through the cells, preventing a contraction (Lowe & King, 2011). Calcium channel blockers have also been associated with maternal hepatotoxicity when administered for preterm labor (Higby, Xenakis, & Pauerstein, 1993). A European comparison of nifedipine and atosiban for preterm labor cessation showed that atosiban had fewer side effects and was warranted for use in women in whom nifedipine is contraindicated (Kashanian, Akbarian, & Soltanzadeh, 2005). A recent meta-analysis of 26 trials compared nifedipine to terbutaline and magnesium sulfate (Conde-Agudelo et al., 2011). Nifedipine was superior to beta-agonists for tocolysis, and there was no difference in efficacy between nifedipine and magnesium sulfate. Nifedipine had significantly fewer maternal side effects than both beta-agonists and magnesium sulfate. Because of nifedipine's pharmacologic properties, it should not be used in women with any cardiovascular compromise, intrauterine infection, multiple pregnancy, maternal hypertension, or cardiac disease (vanGeijn, Lenglet, & Bolte, 2005).

Prostaglandin or Cyclooxygenase (COX) Inhibitors

Prostaglandin is a naturally produced agent that is thought to cause uterine contractions and cervical ripening in term pregnancies. The enzymes COX-1 and COX-2 are essential to the biosynthesis of the prostaglandin that is necessary for labor/birth (Lowe & King, 2011). Because little prostaglandin has been found in women who are not in labor, the use of drugs that inhibit the production of prostaglandin has been hypothesized as a possible treatment for preterm labor. Several types of prostaglandins affect uterine contractions and cervical ripening. The most well-known and well-studied prostaglandin inhibitor for use as a tocolytic agent is indomethacin. Indomethacin competes with other factors in a long-term process whereby prostacyclin is the end product blocking the production of prostaglandin.

Indomethacin is not without fetal effects, however. Although this class of drugs might have some maternal side effects (ACOG, 2012c), after 34 weeks' gestation, indomethacin may cause premature closure of the fetal ductus arteriosus, increasing the risk of fetal pulmonary hypertension (Lowe & King, 2011; Vermillion & Robinson, 2005). Indomethacin also impairs fetal renal function, which may result in oligohydramnios. Systematic reviews published in 2005 concluded that indomethacin was superior to both other tocolytics and placebo in preventing PTB (King et al., 2005) and found no evidence of neonatal adverse effects (Loe et al., 2005). However, the use of indomethacin for prevention of PTB remains controversial because studies regarding its use have tended to be too small to have the power to detect differences in infrequent adverse outcomes. Some in the research community have suggested that the risk to the fetus by using indomethacin is less than the multiple morbidities associated with a birth at less than 32 weeks' gestation (Macones & Robinson, 1998). In a review of the literature regarding its use, Berghella and colleagues (2009) conclude that indomethacin is safe for the fetus when used for no more than 48 hours.

IS THERE ANY GOOD NEWS?

ANTENATAL CORTICOSTEROIDS

Antenatal corticosteroid use for prevention of respiratory distress syndrome in a premature infant has been endorsed by NICHD through its consensus conferences (Gilstrap et al., 1995; NIH, 2000). This class of medication does not prevent PTB; rather, it prevents major complications in the neonate, which is the best outcome possible at this time. Because it is not yet possible to actively prevent PTB, ACOG (2011a, 2012b) has recommended either of the following antenatal corticosteroid courses:

Betamethasone
- 12 mg given intramuscularly (IM) 24 hours apart for two doses

Dexamethasone
- 6 mg given intramuscularly (IM) every 12 hours for four doses

Either medication should be given to any woman at 24 to 34 weeks' gestation at risk for PTB within 7 days. Women with preterm premature rupture of membranes before 32 weeks' gestation should also receive the medication. The greatest benefit occurs between 24 hours and 7 days of administration; however, the medication can still benefit the newborn before 24 hours, so it should be given unless birth is imminent (ACOG, 2011a). Although one additional rescue course may be considered after 2 weeks in women who are <32 6/7 weeks and believed likely to give birth within the next 7 days (ACOG, 2011a; Garite, Kurtzman, Maurel, & Clark, 2009), more research is needed on the risks and benefits of a single rescue course (ACOG, 2011a). However, multiple courses of corticosteroids (more than two) have not shown benefit, and several studies have found decreased birth weight and decreased head circumference (ACOG, 2011a).

NURSING CARE FOR THE PREVENTION OF PRETERM BIRTH

EDUCATION ABOUT SIGNS AND SYMPTOMS OF PRETERM LABOR

Educating women about signs and symptoms of preterm labor has been a hallmark of PTB prevention programs since the early 1980s (Herron et al., 1982). Patient education is one of nursing's core areas of practice and, therefore, nurses are well qualified to teach women about signs and symptoms of preterm labor. At its onset, the woman may think that preterm labor symptoms are a "normal discomfort of pregnancy," in part because physicians, nurse midwives, childbirth educators, and nurses continue to teach women about Braxton-Hicks contractions, expecting the woman to decide whether the contractions experienced are normal or abnormal. Classic nursing research (Patterson, Douglas, Patterson, & Bradle, 1992) has shown that women taught in this fashion experience "diagnostic confusion" when faced with the symptoms of preterm labor and may not notify their healthcare provider because they think that the contractions they are experiencing are normal. If the goal in teaching women is to ensure prompt notification of the provider when early, subtle symptoms of preterm labor appear, use of the term "Braxton-Hicks contractions" for women before 37 weeks' gestation should be removed from prenatal teaching (Hill & Lambertz, 1990).

Because all pregnant women must be considered at risk for preterm labor, it is essential that nurses teach all pregnant women how to detect the early symptoms of preterm labor (Davies et al., 1998; Freda, Damus, & Merkatz, 1991; Freda & Patterson, 2004; Moore & Freda, 1998). Nurses providing care to pregnant women should use the literature to understand the best methods for teaching early recognition of preterm symptoms. Tiedje (2005) has described a model program for teaching women about prematurity in a clinic waiting room. Moore, Ketner, Walsh, and Wagoner (2004) have shown how listening to women can help remove barriers to effective patient education about PTB. Reassessment for symptoms at each subsequent prenatal visit is also essential. Patient education regarding any symptoms of contractions or cramping between 20 and 36 weeks' gestation should include telling the woman that these symptoms are not normal discomforts in pregnancy and that contractions or cramping that do not go away should prompt the woman to contact her healthcare provider.

Although many nurses teach their patients in a one-on-one manner, the use of standardized videotape for teaching women about preterm symptoms has been shown in classic nursing research to be effective in teaching women this information (Freda, Damus, Andersen, Brustman, & Merkatz, 1990). The March of Dimes videotape *Take Action* is one such example of patient education. No matter which method of patient education is used, it is imperative that nurses in prenatal settings make concerted efforts to teach all pregnant women about how to recognize early preterm labor.

Sometimes, patient education cannot be offered in person but can still be effective. A randomized clinical trial demonstrated that education offered by nurses on the telephone can result in a 26% decrease in LBW births and a 27% decrease in PTB among African American women (Moore et al., 1998). This study demonstrates the power of nursing care, nursing support, and patient education in the care of women at highest risk for PTB.

Reinforcement of the signs and symptoms of preterm labor should occur at each subsequent prenatal visit along with a review of any symptoms that may have been experienced since the last visit. Research from the past two decades has shown that some women who experience preterm labor wait for hours or days to call a healthcare provider, significantly delaying their time of entry into the healthcare system when some proactive action could be taken (Freston et al., 1997; Iams, Stilson, Johnson, Williams, & Rice, 1990). Prompt notification of the healthcare provider is essential because the use of antenatal corticosteroids given to hasten fetal lung maturity is the most effective therapy for avoiding neonatal health problems such as respiratory distress syndrome (ACOG, 2011a; Leviton et al., 1999; NIH, 2000).

In addition to teaching the symptoms of preterm labor, it is essential that the nurse in the antepartum or intrapartum setting establish a therapeutic relationship with the pregnant woman so she will feel comfortable reporting vague, nonspecific complaints and will come in or call her primary healthcare provider if she experiences any of the following signs or symptoms of preterm labor:

- Uterine cramping (menstrual-like cramps, intermittent or constant)
- Uterine contractions every 10 to 15 minutes or more frequently
- Low abdominal pressure (pelvic pressure)
- Dull low backache (intermittent or constant)
- Increase or change in vaginal discharge
- Feeling that the baby is "pushing down"
- Abdominal cramping with or without diarrhea

When any of these symptoms is experienced, the woman should be instructed to stop what she is doing, lie down on her side, drink two to three glasses of water or juice, and wait 1 hour. If the symptoms get worse, she should call the healthcare provider. If the symptoms go away, she should tell the healthcare provider at the next visit what happened, and if the symptoms come back, she should call the healthcare provider.

Perinatal nurses must listen carefully when pregnant women between 20 and 37 weeks' gestation complain of these symptoms, assess for cervical effacement or dilation as well as uterine contractions, and encourage them to call their provider or come back to the hospital if the symptoms reappear. It is also important to be sensitive to women who have been identified as at risk for PTB because they may have difficulty balancing concern about bodily symptoms versus overreaction (MacKinnon, 2006), and they may become confused when symptoms that were previously identified as alarming turn out to be "nothing" when they present to the office or hospital for evaluation (MacKinnon, 2006; Palmer & Carty, 2006). If healthcare providers minimize women's symptoms, women may not return early enough for intervention when it is needed.

EDUCATION ABOUT TIMING OF ELECTIVE BIRTH

Perinatal nurses can also offer patient education to prevent elective early term births. Pregnant women are getting mixed messages as to the ideal time for their babies to be born when they are healthy and their pregnancy has been uncomplicated. Many women interpret 9 months to mean that 36 weeks of pregnancy is full term. For a long time, the message from healthcare providers has been that term pregnancy is between 37 and 42 weeks of gestation and that preterm babies are those born before 37 weeks of gestation. This wide time frame is confusing for pregnant women who are considering their options in the last weeks of pregnancy. Recently, there has been education from multiple sources encouraging women to wait until at least 39 completed weeks of gestation before asking their primary care provider for elective labor induction. However well intended, this message implies that 39 weeks is an ideal time for birth. Benefits to the mother and baby of awaiting the onset of spontaneous labor and risks of elective labor induction, especially for nulliparous women with an unfavorable cervix, have been overlooked in some patient education materials. Patient education materials from AWHONN (2012) for pregnant women focuses on 40 weeks of pregnancy as normal and ideal: *40 Reasons to Go the Full 40*. This messaging is clear that at least 40 weeks, rather than 39 weeks, is best for healthy mothers and babies. The emphasis is on finishing pregnancy, labor, and birth healthy and well; managing risks; and enjoying the final weeks of pregnancy (AWHONN, 2012). While the main points of the patient education are serious and targeted to risks of asking to be induced early, there are also light-hearted reasons included for awaiting spontaneous labor. This innovative patient education pamphlet published by AWHONN can be used as part of prenatal visits, prepared childbirth classes, and other patient interactions during the last weeks of pregnancy.

LIFESTYLE MODIFICATION

Evidence exists that some women experience more preterm symptoms when engaged in certain activities. We have known for many years through research that when women are able to modify those lifestyle factors, they have fewer PTBs (Freda, Andersen, et al., 1990; Lynam & Miller, 1992). Activities such as stair climbing, riding long distances in automobiles or public transportation, carrying heavy objects, hard physical work, and inability to rest when tired have been associated with increased PTB (Hobel et al., 1994; Iams et al., 1990; Papiernik, 1989). Nurses who teach women about symptoms of preterm labor should assess whether symptoms increase when these or other activities are performed and work with women to find ways to help them eliminate those activities or at least decrease their frequency.

SMOKING CESSATION

Smoking is a lifestyle factor strongly associated with PTB and LBW. It is one of the few risk factors that can be altered by pregnant women. It is estimated that 20% of women aged between 15 and 44 years in the United States smoke cigarettes (ACOG, 2010). Although the effects of smoking on risk of PTB and LBW have been known for more than 50 years (Simpson, 1957), approximately 13% of women in the United States continue to smoke during their pregnancy (ACOG, 2010).

More women are at risk for secondhand smoke in their homes or public areas. Secondhand smoke is associated with PTB and adverse neonatal outcome, including increased respiratory problems (e.g., bronchitis, pneumonia), ear infections, dying from sudden infant death syndrome, and NICU admission (Ashford et al., 2010; Tong, Jones, Dietz, D'Angelo, & Bombard, 2009). Prenatal smoking remains one of the most common preventable causes of infant morbidity and mortality and is associated with 30% of small-for-gestational-age infants, 10% of preterm infants, and 5% of infant deaths (Tong et al., 2009). Cigarette smoking before conception can cause reduced fertility and conception delay among women (Tong et al., 2009). Maternal cigarette smoking during pregnancy increases the risk for pregnancy complications (e.g., placenta previa, placental abruption, premature rupture of membranes) and poor pregnancy outcomes (e.g., preterm delivery, restricted fetal growth, sudden infant death syndrome). During 2000 to 2004, an estimated 776 babies died annually from causes attributed to maternal smoking during pregnancy (Tong et al., 2009).

It is estimated that there would be a 10% reduction in perinatal mortality and an 11% reduction in LBW if smoking during pregnancy were eliminated. The risk of fetal death for pregnant women who smoke is generally 1.5-fold over that for pregnant nonsmokers (Silver, 2007). We know that even a reduction in smoking could improve perinatal outcome birth weight (England et al., 2001); therefore, it is incumbent on nurses to work toward helping pregnant women stop smoking completely, or at least significantly cut down on the number of cigarettes they smoke.

The physiologic effects of smoking occur as a result of transient intrauterine hypoxemia. When the pregnant woman smokes, carbon monoxide crosses the placenta and binds with maternal and fetal hemoglobin, producing carboxyhemoglobin. Carboxyhemoglobin interferes with the normal binding process of oxygen to the hemoglobin molecule, reducing the ability of the blood to carry adequate levels of oxygen to the fetus (Secker-Walker, Vacek, Flynn, & Mead, 1997). Smoking may also result in an increase in fetal vascular resistance, which can lead to impaired fetal growth and hypoxia (Silver, 2007).

Smoking cessation programs have been widely evaluated. An opportunity to reduce the risk of PTB and LBW exists if education for pregnant women about the effects of smoking on the fetus begins early in pregnancy. One of the most effective interventions to reduce smoking during pregnancy is to encourage the woman to institute a no-smoking policy at home (Mullen, Richardson, Quinn, & Ershoff, 1997). As more employers and cities institute no-smoking policies and restaurants, work environments and public places are becoming off-limits for smokers, a no-smoking policy at home can be even more helpful in eliminating opportunities to smoke. Another effective measure is including partners in the smoking cessation process, since one of the primary barriers to smoking cessation among pregnant women who smoke is having a partner who smokes (Duckworth & Chertok, 2012). It can be extremely challenging to quit smoking without partner support and with the partner continuing to smoke in front of the pregnant woman (Duckworth & Chertok, 2012). Partners influence health behaviors of pregnant women, so nurses should try to include partners whenever possible in all efforts to assist the pregnant woman and postpartum woman to stop smoking.

Jesse, Graham, and Swanson (2006) have shown the importance of including social support and stress-relieving activities in smoking cessation programs. Ferreira-Borges (2005) has described brief counseling programs for smoking cessation with pregnant women, which had positive outcomes. The most recent review in the *Cochrane Database of Systematic Reviews* (Lumley et al., 2009) involved 72 studies, 56 of them randomized trials, of smoking cessation programs during pregnancy and found that smoking cessation interventions in pregnancy reduce the proportion of women who continue to smoke in late pregnancy and reduce LBW and PTB. Smoking cessation interventions in pregnancy need to be implemented in all maternity care settings. Given the difficulty many pregnant women addicted to tobacco have quitting during pregnancy, population-based measures to reduce smoking should be supported (Lumley et al., 2009). ACOG (2011b) has promoted using the 5A's approach—(1) Ask about tobacco use, (2) Advise to quit, (3) Assess willingness to make an attempt, (4) Assist in quit attempt, and (5) Arrange follow-up—to smoking cessation in pregnancy for every pregnant smoker. Although cessation of smoking in pregnancy is important, women should also be taught about the hazards of postpartum smoking for their own health and the health of their children.

When women are successful in stopping or reducing smoking during their pregnancy, this does not necessarily equal permanent positive lifestyle changes. Relapse postpartum is a significant problem. Approximately 40% of women stop smoking when they become pregnant, and abstain for much of the pregnancy (Von Kohorn, Nguyen, Schulman-Green, & Colson, 2012). No other single life event causes so many smokers to stop smoking (Von Kohorn et al., 2012). Unfortunately, approximately 75% of women who stop smoking during pregnancy resume smoking within 1 year postpartum, 50% within the first 6 months (Von Kohorn et al., 2012). Lawrence and colleagues (2005) evaluated a pregnancy smoking cessation program 18 months after birth and found that 86% of women had relapsed at 18 months. Suplee (2005) found 52% of women who stopped smoking during pregnancy had relapsed by 4 weeks postpartum. According to the most recent data available from the Pregnancy Risk Assessment Monitoring System, among women who smoked 3 months before pregnancy, 45% quit during pregnancy; and among women who quit smoking during pregnancy, 50% relapsed within 6 months after giving birth (Tong et al., 2009). Similarity in relapse rates among postpartum women in these studies highlights the significance of this problem. In one study, women who had stopped smoking during pregnancy were interviewed about smoking cessation postpartum (Von Kohorn et al., 2012). Three themes were identified: (1) previous smokers did not intend to return to smoking but doubted whether they would be able to maintain abstinence; (2) they believed that it would be possible to protect their babies from the harms of cigarette smoke; and (3) they felt that they had control over their smoking and did not need help to maintain abstinence after pregnancy (Von Kohorn et al., 2012). Although most participants did not intend to resume smoking, their plans may have been thwarted by their lack of confidence about quitting permanently, perceptions about avoiding second-hand smoke exposure to their baby, and by their overestimation of their control over smoking (Von Kohorn et al., 2012). More research about smoking cessation for childbearing women is greatly needed; this is an opportunity for nurse researchers to make a significant contribution to the health and well-being of women and newborns.

ILLICIT DRUG USE

Although not the major contributors to PTB, women who take illicit drugs in pregnancy are at risk for PTB (Kearney, 2008). It is important, therefore, for nurses to know and understand how to assess for illicit drug use and how to intervene to best help the woman and her baby. These women are frightened and addicted and require specialized care (Hans, 1999). Nurses working in prenatal, intrapartum, or postpartum care should know how to contact social services to ensure that appropriate referrals can be made to the treatment facilities available for drug-using women in their community so women have the best chance to improve the outcome of the pregnancy. It is important to recognize that illicit drug use is generally not an isolated risk behavior; rather, it is often consistent with a life span risk framework for alcohol use problems, childhood abuse, familial alcoholism, and lifetime major depressive disorder (Flynn & Chermack, 2008). Further, alcohol and drug use problems are interrelated (Flynn & Chermack, 2008).

INTIMATE PARTNER VIOLENCE

Parker, McFarlane, and Soeken (1994) were the first to correlate intimate partner violence (domestic violence) with preterm labor and birth. Their work showed that intimate partner violence is a health problem, not a social problem, and that women who are battered have more LBW babies and PTBs than women who are not. Heaman (2005) continued this work, demonstrating again that PTB and intimate partner violence are related. Lederman (2011) has delved further into the psychosocial factors associated with preterm labor and recommends a thorough assessment for all women.

Intimate partner violence is likely to be underreported. Even so, over 300,000 pregnant women are recipients of intimate partner violence each year in the

United States (ACOG, 2012a). Nursing care for women during pregnancy, therefore, should include assessment for family stress and abuse. This can be done easily and quickly with a psychosocial history and the four questions in the *Abuse Assessment Screen*, which can be found in the March of Dimes nursing module *Abuse During Pregnancy: A Protocol for Prevention and Intervention* (McFarlane, Parker, & Moran, 2007). At a minimum, women should be screened at their first prenatal visit, at least once in each trimester, and during the postpartum period, when violence may escalate (ACOG, 2012a). Renker and Tonkin (2006) found that among 519 women screened for abuse in pregnancy, 91% were not offended, embarrassed, or angry because they were asked the questions, and that women wanted to know whether abuse, once disclosed, was reportable to legal authorities. It is important to make screening a routine part of healthcare because women may not disclose intimate partner violence initially.

INTRAPARTUM NURSING CARE OF THE WOMAN IN PRETERM LABOR

The goals of intrapartum care for women with a diagnosis of preterm labor are to achieve a reduction in uterine activity that is long enough to allow for administration of antenatal corticosteroids, transfer of the mother to a facility with the appropriate level of neonatal care for current gestational age, administration of antibiotics for GBS prophylaxis, and consideration of magnesium sulfate for neuroprotection. Nursing care is then delivered by nurses competent to care for the high-risk pregnant woman. Simpson (2004) has described this care, especially the fetal monitoring required for a preterm fetus. See Chapter 15 for a discussion of monitoring the preterm fetus. Although tocolytics have not been found to be successful in preventing PTB, they may contribute to prolonging the pregnancy enough to gain the benefits of antenatal corticosteroid therapy. While the mother is in preterm labor, ongoing monitoring of maternal–fetal status is essential. If the mother is receiving IV tocolytic agents, she should not be considered "stable" or allocated to periodic assessment protocols that preclude vigilant surveillance or transferred to a less intensive level of care (Simpson & Knox, 2004). The recommended nurse-to-patient ratio for women with high-risk obstetrical conditions during labor is one-to-one (AAP & ACOG, 2012; AWHONN, 2010).

Women in preterm labor need emotional support and information about the potential risks to their baby if preterm labor proceeds to PTB. In institutions that provide a special care nursery or neonatal intensive care, a visit from the neonatal nurse practitioner or neonatologist prior to the birth can be helpful in explaining what to expect and how their baby will be cared for in the nursery. This process is preferred over the neonatal resuscitation team rushing in the room at birth without prior introductions and explanations. If the baby's gestational age or condition is such that it is anticipated that an immediate admission to the nursery will be required, every effort should be made to assure that birth occurs in a facility equipped to care for the estimated gestational age of the baby (AAP & ACOG, 2012) and to communicate maternal–fetal status to the neonatal team. See Chapter 13 for details of maternal transfer. Equal effort should be made to allow the mother to see and touch the baby before the neonatal team leaves the birthing room or surgical suite. The father of the baby or other support person should be encouraged to visit the nursery as soon as possible, and the family should be provided visiting policy information. Some nurseries have cameras that can be used to provide the mother with a picture while she is in the postanesthesia recovery period before she is able to visit the nursery. With the widespread use of cell phones and tablets with cameras, mothers will likely be able to see a picture of the baby quickly. Because premature infants benefit tremendously from receiving human milk, nurses need to ensure they engage parents in early discussion of the medical importance of breast milk and support early initiation of pumping. The AAP (2012) considers provision of breast milk a key intervention for preterm infants because of its effects on short-term and long-term health outcomes. See Chapter 20 for a full discussion of breastfeeding.

SUMMARY

Nurses have been extremely active in the research about preterm labor and birth (Freda, 2003). They have studied everything from causes of preterm labor to effects of PTB on families. Because preterm labor and birth are the most pressing problems in perinatal health in the beginning of the 21st century, more research is necessary. Although research has been extensive, it has not yet found a definitive cause nor a cure for preterm labor. The March of Dimes (2011) recommends research to find the causes of premature birth and to identify and test promising interventions; education for healthcare providers and women about risk-reduction strategies; expansion of access to healthcare coverage to improve maternity care and infant health outcomes; provision of information and emotional support to families affected by prematurity; and stimulation of concern and action around the problem.

Nurses have the ability not only to participate in PTB prevention research but also to enhance their clinical knowledge and skills regarding this topic. One of the most important interventions that nurses can implement is their ability to effectively teach pregnant women about the symptoms of preterm labor and birth. This can result in women obtaining the essential antenatal steroids at the earliest time possible. Although we may not yet know how to prevent a PTB, through talking to women, sharing our knowledge, and advocating for women and newborns, nurses can make a big difference in how many babies are born with the devastating sequelae of PTB.

REFERENCES

Africa, C. W., Kayitenkore, J., & Bayingana, C. (2010). Examination of maternal gingival crevicular fluid for the presence of selected periodontopathogens implicated in the pre-term delivery of low birthweight infants. *Virulence, 1*(4), 254–259. doi:org/10.4161/viru.1.4.12004

American Academy of Pediatrics. (2012). Breastfeeding and the use of human milk. *Pediatrics, 129*(3), e827–e841. doi:10.1542/peds.2011-3552

American Academy of Pediatrics & American College of Obstetricians and Gynecologists. (2012). *Guidelines for Perinatal Care* (7th ed.). Elk Grove Village, IL: Author.

American College of Nurse-Midwives. (2010). *Induction of Labor* (Position Statement). Washington, DC: Author. Retrieved from http://www.midwife.org/documents/Induction_of_Labor.pdf

American College of Nurse-Midwives. (2012). *Prevention of Preterm Labor and Preterm Birth* (Position Statement). Washington, DC: Author. Retrieved from http://www.midwife.org/ACNM/files/ACNMLibraryData/UPLOADFILENAME/000000000274/Prevention%20of%20Preterm%20Labor%20and%20Preterm%20Birth%20June%202012.pdf

American College of Obstetricians and Gynecologists. (2001). *Assessment of Risk Factors for Preterm Birth* (Practice Bulletin No. 31; Reaffirmed 2010). Washington, DC: Author.

American College of Obstetricians and Gynecologists. (2005). *The Importance of Preconception Care in the Continuum of Women's Health Care* (Committee Opinion No. 313; Reaffirmed 2009). Washington, DC: Author..

American College of Obstetricians and Gynecologists. (2008a). *Fetal Lung Maturity* (Practice Bulletin No. 97). Washington, DC: Author. doi:10.1097/AOG.0b013e318188d1c2

American College of Obstetricians and Gynecologists. (2008b). *Use of Progesterone to Reduce Preterm Birth* (Committee Opinion No. 419). Washington, DC: Author. doi:10.1097/AOG.0b013e31818b1ff6

American College of Obstetricians and Gynecologists. (2009). *Induction of Labor* (Practice Bulletin No. 107). Washington, DC: Author. doi:10.1097/AOG.0b013e3181b48ef5

American College of Obstetricians and Gynecologists. (2010). *Smoking Cessation During Pregnancy* (Committee Opinion No. 471). Washington, DC: Author. doi:10.1097/AOG.0b013e3182004fcd

American College of Obstetricians and Gynecologists. (2011a). *Antenatal Corticosteroid Therapy for Fetal Maturation* (Committee Opinion No. 475). Washington, DC: Author. doi:10.1097/AOG.0b013e31820eee00

American College of Obstetricians and Gynecologists. (2011b). *Prevention of Early-Onset Group B Streptococcal Disease in Newborns* (Committee Opinion No. 485). Washington, DC: Author. doi:10.1097/AOG.0b013e318219229b

American College of Obstetricians and Gynecologists. (2011c). *Use of Prophylactic Antibiotics in Labor and Delivery* (Practice Bulletin No. 120). Washington, DC: Author. doi:10.1097/AOG.0b013e3182238c31

American College of Obstetricians and Gynecologists. (2012a). *Intimate Partner Violence*. (Committee Opinion No. 518). Washington, DC: Author. doi:10.1097/AOG.0b013e318249ff74

American College of Obstetricians and Gynecologists. (2012b). *Magnesium Sulfate Before Anticipated Preterm Birth for Neuroprotection* (Patient Safety Checklist No. 7). Washington, DC: Author. doi:10.1097/AOG.0b013e318268054c

American College of Obstetricians and Gynecologists. (2012c). *Management of Preterm Labor* (Practice Bulletin No. 127). Washington, DC: Author. doi:10.1097/AOG.0b013e31825af2f0

American College of Obstetricians and Gynecologists & Society for Maternal-Fetal Medicine. (2010). *Magnesium Sulfate Before Anticipated Preterm Birth for Neuroprotection*. (Committee Opinion 455). Washington, DC: Author. doi:10.1097/AOG.0b013e3181d4ffa5

Ashford, K. B., Hahn, E., Hall, L., Ravens, M. K., Noland, M., & Ferguson, J. E. (2010). The effects of prenatal secondhand smoke exposure on preterm birth and neonatal outcomes. *Journal of Obstetric, Gynecologic, and Neonatal Nursing, 39*(5), 525–535. doi:10.1111/j.1552-6909.2010.01169.x

Association of Women's Health, Obstetric and Neonatal Nurses. (2010). *Guidelines for Professional Registered Nurse Staffing for Perinatal Units*. Washington, DC: Author.

Association of Women's Health, Obstetric and Neonatal Nurses. (2012). *40 Reasons to go the Full 40*. Washington, DC: Author. Retrieved from http://www.health4mom.org/a/40_reasons_121611

Audibert, F., Fortin, S., Delvin, E., Djemli, A., Brunet, S., Dubé, J., & Fraser, W. D. (2010). Contingent use of fetal fibronectin testing and cervical length measurement in women with preterm labour. *Journal of Obstetrics and Gynaecology of Canada, 32*(4), 307–312.

Berghella, V., Iams, J. D., Reedy, N. J., Oshiro, B. T., & Wachtel, J. S. (2010). Quality improvement opportunities in prenatal care. In S. D. Berns & A. Kott (Eds.), *Toward Improving the Outcome of Pregnancy III* (pp. 55–64). White Plains, NY: March of Dimes Foundation. Retrieved from http://www.marchofdimes.com/TIOPIII_finalmanuscript.pdf

Berghella, V., & Mackeen, A. D. (2011). Cervical length screening with ultrasound-indicated cerclage compared with history-indicated cerclage for prevention of preterm birth: A meta-analysis. *Obstetrics and Gynecology, 118*(1), 148–155. doi:10.1097/AOG.0b013e31821fd5b0

Berghella, V., Prasertcharoensuk, W., Cotter, A., Rasanen, J., Mittal, S., Chaithongwongwatthana, S., . . . Pereira, L. (2009). Does indomethacin prevent preterm birth in women with cervical dilatation in the second trimester? *American Journal of Perinatology, 26*(1), 13–19. doi:10.1055/s-0028-1091398

Bieber, E., Barfield, W. D., Dowling-Quarles, S., Sparkman, L., & Blouin, A. S. (2010). Systems change across the continuum of perinatal care. In S. D. Berns & A. Kott (Eds.), *Toward Improving the Outcome of Pregnancy III* (pp. 112–122). White Plains, NY: March of Dimes Foundation. Retrieved from http://www.marchofdimes.com/TIOPIII_finalmanuscript.pdf

Bigelow, C., & Stone, J. (2011). Bed rest in pregnancy. *Mount Sinai Journal of Medicine, 78*(2), 291–302. doi:10.1002/msj.20243

Bolt, L. A, Chandiramani, M., De Greeff, A., Seed, P. T., Kurtzman, J., & Shennan, A. H. (2011). The value of combined cervical length measurement and fetal fibronectin testing to predict spontaneous preterm birth in asymptomatic high-risk women. *Journal of Maternal–Fetal and Neonatal Medicine, 24*(7), 928–932. doi:10.3109/14767058.2010.535872

Brown, H. L., Britton, K. A., Brizendine, E. J., Hiett, A. K., Ingram, D., Turnquest, M. A., . . . Abernathy, M. P. (1999). A randomized comparison of home uterine activity monitoring in the outpatient management of women treated for preterm labor. *American Journal of Obstetrics and Gynecology, 180*(4), 798–805. doi:10.1016/S0002-9378(99)70650-2

Burwick, R. M., Lee, G. T., Benedict, J. L., Ross, M. G., & Kjos, S. L. (2009). Blinded comparison of cervical portio length measurements by digital examination vs Cervilenz. *American Journal of Obstetrics and Gynecology, 200*(5), e37–e39. doi:10.1016/j.ajog.2008.11.026

Burwick, R. M., Zork, N. M., Lee, G. T., Ross, M. G., & Kjos, S. L. (2011). Cervilenz assessment of cervical length compared to fetal fibronectin in the prediction of preterm delivery in women with threatened preterm labor. *Journal of Maternal–Fetal and Neonatal Medicine, 24*(1), 127–131. doi:10.3109/14767058.2010.529201

Carroll, J., Slobodzian, R., & Steward, D. K. (2005). Extremely low birthweight infants: Issues related to growth. *MCN: The American Journal of Maternal Child Nursing, 30*(5), 312–318, quiz 319–320.

Centers for Disease Control and Prevention, American Society for Reproductive Medicine, & Society for Assisted Reproductive Technology. (2011). *2009 Assisted Reproductive Technology Success Rates: National Summary and Fertility Clinic Reports.* Atlanta, GA: U.S. Department of Health and Human Services. Retrieved from http://www.cdc.gov/art/ART2009/index.htm

Clark, S. L., Frye, D. R., Meyers, J. A., Belfort, M. A., Dildy, G. A., Kofford, S., . . . Perlin, J. A. (2010). Reduction in elective delivery <39 weeks of gestation: Comparative effectiveness of 3 approaches to change and the impact on neonatal intensive care admission and stillbirth. *American Journal of Obstetrics and Gynecology, 203*(5), 449.e1–449.e6. doi:10.1016/j.ajog.2010.05.036

Clark, S. L., Miller, D. D., Belfort, M. A., Dildy, G. A., Frye, D. K., & Meyers, J. A. (2009). Neonatal and maternal outcomes associated with elective term delivery. *American Journal of Obstetrics and Gynecology, 200*(2), 156.e1–156.e4. doi:10.1016/j.ajog.2008.08.068

Collaborative Group on Preterm Birth Prevention. (1993). Multicenter randomized controlled trial of a preterm birth prevention program. *American Journal of Obstetrics and Gynecology, 169*(2, Pt. 1), 352–366.

Conde-Agudelo, A., Romero, R., & Kusanovic, J. P. (2011). Nifedipine in the management of preterm labor: A systematic review and metaanalysis. *American Journal of Obstetrics and Gynecology, 204*(2), 134.e1–134.e20. doi:10.1016/j.ajog.2010.11.038

Crowther, C. A., Hiller, J. E., & Doyle, L. W. (2002). Magnesium sulphate for preventing preterm birth in threatened preterm labour. *Cochrane Database of Systematic Reviews,* (4), CD001060.

Crowther, C. A., Hiller, J. E., Doyle, L. W., & Haslam, R. R. (2003). Effect of magnesium sulfate given for neuroprotection before preterm birth: A randomized controlled trial. *JAMA: The Journal of the American Medical Association, 290*(20), 2669–2676. doi:10.1001/jama.290.20.2669

Culhane, J. F., & Goldenberg, R. L. (2011). Racial disparities in preterm birth. *Seminars in Perinatology, 35*(4), 234–239. doi:10.1053/j.semperi.2011.02.020

Davidoff, M. J., Dias, T., Damus, K., Russell, R., Bettegowda, V. R., Dolan, S., . . . Petrini, J. (2006). Changes in the gestational age distribution among U.S. singleton births: Impact on rates of late preterm birth, 1992 to 2002. *Seminars in Perinatology, 30*(1), 8–15. doi:10.1053/j.semperi.2006.01.009

Davies, B. L., Stewart, P. J., Sprague, A. E., Niday, P. A., Nimrod, C. A., & Dulberg, C. S. (1998). Education of women about the prevention of preterm birth. *Canadian Journal of Public Health, 89*(4), 260–263.

De Jesus, L. C., Pappas, A., Shankaran, S., Kendrick, D., Das, A., Higgins, R. D., . . . Walsh, M. C. (2012). Risk factors for postneonatal intensive care unit discharge mortality among extremely low birth weight infants. *Journal of Pediatrics, 161*(1), 70–74.e2. doi.org/10.1016/j.jpeds.2011.12.038

de Kieviet, J. F., Zoetebier, L., van Elburg, R. M., Vermeulen, R. J., & Oosterlaan, J. (2012). Brain development of very preterm and very low-birthweight children in childhood and adolescence: A meta-analysis. *Developmental Medicine and Child Neurology, 54*(4), 313–23. doi:10.1111/j.1469-8749.2011.04216.x

Doyle, L. W., Crowther, C. A., Middleton, P., Marret, S., & Rouse, D. (2009). Magnesium sulphate for women at risk of preterm birth for neuroprotection of the fetus. *Cochrane Database of Systematic Reviews, 21*(1), CD004661.

Duckworth, A. L., & Chertok, I. R. (2012). Review of perinatal partner-focused smoking cessation interventions. *MCN: The American Journal of Maternal Child Nursing, 37*(3), 174–181. doi:10.1097/NMC.0b013e31824921b4

Dunlop, A. L., Kramer, M. R., Hogue, C. J., Menon, R., & Ramakrishan, U. (2011). Racial disparities in preterm birth: An overview of the potential role of nutrient deficiencies. *Acta Obstetricia et Gynecologica Scandinavica, 90*(12), 1332–1341. doi:10.1111/j.1600-0412.2011.01274.x

Dyson, D. C., Danbe, K. H., Bamber, J. A., Crites, Y. M., Field, D. R., Maier, J. A., . . . Armstrong, M. A. (1998). Monitoring women at risk for preterm labor. *New England Journal of Medicine, 338*(1), 15–19.

England, L. J., Kendrick, J. S., Wilson, H. G., Merritt, R. K., Gargiullo, P. M., & Zahniser, S. C. (2001). Effects of smoking reduction during pregnancy on the birth weight of term infants. *American Journal of Epidemiology, 154*(8), 694–701. doi:10.1093/aje/154.8.694

Ferreira-Borges, C. (2005). Effectiveness of a brief counseling and behavioral intervention for smoking cessation in pregnant women. *Preventive Medicine, 41*(1), 295–302. doi:10.1016/j.ypmed.2004.11.013

Fisch, J. M., English, D., Pedaline, S., Brooks, K., & Simhan, H. N. (2009). Labor induction process improvement: A patient quality-of-care initiative. *Obstetrics and Gynecology, 113*(4), 797–803. doi:10.1097/AOG.0b013e31819c9e3d

Fleischman, A. R., Oinuma, M., & Clark, S. L. (2010). Rethinking the definition of "term pregnancy." *Obstetrics and Gynecology, 116*(1), 136–139. doi:10.1097/AOG.0b013e3181e24f28

Flynn, H. A., & Chermack, S. T. (2008). Prenatal alcohol use: The role of lifetime problems with alcohol, drugs, depression, and violence. *Journal of Studies on Alcohol and Drugs, 69*(4), 500–509.

Freda, M. C. (2003). Nursing's contributions to the literature on preterm labor and birth. *Journal of Obstetric, Gynecologic, and Neonatal Nursing, 32*(5), 659–667. doi:10.1177/0884217503257530

Freda, M. C., Andersen, H. F., Damus, K., Poust, D., Brustman, L., & Merkatz, I. R. (1990). Lifestyle modification as an intervention for inner city women at risk for preterm birth. *Journal of Advanced Nursing, 15*(3), 364–372. doi:10.1111/j.1365-2648.1990.tb01824.x

Freda, M. C., Damus, K., Andersen, H. F., Brustman, L. E., & Merkatz, I. R. (1990). A "PROPP" for the Bronx: Preterm birth prevention education in the inner city. *Obstetrics and Gynecology, 76*(Suppl. 1), 93S–96S.

Freda, M. C., Damus, K., & Merkatz, I. R. (1991). What do pregnant women know about the prevention of preterm birth? *Journal of Obstetric, Gynecologic, and Neonatal Nursing, 20*(2), 140–145.

Freda, M. C., & DeVore, N. (1996). Should intravenous hydration be the first line of defense with threatened preterm labor? A critical review of the literature. *Journal of Perinatology, 16*(5), 385–389.

Freda, M. C., Moos, M. K., & Curtis, M. (2006). The history of preconception care: Evolving standards and guidelines. *Maternal Child Health Journal, 10*(7), 43–52. doi:10.1007/s10995-006-0087-x

Freda, M. C., & Patterson, E. T. (2004). *Preterm Labor and Birth: Prevention and Management* (Nursing Module). White Plains, NY: March of Dimes Birth Defects Foundation.

Freston, M. S., Young, S., Calhoun, S., Fredericksen, T., Salinger, L., Malchodi, C., & Egan, J. F. (1997). Responses of pregnant women to potential preterm labor symptoms. *Journal of Obstetric, Gynecologic, and Neonatal Nursing, 26*(1), 35–41. doi:10.1111/j.1552-6909.1997.tb01505.x

Garite, T. J., Kurtzman, J., Maurel, K., Clark, R. (2009). Impact of a 'rescue course' of antenatal corticosteroids: A multicenter randomized placebo-controlled trial. *American Journal of Obstetrics and Gynecology, 200*(3), 248.e1–248.e9. doi:10.1016/j.ajog.2009.01.021

Giarratano, G. (2006). Genetic influences on preterm birth. *MCN: The American Journal of Maternal Child Nursing, 31*(3), 169–175.

Gilbert, W. M., Nesbitt, T. S., & Danielsen, B. (2003). The cost of prematurity: Quantification by gestational age and birth weight. *Obstetrics and Gynecology, 102*(3), 488–492.

Gilstrap, L. C., Christensen, R., Clewell, W. H., D'Alton, M. E., Davidson, E. C. Jr., Escobedo, M. B., . . . Hinshaw, A. S. (1995). Effect of corticosteroids for fetal maturation on perinatal outcomes. National Institutes of Health Consensus Development Panel on the effect of corticosteroids for fetal lung maturation and perinatal outcomes. *JAMA: The Journal of the American Medical Association, 273*(5), 413–418. doi:10.1001/jama.1995.03520290065031

Goldenberg, R. L., Cliver, S. P., Bronstein, J., Cutter, G. R., Andrews, W. W., & Mennemeyer, S. T. (1994). Bed rest in pregnancy. *Obstetrics and Gynecology, 84*(1), 131–136.

Goldenberg, R. L., Gravett, M. G., Iams, J., Papageorghiou, A. T., Waller, S. A., Kramer, M., . . . Villar, J. (2012). The preterm birth syndrome: Issues to consider in creating a classification system. *American Journal of Obstetrics and Gynecology, 206*(2), 113–118. doi:10.1016/j.ajog.2011.10.865

Goldenberg, R. L., & Rouse, D. J. (1998). Prevention of premature birth. *New England Journal of Medicine, 339*(5), 313–320.

Green, N. S., Damus, K., Simpson, J. L., Iams, J., Reece, E. A., Hobel, C. J., . . . Schwarz, R. H., and the March of Dimes Scientific Advisory Committee on Prematurity. (2005). Research agenda for preterm birth: Recommendations from the March of Dimes. *American Journal of Obstetrics and Gynecology, 193*(3, Pt. 1), 626–635. doi:10.1016/j.ajog.2005.02.106

Grimes, D. A., & Nanda, K. (2006). Magnesium sulfate tocolysis: Time to quit. *Obstetrics and Gynecology, 108*(4), 986–989. doi:10.1097/01.AOG.0000236445.18265.93

Haas, D. M., Imperiale, T. F., Kirkpatrick, P. R., Klein, R. W., Zollinger, T. W., & Golichowski, A. M. (2009). Tocolytic therapy: A meta-analysis and decision analysis. *Obstetrics and Gynecology, 113*, 585–594. doi:10.1097/AOG.0b013e318199924a

Hack, M. (2006). Young adult outcomes of very-low-birth-weight children. *Seminars in Fetal and Neonatal Medicine, 11*(2), 127–137.

Hack, M., Schluchter, M., Andreias, L., Margevicius, S., Taylor, H. G., Drotar, D., & Cuttler, L. (2011). Change in prevalence of chronic conditions between childhood and adolescence among extremely low-birth-weight children. *JAMA: The Journal of the American Medical Association, 306*(4), 394–401. doi:10.1001/jama.2011.1025

Hack, M., Taylor, H. G., Drotar, D., Schluchter, M., Cartar, L., Andreias, L., . . . Klein, N. (2005). Chronic conditions, functional limitations, and special health care needs of school-aged children born with extremely low-birth-weight in the 1990s. *JAMA: The Journal of the American Medical Association, 294*(3), 318–325. doi:10.1001/jama.294.3.318

Hamilton, B. E., Martin, J. A., & Ventura, S. G. (2011). Births: Preliminary data for 2010. *National Vital Statistics Reports, 60*(2), 1–36.

Han, S., Crowther, C. A., & Moore, V. (2010). Magnesium maintenance therapy for preventing preterm birth after threatened preterm labour. *Cochrane Database of Systematic Reviews, 7*(7), CD000940.

Hans, S. L. (1999). Demographic and psychosocial characteristics of substance-abusing pregnant women. *Clinics in Perinatology, 26*(1), 55–74.

Hassan, S. S., Romero, R., Vidyadhari, D., Fusey, S., Baxter, J., Khandelwal, M., . . . Creasy, G. W. (2011) Vaginal progesterone reduces the rate of preterm birth in women with a sonographic short cervix: A multicenter, randomized, double-blind, placebo-controlled trial. *Ultrasound in Obstetrics and Gynecology, 38*(1), 18–31. doi:10.1002/uog.9017

Heaman, M. I. (2005). Relationships between physical abuse during pregnancy and risk factors for preterm birth among women in Manitoba. *Journal of Obstetric, Gynecologic, and Neonatal Nursing, 34*(6), 721–731. doi:10.1177/0884217505281906

Helderman, J. B., O'Shea, T. M., Kuban, K. C., Allred, E. N., Hecht, J. L., Dammann, O., . . . Leviton, A. (2012). Antenatal antecedents of cognitive impairment at 24 months in extremely low gestational age newborns. *Pediatrics, 129*(3), 494–502. doi:10.1542/peds.2011-1796

Herron, M. A., Katz, M., & Creasy, R. K. (1982). Evaluation of a preterm birth prevention program: A preliminary report. *Obstetrics and Gynecology, 59*(4), 442–446.

Higby, K., Xenakis, E. M., & Pauerstein, C. J. (1993). Do tocolytic agents stop preterm labor? A critical and comprehensive review of efficacy and safety. *American Journal of Obstetrics and Gynecology, 168*(4), 1247–1256.

Hill, W. C., & Lambertz, E. L. (1990). Let's get rid of the term "Braxton-Hicks contractions." *Obstetrics and Gynecology, 75*(4), 709–710.

Hobel, C. J., Ross, M. G., Bemis, R. L., Bragonier, J. Jr., Nessim, S., Sandhu, M., . . . Mori, B. (1994). The West Los Angeles Preterm Birth Prevention Project I: Program impact on high-risk women. *American Journal of Obstetrics and Gynecology, 170*(1, Pt. 1), 54–62.

Huusom, L. D., Secher, N. J., Pryds, O., Whitfield, K., Gluud, C., & Brok, J. (2011). Antenatal magnesium sulphate may prevent cerebral palsy in preterm infants—but are we convinced? Evaluation of an apparently conclusive meta-analysis with trial sequential analysis. *BJOG: An International Journal of Obstetrics and Gynaecology, 118*(1), 1–5. doi:10.1111/j.1471-0528.2010.02782.x

Iams, J. D., Johnson, F. F., O'Shaughnessy, R. W., & West, L. C. (1987). A prospective random trial of home uterine activity monitoring in pregnancies at increased risk of preterm labor. *American Journal of Obstetrics and Gynecology, 157*(3), 638–643.

Iams, J. D., Stilson, R., Johnson, F. F., Williams, R. A., & Rice, R. (1990). Symptoms that precede preterm labor and preterm premature rupture of the membranes. *American Journal of Obstetrics and Gynecology, 162*(2), 486–490.

Institute of Medicine. (1985). *Preventing Low Birth Weight.* Washington, DC: National Academy Press.

Institute of Medicine. (2007). *Preterm Birth: Causes, Consequences, and Prevention.* New York, NY: National Academies Press.

Institute for Safe Medication Practices. (2005). Preventing magnesium toxicity in obstetrics. *ISMP Medication Safety Alert, 10*(21), 1–2.

Institute for Safe Medication Practices. (2006). Preventing magnesium toxicity in obstetrics. *Nurse Advise-ERR: ISMP Medication Safety Alert, 4*(6), 1–2.

Jackson, R. A., Gibson, K. A., Wu, Y. W., & Croughan, M. S. (2004). Perinatal outcome in singletons following in vitro fertilization: A meta-analysis. *Obstetrics and Gynecology, 103*(3), 551–563.

Jesse, E. D., Graham, M., & Swanson, M. (2006). Psychosocial and spiritual factors associated with smoking and substance use during pregnancy in African American and white low-income women. *Journal of Obstetric, Gynecologic, and Neonatal Nursing, 35*(1), 68–77. doi:10.1111/j.1552-6909.2006.00010.x

Johnson, K., Posner, S. F., Biermann, J., Cordero, J. F., Atrash, H. K., Parker, C. S., . . . Curtis, M. G. (2006). Recommendations to improve preconception health and health care—United States. A report of the CDC/ATSDR Preconception Care Work Group and the Select Panel on Preconception Care. *Morbidity and Mortality Weekly Report, 55*(RR06), 1–23.

Kalish, R. B., Vardhana, S., Normand, N. J., Gupta, M., & Witkin, S. S. (2006). Association of a maternal CD14-159 gene polymorphism with preterm premature rupture of membranes and spontaneous preterm birth in multi-fetal pregnancies. *Journal of Reproductive Immunology, 70*(1–2), 109–117. doi:10.1016/j.jri.2005.12.002

Kashanian, M., Akbarian, A. R., & Soltanzadeh, M. (2005). Atosiban and nifedipin for the treatment of preterm labor. *International Journal of Gynaecology and Obstetrics, 91*(1), 10–14. doi:10.1016/j.ijgo.2005.06.005

Kearney, M. H. (2008). *Tobacco, Alcohol and Drug Use in Childbearing Families* (Nursing Module). White Plains, NY: March of Dimes Foundation.

Kent, A. L., Wright, I. M., & Abdel-Latif, M. E. (2012). Mortality and adverse neurologic outcomes are greater in preterm male infants. *Pediatrics, 129*(1), 124–131. doi:10.1542/peds.2011-1578

King, J. F., Flenady, V., Cole, S., & Thornton, S. (2005). Cyclooxygenase (COX) inhibitors for treating preterm labour. *Cochrane Database of Systematic Reviews,* (2), CD001992. doi:10.1002/14651858.CD001992.pub2

Kinney, H. C. (2006). The near-term (late preterm) human brain and risk for periventricular leukomalacia: A review. *Seminars in Perinatology, 30*(2), 81–88. doi:10.1053/j.semperi.2006.02.006

Kramer, M. R., Hogue, C. J., Dunlop, A. L., & Menon, R. (2011). Preconceptional stress and racial disparities in preterm birth: An overview. *Acta Obstetricia et Gynecologica Scandinavica, 90*(12), 1307–1316. doi:10.1111/j.1600-0412.2011.01136.x

Kramer, M. S., Papageorghiou, A., Culhane, J., Bhutta, Z., Goldenberg, R. L., Gravett, M., . . . Villar, J. (2012). Challenges in defining and classifying the preterm birth syndrome. *American Journal of Obstetrics and Gynecology, 206*(2), 108–112. doi:10.1016/j.ajog.2011.10.864

Krans, E. E., & Davis, M. M. (2012). Preventing low birthweight: 25 years, prenatal risk, and the failure to reinvent prenatal care. *American Journal of Obstetrics and Gynecology, 206*(5), 398–403. doi.org/10.1016/j.ajog.2011.06.082

Lawrence, T., Aveyard, P., Cheng, K. K., Griffin, C., Johnson, C., & Croghan, E. (2005). Does stage-based smoking cessation advice in pregnancy result in long-term quitters? 18-month postpartum follow-up of a randomized controlled trial. *Addiction, 100*(1), 107–116. doi:10.1111/j.1360-0443.2005.00936.x

Lederman, R. P. (2011). Preterm birth prevention: A mandate for psychosocial assessment. *Issues in Mental Health Nursing, 32*(3), 163–169. doi:10.3109/01612840.2010.538812

Leviton, L. C., Goldenberg, R. L., Baker, C. S., Schwartz, R. M., Freda, M. C., Fish, L. J., . . . Raczynski, J. M. (1999). Methods to encourage the use of antenatal corticosteroid therapy for fetal maturation: A randomized controlled trial. *JAMA: The Journal of the American Medical Association, 281*(1), 46–52. doi:10.1001/jama.281.1.46

Lewis, J. A. (2006). Genetics: Another nursing specialty. *MCN: The American Journal of Maternal Child Nursing, 31*(3), 142.

Litt, J., Taylor, H. G., Klein, N., & Hack, M. (2005). Learning disabilities in children with very low birthweight: Prevalence, neuropsychological correlates, and educational interventions. *Journal of Learning Disabilities, 38*(2), 130–141. doi:10.1177/00222194050380020301

Lockwood, C. J., Senyei, A. E., Dische, M. R., Casal, D., Shah, K. D., Thung, S. N., . . . Garite, T. J. (1991). Fetal fibronectin in cervical and vaginal secretions as a predictor of preterm delivery. *New England Journal of Medicine, 325*(10), 669–674.

Loe, S. M., Sanchez-Ramos, L., & Kaunitz, A. M. (2005). Assessing the neonatal safety of indomethacin tocolysis: A systematic review with meta-analysis. *Obstetrics and Gynecology, 106*(1), 173–179. doi:10.1097/01.AOG.0000168622.56478.df

Lowe, N. K., & King, T. L. (2011). Labor. In T. King & M. C. Brucker (Eds.), *Pharmacology for Women's Health* (pp. 1086–1116). Sudbury, MA: Jones and Bartlett.

Lu, M. C., Tache V., Alexander, G. R., Kotelchuck, M., & Halfon, N. (2003). Preventing low birth weight: Is prenatal care the answer? *The Journal of Maternal–Fetal and Neonatal Medicine, 13*(6), 362–380.

Luke, B., & Brown, M. B. (2007). Contemporary risks of maternal morbidity and adverse outcomes with increasing maternal age and plurality. *Fertility and Sterility, 88*(2), 283–293. doi:10.1016/j.fertnstert.2006.11.008

Lumley, J., Chamberlain, C., Dowswell, T., Oliver, S., Oakley, L., & Watson, L. (2009). Interventions for promoting smoking cessation during pregnancy. *Cochrane Database of Systematic Reviews, 8*(3), CD001055. doi:10.1002/14651858.CD001055.pub3

Lynam, L. E., & Miller, M. A. (1992). Mothers' and nurses' perceptions of the needs of women experiencing preterm labor. *Journal of Obstetric, Gynecologic, and Neonatal Nursing, 21*(2), 126–136. doi:10.1111/j.1552-6909.1992.tb01731.x

MacDorman, M. F., & Mathews, T. J. (2011). Infant deaths—United States, 2000–2007. *Morbidity and Mortality Weekly Report Supplement, 60*(01), 49–51.

MacKinnon, K. (2006). Living with the threat of preterm labor: Women's work of keeping the baby in. *Journal of Obstetric, Gynecologic, and Neonatal Nursing, 35*(6), 700–708. doi:10.1111/j.1552-6909.2006.00097.x

Macones, G. A., & Robinson, C. A. (1998). Is there justification for using indomethacin in preterm labor? An analysis of neonatal risks and benefits. *American Journal of Obstetrics and Gynecology, 177*(4), 819–824.

Mally, P. V., Bailey, S., & Hendricks-Muñoz, K. D. (2010). Clinical issues in the management of late preterm infants. *Current Problems in Pediatric and Adolescent Health Care, 40*(9), 218–233. doi:10.1016/j.cppeds.2010.07.005

Maloni, J. A. (2010). Antepartum bed rest for pregnancy complications: Efficacy and safety for preventing preterm birth. *Biological Research For Nursing, 12*(2), 106–124. doi:10.1177/1099800410375978

Maloni, J. A., Alexander, G. R., Schluchter, M. D., Shah, D. M., & Park, S. (2004). Antepartum bed rest: Maternal weight change and infant birth weight. *Biological Research for Nursing, 5*(3), 177–186. doi:10.1177/1099800403260307

Maloni, J. A., Chance, B., Zhang, C., Cohen, A. W., Betts, D., & Gange, S. J. (1993). Physical and psychosocial side effects of antepartum hospital bed rest. *Nursing Research, 42*(4), 197–203.

Maloni, J. A., & Park, S. (2005). Postpartum symptoms after antepartum bed rest. *Journal of Obstetric, Gynecologic, and Neonatal Nursing, 34*(2), 163–171. doi:10.1177/0884217504274416

Maloni, J. A., & Schneider, B. S. (2002). Inactivity: Symptoms associated with gastrocnemius muscle disuse during pregnancy. *AACN Clinical Issues, 13*(2), 248–262.

March of Dimes. (2011). *Prematurity Campaign*. White Plains, NY: Author.

March of Dimes. (2012a). Peristats. Infant mortality rates: United States, 1997–2007. Retrieved from http://www.marchofdimes.com/peristats/ViewSubtopic.aspx?reg=99&top=6&stop=91&lev=1&slev=1&obj=1&dv=ms

March of Dimes. (2012b). *Prematurity Prevention Toolkit*. White Plains, NY: Author. Retrieved from https://www.prematurityprevention.org/portal/server.pt

March of Dimes. (2012c). *Preterm Labor Assessment Toolkit*. White Plains, NY: Author. Retrieved from https://www.prematurityprevention.org/portal/server.pt

March of Dimes & California Maternal Quality Care Collaborative. (2010). *Elimination of Non-Medically Indicated (Elective) Deliveries Before 39 Weeks Gestational Age*. White Plains, NY: Author.

Marret, S., Marpeau, L., Zupan-Simunek, V., Eurin, D., Leveque, C., Hellot, M. F., . . . Benichou, J. (2007). Magnesium sulfate given before very-preterm birth to protect infant brain: The randomised controlled PREMAG trial. *BJOG, An International Journal of Obstetrics and Gynaecology, 114*(3), 310–318. doi:10.1111/j.1471-0528.2006.01162.x

Martin, J. A. (2011). Preterm births—United States, 2007. *Morbidity and Mortality Weekly Report, Supplement, 60*(1), 78–79.

Martin, J. A., Hamilton, B. E., Ventura, S. J., Osterman, M. J., Kirmeyer, S., Mathews, T. J., & Wilson, E. C. (2011). Births: Final data for 2009. *National Vital Statistics Report, 60*(1), 1–70.

Martin, J. A., Osterman, M. J. K., & Sutton, P. D. (2010). *Are Preterm Births on the Decline in the United States? Recent Data from the National Vital Statistics System* (NCHS Data Brief No. 39), Hyattsville, MD: National Center for Health Statistics.

McFarlane, J., Parker, B., & Moran, B. A. (2007). *Abuse During Pregnancy: A Protocol for Prevention and Intervention* (Nursing Module, 3rd ed.). White Plains, NY: March of Dimes Foundation.

Medoff-Cooper, B., Bakewell-Sachs, S., Buus-Frank, M. E., & Santa-Donato, A. (2005). The AWHONN Near-Term Initiative: A conceptual framework for optimizing health for near-term infants. *Journal of Obstetric, Gynecologic, and Neonatal Nursing, 34*(6), 666–671. doi:10.1177/0884217505281873

Meis, P. J., Klebanoff, M., Thom, E., Dombrowski, M. P., Sibai, B., Moawad, A. H., . . . Gabbe, S., for the National Institute of Child Health and Human Development Maternal–Fetal Medicine Units Network. (2003). Prevention of recurrent preterm delivery by 17 alpha-hydroxyprogesterone caproate. *New England Journal of Medicine, 348*(24), 2379–2385.

Menon, R., Dunlop, A. L., Kramer, M. R., Fortunato, S. J., & Hogue, C. J. (2011). An overview of racial disparities in preterm birth rates: Caused by infection or inflammatory response? *Acta Obstetricia et Gynecologica Scandinavica, 90*(12), 1325–1331. doi:10.1111/j.1600-0412.2011.01135.x

Mikkola, K., Ritari, N., Tommiska, V., Salokorpi, T., Lehtonen, L., Tammela, O., . . . Fellman, V. (2005). Neurodevelopmental outcome at 5 years of age of a national cohort of extremely low birth weight infants who were born in 1996–1997. *Pediatrics, 116*(6), 1391–1400. doi:10.1542/peds.2005-0171

Moore, M. L., & Freda, M. C. (1998). Reducing preterm and low birthweight births: Still a nursing challenge. *MCN: The American Journal of Maternal Child Nursing, 23*(4), 200–209.

Moore, M. L., Ketner, M., Walsh, K., & Wagoner, S. (2004). Listening to women at risk for preterm birth: Their perceptions of barriers to effective care and nurse telephone interventions. *MCN: The American Journal of Maternal-Child Nursing, 29*(6), 391–397.

Moore, M. L., Meis, P. J., Ernest, J. M., Wells, H. B., Zaccaro, D. J., & Terrell, T. (1998). A randomized trial of nurse intervention to reduce preterm and low birth weight births. *Obstetrics and Gynecology, 91*(5, Pt. 1), 656–661. doi:10.1016/S0029-7844(98)00012-x

Moos, M. K. (2003). *Preconception Health Promotion: A Focus for Women's Wellness* (Nursing Module). White Plains, NY: March of Dimes Birth Defects Foundation.

Moos, M., Badura, M., Posner, S. F., & Lu, M. C. (2011). Quality improvement opportunities in preconception and interconception care. In S. D. Berns (Ed.), *Toward Improving the Outcome of Pregnancy III: Enhancing Perinatal Health Through Quality, Safety and Performance Initiatives. Reissued Edition* (pp. 45–54). Retrieved from http://www2.aap.org/sections/perinatal/pdf/TIOPIII.pdf

Morales, L. S., Staiger, D., Horbar, J. D., Carpenter, J., Kenny, M., Geppert, J., & Rogowski, J. (2005). Mortality among very low-birthweight infants in hospitals serving minority populations. *American Journal of Public Health, 95*(12), 2206–2212. doi:10.2105/AJPH.2004.046730

Moroz, L. A., & Simhan, H. N. (2012). Rate of sonographic cervical shortening and the risk of spontaneous preterm birth. *American Journal of Obstetrics and Gynecology, 206*(3), 234.e1–234.e5. doi:10.1016/j.ajog.2011.11.017

Morse, S. B., Wu, S. S., Ma, C., Ariet, M., Resnick, M., & Roth, J. (2006). Racial and gender differences in the viability of extremely low birth weight infants: A population-based study. *Pediatrics, 117*(1), e106–e112. doi:10.1542/peds.2005-1286

Morsing, E., Asard, M., Ley, D., Stjerngvist, K., & Marsál, K. (2011). Cognitive function after intrauterine growth restriction and very preterm birth. *Pediatrics, 127*(4), e874–e882. doi:10.1542/peds.2010-1821

Mozurkewich, E., Chilimigras, J., Koepke, E., Keeton, K., & King, V. J. (2009). Indications for induction of labour: A best-evidence review. *BJOG: An International Journal of Obstetrics and Gynaecology, 116*(5), 626–636. doi:10.1111/j.1471-0528.2008.02065.x

Muglia, L. J., & Katz, M. (2010). The enigma of spontaneous preterm birth. *New England Journal of Medicine, 362*(6), 529–535.

Mullen, P. D., Richardson, M. A., Quinn, V. P., & Ershoff, D. H. (1997). Postpartum return to smoking: Who is at risk and when. *American Journal of Health Promotion, 11*(5), 323–330.

Murthy, K., Grobman, W. A., Lee, T. A., & Holl, J. L. (2011). Trends in induction of labor at early-term gestation. *American Journal of Obstetrics and Gynecology, 204*(5), 435.e1–435.e6. doi:10.1016/j.ajog.2010.12.023

National Institute of Child Health and Human Development. (2005). *Optimizing Care and Long-Term Outcomes of Near-Term Pregnancy and Near-Term Newborn Infants*. Bethesda, MD: Author.

National Institutes of Health. (2000). *Antenatal Corticosteroids Revisited: Repeat Courses. NIH Consensus Statement, 17*(2), 1–18. Retrieved from http://consensus.nih.gov/2000/2000AntenatalCorticosteroidsRevisted112PDF.pdf

National Institutes of Health. (2006). *State of the Science Conference Statement: Cesarean Delivery on Maternal Request*. Bethesda, MD: Author. Retrieved from http://consensus.nih.gov/2006/cesareanabstracts.pdf

Nightingale, S. L. (1998). From the Food and Drug Administration: Warning on use of terbutaline sulfate for preterm labor. *JAMA: The Journal of the American Medical Association, 279*(1), 9.

Noble, K. G., Fifer, W. P., Rauh, V. A., Nomura, Y., & Andrews, H. F. (2012). Academic achievement varies with gestational age among children born at term. *Pediatrics, 130*(2), e257–e264. doi: 10.1542/peds.2011-2157

Offenbacher, S., Boggess, K. A., Murtha, A. P., Jared, H. L., Lieff, S., McKaig, R. G., . . . Beck, J. D. (2006). Progressive periodontal disease and risk of very preterm delivery. *Obstetrics and Gynecology, 107*(1), 29–36. doi:10.1097/01.AOG.0000190212.87012.96

Orchinik, L. J., Taylor, H. G., Espy, K. A., Minich, N., Klein, N., Sheffield, T., & Hack, M. (2011). Cognitive outcomes for extremely preterm/extremely low birth weight children in kindergarten. *Journal of the International Neuropsychological Society, 17*(6), 1067–1079. doi:10.1017/S135561771100107X

Owen J., Hankins, G., Iams, J. D., Berghella, V., Sheffield, J. S., Perez-Delboy, A., . . . Hauth, J. C. (2009). Multicenter randomized trial of cerclage for preterm birth prevention in high-risk women with shortened midtrimester cervical length. *American Journal of Obstetrics and Gynecology, 201*(4), 375.e1–375.e8. doi:10.1016/j.ajog.2009.08.015

Palmer, L., & Carty, E. (2006). Deciding when it's labor: The experience of women who have received antepartum care at home for preterm labor. *Journal of Obstetric, Gynecologic, and Neonatal Nursing, 35*(4), 509–515. doi:10.1111/j.1552-6909.2006.00070

Papatsonis, D., Flenady, V., Cole S., & Liley, H. (2005). Oxytocin receptor antagonists for inhibiting preterm labour. *Cochrane Database of Systematic Reviews, 20*(3), CD004452.

Papiernik, E. (1989). *Effective Prevention of Preterm Birth: The French Experience at Hagenau*. New York: March of Dimes Birth Defects Foundation.

Parker, B., McFarlane, J., & Soeken, K. (1994). Abuse during pregnancy: Effects on maternal complications and birth weight in adult and teenage women. *Obstetrics and Gynecology, 84*(3), 323–328.

Patterson, E. T., Douglas, A. B., Patterson, P. M., & Bradle, J. B. (1992). Symptoms of preterm labor and self-diagnostic confusion. *Nursing Research, 41*(6), 367–372.

Plunkett, J., Feitosa, M. F., Trusgnich, M., Wangler, M. F., Palomar, L., Kistka, Z. A., . . . Muglia, L. J. (2009). Mother's genome or maternally-inherited genes acting in the fetus influence gestational age in familial preterm birth. *Human Heredity, 68*(3), 209–219. doi:10.1159/000224641

Raju, T. N. K., Higgins, R. D., Stark, A. R., & Leveno, K. J. (2006). Optimizing care and outcome for late-preterm (near-term) infants: A summary of the workshop sponsored by the National Institute of Child Health and Human Development. *Pediatrics, 118*(3), 1207–1214. doi:10.1542/peds.2006-0018

Reisner, D. P., Wallin, T. K., Zingheim, R. W., & Luthy, D. A. (2009). Reduction of elective inductions in a large community hospital. *American Journal of Obstetrics and Gynecology, 200*(6), 674. e1–674.e7. doi:10.1016/j.ajog.2009.02.021

Renker, P. R., & Tonkin, P. (2006). Women's views of prenatal violence screening: Acceptability and confidentiality issues. *Obstetrics and Gynecology, 107*(2, Pt. 1), 348–354. doi:10.1097/01 .AOG.0000195356.90589.c5

Romero, R., Nicolaides, K., Conde-Agudelo, A., Tabor, A., O'Brien, J. M., Cetingoz, E., . . . Hassan, S. S. (2012). Vaginal progesterone in women with an asymptomatic sonographic short cervix in the midtrimester decreases preterm delivery and neonatal morbidity: A systematic review and metaanalysis of individual patient data. *American Journal of Obstetrics and Gynecology, 206*(2), 124.e1–124.e19. doi:10.1016/j.ajog.2011.12.003

Rouse, D. J., Hirtz, D. G., Thom, E., Varner, M. W., Spong, C. Y., Mercer, B. M., . . . Roberts, J. M., for the Eunice Kennedy Shriver NICHD Maternal–Fetal Medicine Units Network. (2008). A randomized, controlled trial of magnesium sulfate for the prevention of cerebral palsy. *New England Journal of Medicine, 359*(9), 895–905. doi:10.1056/NEJMoa0801187

Ross, M. G., & Beall, M. H. (2009). Prediction of preterm birth: Nonsonographic cervical methods. *Seminars in Perinatology, 33*(5), 312–316. doi:10.1053/j.semperi.2009.06.004

Santa-Donato, A. (2005). Near-term infants: What experts say health care providers and parents need to know. *AWHONN Lifelines, 9*(6), 456–461. doi:10.1177/1091592305285274

Sciscione, A. C. (2010). Maternal activity restriction and the prevention of preterm birth. *American Journal of Obstetrics and Gynecology, 202*, 232.e1–232.e5. doi:10.1016/j.ajog.2009.07.005

Sciscione, A. C., Stamilio, D. M., Manley, J. S., Shlossman, P. A., Gorman, R. T., & Colmorgen, G. H. (1998). Tocolysis of preterm contractions does not improve preterm delivery rate or perinatal outcomes. *American Journal of Perinatology, 15*(3), 177–181.

Secker-Walker, R. H., Vacek, P. M., Flynn, B. S., & Mead, P. B. (1997). Smoking in pregnancy, exhaled carbon monoxide, and birth weight. *Obstetrics and Gynecology, 89*(5, Pt. 1), 648–653. doi:10.1016/S0029-7844(97)00103-8

Sibai, B. M. (2002). Hypertension. In S. G. Gabbe, J. R. Niebyl, & J. L. Simpson (Eds.), *Obstetrics: Normal and Problem Pregnancies* (4th ed., pp. 945–1004). New York: Churchill Livingstone.

Silver, R. M. (2007). Fetal death. *Obstetrics and Gynecology, 109*(1), 153–167. doi:10.1097/01.AOG.0000248537.89739.96

Simpson, K. R. (2004). Monitoring the preterm fetus during labor. *MCN: The American Journal of Maternal Child Nursing, 29*(6), 380–390.

Simpson, K. R. (2006). Minimizing risk of magnesium sulfate overdose in obstetrics. *MCN: The American Journal of Maternal Child Nursing, 31*(5), 340.

Simpson, K. R., & Knox, G. E. (2004). Obstetrical accidents involving intravenous magnesium sulfate: Recommendations to promote patient safety. *MCN: The American Journal of Maternal Child Nursing, 29*(3), 161–171.

Simpson, W. J. (1957). A preliminary report on cigarette smoking and the incidence of prematurity. *American Journal of Obstetrics and Gynecology, 73*(4), 808–815.

Society for Maternal–Fetal Medicine. (2012). Progesterone and preterm birth prevention: Translating clinical trials data into clinical practice. *American Journal of Obstetrics and Gynecology, 206*(5), 376–386. doi:10.1016/j.ajog.2012.03.010

Sosa, C., Althabe, F., Belizán, J., & Bergel, E. (2004). Bed rest in singleton pregnancies for preventing preterm birth. *Cochrane Database of Systematic Reviews*, (1), CD003581. doi:10.1002 /14651858.CD003581.pub2

Spong, C. Y., Meis, P. J., Thom, E. A., Sibai, B., Dombrowski, M. P., Moawad, A. H., . . . Gabbe, S., and the National Institute of Child Health and Human Development Maternal Fetal Medicine Units Network. (2005). Progesterone for prevention of recurrent preterm birth: Impact of gestational age at previous delivery. *American Journal of Obstetrics and Gynecology, 193*(3, Pt. 2), 1127–1131. doi:10.1016/j.ajog.2005.05.077

Spong, C. Y., Mercer, B. M., D'Alton, M., Kilpatrick, S., Blackwell, S., & Saade, G. (2011). Timing of indicated late-preterm and early-term birth. *Obstetrics and Gynecology, 118*(2, Pt. 1), 323–333. doi:10.1097/AOG.0b013e3182255999

Stan, C., Boulvain, M., Pfister, R., & Hirsbrunner-Almagbaly, P. (2002). Hydration for treatment of preterm labour. *Cochrane Database of Systematic Reviews*, (2), CD003096. doi:10.1002 /14651858.CD003096

Stoll, B. J., Hansen, N. I., Bell, E. F., Shankaran, S., Laptook, A. R., Walsh, M. C., . . . Higgins, R. D. (2010). Neonatal outcomes of extremely preterm infants from the NICHD Neonatal Research Network. *Pediatrics, 126*(3), 443–456. doi:10.1542 /peds.2009-2959

Straub, H., Adams, M., Kim, J. J., & Silver, R. K. (2012). Antenatal depressive symptoms increase the likelihood of preterm birth. *American Journal of Obstetrics and Gynecology, 207*(4), 329. e1–329.e4. doi.org/10.1016/j.ajog.2012.06.033

Suplee, P. D. (2005). The importance of providing smoking relapse counseling during the postpartum hospitalization. *Journal of Obstetric, Gynecologic, and Neonatal Nursing, 34*(6), 703–712. doi:10.1177/0884217505281861

Thomson Reuters. (2008). *The Cost of Prematurity and Complicated Deliveries to U.S. Employers: Report Prepared for the March of Dimes, October 29, 2008*. Retrieved from http://www.marchofdimes.com/peristats/pdfdocs/cts/ThomsonAnalysis2008_SummaryDocument_final121208.pdf

Tiedje, L. B. (2005). Teaching is more than telling: Education about prematurity in a prenatal clinic waiting room. *MCN: The American Journal of Maternal Child Nursing, 29*(6), 373–379.

Tita, A. T. N., Landon, M. B., Spong, C. Y., Lai, Y., Leveno, K. J., Varner, M. V., . . . Mercer, B. M. (2009). Timing of elective repeat cesarean delivery at term and neonatal outcomes. *New England Journal of Medicine, 360*(2), 111–120.

Tong, V. T., Jones, J. R., Dietz, P. M., D'Angelo, D., & Bombard, J. M. (2009). Trends in smoking before, during, and after pregnancy—Pregnancy Risk Assessment Monitoring System (PRAMS), United States, 31 sites, 2000–2005. *Morbidity and Mortality Weekly Report: Surveillance Summaries, 58*(SS04), 1–29.

U.S. Food and Drug Administration. (2011). *New Warnings Against Use of Terbutaline to Treat Preterm Labor* (FDA Drug Safety Communication). Silver Spring, MD: Author.

vanGeijn, H. P., Lenglet, J. E., & Bolte, A. C. (2005). Nifedipine trials: Effectiveness and safety aspects. *BJOG: An International Journal of Obstetrics & Gynaecology, 112*(Suppl 1), 79–83. doi: 10.1111/j.1471-0528.2005.00591.

Verani, J. R., McGee, L., & Schrag, S. J. (2010). Prevention of perinatal group B streptococcal disease—Revised guidelines from

CDC, 2010. *Morbidity and Mortality Weekly Report, Recommendations and Reports, 59*(RR-10), 1–32.

Vergnes, J. N., Kaminski, M., Lelong, N., Musset, A. M., Sixou, M., & Nabet, C. (2011). Maternal dental caries and pre-term birth: Results from the EPIPAP study. *Acta Odontologica Scandinavica, 69*(4), 248–256. doi:10.3109/00016357.2011.563242

Vermillion, S. T., & Robinson, C. J. (2005). Antiprostaglandin drugs. *Obstetrics and Gynecology Clinics of North America, 32*(3), 501–517. doi:10.1016/j.ogc.2005.04.006

Villar, J., Papageorghiou, A. T., Knight, H. E., Gravett, M. G., Iams, J., Waller, S. A., . . . Goldenberg, R. L. (2012). The preterm birth syndrome: A prototype phenotypic classification. *American Journal of Obstetrics and Gynecology, 206*(2), 119–123. doi:10.1016/j.ajog.2011.10.866

Von Kohorn, I., Nguyen, S. N., Schulman-Green, D., & Colson, E. R. (2012). A qualitative study of postpartum mothers' intention to smoke. *Birth, 39*(1), 65–69. doi:10.1111/j.1523-536X.2011.00514.x

Wang, X., Zuckerman, B., Pearson, C., Kaufman, C., Chen, C., Wang, G., . . . Xu, X. (2002). Maternal cigarette smoking, metabolic gene polymorphism, and infant birth weight. *JAMA: The Journal of the American Medical Association, 287*(2), 195–202. doi:10-1001/pubs.JAMA-ISSN-0098-7484-287-2-joc10264

Ward, K. (2003). Genetic factors in preterm birth. *BJOG: An International Journal of Obstetrics and Gynaecology, 110*(Suppl. 20), 117. doi:10.1046/j.1471-0528.2003.00061.x

Ward, K., Argyle, V., Meade, M., & Nelson, L. (2005). The heritability of preterm delivery. *Obstetrics and Gynecology, 106*(6), 1235–1239. doi:10.1097/01.AOG.0000189091.35982.85

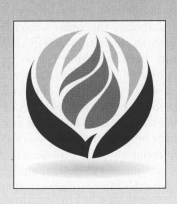

Julie M. Daley

Diabetes in Pregnancy

SIGNIFICANCE AND INCIDENCE

In 2010, 18.8 million people in the United States, or 8.35% of the nation's population, had diabetes. It is estimated that another 7 million people have diabetes that has not yet been diagnosed (Centers for Disease Control and Prevention [CDC], 2011b). About 3.7% of people aged 20 to 44 years have diagnosed or undiagnosed diabetes. There were 465,000 new cases of diabetes in this age group in 2010. People of minority racial and ethnic groups, such as African Americans, Hispanics, American Indians, and Asian/Pacific Islanders, have an 18% to 77% higher risk of diabetes than Caucasians (CDC, 2011b). Approximately 7% of all pregnancies are complicated by gestational diabetes (also known as gestational diabetes mellitus [GDM]) (American Diabetes Association [ADA], 2012).

Although comprehensive obstetric care and intensive metabolic management have reduced perinatal risk in pregnancies complicated by type 1 and type 2 diabetes, morbidity and mortality still remain higher than in the general population. Pregnant women with type 1 and type 2 diabetes have a 2.5-fold increase in risk of fetal death (Silver, 2007). Congenital defects and unexplained fetal death account for the increased fetal and neonatal mortality in women with type 1 and type 2 diabetes (Reece & Homko, 2000) and are likely related to comorbid conditions such as hypertension and obesity (Silver, 2007). Maternal hyperglycemia and disorders of fetal growth, metabolism, and possibly acidosis contribute to risk of fetal mortality (Silver, 2007). Preconception and early pregnancy glycemic control as evidenced by a near-normal glycosylated hemoglobin (A1C) during the period of organogenesis greatly reduces the risk of birth defects (McElvy et al.,

2000; Reece & Homko, 2000; Silver, 2007). Women with poorly controlled preexisting diabetes in the early weeks of pregnancy are three to four times more likely than nondiabetic women to have a baby with a serious malformation, such as a heart defect or neural tube defect. Defects in offspring of women with preexisting diabetes have been found to be more severe, usually multiple, and more often fatal. They also are at increased risk of miscarriage and stillbirth. Glycemic control in women with pregestational diabetes prior to conception reduces these risks as well as the risk of macrosomia (Persson, Norman, & Hanson, 2009; Yang, Cummings, O'Connell, & Jangaard, 2006).

The rate of perinatal mortality with gestational diabetes remains similar to that for nondiabetic women, but when GDM is detected in the first trimester with an elevated A1C and fasting hyperglycemia, the risk for congenital defects has been found to approach that of women with pregestational type 2 diabetes (Schaefer-Graf et al., 2000). It is possible that these data from early diagnosed cases may actually represent type 2 diabetes that was first recognized during pregnancy rather than true gestational diabetes. The ADA (2011) recommends that women who meet standard criteria for diagnosis of type 2 diabetes at the first prenatal visit be referred to as having "overt diabetes," not GDM. According to data using early and appropriate screening criteria, GDM is not associated with an increased risk of fetal death when compared to outcomes of pregnancies of women without diabetes (Silver, 2007).

Women with GDM are at higher risk of perinatal morbidity, such as obesity, gestational hypertension, preeclampsia, and cesarean birth (American College of Obstetricians and Gynecologists [ACOG], 2011; Persson, Pasupathy, Hanson, Westgren, & Norman,

2012). Babies of women with GDM are at higher risk of macrosomia, shoulder dystocia, birth trauma, respiratory distress syndrome, major malformations, hypoglycemia and other metabolic abnormalities, and childhood obesity (ACOG, 2011; Persson et al., 2012). Maintenance of euglycemia throughout pregnancy in GDM reduces the risk of these hyperglycemia-related fetal and neonatal abnormalities. A significant number of pregnant women in the United States are overweight or obese before starting their pregnancy (CDC, 2011c). It is estimated that approximately 30% of pregnant women are obese and 8% are morbidly obese (CDC, 2011c). Being overweight or obese further complicates pregnancies with diabetes. The higher the prepregnancy body mass index of the woman with diabetes, the more risks of adverse outcomes for the mother and fetus (Persson et al., 2012).

Macrosomia has been defined as a weight greater than the 90th percentile for gestational age and sex or a birth weight of 4,000 g (8 lb, 13 oz) to 4,500 g (9 lb, 15 oz) (ACOG, 2000; Hod & Yogev, 2007). Risk of fetal injury sharply increases with birth weights above 4,500 g (ACOG, 2000). Other factors such as morbid maternal obesity and postmaturity are also associated with fetal macrosomia and, when combined with insulin-controlled diabetes, lead to an even higher occurrence. Fetal macrosomia predisposes the mother to a higher risk of postpartum hemorrhage and vaginal lacerations and the newborn to a variety of traumatic injuries such as shoulder dystocia with associated risk for brachial plexus injury and clavicular fracture (ACOG, 2000; Conway, 2007). Shoulder dystocia is the most common injury related to fetal macrosomia but occurs only in approximately 1.4% of all vaginal births (ACOG, 2000). When birth weight exceeds 4,500 g, the risk of shoulder dystocia has been reported to range from 9.2% to 24% (ACOG, 2000). If the woman has diabetes, birth weights greater than 4,500 g are associated with much higher rates of shoulder dystocia: from 19.9% to 50% (ACOG, 2000). Fetal macrosomia contributes to an increased risk of cesarean birth, with resultant increased surgical morbidity in the mother (Conway, 2007).

The Fetal Basis of Adult Disease theory holds that events that occur during fetal development can permanently alter gene expression throughout the lifetime of the individual. A link has emerged between fetal nutrition, birth weight, and metabolic profile in adulthood. Abnormal "programming" of nutrient management increases risk for developing metabolic diseases such as obesity, hypertension, cardiovascular disease, and type 2 diabetes (Barker, 2001). Hyperglycemia in pregnancy is associated with a higher risk of childhood obesity (Hillier et al., 2007) as well as a higher risk of prediabetes and type 2 diabetes in adult offspring of women with diabetes (Clausen et al., 2008).

In addition to the risk of fetal macrosomia for all women with diabetes, the other extreme of weight, intrauterine growth restriction (IUGR), is a significant risk for infants born to women who have vascular complications of diabetes. Retinopathy and nephropathy associated with hypertension and poor renal function may contribute to uteroplacental insufficiency that leads to infants who are small for their gestational age. Gestational hypertension, to which women with diabetes (with or without vascular disease) are predisposed, also decreases uterine blood flow, compromising intrauterine fetal growth. Maintaining excellent control of blood glucose levels and blood pressure can help to avoid IUGR. Mean blood glucose <80 to 90 mg/dL and blood pressure <110/65 mm Hg in pregnancy may be associated with an increased risk of IUGR (Kitzmiller, Jovanovic, Brown, Coustan, & Reader, 2008).

Neonatal metabolic abnormalities occur with a higher frequency in offspring of women with diabetes. Hypoglycemia, whose precise definition may vary by institution, occurs frequently in babies of mothers with uncontrolled diabetes (Straussman & Levitsky, 2010). Preterm and large-for-gestational-age infants are at greatest risk for the development of hypoglycemia in the neonatal period. Chronic maternal hyperglycemia leads to excessive insulin production in the fetus (i.e., fetal hyperinsulinemia), which lowers fetal plasma glucose and inhibits glycogen release from the fetal liver as a normal physiologic response to hypoglycemia. This combination contributes to the risk for hypoglycemia development in the first 24 hours of life when cutting the umbilical cord interrupts transplacental glucose. Early detection and prompt treatment prevent the potential severe neurologic sequelae associated with profound hypoglycemia.

Infants of diabetic mothers may exhibit polycythemia, which is defined as a venous hematocrit of greater than 65%. Chronic hyperglycemia and hyperinsulinemia cause increased oxygen consumption and decreased fetal arterial oxygen content. Erythropoietin production increases, resulting in polycythemia. The elevated red blood cell mass can also result in hyperbilirubinemia (Hatfield, Schwoebel, & Lynyak, 2011). Hypocalcemia and hypomagnesemia are other metabolic abnormalities occasionally seen in infants of women with type 1 and type 2 diabetes, the exact causes of which are unknown.

Strict maternal glycemic control has decreased the incidence of respiratory distress syndrome significantly, but other factors, such as iatrogenic prematurity due to early birth as a result of maternal or fetal compromise, continue to contribute to the risk. Fetal surfactant production is inhibited by hyperinsulinemia, which occurs more frequently in women with poor metabolic control and is the underlying mechanism for respiratory distress syndrome in this group (Hatfield et al., 2011).

Risks during pregnancy for the woman with type 1 or type 2 diabetes include an increased incidence of hypoglycemia (blood glucose less than 60 mg/dL) as a result of stricter control (Kitzmiller, Jovanovic, et al., 2008; Rosenn & Miodovnik, 2000). Hypoglycemia is more common in early pregnancy (41% to 68%), as is nocturnal hypoglycemia (Kitzmiller, Jovanovic, et al., 2008). Hypoglycemia does not seem to cause problems for the fetus unless blood sugar levels are chronically low, but hypoglycemia does threaten the well-being of the mother. Educational efforts focusing on prevention and appropriate management of hypoglycemia can decrease this risk.

Diabetic ketoacidosis (DKA) is a rare complication for women with diabetes. However, the occurrence of DKA carries serious morbidity and mortality for the mother and the fetus and may occur at lower glucose levels (<250 mg/dL; Kitzmiller, Jovanovic, et al., 2008). Acidosis can cause decreased oxygenation of the placenta through decreased uterine blood flow and decreased tissue perfusion (Carroll & Yeomans, 2005; Parker & Conway, 2007). Fetal loss may occur through spontaneous abortion in the first and early second trimesters or as an intrauterine fetal death during an episode of DKA in late second and third trimesters. Improved perinatal management has decreased the fetal loss rate to about 9% (Parker & Conway, 2007), as well as decreased the rate of perinatal mortality.

Women with microvascular complications, poor glycemic control, and a longer duration of diabetes have poorer outcomes. Retinopathy is frequently encountered in women of reproductive age. It may progress during pregnancy, especially in women with elevated first-trimester A1C followed by rapid normalization of blood glucose values. Dilated eye examination should occur in the first trimester with continued surveillance throughout pregnancy. Laser photocoagulation therapy can be performed during pregnancy, if indicated (Kitzmiller, Jovanovic, et al., 2008). Nephropathy is a more serious microvascular complication that has been associated with adverse outcomes, including IUGR, preterm birth, and intrauterine fetal death (Landon, 2007; Rosenn & Miodovnik, 2000). Excellent control of blood glucose levels and hypertension can reduce perinatal complications and preserve kidney function (Kitzmiller, Jovanovic, et al., 2008; Nielsen, Damm, & Mathiesen, 2009).

Hypertensive disorders commonly develop if not present at conception and include chronic hypertension, gestational hypertension, and preeclampsia. Women with hypertensive disorders are at higher risk of preterm birth and cesarean birth, with resultant need for neonatal intensive care. Angiotensin-converting enzyme inhibitors and angiotensin receptor blockers are contraindicated during pregnancy and should be stopped prior to conception or as soon as possible after discovery of pregnancy. Renal failure is a potential complication without meticulous control of blood pressure. Hypertensive disorders of pregnancy also increase the risk of chronic hypertension and cardiovascular events (Kitzmiller, Block, et al., 2008; Sullivan, Umans, & Ratner, 2011). Women with type 1 or type 2 diabetes are at a higher risk of cardiovascular disease than nondiabetic women. Heart failure and ischemic stroke occur more frequently in pregnant women with diabetes. Cardiovascular autonomic neuropathy is associated with increased maternal mortality and poorer pregnancy outcomes (Kitzmiller, Block, et al., 2008).

Gastroparesis or gastropathy is a neuropathic complication that causes delayed gastric emptying and may exacerbate nausea and vomiting. This can result in irregular absorption of nutrients, inadequate nutrition, and poor glycemic control (Kitzmiller, Block, et al., 2008; Rosenn & Miodovnik, 2000). Women who continue pregnancy with gastroparesis may require total parenteral nutrition.

DEFINITIONS AND CLASSIFICATION

Women with diabetes during pregnancy can be divided into two groups. The first group consists of women who have pregestational diabetes (type 1 or type 2 diabetes), *including women diagnosed with diabetes at the first prenatal visit*, and the second group consists of women with gestational diabetes.

PREGESTATIONAL DIABETES (TYPE 1 OR TYPE 2 DIABETES)

Type 1 diabetes is hyperglycemia as a result of absolute insulin deficiency. It occurs as a result of genetic autoimmunity directed at the beta cells of the pancreas after an environmental trigger turns on antibodies that attack the islet cells of the pancreas, resulting in a total lack of insulin production. Exogenous insulin administration and medical nutrition therapy (MNT) are the mainstays of treatment. Type 1 diabetes usually occurs in people younger than 30 years old but can develop at any age.

Insulin resistance and relative insulin deficiency characterize type 2 diabetes. Insulin resistance at the cellular level may exist because of genetic defects in insulin binding to receptor sites or in glucose transport within the cell. This condition demands an increase in insulin secretion from the pancreas to maintain normoglycemia. Eventually, the beta cells exhaust and insulin production is diminished, resulting in hyperglycemia. Type 2 diabetes is the result of either genetic predisposition, environmental factors such as obesity, or a combination of both. To achieve euglycemia, type 2 diabetes may require not only MNT and exercise but also medication. Oral medications that increase the sensitivity of cells to insulin are first-line therapy after diet and exercise for type 2 diabetes, but additional types of medication and/or insulin may be necessary to maintain normoglycemia. Type 2 diabetes is not frequently seen in pregnancy because the age of diagnosis is usually in women beyond the reproductive years (≥45 years old). However, with increasing rates of obesity and type 2 diabetes in women of childbearing age (CDC, 2011a), the number of women with pregnancies complicated by type 2 diabetes now exceeds women with pregnancies complicated by type 1 diabetes (Engelgau, Herman, Smith, German, & Aubert, 1995). In one study, the rate of women with type 2 diabetes giving birth rose 367% from 1994 to 2004 (Albrecht et al., 2010). At our center, the proportion of women with pregestational diabetes who have type 2 diabetes has risen steadily from 54% to 72% in the last 6 years.

Oral antidiabetes medications are not recommended for use during pregnancy in women with type 2 diabetes. Earlier studies with first-generation sulfonylureas, which crossed the placenta, showed profound hypoglycemia in newborns because these drugs caused the fetal pancreas to secrete more insulin (Kemball et al., 1970). Earlier studies also showed an increase in malformations with oral agent use in the first trimester, but these malformations were likely due to hyperglycemia associated with ineffective control of maternal blood glucose. However, in a recent study of women with type 2 diabetes, 61% of the infants with congenital malformations were born to women taking oral antidiabetes agents at conception. Treatment with oral antidiabetes agents was independently associated with congenital anomalies (Roland, Murphy, Ball, Northcote-Wright, & Temple, 2005).

Glucose intolerance diagnosed at a gestational age of 24 weeks or less may represent undiagnosed preexisting type 2 diabetes. The ADA (2011) recommends that women who meet the criteria for diagnosis of type 2 diabetes at the first prenatal visit be referred to has having overt, not gestational, diabetes.

Priscilla White (1949) developed a classification system that was used to determine pregnancy prognosis for women based on the extent of microvascular disease and duration of type 1 or type 2 diabetes. White's classification system is still used for descriptive purposes only because the classification does not consider the level of glycemic control or comprehensive obstetric management, both of which greatly influence perinatal outcome.

GESTATIONAL DIABETES MELLITUS

GDM comprises the second group of women with diabetes during pregnancy and is currently defined as carbohydrate intolerance of any degree with onset or first recognition during pregnancy (ADA, 2004a). GDM has been subdivided further to designate those women whose GDM is diet controlled (GDM A$_1$) or insulin controlled (GDM A$_2$) (Gibson, Waters, & Catalano, 2012).

PATHOPHYSIOLOGY OF DIABETES IN PREGNANCY

Profound metabolic changes occur in normal pregnancy to allow for a continuously feeding fetus in an intermittently feeding mother. These alterations must be understood to comprehend the effects that diabetes has on a progressively changing metabolic state. In early pregnancy, beta-cell hyperplasia results in increased insulin production as a result of progesterone and estrogen increases, which also contributes to increased tissue sensitivity to insulin. This hyperinsulinemic state allows increased lipogenesis and fat deposition in early pregnancy in preparation for the dramatic rise in energy needs of the growing fetus in the latter half of pregnancy. As a result of these changes, along with nausea and vomiting, the mother has an increased risk for episodes of hypoglycemia in the first trimester. In women with type 1 diabetes and insulin-controlled type 2 diabetes, exogenous insulin needs may decrease.

The second half of pregnancy is characterized by accelerated growth of the fetus and rapidly increasing levels of maternal and placental diabetogenic hormones, which include human placental lactogen, cortisol, estrogen, progesterone, and prolactin. Insulin resistance and increased insulin production result from increased circulating levels of insulin-antagonizing hormones (Lain & Catalano, 2007; Parker & Conway, 2007). Increased insulin needs in women with type 1 and type 2 diabetes and the appearance of glucose intolerance in women who have limited pancreatic reserve due to predisposing risk factors are the result of these normal metabolic changes of pregnancy. This constitutes the diabetogenic state of pregnancy—hyperglycemia in the presence of hyperinsulinemia—which allows a continuous supply of glucose to passively diffuse to the fetus transplacentally (Parker & Conway, 2007).

The anabolic phase (i.e., fat storage) of the first 20 weeks of pregnancy is followed by a catabolic phase (i.e., fat breakdown or lipolysis) in the latter half of pregnancy (Lain & Catalano, 2007). This state is referred to as "accelerated starvation" because of the rapid switch from carbohydrate to lipid metabolism during fasting as a fuel source for the mother. Fat breakdown increases circulating fatty acids, triglycerides, and ketones, predisposing the woman with type 1 diabetes to an increased risk for the earlier development of ketoacidosis and starvation ketosis than in women with GDM and type 2 diabetes (Kitzmiller,

Jovanovic, et al., 2008). Hepatic glucose production increases during the latter half of pregnancy to meet the fetal and placental demands during maternal fasting (Lain & Catalano, 2007).

In the absence of vascular disease, the pathologic manifestations of diabetes in pregnancy are usually the result of maternal hyperglycemia. Excessive hyperglycemia, as a result of insulin deficiency with a corresponding increase in counterregulatory hormones (e.g., glucagon, epinephrine, growth hormone, and cortisol), contributes to the development of DKA. Factors in pregnancy that trigger the release of these hormones and development of DKA are fasting hyperglycemia, infection, stress, emesis, dehydration, gastroparesis, and beta-cell-sympathomimetic and steroid administration for the treatment of preterm labor (Carroll & Yeomans, 2005; Kitzmiller, Block, et al., 2008). Continuous subcutaneous insulin infusion (CSII) pump failure and poor patient compliance have also led to the development of DKA during pregnancy. Excessive hyperglycemia results from increased hepatic glucose and ketone production and insulin deficiency. Urinary excretion of potassium, sodium, and water occurs as a result of osmotic diuresis due to excessive plasma glucose. Fat metabolism leads to increased circulating levels of free fatty acids and ketonemia, which quickly overwhelm the maternal buffering system, and metabolic acidosis results (Kitzmiller, Jovanovic, et al., 2008). Maternal hyperglycemia during the time of organogenesis may result in spontaneous abortion or congenital malformations (Correa et al., 2008; Persson et al., 2009). Sustained or intermittent maternal hyperglycemia later in pregnancy stimulates fetal hyperinsulinemia as a normal fetal physiologic response to elevated blood glucose with pathologic consequences. Fetal hyperinsulinemia mediates accelerated fuel use and conversion of glucose to fat. Central fat deposition results in excessive fetal growth (e.g., macrosomia) (Moore, 2004; Sacks, 2007). Maternal hyperglycemia also contributes to fetal hypoxia. Hyperinsulinemia promotes catabolism of the extra fuel, using energy and depleting fetal oxygen stores (Hatfield et al., 2011; Moore, 2004). Fetal hyperinsulinemia also inhibits the release of surfactant that is necessary for pulmonary maturation resulting in respiratory distress syndrome. Maternal hyperglycemia is also associated with other neonatal metabolic abnormalities. Polyhydramnios, hypertension, urinary tract infections, pyelonephritis, and monilial vaginitis are other maternal complications of hyperglycemia.

SCREENING AND DIAGNOSIS OF GESTATIONAL DIABETES MELLITUS

Screening for GDM is recommended between 24 and 28 weeks' gestation, when the diabetogenic hormones

DISPLAY 8-1

Characteristics of Women at Low Risk for Gestational Diabetes Mellitus

- Younger than 25 years old
- Normal body weight
- No history of abnormal glucose tolerance
- No history of poor obstetric outcome
- No known diabetes in first-degree relative
- Not a member of an ethnic or racial group with higher prevalence of type 2 diabetes (e.g., Hispanic, African American, Native American, Asian, or Pacific Islander ancestry)

are exerting a significant influence on insulin performance. Women without risk factors for GDM do not require screening (ACOG, 2001; ADA, 2004a). Display 8–1 lists the characteristics of women who are at low risk for developing GDM. Women younger than 25 years old with any other risk factor for GDM should be tested. Risk factors identifying women who should undergo early screening for GDM at the first prenatal visit (as soon as risk is identified) are listed in Display 8–2. The ADA (2011) recommends testing for type 2 diabetes at the first prenatal visit in populations with a high prevalence of type 2 diabetes, such as Hispanics, African Americans, Native Americans, Southeast Asians, and Pacific Islanders with a fasting blood glucose value and an A1C. If the A1C is ≥6.5 and/or the fasting blood glucose is ≥126 mg/dL, overt diabetes is diagnosed. If the screening at the first prenatal visit is normal, screening is repeated between 24 and 28 weeks of gestation (ADA, 2011).

DISPLAY 8-2

Criteria for Early Screening for Gestational Diabetes Mellitus (Any One of the Following)

- Diabetes symptoms: polydipsia, polyuria, polyphagia, fatigue, sudden weight loss
- Persistent glycosuria
- Obesity
- Polyhydramnios
- Oral beta-mimetic therapy
- Corticosteroid therapy
- Persistent vaginal candidiasis
- Infant with congenital anomalies
- First-degree relative with type 2 diabetes
- Previous glucose intolerance
- Polycystic ovarian syndrome
- History of unexplained fetal death or stillborn
- Multiple spontaneous abortions
- History of fetal macrosomia (>4,000 g)

Evaluation for GDM in the United States is currently performed in a two-step approach (ACOG, 2001). The screening test consists of ingestion of a 50 g glucose solution (glucola) without consideration of time of day or last meal and obtaining a plasma or serum glucose level 1 hour after ingestion. The positive thresholds of 130 and 140 mg/dL have been used for the screening glucola. A value of 130 mg/dL identifies approximately 80% of women with gestational diabetes, whereas a cutoff of 140 mg/dL identifies approximately 90% of women with gestational diabetes (ACOG, 2001). The decision for which cutoff to use should be based on cost-effectiveness and risk factors in the population to be tested. An extremely elevated result on the glucose challenge is considered diagnostic, alleviating the need for an oral glucose tolerance test (OGTT). Some healthcare centers use a value of 200 mg/dL, while others use 180 mg/dL as the diagnostic threshold (Russell, Carpenter, & Coustan, 2007).

If the test result is positive, a diagnostic 3-hour, 100 g oral OGTT is administered after an 8-hour fast preceded by 3 days of unrestricted diet and activity. Women should refrain from smoking or eating and should remain seated during testing. Plasma glucose determinations are made at fasting and at 1-, 2-, and 3-hour intervals after ingestion of the glucose solution. The diagnostic criteria are listed in Table 8–1. Two or more thresholds must be met or exceeded to diagnose GDM (ACOG, 2001).

One abnormal value has been associated with adverse outcomes with 30% of these women exhibiting two abnormal values 1 month later (Neiger &

Coustan, 1991). Women with one abnormal value on the OGTT warrant closer surveillance with MNT and blood glucose monitoring or by repeat testing because of a much higher risk of adverse perinatal outcomes without treatment (Corrado et al., 2009; McLaughlin, Cheng, & Caughey, 2006). In the one-step approach, the screening 50 g test is omitted, and the 75 g, 2-hour OGTT is administered. The one-step approach for diagnosis has widespread use in Europe (Russell et al., 2007) and is endorsed for use in the United States by the ADA (2011) based on the results of the Hyperglycemia and Adverse Pregnancy Outcomes (HAPO) Study and the recommendations of the International Association of the Diabetes and Pregnancy Study Groups.

The HAPO Study was an observational study of 23,325 pregnant women at 15 healthcare centers in 9 countries (HAPO Study Cooperative Research Group, 2008). All women had a 75-g, 2-hour OGTT at 28 weeks of gestation, and the results were blinded unless the fasting value exceeded 105 mg/dL and/or the 2-hour value exceeded 200 mg/dL. The goal of the study was to relate the blood glucose levels on the 75 g, 2-hour OGTT to pregnancy outcomes. The researchers found that the risk of adverse outcome was a continuum, even at levels that were previously considered normal. As blood glucose levels rose, so did the risk of macrosomia, cesarean birth, and neonatal hypoglycemia. The authors concluded that they could not determine what level of blood glucose is clinically important or what level should be considered abnormal (HAPO Study Cooperative Research Group, 2008).

The International Association of Diabetes and Pregnancy Study Groups (IADPSG), a collection of experts on diabetes and pregnancy and representatives from various organizations who have an interest in diabetes and pregnancy, came to a consensus about what criteria should be used to diagnose GDM based on the results of the HAPO Study (IADPSG, 2010). The IADPSG recommends using *only* the 2-hour, 75 g OGTT to diagnose GDM, thus eliminating the two-step process. They do not recommend using an OGTT before 24 weeks of gestation. The recommended threshold values for the diagnosis of GDM are listed in Table 8–1. These values are based on values in the HAPO Study where the odds ratios of birth weight, cord C-peptide, and percent neonatal body fat greater than the 90th percentile reached 1.75 times the odds of these outcomes at mean glucose values. GDM is diagnosed if only one value exceeds the threshold values. Using these threshold values, the rate of GDM in the HAPO Study was 17.8% (IADPSG, 2010). Adopting the IADPSG criteria for the diagnosis of gestational diabetes is expected to significantly increase the rate of GDM.

Table 8–1. DIAGNOSTIC CRITERIA FOR GESTATIONAL DIABETES MELLITUS

| 100-g OGTT | Threshold Glucose Levels (mg/dL) | |
	ACOG[a]	ADA[b]
Fasting	≥95	≥92
1 hr	≥180	≥180
2 hr	≥155	≥153
3 hr	≥140	–

ACOG, American College of Obstetricians and Gynecologists; ADA, American Diabetes Association; OGTT, oral glucose tolerance test.
[a]Two or more values must be met or exceeded to diagnose gestational diabetes mellitus.
[b]One or more values must be met or exceeded to diagnose gestational diabetes mellitus.
Adapted from American College of Obstetricians and Gynecologists. (2011). *Screening and Diagnosis of Gestational Diabetes Mellitus* (Committee Opinion No. 504). Washington, DC: Author. doi:10.1097/AOG.0b013c3182310cc3; American Diabetes Association. (2011). Standards of medical care in diabetes–2011. *Diabetes Care, 34*(Suppl. 1), S11–S61. doi:10.2337/dc11-0174; Carpenter, M. W., & Coustan, D. R. (1982). Criteria for screening tests for gestational diabetes. *American Journal of Obstetrics and Gynecology, 144*(7), 768–773.

CLINICAL MANIFESTATIONS

The clinical manifestations of diabetes occur as a result of hypoglycemia and hyperglycemia. Glycemic goals for pregnancy in women with diabetes reflect the plasma blood glucose values found in pregnant women who do not have diabetes; 60 to 95 mg/dL fasting, 60 to 105 mg/dL before a meal, 140 mg/dL 1 hour after a meal, and 120 mg/dL 2 hours after a meal (ACOG, 2001, 2005). Symptoms of hyperglycemia include polyuria, polydipsia, blurred vision, and polyphagia. Women with gestational diabetes rarely experience these symptoms.

Hypoglycemia is defined as a plasma glucose level of 60 mg/dL, but significant symptoms may occur at higher levels when the patient's average blood glucose level is higher. Autonomic nervous system stimulation by hypoglycemia results in adrenergic and cholinergic symptoms of pallor, diaphoresis, tachycardia, palpitations, hunger, paresthesias, and shakiness. Moderate hypoglycemia causes glucose deprivation in the central nervous system as evidenced by an inability to concentrate, confusion, slurred speech, irrational behavior, slowed reaction time, blurred vision, numbness, somnolence, or extreme fatigue. Disorientation, loss of consciousness, seizures, and coma may result from severe hypoglycemia and is primarily seen in type 1 diabetes and not in gestational or type 2 diabetes.

NURSING ASSESSMENTS AND INTERVENTIONS FOR DIABETES MELLITUS

Evaluation and management of women with diabetes, whether pregestational or gestational, generally occurs on an outpatient basis. Hospital admission may be advisable for uncontrolled diabetes during the period of organogenesis (prior to 8 weeks) or during an episode of illness, DKA, or other obstetric complication. Nurses can have a profound role in educating and monitoring women with diabetes during pregnancy and are vital members of the multidisciplinary diabetes management team. The goal of nursing management focuses on the woman attaining and maintaining self-care behaviors, which result in near-normal blood glucose levels to improve perinatal outcome. Ideally, a team approach should be used to achieve this goal, which includes a physician with expertise in diabetes; MNT by a registered dietitian; exercise; education about self-monitoring of blood glucose and taking medication (as needed) by a registered nurse, preferably a certified diabetes educator; and stress reduction and management by a social worker or behavioral health specialist, as needed.

AMBULATORY AND HOME CARE MANAGEMENT

Ideally, intensive management of diabetes should begin prior to conception in women with pregestational diabetes. Attaining an A1C <1% above normal before pregnancy will decrease the risk of congenital malformations and spontaneous abortion to that of the general population (ADA, 2004c). Unfortunately, about two thirds of pregnancies are unplanned (ADA, 2004c). In one meta-analysis, about 62% of women with type 1 diabetes obtained preconception care, and less than 36% of women with type 2 diabetes had preconception care (Slocum, 2007). In the absence of preconception care, prenatal care should begin immediately on discovery of the pregnancy and continue throughout the perinatal period. The assessment of women with pregestational diabetes should include a thorough history of diabetes type, duration of disease, self-care practices, acute and chronic complication assessment, and a review of current glucose values and a food history of at least 3 days. Knowledge deficits should be identified and an individualized teaching plan outlined during this initial assessment. Psychosocial issues should be explored and evaluated periodically, and appropriate referrals should be made. Display 8–3 lists information that should be discussed with women who have pregestational diabetes.

When women who have type 1 or type 2 diabetes become pregnant, an educational session should be scheduled as soon as possible with the diabetes educator and registered dietitian before or in conjunction with the initial prenatal visit. The session should include all aspects of MNT, self-monitoring of blood glucose levels, and insulin therapy, including a demonstration by the woman of the correct method for drawing up and self-injection of insulin. Injection sites should be observed for correct regional rotation, as well as for identifying evidence of lipohypertrophy or lipoatrophy, bruising, and signs and symptoms of infection.

Women with type 2 diabetes who have been using oral medications for glucose control should be converted to insulin, ideally before conception or as soon as possible thereafter. Because glycemic control is so important to prevent malformations in the first trimester, women on oral antidiabetes agents should not stop those agents until insulin is instituted. These women require more extensive education regarding insulin and additional support with this new aspect of their diabetes management. Display 8–4 lists issues to be reviewed in the educational session about insulin.

TREATMENT OF HYPOGLYCEMIA

Appropriate management of hypoglycemia should be reviewed with women with pregestational diabetes. Signs and symptoms of hypoglycemia are listed in

DISPLAY 8-3

Educational Guidelines for Women with Pregestational Diabetes Mellitus

- **Healthy Eating**
  - Medical nutrition therapy (MNT)
- **Being Active**
  - 30–60 min/day of activity such as brisk walking
- **Monitoring**
  - Self-monitoring of blood glucose levels (SMBG), four to eight times per day
  - Glycemic goals for pregnancy
  - Guidelines for ketone testing
- **Taking Medications**
  - Insulin/oral agent therapy
  - Prenatal vitamins with folic acid
  - Medications for other medical conditions
- **Problem Solving**
  - Sick-day management
  - Appropriate treatment of hypoglycemia (correct amount and composition of snack, use of glucagon by family member)
  - Signs and symptoms of diabetic ketoacidosis and contributing factors
  - When and why to call the healthcare provider
- **Healthy Coping**
  - Psychosocial assessment
  - Barriers to optimal care
- **Reducing Risks**
  - Effect pregnancy has on diabetes
  - Potential for fetal or neonatal complications: intrauterine growth restriction, macrosomia, intrauterine fetal demise, birth trauma, prematurity, respiratory distress syndrome, neonatal metabolic disturbances
  - Potential for maternal complications: preterm birth, hypertensive disorders, cesarean birth
  - Association of hemoglobin A1C to risk congenital anomalies or spontaneous abortion
  - Schedule of antenatal visits and testing

Adapted from American Association of Diabetes Educators. (2012). *AADE7 Self-Care Behaviors*™. Retrieved from http://www.diabeteseducator.org /ProfessionalResources/AADE7

Display 8–5. They need an explanation that the occurrence will increase with intensive management during pregnancy. The level at which symptoms occur should be determined. If women have hypoglycemia unawareness, the risk for a potentially fatal nocturnal episode must be avoided. General guidelines for treatment of hypoglycemia during pregnancy include treatment with one carbohydrate exchange for a blood glucose of 60 mg/dL and treatment with two exchanges (liquid and solid, preferably) at a level of 40 to 60 mg/dL. Blood glucose should be tested again 15 minutes after treatment of hypoglycemia. Retreatment should occur if the blood glucose level has not risen. Including

DISPLAY 8-4

Educational Guidelines for Insulin Therapy

- Glycemic goals for treatment
- Onset, peak, and duration of action of insulins to be administered
- Inspection, storage, and traveling with insulin
- Timing of injections, injection technique, site selection, and regional rotation
- Glucagon use and appropriate administration by family or significant other
- Appropriate sick-day management
- Prevention strategies and appropriate management of hypoglycemia
- Syringe disposal guidelines

protein with the carbohydrate decreases the risk for rebound hypoglycemia and provides a more consistent and stable blood glucose level after treatment. Women with evidence of gastroparesis should use liquids for initial treatment of hypoglycemia because of their slower digestion. Carbohydrates ingested for treatment of hypoglycemia should be in addition to the regularly prescribed diet so that glucagon stores may be replenished. Family members and significant others should be instructed on the use of injectable glucagon, and two kits should be readily available at all times.

SICK–DAY MANAGEMENT

Nurses should also review sick-day management and provide written guidelines. Understanding appropriate self-care strategies during episodes of nausea and vomiting of early pregnancy is vital to prevent the development of ketoacidosis. Display 8–6 contains specific

DISPLAY 8-5

Signs and Symptoms of Hypoglycemia

- Mental confusion and irritability
- Somnolence
- Slowed reaction time
- Pallor
- Diaphoresis
- Tachycardia
- Palpitations
- Hunger
- Paresthesias
- Shakiness
- Cold, clammy skin
- Blurred vision
- Extreme fatigue

DISPLAY 8-6

Sick-Day Management Educational Guidelines

- Insulin should be given even with vomiting.
- Urine ketones should be checked every 4–6 hours and the healthcare provider notified of ≥ moderate results.
- Blood glucose levels should be checked every 1–2 hours.
- Healthcare provider should be notified of blood glucose levels ≥200 mg/dL.
- Liquids or soft foods should be consumed equal to the carbohydrate value of the prescribed diet (sugar-free for blood glucose levels of >120 mg/dL).
- A sipping diet of 15 to 30 g of carbohydrates per hour may be consumed during periods of vomiting.
- Call the healthcare provider if liquids are not tolerated.
- Review signs and symptoms of ketoacidosis to report: abdominal pain, nausea and vomiting, polyuria, polydipsia, fruity breath, leg cramps, altered mental status, and rapid respirations.

information that nurses should review with women about sick-day management.

GESTATIONAL DIABETES MELLITUS

Women who have been diagnosed with GDM need immediate counseling and education. Display 8–7 includes topics that nurses should discuss in the educational session. The diagnosis alone may bring excessive anxiety and fear. Appropriate education and support from the nurse educator should allay the woman's concerns and empower her with the resources she needs to adapt to the diabetic regimen, reducing the risks for perinatal complications. Including family and significant others in the education and care of women with GDM provides another source of support.

MEDICAL NUTRITION THERAPY

MNT is an integral and vital component in the care of women with diabetes and is best provided by a registered dietitian whenever possible. Therapeutic goals for nutritional intervention are blunting of postprandial hyperglycemia and appropriate nourishment of mother and fetus without excessive weight gain or ketosis. Current recommendations for dietary management include 30 to 35 kcal/kg for normal-weight women, 35 to 40 kcal/kg for underweight women, and 25 to 30 kcal/kg for overweight women (Reader, 2007). These calories should be consumed in three meals and three snacks and should contain 40% to 45% carbohydrates, 20% to 25% protein, and 35% to 40% predominately monounsaturated and polyunsaturated fats (Franz et al., 2002). Pregnant women need at least 175 g of carbohydrate per day

DISPLAY 8-7

Educational Guidelines for Women with Gestational Diabetes Mellitus

- **Healthy Eating**
  - Medical nutrition therapy (MNT)
- **Being Active**
  - 30–60 min/day of activity such as brisk walking
- **Monitoring**
  - Technique of meter use
  - Self-monitoring of blood glucose levels (SMBG), four times per day
  - Glycemic goals for pregnancy
  - Guidelines for ketone testing
- **Taking Medications**
  - Insulin/oral agent therapy, as needed
  - Prenatal vitamins
  - Medications for other conditions
- **Problem Solving**
  - Appropriate treatment of hypoglycemia (correct amount and composition of snack)
  - When and why to call the healthcare provider
- **Healthy Coping**
  - Psychosocial assessment
  - Barriers to optimal care
- **Reducing Risks**
  - Explanation of abnormal results from prenatal glucose test
  - Role of glucose and insulin transport and effect of placental hormones
  - Potential for fetal or neonatal complications: intrauterine fetal demise, macrosomia, birth trauma, respiratory distress syndrome, neonatal metabolic disturbances
  - Potential for maternal complications: polyhydramnios, hypertensive disorders, cesarean birth
  - Schedule of antenatal visits and testing

Adapted from American Association of Diabetes Educators. (2012). *AADE7 Self-Care Behaviors*™. Retrieved from http://www.diabeteseducator.org/ProfessionalResources/AADE7

during pregnancy to support fetal growth (Institute of Medicine, 2002).

A 25- to 35-lb weight gain is encouraged for women with normal prepregnancy weight, 15- to 25-lb weight gain for overweight women, 28- to 40-lb weight gain for underweight women, and 11- to 20-lb weight gain for obese women (Institute of Medicine & National Research Council, 2009). Nonnutritive sweeteners, including aspartame, saccharin, acesulfame-K, and sucralose, appear to be safe to use during pregnancy. Saccharin can cross the placenta, although no adverse effects have been found in humans (Franz et al., 2002). Women should take a prenatal vitamin supplement with 400 mcg of folic acid or 4 mg with a positive family history for neural tube defects, additional iron if anemic, and supplemental calcium for those women who do not consume enough dietary calcium.

Nutritional counseling should be individualized and culturally sensitive. Significant others and family members should be included in educational sessions to provide support. The person who prepares the meals must be a part of counseling and financial constraints determined, although a nutritional diet should not pose a financial burden. The registered dietitian should meet with the woman regularly to assess any dietary problems and to reevaluate nutritional needs after the initial session. More frequent visits are required for women with excessive or low weight gain.

EXERCISE THERAPY

Exercise should be used adjunctively with dietary management of diabetes (ADA, 2004b). The glucose-lowering mechanism of exercise is unknown but may be related to increased insulin sensitivity, improved first-phase insulin release, and increased caloric expenditure (Carpenter, 2000; Landon & Gabbe, 2011; Langer, 2000). In one study, only 21.9% of women with GDM who exercised two to three times per week for 30 to 40 minutes required insulin therapy compared to 56% of women in the control group (deBarros, Lopes, Francisco, Sapienza, & Zugaib, 2010). Activity can be divided into 10 to 20-minute sessions after each meal. Women with pregestational diabetes who are poorly controlled or who have vascular disease should avoid vigorous exercise during pregnancy. Walking and swimming are two forms of exercise with minimal risk and may be the exercise of choice for previously sedentary women. Safety considerations before implementing an exercise program should be thoroughly discussed, particularly for women with pregestational diabetes. Display 8–8 lists general guidelines for education of women who plan to exercise during their pregnancy. Women should be counseled to discontinue exercise if uterine activity occurs. The nurse should review the glucose log to evaluate the effect of exercise on blood sugar values and make appropriate food or insulin adjustment recommendations. The feet and lower extremities should be inspected for blisters, bruising, or other evidence of trauma. Exercise change may be required or a change in footwear needed.

METABOLIC MONITORING

Metabolic monitoring during pregnancy is directed at detecting hyperglycemia and hypoglycemia and making pharmacologic, dietary, or activity adjustments to maintain euglycemia. Rather than preprandial values, postprandial blood glucose determinations appear to be the most influential in the development of fetal hyperinsulinemia (ADA, 2004a). Daily self-monitoring of blood glucose in women with gestational diabetes has been found to be superior to intermittent office monitoring (ADA, 2004a). Daily self-monitoring allows the woman to know immediately the effect of food intake or activity on her blood sugar. In women with GDM, blood sugar levels should be checked at a minimum of four times daily: fasting and 1 to 2 hours after the first bite of each meal. Table 8–2 lists the target glycemic values for pregnancy. These values are usually easily attainable in women with GDM and type 2 diabetes but may be unrealistic in women with type 1 diabetes who have hypoglycemia unawareness and are more difficult to control. Women with pregestational diabetes should check their blood sugar levels four to eight times daily, depending on their level of control. These determinations may be obtained fasting, preprandial, postprandial, bedtime, and at 2 to 3 am. for women with a history of nocturnal hypoglycemia. Titration of insulin is smoother when based on multiple blood glucose determinations.

Women with GDM and type 2 diabetes who are on hypocaloric diets (<1,800 kcal/day) should test their urine daily from the first void for ketones to exclude starvation ketosis (ADA, 2004a). Calories should be added at the bedtime snack if ketones are detected. Women with type 1 diabetes are asked to test their urine for ketones daily from the first void and with any blood glucose level of 250 mg/dL or greater because of the increased risk for ketoacidosis (Kitzmiller, Jovanovic, et al., 2008). They should also be instructed

---

DISPLAY 8-8

Exercise Guidelines

- Proper footwear with silica gel or air midsoles
- Polyester or polyester–cotton-blend socks to promote dryness and prevent blisters
- Visible diabetes identification
- Carbohydrate (CHO) consumption when blood glucose <100 mg/dL and CHO snack readily available
- Blood glucose before and after exercise (type 1 diabetes)
- Adequate hydration during and after exercise
- Consult healthcare provider to assist with insulin adjustments

---

Table 8-2. GLYCEMIC GOALS FOR PREGNANCY

Timing	Plasma Glucose Levels (mg/dL)
Fasting	≤90–95
Preprandial	≤100
Postprandial	1 hr: ≤140
	2 hr: ≤120
2 to 6 am	60–100

Adapted from American College of Obstetricians and Gynecologists. (2005). *Pregestational diabetes mellitus* (Practice Bulletin No. 60). Washington, DC: Author.

to call their healthcare provider if they detect moderate levels of ketones.

All women with diabetes are asked to keep a log of their blood sugars, insulin doses, exercise or activity level, food intake with any abnormal values (high or low), and ketone checks when necessary. These logs allow the nurse and healthcare provider to accurately evaluate and make necessary adjustments at office visits. These visits should occur weekly for women having insulin adjustments or for women with identified problems. Telephone contact may be necessary to supplement visits. Visits should occur every other week for women with well-controlled diabetes, whether pregestational or gestational, until the latter half of the third trimester.

The care and use of a blood glucose meter should be reviewed with the woman. Whole blood glucose values are approximately 14% below laboratory plasma glucose determinations. Most meters are calibrated to provide plasma values by increasing the capillary result. Nurses need to know the limits of the meters their patients are using. For women who are newly diagnosed with GDM, a more intensive instructional session should be provided. Meters that have memory capability with date and time are important so that the nurse can correlate the values in the meter to those recorded by the woman. A significant number of patients may falsify blood sugar values, which can be detrimental to perinatal outcome if not detected (Kendrick, Wilson, Elder, & Smith, 2005). If false blood glucose readings have been reported, fears or contributory psychosocial issues should be explored. Sometimes, an underlying fear of insulin by women with GDM contributes to this phenomenon. These women need additional support and education and possibly referral for counseling.

Continuous glucose monitoring is a new development in diabetes care. A sensor is placed in subcutaneous tissue and glucose levels are read from interstitial fluid every 1 to 5 minutes and sent to a screen on a device. Trends in glucose values can be used to adjust insulin therapy. A lag time occurs between blood glucose values and interstitial fluid glucose values, and fingersticks must be done several times daily to calibrate the continuous glucose monitor and with any symptoms of hypoglycemia (Walsh & Roberts, 2006).

PHARMACOLOGIC THERAPY

Insulin is the preferred pharmacologic agent used in conjunction with nutrition therapy in women with pregestational or gestational diabetes (ADA, 2004a, 2004c; Landon & Gabbe, 2011). Insulin requirements during pregnancy increase dramatically from the first to third trimester as the anti-insulin hormones rise and peripheral resistance increases.

Requirements in the first trimester may be slightly reduced because of the nausea and vomiting of pregnancy. The average insulin requirement in the first trimester is 0.7 U/kg of ideal body weight, 0.8 U/kg in the second trimester, and 0.9 to 1.0 U/kg in the third trimester (Homko & Sargrad, 2003; Landon & Gabbe, 2011). These dosages are merely recommended averages requiring titration to blood glucose levels and activity for individualized management.

Glucose control during pregnancy requires intensive insulin management in women with type 1 diabetes, usually three to four injections per day. Women with type 2 diabetes or GDM may require less frequent injections. For example, many women with GDM require only bedtime intermediate-acting insulin to control fasting hyperglycemia. During the day, they are able to use diet and exercise to manage postmeal excursions of glucose. Morbidly obese women with GDM or type 2 diabetes may require more than 1 U/kg to achieve euglycemia.

Several rapid-acting insulin analogs (e.g., lispro, aspart, glulisine) are available for postmeal control. They have a quicker onset of action (10 to 15 minutes) and peak effect (60 minutes) than regular insulin and may help prevent hypoglycemia between meals. Lispro (Boskovic et al., 2003) and aspart (McCance et al., 2008; Pettitt, Ospina, Howard, Zisser, & Jovanovic, 2007) are pregnancy category B medications and are considered safe to use during pregnancy. Intermediate-acting human NPH insulin is used for basal insulin needs. Two long-acting insulin analogs (glargine and detemir) have also been introduced. A recent meta-analysis of studies that examined neonatal outcomes in a total of 702 women with diabetes comparing NPH insulin with glargine found no statistically significant differences in the occurrence of fetal outcomes (Pollex, Moretti, Koren, & Feig, 2011). No information is currently available on the use of detemir during pregnancy.

For women with GDM who fail to achieve euglycemia (see Table 8–2) with diet and exercise, insulin therapy should be initiated. Insulin is initiated when fasting blood sugar (FBS) values are 95 mg/dL or higher, 1-hour postprandial blood glucose values are 130 to 140 mg/dL or higher, or 2-hour postprandial blood glucose values are 120 mg/dL or higher (ACOG, 2001). Approximately 25% to 50% of women with GDM will require insulin therapy (Landon & Gabbe, 2011; Pertot et al., 2011). The insulin regimen should be individualized depending on what time of day blood glucose levels are elevated. Some healthcare centers may calculate doses based on body weight and gestational age, whereas others may use a standard starting dose and make adjustments based on blood glucose values (Biastre & Slocum, 2003). The educational session should follow the guidelines for insulin therapy in women with pregestational diabetes (see Display 8–4).

Women who are injecting insulin for the first time are very fearful and require much support and encouragement from the nurse and family members. They need to be reassured that they have not failed to control their glucose levels.

Occasionally, a woman may not be able to correctly draw up her insulin. In these situations, a home health referral can be made, another family member can be taught, or the nurse can draw the appropriate insulin to be refrigerated before use. Prefilled syringes may be safely refrigerated for up to 30 days. Prefilled insulin pens may be an option for women who have difficulty mixing insulins in one syringe. For women with needle phobias, self-injectors may be used. Women should be educated that insulin requirements normally increase as the pregnancy progresses and reassured that rising insulin needs do not represent a failure in the woman's ability to follow such a complex medical regimen.

CONTINUOUS SUBCUTANEOUS INSULIN INFUSION

Another method for intensive metabolic management in pregnancy is the use of CSII, commonly known as "the insulin pump." An insulin pump involves an electronic device that is programmed to deliver rapid-acting insulin subcutaneously through an implanted catheter. Lispro and aspart insulins are most commonly used in pumps. A continuous low-dose amount of basal insulin is infused, and boluses are given for meals and snacks based on carbohydrate intake. The catheter is changed every 2 to 3 days. The use of CSII in pregnancy requires careful patient selection, and only patients who are very motivated and capable of using a sophisticated electronic device should be chosen. The risk for pump use during pregnancy is pump malfunction, which can lead to the rapid development of DKA. This risk can be reduced by educating the woman to self-inject rapid-acting insulin and check the pump for blood glucose levels of >200 mg/dL.

Switching from conventional insulin therapy to pump therapy can be done on an inpatient or outpatient basis, individualizing the decision according to the level of family support and needs of the woman. The total daily insulin dose is divided between basal insulin and meal boluses; 50% to 60% is given as basal insulin, and the remaining 50% to 40% is given as boluses. Boluses may be given as 30% at breakfast, 25% before lunch, and 25% before dinner, with the remaining 20% before snacks if required (Gabbe, Carpenter, & Garrison, 2007) or calculated using an insulin-to-carbohydrate ratio (Walsh & Roberts, 2006). Another method for determining the insulin dose for CSII is based on patient weight and gestational age. Dosing is based on 0.9 U/kg in the first trimester, 1.0 U/kg in the second trimester, and 1.2 U/kg in the third trimester, and then reduced by 20% (Gabbe et al., 2007). A lower basal rate may be needed during the early nighttime hours to reduce the risk of nocturnal hypoglycemia. However, because of the strong "dawn phenomenon" associated with pregnancy, an increased basal rate may be needed after 3 am.

Self-monitoring of blood glucose should be done often. At a minimum, blood glucose levels should be checked while fasting, before meals, after meals, and at bedtime. Checks are required at 2 to 3 am during nighttime adjustments to avoid hypoglycemia or hyperglycemia. Close contact with the diabetes management team becomes a vital component of successful insulin pump therapy during pregnancy. Continuous glucose monitoring can be very helpful during pregnancy to assess periods of hyperglycemia and hypoglycemia that might not be picked up with intermittent self-monitoring of blood glucose, especially overnight. One pump currently available has continuous glucose monitoring displayed on the pump screen.

ORAL ANTIDIABETES AGENTS

Oral antidiabetes agents are not currently recommended by the ACOG for use during pregnancy because insufficient data are available to recommend for or against their use. Insulin is still the drug of choice to treat diabetes during pregnancy (ACOG, 2001).

However, the use of oral antidiabetes agents has become a focus of controversy, research, and debate. Early studies questioned whether adverse outcomes of pregnancy were due to the medication, usually first-generation sulfonylureas, or poor glycemic control at the time of conception. Many new antidiabetes medications have been introduced in recent years, and research is underway to examine the use, efficacy, and pregnancy outcomes of women using some of these agents (Slocum & Sosa, 2002).

The first randomized controlled trial (Langer, Conway, Berkus, Xenakis, & Gonzales, 2000) compared the use of insulin and glyburide, a second-generation sulfonylurea that stimulates beta cells to produce more insulin, in 404 women with GDM. Both groups had similar rates of macrosomia and cesarean birth, and glyburide was not detected in the cord blood of any infants. The researchers concluded that glyburide was safe to use in women with GDM. Several authors (Conway, Gonzales, & Skiver, 2004; Jacobson et al., 2005) have published their experiences with using glyburide in women with GDM. Many healthcare providers now offer glyburide to women as an alternative to insulin therapy. At the Fifth International Conference–Workshop on GDM, glyburide was recognized as a potentially useful adjunct in the treatment of GDM (ADA, 2007). A more recent pharmacologic study showed that umbilical cord concentration of glyburide was about 70% of maternal plasma concentration (Hebert et al., 2009), so the use of this medication in women with gestational diabetes has declined.

Metformin is a medication that works in the liver to prevent the conversion of glycogen to glucose and prevents its release into the circulation, which helps to decrease fasting glucose levels. It also reduces peripheral insulin resistance, making tissues more sensitive to insulin. Metformin may be used alone or in combination with other antidiabetes agents. If used with insulin, it can decrease the amount of insulin needed to control glucose levels.

Metformin has also been studied for the treatment of gestational diabetes. In the Metformin in Gestational Diabetes (MiG) Study, researchers compared metformin with insulin therapy in the treatment of GDM (Rowan, Hague, Gao, Battin, & Moore, 2008). About 46% of women taking metformin required supplemental insulin. Metformin was not associated with increased perinatal or neonatal complications compared with insulin.

A great deal of research has examined the use of metformin in women with polycystic ovary syndrome (PCOS) (Slocum & Sosa, 2002). PCOS is a condition characterized by hyperinsulinemia, chronic anovulation, oligomenorrhea, and hyperandrogenism. It affects approximately 7% to 8% of women of reproductive age and is a common cause of infertility, early pregnancy loss, and later complications of pregnancy (Legro et al., 2007). Some studies have shown that metformin, by improving insulin sensitivity, can restore ovulatory function and improve pregnancy rates in women with PCOS when used alone or in combination with clomiphene citrate (Kocak, Caliskan, Simsir, & Haberal, 2002; Vandermolen et al., 2001). Other studies (Glueck, Goldenberg, Wang, Loftspring, & Sherman, 2004; Jakubowicz, Iuorno, Jakubowicz, Roberts, & Nestler, 2002) showed that continuing metformin can decrease the rate of first trimester miscarriage and, if continued throughout pregnancy, can decrease the incidence of gestational diabetes in women with PCOS (Glueck, Pranikoff, Aregawi, & Wang, 2008; Nawaz, Khalid, Naru, & Rizvi, 2008). Other studies have not shown better outcomes with the use of metformin (Legro et al., 2007; Vanky et al., 2010). Many women with PCOS present for prenatal care having taken metformin during organogenesis and may be reluctant to discontinue the medication. Some healthcare providers advocate discontinuing metformin on discovery of the pregnancy, whereas others will continue metformin until the end of the first trimester, and still others will continue metformin throughout pregnancy.

Neither glyburide nor metformin are approved for use during pregnancy by the U.S. Food and Drug Administration or the ACOG. There appears to be little to no difference in perinatal and neonatal outcome, but the long-term effects of these medications on the mother and the offspring is still unknown.

FETAL ASSESSMENT

The best method and the appropriate time to begin antepartum fetal assessment for pregnant women with diabetes have yet to be determined. Most recommend beginning some form of fetal assessment in the third trimester for women with pregestational diabetes (ACOG, 2005). Testing of women with GDM controlled by diet may be delayed until near term (Landon & Gabbe, 2011). Women with GDM controlled by insulin should begin earlier in the third trimester—32 to 36 weeks as has been suggested (ACOG, 2005; Landon & Gabbe, 2011). Fetal movement counting is a simple, inexpensive, and appropriate test to begin in all pregnant women with diabetes in the beginning of the third trimester. Women with vascular disease need more intensive fetal and maternal surveillance, requiring a nonstress test, contraction stress testing, or biophysical profile, beginning at 28 weeks of gestation (Kitzmiller, Jovanovic, et al., 2008). Doppler velocimetry of the umbilical artery may also be useful (ACOG, 2005). Table 8–3 provides a sample schedule to consider for fetal testing in women with diabetes. Display 8–9 is a summary of home care management for women with diabetes.

TIMING AND MODE OF BIRTH

The optimal time for birth for a woman with diabetes involves balancing the risk of intrauterine fetal demise with the risks of preterm birth. When glucose control is good, antenatal testing remains reassuring, and no other complications exist, evidence supports awaiting spontaneous labor and birth at 40 weeks of gestation (ACOG, 2001, 2005). The ACOG no longer recommends elective induction of labor before 39 weeks, unless it is for fetal or maternal indications. Parameters for documenting gestational age are an ultrasound at <20 weeks that supports a gestational age of 39 weeks or greater, fetal heart tones that have been documented as present for 30 weeks, or 36 weeks since a positive serum or urine pregnancy test (ACOG, 2009).

Many women with diabetes are able to have a vaginal birth. An estimated fetal weight of >4,500 g may be an indication for cesarean birth without a trial of labor (ACOG, 2001, 2005). Cesarean birth increases maternal risks of morbidity and mortality but decreases risks of shoulder dystocia and brachial plexus injury to the fetus.

Table 8–3. FETAL SURVEILLANCE FOR WOMEN WITH DIABETES

Gestational Age (Weeks)	Type 1 or Type 2 Diabetes: Poorly Controlled or with Vascular Disease	Type 1 or Type 2 Diabetes: Well Controlled, No Vascular Disease	GDM A_1 (Diet Controlled)	GDM A_2 (Insulin Controlled)
6–8	Sonographic estimation of gestational age	Same		
11–13	Nuchal translucency (NT) ultrasound and PAPP-A blood measurement (if available)	Same	Same	Same
15–20	Maternal serum alpha-fetoprotein	Same	Same	Same
20–22	High-resolution sonography, fetal echocardiography	High-resolution sonography, fetal echocardiography		
26–28	Sonographic assessment of interval growth	Same		
28	Twice-daily fetal movement counting (FMC), weekly nonstress test (NST)	Twice-daily FMC	Twice-daily FMC	Twice-daily FMC
32	Twice-weekly NST or weekly biophysical profile, sonographic assessment of interval growth	Weekly NST, then increase to twice weekly at 34–36 weeks		Weekly NST, then increase to twice weekly at 34–36 weeks
36–38	Sonographic estimation of fetal weight	Sonographic estimation of fetal weight	Sonographic estimation of fetal weight, weekly NST	Sonographic estimation of fetal weight
39–40	Elective birth without amniocentesis	Elective birth without amniocentesis	Consider elective birth if cervix favorable and for large-for-gestational-age (LGA) fetus	Consider elective birth if cervix favorable and for LGA fetus

GDM, gestational diabetes; PAPP-A, pregnancy-associated plasma protein A.
Adapted from American College of Obstetricians and Gynecologists. (2001). *Gestational Diabetes* (Practice Bulletin No. 30). Washington, DC: Author; American College of Obstetricians and Gynecologists. (2009). *Induction of Labor* (Practice Bulletin No. 107). Washington, DC: Author. doi:10.1097/AOG.0b013e3181b48ef5; Kitzmiller, J. L., Jovanovic, L. B., Brown, F. M., Coustan, D. R., & Reader, D. M. (Eds.). (2008). *Managing Preexisting Diabetes for Pregnancy: Technical Reviews and Consensus Recommendations for Care.* Alexandria, VA: American Diabetes Association.

INPATIENT MANAGEMENT

Women with diabetes require hospitalization during periods of poor control for intensive insulin adjustment, particularly if they are in the critical time of organogenesis (6 to 8 weeks' gestation). Hospitalization may also be required during periods of illness for women with dehydration and is always required for those in DKA. Women who develop complications of pregnancy, such as preterm labor or preeclampsia, may require hospitalization during the third trimester for more intensive maternal and fetal surveillance.

DIABETIC KETOACIDOSIS

DKA is characterized by severe hyperglycemia, ketosis, acidosis, dehydration, hypovolemia, and electrolyte imbalance (Carroll & Yeomans, 2005). Kussmaul respirations develop in an effort to correct the ensuing metabolic acidosis. Acetone breath develops as ketone bodies are converted to acetone and excreted by the lungs. Dehydration occurs as a result of hyperglycemia. Altered consciousness levels, including coma, are usually present. The diagnosis of DKA is based on the laboratory findings of an elevated blood glucose level, a bicarbonate level below 15 mEq/L, and an arterial pH of less than 7.2 (Montoro, 2004). In pregnant women, DKA may occur with only mild elevations in blood glucose values (Carroll & Yeomans, 2005; Montoro, 2004).

Care of women in DKA should occur in a tertiary care facility with the support services that can provide intensive care. Nurses in community hospitals should be capable of stabilizing the woman in preparation for, and during transport to, an appropriate facility.

Table 8–4 lists specific interventions nurses use in the care of women experiencing DKA. Initial treatment measures focus on rehydration, which improves tissue perfusion, insulin delivery, and a physiologic lowering of blood glucose by hemodilution. After intravenous (IV) access is established, insulin is administered as ordered to lower blood glucose. Caution should be exercised in lowering the blood glucose because too rapid a fall results in the serious complication of cerebral edema. With improvement of the intravascular status, fluid shifts result in a potassium deficit that requires replacement. Nurses should continually assess the woman for signs and symptoms of hypokalemia and monitor electrolyte levels in preparation for replacement. Adequate urinary output must also be maintained with potassium replacement to avoid hyperkalemia. In addition to monitoring laboratory electrolyte status, the complete blood cell count and differential also should be monitored as well as the clinical status for signs and symptoms of infection. Evidence of infection requires prompt and aggressive treatment for DKA treatment to be effective.

Fetal monitoring, even in previable gestations, provides an indication of hydration and perfusion status and should be instituted immediately. Indeterminate fetal status is expected but resolves as the mother is stabilized and should not be an indication for emergent cesarean birth, which could further compromise the mother (Carroll & Yeomans, 2005). Maternal oxygenation status should be monitored continually and oxygen administered based on blood gas determinations, bedside oxygen saturation levels, and fetal

status. Uterine activity also is associated with severe dehydration but resolves in most cases with improved perfusion. Treatment for preterm labor should not be considered in the absence of cervical change because the use of beta-adrenergic agonists or steroids worsens the clinical picture by antagonizing insulin. Magnesium sulfate is the drug of choice for treatment of preterm labor because it does not interfere with the action of insulin.

After DKA has been corrected, the underlying cause—whether infection or poor self-care practices—should be discussed with the mother and family, outlining early detection and prevention strategies. For mothers whose infants did not survive, intensive grief support and follow-up should be provided.

INTRAPARTUM MANAGEMENT: PREGESTATIONAL AND GESTATIONAL DIABETES MELLITUS

Intrapartum management of women with diabetes requires skilled nursing care to prevent maternal and neonatal complications. Plasma glucose levels should be maintained below 110 mg/dL for capillary blood

Table 8-4. NURSING MANAGEMENT OF DIABETIC KETOACIDOSIS

Treatment	Nursing Intervention
Fluid resuscitation	1. Obtain large-bore peripheral access. 2. Anticipate need for hemodynamic monitoring. 3. Administer fluids as ordered, usually 1,000–2,000 mL of normal saline over 1 hr, then 200–500 mL/hr. 4. Assess for signs and symptoms of pulmonary edema—dyspnea, tachypnea, wheezing, cough. 5. Assess for hypovolemia; check vital signs every 15 min; report decrease in blood pressure, increased pulse rate, decrease in central venous and pulmonary capillary wedge pressure, and slow capillary refill. 6. Insert Foley catheter for oliguria or anuria and send specimen for urinalysis, culture, and sensitivity. 7. Hourly intake and output—report output <30 mL/hr. 8. Administer 5% dextrose solution or D5/0.45% normal saline at blood glucose level of 200 mg/dL to prevent hypoglycemia.
Insulin therapy	1. Administer intravenous insulin as ordered: 0.1–0.2 U/kg of regular insulin as bolus, then 0.1 U/kg/hr. Follow hospital insulin/dextrose drip algorithm if established. 2. Hourly capillary blood glucose determinations (lab correlation with each draw). 3. Monitor urine and blood for ketones. 4. Notify physician when blood glucose level of 250 mg/dL is reached, anticipating a decrease in insulin infusion rate to 0.1 U/kg/hr. 5. Monitor for hypoglycemia. 6. Monitor for cerebral edema—headache, vomiting, deteriorating mental status, bradycardia, sluggish pupillary light reflex, widened pulse pressure.
Electrolyte replacement	1. Obtain electrocardiogram and report ST segment depression, inverted T waves, and appearance of U waves after T waves. 2. Obtain laboratory electrolyte levels every 2–4 hr. 3. Anticipate potassium replacement within 2–4 hr.
Oxygenation	1. Establish the airway. 2. Anticipate placement of the peripheral arterial catheter. 3. Obtain initial arterial blood gases, then hourly until pH of 7.20 is maintained. 4. Administer oxygen at 10 L/min by a nonrebreather face mask or as ordered to maintain oxygen saturations of 95% per pulse oximeter. 5. Anticipate the need for intubation/mechanical ventilation. 6. Use continuous pulse oximetry. 7. Administer bicarbonate if ordered for pH of 7.10.
Fetal or uterine monitoring	1. Lateral recumbent position. 2. Apply external fetal or uterine monitoring (EFM). 3. Observe EFM for evidence of fetal compromise. 4. Observe for uterine activity. 5. Administer tocolytics as ordered (magnesium sulfate or drug of choice). 6. Avoid beta-adrenergic agonists and steroids.

Adapted from Jerreat, L. (2010). Managing diabetic ketoacidosis. *Nursing Standard, 24*(34), 49–55; Kitzmiller, J. L., Jovanovic, L. B., Brown, F. M., Coustan, D. R., & Reader, D. M. (Eds.). (2008). *Managing Preexisting Diabetes for Pregnancy: Technical Reviews and Consensus Recommendations for Care.* Alexandria, VA: American Diabetes Association.

determinations (ACOG, 2005). Hyperglycemia in labor contributes to the development of neonatal hypoglycemia. Blood glucose should be assessed on the first laboratory blood draw and then checked at the bedside every 1 to 2 hours for all women who have previously been controlled by insulin. Women with GDM who have been controlled by diet may have their blood glucose levels checked every 2 to 4 hours. Ketones should be checked with every void or every 4 hours if euglycemia is maintained.

IV access should be established early so that hydration can be maintained, and insulin should be administered when necessary. Women with GDM and type 2 diabetes may not require insulin during labor. Laboring women with type 1 diabetes will usually require glucose and insulin at some point. If, on hospital admission, the blood glucose level of a woman with type 1 diabetes is 70 mg/dL or below, an infusion with 5% dextrose should be initiated at a rate of 100 to 125 mL/hr (Coustan, 2005). A main line is required, usually of normal saline, at least to keep open. All glucose-containing solutions and insulin-containing solutions should be piggybacked to the main line at ports closest to the hub of IV insertion. These are basic safety measures. Insulin administration should be initiated according to institutional protocol. Women who present in spontaneous labor and who have taken their intermediate-acting insulin may not require insulin during labor but will need a glucose infusion on admission to avoid hypoglycemia.

A standardized solution of 100 units of regular human insulin (there is no advantage to using analogs when administering IV) to 100 mL of normal saline should be used—again, for safety purposes. When a woman is NPO (nothing per mouth), a rate of 1 U/hr (1 mL/hr) usually is all that is necessary. Most insulin algorithms require IV insulin adjustments according to at least hourly blood glucose levels. Polyvinyl tubing should be flushed thoroughly (at least 50 mL) to allow saturation of the insulin to the tubing, allowing the prescribed dose to be infused consistently. Glucose and insulin should be maintained on pumps to avoid overdosage of either solution. Because of the higher risk for operative birth, no oral intake should be allowed during active labor for women with diabetes.

Insulin is partially catabolized in the kidney, and in women with nephropathy, the action is unpredictable, requiring closer surveillance of blood sugar levels. Prehydration for conduction anesthesia or IV boluses should use non-glucose-containing solutions and be administered more slowly in the presence of vascular disease. Lactated Ringer's solution should be avoided in women with type 1 diabetes because of its gluconeogenic properties (Hirsch, McGill, Cryer, & White, 1991).

Women with diabetes may have scheduled induction or cesarean births. Early morning hospital admissions are preferred, withholding the morning insulin dose, with IV glucose and insulin initiated. Cervical ripening and induction procedures should follow institutional protocols and physician orders. Continuous fetal monitoring should be used and assessed for signs of fetal compromise. Labor abnormalities that would indicate potential cephalopelvic disproportion should be monitored closely. Nurses caring for laboring women with diabetes should prepare for assisted birth and the possibility of shoulder dystocia. The birth of a potentially high-risk newborn should also be anticipated and preparation made for full resuscitation. A neonatal team should be present at the birth or immediately available.

Hypoglycemia during labor is usually avoided with close monitoring but should be recognized and treated aggressively. Observation for signs and symptoms of hypoglycemia should be a continuous nursing assessment. Display 8–5 lists typical signs and symptoms of mild and moderate hypoglycemia. Concentrated dextrose solutions (10% and 50%) should be maintained at the bedside. Treatment should be initiated at a blood glucose level of 70 mg/dL by discontinuing insulin and running only dextrose in the IV to raise the blood glucose level to 80 mg/dL. The insulin drip can then be restarted at an adjusted algorithm or when the blood glucose is 110 mg/dL. The blood sugar should be rechecked hourly, and further treatment should be administered if the blood glucose remains low. If the woman becomes unconscious, the physician should be notified immediately, and 50% dextrose should be infused intravenously. Vital signs should be assessed every 5 to 10 minutes during episodes of hypoglycemia, including blood glucose checks, until a threshold of 80 mg/dL is reached. Insulin should be resumed when the blood glucose level reaches 120 mg/dL according to a laboratory assessment or 110 mg/dL for a capillary blood glucose determination.

POSTPARTUM MANAGEMENT

PREGESTATIONAL DIABETES MELLITUS

Insulin requirements decrease in the immediate postpartum period when the levels of circulating anti-insulin placental hormones drop. Insulin and glucose infusions should be decreased by 50% as insulin sensitivity returns to normal soon after delivery of the placenta (Taylor & Davison, 2007). With oral intake, subcutaneous insulin can be resumed at the prepregnancy dosage or at one half to one third the pregnancy dose for women with type 1 and type 2 diabetes. Strict glycemic control can be relaxed somewhat in the postpartum period.

Women with diabetes have a higher incidence of postpartum infection (e.g., mastitis, endometritis, wound infection). Therefore, nurses should observe for signs and symptoms and notify the physician if they occur. Women who have given birth to a macrosomic infant or have had prolonged or induced labors should be closely monitored for hemorrhage.

Contraceptive options should be explored with the woman and her partner, and pregnancy planning should be encouraged to allow for preconception care to decrease the risks for spontaneous abortion and congenital defects in future pregnancies. Counseling and education should be provided regarding long-term consequences of diabetes and the need for glycemic control to decrease adverse sequelae.

BREASTFEEDING

Breastfeeding is highly recommended for at least 6 months after birth and ideally for 12 months after birth. Mounting evidence indicates that breastfeeding reduces the incidence of childhood obesity and diabetes later in life (Crume et al., 2011; Mayer-Davis et al., 2006; Schaefer-Graf et al., 2006). Evidence also suggests that breastfeeding reduces or delays the onset of type 2 diabetes in women with GDM (Villegas et al., 2008).

Insulin has generally been recommended for women with type 2 diabetes who choose to breastfeed their babies and who cannot achieve normoglycemia by treatment with MNT and exercise alone. Some oral hypoglycemic agents (e.g., glyburide, glipizide, metformin) may be safe for use while breastfeeding (Briggs, Ambrose, Nageotte, Padilla, & Wan, 2005;

Feig et al., 2005). Women with type 2 diabetes who will not be breastfeeding may resume oral hypoglycemic agents.

Caloric needs mandate recalculation based on postpartum body weight and on possible lactation requirements. For obese women, a program for exercise and dietary management for weight loss should be outlined. Breastfeeding should be encouraged with adequate support from the nursing staff. Lactating mothers need assistance to prevent hypoglycemia while nursing, which may require additional snacks. Most breastfeeding mothers require less insulin due to extra calories expended with nursing and the use of maternal glucose to produce the lactase in their milk (Homko & Sargrad, 2003; Stage, Norgard, Damm, & Mathiesen, 2006).

GESTATIONAL DIABETES MELLITUS

Most women revert to normal glucose tolerance in the postpartum period. Reclassification of glycemic status should be obtained at the 6-week postpartum visit for all women with GDM. A fasting plasma glucose may be more convenient and less costly, but a 75 g, 2-hour OGTT will more accurately identify women with impaired glucose tolerance (ACOG, 2001; ADA, 2007; Landon & Gabbe, 2011). If the glucose tolerance test is normal, repeat testing should occur 1 year from the birth of the baby and then every 3 years, or when pregnancy is being considered. Women should also be tested with a FBS annually in any year they are not having a 2-hour OGTT (ADA, 2007). Any abnormal value requires repeat testing on another day (ADA, 2004a). Table 8–5 lists the criteria for diagnosis

of diabetes mellitus from fasting plasma glucose, 75 g OGTT, and random testing. The risk for development of overt diabetes after GDM increases with time. Risk factors related to the development of overt diabetes include gestational age at diagnosis, degree of abnormality of the diagnostic OGTT, level of glycemia at the first postpartum visit, and the presence of obesity (ACOG, 2001).

Counseling should be provided to women with a history of GDM in the postpartum period for risk-reducing strategies such as weight reduction by diet and exercise. The Diabetes Prevention Program Research Group (2002) showed that a lifestyle modification program could decrease the incidence of type 2 diabetes by 58%. Women also need to know the signs and symptoms of hyperglycemia that would warrant testing for diabetes, such as polyuria, polydipsia, polyphagia, persistent vaginal candidiasis, frequent urinary tract infections, excessive fatigue and hunger, or sudden weight loss. Women also should be informed that they have a high risk for development of GDM in subsequent pregnancies. Testing for diabetes is encouraged before conception or at the first prenatal visit, with early prenatal care to allow screening for and intensive management of overt diabetes, which carries a higher perinatal risk than for GDM.

SUMMARY

Diabetes is one of the common medical complications encountered when caring for pregnant women. Diabetes may exist prepregnancy or develop during the pregnancy. Each type of diabetes has specific clinical challenges and the potential for adverse outcomes for the mother and baby. Perinatal nurses should be aware of the required aspects of nursing care for women with diabetes during pregnancy, labor, birth, and postpartum.

Table 8–5. CRITERIA FOR DIAGNOSIS OF DIABETES MELLITUS

Normoglycemia	IFG and IGT (Prediabetes)	Diabetes Mellitus
FPG <100 mg/dL	FPG ≥100 mg/dL and <126 mg/dL (IFG)	FPG ≥126 mg/dL
2-hr plasma glucose <140 mg/dL on a 75-g 2-hr OGTT	2-hr plasma glucose ≥140 mg/dL and <200 mg/dL on a 75-g 2-hr OGTT (IGT)	2-hr plasma glucose ≥200 mg/dL on a 75-g 2-hr OGTT
		Symptoms of diabetes and casual plasma glucose of ≥200 mg/dL

FPG, fasting plasma glucose; IFG, impaired fasting glucose; IGT, impaired glucose tolerance; OGTT, oral glucose tolerance test.
Adapted from American Diabetes Association. (2004a). Gestational diabetes mellitus. *Diabetes Care, 27*(Suppl. 1), S88–S90. doi:10.2337/diacare.27.2007.S88

REFERENCES

Albrecht, S. S., Kuklina, E. V., Bansil, P., Jamieson, D. J., Whiteman, M. K., Kourtis, A. P., . . . Callaghan, W. M. (2010). Diabetes trends among delivery hospitalizations in the U.S., 1994–2004. *Diabetes Care, 33*(4), 768–773. doi:10.2337/dc09-1801

American Association of Diabetes Educators. (2012). *AADE7™ self-care behaviors.* Retrieved from http://www.diabeteseducator.org/ProfessionalResources/AADE7

American College of Obstetricians and Gynecologists. (2000). *Fetal Macrosomia* (Practice Bulletin No. 22). Washington, DC: Author.

American College of Obstetricians and Gynecologists. (2001). *Gestational Diabetes* (Practice Bulletin No. 30). Washington, DC: Author.

American College of Obstetricians and Gynecologists. (2005). *Pregestational Diabetes Mellitus* (Practice Bulletin No. 60). Washington, DC: Author.

American College of Obstetricians and Gynecologists. (2009). *Induction of Labor* (Practice Bulletin No. 107). Washington, DC: Author. doi:10.1097/AOG.0b013e3181b48ef5

American College of Obstetricians and Gynecologists. (2011). *Screening and Diagnosis of Gestational Diabetes Mellitus* (Committee Opinion No. 504). Washington, DC: Author. doi:10.1097/AOG.0b013e3182310cc3

American Diabetes Association. (2004a). Gestational diabetes mellitus. *Diabetes Care, 27*(Suppl. 1), S88–S90. doi:10.2337/diacare.27.2007.S88

American Diabetes Association. (2004b). Physical activity/exercise and diabetes mellitus. *Diabetes Care, 27*(Suppl. 1), S58–S62. doi:10.2337/diacare.27.2007.S58

American Diabetes Association. (2004c). Preconception care of women with diabetes. *Diabetes Care, 27*(Suppl. 1), S76–S78. doi:10.2337/diacare.27.2007.S76

American Diabetes Association. (2007). Proceedings of the Fifth International Workshop—Conference on Gestational Diabetes Mellitus. *Diabetes Care, 30*(Suppl. 2), S105–S261. doi:10.2337/dc07-s225

American Diabetes Association. (2011). Standards of medical care in diabetes—2011. *Diabetes Care, 34*(Suppl. 1), S11–S61. doi:10.2337/dc11-0174

American Diabetes Association. (2012). Diagnosis and classification of diabetes mellitus. *Diabetes Care, 35*(Suppl. 1), S64–S71. doi:10.2337/dc12-s064

Barker, D. J. (2001). A new model for the origins of chronic disease. *Medicine, Health Care & Philosophy, 4*(1), 31–35. doi:10.1023/A:1009934412988

Biastre, S. A., & Slocum, J. M. (2003). Gestational diabetes. In M. J. Franz (Ed.), *A Core Curriculum for Diabetes Education: Diabetes in the Life Cycle and Research* (5th ed., pp. 143–176). Chicago, IL: American Association of Diabetes Educators.

Boskovic, R., Feig, D. S., Derewlany, L., Knie, B., Portnoi, G., & Koren, G. (2003). Transfer of insulin lispro across the placenta: In vitro perfusion studies. *Diabetes Care, 25*(5), 1390–1394. doi:10.2337/diacare.26.5.1390

Briggs, G. G., Ambrose, P. J., Nageotte, M. P., Padilla, G., & Wan, S. (2005). Excretion of metformin into breast milk and the effect of nursing infants. *Obstetrics and Gynecology, 105*(5), 1437–1441.

Carpenter, M. W. (2000). The role of exercise in pregnant women with diabetes mellitus. *Clinical Obstetrics and Gynecology, 43*(1), 56–64.

Carpenter, M. W., & Coustan, D. R. (1982). Criteria for screening tests for gestational diabetes. *American Journal of Obstetrics and Gynecology, 144*(7), 768–773.

Carroll, M. A., & Yeomans, E. R. (2005). Diabetic ketoacidosis in pregnancy. *Critical Care Medicine, 33*(10 Suppl.), S347–S353.

Centers for Disease Control and Prevention. (2011a). *Incidence of Diagnosed Diabetes per 1,000 Population Aged 18–79 years, by Sex and Age, United States, 1997–2010.* Atlanta, GA: Author. Retrieved from http://www.cdc.gov/diabetes/statistics/incidence/fig5.htm

Centers for Disease Control and Prevention. (2011b). *National Diabetes Fact Sheet: National Estimates and General Information on Diabetes and Prediabetes in the United States, 2011.* Atlanta, GA: Author.

Centers for Disease Control and Prevention. (2011c). *Obesity: Halting the Epidemic by Making Health Easier* (At a Glance Report). Atlanta, GA: Author.

Clausen, T. D., Mathiesen, E. R., Hansen, T., Pedersen, O., Jensen, D. M., Lauenborg, J., & Damm, P. (2008). High prevalence of type 2 diabetes and pre-diabetes in adult offspring of women with gestational diabetes mellitus or type 1 diabetes. *Diabetes Care, 31*(2), 340–346. doi:10.2337/dc07-1596

Conway, D. L. (2007). Obstetric management in gestational diabetes. *Diabetes Care, 30*(Suppl. 2), S175–S179. doi:10.2337/dc07-s212

Conway, D. L., Gonzales, O., & Skiver, D. (2004). Use of glyburide for the treatment of gestational diabetes: The San Antonio

experience. *Journal of Maternal-Fetal and Neonatal Medicine, 15*(1), 51–55.

Corrado, F., Benedetto, A. D., Cannata, M. L., Cannizzaro, D., Giordano, D., Indorato, G., . . . D'Anna, R. (2009). A single abnormal value of the glucose tolerance test is related to increased adverse perinatal outcome. *Journal of Maternal–Fetal & Neonatal Medicine, 22*(7), 597–601. doi:10.1080/14767050902801801

Correa, A., Gilboa, S. M., Besser, L. M., Botto, L. D., Moore, C. A., Hobbs, C. A., . . . Reece, E. A. (2008). Diabetes mellitus and birth defects. *American Journal of Obstetrics and Gynecology, 199*(3), 237.e1–237.e9. doi:10.1016/j.ajog.2008.06.028

Coustan, D. R. (2005). Delivery: Timing, mode, and management. In E. A. Reece, D. R. Coustan, & S. G. Gabbe (Eds.), *Diabetes in Women: Adolescence, Pregnancy, and Menopause* (3rd ed., pp. 433–440). Philadelphia: Lippincott Williams & Wilkins.

Crume, T. L., Ogden, L., Maligie, M., Sheffield, S., Bischoff, K. J., McDuffie, R., . . . Dabelea, D. (2011). Long-term impact of neonatal breastfeeding on childhood adiposity and fat distribution among children exposed to diabetes in utero. *Diabetes Care, 34*(3), 641–645. doi:10.2337/dc10-1716

deBarros, M. C., Lopes, M. A., Francisco, R. P., Sapienza, A. D., & Zugaib, M. (2010). Resistance exercise and glycemic control in women with gestational diabetes. *American Journal of Obstetrics and Gynecology, 203*(6), 556.e1–556.e6. doi:10.1016/j.ajog.2010.07.015

Diabetes Prevention Program Research Group. (2002). Reduction in the incidence of type 2 diabetes with lifestyle intervention or metformin. *New England Journal of Medicine, 346*(6), 393–403.

Engelgau, M. M., Herman, W. H., Smith, P. J., German, R. R., & Aubert, R. E. (1995). The epidemiology of diabetes and pregnancy in the U.S., 1988. *Diabetes Care, 18*(7), 1029–1033.

Feig, D. S., Briggs, G. G., Kraemer, J. M., Ambrose, P. J., Moskovitz, D. N., Nageotte, M., . . . Koren, G. (2005). Transfer of glyburide and glipizide into breast milk. *Diabetes Care, 28*(8), 1851–1855. doi:10.2337/diacare.28.8.1851

Franz, M. J., Bantle, J. P., Beebe, C. A., Brunzell, J. D., Chiasson, J. L., Garg, A., . . . Wheeler, M. (2002). Evidence-based nutrition principles and recommendations for the treatment and prevention of diabetes and related complications. *Diabetes Care, 25*(1), 148–198. doi:10.2337/diacare.25.1.148

Gabbe, S. G., Carpenter, L. B., & Garrison, E. A. (2007). New strategies for glucose control in patients with type 1 and type 2 diabetes mellitus in pregnancy. *Clinical Obstetrics and Gynecology, 50*(4), 1014–1024. doi:10.1097/GRF.0b013e31815a6435

Gibson, K. S., Waters, T. P., & Catalano, P. M. (2012). Maternal weight gain in women who develop gestational diabetes mellitus. *Obstetrics and Gynecology, 119*(3), 560–565. doi:10.1097/AOG.0b013e31824758e0

Glueck, C. J., Goldenberg, N., Wang, P., Loftspring, M., & Sherman, A. (2004). Metformin during pregnancy reduces insulin, insulin resistance, insulin secretion, weight, testosterone and development of gestational diabetes: Prospective longitudinal assessment of women with polycystic ovary syndrome from preconception through pregnancy. *Human Reproduction, 19*(3), 510–521.

Glueck, C. J., Pranikoff, J., Aregawi, D., & Wang, P. (2008). Prevention of gestational diabetes by metformin plus diet in patients with polycystic ovary syndrome. *Fertility and Sterility, 89*(3), 625–634. doi:10.1016/j.fertnstert.2007.03.036

HAPO Study Cooperative Research Group. (2008). Hyperglycemia and adverse pregnancy outcomes. *New England Journal of Medicine, 358*(19), 1991–2002.

Hatfield, L., Schwoebel, A., & Lynyak, C. (2011). Caring for the infant of a diabetic mother. *MCN: The American Journal of Maternal Child Nursing, 36*(1), 10–16. doi:10.1097/NMC.0b013e3181fb0b4c

Hebert, M. F., Ma, X., Naraharisetti, S. B., Krudys, K. M., Umans, J. G., Hankins, G. D. V., . . . Vicini, P. (2009). Are we optimizing gestational diabetes treatment with glyburide? The pharmacologic basis for better clinical practice. *Clinical Pharmacology & Therapeutics, 85*(6), 607–614. doi:10.1038/clpt.2009.5

Hillier, T. A., Pedula, K. L., Schmidt, M. M., Mullen, J. A., Charles, M. A., & Pettitt, D. J. (2007). Childhood obesity and metabolic imprinting: The ongoing effects of maternal hyperglycemia. *Diabetes Care, 30*(9), 2287–2292. doi:10.2337/dc06-2361

Hirsch, I. B., McGill, J. B., Cryer, P. E., & White, P. F. (1991). Perioperative management of surgical patients with diabetes mellitus. *Anesthesiology, 74*(2), 346–359.

Hod, M., & Yogev, Y. (2007). Goals of metabolic management of gestational diabetes: Is it all about the sugar? *Diabetes Care, 30*(Suppl. 2), S180–S187. doi:10.2337/dc07-s213

Homko, C. J., & Sargrad, K. R. (2003). Pregnancy with preexisting diabetes. In M. J. Franz (Ed.), *A Core Curriculum for Diabetes Education: Diabetes in the Life Cycle and Research* (5th ed., pp. 97–142). Chicago, IL: American Association of Diabetes Educators.

Institute of Medicine. (2002). *Dietary Reference Intakes: Energy, Carbohydrate, Fiber, Fat, Fatty Acids, Cholesterol, Protein, and Amino Acids.* Washington, DC: The National Academies Press.

Institute of Medicine & National Research Council. (2009). *Weight Gain During Pregnancy: Reexamining the Guidelines.* Retrieved from http://books.nap.edu/openbook.php?record_id=12584

International Association of Diabetes and Pregnancy Study Groups Consensus Panel. (2010). International Association of Diabetes and Pregnancy Study Groups recommendations on the diagnosis and classification of hyperglycemia in pregnancy. *Diabetes Care, 33*(3), 676–682. doi:10.2337/dc09-1848

Jacobson, G. F., Ramos, G. A., Ching, J. Y., Kirby, R. S., Ferrara, A., & Field, D. R. (2005). Comparison of glyburide and insulin for the management of gestational diabetes in a large managed care organization. *American Journal of Obstetrics and Gynecology, 193*(1), 118–124. doi:10.1016/j.ajog.2005.03.018

Jakubowicz, D. J., Iuorno, M. J., Jakubowicz, S., Roberts, K. A., & Nestler, J. E. (2002). Effects of metformin on early pregnancy loss in the polycystic ovary syndrome. *Journal of Clinical Endocrinology & Metabolism, 87*(2), 524–529. doi:10.1210/jc.87.2.524

Jerreat, L. (2010). Managing diabetic ketoacidosis. *Nursing Standard, 24*(34), 49–55.

Kemball, M. L., McIver, C., Milner, R. D., Nourse, C. H., Schiff, D., & Tiernan, J. R. (1970). Neonatal hypoglycemia in infants of diabetic mothers given sulphonylurea drugs in pregnancy. *Archives of Disease in Childhood, 45*(243), 696–701.

Kendrick, J. M., Wilson, C., Elder, R. F., & Smith, C. S. (2005). Reliability of reporting of self-monitoring of blood glucose in pregnant women. *Journal of Obstetric, Gynecologic, & Neonatal Nursing, 34*(3), 329–334. doi:10.1177/0884217505276306

Kitzmiller, J. L., Block, J. M., Brown, F. M., Catalano, P. M., Conway, D. L., Coustan, E. R., . . . Kirkman, M. S. (2008). Managing preexisting diabetes for pregnancy: Summary of evidence and consensus recommendations for care. *Diabetes Care, 31*(5), 1060–1079. doi:10.2337/dc08-9020

Kitzmiller, J. L., Jovanovic, L. B., Brown, F. M., Coustan, D. R., & Reader, D. M. (Eds.). (2008). *Managing Preexisting Diabetes for Pregnancy: Technical Reviews and Consensus Recommendations for Care.* Alexandria, VA: American Diabetes Association.

Kocak, M., Caliskan, E., Simsir, C., & Haberal, A. (2002). Metformin therapy improves ovulatory rates, cervical scores, and pregnancy rates in clomiphene citrate-resistant women with polycystic ovary syndrome. *Fertility and Sterility, 77*(1), 101–106.

Lain, K. Y., & Catalano, P. M. (2007). Metabolic changes in pregnancy. *Clinical Obstetrics and Gynecology, 50*(4), 938–948. doi:10.1097/GRF.0b013e31815a5494

Landon, M. B. (2007). Diabetic nephropathy and pregnancy. *Clinical Obstetrics and Gynecology, 50*(4), 998–1006. doi:10.1097/GRF.0b013e31815a6383

Landon, M. B., & Gabbe, S. G. (2011). Gestational diabetes mellitus. *Obstetrics and Gynecology, 118*(6), 1379–1393. doi:10.1097/AOG.0b013e31823974e2

Langer, O. (2000). Management of gestational diabetes. *Clinical Obstetrics and Gynecology, 43*(1), 106–115.

Langer, O., Conway, D. L., Berkus, M. D., Xenakis, E. M. J., & Gonzales, O. (2000). A comparison of glyburide and insulin in women with gestational diabetes. *New England Journal of Medicine, 343*(16), 1134–1138.

Legro, R. S, Barnhart, H. X., Schalff, W. D., Carr, B. R., Diamond, M. P., Carson, S. A., . . . Myers, E. R. (2007). Clomiphene, metformin, or both for infertility in the polycystic ovary syndrome. *New England Journal of Medicine, 356*(6), 551–566.

Mayer-Davis, E. J., Rifas-Shiman, S. L., Zhou, L., Hu, F. B., Colditz, G. A., & Gillman, M. W. (2006). Breast-feeding and risk for childhood obesity. *Diabetes Care, 29*(10), 2231–2237. doi:10.2337/dc06-0974

McCance, D. R., Damm, P., Mathiesen, E. R., Hod, M., Kaaja, R., Dunne, F., . . . Mersebach, H. (2008). Evaluation of insulin antibodies and placental transfer of insulin aspart in pregnant women with type 1 diabetes mellitus. *Diabetologia, 51*(11), 2141–2143. doi:10.1007/s00125-008-1120-y

McElvy, S. S., Miodovnik, M., Rosenn, B., Khoury, J. C., Siddiqi, T., Dignan, P. S., & Tsang, R. C. (2000). A focused preconceptional and early pregnancy program in women with type 1 diabetes reduces perinatal mortality and malformation rates to general population levels. *Journal of Maternal–Fetal Medicine, 9*(1), 14–20.

McLaughlin, G. B., Cheng, Y. W., & Caughey, A. B. (2006). Women with one elevated 3-hour glucose tolerance test value: Are they at risk for adverse perinatal outcomes? *American Journal of Obstetrics & Gynecology, 194*(5), e16–e19. doi:10.1016/j.ajog.2006.01.028

Montoro, M. N. (2004). Diabetic ketoacidosis in pregnancy. In E. A. Reece, D. R. Coustan, & S. G. Gabbe (Eds.), *Diabetes in Women: Adolescence, Pregnancy, and Menopause* (3rd ed., pp. 345–350). Philadelphia, PA: Lippincott Williams & Wilkins.

Moore, T. R. (2004). Diabetes in pregnancy. In R. K. Creasy & R. Resnik (Eds.), *Maternal-Fetal Medicine: Principles and Practice* (5th ed., pp. 1023–1063). Philadelphia: Saunders.

Nawaz, F. H., Khalid, R., Naru, T., & Rizvi, J. (2008). Does continuous use of metformin throughout pregnancy improve pregnancy outcomes in women with polycystic ovarian syndrome? *Journal of Obstetrics & Gynaecology Research, 34*(5), 832–837. doi:10.1111/j.1447-0756.2008.00856

Neiger, R., & Coustan, D. R. (1991). The role of repeat glucose tolerance tests in the diagnosis of gestational diabetes. *American Journal of Obstetrics and Gynecology, 165*(4, Pt. 1), 787–790.

Nielsen, L. R., Damm, P., & Mathiesen, E. R. (2009). Improved pregnancy outcome in type 1 diabetic women with microalbuminuria or diabetic nephropathy: Effect of intensified antihypertensive therapy? *Diabetes Care, 32*(1), 38–44. doi:10.2337/dc08-1526

Parker, J. A., & Conway, D. L. (2007). Diabetic ketoacidosis in pregnancy. *Obstetrics and Gynecology Clinics of North America, 34*(3), 533–543. doi:10.1016/j.ogc.2007.08.001

Persson, B., Norman, M., & Hanson, U. (2009). Obstetric and perinatal outcomes in type 1 diabetic pregnancies. *Diabetes Care, 32*(11), 2005–2009. doi:10.2337/dc09-0656

Persson, M., Pasupathy, D., Hanson, U., Westgren, M., & Norman, M. (2012). Pre-pregnancy body mass index and the risk of adverse outcome in type 1 diabetic pregnancies: A population-based cohort study. *BMJ Open, 2*(1), e000601. doi:10.1136/bmjopen-2011-000601

Pertot, T., Molyneaux, L., Tan, K., Ross, G. P., Yue, D. K., & Wong, J. (2011). Can common clinical parameters be used to identify patients who will need insulin treatment in gestational diabetes mellitus? *Diabetes Care, 34*(10), 2214–2216. doi:10.2337/dc11-0499

Pettitt, D. J., Ospina, P., Howard, C., Zisser, H., & Jovanovic, L. (2007). Efficacy, safety and lack of immunogenicity of insulin aspart compared with regular human insulin for women with gestational diabetes mellitus. *Diabetic Medicine, 24*(10), 1129–1135. doi:10.1111/j.1464-5491.2007.02247.x

Pollex, E., Moretti, M. E., Koren, G., & Feig, D. S. (2011). Safety of insulin glargine use in pregnancy: A systematic review and meta-analysis. *The Annals of Pharmacotherapy, 45*(1), 9–16. doi:10.1345/aph.1P327

Reader, D. M. (2007). Medical nutrition therapy and lifestyle interventions. *Diabetes Care, 30*(Suppl. 2), S188–S193. doi:10.2337/dc07-s214

Reece, E. A., & Homko, C. J. (2000). Why do diabetic women deliver malformed infants? *Clinical Obstetrics and Gynecology, 43*(1), 32–45.

Roland, J. M., Murphy, H. R., Ball, V., Northcote-Wright, J., & Temple, R. C. (2005). The pregnancies of women with type 2 diabetes: Poor outcomes but opportunities for improvement. *Diabetic Medicine, 22*(12), 1774–1777. doi:10.1111/j.1464-5491.2005.01784.x

Rosenn, B. M., & Miodovnik, M. (2000). Medical complications of diabetes mellitus in pregnancy. *Clinical Obstetrics and Gynecology, 43*(1), 17–31.

Rowan, J. A., Hague, W. M., Gao, W., Battin, M. R., & Moore, M. P. (2008). Metformin versus insulin for the treatment of gestational diabetes. *New England Journal of Medicine, 358*(19), 2003–2015.

Russell, M. A., Carpenter, M. W., & Coustan, D. R. (2007). Screening and diagnosis of gestational diabetes mellitus. *Clinical Obstetrics and Gynecology, 50*(4), 949–958. doi:10.1097/GRF.0b013e31815a5510

Sacks, D. A. (2007). Etiology, detection, and management of fetal macrosomia in pregnancies complicated by diabetes mellitus. *Clinical Obstetrics and Gynecology, 50*(4), 980–989. doi:10.1097/GRF.0b013e31815a6242

Schaefer-Graf, U. M., Buchanan, T. A., Xiang, A., Songster, G., Montoro, M., & Kjos, S. L. (2000). Patterns of congenital anomalies and relationship to initial maternal fasting glucose levels in pregnancies complicated by type 2 and gestational diabetes. *American Journal of Obstetrics and Gynecology, 182*(2), 313–320.

Schaefer-Graf, U. M., Hartmann, R., Pawliczak, J., Passow, D., Abou-Dakn, M., Vetter, K., & Kordonouri, O. (2006). Association of breast-feeding and early childhood overweight in children from mothers with gestational diabetes mellitus. *Diabetes Care, 29*(5), 1105–1107. doi:10.2337/dc05-2413

Silver, R. M. (2007). Fetal death. *Obstetrics and Gynecology, 109*(1), 153–167. doi:10.1097/01.AOG.0000248537.89739.96

Slocum, J. M. (2007). Preconception counseling and type 2 diabetes. *Diabetes Spectrum, 20*(2), 117–123. doi:10.2337/diaspect.20.2.117

Slocum, J. M., & Sosa, M. E. B. (2002). Use of antidiabetes agents in pregnancy: Current practice and controversy. *Journal of Perinatal and Neonatal Nursing, 16*(2), 40–53.

Stage E., Norgard, H., Damm, P., & Mathiesen, E. (2006). Long-term breast-feeding in women with type 1 diabetes. *Diabetes Care, 29*(4), 771–774. doi:10.2337/diacare.29.04.06.dc05-1103

Straussman, S., & Levitsky, L. L. (2010). Neonatal hypoglycemia. *Current Opinion in Endocrinology, Diabetes & Obesity, 17*(1), 20–24. doi:10.1097/MED.0b013e328334f061

Sullivan, S. D., Umans, J. G., & Ratner, R. (2011). Hypertension complicating diabetic pregnancies: Pathophysiology, management, and controversies. *Journal of Clinical Hypertension, 13*(4), 275–284. doi:10.1111/j.1751-7176.2011.00440

Taylor, R., & Davison, J. M. (2007). Type 1 diabetes and pregnancy. *British Medical Journal, 334*(7596), 742–745. doi:10.1136/bmj.39154.700417.BE

Vandermolen, D. T., Ratts, V. S., Evans, W. S., Stovall, D. W., Kauma, S. W., & Nestler, J. E. (2001). Metformin increases the ovulatory rate and pregnancy rate from clomiphene citrate in patients with polycystic ovary syndrome who are resistant to clomiphene citrate alone. *Fertility and Sterility, 75*(2), 310–315.

Vanky, E., Stridsklev, S., Heimstad, R., Romunstad, P., Skogoy, K., Kleggetveit, O., . . . Carlsen, S. M. (2010). Metformin versus placebo from first trimester to delivery in polycystic ovary syndrome: A randomized, controlled multicenter study. *Journal of Clinical Endocrinology & Metabolism, 95*(12), E448–E455. doi:10.1210/jc.2010-0853

Villegas, R., Gao, Y. T., Yang, G., Li, H. L., Elasy, T., Zheng, W., & Shu, X. O. (2008). Duration of breast-feeding and the incidence of type 2 diabetes mellitus in the Shanghai Women's Health Study. *Diabetologia, 51*(2), 258–266. doi:10.1007/s00125-007-0885-8

Walsh, J., & Roberts, R. (2006). *Pumping Insulin* (4th ed). San Diego, CA: Torrey Pines Press.

White, P. (1949). Pregnancy complicating diabetes. *American Journal of Medicine, 7*, 609–616.

Yang, J., Cummings, E. A., O'Connell, C., & Jangaard, K. (2006). Fetal and neonatal outcomes of diabetic pregnancies. *Obstetrics and Gynecology, 108*(3, Pt. 1), 644–650. doi:10.1097/01.AOG.0000231688.08263.47

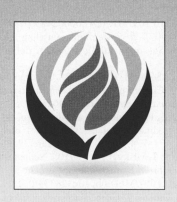

Julie Arafeh

CHAPTER 9

Cardiac Disease in Pregnancy

SIGNIFICANCE AND INCIDENCE

Cardiac disease is a factor in only 1% to 2% of pregnancies, yet it is now the leading cause of indirect pregnancy-related mortality in the United States. Indirect pregnancy-related mortality is defined as deaths from preexisting disease influenced by physiologic changes of pregnancy (Kuklina & Callaghan, 2011; Main, 2010). This trend has been detected in other developed countries, notably the United Kingdom and the Netherlands (Main, 2010). Approximately 10% to 25% of pregnancy-related deaths in the United States are associated with cardiac disease (Foley, Rokey, & Belfort, 2010). The prominence of cardiac disease in maternal mortality and morbidity is attributed to several factors. More women with congenital heart disease (CHD) are reaching childbearing age. Lifestyle trends such as delaying pregnancy until later in life, sedentary routine, obesity, and tobacco use all play a contributory role. The presence of other chronic medical conditions such as diabetes in conjunction with cardiac disease also increases the risk of complications during pregnancy (Bowater & Thorne, 2010; Harris, 2011; Jastrow et al., 2011; Kuklina & Callaghan, 2011). The conditions and complications described above, individually or in combination, place an additional burden on the cardiac muscle during pregnancy, labor, and birth, leading to increased risk.

The incidence of women with cardiac disease in the United States has not changed significantly since 1995; however, the morbidity of pregnant women hospitalized with cardiac disease appears to be increasing (Kuklina & Callaghan, 2011). A cross-sectional review of over 47,800,000 intrapartum and postpartum hospitalizations from across the United States during the years of 1995 to 2006 was undertaken to examine the prevalence

of chronic heart disease and to approximate the impact of chronic heart disease on severe obstetric morbidity. Steady increases were seen in CHD, valvular disease from rheumatic fever, cardiomyopathy and/or congestive heart failure (CHF), and cardiac arrhythmias (Kuklina & Callaghan, 2011). Examination of ICD-9-CM codes for CHD revealed more reports of septal defects, circulatory abnormalities, and valvular disorders while nonspecific congenital disease decreased (Kuklina & Callaghan, 2011). The incidence of cardiac arrest, sepsis, and fluid/electrolyte abnormalities all increased during intrapartum hospitalizations. The number of postpartum hospitalizations tripled, with CHD and cardiac arrhythmias/conduction disorders showing significant increases (Kuklina & Callaghan, 2011).

The impact of maternal cardiac function on the fetus and neonate has also been examined. In a study about the effect of maternal cardiac disease on fetal growth and neonatal outcomes, 331 women with cardiac disease were compared to 662 women without cardiac disease (Gelson et al., 2011). Both groups had similar incidence of maternal hypertension and illicit drug and tobacco use. Perinatal complications in the group with cardiac disease were 50% higher than the control group. The most common complications were small-for-gestational-age neonates and preterm birth. No difference in preterm premature rupture of membranes was seen between the two groups. Maternal characteristics most associated with fetal and neonatal adverse outcomes were decreased cardiac output, cyanosis, or a combination of the two (Gelson et al., 2011).

Earlier studies have also demonstrated the effect reduced maternal cardiac function has on fetal growth. Twenty cases of singleton pregnancies with severe fetal growth restriction were compared to 107 normal singleton pregnancies (Bamfo, Kametas, Turan, Khaw,

& Nicolaides, 2006). Two-dimensional and M-mode echocardiography was used to evaluate maternal cardiac function in both groups. Reduction in cardiac output and stroke volume was seen along with an increase in systemic vascular resistance in the group with severe fetal growth restriction as compared to pregnancies with normal fetal growth (Bamfo et al., 2006). Another study compared 302 pregnancies with cardiac disease to 572 pregnancies without cardiac disease for neonatal complications (Siu et al., 2002). Neonatal complications included small for gestational age (SGA), preterm birth, respiratory distress, intraventricular hemorrhage, and fetal or neonatal death. Neonatal complications occurred over 50% more often in the group with cardiac disease. The subgroup with the highest neonatal complication rate included women with cardiac disease who had the following characteristics: younger than 20 years or older than 35 years, obstetric risk factors, multiple gestation, smoker, anticoagulant therapy, and at least one cardiac risk factor present (Siu et al., 2002).

Despite the significantly increased risk of adverse outcomes, most pregnant women with cardiac disease do well. Careful planning and monitoring prior to, during, and after the pregnancy by an interdisciplinary healthcare team increases the likelihood that the best possible outcome will occur for the mother and baby (Arafeh & Baird, 2006). All members of the team need to possess a thorough understanding of normal cardiac anatomy and physiology, knowledge of how the physiologic changes of pregnancy will influence cardiac function and the mother's cardiac disease, the ability to estimate the risk pregnancy poses to the mother and her baby, and the ability to use the most recent and best knowledge to plan comprehensive care for the duration of the pregnancy, including follow-up in the postpartum period until the effects of pregnancy have resolved.

CARDIOVASCULAR PHYSIOLOGY

ANATOMY

The purpose of the cardiovascular system is to deliver nutrient-rich oxygenated blood and remove waste products in response to the metabolic needs of the body (Darovic, 2002a). The cardiovascular system functions with three components: the heart, an electrical conduction system, and a vascular distribution network. The heart has four muscular chambers: two atria or upper chambers and the lower chambers or ventricles. Chamber walls have three layers: the pericardium or sac that surrounds the heart, the myocardium or the muscular layer, and the endocardium or inner lining of the chambers, which forms the valves of the heart (Darovic, 2002a). Although considered one organ, the heart functions as two pumps. The right side of the heart pumps

deoxygenated blood to the lungs from the venous circulation (i.e., venous return → right atrium → right ventricle → pulmonary artery → pulmonary capillaries → pulmonary vein) (Blackburn, 2007). The left side of the heart receives oxygenated blood from the lungs and pumps it back to the systemic circulation (i.e., pulmonary vein → left atrium → left ventricle → aorta → systemic circulation) (Blackburn, 2007; Torgersen & Curran, 2006). There are four valves located in the heart that allow only forward flow when functioning normally. The two valves that connect the upper and lower chambers of the heart are called atrioventricular valves. The mitral valve is located on the left side of the heart, and the tricuspid valve is located on the right side. Semilunar valves attach the ventricles on each side of the heart to the large arteries they pump into; the pulmonic valve joins the right ventricle and pulmonary artery, and the aortic valve joins the left ventricle and the aorta. Figure 9–1 offers a conceptualization of the conduit of flow through the heart.

Once blood enters the systemic circulation, a fine meshwork of arteries and veins transport blood through the body. Arteries are muscular vessels that regulate blood flow based on cellular metabolic requirements. Veins return blood back to the heart and serve as a reservoir for as much as 70% of the circulating blood volume. Dilation or constriction of the venous bed occurs to accommodate the needs of the circulatory system. For example, in circumstances of low circulating blood volume, constriction of the veins can redistribute volume to augment circulation (Darovic, 2002a). Capillaries are thin-walled vessels with a large cross-sectional area where transfer of nutrients and metabolic waste occurs (Blackburn, 2007). The capillaries also regulate the distribution of extracellular fluid.

The conduction system in the cardiac muscle induces regular coordinated contractions between the upper and lower chambers of the heart to help optimize forward flow of blood. The sinoatrial (SA) node is in the

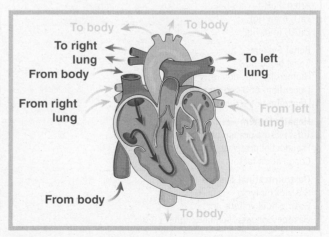

FIGURE 9–1. Linear illustration of blood flow through the heart. (From Association of Women's Health, Obstetric and Neonatal Nurses [AWHONN], 2009. Reprinted with permission.).

right atria and is established as the primary pacemaker of the heart, initiating and setting the pulse (Blackburn, 2007). The atrioventricular node offers backup if conduction through the SA node is impaired or damaged. The heart is innervated or stimulated by the autonomic nervous system (i.e., sympathetic and parasympathetic nervous systems). Nerve receptors in the heart are stimulated by the release of epinephrine and norepinephrine from the sympathetic nervous system. Stimulation of beta-adrenergic receptors results in an increase in discharge from the SA node, augments the automaticity of cells in the heart, and improves contractility of the atria and ventricles (Darovic, 2002a). During pregnancy, the occurrence of arrhythmias is more frequent regardless of the presence of heart disease. For example,

approximately 1.3% of women without heart disease will experience sustained supraventricular tachycardia during pregnancy (Szumowski et al., 2010).

The cardiovascular system undergoes tremendous physiologic change during pregnancy to support the growing fetus and prepare the mother for birth. The tissues of the heart go through a remodeling process during pregnancy that results in enlargement or hypertrophy and expansion of the capillary bed to supply adequate oxygenation for the increased workload. These changes are similar to those seen with endurance training (Cruz, Briller, & Hibbard, 2010; Vitarelli & Capotosto, 2011). Other systems in the body also experience significant physiologic changes. See Table 9–1 for a summary of the major changes associated with normal pregnancy.

Table 9–1. NORMAL PHYSIOLOGIC CHANGES OF PREGNANCY

Body System	Change
Cardiovascular System	
Total blood volume	Increased 30%–50% (1,450–1,750 mL)
Plasma volume	Increased 40%–60% (1,200–1,600 mL)
Red cell volume	Increased 20%–32% (250–450 mL)
Cardiac output	Increased 40%–45% (positional)
Heart rate	Increased 15%–20% (10–20 bpm)
Systolic blood pressure	Unchanged (dependent on patient position and gestation of pregnancy)
Diastolic blood pressure	Decreased 10–15 mm Hg 24–32 weeks
Systemic vascular resistance	Decreased 20%–30%
Central venous pressure	Unchanged
Pulmonary capillary wedge pressure	Unchanged
Ejection fraction	Unchanged
Left ventricular stroke work index	Unchanged
Uterine blood flow	Increased 20%–40% depending on gestation
Respiratory System	
Minute ventilation	Increased 30%–50%
Alveolar ventilation	Increased 50%–70%
Tidal volume	Increased 30%–40% (500–700 mL)
Respiratory rate	Unchanged
Functional residual capacity	Decreased 20%–30%
Residual volume	Decreased 20%–30%
Oxygen consumption	Increased 20% (up to 60% increase during labor)
Arterial pH	Slightly increased (average 7.40–7.45)
PaO_2 (mm Hg)	Increased (101–104 mm Hg)
$PaCO_2$ (mm Hg)	Decreased (27–32 mm Hg)
Renal System	
Renal blood flow	Increased 50% (by fourth month)
Glomerular filtration rate	Increased 50% (by fourth month)
Upper limit of blood urea nitrogen	Decreased 50%
Upper limit of serum creatinine	Decreased 50%
Hepatic System	
Total plasma protein concentration	Decreased 20%
Pseudocholinesterase concentration	Decreased
Coagulation factors	Variable
Gastrointestinal System	
Gastric emptying	Delayed
Gastric fluid volume	Unchanged
Gastroesophageal sphincter tone	Decreased

Data from Bobrowski, R. A. (2010). Maternal–fetal blood gas physiology. In M. Belfort, G. Saade, M. Foley, J. Phelan, & G. Dildy (Eds.), *Critical Care Obstetrics* (5th ed., pp. 53–68). Oxford, UK: Wiley-Blackwell; Norwitz, E. R., & Robinson, J. N. (2010). Pregnancy-induced physiologic alterations. In M. Belfort, G. Saade, M. Foley, J. Phelan, & G. Dildy (Eds.), *Critical Care Obstetrics* (5th ed., pp. 30–52). Oxford, UK: Wiley-Blackwell.

HEMODYNAMICS AND CARDIAC OUTPUT

The movement of blood through the body is essential for life. A major component of the movement of blood or hemodynamics is cardiac output. Cardiac output can be defined as the amount of blood pumped through the heart and is measured in liters per minute (Darovic, Graham, & Pranulis, 2002). Cardiac output is determined by four variables: preload, afterload, contractility, and heart rate. Normal hemodynamic values in pregnancy are listed in Table 9–2. Preload is the volume of blood in the ventricle or tension placed on the myocardial fibers as contraction begins at end-diastole. Preload is primarily influenced by circulating blood volume available to fill the ventricle (Darovic, 2002b). If the volume of blood returning to the heart is diminished, as in hypotension, the subsequent decrease in preload reduces cardiac output. The cardiac muscle has the intrinsic ability to respond to variances in filling pressures, which allows for healthy adaptation to stress. This adaptation is challenged by the 2 to 3 L/min and 40% to 50% overall rise in cardiac output during pregnancy (Bonow et al., 2006). A commensurate increase in cardiac output usually peaks between the midportion of the second and third trimesters (Bonow et al., 2006). Preload is reported as central venous pressure in the right side of the heart and as pulmonary capillary wedge pressure in the left side of the heart (Darovic, 2002b; Darovic & Kumar, 2002).

Afterload is defined as the resistance the ventricle has to overcome to eject blood during systole (Darovic, 2002b). Afterload the right ventricle pumps against is expressed by pulmonary artery pressure or pulmonary vascular resistance. Systemic vascular resistance or the patient's blood pressure provides afterload to the left ventricle. During pregnancy, the influence of progesterone is thought to decrease peripheral vascular resistance, thereby decreasing afterload. As a result, a drop in blood pressure during the second trimester is a common finding (Norwitz & Robinson, 2010).

Contractility is an independent intrinsic ability of the cardiac muscle to shorten aside from influences by preload and afterload (Darovic, 2002b). Contractility is measured indirectly by the left ventricular stroke work index. Heart rate is the final component of cardiac output. The speed at which the cardiac muscle pumps can influence output either positively or negatively. Excessively high heart rates lead to a decrease in filling time of the ventricles and reduction in output. Typically during trauma, dysfunction, or disease, the human heart will alter heart rate (i.e., pulse) prior to detectable influences on any of the other remaining parameters (Belfort, Saade, Foley, Phelan, & Dildy, 2010). In cases of severe hypovolemia, the heart rate may rise appreciably before changes in the peripheral vascular resistance (i.e., blood pressure) are evident. Therefore, blood pressure and pulse are two vital signs reflective of cardiac output and cardiac disease. As a result, accuracy of assessment for both parameters and careful evaluation of trends is a key part of thorough patient assessment.

CARDIAC ADAPTATIONS OF PREGNANCY

Normal pregnancies may precipitate signs and symptoms of dizziness, dyspnea, orthopnea, fatigue, syncope, rales in the lower lung fields, jugular vein distention, systolic murmurs, dysrhythmias, and cardiomegaly (Blanchard & Shabetai, 2004; Torgersen & Curran, 2006). For this reason, it can be difficult to determine whether symptoms experienced by the mother are normal changes found in pregnancy or an indication of cardiac disease. Table 9–3 outlines normal cardiac changes during pregnancy compared to abnormal signs and symptoms of cardiac disease. Symptoms indicative of heart disease include severe dyspnea; syncope with exertion; hemoptysis; paroxysmal nocturnal dyspnea; cyanosis; clubbing; diastolic murmurs; sustained cardiac arrhythmias; loud, harsh systolic murmurs; and chest pain with exertion (Blanchard & Shabetai, 2004). Prompt intervention is warranted if signs or symptoms abnormal for pregnancy are present.

The physiologic changes of pregnancy that tend to be problematic for women with cardiac disease include the increase in blood volume, decrease in systemic vascular resistance, the hypercoagulable state of pregnancy, and fluctuations in cardiac output (Foley et al., 2010). The increase in blood volume may be problematic for women with stenotic heart valves, impaired ventricular function, or congenital artery disease. The inability of the heart to handle the extra volume can lead to failure or an ischemic event. In diseases associated with weakened arterial vessels such as Marfan syndrome or

Table 9–2. NORMAL HEMODYNAMIC VALUES IN LATE PREGNANCY

Parameter	Value and Standard Deviation
Cardiac output (L/min)	6.2 ± 1.0
Systemic vascular resistance (dyne/sec/cm-5)	1,210 ± 266
Pulmonary vascular resistance (dyne/sec/cm-5)	78 ± 22
Mean arterial pressure (mm Hg)	90 ± 6
Pulmonary capillary wedge pressure (mm Hg)	8 ± 2
Central venous pressure (mm Hg)	4 ± 3
Left ventricular stroke index (g/m/m-2)	48 ± 6

Data from Norwitz, E. R., & Robinson, J. N. (2010). Pregnancy-induced physiologic alterations. In M. Belfort, G. Saade, M. Foley, J. Phelan, & G. Dildy (Eds.), *Critical Care Obstetrics* (5th ed., pp. 30–52). Oxford, UK: Wiley-Blackwell.

Table 9-3. NORMAL PREGNANCY SYMPTOMS VERSUS SYMPTOMS OF CARDIAC DISEASE

Pregnancy: May Be Present	Cardiac Disease from Any Cause: May Be Present
• Fatigue • Exertional dyspnea (usually limited to third trimester) • Irregular or infrequent syncope • Palpations (brief, irregular, and asymptomatic) • Jugular venous distention • Mild tachycardia <15% rise • Third heart sound • Grade II/VI systolic murmur • Pedal edema	• Decreased ability to perform activities of daily living • Severe breathlessness, orthopnea, paroxysmal nocturnal dyspnea, cough, or syncope • Chest pain (not normal in pregnancy) • Systemic hypotension • Cyanosis, clubbing • Persistent jugular venous distention • Sinus tachycardia >15% normal heart rate • Fourth heart sound • Ventricular murmurs • Pulmonary edema • Pleural effusion

Data from Curran, C. (2002). Multiple organ dysfunction syndrome (MODS) in the obstetrical population. *Journal of Perinatal & Neonatal Nursing, 15*(4), 37–55; Thorne, S. A. (2004). Pregnancy in heart disease. *Heart, 90*(4), 450–456. doi:10.1136/hrt.2003.027888

coarctation, the pressure from extra blood volume may cause an aneurysm or dissection (Curry, Swan, & Steer, 2009; Foley et al., 2010).

Decrease in systemic vascular resistance is problematic for women with abnormal connections between the right and left heart or shunts. Typically, the left side of the heart is under higher pressure than the right side of the heart due to the task of pumping blood to the large systemic circulation against the pressure of the systemic vascular resistance. In this situation, oxygenated blood will shunt through defects between the two sides of the heart from the left side to the right side. In the short term, this can be tolerated by the heart and the body as oxygenated blood is being recirculated through the lungs. When the systemic vascular resistance drops in pregnancy, this dynamic can change, with potential for blood to shunt from the right side of the heart to the left. In this case, deoxygenated blood is contributing to cardiac output, ultimately resulting in decreased oxygen content in arterial blood (Foley et al., 2010).

The hypercoagulable state of pregnancy increases the risk of clot formation for women with artificial heart valves and some forms of arrhythmia. Particularly in atrial fibrillation, blood can collect and clots can form in the atria due to ineffective emptying from the lack of coordinated atrial and ventricular contractions. The need to achieve anticoagulation can increase the risk of postpartum hemorrhage following birth (Foley et al., 2010). Finally, the dynamic changes in cardiac output throughout pregnancy can precipitate a crisis when disease is present that requires a constant amount of blood volume to maintain output, as in pulmonary hypertension, or when the cardiac output is fixed, as in mitral stenosis.

During pregnancy, cardiac output steadily increases until it is nearly double. The following changes in cardiac output occur during the active phase of labor: increases 17% at ≤3 cm dilated, 23% from 4 to 7 cm

dilated, and 34% at ≥8 cm dilated (Blackburn, 2007). Uterine contractions may enhance cardiac output by as much as 15% to 20% due to the increased metabolic demands (Barth, 2009; Belfort et al., 2010). Uterine contractions can result in marked increases in both systolic and diastolic blood pressure (Bonow et al., 2006). The first 15 minutes following evacuation of the uterus at birth includes a return of approximately 600 to 800 mL of uterine blood to the maternal vascular compartment. Therefore, immediate postpartum is one of the most stressful times (from the standpoint of the cardiovascular system) of all pregnancy, labor, and birth, with a 65% maximum increase in cardiac output (Blackburn, 2007; Foley et al., 2010).

OBSTETRIC OUTCOMES AND ASSESSMENT OF RISK

When the woman with cardiac disease presents prenatally or ideally for preconception counseling, estimating the risk pregnancy and birth poses to her and her baby is an important part of counseling and developing a plan of care. Risk may occur from cardiac disease as well as other factors such as obesity, tobacco use, and presence of other chronic disease states. Assessment of the risk that cardiac disease presents can be evaluated by different methods. While it may seem redundant to routinely use each method, given the relative rarity of cardiac disease in pregnancy and lack of established guidelines to manage cardiac disease in pregnancy, it may be worthwhile to examine risk to the woman from the perspective of each method. The first method is the New York Heart Association (NYHA) Functional Classification (Table 9–4). This is the oldest of the three methods and is based on the functional ability of the person with cardiac disease, regardless of what that disease may be. The patient is assessed either by questioning or direct observation of symptoms in response to activity.

Table 9–4. NEW YORK HEART ASSOCIATION FUNCTIONAL CLASSIFICATION SYSTEM

Class	Description
I	Asymptomatic No limitation of physical activity
II	Asymptomatic at rest; symptomatic with heavy physical activity and exertion Slight limitation of physical activity
III	Asymptomatic at rest; symptomatic with minimal or normal physical activity Considerable limitation of physical activity
IV	Symptomatic at rest; symptomatic with any physical activity Severe limitation of physical activity

American Heart Association, Inc. http://www.heart.org. Reprinted with permission.

Symptoms of interest include dyspnea, chest pain, and shortness of breath. This risk assessment is particularly helpful in pregnancy to document changes in functional status that are expected in response to the physiologic changes of pregnancy. Progression to a higher NYHA classification should prompt further evaluation due to the association with higher maternal mortality. Determining functional classification on a regular basis such as during prenatal visits, frequently during labor, and with each postpartum assessment can uncover a trend that may indicate a decline in status.

Mortality risk can be estimated based on the type of lesion or disease present. In Display 9–1, cardiac disease is divided into three groups based on a combination of several risk estimates and appropriate management by a team knowledgeable in providing care to women with cardiac disease. Group I consists of lesions that generally have a low mortality rate. Group II have moderate risk of an adverse event with a higher mortality rate of 5% to 15%. The risk of complications is considerable in Group III, with an estimated mortality rate in excess of 25%. In the majority of cases, women who are in Group III may be counseled that the risk of achieving or continuing pregnancy is too great to consider (Foley et al., 2010).

In Display 9–2, Siu and colleagues (2001) offer additional guidance regarding potential risk of a cardiac event during pregnancy; 562 women with cardiac disease were followed during pregnancy to determine occurrence of cardiac events. Cardiac events were divided into two groups: primary and secondary. A primary cardiac event was defined as pulmonary edema, persistent symptomatic tachycardia or bradycardia necessitating treatment, stroke, cardiac arrest, or cardiac death. Secondary cardiac events included decrease in functional ability as defined by the NYHA classification and the need for emergent invasive cardiac procedures during pregnancy through 6 months postpartum

DISPLAY 9–1

Mortality Risk Associated with Pregnancy

GROUP I: MORTALITY <1%
- Atrial septal defect
- Ventricular septal defect (uncomplicated)
- Patent ductus arteriosus
- Pulmonic and tricuspid disease
- Corrected Tetralogy of Fallot
- Biosynthetic valve prosthesis (porcine and human allograft)
- Mitral stenosis, New York Heart Association (NYHA) Class I & Class II
- Marfan syndrome (normal aorta)

GROUP II: MORTALITY 5%–15%
- Mitral stenosis with atrial fibrillation
- Mechanical valve prosthesis
- Mitral stenosis, NYHA Class III or NYHA Class IV
- Aortic stenosis
- Coarctation of the aorta (uncomplicated)
- Uncorrected Tetralogy of Fallot
- Previous myocardial infarction

GROUP III: MORTALITY 25%–50%
- Eisenmenger syndrome
- Pulmonary hypertension
- Coarctation of the aorta (complicated)
- Marfan syndrome with aortic involvement

Data from Foley, M. R., Rokey, R., & Belfort, M. A. (2010). Cardiac disease. In M. Belfort, G. Saade, M. Foley, J. Phelan, & G. Dildy (Eds.), *Critical Care Obstetrics* (5th ed., pp. 256–282). Oxford, UK: Wiley-Blackwell.

DISPLAY 9–2

Predictors of Cardiac Events

Prior cardiac event before pregnancy
Heart failure
   Stroke or transient ischemic attack
Arrhythmia
New York Heart Association >Class II
Cyanosis
Obstruction left heart
Gradient >30 peak
Aortic valve <1.5 cm
Mitral valve prolapse <2 cm
Ejection fraction <40%
Number of predictors equals risk of cardiac events during pregnancy: 0 = 5%, 1 = 27%, >1 = 75%

Data from Siu, S. C., Sermer, M., Colman, J. M., Alvarez, A. N., Mercier, L. A., Morton, B. C., & Sorensen, S. (2001). Prospective multicenter study of pregnancy outcomes in women with heart disease. *Circulation*, 104(5), 515–521. doi:10.1161/ hc3001.093437; Thorne, S. A. (2004). Pregnancy in heart disease. *Heart*, 90(4), 450–456. doi:10.1136/hrt.2003.027888.

(Siu et al., 2001). Four predictors of events were identified: previous cardiac complication or arrhythmia, presence of cyanosis or NYHA Class II or greater at the beginning of pregnancy, left heart obstruction, and decreased left ventricle function. As the number of predictors that are present increase, so does the risk of a cardiac event. If the patient's cardiac history has all four predictors, then a healthcare provider should counsel the women to reconsider attempting pregnancy. It should also be noted that even with no predictors present, risk of having an event is assessed at 5% (Siu et al., 2001).

Drenthen and colleagues (2010) used the risk assessment tool just described in 1,302 pregnancies complicated with CHD. Arrhythmias and heart failure were the most common cardiac events noted in this cohort. When comparing the risk assessment tool prediction to outcomes, it was found that risk was overestimated. The authors caution that use of a risk assessment tool be merely one part of a comprehensive evaluation of the woman and her specific cardiac disease (Drenthen et al., 2010). Other types of parameters may be used to determine risk. One such parameter is serum B-type natriuretic peptide (BNP). BNP levels increase in conjunction with worsening heart failure in nonpregnant cardiac patients under circumstances that are similar to pregnancy. A study of 78 pregnant women was conducted, 66 with heart disease and 12 without, that followed BNP levels throughout pregnancy. BNP levels were low throughout pregnancy in the group without heart disease. Elevations in BNP were not conclusively predictive of a cardiac event, but levels of less than 100 pg/mL in women with cardiac disease was found to have a negative predictive value of 100% (Tanous et al., 2010).

The risk of cardiac events late after birth can also be predicted. Balint and colleagues (2010) reviewed 405 pregnancies to determine characteristics predictive of cardiac events that occur more than 6 months after birth. Late events included cardiac arrest/death, pulmonary edema, arrhythmia, and stroke. Characteristics associated with late events were NYHA Class II or higher, presence of cyanosis, subaortic ventricular dysfunction, subpulmonary ventricular dysfunction, pulmonary regurgitation, left heart obstruction, and cardiac complications before pregnancy (Balint et al., 2010). Evaluation for these characteristics can assist in determining how long to carefully assess and hospitalize the woman after birth as well as how to direct home instructions and guide frequency of follow-up after discharge.

CONGENITAL HEART DISEASE IN PREGNANCY

CHD occurs in approximately 0.8% of live births (Harris, 2011). Advances in neonatal care and pediatric cardiac surgery have resulted in a significant improvement in survival rates for babies born with CHD, and 85% of these infants can be expected to survive to adulthood (Gelson, Gatzoulis, Steer, & Johnson, 2009; Kafka, Johnson, & Gatzoulis, 2006). As these infants are coming of age, more women are beginning pregnancy with medical histories of significant cardiac surgical repairs from CHD (Kafka et al., 2006). Women with congenital heart defects are at increased risk of passing the defect to the baby. Maternal conditions (e.g., diabetes, lupus erythematosus, phenylketonuria, drug abuse), medication ingestion (e.g., Lithium, alcohol), genetics, or infections (e.g., rubella, rheumatic fever, viruses) may also result in structural defects in the fetal heart (Blanchard & Shabetai, 2004).

Blood flow is critical to the development of cardiac structures during the embryonic period. If flow through cardiac structures is limited or absent, abnormal development occurs. If flow restriction occurs in early gestation during fetal cardiac development, the specific region and structures "downstream" will become small (hypoplastic) or even completely absent (atretic) (Linker, 2001). As a result, one of four structural defects may develop: hole (defect), narrowing due to stiffness causing obstruction (stenosis), underdevelopment or absence (hypoplasia or atresia), or wrong connection (transposition, inversion, anomalous connection) (Linker, 2001).

For ease of discussion, congenital lesions will be categorized as acyanotic, cyanotic, or aortic.

ACYANOTIC CONGENITAL HEART DISEASE

Acyanotic lesions that involve an abnormal opening in the septum between the right and left side of the heart include atrial septal defect (ASD) and ventricular septal defect (VSD). Since pressures are typically higher on the left side of the heart, blood flows from left to right, as described earlier. Long-term shunting of extra blood volume to the right side of the heart can cause right ventricular hypertrophy. Extension of that enlargement into the right atrium increases the risk of atrial arrhythmias (Harris, 2011). Large septal defects, particularly VSD, can result in hypertension in the pulmonary circulation. Development of pulmonary hypertension can create bidirectional flow or a reverse of the shunt where blood flows from the right to the left side of the heart due to the resistance or afterload exerted by the pulmonary vasculature. This change in shunt flow results in Eisenmenger syndrome and is associated with cyanosis due to deoxygenated blood contributing to cardiac output, leading to poor outcomes during pregnancy. For this reason, large septal defects are usually repaired in childhood (Foley et al., 2010; Harris, 2011). Septal defects also create portals for emboli movement and increase the risk of thromboembolytic injury to the arterial circulation (Linker, 2001). Other acyanotic lesions include pulmonic and aortic stenosis. The degree of stenosis or narrowing of the valve determines the impact on blood flow and cardiac output (Foley et al., 2010; Harris, 2011).

CYANOTIC CONGENITAL HEART DISEASE

Cyanotic cardiac lesions include Tetralogy of Fallot (TOF), transposition of the great vessels, and lesions with a single functioning ventricle (Harris, 2011). TOF consists of four defects: (1) ventricular septal defect (VSD); (2) overriding aorta: dextroposition of the aorta so that the aortic orifice sits astride the VSD and overrides the right ventricle; (3) right ventricular hypertrophy; and (4) pulmonary stenosis (Blanchard & Shabetai, 2004; Foley et al., 2010). The majority of patients with TOF will have correction of the VSD during childhood (Foley et al., 2010; Harris, 2011). Although closure of the VSD will decrease risk during pregnancy, significant arrhythmias and conduction defects may still occur (Harris, 2011). Uncorrected TOF is associated with a higher rate of maternal morbidity and poorer prognosis for the fetus (Foley et al., 2010).

Transposition of the great vessels occurs in two varieties: levo-transposition (L-TGA) and dextro-transposition (D-TGA) (Foley et al., 2010; Harris, 2011). In L–TGA, the vessels along with the atria and ventricles are switched. This type of TGA is described as congenitally corrected. L–TGA may not be detected until later in life, while D–TGA results in cyanosis soon after birth. In D–TGA, only the great vessels are reversed. D– TGA requires surgical intervention to restore delivery of oxygenated blood to the systemic circulation. The original surgical reversal procedure involved an atrial switch, while more recent procedures perform an arterial switch. Prognosis for the mother and fetus depend on the type of TGA, the type of corrective surgery performed, and functional cardiac status (Foley et al., 2010; Harris, 2011). Close collaboration between cardiology and obstetric care providers is required to determine current cardiac function and prognosis.

Congenital defects that result in a single ventricle such as hypoplastic left heart or tricuspid atresia require palliative surgery known as the Fontan procedure. Fontan circulation diverts blood from the venous circulation into the pulmonary circulation and utilizes the single ventricle as the "left" ventricle for systemic circulation. The surgical procedure may vary due to the underlying lesion that requires correction. Due to the altered cardiac circulation and hemodynamics, care of the pregnant woman who has undergone a Fontan procedure should occur in a facility with comprehensive experience in cardiac disease in pregnancy (Foley et al., 2010; Harris, 2011).

AORTIC CONGENITAL HEART DISEASE

Diseases of the aorta include Marfan syndrome (MFS) and coarctation. Coarctation of the aorta is an area of narrowing and is usually associated with hypertension of the upper extremities (Foley et al., 2010; Harris, 2011). Treatment can be challenging when trying to control upper extremity hypertension and still maintain adequate perfusion to the uterus and fetus (Harris, 2011). It is important to determine if the coarctation is complicated or uncomplicated. An uncomplicated coarctation is one that has no aneurysm or other lesion such as VSD that can affect hemodynamics (Foley et al., 2010). While uncomplicated coarctation carries mortality risk during pregnancy of 3% to 4%, the mortality rate for complicated coarctation can reach as high as 15%. The main complications associated with coarctation include aortic dissection, aneurysm, and rupture. If indicated, corrective surgery should precede pregnancy; otherwise, blood pressure titration can be attempted (Foley et al., 2010).

MFS is a connective tissue disorder that is inherited as an autosomal dominant trait. Effect of the disorder on the cardiovascular system is the leading cause of death, although connective tissue from other organ systems may also be affected (Goland, Barakat, Khatri, & Elkayam, 2009). In MFS, connective tissue is weakened and, in the case of the aorta, can expand under the constant pressure of blood being pumped from the left ventricle. The expansion further weakens the aorta, making it vulnerable to dissection or rupture. The alterations in hemodynamics during pregnancy can exacerbate the effect. However, aortic involvement such as aortic root dilation, dissection, and rupture are the most significant complications for any person with MFS (Goland et al., 2009). The risk of aortic dissection is based on the amount of dilation that has occurred. Risk is assessed at 10% when the aorta is 4.0 cm or greater; however, it should be noted that dissection has occurred with a normal-sized aortic root (Goland et al., 2009).

Ideally, the woman with MFS should undergo careful evaluation by a multidisciplinary team prior to pregnancy. The size of the ascending aorta is a key assessment. Usual medical treatment for a patient with a normal-sized aorta is the use of beta-blockers such as atenolol to reduce the velocity of the arterial pulse wave and increase vascular distensibility (Goland et al., 2009). Currently, it is recommended that surgical treatment occur if the diameter of the aorta is greater than or equal to 5.0 cm if the woman is not pregnant and greater than or equal to 4.7 cm in the pregnant woman (Barth, 2009). The size of the ascending aorta should be followed regularly throughout pregnancy because surgery may also be recommended if rapid dilation is noted. Vaginal birth is preferred for women with a normal-sized aorta, and cesarean birth is recommended when the aorta is dilated greater than or equal to 4.0 cm or is unstable (Goland et al., 2009).

CHD varies in pathology and symptomatology with various surgical and medical treatments utilized to improve cardiac function. Therefore, it is the responsibility of healthcare providers to carefully assess the risk of pregnancy and be watchful for signs of deterioration of status. Close collaboration between pediatric cardiology and obstetric care providers supports development of a comprehensive, thorough, and individual plan of care (Gelson et al., 2009).

ACQUIRED CARDIAC DISEASE IN PREGNANCY

Acquired cardiac disease or disease that develops after birth is a growing contributor to maternal mortality and morbidity. In some reports, acquired disease such as myocardial infarction (MI) is one of the leading causes of maternal mortality (Foley et al., 2010; Gelson et al., 2009). Acquired cardiac lesions that will be discussed include valvular disorders, MI, and cardiomyopathy.

VALVULAR DISORDERS

Infection is a leading cause of acquired valvular disease. Etiology includes diseases such as rheumatic fever and endocarditis. In developed countries, by the early 1900s, the incidence of rheumatic cardiac lesions dropped significantly due to better environmental conditions and medical treatment of rheumatic fever; however, this has not occurred in developing countries (Raju & Turi, 2011). In areas with a greater population of women immigrating from developing countries, rheumatic lesions are commonly seen (Bowater & Thorne, 2010; Curry et al., 2009; Foley et al., 2010; Madazli, Sal, Cift, Guralp, & Goymen, 2010). The lesion typically seen on valves from endocarditis is described as a mass of cells on the valve or on the surrounding tissue that includes inflammatory cells, microorganisms, fibrin, and platelets. Endocarditis can occur following intravenous (IV) drug abuse, hospital infections, or invasive medical procedures such as central line placement or hemodialysis (Karchmer, 2011). In fact, IV drug abuse results in a higher risk of infective endocarditis than either presence of a prosthetic valve or rheumatic cardiac disease (Karchmer, 2011). Due to the variety of presentations of valvular disease, thorough evaluation and risk assessment should be accomplished and discussed with the woman (Elkayam & Bitar, 2005a). In cases where valvular disease is advanced, valvular surgery or replacement may be advised before attempting pregnancy or during the course of pregnancy if the woman's clinical condition deteriorates (Barth, 2009; Elkayam & Bitar, 2005a). Replacement valves may be mechanical or bioprosthetic. It was thought that bioprosthetic valves deteriorate more rapidly during pregnancy, but this is currently under debate (Barth, 2009; Curry et al., 2009).

Replacement valves are associated with clot formation and require anticoagulation therapy to decrease this risk. Situations associated with the highest risk of clot formation are presence of older model prosthetic valves such as Starr-Edwards or Bjork Shiley replacing the mitral valve, prior history of clot formation on anticoagulants, or presence of atrial dysrhythmia. Lower risk of clot formation is associated with newer valves such as St. Jude or Medtronic-Hall valves replacing the aortic valve (Barth, 2009). In general, any woman on anticoagulant therapy before pregnancy will need to continue anticoagulation during pregnancy. Unfractionated heparin or low molecular weight heparin are routinely used during pregnancy because they do not cross the placenta and affect the fetus (Bates et al., 2012). However, the majority of patients with artificial heart valves are anticoagulated with warfarin because it is associated with the lowest risk of clot formation (Foley et al., 2010). Warfarin does cross the placenta to the fetus. In pregnancy, warfarin may be used cautiously in women with the highest risk of clot formation due to teratogenic effects early in gestation and risk of fetal hemorrhage late in gestation (Elkayam & Bitar, 2005b; Foley et al., 2010). See Table 9–5 for recommended anticoagulation therapy.

MYOCARDIAL INFARCTION

Acute MI is infrequent during pregnancy, with the highest risk of occurrence in the third trimester and in older (more than 33 years) multigravidas (Blanchard & Shabetai, 2004; Curry et al., 2009; Poh & Lee, 2010; Thorne, 2004). Although rare, MI is now recognized as a growing cause of maternal mortality

Table 9–5. RECOMMENDATIONS FOR ANTICOAGULATION DURING PREGNANCY

Drug Regimens

LMWH bid during pregnancy (dose-adjusted). Adjust dose based on manu'acturer's peak anti-Xa LMWH 4 hr post SC injection

or

UFH during pregnancy (dose-adjusted), given SC every 12 hr with mid-interval aPTT at least twice control or maintain anti-Xa heparin level at 0.35–0.70 U/mL

or

UFH or LMWH as described above until 13 weeks' gestation, then replace with vitamin K antagonist until near delivery when UFH or LMWH is resumed.

anti-Xa, IU/mL; aPTT, activated partial thromboplastin time; LMWH, low molecular weight heparin; SC, subcutaneous; UFH, unfractionated heparin.

Data from Bates, S. M., Greer, I. A., Middeldorp, S., Veenstra, D. L., Prabulos, A., & Vandvik, P. O. (2012). VTE, thrombophilia, antithrombotic therapy, and pregnancy: Antithrombotic therapy and prevention of thrombosis, 9th ed: American College of Chest Physicians evidence-based clinical practice guidelines. *Chest, 141*(2 Suppl.), e691S–e736S. doi:10.1378/chest.11-2300

(Poh & Lee, 2010). Risk factors for MI in pregnancy include typical causes such as high blood pressure, use of tobacco, and diabetes mellitus as well as causes specific to pregnancy such as postpartum infection, presence of thrombophilia, and blood transfusion (Poh & Lee, 2010). The anterior wall is the most frequent lesion site (Foley et al., 2010; Roth & Elkayam, 1996). Mortality risk and frequency is greatest if the MI occurs during the third trimester or if birth occurs within 2 weeks of the infarct (Blanchard & Shabetai, 2004; Foley et al., 2010; Poh & Lee, 2010; Roth & Elkayam, 1996; Thorne, 2004). Cardiac troponin I is unaffected by pregnancy, labor, or birth and therefore is the laboratory measurement of choice in the diagnosis of acute coronary syndrome during pregnancy (Poh & Lee, 2010; Thorne, 2004). The most important therapy for MI is reperfusion of the cardiac muscle as quickly as possible. This may be accomplished by performing percutaneous coronary intervention (PCI), thrombolytic therapy, or coronary artery bypass grafting. Of the three, PCI appears to be the preferred treatment if it can be provided in the appropriate time frame (Barth, 2009; Curry et al., 2009; Poh & Lee, 2010). The major problem with this therapy is the need for anticoagulation following stent placement. Close consultation between obstetric and cardiac providers needs to occur to determine the best course of action for each individual woman (Foley et al., 2010; Poh & Lee, 2010).

CARDIOMYOPATHY

Cardiomyopathy is a disease of the heart muscle resulting in failure. There are different types and causes of cardiomyopathy. Discussion in this chapter will be confined to peripartum cardiomyopathy (PPCM). PPCM is defined as cardiac failure with left ventricular ejection fraction <45% occurring in the last month of pregnancy or within 5 months of delivery, in the absence of any identifiable cause of heart failure; thus, PPCM is a diagnosis of exclusion (Belfort et al., 2010; Cruz et al., 2010; Curry et al., 2009; Foley et al., 2010; Pearson et al., 2000). The cause of PPCM is unknown but has been attributed to viral disease, autoimmune disorder, inflammatory process mediated by cytokines, abnormal apoptosis, genetic inheritance, and excessive levels of prolactin, among others. An occurrence rate of 1:3,000 to 15,000, depending on geographic location, makes this condition rare (Cruz et al., 2010; Pearson et al., 2000; Thorne, 2004). Risk factors include age >30 years, multiparity, twin pregnancy, race (African and African American reported to have higher incidence), and pregnancy-associated hypertension (Cruz et al., 2010; Foley et al., 2010). Diagnosis requires a careful history and physical, NYHA functional classification, electrocardiogram, and echocardiogram. Approximately 30% of women with PPCM will completely recover, with the remaining 70% left with residual effects of varying severity (Cruz et al., 2010; Curry et al., 2009). Management includes optimization of cardiac function with supportive therapies and pharmacologic treatment using diuretics, beta-blockers, vasodilators, and inotropic agents (Cruz et al., 2010; Foley et al., 2010). Vaginal birth is generally well tolerated (Cruz et al., 2010). Due to the delay in disease with occurrence in the third trimester or postpartum, fetal outcomes are usually positive.

CARDIAC TRANSPLANT

Reports of pregnancies in women with cardiac transplant are small in number. However, with maintenance of antirejection medical regimen, the reports are generally of successful pregnancies that have been noted with no reports of maternal mortality. These outcomes require well-coordinated, careful, multidisciplinary care throughout pregnancy (Barth, 2009; Foley et al., 2010).

CLINICAL MANAGEMENT

The underlying cardiac lesion, functional changes imposed by the lesion, maternal and fetal tolerance, and development of pregnancy-related complications affect perinatal morbidity and mortality. Developing baseline status of cardiac function through careful assessment and diagnostic testing such as echocardiography is crucial. Using this baseline for comparison during ongoing evaluation during pregnancy, labor, and the postpartum period guides the clinical management of women with cardiac disease (Vitarelli & Capotosto, 2011). A summary of common cardiac diseases, risk categories, and clinical management is presented in Table 9–6.

The goals of clinical management for a woman whose pregnancy is complicated by cardiovascular disease mirror the goals for optimum uteroplacental perfusion. Stabilization of the mother by maintaining cardiac output stabilizes the fetal compartment. Meeting these goals requires a coordinated multidisciplinary team approach. Management strategies should include estimates of maternal and fetal risk in order for the patient and her family to make an informed decision regarding her pregnancy. The primary practitioner should discuss issues regarding maternal age at the time of pregnancy, estimations of maternal and fetal mortality, potential chronic morbidity, antepartum interventions to minimize risk, and the birth method best suited to her underlying pathology (Arafeh & Baird, 2006; Blanchard & Shabetai, 2004).

The primary focus in cardiac management during pregnancy, labor, and birth maximizes cardiac output while limiting metabolic demand. Careful evaluation of the pregnant woman at each prenatal visit with regular

Table 9–6. CARDIAC DISEASE IN PREGNANCY

Cardiac Disease/Lesion	Risk Category	Description	Clinical Management
Atrial septal defect (ASD)	Small left-to-right shunt = low or minimal risk Large left-to-right shunt = intermediate or moderate risk Assess for pulmonary hypertension, ventricular dysfunction, arrhythmias, thromboembolisms	Most common congenital lesion seen during pregnancy	Physical examination systolic ejection murmur at left sternal border, wide split second heart sound Electrocardiogram (ECG): partial right bundle branch block, right axis deviation; possible right ventricular hypertrophy Common arrhythmias—atrial fibrillation or flutter Optimize preload—avoid hypovolemia or hypervolemia Oxygen during labor Avoid maternal hypotension—may increase left-to-right shunting Avoid maternal tachycardia—may increase left-to-right shunting Labor in lateral recumbent position Pain management: consider narcotic epidural Anticoagulation for thromboembolisms
Ventricular septal defect (VSD)	Small left-to-right shunt = low or minimal risk Large left-to-right shunt = intermediate or moderate risk Assess for presence of pulmonary hypertension, arrhythmias, and endocarditis	Size is the most important prognosticator for pregnancy: • Small → tolerated well • Larger defects → associated with CHF, arrhythmia, and development of pulmonary hypertension • Left-to-right shunt → burdens pulmonary circulation → can lead to pulmonary hypertension	Physical examination: holosystolic thrill and murmur at left sternal border ECG: normal in most patients Echocardiogram findings: left ventricular hypertrophy may suggest large left-to-right shunt; right ventricular hypertrophy may suggest pulmonary hypertension Optimize preload—avoid hypovolemia or hypervolemia Oxygen during labor Labor in lateral recumbent position Avoid maternal hypotension—may increase left-to-right shunting Avoid maternal tachycardia—may increase left-to-right shunting Bacterial endocarditis prophylaxis recommended if uncorrected or cyanotic Pain management: consider narcotic epidural
Eisenmenger syndrome	High or major risk Assess for ventricular dysfunction, arrhythmias	Left-to-right congenital shunt, progressive pulmonary hypertension leads to reversal of shunting Most common cause is large VSD	Avoid hypotension—decrease in systemic vascular resistance causes massive right-to-left shunting leading to hypoxia Avoid excessive blood loss Continuous oxygen therapy: • Keep $PaO_2 \geq 70$ mm Hg • Keep $SaO_2 > 90\%$ Maintain preload—manage on "wet" side Avoid conditions that increase pulmonary vascular resistance (PVR): • Metabolic acidosis • Excess catecholamine • Hypoxemia • Hypercapnia • Vasoconstrictors • Lung hyperinflation High risk for thromboembolism—consider anticoagulation Pain management: consider narcotic epidural Vigilant monitoring for up to 10 days postpartum

Table 9–6. CARDIAC DISEASE IN PREGNANCY (Continued)

Cardiac Disease/Lesion	Risk Category	Description	Clinical Management
Aortic coarctation	Uncorrected, uncomplicated = intermediate or moderate risk Complicated = high or major risk	Congenital narrowing of aorta; most common site is the origin of the left subclavian artery Associated anomalies: • VSD, patent ductus arteriosus (PDA), aortic aneurysm. Intracranial aneurysms of the Circle of Willis are relatively common	Avoid hypotension Consider assisted second stage of labor (vacuum or forceps) and/or "labor down" technique Avoid Valsalva maneuver during pushing Oxygen therapy during labor Bacterial endocarditis prophylaxis recommended Pain management: consider epidural anesthesia
Tetralogy of Fallot	Corrected = low or minimal risk Uncorrected = intermediate or moderate risk Assess for right ventricular obstruction or dysfunction, arrhythmias	Congenital complex of VSD, overriding aorta, right ventricular hypertrophy, and pulmonary stenosis; surgical correction by young adulthood common	Pregnancy discouraged in uncorrected Tetralogy of Fallot and/or with the following: • Hemoglobin level >20 g/L. • Hematocrit >0.65 • History of syncope or congestive heart failure • Cardiomegaly • Right ventricular (RV) pressure <120 mm Hg • Peripheral SaO_2 <85% Maintain preload and blood volume Avoid hypotension—decreased systemic vascular resistance may cause massive right-to-left shunting leading to hypoxia Bacterial endocarditis prophylaxis recommended Pain management: consider epidural anesthesia
Pulmonic stenosis	Low or minimal risk (increased transvalvular pressure gradient may increase risk)	Degree of obstruction rather than site of obstruction is determinant of clinical risk Transvalvular pressure gradient >80 mm Hg considered severe; severe stenosis can cause right-sided heart failure Peak pressure gradient, mm Hg Mild <50 Moderate 50–75 Severe >75	Optimize preload—avoid hypovolemia/hypervolemia Bacterial endocarditis prophylaxis recommended Pain management: consider epidural anesthesia
Mitral stenosis	NYHA Class I or II = Low or minimal risk NYHA Class III or IV = Intermediate or moderate risk Assess for pulmonary hypertension, atrial fibrillation, pulmonary edema	Most common rheumatic valvular lesion in pregnancy (25% of women first present in pregnancy) Scarring and fusion of valve apparatus Area, cm^2 Normal 4–6 Mild 1.5–2.5 Moderate 1.0–1.5 Severe <1 Pressure gradient, mm Hg Mild <5 Moderate 6–12 Severe >12 Left arterial obstruction results in enlargement of left atrium (LA) and right ventricle (RV) and possibly pulmonary hypertension Atrial fibrillation possibility Fixed cardiac output Ventricular diastolic filling obstruction	Physical examination: S1 is accentuated and snapping; low pitch diastolic rumble at the apex: presystolic accentuation Pulmonary artery catheter for NYHA Class III/IV Avoid hypotension—monitor BP with arterial line • Use phenylephrine 20–40 μg/kg/min (ephedrine will cause tachycardia) Optimize preload—pulmonary capillary wedge pressure (PCWP) is not an accurate reflection of left ventricular (LV) filling pressures • May require elevated PCWP to maintain cardiac output: intrapartum PCWP approximately 14 mm Hg; individualize PCWP that optimizes cardiac output • Maintain preload while avoiding pulmonary edema. Prepare for volume shift immediately following delivery—PCWP may rise >15 mm Hg. Avoid maternal tachycardia—may decrease cardiac output by decreasing left ventricular filling time • Consider β-blocker for pulse >90–100 • Avoid β-adrenergic tocolytics and/or other medications that increase heart rate Atrial fibrillation—anticoagulation, digoxin, antiarrhythmics Bacterial endocarditis prophylaxis recommended Assist second stage with vacuum or forceps; consider "labor down" technique Pain management: consider narcotic epidural

(continued)

Table 9–6. CARDIAC DISEASE IN PREGNANCY *(Continued)*

Cardiac Disease/Lesion	Risk Category	Description	Clinical Management

Aortic stenosis	NYHA Class I or II = Low or minimal risk
	NYHA Class III or IV = Intermediate or moderate risk
	Assess for left ventricular dysfunction or failure, arrhythmias
		Critical stenosis with orifice has diminished to one third or less or normal—leads to LV hypertrophy and failure: major issue is fixed cardiac output with critical stenosis; shunt gradients of >100 mm Hg are at the greatest risk
		Area, cm²
		  Normal 3–5
		  Mild 1–2
		  Moderate 0.75–1
		  Severe <0.75
		Maximum pressure gradient, mm Hg
		  Mild 16–36
		  Moderate 36–50
		  Moderate severe 50–75
		  Severe >75
		Mean pressure gradient, mm Hg
		  Mild <20
		  Moderate 20–35
		  Severe >35
			Physical examination: harsh systolic ejection murmur in second right intercostal space
			ECG: left ventricular hypertrophy and left atrial enlargement
			Pulmonary artery catheter prior to labor, during labor, first 24 hr postpartum
			Optimize preload—avoid hypovolemia
			• May require elevated PCWP to maintain cardiac output (intrapartum PCWP approximately 14–17 mm Hg)
			Avoid hypotension—decreased venous return will increase the valvular gradient and decrease cardiac output
			• Avoid/anticipate hemorrhage
			• Avoid supine position—risk of vena cava syndrome
			Avoid maternal tachycardia—may decrease cardiac output by decreasing left ventricular filling time
			• Consider β-blocker for pulse >90
			• Avoid β-adrenergic tocolytics and/or other medications that increase HR
			Oxygen during labor
			Bacterial endocarditis prophylaxis recommended
			Pain management: consider narcotic epidural; avoid spinal block

Idiopathic hypertrophic subaortic stenosis (IHSS)	Intermediate or moderate	Autosomal dominant inheritance Asymmetric LV hypertrophy (especially of septum) Obstruction of LV outflow and secondary mitral regurgitation	Avoid hypotension—decreased venous return will increase the valvular gradient and decrease cardiac output • Avoid/anticipate hemorrhage • Avoid supine position—risk of vena cava syndrome Pulmonary artery catheter prior to labor, during labor, first 24 hr postpartum Optimize preload—avoid hypovolemia • May require elevated PCWP to maintain cardiac output (intrapartum PCWP approximately 14–17 mm Hg) Avoid tachycardia—may worsen obstruction • Avoid β-adrenergic tocolytics and/or other medications that increase HR Consider assisted second stage of labor (vacuum or forceps) and/or "labor down" technique • Avoid Valsalva maneuver during pushing Bacterial endocarditis prophylaxis recommended Pain management: consider narcotic epidural; avoid spinal block
Marfan syndrome	Normal aortic root/<4 cm = low or minimal risk (5%) Enlarged aortic root/≥4 cm or valve involvement = high or major risk (up to 50%)	Autosomal dominant; generalized connective tissue weakness Can result in aneurysm formation, rupture, and dissection Sixty percent may also have mitral or aortic regurgitation	Echocardiogram needed to determine aortic root involvement Avoid maternal tachycardia—may increase shearing force on the aorta • Consider β-blocker if maternal HR >90 beats per minute • Avoid β-adrenergic tocolytics and/or other medications that increase HR Avoid hypertension Avoid positive inotropic medications Bacterial endocarditis prophylaxis recommended with enlarged aortic root Pain management: consider epidural anesthesia

Table 9–6. CARDIAC DISEASE IN PREGNANCY *(Continued)*

Cardiac Disease/Lesion	Risk Category	Description	Clinical Management
Peripartum cardiomyopathy	High or major risk	Cardiac failure developing in pregnancy or in the first 6 mo postpartum without identifiable cause Peak incidence is 2 mo postpartum Higher incidence among older gravidas, multiparas, African-American race, multiple gestations, and patients with preeclampsia Manifests as biventricular failure Fifty percent go on to have dilated cardiomyopathy	Optimize cardiac output Typically requires use of diuretics, antihypertensive agents, and β-blockers in conjunction with a cardiologist Repeat measurement of ejection fraction should be done if change in patient status detected Consider serial B-type natriuretic peptide measurements Consider serial renal and electrolyte measurements Oxygen therapy during labor, vaginal birth preferred Pain management: consider narcotic epidural; keep patient comfortable to decrease oxygen utilization
Myocardial infarction (MI)	Previous MI = intermediate or moderate risk MI during pregnancy = high or major risk	Diagnosis during pregnancy is determined by ECG findings, angina, and elevated cardiac enzymes (Troponin I) Cardiac Troponin I levels are unaffected by pregnancy, labor, and delivery	MI during pregnancy—attempt to delay delivery for 2–3 weeks Previous MI—advise patients to wait at least 1 year after infarction; follow-up coronary angiography recommended Optimize cardiac output Labor in left or right lateral position Consider assisted second stage of labor (vacuum or forceps) and/or "labor down" technique Avoid Valsalva maneuver during pushing Avoid maternal tachycardia and hypertension Bacterial endocarditis prophylaxis recommended Pain management: consider narcotic epidural; keep the patient comfortable to decrease oxygen utilization

BP, blood pressure; CHF, congestive heart failure; HR, heart rate; NYHA, New York Heart Association.
Adapted from Arafeh, J. M., & Baird, S. M. (2006). Cardiac disease in pregnancy. *Critical Care Nursing Quarterly, 29*(1), 32–52; Barth, W. H., Jr. (2009). Cardiac surgery in pregnancy. *Clinical Obstetrics and Gynecology, 52*(4), 630–646. doi:10.1097/GRF.0b013e3181bed9b5; Cruz, M. O., Briller, J., & Hibbard, J. U. (2010). Update on peripartum cardiomyopathy. *Obstetrics and Gynecology Clinics of North America, 37*(2), 283–303. doi:10.1016/j.ogc.2010.02.003.

evaluation by cardiology and coordination of findings to develop and alter the plan of care are required. In the intrapartum period, administration of medications and intravascular volume may be necessary to optimize or minimize preload and afterload in order to maximize cardiac output, depending on the underlying cardiac lesion. If any patient experiences heart failure, traditional treatment methods are used during pregnancy with the exception of use of angiotensin-converting enzyme (ACE) inhibitors. This class of drugs is associated with fetal and neonatal renal agenesis, failure, and death (American College of Obstetricians and Gynecologists, 2012; National High Blood Pressure Education Program, 2000; Thorne, 2004). See Table 9–7 for cardiovascular medications that may be administered to women with cardiac disease.

During the intrapartum period, control of anxiety, pain, and temperature can minimize fluctuation in heart rate (Curran, 2002). Pharmacologic treatment may be needed if cardiac dysrhythmias are present that affect heart rate and cardiac output. Cardioversion, direct pacing, and defibrillation may be required to correct serious dysrhythmias (Blanchard & Shabetai, 2004).

Intrapartum care and birth options need thoughtful consideration to decrease maternal and fetal risk. An interdisciplinary team approach to planning intrapartum care is essential. In the past, cesarean birth under general anesthesia was often chosen as the birth option with the least risk to the mother with heart disease. However, elective cesarean birth increases the risk of hemorrhage, thrombosis, and infection and is associated with 1.2 to 1.4 times the risk of an adverse outcome when compared to vaginal birth (Kafka et al., 2006). Current practice for most cardiac lesions includes a well-planned labor and vaginal birth unless there is a specific obstetric indication for cesarean birth (Earing & Webb, 2005). See Display 9–3 for key aspects of intrapartum management and care. The pain of labor can be managed with epidural anesthesia under the guidance of an anesthesiologist knowledgeable of

Table 9-7. CARDIOVASCULAR MEDICATIONS (DOSES, NURSING CARE, AND MATERNAL–FETAL IMPLICATIONS)

	Generic Name (Trade Name)	Dose	Nursing Care Specific for Pregnancy	Fetal/Neonatal Effects
Anti-arrhythmics	Adenosine (Adenocard)	6 mg intravenous (IV) bolus over 1–3 sec followed by 20–mL saline bolus; may repeat with 12 mg in 1–2 min × 2		No observed fetal or newborn effects reported
	Amiodarone (Cordarone)	5 mg/kg IV over 3 min, then 10 mg/kg/day	Observe for prolonged QT	Electronic fetal monitoring (EFM): Observe for fetal bradycardia • Potential for congenital hypothyroidism • May cause intrauterine growth restriction (IUGR) • Observe for transient bradycardia and prolonged QT in the newborn
	Bretylium	5 mg/kg IV bolus, then 1–2 mg/min infusion	Observe for maternal hypotension	EFM: Potential risks for decreased uterine blood flow, fetal hypoxia, late decelerations, and bradycardia
	Lidocaine	1 mg/kg bolus; repeat one half bolus at 10 min PRN × 4; infusion at 1–4 mg/min; total dose 3 mg/kg		EFM: Rapidly crosses placenta; potential for fetal bradycardia
	Phenytoin (Dilantin)	300 mg IV; then 100 mg every 5 min to a total of 1,000 mg		Teratogenic—fetal hydantoin syndrome; unknown fetal/newborn risk with short-term use.
	Procainamide (Pronestyl)	100 mg over 30 min, then 2–6 mg/min infusion: total dose 17 mg/kg		None reported
	Quinidine	15 mg/kg IV over 60 min, then 0.02 mg/kg/min infusion	Potential oxytocic properties with high doses	Potential for eighth cranial nerve damage and thrombocytopenia.
β-Blockers	Atenolol (Tenormin)	5 mg IV over 5 min; repeat dose in 5 min; total dose 15 mg	Observe for maternal hypotension	EFM: Observe for fetal bradycardia • May cause IUGR and persistent β-blockade in the newborn
	Esmolol (Brevibloc)	500 mcg/kg IV over 1 min with infusion rate of 50–200 mcg/kg/min	Observe for maternal hypotension	EFM: Potential risks for decreased uterine blood flow, fetal hypoxia, late decelerations, and bradycardia
	Labetalol (Normodyne)	10–20 mg IV followed by 20–80 mg IV every 10 min: total dose of 150 mg	Observe for maternal hypotension	EFM: Observe for fetal bradycardia • May cause IUGR
	Metoprolol (Lopressor)	5 mg IV over 5 min; repeat in 10 min		Rapidly enters fetal circulation; fetal serum levels equal to maternal levels; may cause persistent β-blockade in the newborn
	Propranolol (Inderal)	1 mg IV every 2 min PRN	Observe for maternal hypotension	EFM: Observe for fetal bradycardia • May cause IUGR

Table 9–7. CARDIOVASCULAR MEDICATIONS (DOSES, NURSING CARE, AND MATERNAL–FETAL IMPLICATIONS) *(Continued)*

	Generic Name (Trade Name)	Dose	Nursing Care Specific for Pregnancy	Fetal/Neonatal Effects
Calcium Channel Blockers	Diltiazem (Cardizem)	20 mg IV bolus over 2 min; repeat in 15 min		Possible teratogenic effects
	Nifedipine (Procardia)	10 mg PO; repeat every 6 hr	Observe for maternal hypotension and tachycardia. May cause severe hypotension and neuromuscular blockade when given with magnesium sulfate	
	Verapamil (Calan)	2.5–5 mg IV bolus over 2 min; repeat in 5 min and then every 30 min PRN to a maximum dose of 20 mg	Observe for maternal hypotension (5%–10% of patients)	Potential for reduced uterine blood flow and fetal hypoxia
Inotropic Agents	Dobutamine (Dobutrex)	Initial dose of 5 mcg/kg/min; titrate up to 20 mcg/kg/min		
	Digoxin (Lanoxin)	Loading dose 0.5 mg IV over 5 min, then 0.25 IV every 6 hr × 2. Maintenance dose 0.125–0.375 mg IV/PO QD	Because of increased maternal volume and elimination, increased doses are required to obtain therapeutic levels	Fetal toxicity and neonatal death have been reported
	Dopamine	Initial dose 5 mcg/kg/min; titrate by 5–10 mcg/kg/min; to 20 mcg/kg/min		
	Epinephrine	Initial bolus 0.5 mg; follow with 2–10 mcg/kg/min infusion: endotracheal 0.5–1.0 mg every 5 min		
Vasoconstrictors	Ephedrine sulphate	10–25 mg slow IV push; repeat every 15 min PRN × 3	First-line medication in pregnancy (causes peripheral vasoconstriction without reducing uterine blood flow)	EFM: Observe for fetal tachycardia and decreased baseline variability following administration
	Metaraminol (Aramine)	Initial dose of 0.1 mg/min: titrate to 2 mg/min	May interact with oxytocics and ergot medications to produce severe maternal hypertension	Potential for reduced uterine blood flow and fetal hypoxia
	Norepinephrine (Levophed)	Initial dose of 0.05 mcg/kg/min titrate to maximum dose of 1.0 mcg/kg/min	Use only with severe maternal hypotension unresponsive to other agents	May compromise uterine blood flow and cause fetal hypoxia and bradycardia
	Phenylephrine (Neosynephrine)	Initial dose of 0.1 mcg/kg/min; titrate up to 0.7 mcg/kg/min	May interact with oxytocics and ergot medications to produce severe maternal hypertension	Potential for reduced uterine blood flow and fetal hypoxia

(continued)

Table 9–7. CARDIOVASCULAR MEDICATIONS (DOSES, NURSING CARE, AND MATERNAL–FETAL IMPLICATIONS) *(Continued)*

	Generic Name (Trade Name)	Dose	Nursing Care Specific for Pregnancy	Fetal/Neonatal Effects
Vasodilators	Hydralazine (Apresoline)	5–10 mg IV every 20 min; total dose 30 mg	Frequent, small doses preferred to avoid maternal hypotension	EFM: Potential for fetal tachycardia
	Nitroglycerin	IV infusion 10 mcg/min; titrate up by 10–20 mcg/min PRN: 0.4–0.8 mg sublingual; 1–2 in of dermal paste		
	Nitroprusside (Nipride)	Initial dose 0.3 mcg/kg/min; titrate to 10 mcg/kg/min	Monitor serum pH levels	Avoid prolonged use; potential for fetal cyanide toxicity

From Arafeh, J. M., & Baird, S M. (2006). Cardiac disease in pregnancy. *Critical Care Nursing Quarterly, 29*(1), 32–52.

cardiac disease during pregnancy (Kafka et al., 2006; Langesaeter, Dragsund, & Rosseland, 2010). Initiation of epidural anesthesia early in labor inhibits or minimizes the sympathetic response to pain. Labor pain has potentially significant side effects that should be avoided. Cardiac output can be abruptly increased with the pain and tension associated with labor (Bonow et al., 2006). Quality pain management has the benefit of helping avoiding tachycardia (important for cardiac lesions that require adequate diastolic filling or systolic ejection time), reducing myocardial workload, and providing pain relief for operative vaginal birth (Arafeh & Baird, 2006).

Spontaneous labor is preferred to induction of labor; however, in selected cases, labor induction may be the most feasible option to ensure that the required team members are available and present (Kafka et al., 2006). Planned labor also may be chosen for women who live remote from the hospital and thus may not be able to arrive on the labor unit in a timely manner after the initiation of spontaneous labor. Controlled labor or birth may also be necessary due to deterioration of the maternal or fetal condition. Labor should progress at a reasonable pace without tachysystole, which may lead to fetal intolerance and the risk of an urgent surgical birth. A lateral position during labor will minimize the effects of the hemodynamic fluctuations associated with uterine contractions for most women, but position should be individualized to the specific cardiac lesion (Earing & Webb, 2005). See Table 9–8 for changes in cardiac output during labor and birth.

The American College of Cardiology (ACC) and the American Heart Association (AHA) do not recommend routine antibiotic prophylaxis for all patients with heart

disease having an otherwise uncomplicated vaginal or cesarean birth unless infection is suspected (Bonow et al., 2006). Antibiotics are optional for high-risk patients: those with prosthetic heart valves, a previous history of endocarditis, complex CHD, or a surgically constructed systemic–pulmonary conduit (Bonow et al., 2006). Nonetheless, the decision to administer antibiotic therapy should be based on the individual risks of the woman and the mode of birth that is planned (Foley et al., 2010). Antibiotic prophylaxis should be given in two doses. The first dose is given at the start of labor or 30 minutes before cesarean birth. This initial dose is 2.0 g of ampicillin (intramuscular [IM] or IV) plus 1.5 mg/kg of gentamicin (not greater than 120 mg). The second dose is given 6 hours later and is 1.0 g of ampicillin (IM or IV) or 1.0 g of amoxicillin (oral administration). Women allergic to penicillins should be given 1.0 g of vancomycin IV over 1 to 2 hours (Elkayam & Bitar, 2005a).

During the second stage of labor, passive fetal descent, also known as "laboring down," in a lateral position increases oxygenation, limits maternal metabolic demands, and increases uteroplacental perfusion (Mayberry et al., 2000). The management plan for birth should include whether the woman will be allowed to attempt open glottis pushing and how operative birth will be accomplished (by forceps or vacuum) (Kafka et al., 2006). Most cardiac conditions are well tolerated with proper anesthesia, minimal or no pushing, and an operative vaginal birth.

It is important to consider the changes that occur immediately at birth due to relief of caval obstruction and transfusion of blood previously held in the maternal placental bed. This return of blood to the central circulation has the potential to overwhelm the patient's ability

DISPLAY 9-3

Intrapartum Care for Women with Cardiac Disease

An interdisciplinary team should plan and participate in care (nurse and physician representatives from the following special-ties: obstetrics, maternal–fetal medicine, anesthesia, cardiology, neonatology, and pediatrics). Social services and chaplain services should be consulted and available as necessary.

The unit where labor and birth occurs is based on maternal sta-tus. Most women can be managed in the labor unit with personnel from the ICU assisting with assessment of maternal hemodynamic status if invasive hemodynamic monitoring is indicated. Selected women may labor and give birth in the ICU. Personnel with exper-tise in labor management, fetal assessment, and birth are essential.

Labor is the most complex period for many pregnant women with cardiac disease since there are periods of great increases in cardiac output. Therefore, careful monitoring of maternal–fetal status is essential with at least a one-to-one nurse to patient ratio. Patient status and type of cardiac disease provides the basis for selection of monitoring methods.

Invasive hemodynamic monitoring should be considered for women with impaired left ventricular function, NYHA Class III and Class IV, severe mitral stenosis, and pulmonary hypertension.

Noninvasive monitoring includes oxygen saturation via pulse oximetry, blood pressure, heart rate, respirations, careful monitor-ing of fluid status, reassessment of NYHA functional status, fetal status, and use of electrocardiogram (ECG) monitoring for women susceptible to arrhythmias.

Fetal status should be monitored continuously via electronic fetal monitoring (EFM). Fetal status can be an indicator of mater-nal status. A normal fetal heart rate (FHR) can be reflective of ade-quate maternal perfusion. Use of external or internal monitoring of FHR and uterine activity is based on obstetric considerations.

Lateral positioning should be encouraged in most women to avoid risk of venocaval compression.

Adequate and early pain management (usually via epidural anesthesia) will minimize negative effects of pain, anxiety, and tension on maternal hemodynamic parameters. Patients with severe stenotic heart defects will not tolerate sudden decreases in systemic vascular resistance; therefore, epidural anesthesia must be administered by a provider with experience in cardiac disease during pregnancy.

Supportive nursing care along with support from the patient's partner can minimize anxiety. Appropriate preparation with realistic expectations for how the labor and birth will proceed, including potential complications and resultant interventions, can also minimize stress and anxiety.

Labor and vaginal birth is preferred over cesarean birth for most patients because there is less risk of blood loss, fewer postpartum infections, and earlier ambulation with less risk of thrombosis and pulmonary complications.

The second stage should be managed with passive fetal descent, minimal maternal expulsive efforts, and operative (forceps or vacuum) birth as needed.

Uterine contraction after birth should be maintained to prevent postpartum hemorrhage. Women who have received anticoagulation therapy are at greater risk for hemorrhage. Oxytocic drugs have marked hemodynamic effects and should be used at the lowest effective dose. Postpartum hemorrhage should be managed aggressively to prevent hypovolemia, especially important for patients who are preload dependent such as those with severe aortic stenosis or mitral stenosis. Postpartum hemor-rhage should be treated with volume replacement, blood products, and plasma.

Support maternal–infant attachment by encouraging holding, touching, and breastfeeding (if the woman has chosen breast-feeding) as soon as possible.

Data from Arafeh, J. M., & Baird, S. M. (2006). Cardiac disease in pregnancy. *Critical Care Nursing Quarterly, 29*(1), 32–52; Earing, M. G., & Webb, G. D. (2005). Congeni-tal heart disease and pregnancy: Maternal and fetal risks. *Clinics in Perinatology, 32*(4), 913–919. doi:10.1016/j.clp.2005.09.004; Kafka, H., Johnson, M. R., & Gatzoulis, M. A. (2006). The team approach to pregnancy and congenital heart disease. *Cardiology Clinics, 24*(4), 587–605. doi:10.1016/j.ccl.2006.08.009; Klein, L. L., & Galan, H. L. (2004). Cardiac disease in pregnancy. *Obstetrics and Gynecology Clinics of North America, 31*(2), 429–459. doi:10.1016/j.ogc.2004.03.001; Simpson, K. R. (2006). Critical illness during pregnancy: Considerations for evaluation and treatment of the fetus as the second patient. *Critical Care Nursing Quarterly, 29*(1), 20–31.

to cope with the extra volume load. On the other hand, failure of the uterus to contract may result in hemor-rhage and blood loss. Oxytocin can have hemodynamic effects and should be given at the lowest effective dose with close attention to maternal response and effect on blood loss (Kafka et al., 2006).

Table 9-8. INCREASES IN CARDIAC OUTPUT DURING LABOR AND BIRTH

Labor Phase or Stage	Increase Above Pre-labor Values
Latent phase	15%
Active phase	30%
Second stage	45%
Immediately at birth	65%

Risks of decompensation continue during the post-partum period, most notably during the first few hours after birth but depend on the severity of cardiac dis-ease. A period of careful monitoring should follow birth for at least 48 to 72 hours, depending on the type of cardiac disease and maternal condition (Earing & Webb, 2005). Maternal death remains a risk during the postpartum period. The most common compli-cations women with cardiac disease experience after birth include development of pulmonary edema and hemorrhage (Arafeh & Baird, 2006). Risk of pulmo-nary edema can persist for up to 3 to 5 days post-partum due to mobilization of interstitial fluid to the vascular space during the normal diuresis that occurs after birth (Arafeh & Baird, 2006; Blackburn, 2007). Risk of hemorrhage is increased for women who have required anticoagulation during the pregnancy (Klein & Galan, 2004). Because of the large amount of blood flow to the uterus at term (750 to 1,000 mL), significant blood loss can occur in a relative short period if uterine contraction is not maintained during the immediate postpartum period (Arafeh & Baird, 2006). Postpartum hemorrhage should be treated aggressively by efforts to promote hemostasis and with replacement volume, blood products, and plasma to avoid hypovolemia (Arafeh & Baird, 2006; Kafka et al., 2006; Klein & Galan, 2004). See Chapter 17 for a detailed discussion of postpartum hemorrhage.

All women with known underlying cardiac disease and dysfunction should receive care from clinicians who specialize in cardiac disease during pregnancy in a Level III/IV facility due to the risks of preterm labor and birth, SGA fetus, intrauterine growth restriction (IUGR), and potential for fetal or maternal compromise. Although most women with cardiac disease tolerate pregnancy and have a successful outcome, the potential exists to develop significant hemodynamic decompensation, requiring comprehensive management to survive the pregnancy, labor, and birth.

NURSING CARE

Dysrhythmias may accompany pregnancy and often occur with cardiac disease, having an impact on cardiac output if repetitive and prolonged (Blanchard & Shabetai, 2004). Nurses have the most frequent and lengthy patient encounters. Therefore, they must have keen assessment techniques and skills to differentiate normal pregnancy adaptations from cardiac dysfunction and disease (Luppi, 1999). Table 9–3 compares normal adaptations of pregnancy to severe heart disease or heart failure. At any time during the antepartum, intrapartum, or postpartum periods up until 6 months following birth, the nurse should be vigilant for symptoms signaling deterioration. If the pregnant woman reports progressive limitation of physical activity because of worsening dyspnea, chest pain that occurs during exercise or increased activity, or syncope that is preceded by palpitations or physical exertion, underlying cardiac disease should be suspected (Blanchard & Shabetai, 2004). As a part of the multidisciplinary team, the perinatal nurse should maintain knowledge of the unique condition of the woman and the current plan of care prior to each patient encounter.

The woman's history and current physical status are analyzed in relation to cardiovascular physiology and function. The nurse should perform an initial review to include examination of the patient's specific medical, surgical, social, and family history. A current understanding of basic pathophysiology regarding the patient's underlying cardiovascular disorder, previous

therapies (e.g., past hospital admissions for medical stabilization or surgery), current medications, and current NYHA classification are particularly pertinent (Blanchard & Shabetai, 2004). The woman's occupation can also provide useful information about functional status and environmental risk factors.

Knowledge of various methods and tools for cardiac assessment are prerequisites for a complete cardiovascular evaluation. Physical assessments will include a head-to-toe inspection with specific focus on cardiorespiratory indicators. A cardiovascular assessment minimally includes auscultation of the heart and lungs (count both heart rate and respiratory rate with stethoscope for a full minute); identification of pathologic edema; evaluation of respiratory rate and rhythm; evaluation of cardiac rate and rhythm; body weight assessed at the same time of day and on the same scale; assessment of skin color, temperature, and turgor; and capillary refill check. Trending of vital sign data is important because tachypnea, tachycardia, and anxiety are often early signs of edema and may be present before a cough or abnormal breath sounds appear (Mason & Dorman, 2013). Abnormal skin and mucous membrane color may indicate problems with oxygenation and perfusion (Curran, 2002). Assessment of the central nervous system (CNS) may reveal signs of inadequate blood flow. Restlessness, apprehension, anxiety, or changes in level of consciousness may indicate compromised blood flow and oxygenation of the brain (Blackburn, 2007).

Observation for secondary obstetric-specific complications is a primary goal in the treatment of cardiac dysfunction during pregnancy. Hypertension alone may be a secondary complication of pregnancy or may signal worsening of the underlying cardiac disease (Blanchard & Shabetai, 2004). Proper and consistent blood pressure assessment is crucial. Changing from a supine to a left side–lying position may increase blood pressure by 10% to 20%, enhancing cardiac output (Belfort et al., 2010). Maternal positioning, cuff size, auscultation of Korotkoff (K) 4 versus K5 heart sound, device, and timing alter maternal blood pressure results during pregnancy. Electronic blood pressure measures may cause an enhanced widening of pulse pressure compared with manual readings; however, the mean arterial pressure remains unchanged (Marx, Schwalbe, Cho, & Whitty, 1993). It is imperative that the entire perinatal team is consistent in blood pressure technique to ensure accuracy and correct interpretation of data.

Any maternal position that causes aortocaval compression may negatively influence maternal cardiac output and blood pressure; avoidance during all phases of pregnancy, labor, and birth is indicated. Vena caval syndrome may significantly limit maternal cardiac output and promote maternal symptomatology in up to 14% of patients after 36 weeks' gestation (Belfort et al., 2010;

Torgersen & Curran, 2006). Therefore, if improved cardiac output is indicated, lateral recumbent position is optimal in most cases.

Additional noninvasive assessment techniques and equipment necessary for the treatment of cardiac disease in pregnancy should include oxygen saturation (SaO_2) via a pulse oximetry, urinary output, and electronic fetal monitoring (EFM) (in most cases). Other techniques that should be considered include arrhythmia assessment via 5- or 12-lead electrocardiogram (ECG). Pulse oximetry should not be used as the only diagnostic tool if hypoxemia is present. Blood gases offer more complete information when severe pulmonary compromise and systemic color changes exist (Mason & Dorman, 2013). Assessment and documentation of baseline vital signs and condition prior to pregnancy is optimal. All pregnant women with preexisting cardiac disease should have a baseline 12-lead ECG and may require 5-lead cardiac monitoring during labor and birth. Kidney function is also assessed for adequacy of peripheral perfusion. An indwelling Foley catheter with a urometer can assist with assessment of fluid balance and indicate signs of inadequate renal and uterine perfusion (Curran, 2002). Urinary output should be maintained at least 25 to 30 mL/hr (Curran, 2002).

Fetal assessment is a sensitive indicator of adequate cardiac function by affording the perinatal team a means for assessing uteroplacental perfusion (Patton et al., 1990). Antenatal testing (e.g., fetal movement counting, nonstress test, biophysical profile) may assist in the diagnosis of uteroplacental insufficiency during the antepartum period with evidence of SGA, IUGR, or oligohydramnios (Simon, Sadovsky, Aboulafia, Ohel, & Zajicek, 1986). Prior to 23 weeks' gestation, EFM may be used to screen for an early indicator of deterioration in maternal status. Once viability is established, indeterminate (category II) or abnormal (category III) fetal heart rate (FHR) patterns warrant prompt intervention in most cases.

Certain disorders and advanced degrees of cardiovascular illness may require invasive hemodynamic monitoring using pulmonary artery catheters, peripheral arterial catheters, or central venous pressure monitors (Troiano, 1999). Invasive hemodynamic monitoring may be recommended for women designated in the NYHA Class III or Class IV experiencing labor. Many women require continuous cardiac rhythm monitoring during acute events and during prolonged hospitalization (Blanchard & Shabetai, 2004).

Heightened vigilance is warranted in women with cardiac disease throughout pregnancy. Understanding and assessing for variances in normal pregnancy adaptations may signal deterioration. An interdisciplinary approach assists in overall reduction of maternal, fetal, and neonatal morbidity and mortality.

SUMMARY

It is likely that morbidity and mortality from cardiac disease in pregnancy is increasing in either real numbers or in awareness, particularly in the postpartum period. Careful planning of care and vigilance throughout pregnancy is essential. While many women with cardiac disease have favorable outcomes, a low threshold should be established for follow-up of signs and symptoms indicating deteriorating status. The plan of care needs to be flexible to reflect alterations dictated by change in the woman's condition as she continually adapts to the physiologic changes of pregnancy (Kuklina & Callaghan, 2011).

REFERENCES

American College of Obstetricians and Gynecologists. (2012). *Chronic Hypertension in Pregnancy* (Practice Bulletin No. 125). Washington, DC: Author. doi:10.1097/AOG.0b013e318249ff06

Arafeh, J. M., & Baird, S. M. (2006). Cardiac disease in pregnancy. *Critical Care Nursing Quarterly, 29*(1), 32–52.

Association of Women's Health, Obstetric and Neonatal Nurses. (2009). *Perinatal Orientation and Education Program (POEP)* (2nd ed.). Washington, DC: Author.

Balint, O. H., Slu, S. C., Mason, J., Grewal, J., Wald, R., Oechslin, E. N., . . . Silversides, C. K. (2010). Cardiac outcomes after pregnancy in women with congenital heart disease. *Heart, 96*(20), 1656–1661. doi:10.1136/hrt.2010.202838

Bamfo, J. E., Kametas, N. A., Turan, O., Khaw, A., & Nicolaides, K. H. (2006). Maternal cardiac function in fetal growth restriction. *BJOG: An International Journal of Obstetrics and Gynaecology, 113*(7), 784–791. doi:10.1111/j.1471-0528.2006.00945.x

Barth, W. H., Jr. (2009). Cardiac surgery in pregnancy. *Clinical Obstetrics and Gynecology, 52*(4), 630–646. doi:10.1097/GRF.0b013e3181bed9b5

Bates, S. M., Greer, I. A., Middeldorp, S., Veenstra, D. L., Prabulos, A., & Vandvik, P. O. (2012). VTE, thrombophilia, antithrombotic therapy, and pregnancy: Antithrombotic therapy and prevention of thrombosis, 9th ed.: American College of Chest Physicians evidence-based clinical practice guidelines. *Chest, 141*(2 Suppl.), e691S–e736S. doi:10.1378/chest.11-2300

Belfort, M., Saade, G., Foley, M., Phelan, J., & Dildy, G. (Eds.). (2010). *Critical Care Obstetrics* (5th ed.). Oxford, UK: Wiley-Blackwell.

Blackburn, S. (2007). *Maternal, Fetal, & Neonatal Physiology: A Clinical Perspective* (3rd ed.). St. Louis, MO: Saunders.

Blanchard, D., & Shabetai, R. (2004). Cardiac diseases. In R. Creasy, R. Resnick, & J. Iams (Eds.), *Maternal-Fetal Medicine: Principles & Practice* (5th ed., pp. 815–844). Philadelphia, PA: Saunders.

Bobrowski, R. A. (2010). Maternal–fetal blood gas physiology. In M. Belfort, G. Saade, M. Foley, J. Phelan, & G. Dildy (Eds.), *Critical Care Obstetrics* (5th ed., pp. 53–68). Oxford, UK: Wiley-Blackwell.

Bonow, R. O., Carabello, B. A., Chatterjee, K., de Leon, A. C. Jr., Faxon, D. P., Freed, M. D., . . . Shanewise, J. S. (2006). ACC/AHA 2006 guidelines for the management of patients with valvular heart disease: A report of the American College of Cardiology/American Heart Association Task Force on Practice Guidelines (Writing Committee to Revise the 1998 Guidelines for the Management of Patients with Valvular Heart Disease). *Circulation, 114*(5), e84–e231. doi:10.1161/CIRCULATIONAHA.106.176857

Bowater, S. E., & Thorne, S. A. (2010). Management of pregnancy in women with acquired and congenital heart disease. *Postgraduate Medical Journal, 86*(1012), 100–105. doi:10.1136/pgmj.2008.078030

Criteria Committee of the New York Heart Association. (1994). *Nomenclature and Criteria for Diagnosis of Diseases of the Heart and Great Vessels* (9th ed.). New York: New York Heart Association.

Cruz, M. O., Briller, J., & Hibbard, J. U. (2010). Update on peripartum cardiomyopathy. *Obstetrics and Gynecology Clinics of North America, 37*(2), 283–303. doi:10.1016/j.ogc.2010.02.003

Curran, C. (2002). Multiple organ dysfunction syndrome (MODS) in the obstetric population. *Journal of Perinatal & Neonatal Nursing, 15*(4), 37–55.

Curry, R., Swan, L., & Steer, P. J. (2009). Cardiac disease in pregnancy. *Current Opinion in Obstetrics and Gynecology, 21*(6), 508–513. doi:10.1097/GCO.0b013e328332a762

Darovic, G. O. (2002a). Cardiovascular anatomy and physiology. In G. O. Darovic (Ed.), *Hemodynamic Monitoring: Invasive and Noninvasive Clinical Application,* (3rd ed., pp. 57–90). Philadelphia: Saunders.

Darovic, G. O. (2002b). Pulmonary artery pressure monitoring. In G. O. Darovic (Ed.), *Hemodynamic Monitoring: Invasive and Noninvasive Clinical Application,* (3rd ed., pp. 191–243). Philadelphia: Saunders.

Darovic, G. O., Graham, P. G., & Pranulis, M. A. (2002). Monitoring cardiac output. In G. O. Darovic (Ed.), *Hemodynamic Monitoring: Invasive and Noninvasive Clinical Application,* (3rd ed., pp. 245–262). Philadelphia: Saunders.

Darovic, G. O., & Kumar, A. (2002). Monitoring central venous pressure. In G. O. Darovic (Ed.), *Hemodynamic Monitoring: Invasive and Noninvasive Clinical Application,* (3rd ed., pp. 177–190). Philadelphia, PA: Saunders.

Drenthen, W., Boersma, E., Balci, A., Moons, P., Roos–Hesselink, J. W., Mulder, B. J., . . . Pieper, P. G. (2010). Predictors of pregnancy complications in women with congenital heart disease. *European Heart Journal, 31*(17), 2124–2132. doi:10.1093/eurheartj/ehq200

Earing, M. G., & Webb, G. D. (2005). Congenital heart disease and pregnancy: Maternal and fetal risks. *Clinics in Perinatology, 32*(4), 913–919. doi:10.1016/j.clp.2005.09.004

Elkayam, U., & Bitar, F. (2005a). Valvular heart disease and pregnancy: Part I: Native valves. *Journal of the American College of Cardiology, 46*(2), 223–230. doi:10.1016/j.jacc.2005.02.085

Elkayam, U., & Bitar, F. (2005b). Valvular heart disease and pregnancy: Part II: Prosthetic valves. *Journal of the American College of Cardiology, 46*(3), 403–410. doi:10.1016/j.jacc.2005.02.087

Foley, M. R., Rokey, R., & Belfort, M. A. (2010). Cardiac disease. In M. Belfort, G. Saade, M. Foley, J. Phelan, & G. Dildy (Eds.), *Critical Care Obstetrics* (5th ed., pp. 256–282). Oxford, UK: Wiley-Blackwell.

Gelson, E., Curry, R., Gatzoulis, M. A., Swan, L., Lupton, M., Steer, P., & Johnson, M. (2011). Effect of maternal heart disease on fetal growth. *Obstetrics & Gynecology, 117*(4), 886–891. doi:10.1097/AOG.0b013e31820cab69

Gelson, E., Gatzoulis, M. A., Steer, P., & Johnson, M. R. (2009). Heart disease—why is maternal mortality increasing? *BJOG: An International Journal of Obstetrics and Gynaecology, 116*(5), 609–611. doi:10.1111/j.1471-0528.2008.02082.x

Goland, S., Barakat, M., Khatri, N., & Elkayam, U. (2009). Pregnancy in Marfan syndrome: Maternal and fetal risk and recommendations for patient assessment and management. *Cardiology in Review, 17*(6), 253–262. doi:10.1097/CRD.0b013e3181bb83d3

Harris, I. S. (2011). Management of pregnancy in patients with congenital heart disease. *Progress in Cardiovascular Diseases, 53*(4), 305–311. doi:10.1016/j.pcad.2010.08.001

Jastrow, N., Meyer, P., Khairy, P., Mercier, L. A., Dore, A., Marcotte, F., & Leduc, L. (2011). Prediction of complications in pregnant women with cardiac diseases referred to a tertiary center. *International Journal of Cardiology, 151*(2), 209–213. doi:10.1016/j.ijcard.2010.05.045

Kafka, H., Johnson, M. R., & Gatzoulis, M. A. (2006). The team approach to pregnancy and congenital heart disease. *Cardiology Clinics, 24*(4), 587–605. doi:10.1016/j.ccl.2006.08.009

Karchmer, A. W. (2011). Infective endocarditis. In R. O. Bonow, D. L. Mann, D. P. Zipes, & P. Libby (Eds.), *Bonow: Braunwald's Heart Disease–A Textbook of Cardiovascular Medicine* (9th ed., pp. 1540–1557). Philadelphia, PA: Elsevier Saunders.

Klein, L. L., & Galan, H. L. (2004). Cardiac disease in pregnancy. *Obstetrics and Gynecology Clinics of North America, 31*(2), 429–459. doi:10.1016/j.ogc.2004.03.001

Kuklina, E. V., & Callaghan, W. M. (2011). Chronic heart disease and severe obstetric morbidity among hospitalisations for pregnancy in the USA: 1995–2006. *BJOG: An International Journal of Obstetrics and Gynaecology, 118*(3), 345–352. doi:10.1111/j.1471-0528.2010.02743.x

Langesaeter, E., Dragsund, M., & Rosseland, L. A. (2010). Regional anaesthesia for a Caesarean section in women with cardiac disease: A prospective study. *Acta Anaesthesiologica Scandinavica, 54*(1), 46–54. doi:10.1111/j.1399-6576.2009.02080.x

Linker, D. (2001). *Practical Echocardiography of Congenital Heart Disease from Fetal to Adult.* New York: Churchill Livingstone.

Luppi, C. J. (1999). Cardiopulmonary resuscitation in pregnancy. In L. K. Mandeville & N. H. Troiano (Eds.), *AWHONN's High-Risk and Critical Care: Intrapartum Nursing* (2nd ed., pp. 353–379). Philadelphia: Lippincott Williams & Wilkins.

Madazli, R., Sal, V., Cift, T., Guralp, O., & Goymen, A. (2010). Pregnancy outcomes in women with heart disease. *Archives of Gynecology and Obstetrics, 281*(1), 29–34. doi:10.1007/s00404-009-1050-z

Main, E. K. (2010). Maternal mortality: New strategies for measurement and prevention. *Current Opinion in Obstetrics and Gynecology, 22*(6), 511–516. doi:10.1097/GCO.0b013e3283404e89

Marx, G. F., Schwalbe, S. S., Cho, E., & Whitty, J. E. (1993). Automated blood pressure measurements in laboring women: Are they reliable? *American Journal of Obstetrics and Gynecology, 168*(3, Pt. 1), 796–798. doi:10.1016/S0002-9378(12)90822-4

Mason, B. A., & Dorman, K. (2013). Pulmonary disorders in pregnancy. In N. H. Troiano, C. J. Harvey, & B. F. Chez (Eds.), *High Risk and Critical Care Obstetrics.* (3rd ed., pp. 144–162). Philadelphia: Lippincott Williams & Wilkins.

Mayberry, L., Gennaro, S., Strange, L., Lee, L., Heisler, D., & Nielsen-Smith, K. (2000). *Second Stage Labor Management: Promotion of Evidence-Based Practice and a Collaborative Approach to Patient Care* (Practice Monograph). Washington, DC: Association of Women's Health, Obstetric and Neonatal Nurses.

National High Blood Pressure Education Program. (2000). *National High Blood Pressure Education Program Working Group Report on High Blood Pressure in Pregnancy* (NIH Publication No. 00-3029). Bethesda, MD: National Institutes of Health, National Heart, Lung, and Blood Institute, and National High Blood Pressure Education Program.

Norwitz, E. R., & Robinson, J. N. (2010). Pregnancy–induced physiologic alterations. In M. Belfort, G. Saade, M. Foley, J. Phelan, & G. Dildy (Eds.), *Critical Care Obstetrics* (5th ed., pp. 30–52). Oxford, UK: Wiley-Blackwell.

Patton, D. E., Lee, W., Cotton, D. B., Miller, J., Carpenter, R. J. Jr., Huhta, J., & Hankins, G. (1990). Cyanotic maternal heart disease in pregnancy. *Obstetrical and Gynecological Survey, 45*(9), 594–600.

Pearson, G. D., Veille, J. C., Rahimtoola, S., Hsia, J., Oakley, C. M., Hosenpud, J. D., . . . Baughman, K. L. (2000). Peripartum cardiomyopathy: National Heart, Lung, and Blood Institute and Office of Rare Diseases (National Institutes of Health) workshop recommendations and review. *Journal of the American Medical Association, 283*(9), 1183–1188. doi:10.1001/jama.283.9.1183

Poh, C. L., & Lee, C. H. (2010). Acute myocardial infarction in pregnant women. *Annals of the Academy of Medicine, Singapore, 39*(3), 247–253.

Raju, B. S., & Turi, Z. G. (2011). Rheumatic fever. In R. O. Bonow, D. L. Mann, D. P. Zipes, & P. Libby (Eds.), *Bonow: Braunwald's Heart Disease—A Textbook of Cardiovascular Medicine* (9th ed., pp. 1868–1874). Philadelphia, PA: Elsevier Saunders.

Roth, A., & Elkayam, U. (1996). Acute myocardial infarction associated with pregnancy. *Annals of Internal Medicine, 125*(9), 751–762.

Simon, A., Sadovsky, E., Aboulafia, Y., Ohel, G., & Zajicek, G. (1986). Fetal activity in pregnancies complicated by rheumatic heart disease. *Journal of Perinatal Medicine, 14*(5), 331–334.

Simpson, K. R. (2006). Critical illness during pregnancy: Considerations for evaluation and treatment of the fetus as the second patient. *Critical Care Nursing Quarterly, 29*(1), 20–31.

Siu, S. C., Colman, J. M., Sorensen, S., Smallhorn, J. F., Farine, D., Amankwah, K. S., . . . Sermer, M. (2002). Adverse neonatal and cardiac outcomes are more common in pregnant women with cardiac disease. *Circulation, 105*(18), 2179–2184. doi:10.1161/01.CIR.0000015699.48605.08

Siu, S. C., Sermer, M., Colman, J. M., Alvarez, A. N., Mercier, L. A., Morton, B. C., . . . Sorensen, S. (2001). Prospective multicenter study of pregnancy outcomes in women with heart disease. *Circulation, 104*(5), 515–521. doi:10.1161/ hc3001.093437

Szumowski, L., Szufladowicz, E., Orczykowski, M., Bodalski, R., Derejko, P., Przybylski, A, . . . Walczak, F. (2010). Ablation of severe drug-resistant tachyarrhythmia during pregnancy. *Journal of Cardiovascular Electrophysiology, 21*(8), 877–882. doi:10.1111/ j.1540-8167.2010.01727.x

Tanous, D., Siu, S. C., Mason, J., Greutmann, M., Wald, R. M., Parker, J. D., . . . Silversides, C. K. (2010). B–type natriuretic peptide in pregnant women with heart disease. *Journal of the American College of Cardiology, 56*(15), 1247–1253. doi:10.1016/j .jacc.2010.02.076

Thorne, S. A. (2004). Pregnancy in heart disease. *Heart, 90*(4), 450–456. doi:10.1136/hrt.2003.027888

Torgersen, K. L., & Curran, C. A. (2006). A systematic approach to the physiologic adaptations of pregnancy. *Critical Care Nursing Quarterly, 29*(1), 2–19.

Troiano, N. (1999). Invasive hemodynamic monitoring in obstetrics. In L. K. Mandeville & N. H. Troiano (Eds.), *AWHONN's High-Risk and Critical Care: Intrapartum Nursing* (2nd ed., pp. 66–83). Philadelphia: Lippincott Williams & Wilkins.

Vitarelli, A., & Capotosto, L. (2011). Role of echocardiography in the assessment and management of adult congenital heart disease in pregnancy. *International Journal of Cardiovascular Imaging, 27*(6), 843–857. doi:10.1007/s10554–010–9750–9

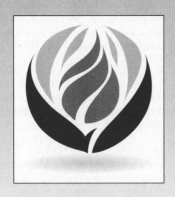

Suzanne McMurtry Baird
Betsy B. Kennedy

CHAPTER 10

Pulmonary Complications in Pregnancy

The frequency and significance of acute and chronic pulmonary complications in pregnant women has increased in recent years, making these complications one of the leading causes of maternal morbidity and mortality (Berg, Callaghan, Syverson, & Henderson, 2010; Clark et al., 2008; Kwon, Triche, Belanger, & Bracken, 2006; MacKay, Berg, Liu, Duran, & Hoyert, 2011). Some of the complications are unique to pregnancy (amniotic fluid embolism [AFE], preeclampsia, and tocolytic-induced pulmonary edema), whereas others are preexisting conditions that may worsen or be exacerbated (cardiomyopathy, thromboembolic disease, asthma, pneumonia, and HIV-related pulmonary complications). When pulmonary complications occur during pregnancy, an understanding of the normal physiologic changes of pregnancy and their implications for assessing maternal–fetal status is essential for developing appropriate interventions and treatment.

ANATOMIC AND PHYSIOLOGIC CHANGES OF PREGNANCY THAT AFFECT THE RESPIRATORY SYSTEM

Pregnant women are susceptible to respiratory compromise and injury for several reasons, including alterations in the immune system that involve cell-mediated immunity and mechanical and anatomic changes involving the chest and abdominal cavities. The cumulative effect is decreased tolerance to hypoxia and acute changes in pulmonary mechanics.

UPPER AIRWAY CHANGES

Increased estrogen levels result in mucosal edema, hyperemia, mucus hypersecretion, capillary congestion, and greater fragility of the upper respiratory tract (Hegewald & Crapo, 2011). These hormonal changes and mucosal changes result in rhinitis of pregnancy, characterized by nasal congestion during 6 or more weeks of pregnancy without other symptoms of respiratory tract infection and no known allergic cause. Rhinitis of pregnancy is experienced by 18% to 42% of pregnant women (Hegewald & Crapo, 2011). Epistaxis, sneezing, voice changes, and mouth breathing also are common (Hegewald & Crapo, 2011).

ANATOMIC CHANGES

Three important changes occur in the configuration of the thorax during pregnancy: (1) an increase in the circumference of the lower chest wall, (2) an elevation of the diaphragm, and (3) a 50% widening of the costal angle (Hegewald & Crapo, 2011; Norwitz & Robinson, 2010). These changes occur to accommodate the increase in uterine size and maternal weight gain, even though they appear in the first trimester prior to significant enlargement of the gravid uterus. The lower rib cage ligaments relax under hormonal influence to allow for a progressive widening of the subcostal angle and increased anterior–posterior and transverse diameters of the chest wall. Increased chest wall circumference accommodates elevation of the diaphragm such that total lung capacity is not reduced (Hegewald & Crapo, 2011).

RESPIRATORY CHANGES

Increased circulating levels of progesterone during pregnancy result in maternal hyperventilation and up to 50% greater tidal volume without corresponding changes in vital capacity or respiratory rate (Hegewald & Crapo, 2011; Norwitz & Robinson, 2010). Oxygen consumption and minute ventilation increase as functional residual capacity (FRC) and residual volume decrease with expanding abdominal girth. Total lung capacity is preserved, however, because of rib flaring and unimpaired diaphragmatic excursion. The overall hemoglobin amount increases and allows for an increase in total oxygen-carrying capacity; however, the increase in blood volume is disproportionate to the increase in hemoglobin concentration, thus resulting in a physiologic anemia (Laibl & Sheffield, 2006).

The increase in minute ventilation that is associated with pregnancy is often perceived as a shortness of breath. Dyspnea usually starts in the first or second trimester and is reported by 60% to 70% of healthy pregnant women by 30 weeks of gestation (Hegewald & Crapo, 2011). Dyspnea occurs secondary to the respiratory stimulation of progesterone, greater hypercapnic ventilatory response, and altered chest wall proprioceptors (Hegewald & Crapo, 2011). Shortness of breath at rest or with mild exertion is so common during pregnancy that it is often referred to as "physiologic dyspnea."

Pregnancy is characterized by a state of chronic compensated respiratory alkalosis. Normal maternal hyperventilation during pregnancy lowers maternal partial pressure of carbon dioxide (PCO_2) and minimally increases blood pH. The increase in blood pH increases the oxygen affinity of maternal hemoglobin and facilitates elimination of fetal carbon dioxide but appears to impair release of maternal oxygen to the fetus. The high levels of estrogen and progesterone during pregnancy facilitate a shift in the oxygen dissociation curve back to the right, thereby stimulating oxygen release to a fetus that has an increased affinity for oxygen. These physiologic adaptations ensure fetal advantage from increased oxygen transfer across the placenta and adequate blood gas exchange.

During labor and birth, hyperventilation is common due to pain, anxiety, and coached breathing techniques (Gei & Suarez, 2011; Hegewald & Crapo, 2011). Narcotics administered during labor and birth will act to decrease minute ventilation. In women with marginal placental reserves, hyperventilation and hypocarbia during labor and birth, leading to uterine vessel vasoconstriction and decreased placental perfusion, can have adverse effects on the fetus. Within 72 hours after birth, the minute ventilation rate decreases significantly with resumption of baseline in a few weeks. Lung volume changes normalize with decompression of the lungs and diaphragm after birth while FRC and residual volume are back to baseline within 48 hours (Hegewald & Crapo, 2011). Chest wall changes of pregnancy return to normal by 24 weeks postpartum, but the subcostal angle remains 20% of pregnancy width (Hegewald & Crapo, 2011).

RECOGNIZING RESPIRATORY COMPROMISE

A significant number of critical events are preceded by early signs of respiratory compromise. However, providers and patients often overlook or deny these signs and symptoms, leading to delays in communication and management. A woman with a pulmonary complication may present with a chief complaint of chest discomfort or tightness, persistant cough, unusual dyspnea or shortness of breath, or hemoptysis. If clinical history indicates a potential pulmonary complication, a thorough physical assessment should be conducted. Evidence-based guidelines that include early warning signs of maternal respiratory compromise should be used to improve communication between nurses and physicians, and to enhance clinical decision making regarding assessment parameters that fall outside defined normal values and that may indicate compromise. Physical signs of maternal respiratory compromise may include anxiety, increasing respiratory rate, wheezing, tachycardia, exertion with minimal activity, decreasing pulse oximetry values (trending below 96%), and/or adventitious breath sounds. Cyanosis, lethargy, agitation, intercostal retractions, and a respiratory rate greater than 30 breaths per minute indicate hypoxia and impending respiratory arrest.

FETAL SURVEILLANCE WITH MATERNAL PULMONARY COMPLICATIONS

In the presence of maternal respiratory compromise, which may include hypoxia, hypocapnia, or alkalosis, the fetus is at risk for impaired maternal–fetal gas exchange. Impaired gas exchange increases the incidence of fetal compromise and, if prolonged, will lead to intrauterine growth restriction (IUGR), oligohydramnios, meconium-stained amniotic fluid, preterm birth, and neonatal mortality (Beckmann, 2003; Coleman & Rund, 1997). The fetus depends on oxygen from maternal arterial oxygen content, venous return, and cardiac output, as well as from uterine artery and placental blood flow. Maternal hypoxia can cause fetal hypoxia directly, or the consequences of poorly controlled pulmonary conditions resulting in hypocapnia and alkalosis can cause fetal hypoxia indirectly by reducing uteroplacental blood flow (Cydulka, 2006). The fetus is sensitive to changes in maternal respiratory status, and decreases in maternal partial pressure of arterial oxygen (P_aO_2) may result in decreased fetal P_aO_2 and cause fetal hypoxia (Meschia, 2011). Rapid and profound decreases in fetal oxygen saturation and resultant fetal hypoxia occur with clinically significant decreases in maternal P_aO_2 below 60 mm Hg (Blaiss, 2004). Despite surviving in an environment of low oxygen tension, the fetus has very little oxygen reserve.

Administration of oxygen to the mother may produce only small increases in fetal P_aO_2, but this may increase fetal oxygen saturation significantly (Gardner & Doyle, 2004; Simpson & James, 2005). Oxygen should be administered as needed to maintain maternal oxygen saturation at 95% or higher (Cydulka, 2006).

Fetal status may offer early warning of maternal pulmonary compromise. Because the uterus is physiologically a nonessential organ, when there is decreased blood volume, decreased cardiac output, or significant hypoxia, oxygenated blood flow will be directed to critical organs such as the brain, heart, and adrenal glands at the expense of uterine blood flow and, therefore, fetal well-being (Frye, Clark, Piacenza, & Shay-Zapien, 2011). Oxygenated blood flow will only be available to the uterus once other critical organs are perfused and oxygenated; therefore, a normal fetal heart rate (FHR) pattern excludes significant maternal hypoxia or hypotension, and an indeterminate or abnormal FHR pattern warrants close evaluation and intervention (Frye et al., 2011). Evaluation of the FHR pattern is an important element of assessment of maternal status and clinical decision making in the context of maternal respiratory disease (Frye et al., 2011).

The frequency of fetal surveillance should be determined by gestational age, current maternal status, and fetal response to illness. If exacerbations of pulmonary complications occur, vigilant fetal surveillance is important. At each prenatal visit, confirmation that fundal height and fetal size are consistent with expected normal values based on current gestational age is crucial. In conjunction with nonstress testing, serial ultrasounds and biophysical profiles (BPPs) are used to monitor fetal status on an ongoing basis (Namazy & Schatz, 2006). Fetal movement counting may also be initiated based on provider preference.

ASTHMA

SIGNIFICANCE AND INCIDENCE

Asthma is the most common chronic medical condition, affecting up to 8% of women during pregnancy (American College of Obstetricians and Gynecologists [ACOG], 2008; Dombrowski et al., 2004). The effects of pregnancy on asthma symptoms vary, with 23% of women improving, 30% experiencing worsening of their symptoms, and 47% remaining unchanged (Dombrowski et al., 2004). Overall, if asthma symptoms worsen, it is more likely to occur between 17 and 24 weeks' gestation, and it is less severe in the last 4 weeks of pregnancy (Belfort & Herbst, 2010; Gluck, 2004). Severe asthmatics, even those under good control prior to pregnancy, are more likely to experience severe exacerbation requiring hospitalization (Belfort & Herbst, 2010; Dombrowski et al., 2004;

Gluck & Gluck, 2006). Exacerbations during labor and birth are unusual (Frye et al., 2011). After birth, 75% of asthmatic women return to their prepregnancy asthmatic status. In most women, asthma severity is the same as prepregnancy status within approximately 3 months postpartum (Gluck & Gluck, 2006).

Asthma has a variable natural history, creating a wide range of symptom expression during pregnancy. History of asthma severity in previous pregnancies may predict the severity of asthma in subsequent pregnancies (Blaiss, 2004). The relationship between asthma and pregnancy outcomes can also be influenced by risk behaviors and demographics. Smoking, age extremes, and Hispanic and African-American races have been shown to increase perinatal risk in asthmatic women (Beckmann, 2003). Maternal complications reported among asthmatics include hyperemesis, vaginal bleeding, placenta previa, preeclampsia, hypertensive disorders, a predisposition to infections, gestational diabetes, preterm rupture of membranes, preterm labor, cesarean birth, an increased length of hospital stay, and having a low-birth-weight infant (ACOG, 2008; Alexander, Dodds, & Armson, 1998; Beckmann, 2003; Cydulka, 2006; Dombrowski, 2006; Gardner & Doyle, 2004; Källén, Rydhstroem, & Aberg, 2000; Kwon et al., 2006; Minerbi-Codish, Fraser, Avnun, Glezerman, & Heimer, 1998; National Asthma Education and Prevention Program [NAEPP], 2005; Pereira & Krieger, 2004). Severe or uncontrolled asthma can be life threatening for a woman and her fetus during pregnancy. Potentially life-threatening complications of severe asthma include pneumothorax, pneumomediastinum, acute cor pulmonale, and respiratory arrest (Belfort & Herbst, 2010; Cydulka, 2006; Gardner & Doyle, 2004). Maternal mortality is reported as high as 40% when a pregnant woman with asthma requires mechanical ventilation (Gardner & Doyle, 2004). Asthma has been associated with a fetal death rate twice that of pregnant women without asthma (Blaiss, 2004; Silver, 2007). However, effective control can optimize pregnancy outcomes close to that of the general population (ACOG, 2008). The NAEPP's (2005) suggested steps for asthma control, as discussed in its publication, *Working Group Report on Managing Asthma During Pregnancy: Recommendations for Pharmacologic Treatment—Update 2004*, are listed in Table 10–1.

PATHOPHYSIOLOGY

Asthma is a chronic inflammatory disease of the airways in which the tracheobronchial tree is hyperresponsive to a multitude of stimuli (Dombrowski & Schatz, 2010). Asthma is one of the specific disease entities that is included in the general category of obstructive lung disease, which is characterized by limitation of airflow that generally is marked more during

Table 10–1. STEPWISE APPROACH FOR THE PHARMACOLOGIC MANAGEMENT OF CHRONIC ASTHMA DURING PREGNANCY

Category	Step Therapy
Mild intermittent	Inhaled β-agonist as needed
Mild persistent	Low-dose inhaled corticosteroid
	Alternative: cromolyn, leukotriene receptor antagonist, or theophylline
Moderate persistent	Low-dose inhaled corticosteroid and long-acting β-agonist
	Alternative: low-dose or (if needed) medium-dose inhaled corticosteroid and either theophylline or leukotriene receptor antagonist
Severe	High-dose inhaled corticosteroid and long-acting β-agonist and (if needed) oral corticosteroids
	Alternative: High-dose inhaled corticosteroid and theophylline

From National Asthma Education and Prevention Program. (2005). *Working Group Report on Managing Asthma during Pregnancy: Recommendations for Pharmacologic Treatment—Update 2004* (NIH Publication No. 05-5236). Bethesda, MD: U.S. Department of Health and Human Services, National Institutes of Health, National Heart, Lung, and Blood Institute.

Table 10–2. COMMON TRIGGERS OF ASTHMA EXACERBATIONS

Allergens	Pollens, molds, animal dander, house-dust mites, cockroach antigen
Irritants	Strong odors, cigarette smoke, wood smoke, occupational dusts and chemicals, air pollution
Medical conditions	Sinusitis, viral upper respiratory infections, esophageal reflux
Drugs, additives	Sulfites, nonsteroidal anti-inflammatory drugs, aspirin, β-blockers, contrast media
Other	Emotional stress, exercise, cold air, menses

expiration than inspiration and results in a prolonged expiratory phase. Asthma has varying degrees of airway obstruction, bronchial hyperresponsiveness, and airway edema that are accompanied by eosinophilic and lymphocytic inflammation (Belfort & Herbst, 2010; Gardner & Doyle, 2004). This results in edema of the bronchial wall, airway diameter reduction, and secretions that are thick and tenacious. Asthma involves a complex interplay of inflammatory cells, cellular mediators, and external triggers (Gluck & Gluck, 2006). It is a chronic disease with acute exacerbations that are characterized by recurrent bouts of wheezing and dyspnea that result from airway obstruction (Frye et al., 2011). The airway of an asthmatic patient is hyperresponsive to stimuli such as allergens, viral infections, air pollutants, smoke, food additives, exercise, cold air, and emotional stress (Dombrowski & Schatz, 2010). Common triggers of asthma exacerbations are listed in Table 10–2.

The precise cause of airway inflammation and hyperresponsiveness is not well understood. When triggered by external stimuli, inflammatory cells infiltrate bronchial tissue and release chemical mediators such as prostaglandins, histamine, cytokines, bradykinin, and leukotrienes. Ultimately, airway smooth muscle responsiveness is increased because of these mediators. Narrowing of the airway lumen and airway hyperresponsiveness may be a result of the development of bronchial mucosal edema, excess fluid and mucus, inflammatory cellular infiltrates, and smooth muscle hypertrophy and constriction. During asthma

exacerbations, there is decreased expiratory airflow, increased FRC, increased pulmonary vascular resistance, hypoxemia, and hypercapnia. The fetus can be negatively affected during acute episodes of asthma in which there is maternal arterial hypoxemia and the potential for uterine artery vasoconstriction (Dombrowski et al., 2004; Frye et al., 2011).

CLINICAL MANIFESTATIONS

Women may have one or a combination of asthma symptoms, which include shortness of breath, wheezing, nonproductive coughing, flaring nostrils, chest tightness, and use of accessory respiratory muscles. There may be scant or copious sputum, which is usually clear. Reports of nocturnal awakenings with asthma symptoms are common. An increase in cough, the appearance of chest tightness, dyspnea, wheezing, decrease in fetal movement, or a 20% decrease in peak expiratory flow rate (PEFR) may signal worsening of asthma and should warrant immediate clinical attention (Cydulka, 2006). Women with the following symptoms should be considered for intubation and mechanical ventilation: (1) worsening pulmonary function tests; (2) decreasing P_aO_2, increasing P_aCO_2, or progressive respiratory acidosis, despite vigorous bronchodilator therapy; (3) declining mental status; and (4) increasing fatigue (Cydulka, 2006).

Guidelines for assessing the severity of asthma before initiating therapy have been developed by the National Heart, Lung, and Blood Institute, a division of the National Institutes of Health (Scheffer, 1991). This classification system, like many others, was developed without specific consideration of pregnancy, but it may be helpful when assessing an adult patient with asthma. Patients are identified as mild, moderate, or severe asthmatics. Mild asthmatics experience exacerbations with coughing and wheezing no more than two times each week. There may be an intolerance of vigorous exercise. Women with moderate asthma experience infrequent exacerbations, with emergent care required

D I S P L A Y 1 0 – 1

Management Plan of Care for Pregnant Women with Exacerbations of Asthma

- Obtain initial blood gas and pulmonary function tests to gather baseline data.
- Continuously monitor maternal pulse oximetry.
- Oxygen therapy to maintain SpO_2 >95%.
- Monitor fetal status as determined by estimated gestational age.
- Tocolytic of choice for preterm labor management is magnesium sulfate. Use of magnesium sulfate therapy may enhance bronchodilation. Nonsteroidal anti-inflammatory medications, such as indomethacin, may exacerbate asthma and are contraindicated.
- β-agonist inhalation therapy is the initial pharmacologic therapy.
- If initial bronchodilator treatments fail to result in adequate response, high-dose intravenous corticosteroids may be considered.
- Antibiotics may be used to cover secondary bacterial infection.
- Measure and record intake and output. Observe for fluid volume imbalances.
- Observe for signs and symptoms of hydrostatic pulmonary edema due to tocolytic therapy and intravenous steroids.
- Ongoing care based on response to initial management.

less than three times each year. Severe asthmatics experience daily wheezing and require emergency treatment more than three times per year. Women with severe asthma have poor exercise tolerance.

Identification of the pregnant woman with severe asthma is important so that a plan of care and intensive treatment can be initiated early. See Display 10–1 for a management plan of care for pregnant women with exacerbations of asthma. Characteristics of maternal history that should alert healthcare providers to an increased risk of a potentially fatal asthma exacerbation are listed in Display 10–2. Nursing evaluation of the symptoms of asthma begins with clinical assessment of signs of respiratory distress. Significant findings include dyspnea, cough, wheezing, chest tightness, nasal flaring, presence of sputum, and tachycardia. Intercostal retractions or a respiratory rate

greater than 30 breaths per minute indicates moderate to severe asthma. Pulsus paradoxus of more than 15 mm Hg is an indication of severe asthma. If pulsus paradoxus is present, blood pressure is audible only during expiration. To make this assessment, carefully observe the woman's breathing, noting when systole first appears, and the millimeter level of mercury until pulsations are heard during inspiration and expiration. Lung auscultation usually reveals bilateral expiratory wheezing. Occasionally, on inspiration or expiration, only rhonchi are heard. Rales are rarely auscultated in asthmatics. Detailed clinical findings are listed in Display 10–3.

The most beneficial tools to determine the severity of asthma is a pulmonary function test such as peak expiratory flow. Predicted values of PEFR are unchanged during pregnancy and range from 380 to 550 L/min. An individual baseline value should be established for each woman when her asthma is under control. Evaluation of exacerbations can be made by comparing baseline values with current peak flow values. Peak expiratory flow values that are more than 50% below personal baseline values require immediate attention.

Evaluations of arterial blood gases can help to establish severity of an asthma attack, with attention focused primarily on the pH and PCO_2 to define severity. A mild attack is characterized by an elevated pH and a PCO_2 below normal for pregnancy. The combination

D I S P L A Y 1 0 – 2

Markers for Potentially Fatal Asthma

- History of systemic steroid therapy >4 weeks
- Three recent emergency room visits for asthma
- History of multiple hospitalizations for asthma
- History of hypoxic seizure, hypoxic syncope, or intubation
- History of admission to an intensive care unit for asthma

D I S P L A Y 1 0 – 3

Clinical Findings in Asthma

SIGNS AND SYMPTOMS
- Shortness of breath, chest tightness, productive or nonproductive cough
- Increased respiratory rate (>20 breaths/min)
- Tachycardia
- Nasal flaring
- Exertion with minimal activity
- Recurrent episodes of symptoms
- Nocturnal awakenings from symptoms
- Waxing and waning of symptoms

AUSCULTATORY FINDINGS
- Diffuse wheezes
- Diffuse rhonchi
- Longer expiratory phase than inspiratory phase

SIGNS OF RESPIRATORY DISTRESS
- Rapid respiratory rate (>30 breaths/min)
- Pulsus paradoxus >15 mm Hg
- Retractions intercostally or supraclavicularly
- Lethargy
- Confusion or agitation
- Cyanosis

of normal pH, low PO_2, and normal PCO_2 for pregnancy indicates a moderate asthma attack. A low PO_2, low pH, and a high PCO_2 are most significant for severe respiratory compromise. When maternal arterial PO_2 falls below 60 mm Hg, the fetus is in severe jeopardy, and risk of fetal demise is increased.

Potentially fatal asthma includes a history of any one of the factors listed in Display 10–2. During pregnancy, monthly evaluations of pulmonary function and asthma history are important. These evaluations should include the following assessments: pulmonary function testing, ideally spirometry; detailed symptom history (symptom frequency, nocturnal asthma, interference with activities, exacerbations, and medication use); and physical examination with specific attention paid to the lungs (Namazy & Schatz, 2006).

CLINICAL MANAGEMENT

The goals when managing the woman with asthma during pregnancy include educational support, maintaining optimal respiratory status and function, objective assessment of maternal and fetal status, avoiding triggers, and pharmacologic treatment to control symptoms and prevent exacerbations and/or adverse effects of medication (ACOG, 2008; NAEPP, 2007). Fetal surveillance for women with asthma begins early in pregnancy. Women who have moderate or severe asthma during pregnancy should have ultrasound examinations and antenatal fetal testing (ACOG, 2008). If possible, first-trimester ultrasound dating should be performed to assist with subsequent evaluations of fetal growth restriction and determine risk of preterm birth. Serial ultrasound examinations to monitor fetal activity and growth should be considered (starting at 32 weeks of gestation) for women who have poorly controlled asthma or moderate to severe asthma and for women recovering from a severe asthma exacerbation (ACOG, 2008).

PATIENT/FAMILY EDUCATION

Education should be designed to assist the woman and her family to gain motivation, confidence, and skills to keep asthma symptoms under control and to understand the potential adverse effects of uncontrolled asthma on the woman and the fetus. Although some women may be reluctant to take prescribed medications for fear they may harm the developing fetus, the woman needs to be reassured that risks to the fetus from hypoxia-related, untreated asthma are greater than risks of medications (ACOG, 2008; Namazy & Schatz, 2006). All patients should be taught to be conscientious of fetal activity and to report concerns to their healthcare provider (ACOG, 2008). Also, it is critically important that the pregnant woman be able to recognize symptoms of worsening asthma and

have the knowledge of how to treat them appropriately. Correct inhaler technique should be reinforced, and the patient should know how to reduce her exposure to, or control, those factors that exacerbate her asthma (Namazy & Schatz, 2006). Educational topics (NAEPP, 2005) include the following:

- Signs and symptoms of asthma
- Airway changes
- Avoiding asthma triggers
- Effects of pregnancy on the disease and the disease on pregnancy
- Peak flow meters and metered dose inhalers
- Role of medications
- Correct use of medications
- Adverse effects of medications
- Managing exacerbations
- Emergency care

Individualized education throughout pregnancy should be guided by assessment of the woman's understanding of her asthma assessment management plan and her level of cooperation. It is essential to highlight the changes that pregnancy has on asthma and treatment. When there is active participation by the healthcare provider, the pregnant woman, and her family, asthma control can be maximized.

NONPHARMACOLOGIC CONTROL

Identification of triggering factors for asthma in each woman is an important aspect of management that may improve clinical status, prevent acute exacerbations, and decrease the need for pharmacologic intervention. Asthma is associated with allergies, with 75% to 85% of patients reporting positive testing to common allergens (Dombrowski, 2006). Historic information and prior skin testing may give important information regarding common triggers such as pollens, molds, house-dust mites, animal dander, and cockroach antigens. Other common asthma irritants include air pollutants, strong odors, food additives, and tobacco smoke. It is particularly important for the pregnant asthmatic woman to stop smoking during her pregnancy (Gluck & Gluck, 2006). Education about the risks of smoking, including an increased severity of her asthma, bronchitis, or sinusitis and the need for increased medication, can be helpful in motivating the woman to stop smoking.

Viral respiratory infections, vigorous exercise, and emotional stress may also cause severe asthma exacerbations. Medications such as aspirin, beta-blockers, nonsteroidal anti-inflammatory drugs (NSAIDs), radiocontrast media, and sulfites have been implicated as asthma triggers as well. Once the woman has been assisted to identify common asthma triggers, exposure to allergens or irritants can be minimized, thereby lessening exacerbations.

PHARMACOLOGIC THERAPY

Pharmacologic therapy plays an essential role in optimizing maternal and fetal outcomes by providing protection for the respiratory system from irritant stimuli, prevention of pulmonary and inflammatory response to allergen exposure, relief of bronchospasm, resolution of airway inflammation to reduce airway hyperresponsiveness, and improvement of pulmonary function. Undertreatment is an ongoing problem in the care of pregnant asthmatic women. Medications commonly used in asthma management are generally considered safe and effective during pregnancy and lactation. It is safer for pregnant women with asthma and their fetuses to take prescribed medications than to experience an exacerbation (ACOG, 2008). The effectiveness of medications for the treatment of asthma during pregnancy is assumed to be the same as in nonpregnant women (NAEPP, 2007). Inhalation therapy is usually more effective than systemic treatment because asthma is an airway disease. Aerosolized medications are ideal because they deliver the drug directly to the airways, minimizing systemic side effects and decreasing exposure to the fetus.

Pharmacologic therapy for asthma is divided into two categories: (1) rescue (medications that provide symptomatic relief of acute bronchospasms without treating the cause of the bronchospasm) and (2) maintenance (medications that control airway hyperreactivity and treat underlying inflammation) (Belfort & Herbst, 2010). Generally, a stepwise approach to the pharmacologic management of chronic asthma is preferred (see Table 10–1).

Rescue Medications

Short-Acting Beta-Agonists

The use of inhaled short-acting beta-2-agonists provides bronchodilation and is recommended for acute and mild intermittent asthma therapy (Chambers, 2006). The onset of action is rapid with demonstrated safety profiles for mother and fetus, making short-acting beta-2-agonists the preferred rescue medication for acute exacerbations of asthma. Medications in this group include metaproterenol (Alupent), terbutaline (Brethine), and albuterol (Ventolin, Proventil). This group of drugs has minimal side effects, such as maternal tachycardia, tremors, restlessness, anxiety, and palpitations (Lehne, 2010). If symptoms disappear and pulmonary function normalizes, these medications can be used indefinitely. Prolonged use may result in rapid tolerance and limited usefulness. Women are candidates for anti-inflammatory therapy if they require the use of a beta-2-agonist more than three times each week. In the management of moderate to severe persistent asthma, long-acting beta-agonists may be added to a regimen of inhaled corticosteroids for greater asthma control (Blaiss, 2004; NAEPP, 2005).

Long-Acting Beta-Agonists

Salmeterol (Serevent Diskus) and formoterol (Foradil) are newer long-acting beta-agonists with limited published data regarding safe use in pregnancy. Therefore, the use of these medications are limited to women with moderate to severe asthma who report relief of symptoms with use of these agents prior to pregnancy or as an add-on therapy for women who are currently on inhaled steroids and need additional therapy for symptom relief.

Anticholinergics

Ipratropium (Atrovent) is an anticholinergic medication that may be used in combination with inhaled beta-agonists to promote bronchodilation. Even though published reports show safe use, the combination of these medications is rarely used in pregnancy (NAEPP, 2005). If prescribed during pregnancy, nebulized forms of anticholinergics may be considered for additional therapy in cases of acute asthma exacerbations that are not controlled after initial beta-agonist therapy (Namazy & Schatz, 2006).

Maintenance Medications

Methylxanthines

Because of the success of inhalation therapy, systemic aminophylline and theophylline are rarely used today. Sustained-release theophylline may be helpful for the pregnant woman whose symptoms are primarily nocturnal because of its long-acting properties. Although safe at recommended doses during pregnancy, theophylline treatment is associated with a higher incidence of maternal side effects than inhaled beta-agonists (NAEPP, 2005).

Cromolyn Sodium

Cromolyn and nedocromil are nonsteroidal anti-inflammatory agents that work by preventing the release of inflammatory mediators through stabilization of mast cells. Neither produces any side effects. Both are FDA category B drugs (Schatz, 2001), and cromolyn data have demonstrated long-term safety (Blaiss, 2004). Neither is as effective as inhaled corticosteroids in preventing asthma symptoms.

Inhaled Corticosteroids

One of the greatest advances in asthma treatment in the past decade has been the availability of inhaled corticosteroids (ACOG, 2008). For women with persistent mild asthma, these medications are currently the treatment of choice because they reduce the risk of asthma exacerbations associated with pregnancy and have not been related to any increases in congenital malformations or other adverse perinatal outcomes (NAEPP, 2005). To minimize systemic effects and improve respiratory tract penetration, inhaled corticosteroids are administered with a spacer. At recommended doses, these medications act without systemic side effects to effectively reduce mucus secretion and airway edema. They may increase bronchodilator responsiveness while inhibiting many of the mediators of inflammation. Studies suggest that beclomethasone or budesonide are the inhaled steroids of choice for use during pregnancy due to reassuring safety data (ACOG, 2008).

Unlike the immediate-acting bronchodilators, the effects of inhaled corticosteroids are gradual. After 2 to 4 weeks of use, full effects of symptom suppression and PEFR improvement are seen. Patient education is vital to ensure that the woman will continue her anti-inflammatory therapy until the medication achieves maximum effectiveness. The most common side effect of inhaled steroids is hoarseness, which disappears when therapy is discontinued. Other uncommon side effects include throat irritation, cough, and oral thrush. Infrequent effects such as easy bruising, skin thinning, and low serum cortisol levels have been reported. Published data have shown no evidence of teratogenicity with use of inhaled corticosteroids (Blaiss, 2004). Intranasal corticosteroids have not been studied during human pregnancy, but because their systemic effects are minimal, continued use during pregnancy appears to be safe (ACOG, 2008; NAEPP, 2005).

Systemic Corticosteroids

Due to associated fetal and pregnancy complications, systemic oral corticosteroids may be prescribed when maximum doses of bronchodilators and anti-inflammatory agents fail to control asthma. Conflicting reports show possible association of increased cleft lip and palate formation with exposure (Park-Wyllie et al., 2000; Reinisch, Simon, Karow, & Gandelman, 1978; Robert et al., 1994). Consistently, reports of pregnancy-associated complication have been shown with corticosteroid use. These complications include gestational hypertension, preeclampsia, gestational diabetes or worsening of diabetes mellitus, preterm birth, and low birth weight (ACOG, 2008; NAEPP, 2005). However, if needed for short-term therapy to control exacerbations of asthma symptoms or long-term management, the benefits of using oral corticosteroids outweigh the risks and are recommended as needed (ACOG, 2008; NAEPP, 2005).

Leukotriene Modifiers

Leukotriene modifiers are a new class of drugs that limit the inflammatory action of leukotrienes—chemical mediators that cause bronchoconstriction and mucus hypersecretion and stimulate microvascular leakage, edema formation, and eosinophil chemotaxis (Belfort & Herbst, 2010). Examples of these drugs include zileuton (Zyflo), zafirlukast (Accolate), and montelukast (Singulair). Due to limited data, ACOG (2008) recommends that, with the exception of zileuton, leukotriene modifiers may be used during pregnancy if women show resistance to other classes of safety-proven medications.

Combination Drugs

Combination drugs, such as Advair Diskus and Combivent, may be prescribed for continued use during pregnancy if symptoms are well controlled. However, because these medications contain a combination of medications, it is not recommended to initiate these drugs during pregnancy unless the benefits outweigh the risks of the individualized medications contained in these combination formulas (ACOG, 2008).

Immunotherapy

Pregnant women with asthma who have allergens responsive to desensitization may benefit from allergen immunotherapy. Pollens, dust mites, and some fungi are aeroallergens that have been effectively suppressed with the use of allergy injections. Maintenance dose injections may continue for a pregnant woman who is not reacting regularly and continues to benefit from the immunotherapy (Blaiss, 2004). Because there is a 6- to 7-month interval before clinical benefits are seen and a significant risk of a systemic reaction, pregnancy is not a time for initiation of immunotherapy.

Other Pharmacologic Therapies

Antihistamines may be useful in the woman with a clear allergic stimulus to her asthma. The safest decongestant for use during pregnancy appears to be pseudoephedrine, although it has recently been linked to the birth defect gastroschisis (ACOG, 2008). Pseudoephedrine has been routinely used in the treatment of rhinitis, although intranasal corticosteroids are currently the most effective medications for this condition and carry a low risk of systemic effects. Avoidance of oral decongestants in the first trimester is suggested unless absolutely necessary. Pregnant women with asthma should be cautioned about use of over-the-counter medications because many of the medications contain vasoconstrictors that may cause fetal abnormalities and decreased uterine blood flow (NAEPP, 2005). The influenza vaccine is indicated for women with chronic asthma after the first trimester. Because it is an inactivated virus, the influenza vaccine poses no risk to the fetus.

LABOR AND BIRTH

Approximately 10% to 20% of women with asthma experience an exacerbation during the intrapartum period (Gluck & Gluck, 2006; Namazy & Schatz, 2006). The risk of dyspnea or wheezing can be minimized through ongoing asthma medication during labor and the postpartum period. An exacerbation during labor is treated no differently than at any other time. Control of the asthma is a priority for safety of the mother and her fetus. Intravenous (IV) access should be established on admission (Gardner & Doyle, 2004). A peak flow rate should be taken on admission and then every 12 hours (Gardner & Doyle, 2004). If the woman develops symptoms of asthma, peak flows should be measured after treatments (Gardner & Doyle, 2004). If a systemic steroid has been administered in the past month prior to birth, additional rescue-dosed steroid therapy should be given during labor to prevent maternal adrenal crisis (Belfort & Herbst, 2010). IV hydrocortisone 100 mg every 6 to 8 hours should be administered for 24 hours or until oral medications are tolerated (Belfort & Herbst, 2010).

Air exchange is enhanced through patient positioning in a semi-Fowler's or high-Fowler's position. Potential for fluid overload can be avoided through strict intake and output measurements. Oxytocin is the drug of choice for the induction of labor because prostaglandin $F_{2\alpha}$ is a known bronchoconstrictor (Frye et al., 2011; Towers, Briggs, & Rojas, 2004). The use of prostaglandin E_2 for cervical ripening intracervically or intravaginally has not been reported to result in a clinical exacerbation of asthma (Namazy & Schatz, 2006). The pain relief method of choice for women in labor with asthma is epidural analgesia (Gardner & Doyle, 2004). Epidural analgesia can reduce oxygen consumption and may enhance the effects of bronchodilators (NAEPP, 2005). Meperidine and morphine sulfate are contraindicated because of their actions on smooth muscle and the potential for respiratory depression, and they may result in bronchospasm through histamine release (Belfort & Herbst, 2010). Butorphanol and fentanyl are appropriate substitutes (Belfort & Herbst, 2010).

A vaginal birth is safest for all women, but particularly for women with asthma. Maternal and fetal hypoxia that is the result of asthma should be managed medically; rarely is cesarean birth indicated. If cesarean birth is necessary for obstetric reasons, regional anesthesia is preferred; however, if general anesthesia is required, propofol is the sedation agent of choice, and ketamine or halogenated anesthetics are preferred due to their bronchodilation effects (Belfort & Herbst, 2010). Use of methylergonovine (i.e., Methergine) and prostaglandin $F_{2\alpha}$ for postpartum hemorrhage can cause bronchoconstriction and should be avoided (Belfort & Herbst, 2010).

POSTPARTUM

Prepregnancy regimens of inhaled medications should be resumed following birth. Women on oral corticosteroid therapy may require IV dosing until oral medications are tolerated (Belfort & Herbst, 2010). Breastfeeding should be encouraged in women with asthma because breast milk confers some immunity to infection to the baby, especially to respiratory and gastrointestinal infections (Gardner & Doyle, 2004). Although breast milk may contain small amounts of the medications used to treat asthma, in general, they are not known to be harmful to the baby (Gardner & Doyle, 2004). Corticosteroids are approximately 90% protein bound in the blood and not secreted in any significant amounts in breast milk. Inhaled beta-2-agonists (terbutaline, metaproterenol, albuterol) by metered dosage are associated with the lowest exposure to the baby. Theophylline, as with caffeine, can cause irritability and wakefulness in the baby and is no longer considered the primary treatment (Gardner & Doyle, 2004).

PNEUMONIA

SIGNIFICANCE AND INCIDENCE

The incidence of pneumonia and spectrum of causative pathogens during pregnancy is similar to that of the nonpregnant population. However, the disease course in pregnancy is often more virulent and less tolerated, and the mortality rates from some pathogens are high (Graves, 2010). Overall, pneumonia is the primary diagnosis for approximately 4.2% of nonobstetric antepartum hospital admissions (Laibl & Sheffield, 2006). Pneumonia is seen more frequently in women with poor health and who postpone childbearing. Also, available rates show higher incidence in large urban hospitals than in community settings (Brito & Neiderman, 2011). Pneumonia has been strongly associated with women with asthma, HIV, cystic fibrosis (CF), anemia, and illicit drug use (Goodnight & Soper, 2005).

Antepartum pneumonia has been associated with the use of tocolytics, as well as with administration of corticosteroids for enhancement of fetal lung maturity (Goodnight & Soper, 2005). Although pneumonia is not gestational-age dependent, the average gestational age at diagnosis is 32 weeks, and hospital admission for pneumonia is highest between 24 and 31 weeks of gestation (Graves, 2010). Pneumonia during the postpartum period is more than twice as high in women who had a cesarean as compared to vaginal birth (Belfort et al., 2010). The higher incidence may be due to associated pain and decreased activity following the cesarean birth or to a disease process that necessitated cesarean birth and/or predisposed the woman to infection (Brito & Neiderman, 2011). Pneumonia is the leading cause of maternal mortality from nonobstetric infection in the peripartum period (Goodnight & Soper, 2005). Maternal conditions and complications that are associated with pneumonia are listed in Display 10–4. Although the introduction of antimicrobial therapy has significantly decreased maternal mortality from 23% to less than 4%, risk of

DISPLAY 10–4

Complications Associated with Pneumonia

- Altered mental status
- Vital sign abnormalities
  - Respirations ≥30 breaths/min
  - Temperature ≥39°C or ≤35°C
  - Hypotension
  - Heart rate >120 bpm
- Laboratory data abnormalities
  - White blood cell count <4,000 mm³ or 30,000 mm³
  - Room air P_aO_2 <60 mm Hg
  - Room air P_aCO_2 >50 mm Hg
  - Serum creatinine >1.2 mg/dL
- Sepsis leading to multiorgan dysfunction/failure
- Radiologic abnormalities
- Multilobe involvement
- Cavitation
- Pleural effusion

maternal and fetal morbidity continues (Laibl & Sheffield, 2006). The majority of maternal deaths resulting from pneumonia are in women with preexisting cardiopulmonary disease (Goodnight & Soper, 2005). Viral pneumonias may be more virulent during pregnancy than in the nonpregnant patient.

Maternal complications of pneumonia include preterm labor, bacteremia, pneumothorax, atrial fibrillation, pericardial tamponade, and respiratory failure requiring intubation (Goodnight & Soper, 2005). Pneumonia has not been related to any congenital syndrome in neonates, but antepartum respiratory infection has been associated with increased incidence of complicated preterm birth. The loss of maternal ventilatory reserve normally seen in pregnancy coupled with maternal fever, tachycardia, respiratory alkalosis, and hypoxemia seen with respiratory infections can be adverse for the fetus. Reports of preterm labor and birth, small-for-gestational-age (SGA) infants, and fetal death have been attributed to pneumonia during pregnancy (Goodnight & Soper, 2005; Lim, Macfarlane, & Colthorpe, 2001; Nolan & Hankins, 1995; Salmon & Bruick-Sorge, 2003).

Fungal pneumonia from environmental organisms is rare in pregnancy, occurring most often in severely immunocompromised patients (Laibl & Sheffield, 2006). In nonimmunosuppressed patients, this disease is frequently mild, self-limiting, and usually resolves with or without treatment in women without other preexisting illnesses. Disseminated disease from *Pneumocystis carinii* develops occasionally in immunocompromised patients and carries a high risk of preterm birth and perinatal and maternal mortality. Symptoms include fever, anorexia, dry cough, and several weeks of dyspnea. Treatment is prolonged and carries risks to the developing fetus.

PATHOPHYSIOLOGY

Pneumonia is an inflammatory infection of the alveoli and distal bronchioles of the lower respiratory tract resulting in consolidation, exudation, and hypoxemia. Pneumonia may be primary or secondary and involve one or both lungs. The microorganisms that give rise to pneumonia are always present in the upper respiratory tract, and unless resistance is lowered, they cause no harm. Most organisms are introduced through inhalation or aspiration of secretions from the nasopharyngeal tract. Bacterial and viral pneumonias and aspiration pneumonitis are the most commonly seen pneumonias during gestation (Salmon & Bruick-Sorge, 2003) (Display 10–5). Alteration in maternal immune status to prevent rejection of the developing fetus is the major factor predisposing women to severe pneumonic infections during pregnancy.

Pneumonia develops when host defenses are overwhelmed by an organism invading the lung parenchyma. Although a number of defense mechanisms protect lower airways from pathogens, infection leads to increased permeability of the capillaries. This causes alveolar and interstitial fluid accumulation, resulting in abnormal chest radiograph findings. Air space pneumonia, interstitial pneumonia, and bronchopneumonia are commonly seen on the chest radiograph of patients with pneumonia. Radiographic patterns differ based on the infective agent and can be helpful in diagnosing the cause of pneumonia.

CLINICAL MANIFESTATIONS

Obtaining a detailed history of the illness, including symptoms, and a physical examination are essential.

DISPLAY 10–5

Causes of Pneumonia in Pregnancy

- *Streptococcus pneumoniae*
- *Haemophilus influenzae*
- *Legionella* species
- *Mycoplasma pneumoniae*
- *Chlamydia pneumoniae*
- *Pneumocystis carinii*
- Viral pathogens
- Influenza A
- Influenza B
- Varicella-zoster virus (VZV)
- Coronavirus (severe acute respiratory syndrome [SARS])
- Aspiration
- Fungi

All pregnant women should be questioned about immunity to varicella during the first prenatal visit. Susceptible women should be counseled to avoid contact with individuals who have chickenpox. If exposure occurs, varicella-zoster immune globulin (VZIG) should be administered within 96 hours in an attempt to prevent maternal infection (Laibl & Sheffield, 2006). Laboratory and radiologic findings are important to help diagnose the type of pneumonia present. Chest X-ray on the majority of patients with pneumonia reflects infiltrates, atelectasis, pleural effusions, pneumonitis, or pulmonary edema. Clinical presentation and laboratory data help to determine whether the pneumonia is classic or atypical. Careful questioning about underlying chronic conditions and prior illness can identify risk factors.

Initially, symptoms of pneumonia may mimic common discomforts in pregnancy and may be overlooked and the woman misdiagnosed with rapid progression of the disease course. Clinical manifestations may assist in diagnosis of pneumonia but lack specificity and sensitivity for causative etiology (Graves, 2010). In one study, 9.3% of pregnant women presented with a productive cough, 32% with shortness of breath, and 27.1% with pleuritic chest pain (Ramsey & Ramin, 2001). Physical examination usually reveals tachypnea and use of accessory muscles for respiration. Lung auscultation may identify inspiratory rales, absent breath sounds over the affected lung field, or a pleural friction rub. A sputum sample with secretions from the lower bronchial tree must be collected for Gram stain and culture. Positive blood culture results are highly specific, although they are infrequently performed, and are rarely positive in women with pneumonia in pregnancy (Yost, Bloom, Richey, Ramin, & Cunningham, 2000). These specimens assist in identifying the pathogen responsible for the pneumonia.

Initial arterial blood gases in the pregnant woman with pneumonia usually reflect significant degrees of hypoxia without hypercapnia or acidosis (Laibl & Sheffield, 2006). The nurse should assess each woman closely for symptoms of hypoxia, including irritability and restlessness, tachycardia, hypertension, cool and pale extremities, and decreased urine output. Confusion, disorientation, and loss of consciousness can result if the hypoxia goes untreated.

Differential diagnosis of pneumonia includes pulmonary embolus and pulmonary edema from tocolysis, hypertension, or vascular leak (Graves, 2010).

BACTERIAL PNEUMONIA

The leading cause of pneumonia in pregnant women is bacterial (Graves, 2010). Risks for acquiring bacterial pneumonia include asthma, smoking, positive HIV status, poor nutrition, anemia, immunosuppressive drugs, binge drinking, and exposure to viral infections (Laibl & Sheffield, 2006). The most common causative bacterial pathogen for pneumonia in pregnancy is *Streptococcus pneumoniae*. It is responsible for approximately one half to two thirds of cases of bacterial pneumonia during pregnancy and approximately two thirds of all pneumonias during pregnancy (Laibl & Sheffield, 2006). Women with bacterial pneumonia during pregnancy most often present with a history of malaise and upper respiratory infection. They frequently have abrupt onset of fever above 100°F with rigors and chills. Pleuritic chest pain, productive cough, dyspnea, and rusty sputum are other common symptoms. Blood cultures are positive in approximately 25% of cases (Neu & Sabath, 1993). *Haemophilus influenzae* is the second most common bacterium identified in women with bacterial pneumonia, and symptoms are similar to those caused by to *S. pneumoniae*. Women with chronic obstructive pulmonary diseases and chronic bronchitis are at greatest risk. There are numerous other uncommon pneumonia pathogens that may be seen in childbearing women, including *Mycoplasma pneumoniae*, *Chlamydia pneumoniae*, *Moraxella catarrhalis*, *Klebsiella pneumoniae*, and *Escherichia coli*. These organisms produce an atypical pneumonia syndrome, which is characterized by gradual onset, less toxicity, lower fever, nonproductive cough, malaise, and a patchy or interstitial infiltrate (Maccato, 1991). *Legionella pneumophila* may cause pneumonia with the typical acute course or the atypical symptoms described with the less common pathogens. Underlying chronic illness, advancing age, and cigarette smoking appear to be significant predisposing factors for bacterial pneumonia. When a superimposed pulmonary infection follows a viral pneumonia, *Staphylococcus aureus* is frequently responsible. This organism may also spread by the hematogenous route related to IV catheters, IV drug abuse, or infective endocarditis. The onset of this pneumonia is usually abrupt, and the course is rapid. Pleuritic chest pain and purulent sputum production are evident.

Aspiration can cause a very serious pneumonia that carries a high mortality rate in spite of respiratory support and aggressive management. Pregnant women are predisposed to gastric aspiration due to the anatomic changes with elevation of the intragastric pressure due to the enlarged gravid uterus, prostaglandin-induced relaxation of the gastroesophageal sphincter, and delayed gastric emptying (Brito & Neiderman, 2011). Aspiration pneumonia usually occurs during induction or emergence from general anesthesia for a cesarean birth. The aspiration of particulate matter and gastric acid causes an immediate chemical pneumonitis, followed in 24 to 48 hours by a secondary anaerobic or gram-negative bacterial infection. The use of nonparticulate antacids (e.g., sodium citrate), regional anesthesia, and rapid sequence induction of general anesthesia with cricoid pressure dramatically reduces the incidence of aspiration-related maternal mortality. Other causes of aspiration pneumonia include anything that may diminish consciousness, such as seizures and drug or alcohol abuse. Acute symptoms of aspiration include cough, significant bronchospasm, and hypoxia. Signs of chemical pneumonitis begin 6 to 24 hours after aspiration and include tachypnea, tachycardia, hypotension, and frothy pulmonary edema. Mechanical ventilation may be necessary and difficult. Resolution usually occurs over 4 to 5 days unless secondary infection develops (Graves, 2010). Prophylactic antibiotics and corticosteroids are not recommended. However, secondary bacterial infection must be identified and treated promptly with antibiotics to minimize significant perinatal morbidity and mortality (Graves, 2010).

VIRAL PNEUMONIAS

Varicella pneumonia occurs in up to 20% of adults with varicella (chickenpox) infection. Because 90% of women are immune due to immunization or previous infection, the incidence of varicella pneumonia during pregnancy is rare (0.7 per 1,000) (Pereira & Krieger, 2004). However, the mortality rate for varicella pneumonia is 25% to 55% due to an increased risk for multiple complications such as bacterial superinfection, acute respiratory distress syndrome (ARDS), endotoxin shock, and bronchiolitis obliterans organizing pneumonia (Chandra, Patel, Schiavello, & Briggs, 1998). Intrauterine infections occur in 8.7% to 26% of cases, exclusively during the first 20 weeks of gestation (Pereira & Krieger, 2004). The neonatal death rate for varicella pneumonia is between 9% and 20% (Grant, 1996). Following the incubation period of 10 to 21 days, symptoms of varicella zoster will begin, which include fever, headache, malaise, and maculopapular-vesicular rash. In a patient with primary varicella symptoms, the diagnosis of varicella pneumonia is confirmed by a chest X-ray that reveals an interstitial, nodular pattern, or focal infiltrates. Varicella pneumonia typically presents with fever, dyspnea, tachypnea, dry cough, pleuritic chest pain, oral mucous lesions, and hemoptysis within 2 to 7 days of the vesicular rash (Ramsey & Ramin, 2001). It is not uncommon to see rapid progression to hypoxia and respiratory failure. In addition to maternal complications, intrauterine infection occurs in up to 26% of varicella pneumonia cases (Pereira & Krieger, 2004). Congenital varicella syndrome may occur if infection occurs in the first trimester and is characterized by cutaneous scars, limb hypoplasia, chorioretinitis, cortical atrophy, cataracts, and other anomalies in the neonate (Balducci et al., 1992; Goodnight & Soper, 2005; Laibl & Sheffield, 2005). Second trimester varicella may result in congenital varicella zoster in some infants. Premature labor and perinatal varicella infection are significant adverse effects that may result from varicella infection during pregnancy. Rubeola during pregnancy may lead to spontaneous abortion and preterm birth. Pneumonia can complicate up to 50% of cases, and bacterial superinfection is also common.

Pregnant women with varicella pneumonia should be hospitalized, and infection control precautions should be implemented. Pharmacologic management should be implemented early with IV acyclovir at a dose of 10 mg/kg every 8 hours for 5 days (Graves, 2010). The addition of corticosteroids may also be given to improve outcomes.

Influenza-mediated viral pneumonia is commonly caused by type A influenza, which is the most virulent strain in humans. Type A influenza attacks the lung parenchyma and causes edema, hemorrhage, and hyaline membrane formation. Chest X-ray demonstrates unilateral patchy infiltrates. Acute onset of dyspnea, tachypnea, wheezing, malaise, headache, high fever, cough, and myalgias are associated symptoms. Frequently, superimposed bacterial pneumonia develops following resolution of influenza symptoms. During pregnancy, fulminant respiratory failure may develop quickly, requiring extended mechanical ventilation and resulting in significant mortality.

Severe acute respiratory syndrome (SARS) is a viral illness first described in 2002. It is transmitted by respiratory droplets or close personal contact and results in an atypical pneumonia that can progress to hypoxemia and respiratory failure. Chest X-ray reveals generalized, patchy, interstitial infiltrates in patients with SARS pneumonia (Graves, 2010). Symptoms that are seen 2 to 7 days after exposure include headache, fever, chills, rigors, malaise, myalgia, dyspnea, and a nonproductive cough (Laibl & Sheffield, 2005). Patients are most infectious during the second week of illness (Laibl & Sheffield, 2005). Based on limited available data, effects on pregnancy from this illness include spontaneous abortion, preterm birth, and SGA fetuses (Wong et al., 2004). The course of SARS and clinical outcomes are worse for pregnant women when compared to nonpregnant women (Lam et al., 2004). The virus does not appear to cross the placenta and infect the fetus (Wong et al., 2004).

INFLUENZA AND H1N1

Physiologic changes cause the pregnant woman to be at increased risk of critical illness from influenza. Five percent of all U.S. H1N1 deaths in 2009 occurred in women who were pregnant. In addition, preterm labor and birth risks are increased in women with influenza (ACOG, 2010a). Vaccination in any trimester is safe and recommended during influenza season (October through May) to prevent morbidity and mortality. Pregnant women should receive inactivated vaccine but should not receive the live attenuated nasal mist (ACOG, 2010a; Creanga et al., 2010). Women who are postpartum can receive either type of vaccination. Both types of vaccination are also safe if the mother is breast-feeding (ACOG, 2010a; Creanga et al., 2010). Another benefit of vaccination during pregnancy is protection in the newborn for up to 6 months of age. Infants younger than 6 months of age have a 10 times higher hospitalization rate for influenza as compared to older children (ACOG, 2010a). Many women do not receive influenza vaccination during pregnancy and postpartum due to a lack of knowledge, awareness, and concerns related to vaccine safety. Obstetric providers should educate and encourage all pregnant and postpartum women to get vaccinated against influenza.

CLINICAL MANAGEMENT

Prevention of pneumonia in pregnancy has been successful through the administration of seasonal influenza and pneumococcus vaccines. These vaccines are safe for administration in pregnancy and should be given to high-risk women. The varicella vaccine is not safe for administration during pregnancy because it is a live vaccine (Laibl & Sheffield, 2006). In pregnant women diagnosed with pneumonia, regardless of the type of pneumonia, interventions focus on close monitoring; oxygen supplementation; antipyretics; adequate hydration; control of pain, fatigue, and anxiety; and ongoing fetal assessment. Positioning the woman in a semi-Fowler's or high-Fowler's position usually is most comfortable and promotes maximum oxygenation. Oxygen supplementation to maintain oxygen saturation of greater than 95% by pulse oximeter is vital to ensure adequate maternal oxygen delivery to the fetus. The most common method of oxygen administration is 2 to 4 L/min through a nasal cannula. If the woman requires more than 4 L of oxygen to maintain adequate hemoglobin oxygen saturation, the use of a nonrebreather mask is more efficacious in delivering a higher fraction of inspired oxygen (FIO_2) (Simpson & James, 2005). Mechanical ventilation is necessary for women who are unable to maintain a P_aO_2 above 60 mm Hg despite high concentrations of inspired oxygen. For women who are unable to cough effectively, postural drainage and tracheal suctioning can be valuable in mobilizing secretions. The use of incentive spirometry may be helpful as well.

The development of preterm labor as a complication of infection may be the result of the response of the uterus to certain mediators of inflammation and infection. Prompt attention to regular uterine contractions and cervical changes is necessary to minimize the risks of preterm birth as a result of significant maternal illness. Conversely, in patients in whom respiratory and cardiovascular statuses continue to deteriorate despite maximum supportive efforts, birth may be necessary for fetal and maternal survival.

PHARMACOLOGIC THERAPY

Antibiotic therapy must be specific to the pathogen present, along with consideration for safety during pregnancy (Table 10–3). Until identification of the causative organism, symptoms, sputum Gram stain, and chest radiography can direct initial antibiotic use. Erythromycin has proven to be successful in treatment of pneumonia in pregnancy and is often administered initially. Ampicillin may be administered if *S. pneumoniae* or *H. influenzae* is the suspected pathogen. With an increase in ampicillin-resistant pathogens, third-generation cephalosporins and trimethoprim-sulfamethoxazole are other choices for most cases of classic pneumonia (Graves, 2010). Varicella pneumonia must be treated promptly with acyclovir, with 8 to 10 mg/kg given intravenously every 8 hours for 5 days to decrease complications and mortality (Graves, 2010). Patients who receive acyclovir early in the course of their illness benefit from lower temperatures and respiratory rates and from improved oxygenation without risk to their fetus. Aggressive treatment of hypoxemia

Table 10–3. ANTIBIOTIC THERAPY FOR PNEUMONIA PATHOGENS

Pathogen	Ampicillin	Cephalosporin	Erythromycin	Trimethoprim-Sulfamethoxazole
Streptococcus pneumoniae	+	+	+	+
Haemophilus influenzae	+	+	−	+
Mycoplasma catarrhalis	−	+	+	+
Chlamydia pneumoniae	−	−	+	−
Legionella pneumophila	−	−	+	−
Mycoplasma pneumoniae	−	−	+	−
Pneumocystis carinii	−	−	−	+

+, antibiotic coverage for bacteria; −, antibiotic not effective to treat bacteria.

and administration of corticosteroids have also shown to improve outcomes in these women (Cheng, Tang, Wu, Chu, & Yuen, 2004; Goodnight & Soper, 2005).

Varicella embryopathy may occur as a result of maternal infection, particularly in the first half of pregnancy, with an incidence of 1% to 2% (Chapman, 1998). Varicella of the newborn is a life-threatening illness that may occur when a newborn is born within 5 days of the onset of maternal illness or after postbirth exposure to varicella. Susceptible newborns should be given VZIG (Chapman, 1998).

Aspiration pneumonia is best treated with broad-spectrum antibiotics to cover gram-negative and gram-positive bacteria that are usually present. Antiviral agents amantadine and ribavirin have been used in the treatment of influenza pneumonia and SARS pneumonia during pregnancy. Although they have shown teratogenicity in some animal studies, both have been effective in decreasing the severity of illness associated with influenza during pregnancy without adverse effects to humans. SARS pneumonia has also been effectively treated with the addition of antibiotics and corticosteroids.

PULMONARY EDEMA

Pulmonary edema is defined as the abnormal accumulation of fluid in the interstitial spaces, alveoli, or cells within the lungs that inhibits adequate diffusion of carbon dioxide and oxygen (Frye et al., 2011). Physiologic changes of the cardiopulmonary system during pregnancy place the pregnant woman at increased risk for developing pulmonary edema (Mason & Dorman, 2012). There are two primary types of pulmonary edema: hydrostatic (cardiogenic) and vascular permeability (noncardiogenic, nonhydrostatic).

HYDROSTATIC

Colloid oncotic pressure (COP) normally pulls excess fluids from the lung tissue into the pulmonary vessels; however, in pulmonary edema, the opposite occurs. Hydrostatic pulmonary edema occurs when the hydrostatic pressure (pushing) within the pulmonary vascular bed exceeds the COP (pulling) of fluid within the vessel. This pressure imbalance causes intravascular fluid to be physically pushed from within the vessel across the semipermeable endothelium; subsequently, interstitial fluid exceeds the pumping capacity of the lymphatic system and alveolar flooding occurs, resulting in interference of gas exchange (Mabie, 2010). Hydrostatic pulmonary edema is related to intravascular hypervolemia. Potential causes in pregnancy include congenital or ischemic heart disease, acquired valvular lesions, tachydysrhythmias, and hypertension, either from chronic disease or

preeclampsia. If a woman has systemic hypertension, the outflow of blood from the left ventricle is impaired, resulting in myocardial dysfunction. Systolic dysfunction is one of the most common causes of hydrostatic pulmonary edema during pregnancy. Cardiomyopathy results in systolic dysfunction (defined as an ejection fraction of less than 45%) and diastolic dysfunction results in impaired ventricular contractility and high filling pressures (Mabie, 2010). Hydrostatic pulmonary edema from beta-agonist and/or magnesium sulfate tocolytic therapy for more than 24 hours is well documented but not completely understood. Several mechanisms have been proposed, including release of antidiuretic hormone from the posterior pituitary causing oliguria and resulting in fluid overload (Mabie, 2010). Multifetal pregnancy with increased intravascular volume and reduced COP predisposes this population to hydrostatic changes.

VASCULAR PERMEABILITY

Vascular permeability (nonhydrostatic) pulmonary edema results from pulmonary capillary or alveolar endothelial injury. The endothelial permeability allows protein-rich (colloid) vascular fluid to leak into the alveoli, pulmonary cells, and interstitial spaces. The resulting hemodynamic values are a decreased COP and decreased intravascular volume (hypovolemia), which results in decreased cardiac output and organ perfusion. The COP in the interstitial spaces increases and will continue to pull intravascular volume (Marini & Wheeler, 2010). Vascular permeability pulmonary edema can lead to acute lung injury (ALI) and ARDS, which carries a maternal mortality rate as high as 24% to 44%, depending upon the etiology and other organ failure (Catanzarite, Willms, Wong, Landers, Cousins, & Schrimmer, 2001). Causes of vascular permeability pulmonary edema in pregnancy include infection leading to sepsis, preeclampsia, blood transfusion reaction, amniotic fluid embolus, aspiration pneumonia, disseminated intravascular coagulopathy, and inhalation injury.

Vascular permeability is caused by several mechanisms. Bacterial or viral infection causes release of prostaglandins, cytokines, and complement components, resulting in endothelium injury and myocardial dysfunction (Mabie, 2010). Aspiration and inhaled toxins cause direct chemical injury to the lung tissues and alveoli.

CLINICAL MANIFESTATIONS

Clinical manifestations of pulmonary edema are the same, regardless of the type and etiology. Symptoms include dyspnea and shortness of breath with a feeling of suffocation. Typically, the woman will want to sit up in bed, demonstrate anxious or agitated behavior, and have tachycardia and tachypnea that progressively increases. Adventitious breath sounds, such as fine crackles, progress to coarse sounds. Wheezing may also be present. Usually, pulmonary edema begins with a nonproductive cough and progresses to a productive state with pink, frothy sputum. As the edema progresses, there will be a downward trend in oxygen saturation (SpO_2) values along with flaring and retractions. An irregular heart rate may occur if cardiac disease is present.

CLINICAL MANAGEMENT

Diagnosis of pulmonary edema is confirmed by history, clinical presentation, and diagnostic testing. The woman's history should be reviewed and include assessment of preexisting or pregnancy-related disease (e.g., preeclampsia), medications, fluid balance, chemical exposure, and anesthetic administration. Also, a complete examination of cardiac, respiratory, and renal function is necessary (Poole & Spreen, 2005).

Some tests that may be included in the diagnostic process of pulmonary edema are chest X-ray, arterial blood gas measurement, assessment of pulse oximetry trends, and electrocardiogram (ECG) monitoring. Echocardiography may show decreased ejection fraction with intravascular volume changes. Invasive hemodynamic monitoring may be required to determine the type of pulmonary edema and management plan. For example, a pregnant woman with preeclampsia is at risk of developing both hydrostatic and vascular permeability pulmonary edema, making it difficult to determine the type of pulmonary edema on the basis of noninvasive assessment. Therefore, if traditional, conservative management does not stop the progression of the symptoms and if signs of decreased cardiac output and oxygen availability are present, pulmonary artery catheterization may be considered to make a definitive diagnosis and develop a plan of care to optimize outcomes for the mother and fetus. These critically ill women require a multidisciplinary team approach to determine an individualized plan.

The management plan is not "one size fits all" for pulmonary edema because the pathophysiology may result in intravascular volume extremes. Noninvasive assessment parameters, such as trends in vital signs and pulse oximetry, urine output, pulse pressure, peripheral pulse quality, venous distention, generalized edema, skin color, and temperature, will assist in determining the woman's intravascular volume status and cardiac output (Poole & Spreen, 2005).

One of the main goals of managing pulmonary edema includes optimizing oxygen delivery. Humidified oxygen should be administered by a nonrebreather face mask. Because one of the diagnostic tools is the evaluation of the woman's arterial blood gas values, an arterial line may be considered to provide the healthcare team with frequent access and capabilities to determine the woman's response to treatment. Decreasing oxygen consumption is an important component of the management of women who are hypoxic. Limiting the woman's movements and providing pain management are necessary. If the SpO_2 value drops in response to activity, limited oxygen reserves may be the cause (Marini & Wheeler, 2010). These women should be monitored in an intensive care environment, and hemodynamic monitoring should be considered.

Position of the mother helps to optimize cardiac output, but the ideal position differs depending on the pathophysiology of pulmonary edema. If the mother has hydrostatic pulmonary edema, she should be placed in a high sitting position, preferably with her feet lower than her torso. This position will decrease return from her lower extremities and decrease volume status while still providing for adequate cardiac output. If vascular permeability pulmonary edema is suspected, if tolerated, the woman should lie on her left or right side. This position will optimize return to the right side of the heart and increase cardiac output.

Management of the woman's fluid intake also differs depending on the type of pulmonary edema. If hydrostatic pulmonary edema is suspected, IV and oral fluids should be restricted because the pathophysiology is related to hypervolemia. All IV fluids should be administered via a controlled infusion pump. If vascular permeability pulmonary edema is confirmed, volume resuscitation may be necessary to maintain cardiac output and organ perfusion. A pulmonary artery catheter may be beneficial to guide treatment according to the woman's hemodynamic responses. All intake and output should be monitored closely, documented, and communicated to the obstetrical care provider (Poole & Spreen, 2005).

PHARMACOLOGIC THERAPY

Pharmacologic therapy to treat pulmonary edema and manage the woman's symptoms may be necessary. When hydrostatic pulmonary edema is suspected, furosemide (Lasix) is administered in small doses (10 to 20 mg IV). A Foley catheter should be placed, and the woman's response to diuretic administration should be observed over the following hour. Serum potassium levels should be monitored closely with repetitive use of diuretics. A woman with left ventricular failure secondary to hypertension may require afterload reduction with antihypertensives to optimize volume status and cardiac output. Hydralazine is the first-line drug of choice to lower systemic vascular resistance. Because of the risk of hydrostatic pulmonary edema, beta-agonist or magnesium sulfate tocolytic therapy should be discontinued. The administration of morphine sulfate in small increments may be beneficial to manage the mother's pain and decrease oxygen consumption. However, morphine sulfate should not be given to women with decreased levels of consciousness or hypotension (Poole & Spreen, 2005).

AMNIOTIC FLUID EMBOLISM

AFE is rare but devastating, with a mortality rate of 61% in developed countries (Clark, 2010). The incidence of AFE is 1 per 13,000 births in the United States and 1 in 50,000 births in the United Kingdom (Abenhaim, Azoulay, Kramer, & Leduc, 2008; Clark, 2010; Knight et al., 2010). In women with AFE and cardiac arrest, less than 10% survive neurologically intact (Clark, 2010).

Understanding of AFE is incomplete; however, AFE classically consists of hypoxia from ALI and transient pulmonary hypertension, hypotension, and cardiac arrest (Clark, 2010). Clinically useful risk factors and preventative measures remain elusive, and perinatal morbidity and mortality continues to be significant. Symptoms of sudden dyspnea, hypotension, and cardiac arrest, with evidence of fetal hypoxia during labor, are the classic presentation of AFE, followed by consumptive coagulopathy (Clark, 2010). AFE can result in ALI by causing pulmonary vascular endothelial damage, complement activation, and direct platelet aggregation effects of amniotic fluid (Wise, Polito, & Krishnan, 2006).

Historically, AFE was thought to be the result of the infusion of amniotic fluid cells or other debris into the maternal circulation during uterine contractions, and the diagnosis was confirmed by the finding of fetal cells in the maternal pulmonary circulation (Clark, 2010). There has been a shift from this view of the pathophysiology of AFE to understanding the process as a systemic inflammatory response syndrome with inappropriate release of endogenous inflammatory mediators (Clark, 2010). It has been proposed that the phenomenon of this abnormal maternal response to fetal antigen exposure be renamed "anaphylactoid syndrome of pregnancy" to better reflect the physiologic underpinnings.

Diagnosis of AFE is made clinically and should be suspected in any pregnant woman who develops profound shock and severe hypoxemic respiratory failure with bilateral pulmonary infiltrates during or immediately after labor. Treatment is mainly supportive with careful monitoring for the development of ARDS and coagulopathy. Basic, advanced, and obstetric cardiac life support protocols are generally followed in initial treatment and resuscitative efforts. Hypoxia is treated with supplemental oxygen and mechanical ventilation, using lung-protective strategies as indicated. Circulatory support is provided with rapid fluid infusion, cardiogenic shock requires use of inotropic and vasoactive agents, and treatment of coagulopathy requires the replacement of coagulation factors (Conde-Agudelo & Romero, 2009; Dobbenga-Rhodes, 2009). Other treatments have been reported in individual cases, but none have been established as a standard of care for women experiencing AFE because there is no data to suggest that any of these treatments improves maternal outcomes (Clark, 2010).

Fetal or newborn outcomes of AFE are directly related to the time between maternal cardiac arrest and birth; however, the relationship is inconsistent due to the variability in onset and intensity of uterine hypoperfusion and maternal decompensation. In the presence of viable fetal gestational age, maternal resuscitative efforts should follow standard cardiac life support with the addition of consideration of birth (Clark, 2010). A perimortem bedside cesarean birth may be indicated in the event of maternal cardiac arrest. Relieving maternal vena caval compression may theoretically enhance maternal resuscitative efforts.

VENOUS THROMBOEMBOLISM

The hypercoagulable state and venous stasis increase the risk for the formation of venous thrombi and pulmonary embolus during pregnancy and the postpartum period (Bates et al., 2012). The majority of women who suffer from venous thromboembolism (VTE) may also be more likely to suffer poor pregnancy outcomes and postthrombotic syndrome, with sequelae ranging from recurrent thromboses, edema, and skin changes to possible ulceration (James, Jamison, Brancazio, & Myers, 2006). Because poor pregnancy outcomes associated with VTE have been reported, such as abruption, preeclampsia, IUGR, and stillbirth, appropriate treatment and prevention of VTE during pregnancy is required to decrease the potential morbidity and mortality for the mother and baby (Lockwood, 2009). VTE is both more common and more complex to diagnose in patients who are pregnant. The incidence is estimated at 0.76 to 1.72 per 1,000 pregnancies, which is four times greater than in the nonpregnant population (Heit et al., 2005; James et al., 2006). Deep venous thrombosis (DVT) and pulmonary embolus are collectively referred to as thromboembolytic diseases. Approximately 75% to 80% of cases of pregnancy-associated venous thrombosis are caused by DVT, and 20% to 25% of cases are caused by pulmonary embolus (James et al., 2006). Regardless of gestational age, VTE may occur at any time, with approximately 40% to 60% of pregnancy-related pulmonary emboli occurring in the postpartum period (James et al., 2006). See Display 10–6 for risk factors for development of VTE during the postpartum period. It is interesting to note that 90% of all DVTs during pregnancy will occur in

DISPLAY   1 0 - 6

Risk Factors for Development of Venous Thromboembolism (VTE) during the Postpartum Period

Major risk factors (odds ratio >6)—Presence of at least one of the following risk factors suggests a risk of postpartum VTE >3%:

- Immobility (strict bed rest for >1 week in the antepartum period)
- Postpartum hemorrhage >1,000 mL with surgery
- Previous VTE
- Preeclampsia with fetal growth restriction
- Thrombophilia
  - Antithrombin deficiency
  - Factor V Leiden (homozygous or heterozygous)
  - Prothrombin G20210A (homozygous or heterozygous)
- Medical conditions
  - Systemic lupus erythematosus
  - Heart disease
  - Sickle cell disease
- Blood transfusion
- Postpartum infection

Minor risk factors (odds ratio >6 when combined)—Presence of at least two of the following risk factors or one of the following risk factors in the setting of emergency cesarean birth suggests a risk of postpartum VTE of >3%:

- Body mass index >30 kg/m^2
- Multiple pregnancy
- Postpartum hemorrhage >1 L
- Smoking >10 cigarettes/day
- Fetal growth restriction (gestational age + sex-adjusted birth weight <25th percentile)
- Thrombophilia
  - Protein C deficiency
  - Protein S deficiency
- Preeclampsia

From Bates, S. M., Greer, I. A., Middeldorp, S., Veenstra, D. L., Prabulos, A. M., & Vandvik, P. O. (2012). VTE, thrombophilia, antithrombotic therapy, and pregnancy: Antithrombotic therapy and prevention of thrombosis, 9th ed: American College of Chest Physicians evidence-based clinical practice guidelines. *Chest, 141*(2 Suppl.), e691s–e736s. doi:10.1378/chest.11-2300

the left lower extremity, which is thought to be caused by compression from the gravid uterus on the left iliac vein (Brown & Hiett, 2010).

The incidence of pulmonary embolus can vary depending on the treatment of DVT. In patients who are adequately treated for DVT with anticoagulants, pulmonary embolus occurs in approximately 4.5%, resulting in death in less than 1%. However, without diagnosis of a DVT or adequate treatment, the incidence of pulmonary embolus increases to 24%, with a resulting mortality rate of 15%. Another factor that increases the incidence of pulmonary embolus is

cesarean birth. Among women who give birth by cesarean, especially emergent cesarean birth, the risk of pulmonary embolus is significantly increased compared with women who have vaginal birth (Bates et al., 2012). This increased incidence is thought to be caused by an increase in tissue trauma and subsequent disruption of the vascular endothelium (Gherman et al., 1999; Weinmann & Salzman, 1994).

RISK FACTORS FOR VTE

There has been inadequate research to validate a specific cause-and-effect relationship between some of the risk factors and thrombus formation. It is likely that a combination of several risk factors causes thrombus formation. The most significant risk factor for VTE in pregnancy is a personal history of thrombosis followed by the presence of an acquired or inherited thrombophilia (ACOG, 2011). Thrombophilia is present in 20% to 50% of all women who experience VTE during pregnancy and postpartum. In an analysis conducted with pregnant women experiencing VTE, women 35 years of age and older had a 38% higher incidence rate (James et al., 2006). This risk may be higher when other risk factors, such as hypertension, obesity, and heart disease, are present. With women delaying childbirth, the risk of VTE may continue to rise. Blood vessel damage, especially in the pelvic region, during vaginal or cesarean birth may cause thrombus formation (Brown & Hiett, 2010). Higher parity increases this risk. Smoking causes blood vessel constriction that potentially damages the endothelial lining and increases the risk for blood clot formation. The risk of VTE is also present for women with mechanical heart valves or who have certain dysrhythmias (e.g., atrial fibrillation) requiring anticoagulant therapy. In one study, the rate of thromboembolism in black women was 64% higher than that for women of other races (James et al., 2006). This risk may be partially explained by an increased incidence of hypertension, heart disease, obesity, and sickle cell trait among blacks. However, genetics and environmental factors are thought to play a role. A significant decrease in the risk for women of Asian and Hispanic origins was also noted in this study (James et al., 2006). Trauma and infection increase the potential for vessel wall damage, which can lead to clot formation. There is a fourfold increase in risk of VTE for women with chorioamnionitis who undergo cesarean birth (Hague & Decker, 2003). Prolonged immobilization in any patient increases the likelihood of clot formation because of venous stasis. Antiphospholipid syndrome is an acquired thrombophilic condition associated with an increased risk for both arterial and venous thrombosis, recurrent fetal loss, and other adverse outcomes during pregnancy.

Obesity increases risks related to hypertension, heart disease, and venous stasis.

PATHOPHYSIOLOGY

A thrombus, which usually arises from a DVT, may dislodge and pass to the lungs. Small thrombi may lodge peripherally in the pulmonary vasculature, preventing blood flow distal to the thrombi and causing the release of inflammatory mediators. These mediators produce a rapid rise in pulmonary vascular resistance, causing symptoms of cough, tachycardia, tachypnea, and rales. If a large thrombus lodges in the pulmonary artery or one of its branches, obstruction of blood flow from the right ventricle occurs. Right ventricular outflow obstruction prevents blood from circulating through the pulmonary vasculature, resulting in deoxygenated blood and hypoxia. The degree of hypoxia and symptoms are related to the size and location of thrombi.

Appropriate and timely assessments for the symptoms of venous thrombosis are essential for early diagnosis and initiation of treatment. Depending on the size of the thrombus, women may be asymptomatic or have symptoms that mimic common conditions of pregnancy. In fact, one half of all DVT is asymptomatic (Colman-Brochu, 2004). Symptoms of DVT include pain, swelling, positive Homans' sign, warmth, redness, thickening, and tenderness over vein (Brown & Hiett, 2010). The pregnant woman undergoes several body changes that can mimic some of these symptoms. Lower extremity aches, pain, and swelling are common, especially in the second and third trimesters. Differentiation between normal and abnormal changes may present challenges. The extremity affected by DVT typically demonstrates the cardinal symptoms of inflammation: pain, swelling, warmth, and redness. A 2-cm difference in calf measurements in the affected and unaffected leg is considered significant. Calf or popliteal pain that occurs with dorsiflexion of the foot is considered a positive Homans' sign (Brown & Hiett, 2010); however, Homans' sign should not be considered diagnostic of DVT and should be followed by additional assessment.

Pulmonary embolus is an acute and potentially life-threatening event. Clinical manifestation of pulmonary embolus depends on the number, size, and location of the emboli; therefore, symptoms may be mild to severe (Brown & Hiett, 2010). Often, the woman will be apprehensive or have feelings of "impending doom" before the presentation of other symptoms. Diagnosis of pulmonary embolus may be considered with the presence of clinical signs and symptoms, including the sudden onset of unexplained dyspnea and tachypnea. Pleuritic chest pain, described by patients as "stabbing" in nature, is common following an embolus. The nurse may also find sudden onset of a productive cough and the presence of rales on auscultation. Tachycardia is a common symptom initially and may continue due to the resulting pain or hemodynamic compromise. The symptoms of pulmonary embolus usually resolve rapidly over a few hours but may last for a few days (Marini & Wheeler, 2009). Following initial assessment, laboratory values and radiologic imaging studies assist the healthcare provider in making the diagnosis.

Because the clinical signs and symptoms are not specific for pulmonary embolus, additional diagnostic testing should be used to rule out other diagnoses, such as pneumonia, myocardial infarction, or pulmonary edema. The diagnosis should be confirmed before initiation of anticoagulant treatment (Lockwood, 2009). Continuous electrocardiography (ECG) is often performed early in the process when the woman reports chest pain. Tachycardia is the most common ECG change. A 12-lead ECG is commonly ordered to rule out other causes of chest pain, such as myocardial infarction. Findings from the 12-lead ECG may include nonspecific T-wave inversion (found in 40% of women) and a right-axis shift in women with a large embolus (Lockwood, 2009).

Obtaining an arterial blood gas analysis on room air is one of the first steps in the diagnosis of a pulmonary embolus. Anticipated changes in maternal arterial blood gases associated with a pulmonary embolus are a decrease in P_aO_2, PCO_2, and SaO_2. If the woman's P_aO_2 value is greater than 80 mm Hg on room air, a pulmonary embolus is not likely. However, if a woman has persistent signs and symptoms of a pulmonary embolus, even with a P_aO_2 greater than 80 mm Hg, additional testing is needed to make a diagnosis (Lockwood, 2009).

A ventilation-perfusion (V/Q) scan requires IV or bronchial administration of a radioactive substance under fluoroscopy. This substance becomes trapped in perfused lung tissue. The radiologic scan will detect areas of decreased perfusion, which will be suspicious for a pulmonary embolus, and will also detect nonperfused areas that may have appeared normal on a chest X-ray (Brown & Hiett, 2010). A determination of high probability, moderate probability, low probability, or normal is made following analysis of the testing data. The term *probability* is added to the interpretation of this test because other diagnoses, such as pulmonary tumors, pneumonia, obstructive lung disease, hypoxic vasoconstriction, atelectasis, and emphysema, can also produce perfusion defects (Marini & Wheeler, 2009). Performing this test is considered to be safe during pregnancy, and it usually is the first-line radiologic testing procedure for the diagnosis of pulmonary embolus. The amount of radiation exposure varies but typically remains at levels considered safe during pregnancy (Lockwood, 2009).

Pulmonary angiography is the definitive procedure to diagnose pulmonary embolus and is advisable when the V/Q scan is indeterminate. For this procedure, contrast dye is injected into lobar or segmental branches of the pulmonary artery, allowing clear visualization of vessels. An emboli would be detected with filling defects or obstructive flow. There is a low risk of an allergic reaction to the contrast dye used for radiographic imaging and vascular damage (pulmonary artery or right ventricular perforation). Mortality rates are reported as 0.01% (Marini & Wheeler, 2009).

CLINICAL MANAGEMENT

Because pulmonary embolus is such a rare event, but one with potentially devastating outcomes, management requires rapid recognition of symptoms, followed by notification and activation of a multidisciplinary team. Aspects of care fall into three management categories: respiratory support, cardiovascular support, and anticoagulation therapy.

Nursing assessments and support of respiratory function should focus on optimization of oxygen exchange. If a pulmonary embolus is suspected, warm, humidified oxygen therapy is administered via a nonrebreather face mask at 10 L per minute during the acute phase. Arterial blood gases should be assessed frequently to evaluate the maternal response to therapy, degree of hypoxemia, and need for ventilatory support. Follow-up evaluation of blood gases after therapy should also be performed. Therefore, an arterial line may facilitate rapid and easy access for blood gas evaluation. Continuous maternal pulse oximetry should be initiated with the first signs of respiratory compromise. A pulmonary embolus will cause SaO_2 to fall dramatically during the acute event, indicating the need for further assessment. If the pulmonary embolus occurs in the antepartum period, maintenance of SaO_2 at 96% or above is optimal to ensure adequate oxygenation of the fetus (Lockwood, 2009).

Analgesics, such as morphine sulfate, may be used to decrease oxygen consumption in women who have pleuritic chest pain. Analgesics help to reduce the work of breathing in women who are feeling anxious or apprehensive. Other nursing measures to increase comfort include elevating the head of the bed and providing emotional support. The potential need for mechanical ventilation should be anticipated with severe maternal compromise in respiratory function or with cardiopulmonary collapse.

The initial treatment is also focused on restoring maternal cardiopulmonary function. Cardiovascular support should be initiated rapidly and include optimizing maternal preload (volume status), decreasing the workload of the heart, and using a positive inotropic agent to increase maternal cardiac contractility. Because of the potential for cardiac dysrhythmias, continuous ECG monitoring should be initiated with the first signs of maternal cardiovascular changes (Lockwood, 2009).

Noninvasive parameters reflecting maternal preload, such as vital signs, breath sounds, jugular venous distention, skin color, turgor and color, and urine output, should be assessed frequently according to the woman's condition and facility protocol. Changes in preload values, hypervolemia, or hypovolemia may decrease maternal cardiac output and organ perfusion. Nursing interventions that focus on decreasing the workload of the heart should be initiated, such as decreasing the woman's activity, eliminating unnecessary procedures, administering pain medication for chest pain, and encouraging relaxation techniques. A positive inotrope, such as dopamine or dobutamine, should be considered to support myocardial contractility and cardiac output if symptoms of shock are present (Lockwood, 2009). Cardiopulmonary resuscitation (CPR) should be initiated as needed.

VENOUS THROMBOPROPHYLAXIS AND ANTICOAGULATION THERAPY

Thromboembolic stockings, use of sequential compression devices (SCDs), and anticoagulation therapy are used for the prevention and treatment of VTE. At present, three types of therapeutic agents are used for anticoagulation in the general population: agents that interfere with platelet aggregation (attraction) and adhesion, agents that interfere with fibrin formation, and agents that facilitate clot lysis (clot breakdown). Anticoagulation during pregnancy requires consideration of both the mother and fetus. The decision for thromboprophylaxis to prevent thrombus formation is based on a previous history of thrombosis, the presence of a diagnosed thrombophilia, and other risk factors, such as race, age, and medical conditions, that may contribute to clot formation. Other risk factors that may indicate treatment to prevent clot formation are age over 35 years, African American race, or medical conditions such as valvular heart disease or antiphospholipid antibodies. Each woman's history should be analyzed to determine the need for thromboprophylaxis.

Heparin

Heparin (also known as UFH) is a large molecule and does not cross the placenta or cause teratogenic effects. Heparin interferes with fibrin formation by binding to AT-III, changing the configuration of AT-III, and neutralizing thrombin and factors Xa, IXa, XIa, and XIIa. Heparin is not absorbed into the gastrointestinal tract, thereby requiring parenteral administration by IV or subcutaneous (SC) injections. Intramuscular (IM) injections are contraindicated because of erratic absorption and risk of hematoma formation (Lockwood, 2009). Pregnant women usually require larger doses of heparin to achieve therapeutic anticoagulation because of increases in plasma volume, heparin-binding proteins, renal clearance, and heparin breakdown by the placenta (Lockwood, 2009).

The primary risk of heparin therapy is hemorrhage, which occurs in approximately 2% of patients. The rate of hemorrhage is related to dosing regimens and prolongation of the activated partial thromboplastin time (aPTT). SC and intermittent IV bolus doses of heparin are associated with higher risks of bleeding. Thrombocytopenia is an immunologic reaction that occurs in less than 3% of patients undergoing heparin anticoagulation for an extended period of time (greater than 4 days) (Murphy, Meadors, & King, 2011). If thrombocytopenia occurs, it is typically 5 to 15 days after initiation of full-dose heparin (Gibson & Powrie, 2009). Patients who undergo prolonged heparin therapy may be at risk for osteoporosis. Changes in bone density have been observed in spine, hip, and femur radiographic tests. Other rare complications of heparin therapy include hypotension, alopecia (hair loss), allergic reaction, and pain at the injection site. Allergic reactions are usually itchy, erythematous plaques that resolve with a switch in medication (Bates, Greer, Hirsh, & Ginsberg, 2004).

Lack of adequate anticoagulation increases the risk of thromboembolus recurrence by 11- to 15-fold (Lockwood, 2009). Continuous IV administration provides a more consistent therapeutic level and results in fewer hemorrhagic events than intermittent IV bolus. Initial treatments for DVT and pulmonary embolus differ slightly. With a diagnosis of DVT only, an initial IV bolus of 100 U/kg of heparin is usually an appropriate treatment plan. For pulmonary embolus, the initial dose of heparin is 150 U/kg. Following initial IV bolus of heparin, an infusion rate between 15 and 25 U/kg/hr may be initiated, depending on the laboratory values and symptoms (Lockwood, 2009).

Low-Molecular-Weight Heparin

Although for many years, unfractionated heparin was the standard anticoagulant used during pregnancy and the postpartum period, current guidelines recommend low-molecular-weight heparin (LMWH) (ACOG, 2011; Bates et al., 2012). LMWH is a fragment of UFH. Its use in pregnancy is considered safe, and it is now the recommended treatment (ACOG, 2011; Bates et al., 2012). Compared with UFH, LMWH has increased bioavailability, half-life, and anticoagulant activity (Murphy et al., 2011). These characteristics make LMWH an attractive alternative to traditional UFH regimens. Venous thrombosis and pulmonary embolus may be effectively treated with LMWH. The benefits of LMWH are ease of administration, predictable dose-response ratios, less frequent need for monitoring, and fewer complications, such as thrombocytopenia, osteoporosis, and bleeding, compared with unfractionated heparin. LMWH is four to six times more costly, but the ability to use this medication in the outpatient setting and the decreased need for strict laboratory monitoring decreases the cost of therapy.

Warfarin

Warfarin (Coumadin) is an oral anticoagulant that antagonizes vitamin K and directly inhibits the coagulation cascade. Warfarin crosses the placenta and has been associated with a risk of fetal hemorrhage and of central nervous system and ophthalmologic abnormalities. When administered between 6 and 12 weeks of gestation, warfarin has been associated with nasal and limb hypoplasia, as well as stippled chondral calcification. Therefore, under most circumstances, warfarin is not the preferred treatment for thromboembolism during pregnancy, and the use of warfarin has been restricted primarily to the postpartum period. However, it may be the drug of choice in high-risk populations, such as women with certain types of mechanical heart valves or with a high risk of thrombosis (ACOG, 2011).

If there is a desire to convert from heparin to warfarin anticoagulation, this switch should be initiated during the postpartum period while the woman is hospitalized. Following birth and maternal stabilization, full heparin anticoagulation is usually reinstituted. Oral warfarin therapy is usually initiated at 5 mg/day for 2 days. Maintenance-dose ranges are adjusted per day depending on the woman's international normalized ratio (INR) or prothrombin time (PT). A goal value for the INR is 2.0 to 3.0. After the woman is anticoagulated, which may take about 3 to 5 days, heparin is discontinued (Whitty & Dombrowski, 2009).

Warfarin anticoagulation is more sensitive to fluctuations and requires close monitoring of clotting-time values. Numerous medications may augment or interfere with absorption and action of warfarin (Murphy et al., 2011). To avoid common drug interactions, nurses and other healthcare providers should review the woman's medication history, be aware of potential medication interactions, and help educate patients to question or avoid medication (prescription or nonprescription) that is not approved by their primary healthcare provider or physician specialist consultant.

LABOR AND BIRTH

It is usually recommended that women receiving UFH or LMWH during pregnancy discontinue these medications 24 hours before elective induction of labor or cesarean birth. If the mother goes into spontaneous labor, aPTT values should be monitored. If the aPTT value is prolonged greater than 1 to 1.5 times the control value, protamine sulfate may be required near birth to reduce the risk of bleeding (Brown & Hiett, 2010). For women in whom anticoagulation therapy has been temporarily suspended, pneumatic compression devices are recommended (ACOG, 2011).

Pain management for labor and birth is an additional concern. Among women who have been taking anticoagulants, there is a concern for potential complications associated with regional anesthesia, including the risk of epidural hematoma formation, which has been linked to use of LMWH. This risk results from the increased half-life of LMWH. The American Society of Regional Anesthesia and Pain Medicine guidelines recommend withholding neuroaxial (spinal and epidural anesthesia) blockade for 10 to 12 hours after the last prophylactic dose of LMWH or 24 hours after the last therapeutic dose of LMWH (Horlocker, Wedel, Rowlingson, & Enneking, 2010). If a woman goes into labor while taking UFH, clearance can be verified with an aPTT. For women who are at increased risk for operative bleeding (e.g., women with placenta previa, accreta, or percreta) and at low risk for clot movement (pulmonary embolus), heparin may be discontinued or the effects reversed with protamine sulfate. Cesarean birth increases the risk of VTE; therefore, placement of pneumatic compression devices before birth is recommended for all women not already receiving thromboprophylaxis (ACOG, 2011). Continued heparin dosing during labor and surgery for high-risk patients, such as those mentioned previously (recent pulmonary embolus, recent ileofemoral thrombosis, and mechanical heart valves), does not significantly increase the risk of hemorrhage during the postpartum period following a normal vaginal birth. Nursing assessments and care should focus on uterine tone and the potential for perineal hematoma following a vaginal birth, according to the healthcare facility's guidelines. If the woman has a cesarean birth, assessments should include signs and symptoms of intra-abdominal bleeding, such as increased abdominal girth, rigid or firm palpation, decreasing blood pressure, and increasing heart rate (James et al., 2006).

The optimal time to restart anticoagulation therapy in the postpartum period is unclear. A reasonable approach to minimize bleeding complications is to resume UFH or LMWH no sooner than 4 to 6 hours following vaginal birth and 6 to 12 hours following cesarean birth, 12 hours after epidural catheter removal (ACOG, 2011; Horlocker et al., 2010). For women who had a thrombotic event during pregnancy, anticoagulation therapy should be continued for 3 to 6 months following birth (James et al., 2006).

The woman may continue to use pneumatic compression devices until she is able to ambulate. Clotting factors that had been increased during pregnancy will normalize in approximately 8 weeks following birth (Lockwood, 2009).

Heparin and LMWH have not been found to be secreted in breast milk in clinically significant amounts and can be safely administered to nursing mothers (Rhode, 2011). Research validates the safety of warfarin use in nursing mothers. Warfarin does not induce an anticoagulant effect in the breastfed infant (Orme et al., 1977). Therefore, women who desire to breastfeed their newborn may be safely treated with any of these medications. Nurses should teach parents to observe and report any signs or symptoms of bleeding in the newborn, such as petechiae, bruising, or bleeding from the gums (Colman-Brochu, 2004). As a general safety precaution, women receiving anticoagulant therapy should consult their physician or primary healthcare provider to confirm that they may take anticoagulants and other medications while breastfeeding.

CYSTIC FIBROSIS

Cystic fibrosis (CF) is a chronic, hereditary, progressive disease involving the exocrine glands and epithelial cells of the pancreas, sweat glands, and mucous glands in the respiratory, digestive, and reproductive tracts (Lomas & Fowler, 2010; Whitty, 2010). Significant improvements in the prognosis and health of women with CF, age of survival into the fourth decade, and more than 45% of individuals (men and women) with CF over 18 years old have led to increasing consideration for management of reproductive issues and pregnancy in this unique group of women (Lau, Moriarty, Ogle, & Bye, 2010; McArdle, 2011; Tsang, Moriarty, & Towns, 2010; Whitty, 2010). As more women with CF achieve pregnancy, taking a multidisciplinary approach to care can optimize maternal and fetal outcomes.

Preconception counseling and planning for pregnancy is optimal for women with CF. Physical and psychosocial issues can be addressed and potential problems identified, and genetic counseling with investigation of paternal carrier status can be offered. The physiologic adaptations of pregnancy may not be tolerated in women with CF. The enlarging uterus causes a change in lung mechanics that may lead to respiratory decompensation in the woman with CF, yet the majority who were considered safe to undergo pregnancy generally tolerate it well without long-term adverse effects (Lau et al., 2010; Whitty, 2010). However, those women with poor clinical status, malnutrition, hepatic dysfunction, and/or advanced lung disease are at increased risk during pregnancy (Whitty, 2010).

Lung function is an important predictor of pregnancy outcomes in women with CF. In women with moderate to severe lung disease, there is risk for preterm birth and decline in lung function (Lau et al., 2010). CF is associated with pulmonary hypertension (cor pulmonale), which carries high maternal mortality risk in pregnancy. Pulmonary infections are aggressively treated with IV antibiotics. Oral antibiotics are frequently used as chronic therapy as well as for exacerbations in CF and are continued in pregnancy with consideration of the type and clearance (Lau et al., 2010; McArdle, 2011; Whitty, 2010). Most routine medications used in CF are safe in pregnancy, but risk of adverse fetal outcomes is weighed against the benefits. Regular chest physiotherapy and drainage are usual and recommended as components of CF treatment for mucus clearance and are continued in pregnancy. Inhaled dornase alpha is the most frequently used mucolytic and, although there is no data on safety in pregnancy, it is used in the absence of reported adverse fetal effects (McArdle, 2011; Whitty, 2010).

Malabsorption and pancreatic insufficiency are frequent issues in CF, resulting in difficulty gaining weight and glucose intolerance that may be exacerbated due to the significant increase in energy costs. Poor nutritional status is usually associated with more severe disease and worse outcomes, including premature birth and low birth weight, whereas proper dietary consultation and attention to diet is associated with greater maternal and fetal weight gain (Lau et al., 2010; McArdle, 2011). Ideally, the woman should be at 90% of optimal weight prior to conception if possible, but that may be difficult to achieve. Enteral and total parenteral feedings have been used to successfully maintain nutritional status and may be considered for support of weight gain (Lau et al., 2010; McArdle, 2011; Whitty, 2010). Rates of gestational diabetes may be higher in pregnant women with CF, with cystic fibrosis–related diabetes (CFRD) present in greater than 50% of patients older than 30 years (McArdle, 2011). Risks of gestational diabetes in pregnancy, including polyhydramnios and preeclampsia, are the same in women with CF; thus, careful monitoring of blood glucose values beginning early in pregnancy, along with initiation of diet modification and insulin therapy as needed, are important components of care. Pancreatic enzyme replacement is required in a large percentage of CF patients and can be continued in pregnancy to optimize nutritional status (McArdle, 2011; Whitty, 2010).

Antenatal testing is utilized in pregnant women with CF due to the risk for uteroplacental insufficiency and IUGR (Whitty, 2010). Antenatal testing is usually initiated at 32 weeks of gestation and possibly earlier if evidence of fetal compromise is demonstrated (Whitty, 2010). Maternal deterioration in lung function may also precipitate early delivery. Vaginal birth is preferable in women with CF, and cesarean birth is reserved for obstetric indications due to higher risk for atelectasis and retained secretions associated with surgery (Lau et al., 2010; Whitty, 2010). The physiologic demands of the labor, birth, and postpartum periods stress the respiratory and cardiovascular systems, placing the woman with CF at risk for pulmonary hypertension, cor pulmonale, and right-sided heart failure (Whitty, 2010). Regional anesthesia to control pain is beneficial in reducing the sympathetic response, reducing tachycardia and hyperventilation.

Lung transplantation is a therapeutic option for improved quality of life in CF patients with end-stage lung disease, with 5-year survival rates of 50% and 10-year survival rates near 40% (Whitty, 2010). There have been extensive reports of pregnancy after other solid-organ transplants with no increased risk of congenital malformation or infections; however, there is a high risk of maternal rejection and mortality (McArdle, 2011; Whitty, 2010).

SPECIAL CONSIDERATIONS FOR THE RESPIRATORY SYSTEM IN PREGNANCY

SLEEP-DISORDERED BREATHING

Sleep disturbances are reported frequently during pregnancy, most notably insomnia and excessive sleepiness associated with the physiologic changes of pregnancy. Sleep-disordered breathing, including obstructive and central sleep apnea, periodic breathing, and nocturnal hypoventilation, is uncommon in otherwise healthy women but occurs at rates higher than the general population in pregnant women (Wise et al., 2006). Despite protective mechanisms in pregnancy protecting against sleep-disordered breathing, including increased minute ventilation, lateral positioning for sleep, and decreased rapid eye movement (REM) sleep, physiologic changes in the upper airway, including mucosal edema and decreased airway patency, may predispose the pregnant woman to sleep-disordered breathing and contribute to adverse outcomes of pregnancy (Bourjeily, Ankner, & Mohsenin, 2011). Weight gain and upper airway resistance due to estrogen effects may cause sleep apnea to develop or worsen during pregnancy. Although regular snoring is usually underreported, it may occur in 14% to 45% of pregnant women (Bourjeily et al., 2011). Snoring during pregnancy is not a benign condition because it has been associated with negative maternal and fetal outcomes such as hypertension, preeclampsia, IUGR, and lower Apgar scores (Bourjeily et al., 2011; Ellegård, 2006).

Pregnancy rhinitis may cause obstructive sleep apnea (OSA) in women who are predisposed to sleep apnea but can normally breathe through their nose (Ellegård, 2006). Women with rhinitis are at greater risk for snoring and OSA. The increase in nocturnal blood pressure that often accompanies snoring and OSA is associated with gestational hypertensive disorders, particularly preeclampsia (Bourjeily et al., 2011; Ellegård, 2006), although the underlying mechanism for this increase is not well understood. Pregnant women often have difficulty breathing in the supine position, but they may unintentionally move into this position during sleep. Nasal congestion occurs while the patient is in the supine position because difficult breathing increases the tendency to resort to mouth breathing and snoring.

Pregnancy rhinitis should be identified and treated to minimize risk of potential adverse outcomes. Women should be asked about symptoms of rhinitis routinely during prenatal care. Diagnostic tools for sleep-disordered breathing may be less predictive in pregnancy, but polysomnography is the gold standard for diagnosis. Criteria for diagnosis may be different in pregnancy because total sleep time is increased with decreased efficiency (Bourjeily et al., 2011). With diagnosis and severity firmly established, the pregnant woman must be aware of risks and treatment options. Weight loss, a typical behavioral modification for individuals with OSA, is not appropriate to initiate during pregnancy, but continued usual advice on lateral positioning for sleep and avoidance of alcohol are appropriate components of therapy (Bourjeily et al., 2011). Positive airway pressure or oral appliances may be used to reduce the frequency of respiratory events during sleep, but surgical procedures are only used in the event of life-threatening apnea (Bourjeily et al., 2011). It is important to note that most studies of sleep-disordered breathing in pregnancy are based on symptoms rather than confirmed sleep-disordered breathing, and there is currently no evidence on the effects of various treatments and outcomes in pregnancy (Bourjeily et al., 2011). Sleep-disordered breathing generally improves in the postpartum period, but repeat sleep-study testing may be indicated in women with preexisting or continuing issues.

SMOKING

Although smoking in women of reproductive age in the United States has decreased, it remains a leading preventable cause of adverse maternal and fetal outcomes (Murin, Rafii, & Bilello, 2011). In studies of smoking during pregnancy, prevalence is likely underestimated by as much as 25% because most information is self-reported (Murin et al., 2011). The prevalence of smoking is highest in women who are young (adolescents and women aged 18 to 24 years), Caucasian, of lower socioeconomic status, and less educated (Murin et al., 2011). Other factors associated with smoking during pregnancy include increased parity and being unmarried, having an unplanned pregnancy, and having a smoking partner (Murin et al., 2011). Pregnancy is usually a strong motivation to quit smoking, but relapse rates both during and after pregnancy are high (U.S. Department of Health and Human Services [USDHHS], 2004).

The adverse effects of smoking during pregnancy have been well documented because umbilical blood flow is altered and toxins in cigarette smoke are delivered to the fetus. Nicotine crosses the placenta and is found in higher amounts in the fetus than in the mother. Smoking tobacco during pregnancy is strongly linked to increased risk for placental abruption, ectopic pregnancy, and preterm premature rupture of membranes (Castles, Adams, Melvin, Kelsch, & Boulton, 1999). In one study, mothers who smoked were 50% more likely to experience intrapartum fetal death than nonsmokers (Schramm, 1997).

It is estimated that the cumulative benefits of all pregnant women stopping smoking would be an 11% reduction in stillbirths and a 12% reduction in all newborn deaths (USDHHS, 2004). The USDHHS (2004) and ACOG (2010b) recommend tailored smoking cessation efforts for pregnant women, and the 5 A's intervention is widely endorsed. The following components comprise the 5 A's approach: (1) *Ask* all pregnant women about their smoking status at every prenatal visit; (2) *Advise* the smoking pregnant woman in a clear, strong, direct, and personalized manner about the advantages of smoking cessation, emphasizing benefits for both mother and fetus, and offer self-help materials; (3) *Assess* the smoking pregnant woman's readiness to quit (within the next 30 days) at each prenatal visit and, if yes, provide assistance; (4) *Assist* pregnant women who express a willingness to quit via counseling and strategies for success; and (5) *Arrange* follow-up visits for assessment and support in cessation efforts (Murin et al., 2011). Evidence for the use of pharmacotherapy for smoking cessation during pregnancy is minimal and includes concerns about nicotine replacement therapy (NRT) and the known risks of nicotine to the fetus. Monitoring maternal nicotine blood levels may benefit the woman's ability to gradually withdraw from nicotine and increase her chance of success. Guidelines for care are based on expert opinion and clinical judgment, with ACOG (2010b) recommending NRT use only when potential benefits outweigh the unknown risks.

HIGH ALTITUDE

The compensatory physiologic changes of pregnancy occur in response to the challenges of oxygen transport and maintenance of uteroplacental circulation. In chronic, high-altitude conditions with limited oxygen availability and hypoxia, these challenges are magnified. High altitude (greater than 2,500 m, P_aO_2 of 60 to 70 mm Hg) is associated with greater incidence of IUGR and preeclampsia, thus increasing the risk for perinatal morbidity and mortality (Julian, 2011).

SUMMARY

As the incidence of pulmonary complications during pregnancy has increased over the past few decades and is associated with potentially adverse outcomes for the mother and baby, perinatal nurses should be able to recognize common pulmonary complications and activate a team response when necessary based on the clinical situation. If the mother continues to show signs of compromise after initial efforts to improve oxygenation, then stabilization and transfer to a higher level of care is necessary. When the condition of the mother necessitates transfer to an off-service intensive-care area, collaboration among healthcare providers is required.

REFERENCES

Abenhaim, H. A., Azoulay, L., Kramer, M. S., & Leduc, L. (2008). Incidence and risk factors of amniotic fluid embolism: A population-based study on 3 million births in the United States. *American Journal of Obstetrics and Gynecology, 199*(1), 49.e1–49.e8. doi:10.1016/j.ajog.2007.11.061

Alexander, S., Dodds, L., & Armson, B. A. (1998). Perinatal outcomes in women with asthma during pregnancy. *Obstetrics and Gynecology, 92*(3), 435–440. doi:10.1016/S0029-7844(98)00191-4

American College of Obstetricians and Gynecologists. (2008). *Asthma in Pregnancy* (Practice Bulletin No. 90). Washington, DC. Author. doi:10.1097/AOG.0b013e3181665ff4

American College of Obstetricians and Gynecologists. (2010a). *Influenza Vaccination During Pregnancy* (Committee Opinion No. 468). Washington, DC. Author. doi:10.1097/AOG.0b013e3181fae845

American College of Obstetricians and Gynecologists. (2010b). *Smoking Cessation During Pregnancy* (Committee Opinion No. 471). Washington, DC. Author. doi:10.1097/AOG.0b013e3182004fcd

American College of Obstetricians and Gynecologists. (2011). *Thromboembolism in Pregnancy* (Practice Bulletin No. 19). Washington, DC: Author. doi:10.1097/AOG.0b013e3182310c4c

Balducci, J., Rodis, J. F., Rosengren, S., Vintzileos, A. M., Spivey, G., & Vosseller, C. (1992). Pregnancy outcome following first-trimester varicella infection. *Obstetrics and Gynecology, 79*(1), 5–6.

Bates, S. M., Greer, I. A., Hirsh, J., & Ginsberg, J. S. (2004). Use of antithrombotic agents during pregnancy: The seventh ACCP conference on antithrombotic and thrombolytic therapy. *Chest, 126*(Suppl. 3), 627S–644S. doi:10.1378/chest.126.3_suppl.627S

Bates, S. M., Greer, I. A., Middeldorp, S., Veenstra, D. L., Prabulos, A. M., & Vandvik, P. O. (2012). VTE, thrombophilia, antithrombotic therapy, and pregnancy: Antithrombotic therapy and prevention of thrombosis, 9th ed: American College of Chest Physicians Evidence-Based Clinical Practice Guidelines. *Chest, 141*(2 Suppl.), e691s–e736s. doi:10.1378/chest.11-2300

Beckmann, C. A. (2003). The effects of asthma on pregnancy and perinatal outcomes. *Journal of Asthma: Official Journal of the Association for the Care of Asthma, 40*(2), 171–180. doi:10.1081/JAS-120017988

Belfort, M. A., Clark, S. L., Saade, G. R., Kleja, K., Dildy, G. A. III, Van Veen, T. R., . . . Kofford, S. (2010). Hospital readmission after delivery: Evidence for an increased incidence of nonurogenital infection in the immediate postpartum period. *American Journal of Obstetrics and Gynecology, 202*(1), 35.e1–35.e7. doi:10.1016/j.ajog.2009.08.029

Belfort, M. A., & Herbst, M. (2010). Severe acute asthma. In M. A. Belfort, G. R. Saade, M. R. Foley, J. P. Phelan, & G. A. Dildy III (Eds.), *Critical Care Obstetrics* (5th ed., pp. 327–337). Hoboken, NJ: Wiley-Blackwell.

Berg, C. J., Callaghan, W. M., Syverson, C., & Henderson, Z. (2010). Pregnancy-related mortality in the United States, 1998 to 2005. *Obstetrics and Gynecology, 116*(6), 1302–1309. doi:10.1097/AOG.0b013e3181fdfb11

Blaiss, M. S. (2004). Management of asthma during pregnancy. *Allergy and Asthma Proceedings: The Official Journal of Regional and State Allergy Societies, 25*(6), 375–379.

Bourjeily, G., Ankner, G., & Mohsenin, V. (2011). Sleep-disordered breathing in pregnancy. *Clinics in Chest Medicine, 32*(1), 175–189. doi:10.1016/j.ccm.2010.11.003

Brito, V., & Neiderman, M. S. (2011). Pneumonia complicating pregnancy. *Clinics in Chest Medicine, 32*(1), 121–132. doi:10.1016/j.ccm.2010.10.004

Brown, H. L., & Hiett, A. K. (2010). Deep vein thrombosis and pulmonary embolism in pregnancy: Diagnosis, complications, and management. *Clinical Obstetrics and Gynecology, 53*(2), 345–359. doi:10.1097/GRF.0b013e3181deb27e

Castles, A., Adams, E. K., Melvin, C. L., Kelsch, C., & Boulton, M. L. (1999). Effects of smoking during pregnancy: Five meta-analyses. *American Journal of Preventive Medicine, 16*(3), 208–215. doi:10.1016/S0749-3797(98)00089-0

Catanzarite, V., Willms, D., Wong, D., Landers, C., Cousins, I., & Schrimmer, D. (2001). Acute respiratory distress syndrome in pregnancy and the puerperium: Causes, courses, and outcomes. *Obstetrics and Gynecology, 97*(5), 760–764.

Chambers, C. (2006). Safety of asthma and allergy medications in pregnancy. *Immunology and Allergy Clinics of North America, 26*(1), 13–28. doi:10.1016/j.iac.2005.10.001

Chandra, P. C., Patel, H., Schiavello, H. J., & Briggs, S. L. (1998). Successful pregnancy outcome after complicated varicella pneumonia. *Obstetrics and Gynecology, 92*(4, Pt. 2), 680–682. doi:10.1016/S0029-7844(98)00237-3

Chapman, S. J. (1998). Varicella in pregnancy. *Seminars in Perinatology, 22*(4), 339–346. doi:10.1016/S0146-0005(98)80023-2

Cheng, V. C., Tang, B. S., Wu, A. K., Chu, C. M., & Yuen, K. Y. (2004). Medical treatment of viral pneumonia including SARS in immunocompetent adult. *Journal of Infection, 49*(4), 262–273. doi:10.1016/j.jinf.2004.07.010

Clark, S. L. (2010). Amniotic fluid embolism. *Clinical Obstetrics and Gynecology, 53*(2), 322–328. doi:10.1097/GRF.0b013e3181e0ead2

Clark, S. L., Belfort, M. A., Dildy, G. A., Herbst, M. A., Meyers, J. A., & Hankins, G. D. (2008). Maternal death in the 21st century: Causes, prevention, and relationship to cesarean delivery. *American Journal of Obstetrics and Gynecology, 199*(1), 36.e1–36.e5. doi:10.1016/j.ajog.2008.03.007

Coleman, M. T., & Rund, D. A. (1997). Nonobstetric conditions causing hypoxia during pregnancy: Asthma and epilepsy. *American Journal of Obstetrics and Gynecology, 177*(1), 1–7.

Colman-Brochu, S. (2004). Deep vein thrombosis in pregnancy. *MCN: The American Journal of Maternal Child Nursing, 29*(3), 186–192. doi:10.1097/00005721-200405000-00010

Conde-Agudelo, A., & Romero, R. (2009). Amniotic fluid embolism: An evidence-based review. *American Journal of Obstetrics and Gynecology, 201*(5), 445.e1–445.e13. doi:10.1016/j.ajog.2009.04.052

Creanga, A. A., Johnson, T. F., Graitcer, S. B., Hartman, L. K., Al-Samarrai, T., . . . Honein, M. A. (2010). Severity of 2009 pandemic influenza A (H1N1) virus infection in pregnant women.

Obstetrics and Gynecology, 115(4), 717–726. doi:10.1097/AOG.0b013e3181d57947

Cydulka, R. K. (2006). Acute asthma during pregnancy. *Immunology and Allergy Clinics of North America, 26*(1), 103–117. doi:10.1016/j.iac.2005.10.006

Dobbenga-Rhodes, Y. A. (2009). Responding to amniotic fluid embolism. *AORN Journal, 89*(6), 1079–1088. doi:10.1016/j.aorn.2009.02.014

Dombrowski, M. P. (2006). Outcomes of pregnancy in asthmatic women. *Immunology and Allergy Clinics of North America, 26*(1), 81–92. doi:10.1016/j.iac.2005.10.002

Dombrowski, M. P., & Schatz, M. (2010). Asthma in pregnancy. *Clinical Obstetrics and Gynecology, 53*(2), 301–310. doi:10.1097/GRF.0b013e3181de8906

Dombrowski, M. P., Schatz, M., Wise, R., Momirova, V., Landon, M., Mabie, W., . . . National Institute of Child Health and Human Development Maternal–Fetal Medicine Units Network and the National Heart, Lung, and Blood Institute. (2004). Asthma during pregnancy. *Obstetrics and Gynecology, 103*(1), 5–12. doi:10.1097/01.AOG.0000103994.75162.16

Ellegård, E. K. (2006). Pregnancy rhinitis. *Immunology and Allergy Clinics of North America, 26*(1), 119–135. doi:10.1016/j.iac.2005.10.007

Frye, D., Clark, S. L., Piacenza, D., & Shay-Zapien, G. (2011). Pulmonary complications in pregnancy: Consideratons for care. *Journal of Perinatal & Neonatal Nursing, 25*(3), 235–244. doi:10.1097/JPN.0b013e3182230e25

Gardner, M. O., & Doyle, N. M. (2004). Asthma in pregnancy. *Obstetrics and Gynecology Clinics of North America, 31*(2), 385–413. doi:10.1016/j.ogc.2004.03.010

Gei, A. F., & Suarez, V. R. (2011). Respiratory emergencies during pregnancy. In M. R. Foley, T. H. Strong, & T. J. Garite (Eds.), *Obstetric Intensive Care Manual* (3rd ed., pp. 145–164). New York: McGraw-Hill.

Gherman, R. B., Goodwin, T. M., Leung, B., Byrne, J. D., Hethumumi, R., & Montoro, M. (1999). Incidence, clinical characteristics, and timing of objectively diagnosed venous thromboembolism during pregnancy. *Obstetrics and Gynecology, 94*(5, Pt.1), 730–734.

Gibson, P. S., & Powrie, R. (2009). Anticoagulants and pregnancy: When are they safe? *Cleveland Clinic Journal of Medicine, 76*(2), 113–127.

Gluck, J. C. (2004). The change of asthma course during pregnancy. *Clinical Reviews in Allergy & Immunology, 26*(3), 171–180. doi:10.1385/CRIAI:26:3:171

Gluck, J. C., & Gluck, P. A. (2006). The effect of pregnancy on the course of asthma. *Immunology and Allergy Clinics of North America, 26*(1), 63–80. doi:10.1016/j.iac.2005.10.008

Goodnight, W. H., & Soper, D. E. (2005). Pneumonia in pregnancy. *Critical Care Medicine, 33*(10 Suppl.), S390–S397. doi:10.1097/01.CCM.0000182483.24836.66

Grant, A. (1996). Varicella infection and toxoplasmosis in pregnancy. *Journal of Perinatal & Neonatal Nursing, 10*(2), 17–29.

Graves, C. R. (2010). Pneumonia in pregnancy. *Clinical Obstetrics and Gynecology, 53*(2), 329–336. doi:10.1097/GRF.0b013e3181de8a6f

Hague, W. M., & Decker, G. A. (2003). Risk factors for thrombosis in pregnancy. *Best Practice and Research Clinical Haematology, 16*(2), 197–210. doi:10.1016/S1521-6926(03)00018-5

Hegewald, M. J., & Crapo, R. O. (2011). Respiratory physiology in pregnancy. *Clinics in Chest Medicine, 32*(1), 1–13. doi:10.1016/j.ccm.2010.11.001

Heit, J. A., Kobbervig, C. E., James, A. H., Petterson, T. M., Bailey, K. R., & Melton, L. J. III. (2005). Trends in the incidence of venous thromboembolism during pregnancy or postpartum: A 30-year population-based study. *Annals of Internal Medicine, 143*(10), 697–706.

Horlocker, T. T., Wedel, D. J., Rowlingson, J. C., & Enneking, F. K. (2010). Executive summary: Regional anesthesia in the patient receiving antithrombotic or thrombolytic therapy: American Society of Regional Anesthesia and Pain Medicine Evidence-Based Guidelines (3rd ed.). *Regional Anesthesia and Pain Medicine, 35*(1), 102–105. doi:10.1097/AAP.0b013e3181c15dd0

James, A. H., Jamison, M. G., Brancazio, L. R., & Myers, E. R. (2006). Venous thromboembolism during pregnancy and the postpartum period: Incidence, risk factors, and mortality. *American Journal of Obstetrics and Gynecology, 194*(5), 1311–1315. doi:10.1016/j.ajog.2005.11.008

Julian, C. G. (2011). High altitude during pregnancy. *Clinics in Chest Medicine, 32*(1), 21–31. doi:10.1016/j.ccm.2010.10.008

Källén, B., Rydhstroem, H., & Aberg, A. (2000). Asthma during pregnancy—A population based study. *European Journal of Epidemiology, 16*(2), 167–171. doi:10.1023/A:1007678404911

Knight, M., Tuffnell, D., Brocklehurst, P., Spark, P., & Kurinczuk, J. J. (2010). Incidence and risk factors for amniotic-fluid embolism. *Obstetrics and Gynecology, 155*(5), 910–917. doi:10.1097/AOG.0b013e3181d9f629

Kwon, H. L., Triche, E. W., Belanger, K., & Bracken, M. B. (2006). The epidemiology of asthma during pregnancy: Prevalence, diagnosis, and symptoms. *Immunology and Allergy Clinics of North America, 26*(1), 29–62. doi:10.1016/j.iac.2005.11.002

Laibl, V. R., & Sheffield, J. S. (2005). Influenza and pneumonia in pregnancy. *Clinics in Perinatology, 32*(3), 727–738. doi:10.1016/j.clp.2005.04.009

Laibl, V. R., & Sheffield, J. S. (2006). The management of respiratory infections during pregnancy. *Immunology and Allergy Clinics of North America, 26*(1), 155–172. doi:10.1016/j.iac.2005.11.003

Lam, C. M., Wong, S. F., Leung, T. N., Chow, K. M., Yu, W. C., Wong, T. Y., . . . Ho, L. C. (2004). A case-controlled study comparing clinical course and outcomes of pregnant and non-pregnant women with severe acute respiratory syndrome. *BJOG: An International Journal of Obstetrics and Gynaecology, 111*(8), 771–774. doi:10.1111/j.1471-0528.2004.00199.x

Lau, E. M., Moriarty, C., Ogle, R., & Bye, P. T. (2010). Pregnancy and cystic fibrosis. *Paediatric Respiratory Reviews, 11*(2), 90–94. doi:10.1016/j.prrv.2010.01.008

Lehne, R. A. (2010). Anticoagulant, antiplatelet, and thrombolytic drugs. In *Pharmacology for Nursing Care* (7th ed., pp. 594–618). St. Louis, MO: Saunders Elsevier.

Lim, W. S., Macfarlane, J. T., & Colthorpe C. L. (2001). Pneumonia and pregnancy. *Thorax: An International Journal of Respiratory Medicine, 56*(5), 398–405. doi:10.1136/thorax.56.5.398

Lockwood, C. J. (2009). Thromboembolic disease in pregnancy. In R. K. Creasy, R. Resnik, J. D. Iams, C. J. Lockwood, & T. R. Moore (Eds.), *Maternal–Fetal Medicine: Principles and Practice* (6th ed., pp. 855–866). Philadelphia: Saunders.

Lomas, P. H., & Fowler, S. B. (2010). Original research: Parents and children with cystic fibrosis. *American Journal of Nursing, 110*(8), 30–37. doi:10.1097/01.NAJ.0000387689.02005.1d

Mabie, W. C. (2010). Pulmonary edema. In M. A. Belfort, G. R. Saade, M. R. Foley, J. P. Phelan, & G. A. Dildy III (Eds.), *Critical Care Obstetrics* (5th ed., pp. 348–357). Hoboken, NJ: Wiley-Blackwell.

Maccato, M. (1991). Respiratory insufficiency due to pneumonia in pregnancy. *Obstetrics and Gynecology Clinics of North America, 18*(2), 289–299.

MacKay, A. P., Berg, C. J., Liu, X., Duran, C., & Hoyert, D. L. (2011). Changes in pregnancy mortality ascertainment: United States, 1999–2005. *Obstetrics and Gynecology, 118*(1), 104–110. doi:10.1097/AOG.0b013e31821fd49d

Marini, J. J., & Wheeler, A. P. (2009). *Critical Care Medicine* (4th ed.). Philadelphia: Lippincott Williams & Wilkins.

Marini, J. J., & Wheeler, A. P. (2010). Oxygen failure, ARDS, and acute lung injury. In *Critical Care Medicine* (4th ed., pp. 430–453). Philadelphia: Lippincott Williams & Wilkins.

Mason, B. A., & Dorman, K. (2012). Pulmonary disorders in pregnancy. In N. H. Troiano, C. J. Harvey, & B. F. Chez (Eds.), *High Risk and Critical Care Obstetrics* (3rd edition, pp. 144–162). Philadelphia: Lippincott Williams and Wilkins.

McArdle, J. R. (2011). Pregnancy in cystic fibrosis. *Clinics in Chest Medicine, 32*(1), 111–120. doi:10.1016/j.ccm.2010.10.005

Meschia, G. (2011). Fetal oxygenation and maternal ventilation. *Clinics in Chest Medicine, 32*(1), 15–19. doi:10.1016/j.ccm.2010.11.007

Minerbi-Codish, I., Fraser, D., Avnun, L., Glezerman, M., & Heimer, D. (1998). Influence of asthma in pregnancy on labor and the newborn. *Respiration, 65*(2), 130–135. doi:10.1159/000029244

Murin, S., Rafii, R., & Bilello, K. (2011). Smoking and smoking cessation in pregnancy. *Clinics in Chest Medicine, 32*(1), 75–91. doi:10.1016/j.ccm.2010.11.004

Murphy, P. J. M., Meadors, B., & King, T. L. (2011). Hematology. In T. L. King & M. C. Brucker (Eds.), *Pharmacology for Women's Health* (pp. 435–461). Sudbury, MA; Jones and Barlett.

Namazy, J. A., & Schatz, M. (2006). Current guidelines for the management of asthma during pregnancy. *Immunology and Allergy Clinics of North America, 26*(1), 93–102. doi:10.1016/j.iac.2005.10.003

National Asthma Education and Prevention Program. (2005). *Working Group Report on Managing Asthma During Pregnancy: Recommendations for Pharmacologic Treatment—Update 2004* (NIH Publication No. 05-5236). Bethesda, MD: U.S. Department of Health and Human Services, National Institutes of Health, National Heart, Lung, and Blood Institute.

National Asthma Education and Prevention Program. (2007). *Expert Panel Report No. 3: Guidelines for the Diagnosis and Management of Asthma* (NIH Publication No. 07-4051). Bethesda, MD: U.S. Department of Health and Human Services, National Institutes of Health, National Heart, Lung, and Blood Institute.

Neu, H. C., & Sabath, L. D. (1993). Criteria for selecting oral antibiotic therapy for community-acquired pneumonia. *Infections in Medicine, 10*(Suppl. 2), 33S–40S.

Nolan, T. E., & Hankins, G. D. (1995). Acute pulmonary dysfunction and distress. *Obstetrics and Gynecology Clinics of North America, 22*(1), 39–54.

Norwitz, E. R., & Robinson, J. N. (2010). Pregnancy-induced physiologic alterations. In M. A. Belfort, G. R. Saade, M. R. Foley, J. P. Phelan, & G. A. Dildy III (Eds.), *Critical Care Obstetrics* (5th ed., pp. 30–52). Hoboken, NJ: Wiley-Blackwell.

Orme, M. L., Lewis, P. J., de Swiet, M., Serlin, M. J., Sibeon, R., Baty, J. D., & Breckenridge, A. M. (1977). May mothers given warfarin breast-feed their infants? *British Medical Journal, 1*(6076), 1564–1565. doi:10.1136/bmj.1.6076.1564

Park-Wyllie, L., Mazzotta, P., Pastuszak, A., Moretti, M. E., Beique, L., Hunnisett, L., . . . Koren, G. (2000). Birth defects after maternal exposure to corticosteroids: Prospective cohort study and meta-analysis of epidemiological studies. *Teratology, 62*(6), 385–392. doi:10.1002/1096-9926(200012)62:6<385::AID-TERA5>3.0.CO;2-Z

Pereira, A., & Krieger, B. P. (2004). Pulmonary complications of pregnancy. *Clinics in Chest Medicine, 25*(2), 299–310. doi:10.1016/j.ccm.2004.01.010

Poole, J. H., & Spreen, D. T. (2005). Acute pulmonary edema in pregnancy. *Journal of Perinatal & Neonatal Nursing, 19*(4), 316–331.

Ramsey, P. S., & Ramin, K. D. (2001). Pneumonia in pregnancy. *Obstetrics and Gynecology Clinics of North America, 28*(3), 553–569.

Reinisch, J. M., Simon, N. G., Karow, W. G., & Gandelman, R. (1978). Prenatal exposure to prednisone in humans and animals retards intrauterine growth. *Science, 202*(4366), 436–438. doi:10.1126/science.705336

Rhode, M. A. (2011). Postpartum. In T. L. King & M. C. Brucker (Eds.), *Pharmacology for Women's Health* (pp. 1117–1145). Boston: Jones and Bartlett.

Robert, E., Vollset, S. E., Botto, L., Lancaster, P. A., Merlob, P., Mastroiacovo, P., . . . Orioli, I. (1994). Malformation surveillance and maternal drug exposure: The MADRE Project. *International Journal of Risk and Safety in Medicine, 6*, 78–118.

Salmon, B., & Bruick-Sorge, C. (2003). Pneumonia in pregnant women. *AWHONN Lifelines, 7*(1), 48–52. doi:10.1177/1091592303251728

Schatz, M. (2001). The efficacy and safety of asthma medications during pregnancy. *Seminars in Perinatology, 25*(3), 145–152. doi:10.1053/sper.2001.24569

Scheffer, A. L. (1991). Guidelines for the diagnosis and management of asthma (National Heart, Lung, and Blood Institute, National Asthma Education Program, Expert Panel Report). *Journal of Allergy and Clinical Immunology, 88*(3, Pt. 2), 427–438.

Schramm, W. F. (1997). Smoking during pregnancy: Missouri longitudinal study. *Paediatric and Perinatal Epidemiology, 11*(Suppl. 1), 73–83. doi:10.1046/j.1365-3016.11.s1.10.x

Silver, R. M. (2007). Fetal death. *Obstetrics and Gynecology, 109*(1), 153–167. doi:10.1097/01.AOG.0000248537.89739.96

Simpson, K. R., & James, D. C. (2005). Efficacy of intrauterine resuscitation techniques in improving fetal oxygen status during labor. *Obstetrics and Gynecology, 105*(6), 1362–1368. doi:10.1097/01.AOG.0000164474.03350.7c

Towers, C. V., Briggs, G. G., & Rojas, J. A. (2004). The use of prostaglandin E2 in pregnant patients with asthma. *American Journal of Obstetrics and Gynecology, 190*(6), 1777–1780. doi:10.1016/j.ajog.2004.02.056

Tsang, A., Moriarty, C., & Towns, S. J. (2010). Contraception, communication and counseling for sexuality and reproductive health in adolescents and young adults with CF. *Paediatric Respiratory Reviews, 11*(2), 84–89. doi:10.1016/j.prrv.2010.01.002

U.S. Department of Health and Human Services. (2004). *The Health Consequences of Smoking: A Report of the Surgeon General*. Washington, DC: Centers for Disease Control and Prevention, National Center for Chronic Disease Prevention and Health Promotion, Office on Smoking and Health.

Weinmann, E. E., & Salzman, E. W. (1994). Deep-vein thrombosis. *New England Journal of Medicine, 331*(24), 1630–1641.

Whitty, J. E. (2010). Cystic fibrosis in pregnancy. *Clinical Obstetrics and Gynecology, 53*(2), 369–376. doi:10.1097/GRF.0b013e3181deb448

Whitty, J. E., & Dombrowski, M. P. (2009). Respiratory diseases in pregnancy. In R. K. Creasy, R. Resnik, J. D. Iams, C. J. Lockwood, & T. R. Moore (Eds.), *Maternal–Fetal Medicine: Principles and Practice* (6th ed., pp. 927–952). Philadelphia: Saunders.

Wise, R. A., Polito, A. J., & Krishnan, V. (2006). Respiratory physiologic changes in pregnancy. *Immunology and Allergy Clinics of North America, 26*(1), 1–12. doi:10.1016/j.iac.2005.10.004

Wong, S. F., Chow, K. M., Leung, T. N., Ng, W. F., Ng, T. K., Shek, C. C., . . . Tan, P. Y. (2004). Pregnancy and perinatal outcomes of women with severe acute respiratory syndrome. *American Journal of Obstetrics and Gynecology, 191*(1), 292–297. doi:10.1016/j.ajog.2003.11.019

Yost, N. P., Bloom, S. L., Richey, S. D., Ramin, S. M., & Cunningham, F. G. (2000). An appraisal of treatment guidelines for antepartum community-acquired pneumonia. *American Journal of Obstetrics and Gynecology, 183*(1), 131–135. doi:10.1067/mob.2000.105743

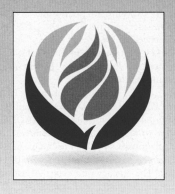

Nancy A. Bowers

CHAPTER 11

Multiple Gestation

During the past 30 years, multiple birth rates have increased dramatically, with the recent numbers of twins, triplets, and other higher order multiples (HOMs) at the highest levels in recorded history. Trends in delayed childbearing and increased use of infertility therapies and assisted reproductive technologies (ARTs) have contributed greatly to these increased rates (Wright, Schieve, Reynolds, & Jeng, 2005). Although multiple births represent a little more than 3% of the total live births in the United States, these births contribute disproportionately to the rates of maternal, fetal, and neonatal morbidity and mortality. Multiple birth infants are at high risk of being born too early and too small and have an impact on national rates of preterm birth (<37 weeks' gestation) and low birth weight (LBW; less than 2,500 g). A key factor is a clear dose–response relationship: Increasing plurality corresponds with higher morbidity and mortality for mothers and their infants. With these high risks, the perinatal team must be alert for potential complications during pregnancy, labor, birth, and the postpartum period.

EPIDEMIOLOGY

Of the more than four million United States live births in 2009, multiple births accounted for 3.32%, with 137,217 infants born as twins, 5,905 as triplets, 355 as quadruplets, and 80 as quintuplets and higher (Martin et al., 2011). Data from the National Center for Health Statistics (Martin et al., 2011) reveal that the multiple birth rate (live births of twins, triplets, and higher/1,000) remains at record levels (see Figures 11–1 and 11–2). The twin birth rate increased by 76% since 1980 and by 47% since 1990 but has now stabilized, rising about

1% annually (Martin et al., 2011). During that same time, the rate of HOMs rose more than 500% but has declined since 2004 (Martin et al., 2011).

A population-based study of births from 1995 to 2000 found mothers of multiples were more likely to be older, white, of lower parity, nonsmokers, married, and to have higher education than mothers of singletons (Luke & Brown, 2007). Shifts in traditional maternal age patterns have occurred along with the rise in multiple births, mirroring the trend of delayed childbearing. Historically, twin birth rates were low for young women, rose through the age group 35 to 39 years, then declined for women in their 40s (Martin & Park, 1999). However, beginning in 1992, multiple birth rates rose steadily for women over age 30, with the highest overall multiple birth rates in 2009 for women in the 45 to 54 age group (237.3/1,000; Martin et al., 2011). Surprisingly, advanced maternal age appears to be associated with better perinatal outcomes for multiple gestations compared to singletons (Delbaere et al., 2008; Kathiresan et al., 2011). This is particularly true for nulliparous women. A variety of explanations have been proposed, including greater use of donor eggs and better socioeconomic status, education, and prenatal care (Zhang, Meikle, Grainger, & Trumble, 2002). Other explanations include older women's healthier lifestyles and higher body mass index (BMI), as well as possible uterine cell proliferation or "remodeling" from prior pregnancies that may improve uterine expansion limits and fetal nourishment (Oleszczuk, Keith, & Oleszczuk, 2005).

There have also been shifts in maternal race patterns for multiple births. Historically, multiple births occurred more often in black women than in white women, but this gap has been overtaken. In 2009, twin birth rates for non-Hispanic white women and

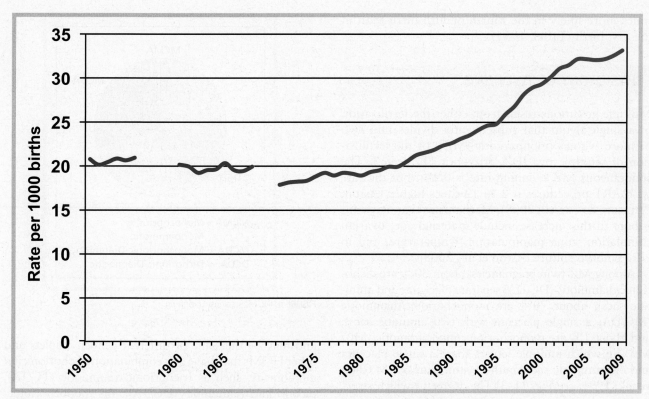

FIGURE 11–1. Twin birth rate: United States 1950–2009. (Based on cumulative natality data from the National Center for Health Statistics.) Break in line represents years in which data were not collected.

non-Hispanic black women were similar (Martin et al., 2011). However, disparities were seen for HOMs. In 2009, the HOM birth rate for non-Hispanic whites (201.4/100,000) was nearly double the rate of non-Hispanic blacks (105.6/100,000)

and was even higher than that of Hispanic mothers (83.5/100,000; Martin et al., 2011). Regardless of maternal age, a prior multiple pregnancy and higher parity increase the likelihood for spontaneous dizygotic (DZ) twin conception. Twinning is about four

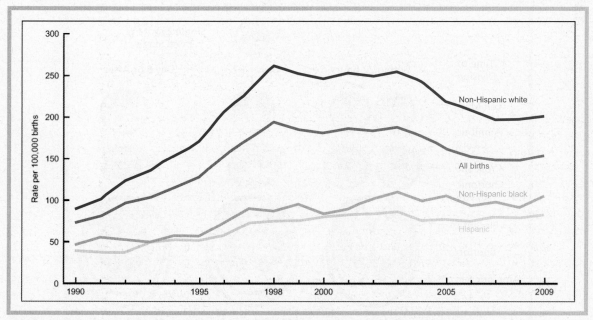

FIGURE 11–2. Higher order multiples birth rate: United States 1990–2009. (From Martin, J. A., Hamilton, B. E., Ventura, S. J., Osterman, M. J. K., Kirmeyer, S., Mathews, T. J., & Wilson, E. C. [2011]. Births: Final data for 2009. *National Vital Statistics Reports, 60*[1], 1–72. Retrieved from http://www.cdc.gov/nchs/data/nvsr/nvsr60/nvsr60_01.pdf. Reprinted with permission.)

times more likely in the fourth or fifth birth than in the first birth (Taffel, 1995).

PHYSIOLOGY OF TWINNING

Multiple gestations result from either the fertilization of a single ovum that subsequently divides into two or more zygotes (monozygotic [MZ]) or the fertilization of multiple ova (DZ, trizygotic [TZ], etc.). The spontaneous MZ twinning rate is 0.4%, but the rate with ART procedures is 2 to 12 times higher (Aston, Peterson, & Carrell, 2008). Mechanisms that may contribute to this increase include maternal age, ovarian stimulation, zona manipulation, temperature, and in vitro embryo culture (Aston et al., 2008).

Among MZ twin pregnancies, about 30% are dichorionic/diamniotic (DC/DA; separate placentas and amniotic sacs); about 70% are monochorionic/diamniotic (MC/DA; a single placenta with two amniotic sacs); and about 1% are monochorionic/monoamniotic (MC/MA), in which multiple fetuses share a single placenta and one amniotic sac (Smith-Levitin, Skupski, & Chervenak, 1999; see Fig. 11–3).The degree to which structures are shared is related to the time of zygotic division after conception; early division (within 72 hours) results in DC/DA, division between days 4 through 7 results in MC/DA, and later division results in MC/MA. Conjoined twins occur following very late and incomplete zygotic splitting, usually after day 13. Because they develop from a single fertilized ovum, MZ twins are always of the same gender. DZ twins are always DC/DA

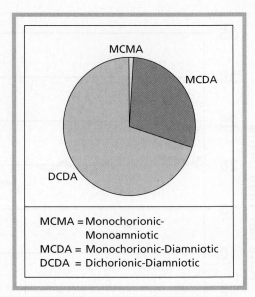

FIGURE 11–3. Monozygotic twinning.

and may be the same or different gender. Triplets and other HOMs may have any combination of chorionicity/amnionicity, such as trichorionic/triamniotic (TC/TA), dichorionic/triamniotic (DC/TA), or monochorionic/triamniotic (MC/TA; see Figs. 11–4 to 11–6).

ROLE OF INFERTILITY AND ASSISTED REPRODUCTIVE TECHNOLOGY

A significant percentage of multiple births in the United States are conceived with some type of infertility therapy,

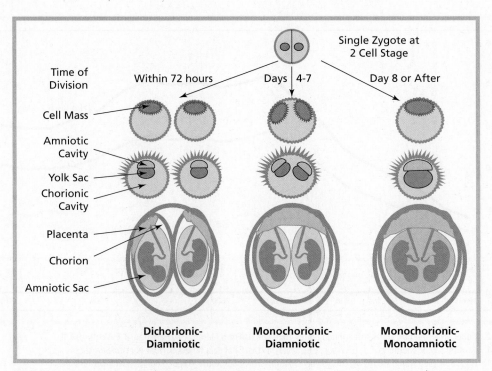

FIGURE 11–4. Monozygotic twins. (Copyright 2006 by Marvelous Multiples, Inc. Used with permission.)

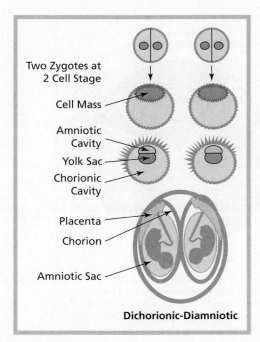

FIGURE 11–5. Dizygotic twins.

or embryos in 2009, 28.9% were twins and 1.6% were HOMs (CDC, ASRM, & SART, 2011; see Fig. 11–7). Among ART births in 2009, 60% of twins and 97.5% of HOMs were born preterm, and 56.1% of twins and 92.1% of HOMs were LBW (CDC et al., 2011).

Fertility-assisted pregnancies, including singletons, appear to have poorer perinatal outcomes than naturally conceived pregnancies. However, the Report cautions against comparing preterm and LBW births between ART's multiple-fetus pregnancies with those of the general population since a substantial proportion of twin births or HOM births are due to infertility treatments (ART and non-ART) (CDC et al., 2011).

The high risk of multiple births with ART and other infertility therapies has generated the creation of policy recommendations and clinical guidelines. In 1998, 2004, 2006, 2009, and again in 2013, SART and the ASRM declared that high-order multiple pregnancy (three or more implanted embryos) is an undesirable consequence of ART and issued guidelines to assist ART programs and patients in determining the appropriate number of embryos to transfer (Practice Committee of ASRM & Practice Committee of SART, 2013). The 2013 guidelines include the following maternal age–based embryo transfer limits for women with a favorable prognosis: transfer of one to two cleavage-stage embryos for women under age 35, two cleavage-stage embryos for women between 35 and 37 years of age, three cleavage-stage embryos for women between ages 38 and 40, and no more than five embryos for women ages 41 to 42. Data are insufficient to recommend a limit for women ≥43 years of age. The guidelines may

including ovulation induction and ART. Although data from the National Summary and Fertility Clinic Report from the Centers for Disease Control and Prevention (CDC), the American Society for Reproductive Medicine (ASRM), and the Society for Assisted Reproductive Technology (SART) provide a fairly accurate estimate of in vitro fertilization (IVF) births, exact numbers of natural conceptions are unknown. Of live births from pregnancies conceived in ART cycles using fresh nondonor eggs

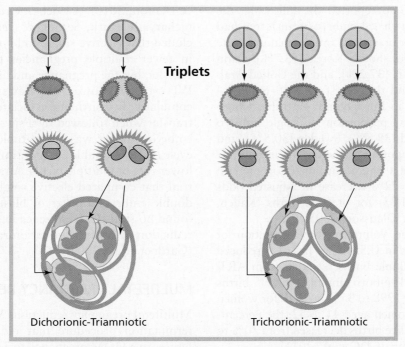

FIGURE 11–6. Triplets. (Copyright 2006 by Marvelous Multiples, Inc. Used with permission.)

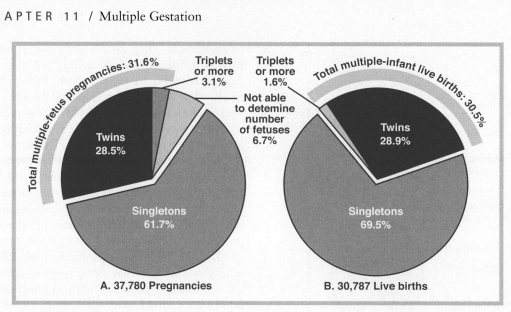

FIGURE 11–7. Risks of having multiple-fetus pregnancies and multiple-infant live births from assisted reproductive technology (ART) cycles using fresh nondonor eggs or embryos, 2009. (From Centers for Disease Control and Prevention, American Society for Reproductive Medicine, & Society for Assisted Reproductive Technology [2011]. *2009 Assisted Reproductive Technology Success Rates: National Summary and Fertility Clinic Reports.* Atlanta, GA: U.S. Department of Health and Human Services. Retrieved from http://www.cdc.gov/art/ART2009/index.htm. Reprinted with permission.)

be individualized based on each woman's clinical condition, prognosis, and circumstances.

In the early 1990s, other countries instituted governmental mandates for IVF clinics to decrease the number of embryos transferred from three to two (Jain, Missmer, & Hornstein, 2004). By 2001, marked declines were seen in the rate of multiple births after IVF, especially in HOMs. The International Committee for Monitoring Assisted Reproductive Technology (ICMART) reported an overall twin rate of 25.7% per delivery and a triplet rate of 2.5% in 2002 for 53 countries (ICMART et al., 2009). The group reported the following: the percentage of cycles with ≥4 embryos transferred had decreased from the prior report, rates remained quite high in some countries (South Korea [53.7%], Latin America [37.9%], India [37.2%], and the United Arab Emirates [37.2%]), and the lowest rates (0 to 0.5%) were in 11 countries in Europe and Australia. Countries with the greatest proportion of single embryo transfers were Finland (38.5%), Sweden (30.5%), and Australia (25.0%). Importantly, the decline in multiple births appears to have a significant impact on preterm births. Sweden had a 72% decrease in adjusted odds ratio (from 4.63 to 1.33) for preterm births (Källen, Finnstrom, Nygren, & Olausson, 2005).

It appears that the voluntary implementation of embryo transfer limits in U.S. clinics has also reduced the occurrence of multiple births resulting from ART. The percentage of live-born multiple-infant births dropped from 42% in 1998 to 35% in 2009 for women <35 years old. For women aged 41 to 42, the percentage of multiple-infant live births decreased from 20% to 16% in those same years (CDC et al., 2011).

A continued decrease in the number of iatrogenic multiple births is challenging. Infertility practices are often motivated by competition for patients, the desire for fertility success, and the need for rapid results (D'Alton, 2004). Infertility patients themselves often desire a multiple pregnancy. A review of the recent literature found that while the majority of IVF patients and their partners showed a desire for twins rather than singletons, elective single embryo transfer could become increasingly acceptable if success rates approached those of double embryo transfers (Leese & Denton, 2010). A Cochrane review (Pandian, Bhattacharya, Ozturk, Serour, & Templeton, 2009) concluded that elective single embryo transfer does result in fewer multiple pregnancies than double embryo transfer, but the pregnancy and live birth rate per fresh IVF cycle was lower. The Review did show that the cumulative live birth rate associated with single embryo transfer when followed by a single frozen and thawed embryo transfer was comparable with that after one cycle of fresh, double embryo transfer yet maintained a lower rate of multiple births. A randomized controlled trial that compared elective single embryo transfer to double embryo transfer of blastocyst stage embryos found no statistical difference in pregnancy rate and a reduction in multiple gestation rate from 47% to 0% (Gardner et al., 2004).

MULTIFETAL PREGNANCY REDUCTION

Multifetal pregnancy reduction (MFPR) is a pregnancy termination procedure that reduces the number of fetuses in a HOM pregnancy to a lower and potentially more viable number, thus increasing the chances for a positive pregnancy outcome. The rise in use of MFPR has paralleled the rising number of HOM pregnancies, particularly in older women using donor eggs (Evans & Britt, 2010). MFPR is typically performed in the late first trimester to terminate one or more fetuses. Nearly all procedures performed today use transabdominal needle insertion under ultrasound guidance. The patient is placed in the lithotomy position, and a 22-gauge needle is inserted transabdominally into the fetal heart. Asystole is achieved following injection of 2 to 3 mL of potassium chloride and is confirmed by ultrasound. Antibiotics are given, and the woman may have abdominal cramping, vaginal spotting, and leaking of amniotic fluid (Little, 2010). Although MFPR is sometimes called selective reduction, the terms are not synonymous. Selective reduction applies to situations in which a specific fetus is targeted for reduction because of a known anomaly, aneuploidy, or a risk identified with nuchal translucency (NT) screening. Reduction of a single fetus in an MC pair requires occlusion of umbilical cord blood flow to prevent interfetal transfusion. Recently, radio frequency ablation has been used to destroy cord tissue for selective reduction of an MC twin (Paramasivam et al., 2010).

There have been many studies comparing pregnancy outcomes following MFPR. The literature is conflicting regarding the outcomes of reduced and unreduced triplets (Wimalasundera, 2010), and a 2009 Cochrane review reconfirmed that there are "insufficient data available to support a policy of pregnancy reduction procedures for women with a triplet or higher order multiple pregnancy" (Dodd & Crowther, 2010). Generally, outcomes following reduction to twins appear comparable to outcomes for twins conceived spontaneously or by ART, but study findings about the risks and benefits associated with reduction procedures are not as clear (Dodd & Crowther, 2005). Complications include procedural complications (e.g., infection or incomplete procedure), total pregnancy loss, and a continued risk for preterm birth. Collaborative data from several centers have shown that higher starting numbers of fetuses (≥ 6) correspond with poorer outcomes after reduction; total pregnancy loss rates prior to 24 weeks' gestation are 4.5% for triplets, 8% for quadruplets, 11% for quintuplets, and 15% for sextuplets or more (Evans, Ciorica, Britt, & Fletcher, 2005). All reduced pregnancies have been shown to have an ongoing increased risk for preterm birth, except for pregnancies reduced to singletons (Evans et al., 2005). Generally, there is an increased risk for lower birth weights in the remaining fetuses post-MFPR, with an inverse correlation to starting numbers (American College of Obstetricians and Gynecologists [ACOG], 2007; Stone et al., 2008). Without prenatal diagnostic testing prior to MFPR, there is the possibility of

terminating a healthy fetus while leaving an abnormal one. Some centers are combining the use of rapid chromosome analysis following chorionic villus sampling (CVS) with MFPR (Evans & Britt, 2010). The ASRM recommends that MFPR should be performed only in specialized centers with fetal medicine practitioners experienced in the procedure (ASRM, 2012).

MFPR presents a difficult dilemma for most couples. They often face conflicting values as they consider reduction after years of desiring fertility and must weigh the medical/obstetric/neonatal risks and the psychosocial/moral/economic impact on their family (Elliott, 2005a). The seemingly (and often actually) arbitrary choice as to which fetus should live and which should die is distressing (Bryan, 2005). Further, the decision for reduction must be made in a short time between diagnosis and the optimal timing for the procedure. The decision has been described as highly stressful, psychologically traumatic, frightening, painful, overwhelming, confusing, and a surreal experience (Bergh, Möller, Nilsson, & Wikland, 1999; Bryan, 2005; Collopy, 2004). The following responses from women indicate their inner conflicts about the decision: "I believe reduction saved one of my children. It's the not knowing that kills me." "If I tried to carry all of the babies, I would most definitely lose them all. I also look at my survivor knowing she probably would have been chosen for reduction. This also wracks me with guilt" (from a mother who spontaneously lost some of her fetuses and did not have to reduce) (Pector, 2004, p. 716). There is also evidence from interviews with patients that viewing fetuses on ultrasound just prior to or during reduction made the reduction more difficult (Maifeld, Hahn, Titler, & Mullen, 2003; Schreiner-Engel, Walther, Mindes, Lynch, & Berkowitz, 1995). Studies have shown that persistent feelings of sadness and guilt may continue after the MFPR procedure; however, most women believe their choice was correct and that reduction was necessary for them to achieve their goal of motherhood (Collopy, 2004). The grief response with MFPR may not fit the classic process and may be more complicated or delayed. Wang and Yu Chao (2006) interviewed six Taiwanese women undergoing MFPR over 8 to 10 weeks. Although the women were able to move past the reduction and adjust to a normal pregnancy experience, the researchers found that MFPR created psychological distress through exposure to moral and ethical dilemmas. More research is needed to determine long-term psychological outcomes, cultural responses, and effects on parent–child bonding and responses of child survivors.

The reduction debate also can be problematic for clinicians. With the improvements in neonatal care and long-term outcomes for preterm infants, some clinicians may be unwilling to accept that medical risks are sufficient grounds for reducing a triplet pregnancy (Bryan, 2005). Another consideration is the first trimester spontaneous loss rate for multiple gestations, which might make MFPR unnecessary. One study found that spontaneous loss of one or more gestational sacs or embryos occurred before the 12th week of gestation in 65% of quadruplet pregnancies, 53% of triplets, and 36% of twins (Dickey et al., 2002). The controversy is likely to continue. Some have proposed that future debates will no longer be over reduction of HOMs and triplets but over a routine offer of reduction of all twins (Evans & Britt, 2010). ACOG concludes that patients should not be given the impression that multifetal pregnancies are without problems because fetal reduction is available (ACOG, 2007).

Nurses have much to contribute in the care of women considering and undergoing MFPR. Establishing a rapport, exploring treatment options, and assisting with decision making with a consistently available primary nurse has been recommended (Collopy, 2004). Patient education includes written instructions, a list of symptoms that would indicate a need for medical care, postprocedure self-care, and grief counseling (Little, 2010).

DIAGNOSIS OF MULTIPLE GESTATIONS

First trimester ultrasound is highly accurate in diagnosing multiple gestations; the earliest gestation for determining chorionicity is 5 gestational weeks; for fetal number, 6 weeks; and for amnionicity, 8 weeks (Shetty & Smith, 2005). Diagnosis is confirmed when multiple embryos or embryonic parts are seen in the gestational sac(s). Women at high risk of conceiving multiples, such as those using infertility therapies, should have an ultrasound early in the first trimester. Thickness and numbers of membrane layers can be counted, and ultrasound markers can be visualized between 6 and 10 gestational weeks (Cleary-Goldman, Chitkara, & Berkowitz, 2007). Membrane thickness of ≤2 mm identifies monochorionicity with a positive predictive value of 90%, and >2 mm identifies dichorionicity with a positive predictive value of 95% (Morin & Lim, 2011). The triangular lambda sign predicts DZ chorionicity, a T-shaped junction is present in MC placentas, and a Y-shaped ipsilon zone is characteristic of the three interfetal membranes of TZ triplet gestations (Shetty & Smith, 2005; Smith-Levitin et al., 1999). First trimester ultrasonography is highly accurate in determining chorionicity, but accuracy decreases as the pregnancy progresses, especially after 14 weeks (Morin & Lim, 2011), and varies with sonographer skill and experience (Menon, 2005). Early identification of MC and MA pregnancies is important in planning appropriate management of these high-risk pregnancies.

Clinical examination may also assist in diagnosis. With an accurate menstrual history, a fundal height 2 cm to 4 cm larger than the expected gestational age suggests multiple gestation. Other signs include palpation during the Leopold maneuver that reveals multiple fetal parts or fetal poles, or when there is more than one fetal heart sound, particularly with a difference of 10 beats per minute (Bowers & Gromada, 2006).

Maternal perceptions may also provide clues to the presence of more than one fetus. These include excessive fatigue, hyperemesis, increased appetite and weight gain (especially in early pregnancy), exaggerated pregnancy discomforts, increased fetal activity, the feeling that the pregnancy is different from previous singleton pregnancies, and peculiar insights about the pregnancy (Bowers & Gromada, 2006).

Not all women are psychologically prepared for the diagnosis of twins, and even fewer for the discovery of HOMs. Ambivalence is normal, even when a pregnancy has been greatly desired or after years of infertility treatments (Klock, 2001). Revealing the diagnosis of multiple pregnancy should be done with sensitivity to each woman's situation, with a factual nonemotional approach and guarded enthusiasm (Bowers & Gromada, 2006). Many couples are at first overwhelmed with joy by the announcement of multiples, then simply overwhelmed by the physical, emotional, and financial demands ahead.

MATERNAL ADAPTATION

Nearly every maternal structure and body system is affected by the physiologic changes that occur in multiple gestation, with symptoms often more exaggerated than with a singleton pregnancy. General complaints of pregnancy such as urinary frequency, constipation, difficulty sleeping, fatigue, and varicose veins tend to be magnified and occur earlier.

GASTROINTESTINAL

Paralleling high human chorionic gonadotropin (hCG) levels in early pregnancy, as many as half of women pregnant with multiples experience nausea and vomiting in the first trimester, with symptoms persisting throughout pregnancy in up to 20% of women. Of these, 1% to 3% suffer with hyperemesis gravidarum (Rohde, Dembinski, & Dorn, 2003); this is approximately double the risk in singletons (Niebyl, 2010). If prolonged, these conditions can affect weight gain and nutritional status of the mother as well as increase the risk for LBW infants (ACOG, 2004b). Interestingly, one study found that women carrying a combination of male and female fetuses have the highest risk for hyperemesis, with risks decreasing for all males followed by all females (Fell, Dodds, Joseph, Allen, & Butler, 2006). Women may also complain of gastroesophageal reflux early in pregnancy, which is consistent with decreased lower esophageal sphincter tone of pregnancy and increasing mechanical pressure due to the rapidly growing uterus and slowed gastrointestinal transit time (Richter, 2003).

HEMATOLOGIC

Plasma volume increases by 50% to 100% with multiple gestations and results in a dilutional anemia (Malone & D'Alton, 2004). Evaluations of iron status in multiple gestations have found lower hemoglobin levels in the first and second trimesters and increased rates of iron-deficiency anemia (Luke, 2005).

CARDIOVASCULAR

Women experience significant cardiovascular changes with a multiple pregnancy. Heart rate and stroke volume are increased over that of singleton gestations, resulting in higher cardiac output and cardiac index in the second and third trimesters (Norwitz, Edusa, & Park, 2005). Total vascular resistance has been found to be lower in uncomplicated twin pregnancies from 20 to 34 gestational weeks when compared to singletons (Kuleva et al., 2011). Combined with increased plasma volume, these cardiovascular changes increase the risk of pulmonary edema in multiple gestations (Rao, Sairam, & Shehata, 2004). A woman's large uterus may increase her susceptibility to supine hypotension syndrome, and aortocaval compression should be avoided.

RESPIRATORY

Respiratory changes with multiple gestation are similar to that in a singleton pregnancy but with greater tidal volumes and oxygen consumption and a more alkalotic arterial pH (Malone & D'Alton, 2004). Increased abdominal distention and loss of abdominal muscle tone may require women to use their accessory muscles during respiration, resulting in greater dyspnea and shortness of breath (Norwitz et al., 2005).

MUSCULOSKELETAL

The rapidly growing uterus of a multiple gestation magnifies typical pregnancy complaints of back and ligament pain, and women often experience symptoms much earlier in their pregnancy. Women may benefit from a pregnancy support garment, and many find that increased rest helps relieve back pain. Women also need instructions in good body mechanics, posture, and placement of supportive pillows while sleeping.

DERMATOLOGIC

Pruritic urticarial papules and plaques of pregnancy (PUPPP) occurs in 2.9% to 16% of multiple gestations (Brzoza, Kasperska-Zajac, Oleś, & Rogala, 2007). This dermatosis is thought to be related to abdominal distention and presents with redness and itching in the abdominal striae and urticarial papules on the lower abdomen. In severe cases, the papules merge into pruritic plaques, extend to the buttocks and thighs, and may be generalized. PUPPP usually responds to treatment with topical antipruritics, topical steroids, or oral antihistamines or steroids and then typically disappears within 2 weeks postpartum. Other causes of abdominal itching should be considered, including normal striae/stretching skin or pruritis secondary to intrahepatic cholestasis, which are both more likely in multiple gestation.

PERINATAL COMPLICATIONS

Despite their overall small numbers and incidence, multiple gestations represent a substantial proportion of poor perinatal outcomes. Compared to their counterparts with singleton gestations, women pregnant with multiples are more likely to experience more frequent and severe pregnancy complications and have infants that are smaller, born earlier, less likely to survive the first year of life, and more likely to suffer lifelong disability.

MATERNAL MORBIDITY AND MORTALITY

Studies have shown significant increases in adverse maternal outcomes in multiple compared with singleton gestations. Women having multiples are six times more likely to have a hospital stay during pregnancy and twice as likely to be admitted to intensive care as women with singletons (Luke & Brown, 2007). The combination of physiologic changes and perinatal pathologies that are unique or more likely in multiple gestations contribute to this increased risk. Increased adverse outcomes include anemia, cardiac morbidity, amniotic fluid embolus, preeclampsia, eclampsia, gestational diabetes, preterm labor (PTL), abruptio placentae, urinary tract infection, cesarean birth, postpartum hemorrhage, puerperal endometritis, prolonged hospital stay, need for obstetric intervention, hysterectomy, and blood transfusion (Conde-Agudelo, Belizan, & Lindmark, 2000; Wen, Demissie, Yang, & Walker, 2004; Walker, Murphy, Pan, Yang, & Wen, 2004). As compared to women with twins, women carrying HOMs are at even greater risk for pregnancy-related morbidities, including anemia, diabetes mellitus, gestational hypertension, eclampsia, abruptio placentae, preterm premature rupture of membranes (PPROM), and increased rate of cesarean birth (Wen et al., 2004). Dose–response relationships of several complications have also been shown with increasing plurality.

There are few studies on maternal deaths in multiple gestations, and national data are likely to be underreported. However, there is a substantially higher risk of maternal death in multiple gestations compared

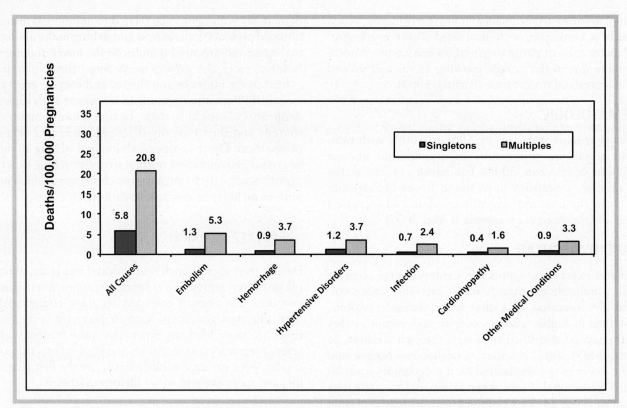

FIGURE 11–8. Maternal mortality in women with multiple gestations, 1979–2000. (Data from MacKay, A. P., Berg, C. J., King, J. C., Duran, C., & Chang, J. [2006]. Pregnancy-related mortality among women with multifetal pregnancies. *Obstetrics & Gynecology, 107*[3], 563–568.)

to singleton pregnancies (MacKay, Berg, King, Duran, & Chang, 2006). The causes of pregnancy-related deaths are similar to that in singleton pregnancies (embolism, hypertensive complications of pregnancy, hemorrhage, and infection), but the risk among women carrying twins and HOMs is 3.6 times higher (20.8/100,000 compared with 5.8/100,000). These increased mortality ratios are consistent with the rising rates of multiple births and the disproportionate share of adverse pregnancy outcomes associated with these pregnancies (see Fig. 11–8).

Preterm Labor

PTL is a significant and frequent complication for multiple gestations, occurring in 50% of twins, 76% of triplets, and 90% of quadruplets (Elliott, 2005b). Although the exact mechanisms are not understood, it is thought that stimuli, including stretch, placental corticotropin-releasing hormone, and lung maturity factors, may be stronger in multiple gestations due to higher fetal and placental mass (Stock & Norman, 2010). In women with twin pregnancies who have symptoms of PTL, approximately 22% to 29% will deliver within 7 days (Chauhan, Scardo, Hayes, Abu-hamad, & Berghella, 2010). Early detection of PTL and potential prevention of preterm birth in multiples may include educating women in signs and symptoms

of PTL, cervical assessment, and reduction of risk factors for PTL. Women should receive formal PTL education by 18 weeks' gestation (Lam & Gill, 2005a) with continual reinforcement at prenatal visits. A recent Cochrane review found no sound evidence to support a policy of routine hospitalization for bed rest in multiple pregnancy, including women with cervical change and signs of PTL (Crowther & Han, 2010). Although historically prescribed for women at risk for preterm labor and birth, evidence is lacking regarding efficacy, and some data suggest bed rest may be associated with potential harm (AAP & ACOG, 2012).

Although some clinicians recommend cessation of sexual activity for women with multiple gestations, particularly those with HOMs, data to support this in the absence of signs of PTL are lacking. One small report of 50 women with twin pregnancy found a decrease in coital frequency from early to late pregnancy. This was especially true in women who had used IVF to achieve pregnancy. There was no association between sexual activity and preterm delivery in the report (Stammler-Safar, Ott, Weber, & Krampl, 2010).

Multiple studies have confirmed that prophylactic beta-mimetic agents do not reduce the incidence of PTL and birth in twins (Dodd & Crowther, 2005). Although use of home uterine activity monitoring (HUAM), along with frequent nurse contact, has been shown to reduce preterm birth in twins, it is not known whether the monitor or the nurse contributes most to preterm birth reduction (Morrison & Chauhan, 2003), and HUAM is not routinely used.

Prophylactic cervical cerclage has not been found to prevent preterm birth of twins (Dodd & Crowther, 2005) nor has it been shown to improve pregnancy or neonatal outcomes in women with triplet pregnancies (Rebarber, Roman, Istwan, Rhea, & Stanziano, 2005). Although cerclage may be indicated for women with a history of cervical incompetence, the use of cerclage for women with second trimester cervical shortening in a triplet pregnancy has not been shown to affect gestational age at delivery or neonatal outcome (Moragianni, Aronis, & Craparo, 2011). The use of a cervical pessary for prevention of preterm birth in women with twins with cervical incompetence is currently being studied (Abdel-Aleem, Shaaban, & Abdel-Aleem, 2010).

Unlike the positive effects for at-risk singleton pregnancies, 17-alpha-hydroxyprogesterone caproate (17P) has not been shown to be effective for prevention of preterm birth in multiple gestations. Randomized controlled trials with 17P in twin and triplet pregnancies have not shown benefit in prolonging gestation or reducing neonatal morbidity (Combs, Garite, Maurel, Das, & Porto, 2010, 2011). Similarly, use of prophylactic vaginal micronized progesterone does not prevent preterm delivery in twin gestations (Rode, Klein, Nicolaides, Krampl-Bettelheim, & Tabor, 2011). The 2011 U. S. Food and Drug Administration (FDA) approval for injectable 17P in the treatment of PTL does not include multiple gestations.

Predicting PTL is difficult as most known risk factors for spontaneous preterm birth in singletons are not significantly associated with spontaneous preterm birth of twins (Goldenberg et al., 1996). In asymptomatic women with a multiple pregnancy, use of transvaginal assessment of cervical length (TVU-CL) in the second trimester is a strong predictor of preterm birth (Lim et al., 2011). For example, cervical length of ≤20 mm at 20 to 24 weeks' gestation appears to be a good predictor of spontaneous preterm birth of twins at <32 and <34 weeks' gestation (Conde-Agudelo, Romero, Hassan, & Yeo, 2010). Fetal fibronectin testing may also be an effective tool in preterm birth prediction for multiple pregnancies, especially in its negative predictive value, but studies are inconsistent (Goldenberg et al.; Gibson et al., 2004).

Cervical length also appears to be predictive of preterm birth risk in triplets. In one study, cervical length of <2.5 mm for triplets between 15 and 20 weeks' gestation had both a specificity and a positive predictive value of 100% for birth at <28 weeks' gestation (Guzman et al., 2000). Despite these findings, it is not known whether identification of a short cervix can help prevent a preterm birth of multiples. A Cochrane review concluded that there is insufficient evidence to recommend routine screening in asymptomatic and symptomatic women for the prevention of preterm birth in multiples (Berghella, Baxter, & Hendrix, 2009).

When cervical assessment is performed, TVU-CL has the advantages of objective measurement as well as visualization of the internal os and proximity of the presenting fetal part and membranes and is a better predictor of spontaneous preterm birth in twin pregnancies than in singleton pregnancies (Conde-Agudelo et al., 2010). Gordon, Robbins, McKenna, Howard, and Barth (2006) found that before 35 weeks' gestation, the preterm delivery rate of twins was significantly lower when the cervical length was measured by transvaginal ultrasound than digital examination alone.

There are several challenges in managing PTL with multiples. These include increased incidence of PTL at earlier gestations, greater tocolytic latency than in singletons, less maternal perception of uterine activity, higher risk of tocolytic-related complications, and failure of therapy resulting in multiple infants affected by potential morbidities and mortality of preterm birth (Lam & Gill, 2005b).

Treatment of PTL in multiples includes use of tocolytics and corticosteroid therapies. However, the application for multiples may be different from singletons. Twin gestations have been shown to have higher mean uterine contraction frequency than singletons throughout the latter half of pregnancy and between 4 pm and 4 am, but this did not predict preterm birth prior to 35 weeks' gestation (Newman et al., 2006). Multiple gestations have also been observed to have different uterine activity patterns, including a significant crescendo in uterine activity 24 hours before the development of clinical PTL, and a higher prevalence of low-amplitude, high-frequency (LAHF) contractions (Morrison & Chauhan, 2003). Lam and Gill (2005a) described a characteristic pattern of recurring PTL in twins in Display 11–1.

DISPLAY 11–1

Pattern of Recurring Preterm Labor in Twins

- Return of excessive levels of LAHF precursor uterine activity patterns
- Return of a circadian, nocturnal pattern of organized, high-amplitude uterine contractions
- Rapidly increasing need for increased frequency and dosage of terbutaline
- Acceleration of frequency of uterine contractions 48–72 hours before the episode of active recurrent preterm labor

LAHF, low-amplitude, high-frequency.
Lam, F., & Gill, P. (2005a). β-Agonist tocolytic therapy. *Obstetrics and Gynecology Clinics, 32*(3), 457–484.

In February 2011, the FDA issued a warning that oral terbutaline should not be used for prevention or any treatment of PTL and further warns that injectable terbutaline should not be used in pregnant women for prevention or prolonged treatment (beyond 48 to 72 hours) of PTL in either the hospital or outpatient setting because of the potential for serious maternal heart problems and death (FDA, 2011).

There is good evidence that magnesium sulfate given before anticipated early preterm birth reduces the risk of cerebral palsy (CP) in surviving infants (ACOG & Society for Maternal-Fetal Medicine, 2010). Women receiving magnesium sulfate should be assessed for signs of neurologic depression by evaluating deep tendon reflexes hourly, monitoring bowel sounds and function, and frequently reviewing the status of each fetal heartbeat. Emergency resuscitation equipment should be easily accessible, and calcium gluconate (10 mL in 10% solution) for magnesium toxicity reversal should be in an easily accessible locked medication cabinet (Lam & Gill, 2005b). Other tocolytic agents include prostaglandin synthetase inhibitors, such as indomethacin, and calcium channel blockers, such as nifedipine. Side effects of indomethacin include increased fetal pulmonary vasculature and ductal constriction and should not be used after 32 weeks' gestation or for treatment >72 hours (Lam & Gill, 2005b). Another side effect of indomethacin is decreased fetal renal function, which can lead to oligohydramnios; thus, twin-to-twin transfusion syndrome (TTTS) is a contraindication for this therapy.

The greatest complication of tocolytic therapy for women with multiple gestation is the high risk for pulmonary edema, particularly if complicated by fluid overload or underlying infection. Maximum fluid administration should not exceed 2,000 mL per 24 hours, and a strict intake and output must be maintained (Lam & Gill, 2005a). Nursing assessments should include signs and symptoms of pulmonary edema by observation (shortness of breath, coughing, or wheezing) and auscultation; daily weights; and metabolic evaluations including blood glucose, complete blood count (CBC), and electrolyte status (Lam & Gill, 2005b).

A single course of corticosteroids for pregnant women between 24 and 34 weeks' gestation who are at risk of preterm delivery within 7 days is recommended by ACOG, including those with premature rupture of membranes before 32 weeks' gestation (ACOG, 2011a). However, the efficacy of steroids is uncertain for multiple gestation, and dosing requirements have not been evaluated. Although concentrations of betamethasone in maternal serum and fetal cord blood were found to be similar in twins and singletons (Gyamfi et al., 2010), steroid administration did not result in a statistically significant reduction in the rate of respiratory distress syndrome (RDS) in twins (Roberts & Dalziel, 2006). Use of repeated corticosteroid dosing is not recommended

(ACOG, 2011a). A single rescue course may be considered if the earlier treatment was given at least 2 weeks prior, the gestational age is less than 32 6/7 weeks, and delivery is anticipated within 1 week (ACOG, 2011a). Increases in uterine contractions following corticosteroid administration have been observed in HOM pregnancies (Elliott & Radin, 1995).

Hypertension

Pregnancy-related hypertensive disease has a dose–response relationship with plurality. National data from 1995 to 2000 showed that pregnancy-associated hypertensive conditions occur in 3.75% of singleton, 8.13% of twin, and 11.1% of triplet pregnancies (Luke & Brown, 2007). Compared to singletons, rates for twins were more than doubled and were nearly three times higher for triplets, and all increased with maternal age.

Preeclampsia tends to develop earlier in a multiple pregnancy and become more severe than in singleton gestations. It is thought that fetal number and placental mass are somehow involved in the pathogenesis of preeclampsia (Gyamfi, Stone, & Eddleman, 2005). Symptoms of severe preeclampsia with laboratory changes may indicate hemolysis, elevated liver enzymes, and low platelet count (HELLP) syndrome. In HOM pregnancies, the signs and symptoms of hypertensive disorders may be atypical, without the classic elevations of blood pressure or proteinuria. In a review of triplet and quadruplet pregnancies, of 16 women delivered for preeclampsia, only 8 had elevated blood pressure, whereas 10 had epigastric pain, visual disturbances, and/or headache; 9 had elevated liver enzymes; and 7 had low platelet counts (Hardardottir et al., 1996). Careful assessment of maternal signs and symptoms, in addition to laboratory evaluations, are important in the diagnosis and early treatment of hypertensive disease. Nurses should also be alert to the often subtle signs of HELLP syndrome (Bowers & Gromada, 2006). When magnesium sulfate is used, fluid balance should be carefully monitored because of the increased risk of pulmonary edema.

Premature Rupture of Membranes

The incidence of premature rupture of membranes (PROM) is increased in multiple gestations, with rates of 6% in twins and 9.61% in triplets compared to 2.68% in singletons (Luke & Brown, 2007). PROM in multiples also has a shorter latency to birth than singletons (Norwitz et al., 2005). Although membrane rupture usually occurs in the presenting sac, rupture of a nonpresenting sac may occur, especially after invasive procedures such as amniocentesis (Norwitz et al., 2005). It is difficult to assess for PROM in a nonpresenting sac, and intermittent leakage of fluid is the typical clinical presentation. Rupture of the separating membrane in a twin gestation is a unique complication in MC/DA twins, creating an MA twin risk scenario. Clinical management of PROM in multiples is similar to that in singletons, with expectant management including antibiotics and delivery for signs and symptoms of chorioamnionitis at 32 to 36 weeks' gestation (Gyamfi et al., 2005).

Gestational Diabetes

The increased placental mass with multiple fetuses and subsequent increase in diabetogenic hormones are thought to influence the incidence of gestational diabetes mellitus (GDM) in multiple gestations (Ben-Haroush, Yogev, & Hod, 2003). Like other maternal complications, gestational diabetes appears to have a dose–response relationship with increasing plurality. A population-based study by Walker and colleagues (2004) found a statistically significant relative risk of 1.12 for twins compared with singletons. The study reported an adjusted odds ratio of 1.56 for GDM in triplets compared to twins and 1.81 in quadruplets compared to twins. In another study, the risk for developing GDM in twin pregnancies was double the risk in singletons, with the highest risk in younger women aged 25 to 30 years and African American women (Rauh-Hain et al., 2009). Diagnosis and management of GDM are similar to that in singleton pregnancies (Norwitz et al., 2005).

Intrahepatic Cholestasis

The incidence of intrahepatic cholestasis in women with a multiple pregnancy is two to five times that of singletons (Rao et al., 2004; Glantz, Marschall, & Mattsson, 2004). The increased risks of preterm birth and fetal death with this condition warrant careful investigation into pruritus without a rash that occurs in the late second and early third trimesters (Nichols, 2005).

Acute Fatty Liver

In a multicenter review of 16 cases of acute fatty liver of pregnancy (AFPL), 18% were multiple gestations, including one triplet pregnancy (Fesenmeier, Coppage, Lambers, Barton, & Sibai, 2005). Nausea and vomiting in the third trimester were the most common symptoms (75%). Although AFPL is very rare, the high associated morbidity and mortality call for careful surveillance. Women with nausea, vomiting, or epigastric pain in the third trimester should be carefully assessed.

Peripartum Cardiomyopathy

Approximately 13% of cases of peripartum cardiomyopathy (PPCM) are twins, and several risk factors for this condition are more likely in multiple gestations, including maternal age >30 years and pregnancy-related hypertension (Elkayam et al., 2005). Women with multiple pregnancy who have dyspnea, orthopnea, persistent weight retention or weight gain, peripheral edema, nocturnal cough, and profound fatigue, especially postpartum, should be carefully assessed for this life-threatening condition (Murali & Baldisseri, 2005). Maternal mortality with PPCM was 9% in one study, and 4% required heart transplantation (Elkayam et al., 2005).

Antepartum Hemorrhage

Placenta previa does not appear to occur more frequently in multiple gestations; however, placental abruption is significantly more common. Salihu, Bekan, and colleagues (2005) found a rate of abruption of 6.2/1,000 in singleton pregnancies and 12.2/1,000 and 15.6/1,000 in twin and triplet gestations, respectively, indicating a dose–response relationship. However, there was an inverse relationship with perinatal mortality and plurality; as the number of fetuses increased from one to three, the risk of placental abruption rose, whereas the risk of abruption-related perinatal mortality declined. Odds ratios for perinatal mortality were 14.3 among singletons, 4.4 for twins, and 3.0 for triplets. The authors suggested this is partly explained by the different circumstances in which abruption is diagnosed in singleton as opposed to multiple gestations, such as more frequent cesarean birth of multiples.

Pulmonary Embolism

Multiple pregnancy is a risk factor for venous thromboembolism, which may lead to pulmonary embolism (Bates et al., 2012). The mechanical obstruction of the enlarged uterus contributes to venous stasis, particularly for women on bed rest. Thromboembolism is associated with cesarean birth, operative vaginal birth, birth before 36 weeks' gestation, hypertension, a BMI of ≥25, and maternal age of ≥35 years (ACOG, 2004a, 2011c), all of which are more common in multiple gestations. Therapeutic levels of anticoagulation may be more difficult to achieve with multiple gestations because of the larger volume of distribution.

FETAL MORBIDITY AND MORTALITY

Zygosity, chorionicity, and fetal growth are important predictors of fetal health and survival in multiples. The inherent physiology associated with the twinning process, along with sharing of uterine space and placental resources, increases the risks for fetal morbidity. Perinatal morbidity and mortality rates for MZ twins are estimated to be 3 to 10 times higher than those for DZ twins (Trevett & Johnson, 2005). Fetal mortality also increases with plurality and late gestational age.

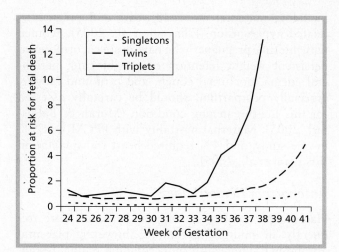

FIGURE 11–9. Prospective risk of fetal mortality by plurality and gestational age. (Data from Kahn, B., Lumey, L. H., Zybert, P. A., Lorenz, J. M., Cleary-Goldman, J., D'Alton, M. E., & Robinson, J. N. [2003]. Prospective risk of fetal death in singleton, twin, and triplet gestations: Implications for practice. *Obstetrics and Gynecology, 102*[4], 685–692.)

Compared to singletons, the risk for delivery before 29 weeks' gestation is 8 times greater for twins and 34 times greater for triplets; the risk for infant mortality is 4 times and 13 times greater for twins and triplets, respectively (Luke & Brown, 2007). Analysis of linked birth and death U.S. population data found that the prospective risk (a proportion of all fetuses still at risk at a given gestational age) of fetal death for singletons, twins, and triplets at 24 weeks' gestation was 0.28/1,000, 0.92/1,000, and 1.30/1,000, respectively (Kahn et al., 2003). In comparison, the corresponding risk was 0.57/1,000 for singletons and 3.09/1,000 for twins at 40 weeks' gestation and 13.18/1,000 for triplets at ≥38 weeks (see Fig. 11–9). Because of the increased risks for fetal death at late gestational ages, some clinicians are electing to deliver multiples at earlier gestations.

Intrauterine Growth Restriction

Overall, the incidence of IUGR is greater in multiple birth infants than in singletons and is likely due to placental insufficiency and competition for nutrients. In one study, nearly half of the women with twin pregnancies had one twin with a birth weight <10th percentile, and 27% had one twin with a birth weight <5th percentile (Fox, Rebarber, Klauser, Roman, & Saltzman, 2011). Interestingly, the IUGR was not significantly associated with any commonly linked maternal risk factors. Studies indicate that slowed or compromised fetal growth in both twins at 20 to 28 weeks' gestation and from 28 weeks to birth is highly associated with very preterm birth (30 to 32 weeks; Hediger et al., 2006). Twins and singletons have similar fetal growth rates until about 32 weeks, triplets

until 29 to 30 weeks, and quadruplets until approximately 27 weeks' gestation (Garite, Clark, Elliott, & Thorp, 2004). Fetal growth and subsequent birth weight are also influenced by zygosity and chorionicity. Birth weights are highest in DZ twins with DC placentas, slightly less in MZ twins with DC placentas, and lowest in MZ twins with an MC placenta (Derom, Derom, & Vlietinck, 1995). IUGR in multiples is associated with increased fetal mortality rates at all gestational ages (Garite et al., 2004). There is disagreement on the use of singleton growth curves or twin-specific growth curves for establishing normal twin growth (Morin & Lim, 2011).

A sizable proportion of multiples have discordant growth, in which the weight of one multiple differs significantly from that of the other(s), usually ≥20% to 25%. Discordancy is more common in MC twins and is characteristic of TTTS. Maternal age, parity, sex discordance, and gestational age may affect the amount of birth weight discordance (Wen et al., 2004). A review of 59,034 Canadian twin births found that 53% had 0% to 9% birth weight difference, 30% had 10% to 19% discordance, 11% had 20% to 29% discordance, and 6% had 30% discordance (Wen et al., 2005). In HOMs, two or more fetuses may be concordant but have discordant co-multiple(s).

Congenital Anomalies

Multiples are more likely to have structural congenital defects as well as chromosomal and genetic anomalies. The most common are cardiovascular, central nervous system, ophthalmic, and gastrointestinal. The overall rate of anomalies in twins is estimated at 1.3 times that of singletons but is three to five times higher in MZ twins (Weber & Sebire, 2010). The rate of anomalies in DZ twins is similar to that in singletons, and the likelihood is small for both co-twins to be affected. Anomalies in MZ twins often result from the twinning process itself or aberrant vascular or placental physiology complications, and the two fetuses may be unequally affected.

Certain abnormalities are unique to multiple gestations. Conjoined twins occur at a rate of 1/50,000 pregnancies (Weber & Sebire, 2010) and are three times more common in female fetuses than in male fetuses (Graham & Gaddipati, 2005). Survival of conjoined twins is usually dependent on the extent of shared organs. Acardiac malformations (defects in which one multiple has no defined cardiac structure and survives using the co-multiple's cardiac pump mechanism) occur exclusively in MZ multiples at a rate of 1/35,000 pregnancies or 1% of MC twins (Weber & Sebire, 2010). This condition is also referred to as twin reversed arterial perfusion (TRAP) sequence because of the reversal of circulation in the acardiac fetus. The acardiac twin of a MZ pair has 100% mortality.

Abnormal Vascular/Placental Changes

TTTS is a condition unique to multiples and develops in about 10% to 20% of MZ pregnancies; the condition is severe in nearly 18% of cases (Habli, Lim, & Crombleholme, 2009). It occurs when there is unequal shunting of blood from donor fetus to the co-twin recipient through vascular connections in a shared (MC) placenta. DC TTTS has also been reported (Malone & D'Alton, 2004). Feto-fetal transfusion can also occur in HOMs with shared placental beds. Vascular anastomoses may be arteriovenous, venovenous, or arterial–arterial and may be balanced or unbalanced (Jackson & Mele, 2009; Habli et al., 2009).

Fetal compromise occurs when there is significant single-direction vascular flow. The recipient twin becomes hypervolemic and polycythemic, progressing to polyhydramnios, congestive heart failure, and death. The donor twin becomes hypovolemic, anemic, and growth restricted. The pathophysiology of TTTS appears to be more complex than just volume shifts between twins. There is evidence that the hypertensive mediators renin and angiotensin also play an important role in TTTS (Harkness & Crombleholme, 2005). The most severe form of TTTS is the stuck twin, when the donor twin is depleted of amniotic fluid. If left untreated, the mortality rate for TTTS is 80% or more, especially when it presents earlier than 28 weeks' gestation (Habli et al., 2009). Up to 30% of survivors have associated neurodevelopmental anomalies (Habli et al., 2009).

Diagnosis of TTTS may include the following sonographic findings: (1) monochorionicity, (2) discrepancy in amniotic fluid between the amniotic sacs with polyhydramnios in one sac (largest vertical pocket >8 cm) and oligohydramnios in the other sac (largest vertical pocket <2 cm), (3) discrepancy in umbilical cord size, (4) presence of cardiac dysfunction in the polyhydramniotic twin, (5) abnormal umbilical artery or ductus venosus Doppler velocimetry, and (6) significant growth discordance (often >20%; Habli et al., 2009). At least four staging systems are currently used to describe cases and vary according to the assessment techniques, such as ultrasound for Doppler waveform changes with disease progression and fetal echocardiographic findings.

The most common treatments for TTTS are serial amnioreduction and selective fetoscopic laser photocoagulation (SFLP). Other interventions, such as intertwin amniotic membrane septostomy and umbilical cord coagulation, have fallen out of favor due to ineffectiveness or risk. Serial amnioreduction is a simple outpatient procedure, easily performed by a trained obstetrician. The procedure involves removal of large amounts of amniotic fluid, often more than 1 to 2 L, on a recurring basis. In addition to the paradoxical effect of fluid increasing in the oligohydramniotic sac, side benefits of this therapy include prevention of PTL related to polyhydramnios, improved fetal hemodynamics, and uteroplacental blood flow (Harkness & Crombleholme, 2005). Yet the procedure is not without problems. Survivors have poorer long-term neurodevelopmental outcomes compared to those treated with SFLP (van Klink, Koopman, Oepkes, Walther, & Lopriore, 2011).

Once considered experimental, SFLP is now a widely accepted treatment for TTTS (Jackson & Mele, 2009). This procedure uses fetoscopy to visualize and laser to coagulate the vascular anastomoses at the intertwin membrane that are contributing to the syndrome. A Cochrane review determined that SFLP should be considered in the treatment of all stages of TTTS to improve perinatal and neonatal outcome, but it is unclear whether SFLP increases or reduces the risk of neurodevelopmental delay or intellectual impairment in childhood compared to other therapies (Roberts, Gates, Kilby, & Neilson, 2008). Some have suggested a sequential approach, with amnioreduction used initially, followed by SFLP with onset of echocardiographic progression (Habli et al., 2009). Patient education is critical to meet complex learning needs regarding the syndrome, treatment options, and outcome expectations and to assist the family to make informed decisions regarding care (Jackson & Mele, 2009).

Abnormal umbilical cord insertion is a common finding in multiple gestations, especially in those with MC placentas. Marginal insertions are twice as likely and velamentous insertions (directly into the membranes) are five times more likely in twin pregnancies compared with singleton pregnancies; a noncentral insertion site is twice as common in MC (31.5%) as DC (17.1%) placentas (Kent et al., 2011). Velamentous insertion is estimated to occur in 25% of triplet pregnancies and represents a 25- to 50-fold increase compared to singleton gestations (Feldman et al., 2002). Abnormal cord insertions contribute to poor uteroplacental perfusion, and an 80% higher risk of ≥20% birth weight discordance has been shown for twins with a noncentral cord insertion (Kent et al., 2011).

Fetal Loss

Spontaneous loss of gestational sacs or embryos after documentation of fetal heart rate (FHR) in a multiple pregnancy is termed the "vanishing twin" and is estimated to occur in 30% of pregnancies (van Oppenraaij et al., 2009). Exact rates are not known, and there may be no visual or pathologic evidence at delivery. In known cases, preterm birth, LBW, and small for gestational age (SGA) appear to be associated with the remaining fetuses, particularly when losses occur after 8 weeks' gestation (van Oppenraaij et al., 2009).

Later intrauterine death of one fetus in a set of multiples poses both physiologic and psychologic risks. Fetal death at 20 weeks or later occurs in 2.6% of twin and 4.3% of triplet gestations (Johnson & Zhang, 2002). The surviving twin is at increased risk of fetal death, neonatal death, and severe long-term morbidity. Risks for MC and DC twin deaths following a co-twin demise are, respectively, death, 12% and 4%; neurological abnormality, 18% and 1%; preterm delivery, 68% and 57%; and the risk of neurologic abnormality (including CP) is four times higher for MC compared to DC pregnancies (Ong, Zamora, Khan, & Kilby, 2006).

Although MA twins are rare (1% of MZ twins), these fetuses have an extremely high risk of death during pregnancy and at birth, primarily due to cord entanglement and knotting. Historically, perinatal mortality rates for MA twins have ranged from 40% to 70%, but more recent reports have found fetal mortality rates of 10% to 20% with intensive surveillance (Hack et al., 2009).

Management of single fetal death depends on multiple factors, including chorionicity, gestational age, and condition of the surviving fetus(es) and may include monitoring of the remaining fetuses for evidence of hemodynamic instability and of the mother for coagulopathy, PTL, and preeclampsia (Hillman, Morris, & Kilby, 2010). Fetal magnetic resonance imaging may provide information about brain abnormalities in the MZ co-twin survivor (Cleary-Goldman et al., 2007).

ANTEPARTUM MANAGEMENT

Antepartum management of multiple pregnancy should be a collaborative effort of the members of the perinatal healthcare team, including perinatologists, obstetricians, nurse midwives, registered nurses, advanced practice nurses, perinatal educators, ultrasonographers, social workers, and dietitians.

PRENATAL DIAGNOSIS AND GENETIC TESTING

As with all women, prenatal diagnostic screening should be offered to women with a multiple gestation. However, the assessment and calculations are more complex. The maternal age–related risk for aneuploidy is approximately the same for MZ twins as for singletons (Rustico, Baietti, Coviello, Orlandi, & Nicolini, 2005). However, for DZ twins, the risk of aneuploidy in one of the twins is double that of singletons because the independent risk for each twin is additive. The risk of aneuploidy occurring in both DZ twins is the singleton risk squared (Bush & Malone, 2005). In practical terms, a 33-year-old woman with twins has the same risk of Down syndrome as a 35-year-old woman with a singleton (ACOG, 2004a). In a 28-year-old woman with triplets, the risk of at least one fetus having

Down syndrome is similar to the risk of a 35-year-old with a singleton (Malone & D'Alton, 2004). Referral to a genetic counselor is also recommended for women of advanced maternal age who are pregnant with multiples (Cleary-Goldman et al., 2007).

First trimester NT screening for aneuploidy is highly sensitive in multiple pregnancies (Sepulveda, Wong, & Casasbuenas, 2009).The addition of nasal bone assessment has been shown to lower the false-positive rate of NT screening in triplet pregnancies (Krantz, Hallahan, He, Sherwin, & Evans, 2011). For these tests, each fetus is individually assessed and the pregnancy risk is calculated.

Second-trimester maternal serum screening in twin gestations is associated with a high false-positive rate, particularly in ART pregnancies (Maymon, Neeman, Shulman, Rosen, & Herman, 2005), as an unaffected co-twin may mask the abnormal maternal serum levels associated with an aneuploid fetus. Even if screening suggests the presence of an affected fetus, biochemical markers cannot specify which twin is abnormal (Bush & Malone, 2005). Because ultrasound is needed to confirm which fetus is affected following a positive result, many centers are not routinely offering serum screening for multiples (Cleary-Goldman, D'Alton, & Berkowitz, 2005). Regardless of other screening tests, a targeted ultrasound examination for fetal anomaly detection is suggested for all multiples between 18 and 20 weeks' gestation (Dodd & Crowther, 2005).

Invasive prenatal diagnostic techniques may be indicated when prenatal screening tests identify increased risks for genetic or chromosomal abnormalities. Genetic amniocentesis between 15 and 20 weeks' gestation has been found to be accurate in twin gestations. Use of a marker dye, such as indigo carmine, helps prevent cross-contamination of fluids when tapping multiple sacs. There appears to be an increased procedure-related loss rate compared to that in singletons (Chauhan et al., 2010).

CVS appears to be safe in multiple gestations, although there are technical difficulties in accessing multiple fetuses, a higher risk of uncertain results compared to singletons, and risks for sample cross-contamination (Cleary-Goldman et al., 2005).

Prenatal diagnosis presents unique challenges for parents, especially if one fetus is abnormal, as they may face the dilemma of selective reduction. Parents may also worry about the status of the unaffected twin throughout pregnancy, highlighting a potential need for regular prenatal and postnatal examination and ongoing reassurance, or invasive prenatal testing in the surviving fetuses after reduction (Bryan, 2005).

PRENATAL CARE

The *Guidelines for Perinatal Care* (AAP & ACOG, 2012) recommend referral of twin gestations to a board-certified obstetrician and consultation with a maternal–fetal specialist if necessary. These specialists typically coordinate care with the primary obstetrician or may provide primary obstetrical care. Although most clinicians increase the number of antenatal care visits for women with multiple pregnancy, there is no consensus as to the frequency of visits that constitutes optimal care (Dodd & Crowther, 2005). However, in light of the higher risks for perinatal complications in these pregnancies, regular and frequent antenatal visits increase the likelihood for early detection and treatment.

Specialized multiple birth clinics (twin clinics) have reported improved perinatal morbidity and neonatal outcomes (Knox & Martin, 2010; Luke, Brown et al., 2003; Ruiz, Brown, Peters, & Johnston, 2001); however, there have been no randomized controlled trials to show that this intervention is superior to standard antenatal care (Dodd & Crowther, 2007). Interventions in such clinics include consistent care providers, intensive education about prevention of preterm birth, individualized modification of maternal activity, increased attention to nutrition, ultrasonography, tracking of clinic nonattendees, and a supportive clinical environment. Cited benefits include improved maternal education; increased maternal weight gain and birth weights; longer gestations; lowered rates of very low birth weight (VLBW), neonatal intensive care unit (NICU) admissions, and perinatal mortality; shortened hospital stays; and lower hospital charges.

Management of HOM gestations involves more intensive surveillance, attention, and interventions. Although there is no consensus as to content or frequency of prenatal care for these high-risk pregnancies, some suggested strategies for prenatal management of HOMs are listed in Table 11–1.

PRENATAL EDUCATION

Parents expecting multiples have unique perinatal educational needs. The high-risk nature and extraordinary aspects of their pregnancy, along with the unknowns of parenting multiple infants, present a need for specialized education (Bryan, 2002). As the goal of patient education for women with high-risk pregnancies is to assist them in the improvement of their own health (Freda, 2000), providing education about their condition and healthcare options allows women expecting multiples to make informed decisions concerning treatment. The increasing number of multiple gestations makes providing specialized multiple birth classes both feasible and practical. Such classes offer detailed information about the differences in multiple pregnancy and birth, educate about potential complications, enhance coping skills, teach parenting skills, and provide an immediate support system for expectant families with other parents of multiples (Bowers & Gromada, 2006). Multiple birth class

Table 11–1. SUGGESTED COMPONENTS OF ROUTINE ANTEPARTUM CARE OF TWINS	
Conception to 12 wk	Early diagnosis Confirm viability Determine placentation Patient education
12–20 wk	Identify anomalies Prenatal diagnostic testing Cervical length and integrity Nutritional counseling
20–26 wk	Cervical length and score Fetal fibronectin Activity modification as needed BMI-specific weight gain Serial ultrasound assessment
26–32 wk	Preterm birth prevention efforts Serial ultrasound assessment Screening for GDM BMI-specific weight gain
32–38 wk	Preeclampsia surveillance Weekly fetal testing Serial ultrasound assessment Determine fetal positions Determine optimal birth time

BMI, body mass index; GDM, gestational diabetes mellitus. Newman, R. B. (2005). Routine antepartum care of twins. In I. Blickstein & L. G. Keith (Eds.), *Multiple Pregnancy: Epidemiology, Gestation and Perinatal Outcome* (2nd ed., pp. 405–419). New York: Taylor and Francis.

topics include physical and emotional changes; variations in labor, birth, and postpartum care; and detailed education about nutrition. Common pregnancy complications, especially PTL, should also be included, with a focus on preventive measures and monitoring actions (Montgomery et al., 2005). Parents will need advice in practical skills for coping with more than one newborn, breastfeeding multiples, and choosing appropriate layette and infant equipment (Bowers & Gromada, 2006). A hospital tour should include the NICU, optimally allowing couples to meet neonatologists and nurses and see premature infants in intensive care (Bryan, 2002). Because so many women with multiples are at risk for complications and potential bed rest, they should attend classes in their early second trimester, by 24 weeks' gestation (Leonard & Denton, 2006). Options include a mini-class to supplement standard childbirth classes, offering tips and practical advice on handling multiple newborns, or a complete multiples-specific prenatal education curriculum.

NUTRITION AND WEIGHT GAIN

Luke (2005) described a multiple pregnancy as "a state of magnified nutritional requirements, resulting in a greater nutrient drain on maternal resources and an accelerated depletion of nutritional reserves" (p. 348). Evidence is growing that optimal maternal nutrition and weight gain are linked with positive perinatal outcomes for multiples, including reduced incidence of LBW and VLBW infants (Roem, 2003). The shortened length of gestation for most multiples limits the time for intrauterine growth, and the more rapid aging of multiple birth placentas shortens the period for effective transfer of nutrients to the developing fetuses. Thus, higher weight gains during early gestation may influence the structural and functional development of the placenta and subsequently augment fetal growth through more effective placental function as well as the transfer of a higher level of nutrients (Luke, 2005). Goodnight and Newman (2009) have described four objectives for maternal nutrition in multiple gestations: (1) optimizing fetal growth and development, (2) reducing incidence of obstetric complications, (3) increasing gestational age at delivery, and (4) avoiding excess maternal weight gain that may result in unnecessary weight retention postdelivery.

Women with multiple gestation require additional calories, micronutrient supplementation, and a higher gestational weight gain than women with singletons (Brown & Carlson, 2000; Luke, 2005; Roem, 2003; Rosello-Soberon, Fuentes-Chaparro, & Casanueva, 2005). Energy expenditures are increased in women carrying multiples as evidenced by significantly higher resting basal metabolic rates in twin pregnancies compared to singletons (1,636 ± 174 kcal/day and 1,456 ± 158 kcal/day, respectively; Shinagawa et al., 2005). The increased body mass in maternal breasts, uterus, body fat, and muscle, along with greater blood volume, can result in a 40% increase in caloric requirements for twin pregnancies (Goodnight & Newman, 2009). Official dietary standards for nutrient and energy intake for multiple gestations have not been established, but guidelines for caloric intake for twin pregnancy have been proposed. The following recommended daily caloric intakes are based on a woman's prepregnant BMI: underweight, 4,000 kcal; normal BMI, 3,000 to 3,500 kcal; overweight, 3,250 kcal; obese, 2,700 to 3,000 kcal (Goodnight & Newman, 2009). One nutritional intervention program for twin and triplet pregnancies recommends a diet with 20% of calories from protein, 40% of calories from carbohydrates, and 40% of calories from fat to provide additional calories with less bulk (Luke, 2004). This diet emphasizes low glycemic index carbohydrates to prevent wide fluctuations in blood glucose concentrations. Compared to singleton pregnancies, multiple gestations have a faster depletion of glycogen stores and increased metabolism of fat between meals and overnight (Luke, 2005). Women should be counseled to eat frequent, small meals, similar to a diabetic diet; this may also aid digestion as the rapidly growing uterus crowds the stomach.

Studies have shown that pregravid maternal weight, weight gain patterns, and total amounts of gain in multiple pregnancy are linked to fetal weight gain, length of gestation, and eventual infant birth weights (Luke et al., 2003; Brown & Carlson, 2000; Luke, 2005; Rosello-Soberon et al., 2005). Maternal nutrient stores deposited in early pregnancy are utilized in late pregnancy for placental growth. This is demonstrated in studies showing that poor early maternal weight gain is associated with inadequate intrauterine growth and increased perinatal morbidity in twins (Rosello-Soberon et al., 2005). Early maternal weight gain in multiple gestations appears to have a stronger effect on infant birth weights than do mid- and late-pregnancy gains (Luke, 2004).

In 2009, the Institute of Medicine (IOM) established provisional guidelines for weight gain in twin pregnancy based on maternal pregravid BMI status (IOM, 2009). Women with a normal BMI should aim to gain 37 to 54 lb; overweight women, 31 to 50 lb; and obese women, 25 to 42 lb. No recommendations were made for underweight women with twins, but higher gains are prudent for these women. One study of nearly 300 women with twin pregnancies and normal starting BMIs found that pregnancy weight gain consistent with the IOM guidelines was significantly associated with improved outcomes, including a decreased risk of prematurity and higher birth weights (Fox et al., 2010). In a subsequent report, the researchers examined a cohort of women with twin pregnancies and normal starting BMIs who delivered at ≥37 weeks' gestation. Those who gained more than 54 lb had significantly larger newborns and a decreased rate of LBW compared to women with normal or poor weight gain. Despite their weight gain exceeding the IOM recommendations, these women did not have a higher incidence of gestational diabetes, gestational hypertension, or preeclampsia (Fox, Saltzman, Kurtz, & Rebarber, 2011).

Few studies have examined weight gain and nutritional recommendations for HOM pregnancies. A 50-lb total weight gain for triplet pregnancy, approximately 1.5 lb/week, has been suggested (Brown & Carlson, 2000). Available data indicate that the associations of maternal weight gain with fetal growth and infant birth weights are even more important for these pregnancies, as early pregnancy weight gain and higher total gain in underweight women with HOMs appear to have an even greater effect on outcomes (Luke, 2005). Eddib and colleagues (2007) found that for triplets, higher maternal weight gain is associated with better neonatal outcomes, without an increase in adverse pregnancy outcomes, compared to singleton gestations. As with all pregnant women, high prepregnancy BMI increases risk for many maternal complications, including diabetes and hypertension. Nutrition

DISPLAY 11–2

Nutrition and Weight Gain in Multiple Gestation[a, b]

Optimal maternal nutrition and weight gain are linked with positive perinatal outcomes for multiples.

Women pregnant with multiples need:

- Increased caloric intake
- Daily micronutrient supplementation (Goodnight & Newman, 2009)
  - 15 mg zinc (increased to 30 mg in second and third trimesters)
  - 1 multivitamin with 30 mg iron
  - 1,500 mg calcium (increased to 2,500 mg in second and third trimesters)
  - 2 mg vitamin B_6
  - 1 mg folic acid
  - 500–1,000 mg vitamin C
  - (1,000 IU) vitamin D
  - 300–500 mg DHA/EPA
  - 400 mg magnesium (increased to 800 mg in second and third trimesters)
  - Nutrition education, counseling, referral to services for basic food supplements

Weight gain counseling in multiple gestation includes:

- Higher weight gains than for singleton pregnancies
- Early (first-trimester) weight gain to build maternal stores for later placental growth
- Assessment of pregravid weight status and adjustment of weight gain goals

Provisional weight gain recommendations for twin pregnancy (IOM, 2009):

- Normal (BMI 18.5–24.9): 37–54 lb
- Overweight (BMI 25.0–29.9): 31–50 lb
- Obese (BMI >30.0): 25–42 lb.

[a]Goodnight & Newman, 2009
[b]IOM, 2009

---

and weight gain recommendations for multiple gestation are listed in Display 11–2.

Bed rest appears to have a negative effect on maternal weight gain; women lost or did not gain weight while on antepartum bed rest in three studies (Maloni, 2010). However, in one of the studies, twins and triplets had birth weights appropriate for gestational age despite maternal weight loss. It is unknown whether nutritional interventions are effective in countering weight loss for women on bed rest, either at home or in the hospital, and additional studies are needed.

Nutrition counseling and weight gain advice is a simple, low-cost, and effective intervention for improving perinatal outcome in multiple gestations (Brown & Carlson, 2000). Surveys showed that more than one fourth of pregnant women, including those with twins, received no advice regarding weight gain, and among women who did receive guidance, more than one third received inappropriate advice (Luke, 2004). A consult with a registered dietitian specializing in perinatal nutrition is helpful for all expectant mothers of multiples, especially for those who are underweight for height, vegetarian (particularly vegans, who consume no animal proteins), and pregnant with HOMs (Goodnight & Newman, 2009; Bowers & Gromada, 2006).

FETAL SURVEILLANCE

Due to the increased incidence of fetal morbidity and mortality in multiples, assessment of fetal well-being is often incorporated into routine antenatal care. However, there is no clear consensus on the timing or frequency of antenatal testing for multiple gestations. There is possible benefit for serial antenatal surveillance for abnormal growth, abnormal amniotic fluid volumes, fetal anomaly, single surviving twin, MA twins, TTTS, and other medical/obstetric complications (Devoe, 2008; Cleary-Goldman et al., 2007). Doppler velocimetry is useful in the diagnosis and assessment of growth discordancy and has been associated with improved perinatal outcomes (Dodd & Crowther, 2005). A suggested plan for antenatal surveillance is listed in Display 11–3. Fetal movement counting may be a useful adjunct with other antepartum fetal surveillance (AAP & ACOG, 2012). Emphasis should be placed on a woman's perception of a decrease in fetal activity relative to previous levels rather than on a precise number of movements. However, some women may have difficulty differentiating movement among fetuses.

For all surveillance techniques, fetal positions should be consistently documented using a uterine mapping system. This allows comparisons with prior assessments and accurate clinical reporting. The presenting fetus is always "A," and remaining fetuses ("B," "C," etc.) are identified by relative ascending positions (Bowers & Gromada, 2006). Notations should also be made of fetal position changes, such as when female fetus B moves to C position, and when male fetus C moves to B position.

INTRAPARTUM MANAGEMENT

The high risks of twin and HOM pregnancies require a hospital-based birth in a facility that is capable of emergent cesarean birth and neonatal resuscitation. Antepartum transfer to a specialty- or subspecialty-level care facility ensures access to appropriate neonatal care (AAP & ACOG, 2012). This also assures that mother and babies stay together. Ideally, births prior to 34 to 35 weeks' gestation occur in a facility with a level III NICU. Despite some proponents of home birth for multiples, this alternative lacks the obstetric,

DISPLAY 11–3

Suggested Plan for Fetal Surveillance of Multiples

- First-trimester ultrasound for all women suspected or at risk for twin pregnancy[b]
- First-trimester ultrasound for fetal number and chorionicity; offer NT assessment at 10–14 weeks' gestation[a, b]
- Gestational dating using first-trimester ultrasound[b]
- Targeted ultrasound at 18–20 weeks' gestation for gestational age, amniotic fluid assessment, and anatomic survey for anomalies[a] (18–22 weeks[b])

- DC/DA twins with normal prior scans: subsequent ultrasound every 3–4 weeks if no problems[a]
- MC placentation: subsequent ultrasounds every 2–3 weeks[a]
- MC/MA: daily NSTs from 24–26 weeks' gestation; continuous monitoring for variable deceleration[a]
- IUGR, growth or fluid discordance, intensified fetal surveillance with nonstress test (NST), biophysical profile (BPP), and Doppler velocimetry studies[a, b]
- Further testing for any nonreassuring result[a]
- When ultrasound is used for preterm birth screening, use endovaginal ultrasound cervical length measurement.[b]
- Umbilical artery Doppler should not be routinely offered.[b]

BPP, biophysical profile; DC/DA, dichorionic/diamniotic; IUGR, intrauterine growth restriction; MA, monoamniotic; MC, monochorionic; NST, nonstress test; NT, nuchal translucency.
[a]Chitkara, U., & Berkowitz, R. L. (2007). Multiple gestations. In S. G. Gabbe, J. R. Niebyl, & J. L. Simpson (Eds.), *Obstetrics: Normal and Problem Pregnancies* (5th ed., pp. 733–763. Philadelphia: Churchill Livingstone.
[b]Morin L., & Lim K. (2011). Ultrasound in twin pregnancies. *Journal of Obstetrics and Gynaecology Canada, 33*(6), 643–656.

---

anesthetic, and surgical care needed for emergency interventions. Multiples, including twins, do not meet home birth selection criteria and are associated with a higher risk of perinatal death (ACOG, 2011b).

On admission, ultrasound should be used to confirm viability, placental location, and fetal presentation. Although there is excellent correlation between fetal presentations at 32 to 36 weeks and those at birth, some twins undergo spontaneous version in the third trimester. Cephalic-presenting twins at 28 weeks are fairly stable, but non–vertex-presenting twins are more likely to spontaneously convert to a vertex presentation before birth (Chasen, Spiro, Kalish, & Chervenak, 2005).

Expectant parents' birth plans and desires should be respected as much as possible, acknowledging the unique aspects of the birth for many of these families. They should be given anticipatory guidance for all labor and birth procedures. Many are surprised at the large perinatal team that typically attends the birth of multiples. For a preterm cesarean birth of twins, it is not uncommon for as many as 15 people to be present: 2 obstetricians, 2 to 3 labor and delivery nurses, 1 or 2 neonatologists, a NICU team for each infant, 1 or 2 anesthesia staff, and the parents (Bowers & Gromada, 2006). Essential personnel for intrapartum management of multiple births include experienced obstetricians, nurses, anesthesiologists, operating room technicians, and neonatal staff. Women may labor in labor rooms/labor-delivery-recovery rooms, but vaginal births should be performed in a surgical suite with a double setup in case of emergent cesarean birth (Healy & Gaddipati, 2005; Simpson, 2004). The increased risk for cesarean birth of multiples warrants interventions such as a large-bore intravenous (IV), withholding oral liquids and solid food, evaluating the woman's airway, and providing an antacid to prevent gastric aspiration (Bowers & Gromada, 2006). Recommendations for labor and birth procedures and management are listed in Display 11–4.

TIMING OF BIRTH

There is current debate over the optimal timing for birth of multiples. The lowest perinatal mortality rates are at 37 and 35 completed weeks' gestation for twins and triplets, respectively; fetal and neonatal morbidity and mortality increase after 37 weeks in twin gestations and after 35 weeks in triplet pregnancies (AAP & ACOG, 2012). However, there is limited evidence to support elective delivery to decrease perinatal mortality and morbidity in twins. Results are awaited from a multicenter randomized trial designed to determine whether elective birth at 37 weeks' gestation compared with standard care in women with a twin pregnancy affects the risk of perinatal death and serious infant complications (Dodd, Crowther, Haslam, & Robinson, 2010).

A 2011 workshop of the National Institute of Child Health and Human Development (Spong et al., 2011) proposed guidelines for medically indicated birth at or after 34 weeks of gestation. Recommendations for otherwise uncomplicated multiple pregnancies were delivery at 38 completed weeks for DC/DA and 34 to 37 completed weeks for MC/DA. See Display 11–5 for other recommendations. In conjuction with these guidelines, consideration must be given to each clinical situation, weighing the risks of continuing the pregnancy for mother and fetuses against the risks to the infants once they are born. Evidence of appropriate fetal size for gestational age and sustained intrauterine growth, with normal amniotic fluid volume and reassuring tests of fetal well-being, in the absence of maternal complications, warrant allowing the pregnancy

DISPLAY 11-4

Labor and Birth Recommendations for Multiple Births

- Hospital birth with a level II or III NICU
- Antenatal maternal transport if appropriate maternal or neonatal services are not available
- Two experienced obstetricians or an obstetrician and a certified nurse-midwife
- Obstetric nurses to circulate and assist and provide support to the woman
- Anesthesiologist and assistant to provide epidural and general anesthesia
- Neonatal team with nurses and respiratory care personnel sufficient for all infants—pediatricians/neonatologists available if fetal problems occur or birth is preterm or operative
- Delivery in room large enough to accommodate personnel and equipment
- Cesarean birth access immediately available
- Neonatal resuscitation beds available with individual oxygen and suction supplies
- Neonatal transport protocol in place
- Forceps or vacuum extraction immediately available
- Qualified ultrasonographer present with real-time ultrasound
- Continuous electronic fetal monitoring of all fetuses; scalp electrode on each presenting fetus, when possible
- Large-bore (16- to 18-gauge) IV access
- Oxytocin infusion, premixed
- Typed and cross-matched blood immediately available
- Agents for hemorrhage management available
- Cord blood samples for blood gas analysis obtained routinely
- All placentas sent for pathological examination

From Bowers, N. A., & Gromada, K. K. (2006). *Care of the Multiple-Birth Family: Pregnancy and Birth* (Nursing Module). White Plains, NY: March of Dimes Birth Defects Foundation.

DISPLAY 11-5

Proposed Guidelines for Timing of Birth for Multiple Gestation

CHORIONICITY AND COMPLICATION	GESTATIONAL AGE AT DELIVERY (COMPLETED WEEKS)
Uncomplicated DC/DA	38 weeks
Uncomplicated MC/DA twins	34–37 weeks
MC/MA	32–34 weeks
Fetal growth restriction—twins	
DC/DA twins with isolated fetal growth restriction	36–37 weeks
MC/DA twins with isolated fetal growth restriction	32–34 weeks
Concurrent conditions: oligohydramnios, abnormal Doppler studies, maternal risk factors, comorbidity	32–34 weeks
Single fetal death	If death ≥34 weeks, consider delivery.
DC/DA or MC/DA	If <34 weeks, individualize.
MC/MA	Consider delivery: individualize based on gestational age and coexisting complications

DA, diamniotic; DC, dichorionic; MA, monoamniotic; MC, monochorionic.
Spong, C. Y., Mercer, B. M., D'Alton, M., Kilpatrick, S., Blackwell, S., & Saade, G. (2011). Timing of indicated late-preterm and early-term birth. *Obstetrics and Gynecology, 118*(2, Pt. 1), 323–333. doi:10.1097/AOG.0b013e3182255999

to continue (ACOG, 2004a). However, effecting an early birth exclusively for maternal and/or physician convenience risks iatrogenic complications related to induction and prematurity (Ramsey & Repke, 2003).

Fetal pulmonary maturity should be documented if prenatal care is uncertain for both scheduled births and cases with PTL or PPROM (ACOG, 2004a). Tapping of both sacs is recommended due to inconsistent lecithin/sphingomyelin levels between twins, and especially if lung maturity testing will affect clinical management (Cleary-Goldman et al., 2007).

LABOR WITH MULTIPLES

Labor in multiple gestations appears to differ in length from that of singletons. Most data are from twin labors, with limited information from triplets. Early studies evaluated cervical dilatation on admission and found significant differences between twins and singletons (Friedman & Sachtleben, 1964). However,

preterm contractions can lead to advanced cervical dilatation long before a woman enters active labor. Later reports evaluated the length of labor from the onset of the active phase at 4 or 5 cm. One study of 1,821 twin births in a single institution found that cervical effacements and vertex stations on admission were similar for twins and matched singleton controls (Schiff et al., 1998). Interestingly, women with twins had less cervical dilatation on admission. In this study, the time for cervical progression from 4 to 10 cm was less in nulliparous women with twins (3.2 ± 1.3 hours) than those with singletons (4.7 ± 2.6 hours; $P < .001$), but there were no differences for multiparous women. No significant differences in the mean length of the second stage of labor were observed for twins (0.8 hours) and singletons (0.7 hours). Silver and colleagues (2000) reported similar findings and included triplets in their analysis (32 triplets, 64 twins, and 64 singletons—all at approximately 34 weeks' gestation). The mean rate of cervical dilatation in hours from 5 cm to complete was 1.8 ± 1.2 for triplets, 1.7 ± 1.3 for twins, and 2.3 ± 1.5 for singletons ($P < .05$). Factors affecting labor progress may include fetal weights, presentations, and use of epidural anesthesia.

FETAL MONITORING

All women with high-risk conditions such as multiples should have continuous FHR monitoring during labor (ACOG, 2005, 2009). Dual-channel electronic fetal monitors allow simultaneous heart rate recordings, eliminating the need to synchronize several monitors for tracing comparisons. Monitors may display each FHR in a different color and/or by printing one in a bold line and the other in a faint line. Each FHR should be clearly labeled to indicate the corresponding ultrasound transducer and fetus that is being monitored. For example, the nurse should monitor one fetus long enough to get a tracing and then identify on the tracing (either electronically or directly on the paper version) and nurses' notes, "Bold line = fetus in LLQ or A" (Bowers & Gromada, 2006). Ultrasound may be helpful in locating fetal hearts for transducer placement. A fetal scalp electrode should be applied to the presenting fetus in early labor if membranes are already ruptured (Chitkara & Berkowitz, 2007; Rao et al., 2004).

Eganhouse and Peterson (1998) explained the phenomenon of fetal synchrony in multiples. This is a similarity in frequency and timing of FHR accelerations, baseline oscillations, and periodic changes with contractions that occur in healthy twins more than 50% of the time. Some electronic monitors address synchrony with discrimination technology that uses printing of signal marks on the tracing, separate monitoring scales, or artificial separation of single-scale tracings into two separate tracings (Bowers & Gromada, 2006). However, these system cues do not replace careful nursing assessment of each FHR pattern (Simpson, 2004). Bakker, Colenbrander, Verstraeten, and Van Geijn (2004) reported a higher incidence of signal loss in twins compared to singletons and cited abnormal twin positions, polyhydramnios, and twin–twin interactions as factors contributing to signal loss. Caution is also needed to ensure that maternal heart rate is not mistakenly recorded as the second twin (Hanson, 2010).

Clinicians must be familiar with principles of monitoring preterm fetuses because many multiples present in labor before 37 weeks' gestation. Preterm fetuses typically have baseline FHR in the upper range of normal (150 to 160 beats per minute), and accelerations are shorter in duration and of lower amplitude than in more mature fetuses (Eganhouse & Peterson, 1998). Indeterminate or abnormal FHR patterns, including decelerations, bradycardia, tachycardia, and minimal to absent variability may occur in up to 60% of preterm fetuses, and variable decelerations are more common among preterm than term births (ACOG, 2005). However, published data are limited to monitoring preterm twins during antepartum testing, so these conditions and FHR patterns may or may not be applicable to intrapartum monitoring (Simpson, 2004). A full discussion of fetal assessment during labor, including specific details regarding monitoring the preterm fetus, is presented in Chapter 15.

After birth of the first infant, ultrasound should be used to assess presentation of the second twin and to exclude a funic presentation (cord between the fetal vertex and the internal cervical os; Malone & D'Alton, 2004). Membrane rupture of the second twin should be delayed until contractions are reestablished and the presenting part is engaged in the pelvis to minimize the risk of cord prolapse (Rao et al., 2004). Once the presenting part of the next fetus is accessible and membranes are ruptured, a scalp electrode should be applied. An intrauterine pressure catheter may be used for accurate monitoring of uterine contraction activity (Bowers & Gromada, 2006).

LABOR INDUCTION AND AUGMENTATION

There are limited data pertaining to the safety and efficacy of labor induction methods, including prostaglandins, mechanical dilators, and medications to stimulate uterine contractions in twin pregnancies (Healy & Gaddipati, 2005). However, standard protocols for cervical ripening and labor induction appear to be appropriate for twin pregnancies (Ramsey & Repke, 2003; Malone & D'Alton, 2004). Oxytocin is often used for uterine inertia following the birth of the first twin (Rao et al., 2004).

MODE OF BIRTH

There are three routes for twin birth: vaginal delivery for both, cesarean delivery for both, or a combined vaginal/cesarean birth. The choice of birth mode varies with fetal presentations, estimated fetal weights, and maternal and fetal health, as well as clinician experience and preferences of mother and clinician. Perinatal outcomes for vaginal and cesarean births also vary depending on gestational age and birth weight, as well as fetal presentation. Some studies have shown higher rates of adverse perinatal outcome for the second twin in a vaginal birth and for twins at or near term with vaginal birth, especially for those weighing >3,000 g, when compared with twins born via cesarean (Barrett, 2004). Twins born via cesarean between 36 and 38 weeks' gestation have a greater incidence of neonatal respiratory disease compared with twins born vaginally between 38 and 40 weeks' gestation and have a greater risk of death due to RDS following cesarean birth (Dodd & Crowther, 2005).

In 2008, 75% of twins were delivered by cesarean, more than double the rate for singletons (CDC et al., 2011). A cross-sectional study examined trends in cesarean delivery for twins in the United States from 1995 to 2008 and found a significant increase that could not be explained by increases in breech presentation of either twin (Lee, Gould, Boscardin, El-Sayed, & Blumenfeld, 2011). Cesarean birth rates increased 38.4% for twins born at term and nearly 40% for twins born preterm. This trend was most prominent in twins with lower risk conditions including no prior cesarean delivery, vertex presentation, no fetal distress or cephalopelvic disproportion, and mother with no diabetes.

Twin A Vertex/Twin B Vertex

Approximately 43% to 45% of twins present vertex–vertex, and the general recommendation is for vaginal birth, including those with estimated fetal weights <1,500 g (Chitkara & Berkowitz, 2007; Dodd & Crowther, 2005; Robinson & Chauhan, 2004). In one large population-based study, the vaginal/vaginal route carried the lowest neonatal and postneonatal mortality rates for vertex–vertex twins ≥34 weeks' gestation (Kontopoulos, Ananth, Smulian, & Vintzileos, 2004). In this study, combined vaginal/cesarean birth for vertex–vertex twin pairs had the highest neonatal, postneonatal, and infant mortality rates (IMRs). This is consistent with the potential for prolonged fetal heart rate deceleration, cord prolapse, vaginal bleeding, or placental abruption in the second twin that may require cesarean birth. These complications may also explain the increased IMRs in this subset of twins (Kontopoulos et al., 2004).

A trend is emerging for elective/non–medically indicated cesarean birth of vertex–vertex presenting twins despite the estimate that 70% to 86% of vertex–vertex twins may be safely born vaginally (ACOG, 2000; Healy & Gaddipati, 2005; Spong et al., 2011). Kontopoulos and colleagues (2004) found that 87.4% of cesarean twin births had vertex–vertex presentations. Just as with the trend toward elective cesarean birth for singleton births (Meikle, Steiner, Zhang, & Lawrence, 2005), consumer choice may play a role in the increase in cesarean births of twins. Clinicians may be turning to non–medically indicated cesarean births of vertex–vertex twins due to concerns over possible intrapartum changes in fetal presentation and subsequent fetal compromise (ACOG, 2000; Barrett, 2004) as well as fears over potential malpractice litigation. However, spontaneous version of the second twin has been reported to occur following birth of the first twin in only 2% of vertex–vertex twins (Robinson & Chauhan, 2004). It has been suggested that obstetric practitioners not comfortable with vaginal birth of the second twin should consider referral to or co-management with an experienced obstetrician (ACOG, 2000).

Twin A Vertex/Twin B Nonvertex

Approximately 34% to 38% of twins present vertex–nonvertex (Chitkara & Berkowitz, 2007; Robinson & Chauhan, 2004). There is no consensus for the mode of birth for vertex–nonvertex (breech or transverse) twins (ACOG, 2000; Dodd & Crowther, 2005). Options for delivery include cesarean for both, vaginal birth of twin A and version of twin B, vaginal birth of twin A and breech extraction of twin B, or vaginal birth of twin A with emergent cesarean birth of twin B. Outcomes for management of vertex–nonvertex twins are not clear. Cesarean delivery performed for a nonvertex second twin is associated with increased maternal febrile morbidity and no identified improvements in neonatal outcome (Crowther, 2009). Vaginal delivery with active management of the second twin appears to be a reasonable approach for twin pregnancies with no other complications (D'Alton, 2010). However, this requires that obstetricians are skilled in the maneuvers for a nonvertex or unengaged second twin (such as internal podalic version), and the delivery must be in a center with appropriate monitoring protocols and anesthesia. Women who had experienced labor and had a combined delivery (vaginal birth of twin A and cesarean birth of twin B) had an increased risk for maternal endometritis and neonatal sepsis over laboring women who had cesarean delivery for both babies (Alexander et al., 2008).

Twin A Nonvertex

The first twin presents as nonvertex in approximately 19% to 21% of cases (Chitkara & Berkowitz, 2007; Robinson & Chauhan, 2004). Although rare, the primary risk is interlocking of the heads of breech–vertex twins during a vaginal birth. Cesarean birth is generally recommended for this presentation in the United States (ACOG, 2000; Healy & Gaddipati, 2005). However, experience in other countries indicates that a vaginal delivery for a breech-first twin may be appropriate in carefully selected cases (Sentilhes et al., 2007). Planned cesarean section may not only decrease the risk of a low 5-minute Apgar score when twin A is breech (Hogle, Hutton, McBrien, Barrett, & Hannah, 2003) but may also increase the risk for deep vein thrombophlebitis and pulmonary embolism (Sentilhes et al., 2007).

Triplet Birth

Although 94.2% of U.S. triplets were delivered by cesarean in 2008 (CDC et al., 2011), vaginal birth may be an option for select triplet pregnancies (AAP & ACOG, 2012). Some prospective studies using a standardized protocol have reported improved or similar Apgar scores, cord pH, and length of maternal and neonatal stays compared to cesarean births (Ramsey & Repke, 2003). In addition to standard considerations for a safe birth of multiples, criteria for vaginal birth of triplets include gestational age ≥28 weeks, the presenting triplet positioned vertex, fetal monitoring for all three fetuses, no obstetric contraindications, and informed consent (Ramsey & Repke, 2003). In contrast, a review of U.S. triplet births for 1995 to 1998 found that vaginal birth was associated with the highest gestational age–adjusted relative risks for stillbirth (6.04), neonatal death (2.92), and infant death (2.38 compared to cesarean birth of all three triplets (1.0; Vintzileos, Ananth, Kontopoulos, & Smulian, 2005). There was no association between birth order and mortality rates, except that the stillbirth rate was increased for the third fetus regardless of the mode of birth.

INTERDELIVERY INTERVAL

No clear guidelines are established for the interdelivery interval between births of twins. However, with increasing time, risks increase in the second twin for complications such as umbilical cord prolapse, abruption, and malpresentation (Healy & Gaddipati, 2005). The risk for asphyxia-related mortality increases if the birth interval between twins is greater than 30 minutes (Dodd & Crowther, 2005). Umbilical cord arterial and venous pH of the second twin has been found to decline in a continuous linear fashion with increasing intertwin birth interval time (McGrail & Bryant, 2005). Lengthy interdelivery intervals also increase the chances of a fully dilated cervix to contract down, limiting birth options for the second fetus (Malone & D'Alton, 2004). It has been suggested that with normal fetal status, progressive descent, and stable maternal condition, an interval beyond 30 minutes may be reasonable with judicious oxytocin use (Healy & Gaddipati, 2005). Continuous fetal monitoring of the remaining fetus(es) is essential in the interdelivery interval.

DELAYED–INTERVAL BIRTH

Delayed-interval birth, or asynchronous birth, occurs when one or more very preterm multiples are vaginally delivered, and births of the remaining fetus(es) are delayed in hopes of improving neonatal survival and decreasing neonatal morbidity. Lengthy interdelivery time intervals (up to 153 days) have been reported in the literature, with a median ranging from 6 to 31 days (Cristinelli, Fresson, André, & Monnier-Barbarino, 2005; Zhang, Hamilton, Martin, & Trumble, 2004). Population-based reviews of multiple births from 1995 to 1998 found that 56% had delays from 2 to 7 days (Zhang et al., 2004), whereas 6.0% of twins had delayed birth ≥1 week (Oyelese, Ananth, Smulian, & Vintzileos, 2005).

Perinatal outcomes appear to be improved for second twins whose delivery is delayed when the first co-twin is delivered between 20 and 29 weeks' gestation (Arabin & van Eyck, 2009). The optimal clinical management of delayed-interval births is unknown. Fetal pathology, monochorionicity, placenta previa, placental abruption, and preeclampsia have been cited as contraindications (Cristinelli et al., 2005). Clinical reports include use of aggressive tocolysis, cervical cerclage, corticosteroids, and prophylactic and therapeutic antibiotics (Arabin & van Eyck, 2009; Oyelese et al., 2005; Zhang et al., 2004). Although there appear to be benefits for the remaining fetuses, this practice bears substantial risk. Maternal complications frequently associated with delayed-interval birth include chorioamnionitis, postpartum hemorrhage, retained placenta, and abruption (Arabin & van Eyck, 2009).

VAGINAL BIRTH AFTER CESAREAN

For women with a prior cesarean birth, a trial of labor may be a reasonable option for appropriately selected twin pregnancies at or near term (Varner, et al., 2005). In one study, VBAC was successful in 64.5% of women, but nearly half of those who had a failed trial of labor had a vaginal delivery for twin A and cesarean birth for twin B. Maternal morbidities were no more likely than with singleton births, and fetal and neonatal complications were uncommon in either group at ≥34 weeks' gestation. Women desiring VBAC should be evaluated with criteria and counseling similar to that used for women with singleton gestations.

ANESTHESIA

The choice of anesthesia should be made with anticipation of the potential need for uterine manipulation, operative birth, version of the second twin, emergent cesarean birth, and the increased risks for uterine atony and postpartum hemorrhage (Dodd & Crowther, 2005; Ramsey & Repke, 2003). Epidural anesthesia is commonly used for vaginal and cesarean births of twins. Both epidural and spinal anesthesia are safely used for triplet cesarean births, but spinal anesthesia has been associated with a larger initial decrease in systolic blood pressure in these pregnancies (Marino, Goudas, Steinbok, Craigo, & Yarnell, 2001). Sublingual or IV nitroglycerin may be used for acute uterine relaxation for situations such as head entrapment of the second breech twin or retained placenta (Ramsey & Repke, 2003).

Although nonmedicated vaginal births of twins are uncommon, the woman's preferences must be balanced with potential risks and need for interventions. For example, an option for a woman desiring a nonmedicated birth is to have an epidural catheter placed but not have medication infused through the catheter (Bowers & Gromada, 2006).

POSTPARTUM MANAGEMENT

HEMORRHAGE

Blood loss with twin vaginal births is approximately 1,000 mL, similar to that of singleton cesarean birth; blood loss with triplet cesarean birth is typically much greater than 1,000 mL due to increased risk of uterine atony (Klein, 2002). The risk of bleeding from factors including abruptio placentae, placenta previa, and other excessive bleeding during labor and delivery was found to be two times higher in twin and three times higher in triplet pregnancies compared to singleton gestations (Luke & Brown, 2007). Mothers of multiples were 1.66 times more likely to need blood transfusion than mothers of singletons (1.0; Walker et al., 2004) and the risk of maternal death from hemorrhage is 4 times higher (MacKay et al., 2006).

Uncontrollable hemorrhage may lead to hysterectomy. A historical review of 100 peripartum hysterectomies performed in one clinical center found a significant increase in risk for twin (0.44%) and HOM (3.48%) gestations compared to singleton pregnancies (0.15%; Francois, Ortiz, Harris, Foley, & Elliott, 2005). Others have found similar rates (Walker et al., 2004). In the review by Francois and colleagues (2005), all the hysterectomies in multiple gestations were performed emergently, and all but one were for uterine atony.

Hemorrhage prevention includes anticipation of risk, recognition of uterine atony, and use of uterotonic agents in the third stage of labor. Type and cross-matched blood and blood products should be on hand. Immediately after birth, nurses should make careful postpartum assessments of bleeding, uterine tone, and vital signs every 15 minutes for at least 2 hours to detect later hemorrhage (AAP & ACOG, 2012). The nurse providing recovery care should have no other responsibilities so full attention can be devoted to the immediately postpartum woman until she is determined to be in stable condition (AAP & ACOG, 2012). A comprehensive discussion of risks, prevention, and treatment of postpartum hemorrhage is presented in Chapter 17.

MATERNAL RECOVERY

Multiple pregnancy and birth increase stresses on a woman's body, and these are intensified by antepartum, intrapartum, and postpartum complications (Gromada & Bowers, 2005). Having an infant in the NICU or caretaking responsibilities for multiple infants at home can also increase physical and emotional stress. In particular, women who have had extended antepartum bed rest may have difficulty recuperating after birth. A study of 31 women with twins and triplets who had been hospitalized during pregnancy reported a higher mean number and longer duration of postpartum symptoms than women with singleton pregnancies (Maloni, Margevicius, & Damato, 2006). Although many symptoms decreased over the days and weeks after birth, a high percentage persisted at 6 weeks' postpartum, including back muscle soreness, dry skin, fatigue, tenseness, mood changes, and difficulty concentrating. Muscle atrophy was also present, particularly in the weight-bearing muscles of the legs and back (Maloni & Schneider, 2002). These continuing symptoms increase the difficulty for these mothers as they remobilize after birth to care for themselves and their infants. Women need anticipatory guidance that their recovery will be slower than expected. Some may also benefit from a physical therapy assessment and rehabilitation plan for their physical limitations due to bed rest–induced muscle atrophy and cardiovascular deconditioning.

MULTIPLE BIRTH INFANTS

INFANT MORBIDITY AND MORTALITY

Gestational age and birth weight are important predictors of subsequent infant health and survival (Mathews & MacDorman, 2012). In 2009, preterm birth occurred in 10.4% of singletons, 58.8% of twins, 94.4% of triplets, and 98.3% of quadruplets (Martin et al., 2011; see Fig. 11–10).The gestational age distribution by plurality is shown in Figure 11–11. Compared to only 1% of singletons, 10% of twins, 35% of triplets, and 68% of quadruplets were born VLBW (less than 1,500 g) in 2009 (see Table 11–2; Martin et al., 2011).

Increased use of labor induction and/or cesarean birth in recent years has increased the rate of preterm birth among twins, especially at 34 to 36 weeks' gestation (Ananth, Joseph, & Kinzler, 2004). In one study, investigators found a 235% increase in the rate of PTL induction (from 1.7% to 5.7%) and a 40% increase in the rate of preterm cesarean delivery of twins (from 23.5% to 33.0%; Ananth et al., 2004).

Several studies have found no differences in neonatal outcomes among singletons, twins, and triplets. Ballabh and colleagues (2003) analyzed outcomes of 116 sets of triplets matched with the same number of twins and singletons over 7 years in a tertiary center. Of 9 respiratory and 22 nonrespiratory outcome variables, there were no statistically significant differences among triplets, twins, and singletons. This study had several limitations, including use of a single tertiary center and inclusion of only those infants admitted to the NICU. Infants were matched only for gestational age and not for race, use of ART,

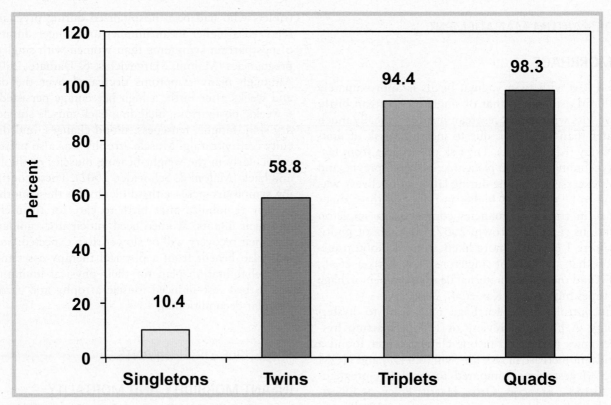

FIGURE 11-10. Preterm births by plurality: United States, 2009.

or mode of birth. Another analysis of 36,931 singletons, 12,302 twins, and 2,155 triplets in a prospectively recorded database from 24 NICUs from 1997 to 2002 also found no significant differences in neonatal outcomes (Garite et al., 2004). Although this study drew from a large and diverse database, the infants studied were all in NICUs and did not include multiple birth infants who died, were stillborn, or were not admitted to the NICU because of stable health.

According to national data for 2008, multiples accounted for 3% of all live births but 15% of all infant deaths in the United States (Mathews & MacDorman, 2012). The infant mortality rate (IMR) increases with plurality; the rate for twins (27.33/1,000) was nearly 5 times higher and the rate for triplets (59.70/1,000) was 10 times higher than the rate for singletons (5.83/1,000). IMR also differs by race. Black infants have the highest IMR for all pluralities compared to whites and Hispanics (Salihu, Garces, et a1., 2005). Interestingly, Hispanic singletons and twins have slightly improved survival over whites, but infant mortality for Hispanic triplets is 20% higher. The association of maternal age with infant mortality

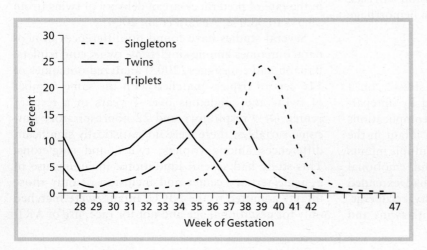

FIGURE 11-11. Gestational age distribution by plurality: United States, 2002. (Data from Martin, J. A., Hamilton, B. E., Sutton, P. D., Ventura, S. J., Menacker, F., & Munson, M. L. [2003]. Births: Final data for 2002. *National Vital Statistics Reports, 55* [1], 1–102.)

Table 11–2. GESTATIONAL AGE AND BIRTHWEIGHT CHARACTERISTICS BY PLURALITY: UNITED STATES, 2009

	All births	Singletons	Twins	Triplets	Quadruplets	Quintuplets and higher-order multiples[1]
Number	4,130,665.0	3,987,108.0	137,217.0	5,905.0	335	80.0
Percent very preterm[2]	2.0	1.6	11.4	36.8	64.5	95.0
Percent preterm[3]	12.2	10.4	58.8	94.4	98.3	96.3
Mean gestational age in weeks (standard deviation)	38.6 (2.5)	38.7 (2.4)	35.3 (3.6)	31.9 (3.9)	29.5 (4.0)	26.6 (4.6)
Percent very low birthweight[4]	1.5	1.1	9.9	35.0	68.1	86.5
Percent low birthweight[5]	8.2	6.4	56.6	95.1	98.6	94.6
Mean birthweight in grams (standard deviation)	3,262.0 (591)	3,296.0 (560)	2,336.0 (626)	1,660.0 (558)	1,291.0 (520)	1,002.0 (672)

[1]Quintuplets, sextuplets, and higher-order multiple births are not differentiated in the national data set.
[2]Very preterm is less than 32 completed weeks of gestation.
[3]Preterm is less than 37 completed weeks of gestation.
[4]Very low birthweight is less than 1,500 grams.
[5]Low birthweight is less than 2,500 grams.
From Martin, J. A., Hamilton, B. E., Ventura, S. J., Osterman, M. J. K., Kirmeyer, S., Mathews, T. J., & Wilson, E. C. (2011). Births: Final data for 2009. *National Vital Statistics Reports, 60*(1), 1–72. http://www.cdc.gov/nchs/data/nvsr/nvsr60/nvsr60_01.pdf. Reprinted with permission.

in multiple births is a paradox. In singletons, infant mortality is higher at the extremes of maternal age, producing a U-shaped curve; but in multiples, IMRs are highest at young maternal ages but continue to decrease with rising maternal age (Luke & Brown, 2007). See Figure 11–12.

LONG-TERM MORBIDITIES

Although early studies showed lower cognitive abilities of twins compared to singletons, when matched for birth weight and gestation, cognitive abilities of twins are not different (Ingram Cooke, 2010). However, multiple birth infants are more likely than singletons

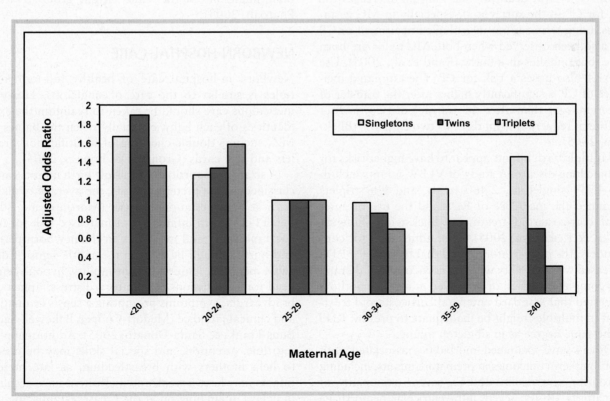

FIGURE 11–12. Maternal age–specific infant mortality by plurality, United States, 1995–2000. (Data from Luke, B., & Brown, M. B. [2007]. Contemporary risks of maternal morbidity and adverse outcomes with increasing maternal age and plurality. *Fertility and Sterility, 88*[2], 283–293.)

to suffer long-term serious morbidities, including CP, severe learning disabilities (LDs), behavioral difficulties, and chronic respiratory disease (Pharoah, 2002; Rand, Eddleman, & Stone, 2005).

Overall, the prevalence of CP in twins is six times higher than in singletons (O'Callaghan et al., 2011). In the United States, it is estimated that 8% of the increase in the prevalence of CP is due solely to the rise in multiple births, with rates for CP in singletons, twins, and triplets of 1.6 to 2.3, 7.3 to 12.6, and 28 to 44.8 per 1,000, respectively (Blickstein, 2001).

The increased prevalence of CP is due in part to a combination of a higher proportion of LBW infants among twins and the significantly higher prevalence of CP in normal birth weight twins (Pharoah, 2002). However, multiple birth appears to be an independent risk factor for CP, as the excess risk for death and severe morbidity in twins cannot be explained by their greater rates of prematurity and LBW alone (Rand et al., 2005). A large, multicenter study found that extremely LBW (<1,000 g) twins and HOMs have an increased risk of death or neurodevelopmental impairment at 18 to 22 months' corrected age when compared to extremely LBW singletons (Wadhawan et al., 2011). It has been suggested that cerebral impairment occurring during intrauterine development and attributable to the twinning process may lead to preterm birth. Or, preterm birth of a vulnerable infant might lead to an impairment that occurred in the perinatal period (Pharoah, 2002). The fetal death of one multiple increases the risk for CP in the survivor(s), especially in MC gestations. Long-term serious neurologic impairment or CP has also been observed when both MC twins are born alive, but one dies in infancy (Rand et al., 2005). Use of ART also poses a risk for CP. The estimated incidence of CP is significantly higher after the transfer of three embryos than after the transfer of two or after multifetal reduction from three to two embryos (Blickstein, 2005).

Multiple birth infants appear to have higher risks for chronic lung disease. A study of VLBW infants including 4,754 singletons, 2,460 twins, and 906 triplets examined the incidence of RDS and the use of antenatal corticosteroid treatment (Blickstein, Shinwell, Lusky, & Reichman, 2005). After adjustment for confounders, the investigators found that the risk for RDS increased with plurality whether corticosteroid therapy was complete, partial, or not given at all. The authors suggested that standard antenatal corticosteroid treatment in multiples might be inadequate to prevent RDS to the same degree as in singleton infants.

Others have examined morbidities associated with poor long-term outcomes in premature infants, including necrotizing enterocolitis (NEC), severe retinopathy of prematurity (ROP), severe intraventricular hemorrhage (IVH), and the need for ventilator use and respiratory support at 28 days of age, but found no differences in these morbidities at any gestational age among singletons, twins, and triplets (Blickstein et al., 2005).

Deformational plagiocephaly (asymmetrically shaped head) has been found to occur more frequently in newborn twins than in singletons (56% vs. 13%; Peitsch, Keefer, LaBrie, & Mulliken, 2002). It has been suggested that positioning in utero may be the initial cause of plagiocephaly, with sleep positions worsening the condition (positional plagiocephaly) (Langkamp & Girardet, 2006). Vertex-presenting first twins, identical twins, and the smaller of a twin pair appear to have more severe involvement.

Studies conflict on the risk of sudden infant death syndrome (SIDS) in twins. Analysis of linked birth and infant death files for 1995 to 1998 found that twins are at higher risk for SIDS than are singletons, and that the epidemiology of SIDS in twins was similar to that seen in singletons (Getahun, Demissie, Lu, & Rhoads, 2004). A similar analysis of an earlier data set (1987 to 1991) found that although the incidence of SIDS in twins is higher than in singletons, independent of birth weight, twins do not appear to be at greater risk for SIDS compared to singletons (Malloy & Freeman, 1999). The authors concluded that the increased risk is a function of the higher prevalence of LBW infants among twins. A review of 2,349 British SIDS cases observed that heavier twins (birth weight >3,000 g) were at significantly greater risk of SIDS than singletons of the same weight group (Platt & Pharoah, 2003).

NEWBORN HOSPITAL CARE

Newborn in-hospital care of healthy full-term multiples is similar to the care of singletons. However, meticulous care should be taken to maintain the exact identities of each baby, especially when the babies are MZ, such as double-checking of identification bracelets and crib cards (Gromada & Bowers, 2005).

A sizable proportion of multiple birth infants can be classified as late preterm infants; the average twins are born at 35.3 gestational weeks (Martin et al., 2011; Fig. 11–13).Such infants are at increased risk for neonatal mortality and morbidity in the newborn period, and nurses should be alert to the subtle signs of difficulty, including temperature instability, hypoglycemia, need for IV infusions, respiratory distress, apnea and bradycardia, symptoms prompting a sepsis evaluation, and clinical jaundice (Medoff-Cooper, Bakewell-Sachs, Buus-Frank, & Santa-Donato, 2005). Additional nursing time, attention, and special skills may be needed to help mothers with breastfeeding, as late preterm infants may have a weak and ineffective suck, resulting in delays in latching on at the breast, establishing successful nutritive breastfeeding, or achieving adequate

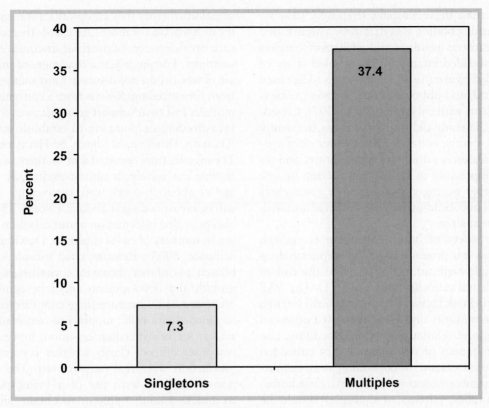

FIGURE 11-13. Late preterm births by plurality: United States, 2008.

oral intake from either the breast or bottle (Medoff-Cooper et al., 2005).

Rooming-in with newborn multiples is optimal, as long as a support person is with the new mother in her hospital room. As some mothers may not be physically ready or will be overwhelmed with all the infants at once, having only one infant in the room at a time may be helpful at first. However, a mother should be encouraged to assume care for all healthy infants together as soon as she is able before discharge (Gromada & Bowers, 2005).

COBEDDING MULTIPLE NEONATES

Cobedding is the practice of placing multiple birth infants together in the same bed based on the concept of continuing the womb-sharing experience. Cobedding allows prenatal interaction to continue, thus providing comfort and decreasing stress to the co-multiples. It is a form of developmentally supportive care and one way to foster the continuity between the intrauterine and extrauterine life of multiple birth infants (Leonard, 2002). Cobedding literature and research are limited, often anecdotal, and most studies are of preterm multiples, but currently there are no demonstrated indications that cobedding in the NICU increases risk for poor outcomes (AAP, 2007). The National Association of Neonatal Nurses (NANN) states that while the

underlying principles of cobedding may be reasonable, cobedding hospitalized infants cannot be endorsed or refuted until further research is available, and that neonatal units choosing to use cobedding should develop a clinical evaluation protocol to assess the safety and benefits of the practice (NANN, 2009). A Cochrane protocol has been developed for reviewing studies to assess the effectiveness of cobedding for stable preterm twins in the neonatal nursery (Lai, Foong, Foong, & Tan, 2010).

Nurses need information on how to respond to parent questions about cobedding at home and provide anticipatory guidance before discharge. Parents of multiples may desire cobedding at home for various reasons, such as convenience, sleep synchronicity, cost savings, ability to have the babies in the parents' room, or because the infants were cobedded in the NICU. There are limited data on home cobedding practices, and studies are largely observational. In one report, 54% of 109 mothers of twins in New Zealand cobedded their infants at 6 weeks of age, with 31% and 10% still cobedding at 4 and 8 months, respectively (Hutchison, Stewart & Mitchell, 2010). In a British study of 60 twin pairs, 60% of twins were cobedded in eight cobedding configurations (Ball, 2006). No significant differences were found in duration of parent or infant sleep between the cobedded and separate sleeping groups. The study did find that cobedded twins were less likely to be moved from their parents' room than those sleeping separately (9% vs. 33%). A concerning finding was that some parents used potentially hazardous bedding and makeshift barriers between the cobedded infants. Another small study of healthy cobedded twin pairs under 3 months of age used video, behavioral, and physiologic monitoring to assess potential problems with cobedding (Ball, 2007). Cobedded infants in the study did not wake more frequently than separated infants, and there was greater sleep synchrony, no increases in core body temperature, and no evidence of compression or airway obstruction by one twin on the other during cobedding. The researchers advised caution in cobedding babies with fever and with babies of different sizes.

Because the safety of home cobedding is unclear, the AAP believes it is prudent to provide separate sleep areas for multiple birth infants to decrease the risk of SIDS and accidental suffocation (AAP, 2011). The AAP cites the following risk factors for multiple birth infants: frequency of prematurity and LBW, increased potential for overheating and rebreathing while cobedding, size discordance, frequency of side placement of cobedded twins, and hospital practice of cobedding as an encouragement for parents to continue this practice at home. As with all families, parents of multiples should be taught SIDS risk-reduction practices including supine positioning; firm sleep surface; breastfeeding; room sharing without bed sharing; routine immunizations; consideration of pacifier use; and avoidance of soft bedding, overheating, and exposure to tobacco smoke, alcohol, and illicit drugs (AAP, 2011).

DISCHARGE PLANNING

Multiple babies, particularly those born preterm, frequently cannot be discharged at the same time due to illness or differences in growth and feeding abilities. This can place a physical and emotional burden on parents, especially on postpartum mothers recuperating from multiple pregnancy and often a surgical or complicated vaginal birth who must travel back and forth to the hospital (Gromada & Bowers, 2005). Parents will need a place for daytime visits and privacy for breastfeeding, and ideally, rooms are available for overnight stays. Policies should be in place to clarify issues such as bringing the well multiple(s) back to the hospital. Discharging infants separately may be easier for families with HOMs. When infants go home one or two at a time, the parents can become acquainted with each infant individually before facing the overwhelming tasks of caring for all of the infants together (Gromada & Bowers, 2005).

FEEDING MULTIPLES

Just as for singleton infants, breast milk is the ideal food for multiple birth infants, especially those who are born preterm. However, it is common for mothers of multiples to be unaware that breastfeeding is an option, and many question whether they can produce enough milk to meet the needs of two or more infants. Mothers also report that care providers are unaware or discourage breastfeeding multiples. Fortunately, the challenges of managing multiple newborns do not dissuade most mothers of multiples from breastfeeding. Results from a convenience sample of mothers in a twin support group showed 89.4% initiated breastfeeding or pumping to establish milk production (Damato, Dowling, Madigan, & Thanattherakul, 2005). The investigators reported that mothers who were breastfeeding exclusively or almost exclusively at an average age of about 9 weeks were significantly more likely to still be breastfeeding at about 28 weeks. The same sample also provided information about cessation of breastfeeding in mothers of twins (Damato, Dowling, Standing, & Schuster, 2005). Reasons cited included unique issues related to infants' behaviors, challenges presented by growth and development, and time commitments that interfered with breastfeeding continuation. In particular, inadequate milk supply was reported as a leading reason for breastfeeding cessation; however, the survey responses did not clarify whether concerns about milk production were real or perceived. The study authors noted that long-term use of a breast pump, whether to initiate a milk supply or to obtain milk to store for future use, was beneficial in prolonging the provision of breast milk. However, this practice had the potential to become an extreme burden for a mother who was also breastfeeding or bottle-feeding two infants. These reports emphasize the need for ongoing lactation support after birth to manage challenges of new breastfeeding issues with twin growth and development.

Several breastfeeding principles must be recognized and communicated to mothers of multiples. First, mothers need to be informed early in pregnancy that breastfeeding is not only an option for feeding multiple infants but also the recommended feeding method. Second, establishing adequate milk production for multiple babies begins as soon as possible after birth with babies effectively removing milk at the breast or initiating milk expression/breast-pumping when babies are preterm and/or ineffective at adequate milk removal. Third, maintenance of adequate milk production is dependent on frequent feedings or pumpings that effectively remove milk from the breasts; ineffective milk removal is associated with inadequate milk production. Fourth, meeting a mother's goal of successful breastfeeding requires support from everyone around her, including her care providers. The British Columbia Reproductive Care Program (2007) has developed guidelines for breastfeeding multiples for use by healthcare providers. The guidelines describe best practices based on current research as well as empirical and anecdotal evidence from professionals and multiple birth families and are listed in Display 11–6. Mothers should also be provided with community breastfeeding support resources, such as lactation consultants, mother-to-mother support groups, and parents of multiples clubs.

D I S P L A Y   1 1 – 6

Guidelines for Breastfeeding Multiples

1. Families need opportunities to become informed about and prepared for breastfeeding term and preterm multiple birth infants.
2. Families require access to multiple-specific and general breast-feeding resources.
3. Families should be supported to initiate lactation and provide breast milk to their infants at the earliest opportunity.

4. Families should be assisted in the ongoing development of a breastfeeding plan that considers the needs of the mother, each infant, and the family as a whole.
5. Families should receive evidence-based and skilled breastfeeding assistance throughout the postpartum and early childhood periods.
6. Families should receive coordinated, comprehensive, consistent, and seamless breastfeeding care throughout pregnancy and early childhood.

Perinatal Services British Columbia (formerly British Columbia Reproductive Care Program). (2007). *Breastfeeding multiples, nutrition, part III*. Retrieved from http://www.perinatalservicesbc.ca/NR/rdonlyres/D72E27F9-11A1-4E97-8E7D-DF60B5EFE57C/0/BFGuidelinesBreastfeedingMultiplesPartIII3.pdf

Breastfeeding management of healthy newborn multiples born at term is similar to singleton care. Usually, mothers begin with one infant at a time in order to monitor for effective breastfeeding behaviors (latch on and active suckling [for ≥10 minutes]) by each infant as both learn to breastfeed. Breasts can be alternated on a per-feeding or daily basis. Once one infant is able to achieve a deep, comfortable latch and is feeding effectively, the second infant can be positioned for simultaneous feedings. Mothers and/or infants may not be ready for simultaneous feedings in the first few days, or even weeks. However, nurses or lactation consultants should help mothers with positioning options by demonstration before they leave the hospital. These positions include the double football, parallel/cradle-clutch combo, and double cradle/criss-cross holds (see Fig. 11–14). At home, infants can be fed on cue, feeding each when he or she demonstrates feeding cues, or feeding together, with the mother actively waking the second twin when the first one shows feeding cues. This method of feeding takes less time than feeding the infants separately or based solely on individual infant feeding cues. Many mothers use a combination of individual and simultaneous feedings. For HOMs, a mother may rotate infants and breasts so that each has the optimal time at the breast, or she may have a helper bottle-feed one or two infants while she breastfeeds the other two (Gromada & Bowers, 2005).

Breastfeeding premature or sick multiples is more complex, yet there are clear benefits of providing breast milk for these infants. Mothers whose infants are unable to breastfeed should begin pumping as soon as possible, within hours after birth (Biancuzzo, 2003). This provides sick infants with antibody-rich colostrum, may have a long-term impact on milk production and volumes obtained, and facilitates the establishment of a pumping routine. Pumped colostrum or milk should be distributed among the infants; however, priority is often given to the sickest of the infants (Gromada & Bowers, 2005). Mothers will need instructions about pumping and storage of breast milk, as well as resources for obtaining a hospital-grade breast pump after discharge. A plan for breastfeeding well and sick or premature multiples is provided in Table 11–3.

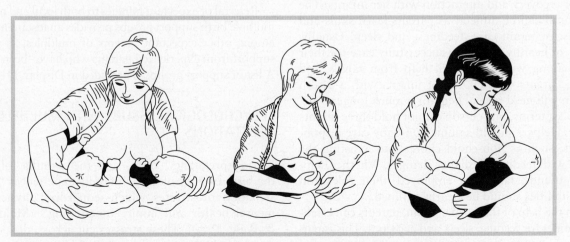

FIGURE 11–14. Breastfeeding positions for mothers of multiples. (Copyright 2006 by Marvelous Multiples, Inc. Used with permission.)

Table 11–3. PLAN FOR BREASTFEEDING MULTIPLES (INFORMATION FOR MOTHERS)

For Well Newborns	For Preterm or Sick Newborns
• After birth (vaginal or cesarean), put each baby to breast within the first 30–90 min or as soon as any baby cues to feed. (Initiate skin-to-skin contact immediately after birth.)	• Begin breast pumping using an electric breast pump with double-collection kit setup as soon as possible after delivery (vaginal or cesarean). Ideally, begin within 6 hr.
• Avoid using bottles, pacifiers, and other intraoral objects if possible.	• Apply the pump to both breasts at least eight times each 24 hr. Nighttime pumping can be limited if babies' discharge is unlikely, but do not allow more than 5–6 hr between pumpings. Pump more often during the day to achieve at least eight pumping sessions per 24 hr.
• Room-in with your babies at least 8 hr each day. (You may need a support person to stay with you.)	
• Ask your nurse or lactation consultant to help you the first few times you breastfeed.	• Pump on a regular schedule. As your babies' discharge nears, pump more often and add night pumping to achieve up to 10–12 times in 24 hr.
• Initially feed each baby separately. Make sure each baby can latch-on to the breast and has correct tongue placement and suck.	
• Nurse each baby when any demonstrates feeding cues, which should be 8–12 times over 24 hr by their second 24 hr after birth.	• Learn how to safely collect, store, and transport your beast milk.
• Alternate breasts at each feeding or daily for each baby or offer your fullest breast to the hungriest baby.	• Let your babies' nurses and doctors know that you want to start kangaroo care (KC) skin-to-skin as soon as possible. Let each baby have mouth/nose-to-nipple contact as soon as possible. Allow the babies to progress to breastfeeding as soon as medically possible.
• If babies are nursing well, you can feed them together. Your nurse or lactation consultant can show you different positions. Practice with all babies before discharge.	
• If you are concerned about your milk supply, call a lactation consultant or breastfeeding support leader, feed your babies more frequently, and use an electric breast pump after feedings, between feedings, or as needed to help increase milk supply.	• Preterm babies must physically mature before they can sustain effective breastfeeding. Gradually, they will improve so you can nurse your babies as with well babies.
	• Use your breast pump at home after feedings if needed to help with milk supply.
• Know the number of your lactation consultant breastfeeding support leader if you need help at home.	• Know the number of your lactation consultant or breastfeeding support leader if you need help at home.

Marvelous Multiples, Inc., used with permission.

PARENTING NEWBORN MULTIPLES

Multiple births have been shown to have a five times greater risk of severe parenting stress and double the risk of lower quality of life, social stigma, and maternal depression (Luke & Brown, 2007). In addition to the physical demands of their own recovery, mothers of multiple newborns face challenges in parenting several babies at once. In the first weeks at home, it is essential that tasks of housekeeping, laundry, cooking, grocery shopping, and sibling care are delegated to friends and family so that the mother is permitted time for recovery and interaction with her infants. The first month can be difficult as parents learn skills and routines for infant care, feedings, and sleep. Usually, parents of healthy twins can successfully care for their infants along with occasional help from family and friends. Parents with HOMs or infants with a health problem will need formal help for a much longer time. In simplest terms, one person cannot hold three infants at once. Helpers should assume non-baby care responsibilities, such as household chores and assisting the mother with feedings or diaper changes. Whether helpers are friends, family, or employed, their roles and responsibilities should be clearly outlined.

With the help of their pediatrician, parents can establish routines for feeding, sleep, and activities. This is particularly important for preterm infants who may need frequent feedings. Simultaneous feeding can be helpful but requires waking a sleeping infant when another is ready to eat. This may be challenging as the other multiple(s) may not always cooperate, especially when in a deep sleep state. Feeding routines also help develop similar sleep/waking patterns. Nurses should stress flexible routines, allowing for differences in each infant's temperament and needs. Some infants are high need, requiring constant cuddling or touch, whereas others are content with a feeding and a few visual toys. A daily log of feedings and diaper counts for each infant is important until growth and weight gain are well established (Gromada & Bowers, 2005).

Referral of expectant families to both local and national multiple birth support groups provides an instant network among other expectant parents of multiples, as well as support from experienced parents who have "been there." A list of support groups is provided in Display 11–7.

PSYCHOLOGICAL ISSUES WITH MULTIPLE GESTATIONS

During pregnancy, birth, and the months following the birth of multiples, each family experiences "a constellation of stresses which jeopardize physical and mental health and family functioning" (Malmstrom & Biale, 1990). These stresses cut across all socioeconomic and educational levels and include increases in child abuse, marital troubles, and family dysfunction.

Four interrelated principles have been proposed to guide the care of multiple birth families: interdisciplinary involvement, provision of multiples-focused care, coordinated services, and the building of family competency (Leonard & Denton, 2006). These are illustrated in Figure 11–15.

PRENATAL ATTACHMENT

The prenatal attachment process for multiples is complex, with maternal/fetal interactions woven together with interfetal interactions. Just as an expectant mother relates to her fetuses through fetal movement, intrauterine tactile stimulation between multiples plays a role in attachment among infants. Each multiple develops an individual temperament, and each set of multiples establishes their own patterns of tactile communication. The same behaviors, traits, and intermultiple interactions seen in pregnancy also have been observed in infancy and beyond (Leonard, 2002).

Maternal attachment with multiples is similar to attachment processes in singleton pregnancies. Interestingly, women who were younger, with lower income, a history of infertility, greater self-esteem, who had experienced quickening, and who were further along in their pregnancy reported greater prenatal attachment to their twins (Damato, 2004b). Postpartum depression, cesarean birth, and the experience of a NICU admission for one or both twins negatively influenced mothers' postnatal attachment compared to their prenatal attachment (Damato, 2004a).

Fetal movements enable a woman expecting multiples to relate to her unborn children, affirm that each one is alive and healthy, and attach to them individually and as a unit (Leonard, 2002). Nurses can promote prenatal attachment by encouraging expectant mothers to observe fetal movements and patterns, differentiate between individual multiples, identify behavioral similarities and differences, recognize intermultiple contacts (during ultrasound examinations and fetal monitoring), and ask questions during fetal testing (Leonard, 2002). Nurses should provide support and follow-up, especially for older, higher-income women with low self-esteem, and provide prenatal education and counseling to help build confidence and develop effective parenting strategies (Damato, 2004b). Postnatal attachment can be supported by implementing measures to increase a mother's opportunities for proximity with her twins, such as promotion of breastfeeding, skin-to-skin contact, and encouraging complete access to and participation in her infants' NICU care (Damato, 2004a).

PRENATAL FAMILY ADJUSTMENTS

Preparation for multiple infants requires significant adjustments for families even before the babies are born. Depending on the pregnancy, women may need to reduce or stop working, be limited in activities, or be placed on bed rest at home or in the hospital. There is evidence that women on bed rest with multiples may have even greater emotional and physical needs than those with singletons. Women with multiple gestations in one study had many more antepartum symptoms during hospitalization and treatment with bed rest than women with singleton gestations

---

DISPLAY 11-7

Recommendations to Help Grieving Parents of Multiples

- Provide opportunities for parents to see and/or hold all babies of a set, together, and separately.
- Mementos such as photographs, videos, monitor strips, locks of hair, and footprints should be collected for all babies.
- Do not place beds of surviving multiples beside intact sets in the nursery or NICU.
- After a prenatal loss or multifetal reduction, ask how parents want to refer to the pregnancy: by the number conceived or by the number remaining.
- After neonatal loss, most parents consider living children to be survivors and are comfortable with saying they had triplets or twins.
- Parents should have input into labeling for two or more remaining multiples; generally, triplets B and C should retain their designation of B & C after triplet A's death.

- Allow mothers to wear all their infants' bracelets throughout the hospital stay.
- **Suggested helpful and healing responses include:**
- This must be very hard for you.
- I'm so sorry your twins died.
- I have no idea how you must feel.
- How are you feeling? What would help your family through this?
- How are you coping with everything?
- **Hurtful responses to be avoided include:**
- You're young, you could have other multiples.
- You couldn't handle them all.
- At least it happened before you were too attached.
- It's for the best. They would have been severely disabled.
- Set your grief aside. You must be strong for your survivors.
- At least you have two living babies. Some parents can't have any!
- Multiples are so expensive. Think of the money you'll save.

From Gromada, K. K., & Bowers, N. A. (2005). *Care of the Multiple-Birth Family: Postpartum Through Infancy* (Nursing Module). New York: March of Dimes Birth Defects Foundation; Pector, E. A., & Smith-Levitin, M. (2002). Mourning and psychological issues in multiple birth loss. *Seminars in Neonatology, 7*(3), 247-256.

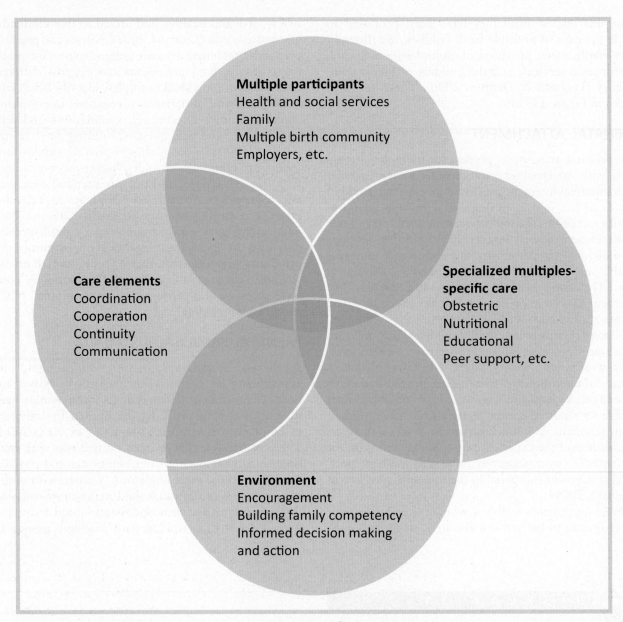

Multiple participants
Health and social services
Family
Multiple birth community
Employers, etc.

Care elements
Coordination
Cooperation
Continuity
Communication

Specialized multiples-specific care
Obstetric
Nutritional
Educational
Peer support, etc.

Environment
Encouragement
Building family competency
Informed decision making
and action

FIGURE 11–15. Framework of care during multiple pregnancy and parenthood. (From Leonard, L. G., & Denton, J. [2006]. Preparation for parenting multiple birth children. *Early Human Development, 82*[6], 371–378.)

(Maloni et al., 2006). The number of symptoms reported by women with multiples appears to be higher than those reported by women with singleton gestations. Over half of the women in the study had very high depressive symptom scores on admission, and they identified concerns for their family and being separated as major stressors. The average number and persistence of postpartum symptoms reported during the first weeks also appear to be higher than those for women with singleton pregnancies. The authors concluded that women have many physical and psychological discomforts during a multiple gestation and experience continuing symptoms indicative of underlying postpartum morbidity that are not completely recovered by 6 weeks.

Families with a mother on bed rest often experience difficulty assuming maternal responsibilities, anxiety about outcomes for mother and infants, and adverse emotional effects on the children (Maloni, Brezinski-Tomasi, & Johnson, 2001). Expectant fathers often receive the brunt of family and household responsibilities during a multiple pregnancy and are often required to "be all things to all family members, including father and mother, financial provider, cook, maid and the emotional support system" (Bowers & Gromada, 2006, p. 36). In addition to their concerns about the health of the mother and fetuses, fathers must cope with the effects of increased family responsibilities and emotional pressures in their own lives. If a mother's income is eliminated due to pregnancy complications, finances may become a concern, even in economically advantaged families. Fathers may be at increased risk for depression, especially those who have a history of depression, are unemployed, and have an unsupportive partner or one with perinatal depression (Leonard, 1998).

Children may be affected by the strains of a high-risk pregnancy as well. Young children whose mothers are on bed rest may be unable to fully comprehend maternal restrictions, the need to reallocate childcare, or maternal absence during hospitalization (Maloni et al., 2001).

Nurses play an integral role in providing psychosocial support for families expecting multiples. Anticipatory guidance includes the expected physical and emotional changes of a multiple pregnancy; the need for contingency planning at home for children and household management; nutritional assessment and counseling; plans for testing, interventions, and treatment options; referrals to support organizations such as local parents of twins groups; and information about multiple birth prenatal education classes. It is also important to ensure that hospitalized women and those on bed rest at home have access to education; this may include provision of in-home or online classes, videos, reading materials, and resources. Measures to decrease the stressors of hospitalization may include liberal visitation with husband and other children; home-cooked food from family and friends; provision of technology for in-room videos, music, and Internet access; and opportunities for networking with other expectant mothers of multiples (Bleyl, 2002).

POSTNATAL ATTACHMENT

Parent–infant attachment with multiple infants is complex and evolves through various processes. Ultimately, parents need to view each infant as an individual with a unique personality and characteristics. Initially, a unit attachment is formed, with parents focusing on the concept of the set of twins or triplets prenatally and after birth (Damato, 2004b). Individual attachments follow, often with brief periods of attachment to one infant before shifting to another (Gromada & Bowers, 2005). Some parents develop preferential feelings for a particular infant. If this is consistently demonstrated, there can be long-term cognitive and behavioral effects for all the infants. Unequal attachments are more likely when one infant is healthier than the other, or one is more responsive (Gromada & Bowers, 2005). Nurses should observe parent–infant interactions, noting behaviors indicative of progression toward individualization. Signs of positive attachment/individualization behaviors include acknowledgment and response to each infant's cues; initiating verbalization, touching, soothing, cuddling, and so forth with each infant; alternating eye contact among infants; and referring to each infant by name (Gromada & Bowers, 2005).

The demands of multiple infants can limit parent–infant interactions. Frequent, slow feedings, repeated diaper changes, and constant cries of multiple infants are exhausting. To compensate, parents may focus more on physical care than on their infants' emotional needs. This exposes multiple birth infants to a unique risk—the deprivation of the parents' exclusive focus and involvement (Feldman & Eidelman, 2004). A study of preterm twins and singletons found that mothers of twins exhibited fewer initiatives toward their infants and were less responsive to both positive signals and to crying (Ostfeld, Smith, Hiatt, & Hegyi, 2000). The twin mothers lifted or held, touched, patted, and talked to their infants less, and their infants had lower cognitive scores at 18 months than singletons. The child who is less effective in eliciting parental care or who may be less rewarding during interactions appears to be at an especially high risk. A study of social–emotional development of triplets found that the infant with birth weight discordance >15% received the lowest levels of parent response and displayed the poorest behavior outcomes among the set. Parenting difficulties appeared to be related to the lack of emotional resources for adapting to each infant's individual patterns (Feldman & Eidelman, 2004). Multiple birth children also appear to be at increased risk for child abuse. One long-standing study found a nine-fold higher risk of reported abuse/neglect among twins compared to singletons (Groothuis et al., 1982).

ANXIETY AND DEPRESSION

The very nature of a high-risk pregnancy increases stress and anxiety for expectant mothers and may be intensified by the unknowns of a multiple pregnancy. Around-the-clock needs of multiple infants, sleep deprivation, inconsistent support, and a sense of isolation may contribute to maternal stress (Gromada & Bowers, 2005). It has been estimated that as many as 25% of multiple birth parents are affected by perinatal depression and anxiety disorders (Leonard, 1998). Compared to parents of singletons, both mothers and fathers of twins experience significantly greater depression, anxiety, sleeping difficulties, and social dysfunction (Vilska et al., 2009). Evidence indicates that stress and depression in pregnant and postpartum women are of considerable concern due to the association with adverse obstetrical outcomes, postpartum depression, and emotional and behavioral problems in the children (Mian, 2005). The additive effects of infertility history, multiple birth, and first-time parenting may increase the risk for psychological resource depletion (Klock, 2004). Other researchers found that regardless of whether multiples were the result of ART or spontaneous conception, families had increased need for material goods, higher social stigma, lower marital satisfaction, more depression, and lower quality of life, which included health and social and psychological aspects (Roca-de Bes, Gutierrez-Maldonado, & Gris-Martínez, 2011). Nurses have a key role in identifying parents at risk; early recognition and support of women and families affected by these disorders; and providing prevention-focused health, education, and social support programs at the family and community levels (Leonard, 1998).

Beck (2002) found that "life on hold" was the basic social psychological problem during the first year for mothers of twins in a multiple birth support group. Mothers in the study experienced four phases: (1) draining power, a demanding, sleep-deprived period when mothers had no time and were torn between infants' needs; (2) pausing own life, which involved a blurring of days and nights with confinement and self-surrender; (3) striving to reset, when mothers began to develop coping strategies such as routines, schedules, prioritizing tasks, recruiting family help, and problem solving; (4) resuming own life, which was achieved when mothers felt their lives were more manageable, and when milestones such as sleeping through the night or twins beginning to self-feed were reached. It was in this last phase that mothers were able to relate the blessings of having twins. Beck (2002) concluded that the most vulnerable period for these mothers was 3 months postpartum.

A study of mothers of multiples who conceived with ART identified children's health, unmet family needs, maternal depression, and parental stress as key areas of concern (Ellison & Hall, 2003). The study revealed that the inordinate stresses of raising multiple birth infants strengthened some marriages when there was greater paternal participation in childcare and household tasks. Marriages weakened when couples were unable to equitably divide family and household labor or were unable to work together as a team. The psychosocial risks associated with iatrogenic multiple births appear to increase with plurality. In another study, parents of ART multiples reported significant difficulty in providing basic material needs for their families, decreased quality of life, social stigma, and maternal depression (Ellison et al., 2005). Such distress may decrease their willingness to seek help or admit their distress to their care providers. A review of the research related to parenting after assisted reproduction concluded that supportive nursing interventions should include strategies to reduce parental anxiety, increase parental self-esteem, and foster healthy parent–infant relationships, (McGrath, Samra, Zukowsky, & Baker, 2010). Interventions for improving parenting sense of competence and parenting distress may include attendance at specialized prenatal clinics, postpartum home visits, maternal involvement in neonatal care activities, and assisting women to reframe their expectations for the demands of caring for twins and maintaining a household (Damato, Anthony, & Maloni, 2009).

GRIEF AND LOSS

Parents who experience the death of a complete set of multiples have been found to grieve more intensely than parents who lose a singleton; they are at significant risk for depression and may experience grief 6 months longer (Pector & Smith-Levitin, 2002). However, the grieving process becomes more complex with the death of part of a set of multiples. These parents experience the difficult paradox of grieving for the infants that died while feeling joy for their living infants. Grieving multiple birth families with a surviving twin have been described as having "special and complex characteristics that affect them in ways greater than, or different from, bereaved single birth families" (Swanson, Kane, Pearsall-Jones, Swanson, & Croft, 2009). Studies have shown that grief is often delayed for 1 to 3 years while parents focus on survivors, bonding is sometimes impaired, and some parents may even resent the survivors (Pector & Smith-Levitin, 2002). The intensity of grief after a multiple's death equals that with a singleton, yet parents rarely receive as much sympathy (Pector & Smith-Levitin, 2002). In one study, mothers experienced significantly more depression and grief than fathers at the time of loss (Swanson et al., 2009). A fundamental concept with loss in multiple births is that no matter how many infants survive, the parents remain parents of multiples (Gromada & Bowers, 2005). It is important to validate parents' loss with healing actions and responses; parents wished that clinicians had been more sensitive and compassionate to them at the time of the loss (Swanson et al., 2009). Recommendations for clinicians to help grieving parents of multiples are listed in Display 11–7. Peer support can be especially helpful at the time of the loss. Multiple birth organizations such as Center for Loss in Multiple Birth (CLIMB) and the Triplet Connection have information and support to help parents cope with the death of one or more multiples.

MULTIPLE BIRTH RESOURCES AND SUPPORT ORGANIZATIONS

Organizations for multiple birth families provide a supportive environment for parents to network and learn from others (see Display 11–8). National organizations often offer free brochures and handouts that can be included in packets created especially for the expectant parents of multiples. See Figure 11–16 for pictures of twins in utero, at birth, and at 3 years old.

SUMMARY

With the incidence of multiples at an all-time high in the United States, perinatal nurses will frequently have the opportunity to care for women pregnant with more than one fetus. A thorough knowledge of the special care needs of women with multiple gestation is requisite for safe care for mothers and their babies.

DISPLAY 11-8

Multiple Birth Resources and Support Organizations

Center for Loss in Multiple Birth, Inc. (CLIMB)
PO Box 91377
Anchorage, AK 99509
907-222-5321
E-mail: climb@pobox.alaska.net
http://www.climb-support.org

International Society for Twin Studies (ISTS)
http://www.ists.qimr.edu.au

Marvelous Multiples, Inc.
PO Box 381164
Birmingham, AL 35238-1164
205-437-3575
Fax: 205-437-3574
E-mail: marvmult@aol.com
http://www.marvelousmultiples.com

Monoamniotic Monochorionic Support Site
http://www.monoamniotic.org

MOST (Mothers of Supertwins)
PO Box 306
East Islip, NY 11730
631-859-1110
E-mail: info@MOSTonline.org
http://www.mostonline.org

Multiple Births Canada (MBC)/Naissances Multiples Canada
(formerly Parents of Multiple Births Association [POMBA] Canada)
PO Box 432
Wasaga Beach, Ontario, Canada L9Z 1A4
613-834-8946, 866-228-8824 (toll-free in Canada)
Fax: 705-429-9809
E-mail: office@multiplebirthscanada.org
http://www.multiplebirthscanada.org

National Organization of Mothers of Twins Clubs, Inc. (NOMOTC)
NOMOTC Executive Office
2000 Mallory Lane, Suite 130-600
Franklin, TN 37067-8231
248-231-4480
877-540-2200
E-mail: info@nomotc.org
http://www.nomotc.org

The Triplet Connection
PO Box 429
Spring City, UT 84662
435-851-1105
Fax: 435-462-7466
E-mail: TC@tripletconnection.org
http://www.tripletconnection.org

***TWINS* Magazine**
30799 Pinetree Road, #256
Cleveland, OH 44124
888-55-TWINS
Fax: 866-586-7683
http://www.twinsmagazine.com

The Twin to Twin Transfusion Syndrome (TTTS) Foundation, Inc.
411 Longbeach Parkway
Bay Village, OH 44140
440-899-TTTS (8887)
800-815-9211
Fax: 440-899-1184
E-mail: info@tttsfoundation.org
http://www.tttsfoundation.org

Twinless Twins Support Group
PO Box 980481
Ypsilanti, MI 48198
888-205-8962
E-mail: contact@twinlesstwins.org
http://www.twinlesstwins.org

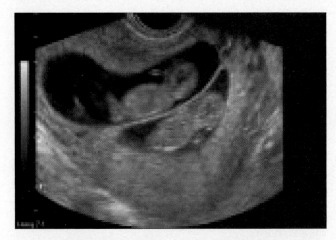

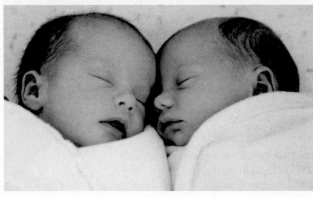

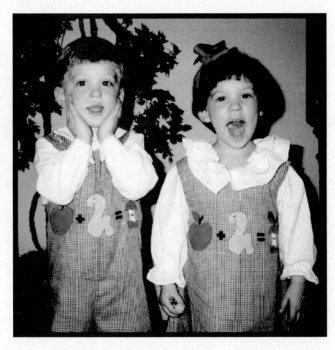

FIGURE 11–16. Twins from pregnancy, birth, and as toddlers. (Courtesy of photographer [and proud new father] Robert Hammer. Used with permission.)

REFERENCES

Abdel-Aleem, H., Shaaban, O. M., & Abdel-Aleem, M. A. (2010). Cervical pessary for preventing preterm birth. *Cochrane Database of Systematic Reviews*, (9), CD007873. doi:10.1002/14651858.CD007873.pub2

Alexander, J. M., Leveno, K. J., Rouse, D., Landon, M. B., Gilbert, S. A., Spong, C. Y., . . . Gabbe, S. G. (2008). Cesarean delivery for the second twin. *Obstetrics and Gynecology, 112*(4), 748–752. doi:10.1097/AOG.0b013e318187ccb2

American Academy of Pediatrics. (2007). Cobedding twins and higher-order multiples in a hospital setting. *Pediatrics, 120*(6), 1341–1367. doi:10.1542/peds.2011-2285.

American Academy of Pediatrics. (2011). SIDS and other sleep-related infant deaths: Expansion of recommendations for a safe infant sleeping environment. *Pediatrics, 128*(5), 1030–1039. doi:10.1542/peds.2011-2284.

American Academy of Pediatrics & American College of Obstetricians and Gynecologists. (2012). *Guidelines for Perinatal Care* (7th ed.). Elk Grove Village, IL: Author.

American College of Obstetricians and Gynecologists. (2000). *Evaluation of Cesarean Delivery*. Washington, DC: Author.

American College of Obstetricians and Gynecologists. (2004a). *Multiple Gestations: Complicated Twin, Triplet, and High-Order Multifetal Pregnancy* (Practice Bulletin No. 56). Washington, DC: Author.

American College of Obstetricians and Gynecologists. (2004b). *Nausea and Vomiting of Pregnancy*. (Practice Bulletin No. 52). Washington, DC: Author.

American College of Obstetricians and Gynecologists. (2005). *Intrapartum Fetal Heart Rate Monitoring*. (Practice Bulletin No. 70). Washington, DC: Author.

American College of Obstetricians and Gynecologists. (2007). *Multifetal Pregnancy Reduction*, (Committee Opinion No. 369). Washington, DC: Author.

American College of Obstetricians and Gynecologists. (2009). *Intrapartum Fetal Heart Rate Monitoring: Nomenclature, Interpretation, and General Management Principles* (Practice Bulletin No. 106). Washington, DC: Author. doi:10.1097/AOG.0b013e3181aef106

American College of Obstetricians and Gynecologists. (2011a). *Antenatal Corticosteroid Therapy for Fetal Maturation* (Committee Opinion No. 475). Washington, DC: Author. doi:10.1097/AOG.0b013e31820eee00

American College of Obstetricians and Gynecologists. (2011b). *Planned Home Birth* (Committee Opinion No. 476). Washington, DC: Author. doi:10.1097/AOG.0b013e31820eee20

American College of Obstetricians and Gynecologists. (2011c). *Thromboembolism in Pregnancy* (Practice Bulletin No. 123). Washington, DC: Author. doi:10.1097/AOG.0b013e3182310c4c

American College of Obstetricians and Gynecologists & Society for Maternal-Fetal Medicine. (2010). *Magnesium Sulfate Before Anticipated Preterm Birth for Neuroprotection* (Committee Opinion No. 455). Washington, DC: Author. doi:10.1097/AOG.0b013e3181d4ffa5

Ananth, C. V., Joseph, K. S., & Kinzler, W. L. (2004). The influence of obstetric intervention on trends in twin stillbirths: United States, 1989–99. *The Journal of Maternal-Fetal & Neonatal Medicine, 15*(6), 380–387.

Arabin, B., & van Eyck, J. (2009). Delayed-interval delivery in twin and triplet pregnancies: 17 years of experience in 1 perinatal center. *American Journal of Obstetrics and Gynecology, 200*(2), 154.e1–8. doi:10.1016/j.ajog.2008.08.046

Aston, K. I., Peterson, C. M., & Carrell, D. T. (2008). Monozygotic twinning associated with assisted reproductive technologies: A review. *Reproduction, 136*(4), 377–386.

Bakker, P. C., Colenbrander, G. J., Verstraeten, A. A., & Van Geijn, H. P. (2004). Quality of intrapartum cardiotocography in twin deliveries. *American Journal of Obstetrics and Gynecology, 191*(6), 2114–2119.

Ball, H. (2006). Caring for twin infants: Sleeping arrangements and their implications. *Evidence Based Midwifery, 4*(1), 10–16.

Ball, H. L. (2007). Together or apart? A behavioural and physiological investigation of sleeping arrangements for twin babies. *Midwifery, 23*, 404–412.

Ballabh, P., Kumari, J., AlKouatly, H. B., Yih, M., Arevalo, R., Rosenwaks, Z., & Krauss, A. N. (2003). Neonatal outcome of triplet versus twin and singleton pregnancies: A matched case control study. *European Journal of Obstetrics, Gynecology, and Reproductive Biology, 107*(1), 28–36.

Barrett, J. F. R. (2004). Delivery of the term twin. *Best Practice & Research Clinical Obstetrics & Gynaecology, 18*(4), 625–630.

Bates, S. M., Greer, I. A., Middeldorp, S., Veenstra, D. L., Prabulos, A., & Vandvik, P. O. (2012). VTE, thrombophilia, antithrombotic therapy, and pregnancy: Antithrombotic therapy and prevention of thrombosis, 9th ed: American College of Chest Physicians Evidence-Based Clinical Practice Guidelines. *Chest, 141*(2 Suppl.), e691s–e736s. doi:10.1378/chest.11-2300

Beck, C. T. (2002). Releasing the pause button: Mothering twins during the first year of life. *Qualitative Health Research, 12*(5), 593–608.

Ben-Haroush, A., Yogev, Y., & Hod, M. (2003). Epidemiology of gestational diabetes mellitus and its association with Type 2 diabetes. *Diabetic Medicine, 21*(2), 103–113.

Bergh, C., Möller, A., Nilsson, L., & Wikland, M. (1999). Obstetrical outcome and psychological follow-up of pregnancies after embryo reduction. *Human Reproduction, 14*(8), 2170–2175.

Berghella, V., Baxter, J. K., & Hendrix, N. W. (2009). Cervical assessment by ultrasound for preventing preterm delivery. *Cochrane Database Systematic Reviews*, (3), CD007235.

Biancuzzo, M. (2003). *Breastfeeding the Newborn: Strategies for Nurses* (2nd ed.). St. Louis, MO: Mosby.

Bleyl, J. (2002). Familial and psychological reaction in triplet families. In L. G. Keith & I. Blickstein (Eds.), *Triplet Pregnancies and Their Consequences* (pp. 361–369). New York: The Parthenon Publishing Group.

Blickstein, I. (2001). The risk of cerebral palsy after assisted reproductive technologies. In I. Blickstein & L. G. Keith (Eds.), *Iatrogenic Multiple Pregnancy: Clinical Implications* (pp. 21–33). New York: The Parthenon Publishing Group.

Blickstein, I. (2005). Estimation of iatrogenic monozygotic twinning rate following assisted reproduction: Pitfalls and caveats. *American Journal of Obstetrics and Gynecology, 192*(2), 365–368.

Blickstein, I., Shinwell, E. S., Lusky, A., & Reichman, B. (2005). Plurality-dependent risk of respiratory distress syndrome among very-low-birth-weight infants and antepartum corticosteroid treatment. *American Journal of Obstetrics and Gynecology, 192*, 360–364.

Bowers, N. A., & Gromada, K. K. (2006). *Care of the Multiple-Birth Family: Pregnancy and Birth* (Nursing Module). White Plains, NY: March of Dimes Birth Defects Foundation.

Brown, J. E., & Carlson, M. (2000). Nutrition and multifetal pregnancy. *Journal of the American Dietetic Association, 100*(3), 343–348.

Bryan, E. (2002). Educating families, before, during and after a multiple birth. *Seminars in Neonatology, 7*(3), 241–246.

Bryan, E. (2005). Psychological aspects of prenatal diagnosis and its implications in multiple pregnancies. *Prenatal Diagnosis, 25*(9), 827–834.

Brzoza, Z., Kasperska-Zajac, A., Oleś, E., & Rogala, B. (2007). Pruritic urticarial papules and plaques of pregnancy. *Journal of Midwifery and Women's Health, 52*(1), 44–48.

Bush, M. C., & Malone, F. D. (2005). Down syndrome screening in twins. *Clinics in Perinatology, 32*(2), 373–386.

Centers for Disease Control and Prevention, American Society for Reproductive Medicine, & Society for Assisted Reproductive Technology. (2011). *2009 Assisted Reproductive Technology Success Rates: National Summary and Fertility Clinic Reports.* Atlanta, GA: U.S. Department of Health and Human Services. http://www.cdc.gov/art/ART2009/index.htm

Chasen, S. T., Spiro, S. J., Kalish, R. B., & Chervenak, F. A. (2005). Changes in fetal presentation in twin pregnancies. *The Journal of Maternal-Fetal and Neonatal Medicine, 17*(1), 45–48.

Chauhan, S. P., Scardo, J. A., Hayes, E., Abuhamad, A. Z., & Berghella, V. (2010). Twins: Prevalence, problems, and preterm births. *American Journal of Obstetrics and Gynecology, 203*(4), 305–315. doi:10.1016/j.ajog.2010.04.031

Chitkara, U., & Berkowitz, R. L. (2007). Multiple gestations. In S. G. Gabbe, J. R. Niebyl, & J. L. Simpson (Eds.), *Obstetrics: Normal and Problem Pregnancies* (5th ed., pp. 733–763). Philadelphia: Churchill Livingstone.

Cleary-Goldman, J., Chitkara, U., & Berkowitz, R. L. (2007). Multiple gestations. In S. G. Gabbe, J. R. Niebyl, & J. L. Simpson (Eds.), *Obstetrics: Normal and Problem Pregnancies* (5th ed., pp. 733–763). Philadelphia: Churchill Livingstone.

Cleary-Goldman, J., D'Alton, M. E., & Berkowitz, R. L. (2005). Prenatal diagnosis and multiple pregnancy. *Seminars in Perinatology, 29*(5), 312–320.

Collopy, K. S. (2004). "I couldn't think that far": Infertile women's decision making about multifetal reduction. *Research in Nursing & Health, 27*(2), 75–86.

Combs, C. A., Garite, T., Maurel, K., Das, A., & Porto, M. (2010). Failure of 17-hydroxyprogesterone to reduce neonatal morbidity or prolong triplet pregnancy: A double-blind, randomized clinical trial. *American Journal of Obstetrics and Gynecology, 203*(3), 248.e1–9. doi:10.1016/j.ajog.2010.06.016

Combs, C. A., Garite, T., Maurel, K., Das, A., & Porto, M. (2011). 17-hydroxyprogesterone caproate for twin pregnancy: A double-blind, randomized clinical trial. *American Journal of Obstetrics and Gynecology, 204*(3), 221.e1–8. doi.org/10.1016/j.ajog.2010.12.042

Conde-Agudelo, A., Belizan, J. M., & Lindmark, G. (2000). Maternal morbidity and mortality associated with multiple gestations. *Obstetrics and Gynecology, 95*(6 Pt. 1), 899–904.

Conde-Agudelo, A., Romero, R., Hassan, S. S., & Yeo, L. (2010). Transvaginal sonographic cervical length for the prediction of spontaneous preterm birth in twin pregnancies: A systematic review and metaanalysis. *American Journal of Obstetrics and Gynecology, 203*(2), 128.e1–12. doi.org/10.1016/j.ajog.2010.02.064

Cristinelli, S., Fresson, J., André, M., & Monnier-Barbarino, P. (2005). Management of delayed-interval delivery in multiple gestations. *Fetal Diagnosis and Therapy, 20*(4), 285–290.

Crowther, C. A. (2009). Caesarean delivery for the second twin. *Cochrane Database of Systematic Reviews*, (1), CD000047. doi:10.1002/14651858.CD000047.

Crowther, C. A., & Han, S. (2010). Hospitalisation and bed rest for multiple pregnancy. *Cochrane Database Systematic Reviews*, (7), CD000110. doi:10.1002/14651858.CD000110.pub2

D'Alton, M. (2004). Infertility and the desire for multiple births. *Fertility and Sterility, 81*(3), 523–525.

D'Alton, M. E. (2010). Delivery of the second twin: Revisiting the age-old dilemma. *Obstetrics and Gynecology, 115*(2 Pt. 1), 221–222. doi:10.1097/AOG.0b013e3181cd3380

Damato, E. G. (2004a). Predictors of prenatal attachment in mothers of twins. *Journal of Obstetric, Gynecologic and Neonatal Nursing, 33*(4), 436–445.

Damato, E. G. (2004b). Prenatal attachment and other correlates of postnatal maternal attachment to twins. *Advances in Neonatal Care, 4*(5), 274–291.

Damato, E. G., Anthony, M. K., & Maloni, J. A. (2009). Correlates of negative and positive mood state in mothers of twins. *Journal of Pediatric Nursing, 24*(5), 369–377. doi:10.1016/j.pedn.2008.05.003

Damato, E. G., Dowling, D. A., Madigan, E. A., & Thanattherakul, C. (2005). Duration of breastfeeding for mothers of twins. *Journal of Obstetric, Gynecologic and Neonatal Nursing, 34*(2), 201–209.

Damato, E. G., Dowling, D. A., Standing, T. S., & Schuster, S. D. (2005). Explanation for cessation of breastfeeding in mothers of twins. *Journal of Human Lactation, 21*(3), 296–304.

Delbaere, I., Verstraelen, H., Goetgeluk, S., Martens, G., Derom, C., De Bacquer, D., . . . Temmerman, M. (2008). Perinatal outcome of twin pregnancies in women of advanced age. *Human Reproduction, 23*(9), 2145–2150. doi:10.1093/humrep/den134

Derom, R., Derom, C., & Vlietinck, R. (1995). Placentation. In L. G. Keith, E. Papiernik, D. M. Keith, & B. Luke (Eds.), *Multiple Pregnancy: Epidemiology, Gestation and Perinatal Outcome.* (pp. 113–128). New York: The Parthenon Publishing Group.

Devoe, L. D. (2008). Antenatal fetal assessment: Multifetal gestation—An overview. *Seminars in Perinatology, 32*(4), 281–287. doi:10.1053/j.semperi.2008.04.011

Dickey, R. P., Taylor, S. N., Lu, P. Y., Sartor, B. M., Storment, J. M., Rye, P. H., . . . Matulich, E. M. (2002). Spontaneous reduction of multiple pregnancy: Incidence and effect on outcome. *American Journal of Obstetrics and Gynecology, 186*(1), 77–83.

Dodd, J. M., & Crowther, C. A. (2005). Evidence-based care of women with a multiple pregnancy. *Best Practice & Research Clinical Obstetrics and Gynaecology, 19*(1), 131–153.

Dodd, J. M., & Crowther, C. A. (2007). Specialised antenatal clinics for women with a multiple pregnancy for improving maternal and infant outcomes. *Cochrane Database of Systematic Reviews,* (2), CD005300. doi:10.1002/14651858.CD005300.pub2

Dodd, J. M., & Crowther, C. A. (2010). Reduction of the number of fetuses for women with triplet and higher order multiple pregnancies. *Cochrane Database of Systematic Reviews,* (2), CD003932. doi:10.1002/14651858.CD003932.

Dodd, J. M., Crowther, C. A., Haslam, R. R., & Robinson, J. S. (2010). Timing of birth for women with a twin pregnancy at term: A randomised controlled trial. *BMC Pregnancy Childbirth, 10,* 68. doi:10.1186/1471-2393-10-68

Eddib, A., Penvose-Yi, J., Shelton, J.A., & Yeh, J. (2007). Triplet gestation outcomes in relation to maternal prepregnancy body mass index and weight gain. *Journal of Maternal, Fetal, and Neonatal Medicine, 20*(7), 515–519.

Eganhouse, D. J., & Peterson, L. A. (1998). Fetal surveillance in multifetal pregnancy. *Journal of Obstetric, Gynecologic and Neonatal Nursing, 27*(3), 312–321.

Elkayam, U., Akhter, M. W., Singh, H., Khan, S., Bitar, F., Hameed, A., & Shotan, A. (2005). Pregnancy-associated cardiomyopathy: Clinical characteristics and a comparison between early and late presentation. *Circulation, 111*(16), 2050–2055.

Elliott, J. P. (2005a). Management of high-order multiple gestations. *Clinics in Perinatology, 32*(2), 387–402.

Elliott, J. P. (2005b). Preterm labor in twins and high-order multiples. *Obstetrics and Gynecology Clinics, 32*(3), 429–439.

Elliott, J. P., & Radin, T. G. (1995). The effect of corticosteroid administration on uterine activity and preterm labor in high-order multiple gestations. *Obstetrics and Gynecology, 85*(2), 250–254.

Ellison, M. A., & Hall, J. E. (2003). Social stigma and compounded losses: Quality-of-life issues for multiple-birth families. *Fertility and Sterility, 80*(2), 405–414.

Ellison, M. A., Hotamisligil, S., Lee, H., Rich-Edwards, J. W., Pang, S. C., & Hall, J. E. (2005). Psychosocial risks associated with multiple births resulting from assisted reproduction. *Fertility and Sterility, 83*(5), 1422–1428.

Evans, M. I., & Britt, D. W. (2010). Multifetal pregnancy reduction: Evolution of the ethical arguments. *Seminars in Reproductive Medicine, 28*(4), 295–302.

Evans, M. I., Ciorica, D., Britt, D. W., & Fletcher, J. C. (2005). Update on selective reduction. *Prenatal Diagnosis, 25*(9), 807–813.

Feldman, D. M., Borgida, A. F., Trymbulak, W. P., Barsoom, M. J., Sanders, M. M., & Rodis, J. F. (2002). Clinical implications of velamentous cord insertion in triplet gestations. *American Journal of Obstetrics and Gynecology, 186*(4), 809–811.

Feldman, R., & Eidelman, A. I. (2004). Parent–infant synchrony and the social–emotional development of triplets. *Developmental Psychology, 40*(6), 1133–1147.

Fell, D. B., Dodds, L., Joseph, K. S., Allen, V. M., & Butler, B. (2006). Risk factors for hyperemesis gravidarum requiring hospital admission during pregnancy. *Obstetrics and Gynecology, 107*(2, Pt. 1), 277–284.

Fesenmeier, M. F., Coppage, K. H., Lambers, D. S., Barton, J. R., & Sibai, B. M. (2005). Acute fatty liver of pregnancy in 3 tertiary care centers. *American Journal of Obstetrics and Gynecology, 192*(5), 1416–1419.

Fox, N. S., Rebarber, A., Klauser, C. K., Roman, A. S., & Saltzman, D. H. (2011). Intrauterine growth restriction in twin pregnancies: Incidence and associated risk factors. *American Journal of Perinatology, 28*(4), 267–272. doi: http://dx.doi.org/10.1055/s-0030-1270116

Fox, N. S., Rebarber, A., Roman, A. S., Klauser, C. K., Peress, D., & Saltzman, D. H. (2010). Weight gain in twin pregnancies and adverse outcomes: Examining the 2009 Institute of Medicine guidelines. *Obstetrics and Gynecology, 116*(1), 100–106. doi:10.1097/AOG.0b013e3181e24afc

Fox, N. S., Saltzman, D. H., Kurtz, H., & Rebarber, A. (2011). Excessive weight gain in term twin pregnancies: Examining the 2009 Institute of Medicine definitions. *Obstetrics and Gynecology, 118*(5):1000-1004. doi:10.1097/AOG.0b013e318232125d.

Francois, K., Ortiz, J., Harris, C., Foley, M. R., & Elliott, J. P. (2005). Is peripartum hysterectomy more common in multiple gestations? *Obstetrics and Gynecology, 105*(6), 1369–1372.

Freda, M. C. (2000). Educational interventions in high-risk pregnancy. In W. R. Cohen (Ed.), *Cherry and Merkatz's Complications of Pregnancy* (pp. 177–184). Philadelphia: Lippincott Williams & Wilkins.

Friedman, E. A., & Sachtleben, M. R. (1964). The effect of uterine overdistention on labor: Multiple pregnancy. *Obstetrics and Gynecology, 23,* 164–172.

Gardner, D. K., Surrey, E., Minjarez, D., Leitz, A., Stevens, J., & Schoolcraft, W. B. (2004). Single blastocyst transfer: A prospective randomized trial. *Fertility and Sterility, 81*(3), 551–555.

Garite, T. J., Clark, R. H., Elliott, J. P., & Thorp, J. A. (2004). Twins and triplets: The effect of plurality and growth on neonatal outcome compared with singleton infants. *American Journal of Obstetrics and Gynecology, 191*(3), 700–707.

Getahun, D., Demissie, K., Lu, S. E., & Rhoads, G. G. (2004). Sudden infant death syndrome among twin births: United States, 1995–1998. *Journal of Perinatology, 24*(9), 544–551.

Gibson, J. L., Macara, L. M., Owen, P., Young, D., Macauley, J., & Mackenzie, F. (2004). Prediction of preterm delivery in twin pregnancy: A prospective, observational study of cervical length and fetal fibronectin testing. *Ultrasound in Obstetrics & Gynecology, 23*(6), 561–566.

Glantz, A., Marschall, H. U., & Mattsson, L. A. (2004). Intrahepatic cholestasis of pregnancy: Relationships between bile acid levels and fetal complication rates. *Hepatology, 40*(2), 467–474.

Goldenberg, R. L., Iams, J. D., Miodovnik, M., Van Dorsten, J. P., Thurnau, G., Bottoms, S., . . . McNellis, D. (1996). The preterm prediction study: Risk factors in twin gestations. National Institute of Child Health and Human Development Maternal-Fetal Medicine Units Network. *American Journal of Obstetrics and Gynecology, 175*(4 Pt. 1), 1047–1053.

Goodnight, W., & Newman, R. (2009). Optimal nutrition for improved twin pregnancy outcome. *Obstetrics and Gynecology, 114*(5), 1121–1134. doi:10.1097/AOG.0b013e3181bb14c8

Gordon, M., Robbins, A., McKenna, D., Howard, B., & Barth, W. (2006). Cervical length assessment as a resource to identify twins at risk for preterm delivery (clarity study). *American Journal of Obstetrics and Gynecology, 195*(6 Suppl. 1), S55.

Graham, G. M. III, & Gaddipati, S. (2005). Diagnosis and management of obstetrical complications unique to multiple gestations. *Seminars in Perinatology, 29*(5), 282–295.

Gromada, K. K., & Bowers, N. A. (2005). *Care of the Multiple-Birth Family: Postpartum Through Infancy* (Nursing Module). New York: March of Dimes Birth Defects Foundation.

Groothuis, J. R., Altemeier, W. A., Robarge, J. P., O'Connor, S., Sandler, H., Vietze, P., & Lustig, J. V. (1982). Increased child abuse in families with twins. *Pediatrics, 70*(5), 769–773.

Guzman, E. R., Walters, C., O'Reilly-Green, C., Meirowitz, N. B., Gipson, K., Nigam, J., & Vintzileos, A. M. (2000). Use of cervical ultrasonography in prediction of spontaneous preterm birth in triplet gestations. *American Journal of Obstetrics and Gynecology, 183*(5), 1108–1113.

Gyamfi, C., Stone, J., & Eddleman, K. A. (2005). Maternal complications of multifetal pregnancy. *Clinics in Perinatology, 32*(2), 431–442.

Gyamfi, C., Mele, L., Wapner, R. J., Spong, C. Y., Peaceman, A., Sorokin, Y., . . . Sibai, B. (2010). The effect of plurality and obesity on betamethasone concentrations in women at risk for preterm delivery. *American Journal of Obstetrics and Gynecology, 203*(3), 219.e1–5. doi:10.1016/j.ajog.2010.04.047

Habli, M., Lim, F. Y., & Crombleholme, T. (2009). Twin-to-twin transfusion syndrome: A comprehensive update. *Clinics in Perinatology, 36*(2), 391–416. doi:10.1016/j.clp.2009.03.003

Hack, K. E., Derks, J. B., Schaap, A. H., Lopriore, E., Elias, S. G., Arabin, B., . . . Visser, G. H. (2009). Perinatal outcome of monoamniotic twin pregnancies. *Obstetrics and Gynecology, 113* (2 Pt. 1), 353–360. doi:10.1097/AOG.0b013e318195bd57

Hanson, L. (2010). Risk management in intrapartum fetal monitoring: Accidental recording of the maternal heart rate. *Journal of Perinatal & Neonatal Nursing, 24*(1), 7–9. doi:10.1097/JPN.0b013e3181cc3a95

Hardardottir, H., Kelly, K., Bork, M. D., Cusick, W., Campbell, W. A., & Rodis, J. F. (1996). Atypical presentation of preeclampsia in high-order multifetal gestations. *Obstetrics and Gynecology, 87*(3), 370–374.

Harkness, U. F., & Crombleholme, T. M. (2005). Twin–twin transfusion syndrome: Where do we go from here? *Seminars in Perinatology, 29*(5), 296–304.

Healy, A. J., & Gaddipati, S. (2005). Intrapartum management of twins: Truths and controversies. *Clinics in Perinatology, 32*(2), 455–473.

Hediger, M. L., Luke, B., Gonzalez-Quintero, V. H., Martin, D., Nugent, C., Witter, F. R., . . . Newman, R. B. (2006). Fetal growth rates and the very preterm delivery of twins. *American Journal of Obstetrics and Gynecology, 193*(4), 1498–1507.

Hillman, S. C., Morris, R. K., & Kilby, M. D. (2010). Single twin demise: Consequence for survivors. *Seminars in Fetal and Neonatal Medicine, 15*(6), 319–326. doi.org/10.1016/j.siny.2010.05.004,

Hogle, K. L., Hutton, E. K., McBrien, K. A., Barrett, J. F., & Hannah, M. E. (2003). Cesarean delivery for twins: A systematic review and meta-analysis. *American Journal of Obstetrics and Gynecology, 188*(1), 220–227.

Hutchison, B. L, Stewart, A. W., & Mitchell, E. A. (2010). The prevalence of cobedding and SIDS-related child care practices in twins. *European Journal of Pediatrics, 169*(12), 1477–1485. doi:10.1007/s00431-010-1246-z

Ingram Cooke, R. W. (2010). Does neonatal and infant neurodevelopmental morbidity of multiples and singletons differ? *Seminars in Fetal & Neonatal Medicine, 15*(6), 362–366. doi:10.1016/j.siny.2010.06.003

Institute of Medicine. (2009). *Weight Gain During Pregnancy: Reexamining the Guidelines*. Washington, DC: The National Academies Press.

International Committee for Monitoring Assisted Reproductive Technology, de Mouzon, J., Lancaster, P., Nygren, K. G., Sullivan, E., Zegers-Hochschild, F., . . . Adamson, D. (2009). World collaborative report on Assisted Reproductive Technology, 2002. *Human Reproduction, 24*(9), 2310–2320. doi:10.1093/humrep/dep098

Jackson, K. M., & Mele, N. L. (2009). Twin-to-twin transfusion syndrome: What nurses need to know. *Nursing for Women's Health, 13*(3), 224–233. doi:10.1111/j.1751-486X.2009.01423.x

Jain, T., Missmer, S. A., & Hornstein, M. D. (2004). Trends in embryo-transfer practice and in outcomes of the use of assisted reproductive technology in the United States. *New England Journal of Medicine, 350*(16), 1639–1645.

Johnson, C. D., & Zhang, J. (2002). Survival of other fetuses after a fetal death in twin or triplet pregnancies. *Obstetrics and Gynecology, 99*(5 Pt. 1), 698–703.

Kahn, B., Lumey, L. H., Zybert, P. A., Lorenz, J. M., Cleary-Goldman, J., D'Alton, M. E., & Robinson, J. N. (2003). Prospective risk of fetal death in singleton, twin, and triplet gestations: Implications for practice. *Obstetrics and Gynecology, 102*(4), 685–692.

Källen, B., Finnstrom, O., Nygren, K. G., & Olausson, P. O. (2005). Temporal trends in multiple births after in vitro fertilisation in Sweden, 1982–2001: A register study. *British Medical Journal, 331*(7513), 382–383.

Kathiresan, A. S., Roca, L. E., II, Istwan, N., Desch, C., Cordova, Y. C., Tudela, F. J., & Gonzalez-Quintero, V. H. (2011). The influence of maternal age on pregnancy outcome in nulliparous women with twin gestation. *American Journal of Perinatology, 28*(5), 355–360. doi:http://dx.doi.org/10.1055/s-0030-1270117

Kent, E. M., Breathnach, F. M., Gillan, J. E., McAuliffe, F. M., Geary, M. P., Daly, S., . . . Malone, F. D. (2011). Placental cord insertion and birthweight discordance in twin pregnancies: Results of the national prospective ESPRiT Study. *American Journal of Obstetrics and Gynecology, 205*(4), 376.e1–376.e7. doi:10.1016/j.ajog.2011.06.077

Klein, V. R. (2002). Maternal complications. In L. G. Keith & I. Blickstein (Eds.), *Triplet Pregnancies and Their Consequences* (pp. 215–224). New York: The Parthenon Publishing Group.

Klock, S. C. (2001). The transition to parenthood. In I. Blickstein & L. G. Keith (Eds.), *Iatrogenic Multiple Pregnancy: Clinical Implications* (pp. 225–234). New York: The Parthenon Publishing Group.

Klock, S. C. (2004). Psychological adjustment to twins after infertility. *Best Practice & Research Clinical Obstetrics & Gynaecology, 18*(4), 645–656.

Knox, E., & Martin, W. (2010). Multiples clinic: A model for antenatal care. *Seminars in Fetal and Neonatal Medicine, 15*(6), 357–361. doi.org/10.1016/j.siny.2010.07.001

Kontopoulos, E. V., Ananth, C. V., Smulian, J. C., & Vintzileos, A. M. (2004). The impact of route of delivery and presentation on twin neonatal and infant mortality: A population-based study in the USA, 1995–97. *Journal of Maternal-Fetal & Neonatal Medicine, 15*(4), 219–224.

Krantz, D. A., Hallahan, T., He, K., Sherwin, J., & Evans, M. I. (2011). First trimester screening in triplets. *American Journal of Obstetrics & Gynecology, 205*(4), 364.e1–364.e5. doi:10.1016/j.ajog.2011.06.107

Kuleva, M., Youssef, A., Maroni, E., Contro, E., Pilu, G., Rizzo, N., . . . Ghi, T. (2011). Maternal cardiac function in normal twin pregnancy: A longitudinal study. *Ultrasound in Obstetrics & Gynecology, 38*(5), 575–580. doi:10.1002/uog.8936

Lai, N. M., Foong, S. C., Foong, W. C., & Tan, K. (2010). Co-bedding in neonatal nursery for promoting growth and neurodevelopment in stable preterm twins. *Cochrane Database of Systematic Reviews*, (1), CD008313. doi:10.1002/14651858.CD008313

Lam, F., & Gill, P. (2005a). β-Agonist tocolytic therapy. *Obstetrics and Gynecology Clinics, 32*(3), 457–484.

Lam, F., & Gill, P. (2005b). Inhibition of preterm labor and subcutaneous terbutaline therapy. In I. Blickstein & L. G. Keith (Eds.), *Multiple Pregnancy: Epidemiology, Gestation and Perinatal Outcome* (2nd ed., pp. 601–620). New York: Taylor and Francis.

Langkamp, D. L., & Girardet, R. G. (2006). Primary care for twins and higher order multiples. *Current Problems in Pediatric and Adolescent Health Care, 36*(2), 47–67.

Lee, H. C., Gould, J. B., Boscardin, W. J., El-Sayed, Y. Y., & Blumenfeld, Y. J. (2011). Trends in cesarean delivery for twin births in the United States: 1995–2008. *Obstetrics and Gynecology, 118*(5), 1095–1101. doi:10.1097/AOG.0b013e3182318651

Leese, B., & Denton, J. (2010). Attitudes towards single embryo transfer, twin and higher order pregnancies in patients undergoing infertility treatment: A review. *Human Fertility: Journal of the British Fertility Society, 13*(1) 28–34. doi:10.3109/14647270903586364

Leonard, L. G. (1998). Depression and anxiety disorders during multiple pregnancy and parenthood. *Journal of Obstetric, Gynecologic and Neonatal Nursing, 27*(3), 329–337.

Leonard, L. G. (2002). Prenatal behavior of multiples: Implications for families and nurses. *Journal of Obstetric, Gynecologic and Neonatal Nursing, 31*(3), 248–255.

Leonard L. G., & Denton, J. (2006). Preparation for parenting multiple birth children. *Early Human Development, 82*(6), 371–378.

Lim, A. C., Hegeman, M. A., Huis In 't Veld, M. A., Opmeer, B. C., Bruinse, H. W., & Mol, B. W. (2011). Cervical length measurement for the prediction of preterm birth in multiple pregnancies: A systematic review and bivariate meta-analysis. *Ultrasound in Obstetrics & Gynecology, 38*(1), 10–17. doi:10.1002/uog.9013

Little, C. M. (2010). Nursing considerations in the case of multifetal pregnancy reduction. *MCN, The American Journal of Maternal/Child Nursing, 35*(3), 166–171. doi:10.1097/NMC.0b013e3181d765bc

Luke, B. (2004). Improving multiple pregnancy outcomes with nutritional interventions. *Clinical Obstetrics and Gynecology, 47*, 146–162.

Luke, B. (2005). Nutrition and multiple gestations. *Seminars in Perinatology, 29*(5), 349–354.

Luke, B., & Brown, M. B. (2007). Contemporary risks of maternal morbidity and adverse outcomes with increasing maternal age and plurality. *Fertility and Sterility, 88*(2), 283–293.

Luke, B., Brown, M. B., Misiunas, R., Anderson, E., Nugent, C., van de Ven, C., . . . Gogliotti, S. (2003). Specialized prenatal care and maternal and infant outcomes in twin pregnancy. *American Journal of Obstetrics and Gynecology, 189*(4), 934–938.

MacKay, A. P., Berg, C. J., King, J. C., Duran, C., & Chang, J. (2006). Pregnancy-related mortality among women with multifetal pregnancies. *Obstetrics & Gynecology, 107*(3), 563–568.

Maifeld, M., Hahn, S., Titler, M. G., & Mullen, M. (2003). Decision making regarding multifetal reduction. *Journal of Obstetric, Gynecologic, and Neonatal Nursing, 32*(3), 357–369.

Malone, F. D., & D'Alton, M. E. (2004). Multiple gestations: Clinical characteristics and management. In R. K. Creasy & R. Resnik (Eds.), *Maternal–Fetal Medicine* (5th ed., pp 513–538). Philadelphia: WB Saunders

Malloy, M. H., & Freeman, D. H. Jr. (1999). Sudden infant death syndrome among twins. *Archives of Pediatrics & Adolescent Medicine, 153*(7), 736–740.

Maloni, J. A. (2010). Antepartum bed rest for pregnancy complications: Efficacy and safety for preventing preterm birth. *Biological Research for Nursing, 12*(2), 106–124. doi:10.1177/1099800410375978

Maloni, J. A., Brezinski-Tomasi, J. E., & Johnson, L. A. (2001). Antepartum bedrest: Effect upon the family. *Journal of Obstetrics, Gynecologic and Neonatal Nursing, 30*(2), 165–173.

Maloni, J. A., Margevicius, S. P., & Damato, E. G. (2006). Multiple gestations: Side effects of antepartum bed rest. *Biological Research for Nursing, 8*(2), 115–128.

Maloni, J. A., & Schneider, B. S. (2002). Inactivity: Symptoms associated with gastrocnemius muscle disuse during pregnancy. *AACN Clinical Issues, 13*(2), 248–262.

Malmstrom, P. M., & Biale, R. (1990). An agenda for meeting the special needs of multiple birth families. *Acta Geneticae Medicae et Gemellolgiae, 39*(4), 507–514.

Marino, T., Goudas, L. C., Steinbok, V., Craigo, S. D., & Yarnell, R. W. (2001). The anesthetic management of triplet cesarean delivery: A retrospective case series of maternal outcomes. *Anesthesia and Analgesia, 93*(4), 991–995.

Martin, J. A., Hamilton, B. E., Ventura, S. J., Osterman, M. J. K., Kirmeyer, S., Mathews, T. J., & Wilson, E. C. (2011). Births: Final data for 2009. *National Vital Statistics Reports, 60*(1), 1–72. http://www.cdc.gov/nchs/data/nvsr/nvsr60/nvsr60_01.pdf

Martin, J. A., & Park, M. M. (1999). Trends in twin and triplet births: 1980–97. *National Vital Statistics Reports, 47*(24), 1–16.

Mathews, T. J., & MacDorman, M. F. (2008). Infant mortality statistics from the 2005 period linked birth/infant death data set. *National Vital Statistics Reports, 57*(2), 1–31.

Maymon, R., Neeman, O., Shulman, A., Rosen, H., & Herman, A. (2005). Current concepts of Down syndrome screening tests in assisted reproduction twin pregnancies: Another double trouble. *Prenatal Diagnosis, 25*(9), 746–750.

McGrail, C., & Bryant, D. (2005). Intertwin time interval: How it affects the immediate neonatal outcome of the second twin. *American Journal of Obstetrics and Gynecology, 192*(5), 1420–1422.

McGrath, J. M., Samra, H. A., Zukowsky, K., & Baker, B. (2010). Parenting after infertility: Issues for families and infants. *MCN. The American Journal of Maternal Child Nursing, 35*(3), 156–164. doi:10.1097/NMC.0b013e3181d7657d

Medoff-Cooper, B., Bakewell-Sachs, S., Buus-Frank, M. E., & Santa-Donato, A. (2005). The AWHONN Near-Term Infant Initiative: A conceptual framework for optimizing health for near-term infants. *Journal of Obstetric, Gynecologic and Neonatal Nursing, 34*(6), 66–671.

Meikle, S. F., Steiner, C. A., Zhang, J., & Lawrence, W. L. (2005). A national estimate of the elective primary cesarean delivery rate. *Obstetrics and Gynecology, 105*(4), 751–756.

Menon, D. K. (2005). A retrospective study of the accuracy of sonographic chorionicity determination in twin pregnancies. *Twin Research and Human Genetics, 8*(3), 259–261.

Mian, A. I. (2005). Depression in pregnancy and the postpartum period: Balancing adverse effects of untreated illness with treatment risks. *Journal of Psychiatric Practice, 11*(6), 389–396.

Montgomery, K. S., Cubera, S., Belcher, C., Patrick, D., Funderburk, H., Melton, C., & Fastenau, M. (2005). Childbirth education for multiple pregnancy: Part 1: Prenatal considerations. *Journal of Perinatal Education, 14*(2), 26–35.

Moragianni, V. A., Aronis, K. N., & Craparo, F. J. (2011). Biweekly ultrasound assessment of cervical shortening in triplet pregnancies and the effect of cerclage placement. *Ultrasound in Obstetrics & Gynecology, 37*(5), 617–618. doi:10.1002/uog.8905

Morin, L., & Lim, K. (2011). Ultrasound in twin pregnancies. *Journal of Obstetrics and Gynaecology Canada, 33*(6), 643–656.

Morrison, J. C., & Chauhan, S. P. (2003). Current status of home uterine activity monitoring. *Clinics in Perinatology, 30*(4), 757–801.

Murali, S., & Baldisseri, M. R. (2005). Peripartum cardiomyopathy. *Critical Care Medicine, 33*(Suppl. 10), 340–346.

National Association of Neonatal Nurses. (2009). NANN Position Statement 3045: Cobedding of twins or higher-order multiples. *Advances in Neonatal Care, 9*(6), 307–313.

Newman, R. B., Iams, J. D., Das, A., Goldenberg, R. L., Meis, P., Moawad, A., . . . Fischer, M. (2006). A prospective masked observational study of uterine contraction frequency in twins. *American Journal of Obstetrics and Gynecology, 195*(6), 1564–1570.

Nichols, A. A. (2005). Cholestasis of pregnancy: A review of the evidence. *Journal of Perinatal & Neonatal Nursing, 19*(3), 217–226.

Niebyl, J. R. (2010). Clinical practice. Nausea and vomiting in pregnancy. *New England Journal of Medicine, 363*(16), 1544–1550.

Norwitz, E. R., Edusa, V., & Park, J. S. (2005). Maternal physiology and complications of multiple pregnancy. *Seminars in Perinatology, 29*(5), 338–348.

O'Callaghan, M. E., Maclennan, A. H., Gibson, C. S., McMichael, G. L., Haan, E. A., Broadbent, J. L., . . . Dekker, G. A. (2011). Epidemiologic associations with cerebral palsy. *Obstetrics and Gynecology, 118*(3), 576–582. doi:10.1097/AOG.0b013e31822ad2dc

Oleszczuk, J. J., Keith, L. G., & Oleszczuk, A. K. (2005). The paradox of old maternal age in multiple pregnancies. *Obstetric and Gynecologic Clinics of North America, 32*(1), 69–80.

Ong, S. S., Zamora, J., Khan, K. S., & Kilby, M. D. (2006). Prognosis for the co-twin following single-twin death: A systematic review. *British Journal of Obstetrics and Gynaecology, 113,* 992e8.

Ostfeld, B. M., Smith, R. H., Hiatt, M., & Hegyi, T. (2000). Maternal behavior toward premature twins: Implications for development. *Twin Research, 3*(4), 234–241.

Oyelese, Y., Ananth, C. V., Smulian, J. C., & Vintzileos, A. M. (2005). Delayed interval delivery in twin pregnancies in the United States: Impact on perinatal mortality and morbidity. *American Journal of Obstetrics and Gynecology, 192*(2), 439–444.

Pandian, Z., Bhattacharya, S., Ozturk, O., Serour, G., & Templeton, A. (2009). Number of embryos for transfer following in-vitro fertilisation or intra-cytoplasmic sperm injection. *Cochrane Database of Systematic Reviews,* (2), CD003416. doi:10.1002/14651858.CD003416.pub3

Paramasivam, G., Wimalasundera, R., Wiechec, M., Zhang, E., Saeed, F., & Kumar, S. (2010). Radiofrequency ablation for selective reduction in complex monochorionic pregnancies. *British Journal of Obstetrics and Gynaecology, 117*(10), 1294–1298. doi:10.1111/j.1471-0528.2010.02624.x

Pector, E. A. (2004). How bereaved multiple-birth parents cope with hospitalization, homecoming, disposition for deceased, and attachment to survivors. *Journal of Perinatology, 24*(11), 714–722.

Pector, E. A., & Smith-Levitin, M. (2002). Mourning and psychological issues in multiple birth loss. *Seminars in Neonatology, 7*(3), 247–256.

Peitsch, W. K., Keefer, C. H., LaBrie, R. A., & Mulliken, J. B. (2002). Incidence of cranial asymmetry in healthy newborns. *Pediatrics, 110*(6), e72.

Perinatal Services British Columbia (formerly British Columbia Reproductive Care Program). (2007). Breastfeeding multiples, nutrition, part III. Retrieved from http://www.perinatalservicesbc.ca/NR /rdonlyres/D72E27F9-11A1-4E97-8E7D-DF60B5EFE57C/0 /BFGuidelinesBreastfeedingMultiplesPartIII3.pdf

Pharoah, P. O. (2002). Neurological outcome in twins. *Seminars in Neonatology, 7*(3), 223–230.

Platt, M. J., & Pharoah, P. O. (2003). The epidemiology of sudden infant death syndrome. *Archives of Disease in Childhood, 88*(1), 27–29.

Practice Committee of the American Society for Reproductive Medicine. (2012). Multiple gestation associated with infertility therapy: An American Society for Reproductive Medicine Practice Committee opinion. *Fertility and Sterility, 97*(4), 825–834.

Practice Committee of the American Society for Reproductive Medicine & Practice Committee of the Society for Assisted Reproductive Technology. (2013). Criteria for number of embryos to transfer: A committee opinion. *Fertility and Sterility, 99*(1), 44–46. doi:10.1016/j.fertnstert.2012.09.038

Ramsey, P. S., & Repke, J. T. (2003). Intrapartum management of multifetal pregnancies. *Seminars in Perinatology, 27*(1), 54–72.

Rand, L., Eddleman, K. A., & Stone, J. (2005). Long-term outcomes in multiple gestations. *Clinics in Perinatology, 32*(2), 495–513.

Rao, A., Sairam, S., & Shehata, H. (2004). Obstetric complications of twin pregnancies. *Best Practice & Research Clinical Obstetrics & Gynaecology, 18*(4), 557–576.

Rauh-Hain, J. A., Rana, S., Tamez, H., Wang, A., Cohen, B., Cohen, A., . . . Thadhani, R. (2009). Risk for developing gestational diabetes in women with twin pregnancies. *Journal of Maternal-Fetal & Neonatal Medicine, 22*(4), 293–299. doi:10.1080/14767050802663194

Rebarber, A., Roman, A. S., Istwan, N., Rhea, D., & Stanziano, G. (2005). Prophylactic cerclage in the management of triplet pregnancies. *American Journal of Obstetrics and Gynecology, 193* (3 Pt. 2), 1193–1196.

Richter, J. E. (2003). Gastroesophageal reflux disease during pregnancy. *Gastroenterology Clinics of North America, 32*(1), 235–261.

Roberts, D., & Dalziel, S. (2006). Antenatal corticosteroids for accelerating fetal lung maturation for women at risk of preterm birth. *Cochrane Database Systematic Reviews,* (3), CD004454.

Roberts, D., Gates, S., Kilby, M., & Neilson, J. P. (2008). Interventions for twin-twin transfusion syndrome: A Cochrane review *Ultrasound in Obstetrics & Gynecology, 31*(6), 701–711.

Robinson, C., & Chauhan, S. P. (2004). Intrapartum management of twins. *Clinical Obstetrics and Gynecology, 47*(1), 248–262.

Roca-de Bes, M., Gutierrez-Maldonado, J., Gris-Martínez, J. M. (2011). Comparative study of the psychosocial risks associated with families with multiple births resulting from assisted reproductive technology (ART) and without ART. *Fertility and Sterility, 96*(1), 170–174. doi:10.1016/j.fertnstert.2011.05.007

Rode, L., Klein, K., Nicolaides, K., Krampl-Bettelheim, E., & Tabor, A. (2011). Prevention of preterm delivery in twin gestations (PREDICT): A multicentre randomised placebo-controlled trial on the effect of vaginal micronised progesterone. *Ultrasound in Obstetrics & Gynecology, 38* (3), 272–280. doi:10.1002/uog.9093

Roem, K. (2003). Nutritional management of multiple pregnancies. *Twin Research, 6*(6), 514–519.

Rohde, A., Dembinski, J., & Dorn, C. (2003). Mirtazapine (Remergil) for treatment resistant hyperemesis gravidarum: Rescue of a twin pregnancy. *Archives of Gynecology and Obstetrics, 268*(3), 219–221.

Rosello-Soberon, M. E., Fuentes-Chaparro, L., & Casanueva, E. (2005). Twin pregnancies: Eating for three? Maternal nutrition update. *Nutrition Reviews, 63*(9), 295–302.

Ruiz, R. J., Brown, C. E., Peters, M. T., & Johnston, A. B. (2001). Specialized care for twin gestations: Improving newborn outcomes and reducing costs. *Journal of Obstetric, Gynecologic and Neonatal Nursing, 30*(1), 52–60.

Rustico, M. A., Baietti, M. G., Coviello, D., Orlandi, E., & Nicolini, U. (2005). Managing twins discordant for fetal anomaly. *Prenatal Diagnosis, 25*(9), 766–771.

Salihu, H. M., Bekan, B., Aliyu, M. H., Rouse, D. J., Kirby, R. S., & Alexander, G. R. (2005). Perinatal mortality associated with abruptio placenta in singletons and multiples. *American Journal of Obstetrics and Gynecology, 193*(1), 198–203.

Salihu, H. M., Garces, I. C., Sharma, P. P., Kristensen, S., Ananth, C. V., & Kirby, R. S. (2005). Stillbirth and infant mortality among Hispanic singletons, twins, and triplets in the United States. *Obstetrics and Gynecology, 106*(4), 789–796.

Schreiner-Engel, P., Walther, V. N., Mindes, J., Lynch, L., & Berkowitz, R. L. (1995). First-trimester multifetal pregnancy reduction: Acute and persistent psychologic reactions. *American Journal of Obstetrics and Gynecology, 172*(2 Pt. 1), 541–547.

Schiff, E., Cohen, S. B., Dulitzky, M., Novikov, I., Friedman, S. A., Mashiach, S., & Lipitz, S. (1998). Progression of labor in twin versus singleton gestations. *American Journal of Obstetrics and Gynecology, 179*(5), 1181–1185.

Sentilhes, L., Goffinet, F., Talbot, A., Diguet, A., Verspyck, E., Cabrol, D., & Marpeau, L. (2007). Attempted vaginal versus planned cesarean delivery in 195 breech first twin pregnancies. *Acta Obstetricia et Gynecologica Scandinavica, 86*(1), 55–60.

Sepulveda, W., Wong, A. E., & Casasbuenas, A. (2009). Nuchal translucency and nasal bone in first-trimester ultrasound screening for aneuploidy in multiple pregnancies. *Ultrasound in Obstetrics & Gynecology, 33*(2), 152–156. doi:10.1002/uog.6222

Shetty, A., & Smith, A. P. (2005). The sonographic diagnosis of chorionicity. *Prenatal Diagnosis, 25*(9), 735–739.

Shinagawa, S., Suzuki, S., Chihara, H., Otsubo, Y., Takeshita, T., & Araki, T. (2005). Maternal basal metabolic rate in twin pregnancy. *Gynecologic and Obstetric Investigation, 60*(3), 145–148.

Silver, R. K., Haney, E. I., Grobman, W. A., MacGregor, S. N., Casele, H. L., & Neerhof, M. G. (2000). Comparison of active phase labor between triplet, twin and singleton gestations. *Journal of the Society for Gynecologic Investigation, 7*(5), 297–300.

Simpson, K. R. (2004). Monitoring the preterm fetus during labor. *MCN The American Journal of Maternal Child Nursing, 29*(6), 380–388.

Smith-Levitin, M., Skupski, D. W., & Chervenak, F. A. (1999). Multifetal pregnancies: Epidemiology, clinical characteristics and management. In E. A. Reece & J. C. Hobbins (Eds.), *Medicine of the Fetus and Mother* (2nd ed., pp. 243–264). Philadelphia: Lippincott-Raven

Spong, C. Y., Mercer, B. M., D'Alton, M., Kilpatrick, S., Blackwell, S., & Saade, G. (2011). Timing of indicated late-preterm and early-term birth. *Obstetrics and Gynecology, 118*(2, Pt. 1), 323–333. doi:10.1097/AOG.0b013e3182255999

Stock, S., & Norman, J. (2010). Preterm and term labour in multiple pregnancies. *Seminars in Fetal & Neonatal Medicine, 15*(6), 336–341. doi.org/10.1016/j.siny.2010.06.006

Stone, J., Ferrara, L., Kamrath, J., Getrajdman, J., Berkowitz, R., Moshier, E., & Eddleman, K. (2008). Contemporary outcomes with the latest 1000 cases of multifetal pregnancy reduction (MPR). *American Journal of Obstetrics & Gynecology, 199*(4), 406.e1–4. doi:10.1016/j.ajog.2008.06.017

Stammler-Safar, M., Ott, J., Weber, S., & Krampl, E. (2010). Sexual behaviour of women with twin pregnancies. *Twin Research and Human Genetics, 13*(4), 383–388.

Swanson, P. B., Kane, R. T., Pearsall-Jones, J. G., Swanson, C. F., & Croft, M. L. (2009). How couples cope with the death of a twin or higher order multiple. *Twin Research and Human Genetics, 12*(4), 392–402.

Taffel, S. M. (1995). Demographic trends: USA. In L. G. Keith, E. Papiernik, D. M. Keith, & B. Luke (Eds.), *Multiple Pregnancy: Epidemiology, Gestation and Perinatal Outcome* (pp. 133–144). New York: The Parthenon Publishing Group.

Trevett, T., & Johnson, A. (2005). Monochorionic twin pregnancies. *Clinics in Perinatology, 32*(2), 475–494.

U.S. Food and Drug Administration. (2011). *New Warnings Against Use of Terbutaline to Treat Preterm Labor* (Safety Announcement. FDA Drug Safety Communication). Retrieved from http://www.fda.gov/Drugs/DrugSafety/ucm243539.htm

van Klink, J. M., Koopman, H. M., Oepkes, D., Walther, F. J., & Lopriore, E. (2011). Long-term neurodevelopmental outcome in monochorionic twins after fetal therapy. *Early Human Development, 87*(9), 601–606. doi:10.1016/j.earlhumdev.2011.07.007

van Oppenraaij, R. H., Jauniaux, E., Christiansen, O. B., Horcajadas, J. A., Farquharson, R. G., & Exalto, N. (2009). Predicting adverse obstetric outcome after early pregnancy events and complications: A review. *Human Reproduction Update, 15*(4), 409–421. doi:10.1093/humupd/dmp009

Varner, M. W., Leindecker, S., Spong, C. Y., Moawad, A. H., Hauth, J. C., Landon, M. B., . . . Gabbe, S. G. (2005). The Maternal-Fetal Medicine Unit cesarean registry: Trial of labor with a twin gestation. *American Journal of Obstetrics and Gynecology, 193*(1), 135–140.

Vilska, S., Unkila-Kalliom, L., Punamäkim, R. L., Poikkeusm, P., Repokari, L. M., Sinkkonenm, J., . . . Tulppalam, M. (2009). Mental health of mothers and fathers of twins conceived via assisted reproduction treatment: A 1-year prospective study. *Human Reproduction, 24*(2), 367–377. doi:10.1093/humrep/den427

Vintzileos, A. M., Ananth, C. V., Kontopoulos, E., & Smulian, J. C. (2005). Mode of delivery and risk of stillbirth and infant mortality in triplet gestations: United States, 1995 through 1998. *American Journal of Obstetrics and Gynecology, 192*(2), 464–469.

Wadhawan, R., Ohm, W., Vohrm, B. R., Wragem, L., Dasm, A., Bellm, E. F., . . . Higgins, R. D. (2011). Neurodevelopmental outcomes of triplets or higher-order extremely low birth weight infants. *Pediatrics, 127*(3), e654–660. doi:10.1542/peds.2010-2646

Walker, M. C., Murphy, K. E., Pan, S., Yang, Q., & Wen, S. W. (2004). Adverse maternal outcomes in multifetal pregnancies. *BJOG: An International Journal of Obstetrics and Gynaecology, 111*(11), 1294–1296.

Wang, H. L., & Yu Chao, Y. M. (2006). Lived experiences of Taiwanese women with multifetal pregnancies who receive fetal reduction. *The Journal of Nursing Research, 14*(2), 143–154.

Weber, M. A., & Sebire, N. J. (2010). Genetics and developmental pathology of twinning. *Seminars in Fetal & Neonatal Medicine, 15*(6), 313–318. doi.org/10.1016/j.siny.2010.06.002

Wen, S. W., Demissie, K., Yang, Q., & Walker, M. C. (2004). Maternal morbidity and obstetric complications in triplet pregnancies and quadruplet and higher-order multiple pregnancies. *American Journal of Obstetrics and Gynecology, 191*(1), 254–258.

Wen, S. W., Fung, K. F., Huang, L., Demissie, K., Joseph, K. S., Allen, A. C., & Kramer, M. S. (2005). Fetal and neonatal mortality among twin gestations in a Canadian population: The effect of intrapair birth weight discordance. *American Journal of Perinatology, 22*(5), 279–286.

Wimalasundera, R. C. (2010). Selective reduction and termination of multiple pregnancies. *Seminars in Fetal & Neonatal Medicine, 15*(6), 327–335. doi.org/10.1016/j.siny.2010.08.002

Wright, V. C., Schieve, L. A., Reynolds, M. A., & Jeng, G. (2005). Assisted reproductive technology surveillance–United States, 2002. *Morbidity and Mortality Weekly Report. Surveillance Summaries, 54*(2), 1–24.

Zhang, J., Hamilton, B., Martin, J., & Trumble, A. (2004). Delayed interval delivery and infant survival: A population-based study. *American Journal of Obstetrics and Gynecology, 191*(2), 470–476.

Zhang, J., Meikle, S., Grainger, D. A., & Trumble, A. (2002). Multifetal pregnancy in older women and perinatal outcomes. *Fertility and Sterility, 78*(3), 562–568.

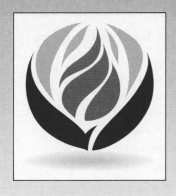

CHAPTER 12

Obesity in Pregnancy

Mary Ann Maher

SIGNIFICANCE AND INCIDENCE

Obesity is characterized by having very high body fat content relative to lean body mass. The National Heart, Lung, and Blood Institute (NHLBI), in cooperation with the National Institute of Diabetes and Digestive and Kidney Diseases (NIDDK) (NHLBI, 1998) and the World Health Organization (WHO; 2011), define obesity as a body mass index (BMI) of ≥ 30 kg/m^2. Normal body weight is defined as a BMI or weight (kg)/height (m^2) of 18.5 to 24.9, overweight as BMI of 25.0 to 29.9, obese as BMI of 30.0 to 39.9, and extremely (morbidly) obese as BMI ≥ 40.0 (NHLBI, 1998; WHO, 2011). See Table 12–1 for a summary of BMI criteria for classifying weight status.

Obesity has become a worldwide public health problem, prevalent in both developed and developing countries (Knight, Kurinczuk, Spark, & Brocklehurst, 2010). There are more than 1.5 billion overweight adults in the world; 300 million meet criteria for obesity (WHO, 2011). Approximately 65% of the world's population live in countries where overweight and obesity are responsible for more deaths than underweight (WHO, 2011). The global epidemic of obesity is of great concern, especially in the United States, where two thirds of adults are either overweight or obese as compared to slightly under half of adults in developing countries with weight problems (Berrington de Gonzalez et al., 2010). Based on data from the 2009 to 2010 National Health and Nutrition Examination Survey (Ogden, Carroll, Kit, & Flegal, 2012), it is estimated that 68% of adults 20 years of age or older in the United States are overweight, 35.7% are obese, and 5.7% are extremely obese. There are currently more obese adults in the United States than at any other time in our history. Over the last 30 years, the rate of obesity has doubled for adults and tripled for children (Gunatilake & Perlow, 2011). There now appears to be a slowing of the rate of increase or even a leveling off of obesity, particularly for women (Flegal, Carroll, Ogden, & Curtin, 2010). While there has been a considerable increase in obesity among men and boys of the last decade, prevalance of obesity among women and girls has remained essentially the same (Flegal et al., 2010). Based on comparison of data from 1999 to 2000 and 2009 to 2010, differences in prevalence of obesity between men and women have diminished significantly (Flegal et al., 2010; Ogden et al., 2012). There was no change in the prevalence of obesity in the United States among adults or children from 2007–2008 to 2009–2010 (Ogden et al., 2012). In the United States, risk of becoming overweight is approximately 50%; risk of obesity is estimated to be 25% (Duran, 2011). See Display 12–1 for a list of risk factors for developing obesity (Duran, 2011).

While the etiology of obesity may be very basic, for example, an energy imbalance due to taking in more calories than energy expended, there are multiple complex factors contributing to the increase in obesity in the United States. These factors occur at all social, economic, and environmental levels (Centers for Disease Control and Prevention [CDC], 2011). Body weight is the result of genes, metabolism, behavior, environment, culture, and socioeconomic status (Chescheir, 2011). A significant factor related to the current prevalence of obesity is the evolution of the human species, which occurred in an environment where few calories were available and a significant expenditure of energy

Table 12–1. BODY MASS INDEX CRITERIA FOR CLASSIFYING WEIGHT STATUS

BMI Formulas

weight (lb)/height (in^2 × 703) or weight (kg)/height (m^2)

NHLBI Terminology	BMI Categories	WHO Classification
Obesity class 3	>40	Morbidly obese (obese class 3)
Obesity class 2	35.0–39.9	Obesity (obese class 2)
Obesity class 1	30.0–34.9	Obesity (obese class 1)
Overweight	25.0–29.9	Pre-obese
Normal	20.0–24.9	Normal range
Lean	<20	Underweight

NHLBI, National Heart, Lung, and Blood Institute;
WHO, World Health Organization.
From James, D., & Maher, M. (2009). Caring for the extremely obese woman during pregnancy and birth. *MCN: The American Journal of Maternal Child Nursing*, *34*(1), 24–30.

DISPLAY 12–1

Risk Factors for Obesity

Low metabolic rate
Increased carbohydrate, oxidation, and insulin resistance
Polycystic ovarian syndrome
Cushing syndrome
Mother smoked during pregnancy
Mother had diabetes during pregnancy
Born of a multiple pregnancy
Born premature
Born small-for-gestational-age babies
Born large-for-gestational-age babies
Breastfed less than 3 months
Recent marriage
Smoking cessation
Lower socioeconomic status
Low education level
Overweight parents
Overweight during childhood or adolescence
Mother's lack of monitoring of child's eating habits
Low level of physical activity
High dietary intake of fat
Sedentary lifestyle
Lack of regular exercise
Pregnancy
Menopause

Adapted from Duran, E. H. (2011). Obesity as an epidemic: Causes, morbidities and reproductive performance. *Proceedings in Obstetrics and Gynecology, 1*(3), 8–16.

was needed to acquire those calories (Phelan, 2010). To ensure survival of the species, humans needed to store fat for times when resources were limited. Women specifically needed to have adequate stores of fat to sustain a pregnancy and breastfeed their newborns (Phelan, 2010). As a result, the human body is quite efficient in using calories and has no limit in storing excessive caloric intake in the form of fat. Humans may be predisposed to preferring sweet foods that are calorie dense and require a relatively low expenditure of energy to obtain (Phelan, 2010). Some scientists hypothesize that certain DNA are responsible for consumption of sugary foods and are linked to obesity-related illnesses such as diabetes (Daniels, 2006). Storing unlimited amounts of fat may have been a useful trait in the early days of evolution when humans were hunters and gatherers, but it has not been shown to be advantageous in today's environment where many occupations are sedentary, physical activity is limited, and minimal energy is required to acquire high-calorie food (Phelan, 2010). American society has become characterized by environments that promote physical inactivity and increased consumption of less-healthy food (CDC, 2011; Chescheir, 2011). The increased intake of energy-dense foods that are high in fat, salt, and sugars but low in vitamins, minerals, and other micronutrients combined with the decrease in physical activity due to the increasingly sedentary nature of many forms of work, changing modes of transportation, and increasing urbanization have not been beneficial in promoting human health (WHO, 2011).

Costs and availability of healthy foods are other factors contributing to obesity (CDC, 2011; Phelan, 2010). Healthy foods, including lean meats, fish, fresh fruits, and vegetables, cost more than fast food meals, which can easily exceed 1,000 calories for $5 or less.

Energy-dense foods with increased calorie, fat, and sugar content are associated with poverty as they are less expensive (Black, 2009). Grocery stores in which fresh foods are available are often not located in the most economically depressed areas, leaving some members of society with few options for good nutrition on a routine basis (American College of Obstetricians and Gynecologists [ACOG], 2010; CDC, 2011). Therefore, women of lower income and certain racial and ethnic groups have higher rates of obesity (Ogden & Carroll, 2010).

As a chronic disease, obesity represents a significant economic burden to society. It is estimated that obesity is responsible for an annual cost of $198 billion in the United States, with an additional $72 billion related to those who are overweight but not obese (Society of Actuaries [SOA], 2011). These economic costs include medical care ($127 billion), loss of worker productivity due to higher rates of death ($49 billion), loss of productivity due to disability of active workers ($43 billion), and loss of productivity due to total disability ($72 billion) (SOA, 2011). The high health-care costs are related to the comorbidities and medical complications associated with obesity and the sheer number of obese individuals. Obesity is linked to many significant diseases, such as hypertension, coronary heart disease, type 2 diabetes, gastroesophageal reflux disease, gallbladder disease, asthma, osteoarthritis, stroke, sleep apnea, thromboembolic events, elevated lipids, certain cancers (endometrial, breast, and colon) and psychological disorders such as depression (Reece, 2008; Vallejo, 2007). See Figure 12–1. Obesity-related deaths are mostly the result of diabetes, heart disease, hypertension, and cancer and estimated to account for 100,000 to 300,000 U.S. deaths every year (Duran, 2011).

Ethnicity and U.S. geographic region are factors that influence risk of obesity, based on a summary of data from 2006 to 2008 from the CDC (Odgen & Carroll, 2010). Obesity disproportionally affects minority women. Non-Hispanic blacks have a 51% higher prevalence of obesity compared with non-Hispanic whites. Hispanics have a 21% higher prevalence of obesity compared with non-Hispanic whites. The highest rate of obesity is among non-Hispanic black women at 49.6%, followed by 45.1% of Mexican American women, 36.8% of all Hispanic women, and 33.0% of non-Hispanic white women (Ogden & Carroll, 2010). Obesity in each of these groups has increased over the last 20 years (Ogden & Carroll, 2010). The prevalence of obesity for non-Hispanic whites as well as non-Hispanic blacks is highest in the Midwest and South (Ogden & Carroll, 2010). The highest prevalence for obesity in the Hispanic population is in the Midwest, South, and West (Ogden & Carroll, 2010). There are 39 states with obesity prevalence ≥25% and 9 states (Alabama, Arkansas, Kentucky, Louisiana, Mississippi, Missouri, Oklahoma, Tennessee, and West Virginia)

with ≥30% (Ogden & Carroll, 2010). Only Colorado and the District of Columbia have obesity prevalence less than 20%. In the United States, obesity is rapidly approaching tobacco as the leading cause of preventable death (Rahman & Berenson, 2010).

It is estimated that 31.9% of U.S. reproductive age women from 20 to 39 years old are obese; 7.6% of these women are morbidly obese, defined as a BMI of ≥40 (CDC, 2011; Wolfe, Rossi, & Warshak, 2011). Obesity in pregnancy has increased concurrently with obesity in the general population. Approximately 30% of pregnant women are obese (CDC, 2011). Further, it is estimated that 8% of pregnant women meet criteria for morbid obesity (Gunatilake & Perlow, 2011).

During the reproductive years, women are usually at peak health, which can accommodate the dramatic physiologic changes of pregnancy and the physical challenges of birth. However, more women are becoming pregnant who have preexisting medical conditions such as obesity. Pregnancy can exacerbate obesity-related comorbidities such as hypertension and/or diabetes as well as result in the development of additional maternal complications during pregnancy, labor, and birth (Wolfe et al., 2011). Maternal morbidity and mortality increase with increasing BMI (Mantakas & Farrell, 2010; Vallejo, 2007). Women may develop lifelong obesity as a result of excessive pregnancy weight gain and postpartum weight retention (Davis & Olson, 2009).

OBESITY-RELATED RISKS TO THE MOTHER AND FETUS

Obesity during pregnancy increases the risk of morbidity and mortality for both the mother and baby (see Display 12–2). The obese woman has an increased risk of spontaneous abortion, gestational diabetes, preeclampsia, labor abnormalities, operative vaginal or cesarean birth, anesthesia complications, wound infections, deep vein thrombosis, respiratory complications such as asthma and obstructive sleep apnea, medically indicated preterm birth, postterm pregnancy, urinary tract infections, and birth trauma related to macrosomic infants and fourth-degree lacerations (ACOG, 2013a; Blomberg, 2011; Catalano, 2007; Chescheir, 2011; Ehrenberg, 2011; Hendler et al., 2005; Jungheim & Moley, 2010; Ovesen, Rasmussen, & Kesmodel, 2011; Stream & Sutherland, 2012; Tan & Sia, 2011; Thornburg, 2011; Vidarsdottir, Geirsson, Hardardottir, Valdimarsdottir, & Dagbjartsson, 2011). An obese pregnant woman is much more likely to develop gestational diabetes than a woman of normal weight (Chu et al., 2007; Davis & Olson, 2009; Saldana, Siega-Riz, Adair, & Suchindran, 2006). Hypertensive disorders of pregnancy are more common in obese women. An increase of 5 to 7 kg/m^2 BMI nearly doubles the risk

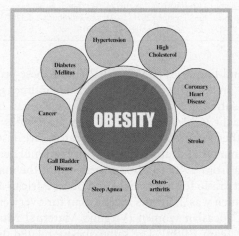

FIGURE 12–1. Obesity: A vicious cycle. (From Reece, E. A. [2008]. Perspectives on obesity, pregnancy and birth outcomes in the United States: The scope of the problem. *American Journal of Obstetrics and Gynecology, 198*[1], 23–27.)

DISPLAY 12-2

Risks Associated with Maternal Obesity during Pregnancy, Labor, and Birth

MATERNAL

Spontaneous abortion

Antepartum hospitalization

Hypertensive diseases, both preexisting and gestational; preeclampsia

Diabetes, both preexisting and gestational

Ischemic heart disease

Sleep apnea

Multiple pregnancy

Medically indicated preterm birth

Postterm pregnancy

Labor and birth abnormalities (labor dystocia, prolonged labor, labor induction and augmentation, unsuccessful vaginal birth after cesarean [VBAC], fetal compromise, shoulder dystocia, operative vaginal birth, fourth-degree lacerations, postpartum hemorrhage, cesarean birth)

Labor anesthesia complications (difficult epidural catheter placement, inadvertent dural puncture, failure to establish regional anesthesia, insufficient duration of regional anesthesia, hypotension, postdural headaches)

Complications of cesarean birth (increased time from decision to incision, increased time from incision to birth, increased intraoperative time, general anesthesia, failed intubation, aspiration, intraoperative hypotension, increased blood loss, venous thrombo-embolism, surgical site infection, wound dehiscence)

Infection (urinary tract infection, episiotomy infection, endometritis, wound infection)

Increased length of stay

Breastfeeding difficulties

Short duration of breastfeeding

Postpartum maternal rehospitalization

Maternal death

FETAL AND INFANT

Congenital anomalies (neural tube defects, cardiovascular anomalies, diaphragmatic hernia, cleft lip and palate, anorectal atresia, hydrocephaly, limb reduction)

Intrauterine growth restriction

Prematurity related to medically indicated preterm birth due to maternal complications and co-morbidities

Conditions associated with prematurity (intracranial hemorrhage, respiratory distress, vision, gastrointestinal and cardiac problems)

Neonatal macrosomia

Fetal death

Stillbirth

Low Apgar scores

Birth trauma

Neonatal acidosis

Neonatal intensive care unit admission

Neonatal respiratory complications

Childhood, adolescent, and adult obesity

Adapted from American College of Obstetricians and Gynecologists. (2013a). *Obesity in Pregnancy* (Committee Opinion No. 549). Washington, DC: Author; Blomberg, M. (2011). Maternal obesity and risk of postpartum hemorrhage. *Obstetrics and Gynecology, 118*(3), 561–568. doi:10.1097/AOG.0b013e31822a6c59; Chescheir, N. (2011). Global obesity and the effect on women's health. *Obstetrics and Gynecology, 117*(5), 1213–1222. doi:10.1097.AOG.0b013e3182161732; Ehrenberg, H. M. (2011). Intrapartum considerations in perinatal care. *Seminars in Perinatology, 35*(6), 324–329. doi:10.1053/j.semperi.2011.05.016; Jungheim, E. S., & Moley, K. H. (2010). Current knowledge of obesity's effects in the pre- and periconceptional periods and avenues for future research. *American Journal of Obstetrics and Gynecology, 203*(6), 525–530. doi:10.1016/j.ajog.2010.06.043; Ovesen, P., Rasmussen, S., & Kesmodel, U. (2011). Effect of prepregnancy maternal overweight and obesity on pregnancy outcome. *Obstetrics and Gynecology, 118*(2, Pt. 1), 305–312. doi:10.1097/AOG.0b013e3182245d49; Tan, T., & Sia, A. T. (2011). Anesthesia considerations in the obese gravida. *Seminars in Perinatology, 35*(6), 350–355. doi:10.1053/j.semperi.2011.05.021; and Thornburg, L. L. (2011). Antepartum obstetrical complications associated with obesity. *Seminars in Perinatology, 35*(6), 317–323. doi:10.1053/j.semperi.2011.05.015

of preeclampsia (O'Brien, Ray, & Chan, 2003). Operative and postoperative complications are increased with maternal obesity as well, including as a longer operative time; prolonged time from incision to birth of the baby; and increased blood loss, wound infection, and uterine dehiscence (Duran, 2011).

Maternal death is also associated with obesity (Goffman, Madden, Harrison, Merkatz, & Chazotte, 2007). Overweight and obese women are overrepresented among women who die during or within 1 year of a pregnancy. More than half of women who died during or after pregnancy between 2003 and 2005 in the United Kingdom were overweight or obese; 15% were morbidly or extremely obese (Centre for Maternal

and Child Enquiries [CMACE], 2011). Obese pregnant women are estimated to be at four to five times greater risk of suffering maternal death than a woman of normal weight (CMACE, 2011). Racial disparities found with other health and illness indicators are also present in maternal deaths. A review of maternal deaths in Virginia from 1999 to 2002 revealed that the maternal mortality ratio for overweight and obese African American women was 2.2 times higher than for overweight or obese Caucasian women (Virginia Maternal Mortality Review Team, 2009). The same obesity-related diseases that are associated with death in the general population are also associated with maternal mortality. Many of the obese women who died in the Virginia case series report had other chronic health conditions that are caused or exacerbated by obesity (Virginia Maternal Mortality Review Team, 2009). Nearly one third of overweight and obese women who died had cardiac disorders or gestational hypertension, preeclampsia, or eclampsia (Virginia Maternal Mortality Review Team, 2009).

The risk of spontaneous abortion and recurrent spontaneous abortion in the obese population is twice that of their non-obese counterparts (Thornburg, 2011). Extremely obese women may be at 40% greater risk of stillbirth than a normal weight woman (Salihu et al., 2007; Salihu, 2011). It is hypothesized that hyperlipidemia of obesity may lead to atherosclerotic changes in the placental vessels. This change combined with sleep apnea, leading to desaturation and decreased perception of fetal movement due to body habitus, may contribute to the increased rate of stillbirth in this population (Society of Obstetricians and Gynaecologists of Canada [SOGC], 2010).

The fetus of an obese woman is at increased risk for congenital anomalies, macrosomia, and fetal death. Excessive maternal weigh and obesity have a negative effect on uterine contractility (Zhang, Bricker, Wray, & Quenby, 2007), which may explain why these women have a lower rate of spontaneous preterm birth (Hendler et al., 2005). However, the comorbidites associated with overweight and obesity such as hypertensive disorders and diabetes predispose overweight and obese women to medically indicated preterm birth and their babies to the sequelae of prematurity (Hendler et al., 2005). Multiple congenital anomalies have been associated with maternal obesity, such as neural tube defects, cardiovascular anomalies, cleft lip and palate, diaphragmatic hernia, and gastroschisis (Gunatilake & Perlow, 2011). Evidence suggests that the risk of malformations increases proportionate to the level of obesity (Gunatilake & Perlow, 2011). Macrosomic infants are exposed to an increased risk of birth trauma from shoulder dystocia. Due to the increased risk of medically indicated preterm birth associated with the comorbidities of obesity such as diabetes and hypertensive disorders, babies of obese women are at increased risk for the neonatal complications related to prematurity, including respiratory distress, cardiac problems, intracranial hemorrhage, and vision and intestinal problems (James & Maher, 2009).

Excessive weight gain during pregnancy appears to create an intrauterine environment that promotes larger babies with more fat cells, which in turn puts the baby at higher risk for obesity during childhood and as an adult with all the long-term consequences (Phelan, 2010). There is evolving evidence about the developmental origins of disease that has implications for fetuses of women who gain excessive weight during pregnancy. When the fetus is subjected to an environment during pregnancy characterized by nutritional factors contributing to excessive maternal weight gain,

fetal programming, that is, the process in which a stimulus in utero establishes a permanent response in the fetus, can lead to increased susceptibility to disease in childhood and throughout life (Catalano, 2007). Children born to obese mothers are twice as likely to develop obesity at 2 to 4 years of age (Whitaker, 2004). Primarily due to the obesity epidemic, U.S. children born now are projected to have a shorter life span than their parents (Phelan, 2010). Excessive weight gain during pregnancy results in a negative cycle of adverse health as obese women give birth to macrosomic daughters who are more likely to become obese themselves and deliver large babies (Artal, Lockwood, & Brown, 2010).

The risk for offspring of obese women extends past the pregnancy. Children born of obese mothers are at increased risk for diabetes, heart disease, and long-term obesity (Gunatilake & Perlow, 2011). Several studies have noted an association between birth weight and childhood obesity (Baird et al., 2005; Hui et al., 2008; Phelan et al., 2011). Research has shown a close association between large-for-gestational-age (LGA) babies and childhood obesity in African American, inner city single mothers of low income and education, putting this population at high risk (Mehta, Kruger, & Sokol, 2011). The United States has launched programs to address childhood obesity. These efforts are aimed at school foods and activity level of schoolchildren, food marketing, taxation, and reducing sedentary time at a computer or television (Ogden, Carroll, Curtin, Lamb, & Flegal, 2010). Since the antenatal period is further implicated in contributing to the obesity of children, more emphasis is needed on counseling mothers on the association between the effects of pregnancy and obesity to address some of the modifiable risk factors before pregnancy occurs (Mehta et al., 2011).

PRECONCEPTION CARE

Weight loss and modification of nutritional intake before pregnancy reduce risk of obesity and the related potential complications for the mother and baby (American Academy of Pediatrics [AAP] & ACOG, 2012; CDC, 2006). Preconception care that includes risk screening, health promotion counseling, and interventions based on individual patient status enables women to enter pregnancy in optimal health (CDC, 2006). Therefore *all* pregnant women, including those that are overweight or obese, should have a preconception visit to their obstetrical care provider to assess health status; evaluate physical, emotional, and nutritional readiness for pregnancy; and allow for modification of potential risk factors and behaviors (CDC, 2006). Obesity increases risk of early miscarriage by twofold to threefold and decreases success of fertility treatments; therefore, obese women planning pregnancy should be counseled that achieving a successful pregnancy may be more difficult (Jungheim

& Moley, 2010; Thornburg, 2011). Women who have had bariatric surgery should be advised to wait 12 to 24 months before attempting pregnancy as this time frame is the period of the most rapid weight loss, which can be detrimental to the growing fetus (ACOG, 2009a). During the preconception visit, the woman's height and weight should be recorded so BMI can be calculated (AAP & ACOG, 2012).

Counseling an obese woman who is planning pregnancy should include information regarding maternal and fetal risks associated with obesity, screening for diabetes and hypertension, nutrition counseling, encouragement of exercise, and consultation with a weight loss specialist before attempting pregnancy. This counseling should take into consideration the woman's food preferences, eating patterns, cultural beliefs, and access to healthy food (AAP & ACOG, 2012). Referral to a dietitian may be indicated for women who are overweight or obese. Obese women considering pregnancy should be encouraged to follow an exercise program (AAP & ACOG, 2012). Follow-up visits with healthcare providers to monitor lifestyle changes in nutrition and physical activity prior to pregnancy may be warranted.

Preconception weight loss with possible resolution of hypertension, hyperlipidemia, and diabetes most likely will improve both maternal and fetal outcomes during pregnancy, labor, birth, and the postpartum period (CDC, 2006). Establishing a healthy diet and physical activity program prior to pregnancy may translate into maintaining these beneficial lifestyle changes during the pregnancy and beyond. The fetus and newborn may have less risk of maternal obesity–related problems when the mother adopts a healthier lifestyle. Weight loss will also decrease the lifelong disease burden for the woman (Gunatilake & Perlow, 2011).

ANTENATAL CARE

Every pregnant woman should be provided information about a balanced diet, ideal calorie intake, and recommended weight gain (AAP & ACOG, 2012;

ACOG, 2013b). The Institute of Medicine (IOM, 2009) and ACOG (2013b) recommend that pregnant women gain weight based on their prepregnancy BMI. See Table 12–2 for IOM recommendations for weight gain during pregnancy. Data were insufficient to offer specific guidelines for women with class II and class III obesity; therefore, the recommendations for weight gain for obese women include all classes of obesity (IOM, 2009). The IOM (2009) recommendations on weight gain during pregnancy advise a narrow margin of weight gain for the obese pregnant woman in the United States of 11 to 20 lb. Overweight women should gain about 15 to 25 lb during pregnancy (March of Dimes [MOD], 2011). There is controversy as to whether obese women should limit weight gain during pregnancy to lower levels than recommended by the IOM (2009), especially those in obesity class II and class III (Artal et al., 2010). Some studies have shown that limited or no weight gain during pregnancy for obese women is associated with favorable outcomes for the baby and less risk of maternal adverse outcomes (Cedergen, 2007; Kiel, Dodson, Artal, Boehmer, & Leet, 2007). Artal and colleagues (2010) recommend a nutrient-dense diet of 2,000 to 2,500 calories per day for obese pregnant women, which should result a gestational weight gain of 10 lb or less. For some women, this may represent a net negative weight gain. More research is needed regarding optimal weight gain targets for obese women.

The weight gain of pregnancy is a combination of the baby (7 to 9 lb), placenta (1 to 2 lb), amniotic fluid (2 lb), uterus (2 lb), breasts (1 to 2 lb), increase in blood volume (2 to 4 lb), increase in fluid volume (2 to 4 lb), and fat stores (6 to 8 lb) (Johnson, Gregory, & Niebyl, 2007). Generally, women can be expected to gain 3 to 6 lb during the first trimester and 0.5 to 1 lb each week thereafter until birth; however, for obese women, it is important to try to avoid gaining more than the recommended weight. Proper maternal nutrition can have a positive influence on improving the woman's overall health and birth of healthy baby of an appropriate weight (AAP & ACOG, 2012). Weight gain during pregnancy should be assessed and recorded at each

Table 12–2. RECOMMENDATIONS FOR TOTAL AND RATE OF WEIGHT GAIN DURING PREGNANCY, BY PREPREGNANCY BODY MASS INDEX (BMI)

Prepregnancy BMI	BMI (kg/m²) (WHO)	Total Weight Gain Range (lb)	Rates of Weight Gain 2nd and 3rd Trimesters (Mean Range in lb/wk)
Underweight	<18.5	28–40	1 (1–1.3)
Normal weight	18.5–24.9	25–35	1 (0.8–1)
Overweight	25.0–29.9	15–25	0.6 (0.5–0.7)
Obese (includes all classes)	≥30.0	11–20	0.5 (0.4–0.6)

From Institute of Medicine. (2009). *Weight Gain During Pregnancy: Reexamining the Guidelines* (Report Brief). Washington, DC: National Academies Press.

prenatal visit to allow for immediate feedback to the woman regarding potential modifications in diet and exercise. As during the preconception period, prenatal nutrition counseling should take into consideration the woman's food preferences, eating patterns, cultural beliefs, and access to healthy food (AAP & ACOG, 2012). If financial resources are a barrier to proper nutritional needs, the woman should be referred to federal food and nutrition programs such as the Special Supplemental Food Program for Women, Infants and Children (WIC) (AAP & ACOG, 2012).

Nutrition counseling is an essential component of prenatal care for all women (AAP & ACOG, 2012). Dieticians and nutritionists may be enlisted to help the overweight or obese woman achieve appropriate gestational weight goals. It may be advisable for some obese women to participate in a session with a dietician during each prenatal visit to offer suggestions for success, answer questions, and monitor progress. Obese pregnant women can benefit from a healthy, well-balanced nutrition monitoring program (Thornton, Smarkola, Kopacz, & Ishoof, 2009). If there are no medical or obstetric contraindications, 30 minutes or more of exercise per day is recommended for pregnant women (AAP & ACOG, 2012). Moderate exercise is safe during pregnancy; however, each activity should be reviewed with the woman by the healthcare provider for potential risk of injury, and those with high risk of falling or abdominal trauma should be avoided (AAP & ACOG, 2012; Szymanski & Satin, 2012).

Insulin resistance is associated with pregnancy; however, overweight and obesity exacerbates insulin resistance, and these patients often develop high blood glucose levels when their metabolism does not respond properly to insulin. Obese and overweight pregnant women are six times more likely to have gestational diabetes than normal weight women (Davis & Olson 2009; Saldana et al., 2006). Early screening for gestational diabetes is recommended at the first presentation for prenatal care (ACOG, 2013a). If the initial screening is negative, repeat testing is recommended in the third trimester (ACOG, 2013a). A thorough history and physical should occur upon entry into prenatal care to determine if there are any comorbid conditions prior to pregnancy. Some experts recommend baseline blood chemistry as well as uric acid, liver enzymes, creatinine, and a 24-hour urine test for protein, which can be used for comparison if hypertensive disorders arise or to screen for other conditions (Gunatilake & Perlow, 2011).

Overweight and obese pregnant women are at risk for developing sleep-disordered breathing, including the most severe form, obstructive sleep apnea, which is characterized by repeated episodes of partial or complete upper airway obstruction accompanied by oxygen desaturation during sleep. Obstructive sleep apnea can result in disruption of normal ventilation,

intermittent hypoxemia, and arousals from sleep (Izci-Balserak & Pien, 2010). Physiologic and hormonal changes occur during pregnancy that increase the likelihood of developing sleep-disordered breathing and exacerbate its effects, including pregnancy weight gain, pregnancy-associated nasopharyngeal edema, decreased functional reserve capacity, and increased arousals from sleep (Izci-Balserak & Pien, 2010). The mother may experience pauses in breathing for several seconds followed by gasps of air while she is sleeping during the night. The nighttime breathing disturbances can result in daytime sleepiness, chronic fatigue, and difficulty concentrating. Risk of sleep apnea is higher for those that are overweight because of excess fat stored in the neck area, which may make the airway smaller and make breathing difficult, loud such as snoring, or stop intermittently (Facco, 2011). If the woman is symptomatic, a sleep apnea study should be conducted. Treatment often leads to improved sleep quality and daytime functioning. The most common treatment for obstructive sleep apnea is continuous positive airway pressure via a device worn while sleeping, which appears to be a safe treatment with minimal adverse effects (Chen et al., 2012; Facco, 2011). Obstructive sleep apnea during pregnancy has been linked to an increased risk of developing gestational hypertension, preeclampsia, and gestational diabetes (Bourjeily, Ankner & Mohsenin, 2011; Chen et al., 2012; Izci-Balserak & Pien, 2010; Olivarez et al., 2011).

An ultrasound to determine fetal anatomy may be more difficult due to the abdominal contour (Khoury, Ehrenberg, & Mercer, 2009). Frequency of suboptimal visualization of detailed fetal anatomy is significantly increased for obese women, particularly for the cardiovascular system, facial soft tissue, and abdominal wall (Khoury et al., 2009). For this reason, some experts have reported better results when this examination was done at 20 to 22 weeks of gestation (Gunatilake & Perlow, 2011; SOGC, 2010). Serial ultrasound to monitor fetal growth may be performed as routine fundal height measurement may be difficult due to body habitus. Frequent ultrasound may be indicated since macrosomia is twice as common in obese women and growth restriction can occur due to hypertensive disorders of pregnancy associated with obesity. Extremely obese women should be aware of the risk of the need for induction of labor as well as the decreased risk of success (Wolfe et al., 2011).

INTRAPARTUM CARE

Approximately 30% of pregnant women are obese (CDC, 2011); therefore, every perinatal service should have policies and practices in place specifically for this patient population. Potential peripartum

Table 12–3. OBESITY-RELATED PERIPARTUM COMPLICATIONS AND POSSIBLE INTERVENTIONS

Obesity-Related Peripartum Complications	
Problem/Risk	Potential Intervention
Increased respiratory work and myocardial oxygen requirement	Epidural anesthesia, supplemental oxygen, left-lateral laboring position
Difficult peripheral intravenous access	Central intravenous catheter
Inaccurate blood pressure monitoring	Appropriate-sized cuff, arterial line
Increased risk of general anesthesia	Anesthesia consultation, early epidural
Anticipated difficulty with intubation	Capability for awake/fiber-optic intubation
Difficulty with patient transfers	Bariatric lifts and inflatable mattresses, additional personnel
Prolonged cesarean operative time	Combined spinal-epidural anesthesia
Poor operative exposure	Evaluation of maternal anthropometry, panniculus retraction, periumbilical skin incision, atraumatic self-retaining retractor
Enhanced risk of hemorrhage	Blood typed and crossed for transfusion, ligate large subcutaneous vessels, meticulous surgical technique
Enhanced aspiration risk	Prophylactic epidural, H_2 antagonist, sodium citrate with citric acid, metoclopramide, nothing by mouth in labor
Enhanced thromboembolic risk	Early postoperative ambulation, sequential pneumatic compression, heparin until fully ambulatory
Enhanced risk of infectious morbidity	Thorough skin preparation, adequate antimicrobial prophylaxis, avoidance of subpannicular incision, meticulous surgical technique, consideration of subcutaneous drain
Enhanced risk of cesarean delivery	Informed consent, monitoring of labor curve, and intervention for labor dystocia
Enhanced risk of shoulder dystocia	Near-term sonographic fetal weight, caution with operative delivery

From Gunatilake, R., & Perlow, J. (2011). Obesity and pregnancy: Clinical management of the obese gravida. *American Journal of Obstetrics and Gynecology, 204*(2), 106–119. doi:10:1016/j.ajog.2010.10.002

complications for obese pregnant women are numerous (see Table 12–3); however, advance planning and anticipation of problems may be able to mitigate risk of an adverse outcome. Consultation with anesthesia providers is recommended due to many possible anesthesia-associated complications (see section on intraoperative care) (Tan & Sia, 2011). For the extremely obese patient, this consultation should occur prior to admission for labor and birth.

Advance planning for birth for women who are extremely obese is prudent. Ideally, the obstetrical care provider will notify the clinical leadership team of the perinatal service by at least 34 weeks' gestation when they have an extremely obese patient in prenatal care if she is expected to give birth at term. Earlier notification is warranted if complications are developing that may result in preterm labor and birth. Advance notice will give the perinatal team in the inpatient setting time to evaluate the unit's capability to provide safe care by planning for additional personnel as needed and ordering special equipment to accommodate the woman's excess weight. Advance evaluation of the unit's capabilities may reveal that the patient's needs for labor and birth may be best served elsewhere, which should prompt instructions to the patient regarding where to go when labor begins and plans for transfer if she presents to the unit in early labor but is stable enough for transport. When the facility is unable to provide necessary resources, transfer to a tertiary facility should be considered to provide the safest care possible for both the mother and the baby

(see Chapter 13). However, there may be times when the best plans do not become reality, as may be the situation when an extremely obese pregnant patient presents for care but is unstable for transport due to labor status or her clinical condition. In this case, necessary resources and equipment need to be assembled as quickly as possible based on availability.

After notification from the obstetrical care provider and determination that the perinatal service can safely handle care of the extremely obese pregnant patient for her labor and birth, clinical care conferences can be scheduled so all members of the team can be involved and develop a plan to provide the best care possible. Participation by the obstetrical care provider in these conferences is very useful in anticipating special clinical needs and securing adequate resources. See Display 12–3 for suggestions for clinical, operational, and equipment issues that should be considered in planning for inpatient care of the extremely obese pregnant woman (James & Maher, 2009). Extra time and attention is necessary to make sure appropriate specialty equipment is ordered and available, including a bariatric bed with 1,000-lb weight capacity and an expandable frame, lift equipment, a hover mat to assist with transfer after regional anesthesia, a commode and/or toilet that will support 500+ lb, extra large gowns, appropriate size blood pressure cuffs, extra large pneumatic compression devices, extra wide wheelchairs, and a method to weigh a person who is extremely obese. Surgical equipment to care for the extremely obese person should be available,

---

DISPLAY 12 - 3

Advance Preparations When an Extremely Obese Pregnant Woman Will Be Admitted to the Hospital for Childbirth

The following factors should be evaluated and considered for advance unit preparations for pregnant women with extreme obesity:

Evaluation of Unit Capabilities
What is the best location for patient's care?
Can the facility manage these special needs?
Is referral to a tertiary or other center necessary?

Preadmission Planning
Develop plan of care for labor, vaginal and cesarean birth, postpartum period
Conduct pre-anesthesia evaluation and airway evaluation
Develop plans for pain relief during labor, birth, and postoperative period
Practice drills for using and moving special equipment
Conduct tabletop rehearsals before and during the mother's stay
Plan for additional time for epidural placement, repositioning for intrauterine resuscitation, and emergent movement to operating room (OR) and/or birthing suite

Equipment and Supplies Needs and Evaluation
Bariatric scale
Extra-wide wheelchair
Evaluate weight limits of labor bed, the OR table in the perinatal unit and the OR table in the main surgical department in flat and in semi-Fowler's position and with use of stirrups
Evaluate need to order a bariatric bed and/or hover mat

Evaluate weight limits of labor, delivery, and recovery (LDR) and mother-baby (MB) room furniture, including visitor chairs if partner/family are persons of size
Evaluate weight limits of commode in LDR and MB rooms
Obtain extra large gowns, appropriate size blood pressure cuffs, extra large pneumatic compression devices
Practice use of hover mat for transfer of patient to OR table
Practice application of stirrups to bariatric bed
Practice application and removal of bed extenders
Practice movement of a large bed throughout department, for example, from labor room to the OR (conduct drills for emergent cesarean birth)
Practice positioning for possible shoulder dystocia
Plan for supplies and equipment for potential cesarean birth, including extra deep abdominal instruments and Montgomery straps for visualization
Obtain bariatric OR table extensions that provide an additional 6 to 8 in on each side of the table, if needed based on patient size
Contact information for equipment suppliers for each item needed should be included in the patient's file and readily available to the clinical leadership team

Roles of Additional Personnel
At a minimum, anticipate one-to-one nursing care; however, more than one nurse may be needed at various stages of labor, birth, and the immediate postpartum period
Assisting with holding external ultrasound and toco for continuous EFM during labor
Assisting with positioning during epidural placement
Assisting with repositioning during labor
Assisting with holding legs during vaginal birth
Retraction during vaginal birth
Assisting with transfer
Assisting with holding extra tissue and the panniculus adiposis away from the field during cesarean birth

EFM, electronic fetal monitoring
Adapted from James, D., & Maher, M. (2009). Caring for the extremely obese woman during pregnancy and birth. *MCN: The American Journal of Maternal Child Nursing, 34*(1), 24–30.

---

including an operating room (OR) table with a 1,000-lb capacity, extension devices to increase the width of the table, and extra-long surgical instruments and retractors.

There can be many challenges for nurses caring for extremely obese women in labor. Intravenous (IV) access may be more difficult. External fetal monitoring may be more complex due to abdominal girth, so frequent adjustments may be necessary to continually assess both the mother and fetus. One-to-one nursing care may be necessary to maintain a continuous fetal heart rate (FHR) and uterine activity tracing. It is important to avoid confusing the maternal heart rate with the FHR. Clinical conditions that increase risk of confusion include low FHR baseline, maternal pushing efforts during second-stage labor, maternal repositioning, maternal obesity, and maternal tachycardia, which may be associated with an elevated temperature, anxiety, or medications (Neilson, Freeman, & Mangan, 2008; Simpson, 2011). An abrupt change in

the characteristics of the FHR tracing or FHR accelerations consistently coincident with uterine contractions or coincident with maternal pushing efforts should be evaluated to confirm that the tracing is of fetal origin. In the case of fetal demise, a recording may be produced of the maternal heart rate either via the external ultrasound transducer detecting maternal aortic pulsations or via the fetal scalp electrode (FSE) detecting the maternal ECG. When there are two sources of data, for example, maternal heart rate via pulse oximetry and fetal or maternal heart rate via external ultrasound or via FSE, the fetal monitor may display coincidence alerts to suggest that both data sources are detecting the same heart rate. When these alerts are displayed, confirmation of two distinct heart rates, one from the fetus and one from the mother, should be undertaken. Coincidence alerts may not be displayed if the data from the automatic blood pressure device indicates a maternal pulse in the same range as the

FHR. It may be helpful to confirm maternal heart rate by palpating maternal pulse during initiation of electronic fetal monitoring (EFM), comparing with FHR, and repeating this confirmation periodically during first- and second-stage labor when caring for an obese laboring woman (Simpson, 2011).

More nurses may be needed for prolonged periods of time as the overweight or obese mother has a longer labor. The unit will likely need to provide additional personnel to transfer the patient, to position and turn her, and to assist with her legs for procedures such as catheterization, internal lead placement, and during the active pushing phase of the second stage of labor. Adequate personnel are required for both for the woman's safety and the safety of the staff. Caregivers should be mindful of proper body mechanics to protect themselves from injury; however, good body mechanics may not be sufficient to prevent injury. Equipment for transferring and moving the extremely obese woman is required. Transporting the extremely obese mother will take more time than usual, so it may be necessary to rehearse with unfamiliar equipment and practice movement through the department in order to provide safe care, especially in the case of an unplanned cesarean birth.

A sensitive and empathetic environment should be provided for the mother and her partner. When there are challenges in care due to the patient's weight status, such as IV access, epidural catheter placement, and external fetal monitoring, and extra steps or equipment are required for patient transfer and anesthesia management, it is important to avoid reminding the woman that these additional clinical issues are related to her obesity. The woman and her support person will appreciate the time and effort devoted to her special needs in the context of a care environment that does not cause embarrassment, guilt, or self-esteem problems. The focus of the care should be centered on her safety and clinical needs as it is with women with other chronic diseases.

Due to the increased rate of complications associated with obesity, such as diabetes, hypertension, and postdates, obese women are more likely to have an induction or augmentation of labor. Wolfe and colleagues (2011) found that obese women experience two times the rate of failure of induction of labor as mothers of normal weight and that rate of induction failure is associated with the degree of obesity. This risk is highest for women in obesity class III (see Table 12–1), obese nulliparous women with a macrosomic fetus, and obese women without a previous successful vaginal birth (Wolfe et al., 2011). Labor proceeds more slowly as BMI increases, suggesting that labor management be altered to allow longer time for these differences (Kominiarek et al., 2011; Vahratian, Zhang, Troendle, Savitz, & Siega-Riz, 2004). Uterine contractility may be diminished in overweight and obese women (Zhang et al., 2007), which can cause prolonged or dysfunctional labor and may be attributed

to an increased level of serum cholesterol, which is more common in obese women than their normal weight counterparts (Wolfe et al., 2011). Regional anesthesia complications are more common in labor of morbidly obese women, including more frequent and prolonged systolic and diastolic hypotension and subsequent late FHR decelerations (Vricella, Louis, Mercer, & Bolden, 2011). These risks increase proportionally with higher BMIs (Vricella et al., 2011). All women are at greater risk for morbidity with cesarean birth following a long labor, but obese women have a significantly increased risk of complications following a cesarean birth after a prolonged labor or ruptured membranes when compared to normal weight women (Goffman et al., 2007).

INTRAOPERATIVE CARE

Obese women have an increased risk for cesarean birth (ACOG, 2013a; Dietz, Callaghan, Morrow, & Cogswell, 2005; Ehrenberg, 2011; Fyfe et al., 2011; Kominiarek et al., 2010; Ovesen et al., 2011; Sarkar et al., 2007; SOGC, 2010). A cesarean birth rate of nearly 50% has been reported for extremely obese women (Ehrenberg, 2011; Gunatilake & Perlow, 2011). Excessive weight gain in pregnancy above the IOM recommendations is also an independent risk factor for cesarean birth even in non-obese women (Stotland, Hopkins, & Caughey, 2004). It is estimated that over 20% of cesarean births of nulliparous women could be prevented if pregnant women limited their gestational weight gain to within the IOM recommendations (Stotland et al., 2004).

Obese women should be counseled prior to birth that cesarean birth for emergent conditions may be more difficult (ACOG, 2013a). The time interval from decision to incision may be longer for the obese mother due to difficulty with anesthesia and challenges with transfer and transport. The time from incision to birth may also be prolonged due to operative difficulty as a result of excessive abdominal adipose tissue. Prolonged time from incision to birth may result in a depressed baby at birth if the medications given to the mother for induction anesthesia or sedation are transferred to the baby before birth and/or if the fetus becomes hypoxemic due to difficulties in getting the baby out of the uterus in a timely manner because of excess maternal fat and tissue. The challenge may be increased with extremely obese mothers because pressure on the fundus to assist in delivering the baby may dissipate due to the adipose tissue. If operative table width extenders are used, it may be more difficult for the surgeon to reach the operative site. Therefore, presence of a neonatal resuscitation team at the birth involving an extremely obese woman is advised.

Both surgical site infection and endometritis are increased in this population, so preoperative prophylactic antibiotics are especially important (ACOG, 2013a).

Wound breakdown and dehiscence is also more common in the obese mother who has had a cesarean birth. A major determinant of cesarean wound morbidity is likely due to depth of the incision (Ehrenberg, 2011). Closure of the subcutaneous layer has been found to decrease wound dehiscence and is recommended (ACOG, 2013a; Gunatilake & Perlow, 2011). Depending on the abdominal contour and deposition of fat in the extremely obese mother, there may be variations in the type of cesarean incision (ACOG, 2013a).

Choice of incision direction is based on individual clinical situations and surgeon preference. Vertical skin incision is often used for the more profoundly obese patient though there is no conclusive evidence supporting use of either the Pfannenstiel or vertical skin incision for obese patients requiring cesarean birth. In one study, risk of postoperative complications requiring the reopening of the wound were found to be 12-fold greater in vertical skin incisions than in the Pfannenstiel incision; however, in this study, patients that had a vertical incision had higher BMIs than those with the Pfannenstiel incision (Ehrenberg, 2011). Vertical abdominal incisions and closed suction subcutaneous drains are commonly used to reduce postoperative wound complications for obese patients having cesarean birth, though evidence suggests that these two practices have a negligible or even negative impact on the incidence of wound complications (Alanis, Villers, Law, Steadman, & Robinson, 2010). Each type of incision holds separate theoretic benefits and risks to the patient, but these risks have not yet been adequately studied (Ehrenberg, 2011). Typically, low transverse incisions afford less pain postoperatively, which can improve postoperative mobility and prevent atelectasis and respiratory complications, which are more common in this population. There are generally fewer cases of wound breakdown with this type of incisions.

Exposure may be difficult with low transverse approach and a dependent panniculus. Montgomery straps may be used to retract the panniculus superiorly, but this maneuver can cause difficulties in ventilation, hypotension, and cardiovascular and respiratory compromise from the weight of the tissue on the chest. The fetus may be negatively affected as well due to maternal compromise related to cephalad retraction of the panniculus for surgical access (Tan & Sia, 2011). Depending on the abdominal contour, the panniculus can be retracted downward as well. A low transverse incision could lead to wound infection because the surgical wound is covered by tissue and maintains moisture. A vertical skin incision, placed in a periumbilical fashion, can accommodate rapid entry into the abdomen and allow for extension of the incision if necessary, but it is also associated with more hernias, increased operative time, increased blood loss, increased postoperative discomfort, and more wound separation (Alanis et al., 2010; Gunatilake &

Perlow, 2011). Maintaining normothermia intraoperatively may help reduce incidence of postoperative wound complications for obese women after cesarean birth (Tipton, Cohen, & Chelmow, 2011).

There are multiple anesthesia risks for the obese pregnant woman, both for general and regional anesthesia (Duran, 2011). These include difficulties in epidural catheter placement, failure to establish regional anesthesia, insufficient duration of regional anesthesia, postdural headaches, a higher rate of general anesthesia, and intraoperative hypotension (Vricella, Louis, Mercer, & Bolden, 2010). Regional anesthesia may be difficult due to decreased ability to identify landmarks because of adipose tissue and difficulty with positioning, so adequate time should be allowed as multiple attempts at catheter placement may be necessary. Morbidly obese women not only have a higher initial epidural failure rate, but they also have a higher rate of catheter migration, probably from increased subcutaneous tissue causing the skin to slide and dislodge the catheter (Vallejo, 2007). For these reasons, and because of the increased risk of cesarean, early epidural placement in labor is suggested (SOGC, 2010).

Aspiration is the number one cause of anesthesia-related death in the obstetric population (Tan & Sia, 2011). Obese pregnant women are at increased risk for aspiration and should ideally be given nothing by mouth in active labor and 8 hours prior to cesarean birth (Gunatilake & Perlow, 2011). Physiologic changes in pregnancy that increase the risk of aspiration such as relaxed esophageal sphincter, increased abdominal pressure, increased acidity, and decreased gastrointestinal motility are all amplified with the morbidly obese patient (Vallejo, 2007). There is a higher rate of difficult intubation with obese mothers (Tan & Sia, 2011). During the pre-anesthesia assessment, particular attention must be devoted to neck circumference rather than BMI alone when evaluating a patient with respect to intubation (Bell & Rosenbaum, 2005; Vallejo, 2007). Plans for intubation while awake may be necessary along with other tools to secure a difficult airway (Gunatilake & Perlow, 2011; SOGC, 2010) if general anesthesia is planned.

POSTPARTUM CARE

Obese mothers are at risk postoperatively for atelectasis, pneumonia, hypoxemia, postpartum cardiomyopathy, infection and wound complications, thromboembolism, uterine atony, and postpartum hemorrhage (Blomberg, 2011; Saravanakumar, Rao, & Cooper, 2006). There is an increased incidence of infection and wound complications for obese women, regardless of method of birth, including episiotomy infection and breakdown after vaginal birth and surgical site infection, wound dehiscence, and endometritis after cesarean birth. Postoperative morbidity is high in obese women after cesarean birth, thus postoperative care issues, such as supplementary monitoring, thromboprophylaxis, and additional respiratory support devices, must planned for in advance (Tan & Sia, 2011). Mothers with a history of obstructive sleep apnea should have oxygen administered continuously and be monitored closely until they can maintain oxygen saturation on room air. A lateral or upright position is advised rather than supine, which can exacerbate obstructive sleep apnea. Opiods given for pain relief may blunt the arousal response and result in hypoxemia while sleeping; therefore, alternative analgesics such as nonsteroidal anti-inflammatory medications should be considered. For extremely obese mothers who have had a cesarean birth, it may be more appropriate to observe them in the post-anesthesia care unit for 24 hours (American Society of Anesthesiologists [ASA], 2006). If the woman is cared for on the postpartum unit after being discharged from post-anesthesia care, careful monitoring is required. Placing patient in a monitored bed with specific vital signs observed at a central station with 24/7 surveillance rather than relying on in-room alarms may allow any negative changes in patient status to be identified in a timely manner. End tidal CO_2 monitoring during postoperative pain relief with narcotics is possible with use of smart pumps with this option.

Careful assessment of the wound for signs of infection, use of incentive spirometry to prevent respiratory complications, and accurate assessment of vital signs and intake and output are warranted. Precise assessment of bleeding and uterine tone may be difficult due to maternal size. Due to the increased risk for atonic postpartum hemorrhage, administration of prophylactic postpartum uterotonic drugs should be considered for obese women in the immediate postpartum period (Blomberg, 2011). Since the risk of venous thromboembolism (VTE) is increased with obesity above the risks related to pregnancy (ACOG, 2011; SOGC, 2010; Vallejo, 2007), use of intermittent pneumatic pressure stockings prior to cesarean birth and continued until the mother is fully ambulatory is recommended (ACOG, 2011; Gunatilake & Perlow, 2011). Adequate fluid intake and early ambulation after cesarean birth can decrease risk of VTE (Bates et al., 2012).

Obese mothers should be encouraged to breastfeed for the health benefits to themselves as well as their babies, yet obese women tend to have more difficulties. Obese women are less likely to initiate breastfeeding, experience delayed lactogenesis more frequently, and breastfeed for shorter durations than women of normal weight (Baker, Michaelsen, Rasmussen, & Sorensen, 2004; Donath & Amir, 2008). Since women that breastfeed tend to lose their pregnancy weight gain more quickly than non-breastfeeding mothers and breastfed infants are less likely to become obese as adults, every effort should be given to support her

in this effort (Chescheir, 2011). All women with gestational diabetes should be screened at 6 to 12 weeks postpartum (ACOG, 2009b). Generally, carbohydrate intolerance and insulin resistance related to gestational diabetes resolves in the postpartum period; however, up to one third of women with gestational diabetes will have evidence of abnormal glucose metabolism during postpartum screening, and up to 50% of those women will develop diabetes in the decades after the pregnancy (ACOG, 2009b).

One of the most important interventions in the later postpartum period is discussion of prevention strategies. Excessive pregnancy weight gain, retention of gestational weight, and high prepregnancy weight are predictors of obesity during the postpartum period and into the midlife years with associated comorbidities of diabetes, hypertension, and heart disease (Gore, Brown, & Smith, 2003; Rooney, Schauberger, & Mathiason, 2005; Viswanathan et al., 2008). Excessive postpartum weight retention is especially prevalent among minority women (Gore et al., 2003). Women who gain more than the IOM (2009) recommended weight are more likely to retain that excessive weight both short term and long term (Viswanathan et al., 2008). Further, it is estimated that up to 40% of women who were not obese prior to pregnancy retain at least 14 lb past the postpartum period (Ohlendorf, Weiss, & Ryan, 2012). More than 60% of women become overweight in subsequent pregnancies (Artal et al., 2010). Obese women should be encouraged to lose the weight gained in pregnancy to prevent incremental gains with subsequent pregnancies. Excessive gestational weight gain and the effect on the next pregnancies cause a permanent increase in weight for every BMI category, and this increase is a significant contributor to the obesity epidemic and associated comorbidities in the United States (Artal et al., 2010).

The ideal time for intervention for obese women to optimize their health and the health of their future children is preconception (ACOG, 2013a; CDC, 2006; Davis & Olson, 2009; Gunatilake & Perlow, 2011); however, the interconception period prior to the next pregnancy is an additional opportunity to develop healthy behaviors and eating patterns that will promote well-being (Ohlendorf et al., 2012). During the postpartum hospitalization and postpartum outpatient visit, it is important to discuss plans for postpartum weight loss, offering specific examples and resources as to how this might be accomplished (Ohlendorf et al., 2012). Many postpartum women are seeking quality information on this topic during their hospital stay. In one study, over 50% of normal weight women, 75% of overweight women, and 82% of obese postpartum women indicated they were planning to search for information about losing their pregnancy weight (Ohlendorf et al., 2012). Referral to weight management healthcare professionals, including hospital or community-based services, is appreciated by postpartum women (Ohlendorf et al., 2012). Hospitals may consider offering postpartum exercise classes as part of their women's services program.

BARIATRIC SURGERY AND PREGNANCY

A number of morbidly obese women have chosen to have bariatric surgery to lose weight and control their obesity. Patients are considered eligible for weight-loss surgery if they have a BMI >40 kg/m^2 or a BMI >35 kg/m^2 with other comorbid conditions (Kominiarek, 2011). There was an 800% increase in bariatric procedures in the United States from 1998 to 2005 (Maggard et al., 2008; Shekelle et al., 2008). In 2005, approximately 113,500 patients in the United States elected to have weight reduction surgery; approximately 80% of patients were women (ACOG, 2009a; Edwards, 2006). Between 2004 and 2007, there was a trend of more men having this type of surgery so that the differences based on gender are gradually diminishing (Shekelle et al., 2008). More than one half of bariatric surgeries are performed on reproductive-age women (ACOG, 2009a; Maggard et al., 2008). An evaluation of bariatric surgery in both the inpatient and outpatient setting in the United States from 1993 to 2007 suggests the incidence of bariatric surgery appears to have plateaued at approximately 113,000 cases per year while complication rates have fallen from 10.5% in 1993 to 7.6% of all cases in 2006 (Livingston, 2010). It is estimated that bariatric surgery costs in the United States are at least $1.5 billion annually (Livingston, 2010). There are variations in insurance coverage for bariatric surgery; all costs may not be covered under some plans.

There are various methods for bariatric surgery. In general, bariatric surgery is either purely restrictive in nature, for example, reducing the size of the stomach, or a combination of restrictive and malabsorptive methods in which in addition to a smaller stomach, a bypass of part of the intestine adds the aspect of less area for food to be absorbed. These procedures can be performed either via laparoscopy or laparotomy based on the method selected and the individual clinical situation (Kominiarek, 2011). Restrictive surgery may involve laparoscopic adjustable gastric banding (LAGB) or vertical banded gastroplasty (Conrad, Russell, & Keister, 2011). With this type of procedure, a band is placed around the upper portion of the stomach and the physician is able to change the amount of restriction by injecting saline into or removing saline from a tube with a connection port to the circular band (Conrad et al., 2011; Kominiarek, 2011). With the LAGB procedure, the gastric pouch is usually limited to 50 mL initially (Kominiarek, 2011). Nutritional deficiencies are less common with LAGB surgery when compared to procedures that involve restrictive and malabsorption techniques. In the United States, the most common method performed that is categorized as both restrictive and malabsorptive is the Roux-en-Y gastric bypass (RYGB) procedure, in which a small section of the stomach is sectioned off to contain <30 mL and reconnected to the jejunum (Conrad et al., 2011; Kominiarek, 2011). Food bypasses a large portion of the stomach and the duodenum, thereby allowing a smaller area of the intestine for absorption of calories and also stimulating a full feeling so patients eat less (Conrad et al., 2011). Various levels of success of each procedure have been reported. The surgery in isolation is not guaranteed to produce long-term results. To maintain weight loss, it is important that patients are aware that significant lifestyle changes, including modifications of eating habits and exercise, are required. Close supervision before, during, and after pregnancy that follows bariatric surgery and nutrition supplementation adapted to the individual needs of the woman is necessary to prevent nutrition-related complications (Magdaleno, Pereira, Chaim, & Turato, 2012).

The woman contemplating pregnancy after bariatric surgery has special nutritional needs. Preconception counseling is especially important for these patients as deficiencies in vitamins B$_{12}$, A, and K; iron; folate; and calcium may occur and can result in maternal and fetal complications (Magdaleno et al., 2012). Vitamin supplementation is recommended (ACOG, 2009a). Laboratory tests to evaluate potential deficiencies should be considered each trimester and, if identified, treated with oral or parental therapy (ACOG, 2009a). Recommendations for the nutritional management including supplementation and laboratory testing of the postbariatric surgery patient from a task force of the American Association of Clinical Endocrinologists, the Obesity Society, and the American Society for Metabolic and Bariatric Surgery (Mechanick et al., 2009) are listed in Table 12–4. Some obstetric care providers recommend waiting at least 1 to 2 years after bariatric surgery to conceive as the resultant initial rapid weight loss can be harmful to the growing fetus (ACOG, 2009a; Edwards, 2006; MOD, 2011). This waiting period may allow for the woman to fully meet her weight loss goal. Women who have had bariatric surgery but are not planning immediate pregnancy should be aware that there is an increased risk of failure of oral contraceptives due to gastric malabsorption (ACOG, 2009a). Other types of contraceptives rather than oral hormones should be considered for this patient population (ACOG, 2009a).

Small, frequent meals consisting of calorie-dense foods high in protein and low in fat and carbohydrates are advised (James & Maher, 2009). Generally, 60 g of protein per day is recommended (Kominiarek, 2011).

Table 12–4. GUIDELINES FOR SUPPLEMENTATION AND LABORATORY TESTING OF THE POSTBARIATRIC SURGERY PATIENT

Deficiency	Laboratory Testing	Treatment if Deficient or Not Responsive to Oral Supplements	Routine Supplementation in Pregnancy
Protein	Serum albumin	Protein supplements	60-g protein/day in balanced diet
Calcium	Total and ionized calcium, parathyroid hormone		1,200 mg/d calcium citrate in addition to prenatal vitamin 400 μg/d contained in prenatal vitamin
Folic acid	Complete blood count, folic acid level	Oral folate 1,000 μg/d	400 μg/d contained in prenatal vitamin
Iron	Complete blood count, serum, iron, ferritin, total iron binding capacity	Parental iron; consult with nutritionist or hematologist	Ferrous sulfate, 300 mg two to three times per day with vitamin C in addition to prenatal vitamin 4,000 IU/d contained in prenatal vitamin
Vitamin A	Vitamin A levels	Vitamin A supplements should not exceed 10,000 IU/d in pregnancy	4,000 IU/d contained in prenatal vitamin
Vitamin B$_{12}$	Complete blood count, vitamin B$_{12}$ levels	Oral crystalline B$_{12}$ 350 μg/d or 1,000–2,000 μg intramuscularly every 2–3 mo; consult with nutritionist or hematologist	4 μg/d contained in prenatal vitamin
Vitamin D	25-hydroxyvitamin D	Calcitriol oral vitamin D 1,000 IU/d	400-800 IU/d contained in prenatal vitamin

Adapted from Mechanick, J. I., Kushner, R. F., Sugerman, H. J., Gonzalez-Campoy, J. M., Collazo-Clavell, M. L., Spitz, A. F., . . . Dixon, J. (2009). American Association of Clinical Endocrinologists, the Obesity Society, and American Society for Metabolic and Bariatric Surgery: Medical guidelines for clinical practice for the perioperative nutritional, metabolic, and nonsurgical support of the bariatric surgery patient (Perioperative bariatric guidelines). *Obesity, 17* (Supp.), S1–S70. doi:10.1038/oby.2009.28

After RYGB bariatric surgery, it is important to minimize or eliminate intake of simple carbohydrate-dense foods and beverages as their ingestion can result in dumping syndrome (a group of symptoms, including abdominal pain, cramping, nausea, diarrhea, light-headedness, flushing, tachycardia, and syncope) thought to be caused as gut peptides are released when food bypasses the stomach and enters the small intestine directly (Kominiarek, 2011). This potential problem has implications for screening for gestational diabetes during pregnancy. A substitute for the 50 g of glucola for gestational diabetes screening is recommended, such as home glucose monitoring with fasting and postprandial values during 1 week in the 24 to 28-week period (Kominiarek, 2011). When a woman has had LAGB surgery, one concern is how to manage the band during pregnancy. Some experts advocate deflating the band either before or early in the pregnancy to lessen complications, such as band migration and nausea and vomiting in pregnancy, while others prefer to wait and see if complications such as vomiting or lack of weight gain occur before releasing the band (Kominiarek, 2011). If complications arise, care should be individualized and provided in consultation with a bariatric surgeon.

Weight loss afforded by bariatric surgery will reduce many obstetrical complications associated with maternal obesity, including diabetes, hypertensive disorders, and birth of a macrosomic baby (Aricha-Tamir, Weintraub, Levi, & Sheiner, 2011; Maggard et al., 2008). The incidence of intrauterine growth restriction and small for gestational age are increased, particularly with malabsorptive methods (Magdaleno et al., 2012). Weight loss may decrease risk of labor abnormalities, failed labor induction, shoulder dystocia, cesarean birth, and low Apgar scores (Fyfe et al., 2011; Ovesen et al., 2011; Wolfe et al., 2011).

Bariatric surgery can increase the risk for gallstones, abdominal hernias, herniation of the bowel, changes in metabolism, and organ displacement caused by increased uterine size (NIDDK, 2004). Intestinal obstruction can occur after bariatric surgery and is most common when the uterus becomes an abdominal organ, when the presenting part descends into the birth canal, and during uterine involution (Cunningham et al., 2009). During pregnancy, diagnosis of bariatric-related operative complications may be delayed (ACOG, 2009a). These include anastomotic leaks, bowel obstruction, internal hernias, ventral hernias, band erosion, and band migration. Care providers should be alert for complaints of abdominal pain, nausea, vomiting, and fever, which could signify intestinal obstruction or other complications in pregnant women with a history of bariatric surgery. When these types of patients present with abdominal pain, consultation with the bariatric surgeon is indicated as the underlying pathology may be related to the bariatric surgery (ACOG, 2009a).

SUMMARY

Obesity is an epidemic that affects women of child-bearing age. This population has a significantly greater chance for complications during pregnancy, labor, birth, and the postpartum period. Obesity is a preventable disease with lifelong implications for both the mother and her baby. Preconception counseling may encourage changes in nutrition and lifestyle modifications that can mitigate risks by promoting weight loss prior to pregnancy. Care of the obese woman during childbirth can be challenging. Advance planning by the interdisciplinary perinatal team, knowledge of how to manage complications, and adequate resources can promote safe care for the obese woman and her baby.

REFERENCES

Alanis, M. C., Villers, M. S., Law, T. L., Steadman, E. M., & Robinson, C. J. (2010). Complications of cesarean delivery in the massively obese parturient. *American Journal of Obstetrics and Gynecology, 203*(3), 271.e1–271.e7. doi:10.1016/j.ajog.2010.06.049

American Academy of Pediatrics & American College of Obstetricians and Gynecologists. (2007). *Guidelines for Perinatal Care* (6th ed.). Elkgrove Village, IL: Author.

American College of Obstetricians and Gynecologists. (2013a). *Obesity in Pregnancy* (Committee Opinion No. 549). Washington, DC: Author.

American College of Obstetricians and Gynecologists. (2013b). *Weight Gain During Pregnancy* (Committee Opinion No. 548). Washington, DC: Author.

American College of Obstetricians and Gynecologists. (2009a). *Bariatric Surgery and Pregnancy* (Practice Bulletin No. 105). Washington, DC: Author.

American College of Obstetricians and Gynecologists. (2009b). *Postpartum Screening for Abnormal Glucose Tolerance in Women Who Had Gestational Diabetes Mellitus* (Committee Opinion No. 435). Washington, DC: Author.

American College of Obstetricians and Gynecologists. (2010). *Challenges for Overweight and Obese Urban Women* (Committee Opinion No. 470). Washington, DC: Author.

American College of Obstetricians and Gynecologists. (2011). *Thromboembolism in Pregnancy* (Practice Bulletin No. 123). Washington, DC: Author.

American Society of Anesthesiologists. (2006). Practice guidelines for the perioperative management of patients with obstructive sleep apnea. *Anesthesiology, 104*(5), 1081–1093.

Aricha-Tamir, B., Weintraub, A. Y., Levi, I., & Sheiner, E. (2011). Downsizing pregnancy complications: A study of paired pregnancy outcomes before and after bariatric surgery. *Surgery for Obesity and Related Diseases.* Advance online publication.

Artal, R., Lockwood, C. J., & Brown, H. L. (2010). Weight gain recommendations in pregnancy and the obesity epidemic. *Obstetrics and Gynecology, 115*(1), 152–155. doi:10.1097/AOG.0b013e3181c51908

Baird, J., Fisher, D., Lucas, P., Kleijnen, J., Roberts, H., & Law, C. (2005). Being big or growing fast: Systematic review of size and growth in infancy and later obesity. *British Medical Journal, 331*(7522), 929. doi:10.1136/bmj.38586.411273.EO

Baker, J. L., Michaelsen, K. F., Rasmussen, K. M., & Sorensen, T. I. A. (2004). Maternal prepregnant body mass index, duration of breastfeeding and timing of complementary food introduction are associated with infant weight gain. *American Journal of Clinical Nutrition, 80*(6), 1579–1588.

Bates, S. M., Greer, I. A., Middeldorp, S., Veenstra, D. L., Prabulos, A. M., & Vandvik, P. O. (2012). VTE, thrombophilia, antithrombotic therapy, and pregnancy (Evidence-Based Clinical Practice Guidelines, 9th ed.). *Chest, 141*(Suppl.), e691S– e736S. doi:10.1378/chest.11-2300

Bell, R. L., & Rosenbaum, S. H. (2005). Postoperative considerations for patients with obesity and sleep apnea. *Anesthesiology Clinics of North America, 23*(3), 493–500.

Berrington de Gonzalez, A., Hartge, P., Cerhan, J. R., Flint, A. J., Hannan, L., MacInnis, R. J., . . . Thun, M. J. (2010). Body-mass index and mortality among 1.46 million white adults. *New England Journal of Medicine, 363*(23), 2211–2219. doi:10.1056/NEJMoa1000367

Black, P. (2009). Obesity and diabetes: Time to act. *British Journal of Nursing, 18*(18), 1089.

Blomberg, M. (2011). Maternal obesity and risk of postpartum hemorrhage. *Obstetrics and Gynecology, 118*(3), 561–568. doi:10.1097/AOG.0b013e31822a6c59

Bourjeily, G., Ankner, G., Mohsenin, V. (2011). Sleep-disordered breathing in pregnancy. *Clinics in Chest Medicine, 32*(1), 175–189. doi:10.1016/j.ccm.2010.11.003

Catalano, P. M. (2007). Management of obesity in pregancy. *Obstetrics and Gynecology, 109*(2, Pt. 1), 419–433. doi:10.1097/01.AOG.0000253311.44696.85

Cedergen, M. I. (2007). Optimal gestational weight gain for body mass index categories. *Obstetrics and Gynecology, 110*(4), 759–764. doi:10.1097/01.AOG.0000279450.85198.b2

Centers for Disease Control and Prevention. (2006). Recommendations to improve preconception health and health care—United States: A report of the CDC/ATSDR Preconception care work group and the select panel on preconception care. *Morbidity and Mortality Weekly Report, 55*(RR06), 1–23.

Centers for Disease Control and Prevention. (2011). *Obesity: Halting the Epidemic by Making Health Easier* (At a Glance Report). Atlanta, GA: Author.

Centre for Maternal and Child Enquirie (2011). Saving Mothers' Lives: Reviewing maternal deaths to make motherhood safer: 2006–08. The eighth report on confidential enquiries into maternal deaths in the United Kingdom. *British Journal of Obstetrics and Gynaecology, 118* (Suppl. 1):1–203.

Chen, Y. H., Kang, J. J., Lin, C. C., Wang, I. T., Keller, J. J., & Lin, H. C. (2012). Obstructive sleep apnea and the risk of adverse pregnancy outcomes. *American Journal of Obstetrics and Gynecology, 206*(2), 136.e1– 136.e5. doi:10.1016/j.ajog.2011.09.006

Chescheir, N. (2011). Global obesity and the effect on women's health. *Obstetrics and Gynecology, 117*(5), 1213–1222. doi:10.1097/AOG.0b013e3182161732

Chu, S. Y., Callaghan, W. H., Kim, S. Y., Schmid, C. H., Lau, J., England, L. J., & Dietz, P. M. (2007). Maternal obesity and risk of diabetes mellitus. *Diabetes Care, 30*(8), 2070–2076.

Conrad, K., Russell, A. C., & Keister, K. J. (2011). Bariatric surgery and its impact on childbearing. *Nursing for Women's Health, 15*(3), 226–233. doi:10.111/j.1751-486X.2011.01637.x

Cunningham, F. G., Leveno, K. J., Bloom, S. K., Hauth, J. C., Rouse, D. J., & Spong, C. Y. (Eds.). (2009). Obesity. In *Williams Obstetrics* (23rd ed., pp. 946–957). New York: McGraw-Hill.

Daniels, J. (2006). Obesity: America's epidemic. *American Journal of Nursing, 106*(1), 40–50.

Davis, E., & Olson, C. (2009). Obesity in pregnancy. *Primary Care: Clinics in the Office Practice, 36*(2), 341–356. doi:10.1016/j.pop.2009.01.005.

Dietz, P. M., Callaghan, W. M., Morrow, B., & Cogswell, M. E. (2005). Population-based assessment of the risk of primary cesarean delivery due to excess pre-pregnancy weight among nulliparous women delivering term infants. *Maternal Child Health Journal, 9*(3), 237–244.

Donath, S. M., & Amir, L. H. (2008). Maternal obesity and initiation and duration of breastfeeding: Data from the longitudinal study of Australian children. *Maternal and Child Nutrition, 4*(3), 163–170.

Duran, E. H. (2011). Obesity as an epidemic: Causes, morbidities and reproductive performance. *Proceedings in Obstetrics and Gynecology, 1*(3), 8–16.

Edwards, J. (2005). Pregnancy after bariatric surgery. *AWHONN Lifelines, 9*(5), 388–393.

Ehrenberg, H. M. (2011). Intrapartum considerations in perinatal care. *Seminars in Perinatology, 35*(6), 324–329. doi:10.1053/j.semperi.2011.05.016

Facco, F. L. (2011). Sleep-disordered breathing and pregnancy. *Seminars in Perinatology, 35*(6), 335–339. doi:10.1053/j.semperi.2011.05.018

Flegal, K. M., Carroll, M. D., Ogden, C. L., & Curtin, L. R. (2010). Prevalence and trends in obesity among US adults, 1999–2008. *Journal of the American Medical Association, 303*(3), 235–241. doi:10.1001/jama.2009.2014

Fyfe, E. M., Anderson, N. H., North, R. A., Chan, E. H. Y., Taylor, R. S., Dekker, G. A., & McCowan, L. M. E. (2011). Risk of first-stage and second-stage cesarean delivery by maternal body mass index among nulliparous women in labor at term. *Obstetrics and Gynecology, 117*(6), 1315–1322. doi:10.1097/AOG.0b013e318217922a

Goffman, D., Madden, R. C., Harrison, E. A., Merkatz, I. R., & Chazotte, C. (2007). Predictors of maternal mortality and near-miss maternal morbidity. *Journal of Perinatology, 27*(10), 597–601.

Gore, S. A., Brown, D. M., & Smith, D. (2003). The role of postpartum weight retention in obesity among women: A review of the evidence. *Annals of Behavioral Medicine, 26*(2), 149–159.

Gunatilake, R., & Perlow, J. (2011). Obesity and pregnancy: Clinical management of the obese gravida. *American Journal of Obstetrics and Gynecology, 204*(2), 106–119. doi:10.1016/j.ajog.2010.10.002

Hendler, I., Goldenberg, R. L., Mercer, B. M., Iams, J. D., Meis, P. J., Moawad, A. H., . . . Sorokin, Y. (2005). The preterm prediction study: Association between maternal body mass index and spontaneous and indicated preterm birth. *American Journal of Obstetrics and Gynecology, 192*(2), 882–886. doi:10.1016/ajog.2004.009.021

Hui, L. L., Schooling, C. M., Leung, S. S., Mak, K. H., Ho, L. M., Lam, T. H., & Leung, G. M. (2008). Birth weight, infant growth, and childhood body mass index. *Archives in Pediatric Adolescent Medicine, 162*(3), 212–218.

Institute of Medicine. (2009). *Weight Gain During Pregnancy: Reexamining the Guidelines* (Report Brief). Washington, DC: National Academies Press.

Izci-Balserak, B., & Pien, G. W. (2010). Sleep-disordered breathing and pregnancy: Potential mechanisms and evidence for maternal and fetal morbidity. *Current Opinion in Pulmonary Medicine, 16*(6), 574–582. doi:10.1097/MCP.Ob013e32833f0d55

James, D., & Maher, M. (2009). Caring for the extremely obese woman during pregnancy and birth. *MCN: The American Journal of Maternal Child Nursing, 34*(1), 24–30.

Johnson, T. R. B., Gregory, K. D., & Niebyl, J. R. (2007). Preconception and prenatal care: Part of the continuum. In S. G. Gabbe, J. R. Niebyl, & J. L. Simpson (Eds.), *Obstetrics: Normal and Problem Pregnancies* (pp. 11–151). Philadelpia: Churchill Livingstone.

Jungheim, E. S., & Moley, K. H. (2010). Current knowledge of obesity's effects in the pre- and periconceptional periods and avenues for future research. *American Journal of Obstetrics and Gynecology, 203*(6), 525–530. doi:10.1016/j.ajog.2010.06.043

Khoury, F. R., Ehrenberg, H. M., & Mercer, B. M. (2009). The impact of maternal obesity on satisfactory detailed ultrasound image acquisition. *Journal of Maternal Fetal and Neonatal Medicine, 22*(4), 337–341. doi:10.1080/14767050802524586

Kiel, D. W., Dodson, E. A., Artal, R., Boehmer, T. K., & Leet, T. L. (2007). Gestational weight gain and pregnancy outcomes in obese women:

How much is enough? *Obstetrics and Gynecology, 110*(4), 752–758. doi:10.1097/01.AOG.0000278819.17190.87

Knight, M., Kurinczuk, J., Spark, P., & Brocklehurst, P. (2010). Extreme obesity in pregnancy in the United Kingdom. *Obstetrics and Gynecology, 115*(5), 989–997. doi:10.1097/AOG.0b013e3181da8f09

Kominiarek, M. A. (2011). Preparing for and managing a pregnancy after bariatric surgery. *Seminars in Perinatology, 35*(6), 356–361. doi:10.1053/j.semperi.2011.05.022

Kominiarek, M. A., VanVeldhuisen, P., Hibbard, J., Landy, H., Haberman, S., Learman, L., . . . Zhang, J., for the Consortium on Safe Labor. (2010). The maternal body mass index: A strong association with delivery route. *American Journal of Obstetrics and Gynecology, 203*(3), 264.e1–264.e7. doi:10.1016/j.ajog.2010.06.024

Kominiarek, M. A., Zhang, J., VanVeldhuisen, P., Troendle, J., Beaver, J., & Hibbard, J. (2011). Contemporary labor patterns: The impact of maternal body mass. *American Journal of Obstetrics and Gynecology, 205*(3), 244.e1–244.e8. doi:10.1016/j.ajog.2011.06.014

Livingston, E. H. (2010). The incidence of bariatric surgery has plateaued in the U.S. *American Journal of Surgery, 200*(3), 378–385. doi:10.1016/j.amjsurg.2009.11.007

Magdaleno, R., Pereira, B. G., Chaim, E. A., & Turato, E. R. (2012). Pregnancy after bariatric surgery: A current view of maternal, obstetrical and perinatal challenges. *Archives of Gynecology and Obstetrics, 285*(3), 559–566. doi:1007/DD4D4-011-2187-0

Maggard, M. A., Yermilov, I., Li, Z., Maglinone, M., Newberry, S., Suttorp, M., . . . Shekelle, P. G. (2008). Pregnancy and fertility following bariatric surgery: A systematic review. *Journal of the American Medical Association, 300*(19), 2286–2296.

Mantakas, A., & Farrell, T. (2010). The influence of increasing BMI in nulliparous women on pregnancy outcome. *European Journal of Obstetrics & Gynecology and Reproductive Biology, 153*(1), 43–46. doi:10.1016/j.ejogrb.2010.06.021

March of Dimes. (2011). Overweight and obesity during pregnancy. Retrieved from http://www.marchofdimes.com/pregnancy/complications_obesity.html

Mechanick, J. I., Kushner, R. F., Sugerman, H. J., Gonzalez-Campoy, J. M., Collazo-Clavell, M. L., Spitz, A. F., . . . Dixon, J. (2009). American Association of Clinical Endocrinologists, the Obesity Society, and American Society for Metabolic and Bariatric Surgery: Medical guidelines for clinical practice for the perioperative nutritional, metabolic, and nonsurgical support of the bariatric surgery patient (Perioperative bariatric guidelines). *Obesity, 17*(Suppl.), S1–S70. doi:10.1038/oby.2009.28

Mehta, S. H., Kruger, M. S., & Sokol, R. J. (2011). Being too large for gestational age precedes childhood obesity in African Americans. *American Journal of Obstetrics and Gynecology, 204*(3), 265.e1–265.e5. doi:10.1016/j.ajog.2010.12.009

National Heart, Lung, and Blood Institute. (1998). *Clinical Guidelines on the Identification, Evaluation, and Treatment of Overweight and Obesity in Adults* (Evidence Report). (NIH Publication No. 98-4083). Washington, DC: National Institutes of Health.

National Institute of Diabetes and Digestive and Kidney Diseases. (2004). *Gastrointestinal Surgery for Severe Obesity*. Bethesda, MD: Author.

Neilson, D. R. Jr., Freeman, R. K., & Mangan, S. (2008). Signal ambiguity resulting in unexpected outcome with external fetal heart rate monitoring. *American Journal of Obstetrics and Gynecology, 198*(6), 717–724. doi:10.1016/j.ajog.2008.02.030

O'Brien, T. E., Ray, J. G., & Chan, W. S. (2003). Maternal body mass index and the risk of preeclampsia: A systematic overview. *Epidemiology, 14*(3), 368–374.

Ogden, C. L., & Carroll, M. D. (2010). *Prevalence of Obesity, and Extreme Obesity Among Adults: United States, Trends 1976–1980 Through 2007–2008* (National Center for Health Statistics E-Stats). Atlanta, GA: Centers for Disease Control and Prevention.

Ogden, C. L., Carroll, M. D., Curtin, L. R., Lamb, M. M., & Flegal, K. M. (2010). Prevalence of high body mass index in US children and adolescents, 2007–2008. *Journal of the American Medical Association, 303*(3), 242–249. doi:10.1001/jama.2009.2012

Ogden, C. L., Carroll, M. D., Kit, B. K., & Flegal, K. M. (2012). *Prevalence of Obesity in the United States: 2009–2010* (National Center for Health Statistics Data Brief No. 82). Atlanta, GA: National Centers for Disease Control and Prevention.

Ohlendorf, J. M., Weiss, M. E., & Ryan, P. (2012). Weight-management information needs of postpartum women. *MCN: The American Journal of Maternal Child Nursing, 37*(1), 56–63. doi:10.1097/NMC.Ob013e1823851ee

Olivarez, S. A., Ferres, M., Antony, K., Mattewal, A., Maheshwari, B., Sangi-Hagjpeykar, H., & Aagaard-Tillery, K. (2011). Obstructive sleep apnea screening in pregnancy, perinatal outcomes, and impact of maternal obesity. *American Journal of Perinatology, 28*(6), 651–658. doi:10.1055/s-0031-1276740

Ovesen, P., Rasmussen, S., & Kesmodel, U. (2011). Effect of prepregnancy maternal overweight and obesity on pregnancy outcome. *Obstetrics and Gynecology, 118*(2, Pt. 1), 305–312. doi:10.1097/AOG.0b013e3182245d49

Phelan, S. (2010). Obesity in the American populations: Calories, cost, and culture. *American Journal of Obstetrics and Gynecology, 203*(6), 522–524. doi:10.1016/j.ajog.2010.07.026

Phelan, S., Hart, C., Phipps, M., Abrams, B., Schaffner, A., Adams, A., & Wing, R. (2011). Maternal behaviors during pregnancy impact offspring obesity risk. *Experimental Diabetes Research, 2011*(10), e1–e9. doi:10.115/2011/985139

Rahman, M., & Berenson, A. (2010). Accuracy of current body mass index obesity classification for white, black, and Hispanic reproductive-age women. *Obstetrics and Gynecology, 115*(5), 982–988. doi:10.1097/AOG.0b013e3181da9423

Reece, E. A. (2008). Perspectives on obesity, pregnancy and birth outcomes in the United States: The scope of the problem. *American Journal of Obstetrics and Gynecology, 198*(1), 23–27. doi:10.1016/j.ajog.2007.06.076

Rooney, B. L., Schauberger, C. W., & Mathiason, M. A. (2005). Impact of perinatal weight change on long-term obesity and obesity-related illnesses. *Obstetrics and Gynecology, 106*(6), 1349–1356.

Saldana, T. M., Siega-Riz, A. M., Adair, L. S., & Suchindran, C. (2006). The relationship between pregnancy weight gain and glucose tolerance status among black and white women in central North Carolina. *American Journal of Obstetrics and Gynecology, 195*(6), 1629–1635.

Salihu, H. M. (2011). Maternal obesity and stillbirth. *Seminars in Perinatology, 35*(6), 340–344. doi:10.1053/j.semperi.2011.05.019

Salihu, H. M., Dunlop, A.-L., Hedayatzadeh, M., Alio, A. P., Kirby, R. S., & Alexander, G. R. (2007). Extreme obesity and risk of stillbirth among black and white gravidas. *Obstetrics and Gynecology, 110*(3), 552–557.

Saravanakumar, K., Rao, S. G., & Cooper, G. M. (2006). The challenges of obesity and obstetric anesthesia. *Current Opinion in Obstetrics and Gynecology, 18*(6), 631–635.

Sarkar, R., Cooley, S., Donnelly, J., Walsh, T., Collins, C., & Geary, P. (2007). The incidence and impact of increased body mass index on maternal and fetal morbidity in the low-risk primigravid population. *Journal of Maternal-Fetal and Neonatal Medicine, 20*(120), 879–883. doi:10.1080/14767050701713090

Shekelle, P. G., Newberry, S., Maglione, M., Li, Z., Yermilov, I., Hilton, L., . . . Chen, S. (2008). Bariatric surgery in women of reproductive age: Special concerns for surgery. *Evidence Report/Technology Assessment, 11*(169), 1–51.

Simpson, K. R. (2011). Avoiding confusion of maternal heart rate with fetal heart rate during labor. *MCN: The American Journal of Maternal Child Nursing, 36*(4), 272. doi:10.1097/NMC.0b013e318217a61a

Society of Actuaries. (2011). *Cost of Obesity Approaching $300 Billion a Year.* Schaumburg, IL: Author.

Society of Obstetricians and Gynaecologists of Canada. (2010). *Obesity in Pregnancy* (Clinical Practice Guideline No. 239). Vancouver, BC: Author.

Stotland, N. E., Hopkins, L. M., & Caughey, A. B. (2004). Gestational weight gain, macrosomia, and risk of cesarean birth in nondiabetic nulliparas. *Obstetrics and Gynecology, 104*(4), 671–677. doi:10.1097/01.aog.0000139515.97799.fg

Stream, A. R., & Sutherland, E. R. (2012). Obesity and asthma disease phenotypes. *Current Opinion in in Allergy & Clinical Immunology, 12*(1), 76–81. doi:10.1097/ACI.0b013e32834eca41

Szymanski, L. M., & Satin, A. J. (2012). Exercise in pregnancy: Fetal responses to current public health guidelines. *Obstetrics and Gynecology, 119*(3), 603–610. doi:10.1097/AOG.0b013e31824760b5

Tan, T., & Sia, A. T. (2011). Anesthesia considerations in the obese gravida. *Seminars in Perinatology, 35*(6), 350–355. doi:10.1053/j.semperi.2011.05.021

Thornburg, L. L. (2011). Antepartum obstetrical complications associated with obesity. *Seminars in Perinatology, 35*(6), 317–323. doi:10.1053/j.semperi.2011.05.015

Thornton, Y. S., Smarkola, C., Kopacz, S. M., & Ishoof, S. B. (2009). Perinatal outcomes in nutritionally monitored obese pregnant women: A randomized trial. *Journal of the National Medical Association, 101*(6), 569–577.

Tipton, A. M., Cohen, S. A., & Chelmow, D. (2011). Wound infection in the obese pregnant woman. *Seminars in Perinatology, 35*(6), 345–349. doi:10.1053/j.semperi.2011.05.020

Vahratian, A., Zhang, J., Troendle, J. F., Savitz, D. A., & Siega-Riz, A. M. (2004). Maternal prepregnancy overweight and obesity and the pattern of labor progression in term nulliparous women. *Obstetrics and Gynecology, 104*(5, Pt. 1), 943–951. doi:10.197/01.AOG.0000142712.53197.91

Vallejo, M. C. (2007). Anesthetic management of the morbidly obese parturient. *Current Opinion in Anaesthesiology, 20*(3), 175–180. doi:10.1097/ACO.0b013e328014646b

Vidarsdottir, H., Geirsson, T., Hardardottir, H., Valdimarsdottir, U., & Dagbjartsson, A. (2011). Obstetric and neonatal risks among extremely macrosomic babies and their mothers. *American Journal of Obstetrics and Gynecology, 204*(5), 423.e1–423.e6. doi:10.1016/j.ajog.2010.12.036

Virginia Maternal Mortality Review Team. (2009). *Obesity and Maternal Death in Virginia 1999–2002.* Richmond, VA: Virginia Department of Health, Office of the Chief Medical Examiner.

Viswanathan, M., Siega-Riz, A. M., Moos, M. K., Deierlein, A., Mumford, S., Knaack, J., . . . Lohr, K. N. (2008). *Outcomes of Maternal Weight Gain* (Evidence Report/Technology Assessment No. 168). Rockville, MD: Agency for Healthcare Research and Quality.

Vricella, L. K., Louis, J. M., Mercer, B. M., & Bolden, N. (2010). Anesthesia complications during scheduled cesarean delivery for morbidly obese women. *American Journal of Obstetrics and Gynecology, 203*(3), 276.e1–276.e5. doi:10.1016/j.ajog.2010.06.022

Vricella, L. K., Louis, J. M., Mercer, B. M., & Bolden, N. (2011). Impact of morbid obesity on epidural anesthesia complications in labor. *American Journal of Obstetrics and Gynecology, 205*(4), 370.e1–370.e6. doi:10.1016/j.ajog.2011.06.085

Whitaker, R. C. (2004). Predicting preschooler obesity at birth: The role of maternal obesity in early pregnancy. *Pediatrics, 114*(1), 29–36.

Wolfe, K. B., Rossi, R. A., & Warshak, C. (2011). The effect of maternal obesity on the rate of failed induction of labor. *American Journal of Obstetrics and Gynecology, 205*(2), 128.e1–128.e7. doi:10.1016/j.ajog.2011.03.051 1.e1–1.e7

World Health Organization. (2011). *Obesity and Overweight* (Fact Sheet No. 311). Geneva, Switzerland: Author.

Zhang, J., Bricker, L., Wray, S., & Quenby, S. (2007). Poor uterine contractility in obese women. *BJOG: International Journal of Obstetrics and Gynaecology, 114*(3), 343–348. doi:10.1111/j.1471-0528.2006.01233.x

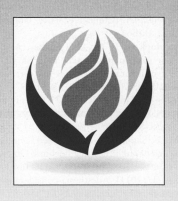

Judy Wilson-Griffin

CHAPTER 13

Maternal–Fetal Transport

Maternal transport is a fundamental component of regionalized perinatal care. Perinatal regionalization through a structured designated method guarantees that hospitals and healthcare systems provide a full range of services for pregnant women and their babies within in a specified geographic region (American Academy of Pediatrics [AAP] & American College of Obstetricians and Gynecologists, 2012). In a seminal document published in 1976, *Toward Improving the Outcome of Pregnancy*, the March of Dimes (MOD; 1976) proposed a model system for regionalization of perinatal care including definitions for levels of care (e.g., levels I to III) in hospitals that provided perinatal services. The goal was to promote transfer of high-risk mothers to hospitals with the appropriate level of care based on gestational age of the fetus. This model was adopted across the United States and resulted in perinatal regionalization and improved perinatal outcomes as more preterm babies and babies with high-risk conditions were born at centers that had the skilled personnel and additional resources for their stabilization and ongoing care (MOD, 1993). High-risk pregnant women also benefited by being cared for in level II and level III perinatal centers. Since the 1970s, regionalized care has proven to be a useful service that can improve both maternal and/or fetal outcome (MOD, 1993). Due to the evidence of significant improvements in outcomes for these patients when transferred appropriately when stable, in 2009, the National Quality Forum (NQF; 2009) in their *National Voluntary Consensus Standards for Perinatal Care* recommended using *babies under 1,500 g born at a hospital with the appropriate level of care* as a quality care indicator.

Neonatal transport has been active in the United States since the 1960s after the establishment of neonatal intensive care units (NICUs) (Glass, 2004). However, even with the development of well-trained neonatal transport teams, evidence has shown that in most cases, the mother proves to be the best transport vehicle for the fetus (MacDonald, 1989). Thus, maternal, instead of neonatal, transport is preferred when feasible. As with any procedure, transport has advantages and disadvantages. While there may be advantages to the health of both the mother and her unborn fetus, it can be less than ideal to have women give birth sometimes far from their home, family, and friends and without their primary obstetrician who they have become accustomed to for continued care. Indications for maternal–fetal transport are listed in Display 13–1.

EMTALA

When discussing maternal–fetal transport, it is important to review the Emergency Medical Treatment and Active Labor Act (EMTALA) regulations as they relate to appropriate transfers. EMTALA originated in 1985 as part of the Consolidated Omnibus Budget Reconciliation Act (COBRA; 1985), to protect patients during an emergency regardless of their ability to pay for care or insurance status. The law requires that all patients, including those in labor, be assessed, stabilized, and treated at the hospital where they present regardless of their ability to pay for care or insurance status. EMTALA (U.S. Department of Health and Human Services & Centers for Medicare & Medicaid Services, 2003, 2009) requires that hospitals perform a medical screening exam (MSE) for anyone who presents with an emergency medical condition (EMC). The goal for the patient who presents is to either be stabilized and treated or transferred to a facility that can better meet the medical needs of the patient based

DISPLAY 13-1

Indications for Maternal–Fetal Transport

Medical
- Anemia
- Autoimmune
- Cardiac disease
- Chemical abuse
- Diabetes
- Hematologic disorder
- Infection
- Malignancy
- Neurologic disorder
- Obesity
- Psychiatric disorder
- Pulmonary disease
- Renal disease
- Sepsis
- Surgical emergencies
- Thromboembolic disease

Obstetric
- Amniotic fluid abnormalities
- Fetal demise
- Hemorrhagic disorders of pregnancy
- Hypertensive disorders in pregnancy
- Multiple gestation
- Premature labor
- Premature rupture of membranes
- Vaginal bleeding

Fetal/newborn
- Fetal anomalies
- Fetal growth restriction
- Placental abnormalities
- Congenital abnormalities
- Isoimmunization

on her individual clinical situation. Pregnant women who present with contractions and/or who may be in labor are considered unstable. Caregivers must consider many factors in their decision regarding when it is appropriate to transfer a pregnant woman to another facility. A pregnant woman who is having contractions is not considered to be having an EMC if it is determined that there is adequate time to safely transfer her before she gives birth or if the transfer will not pose a threat to the safety of the patient. Caregivers must evaluate whether the woman and her fetus will be better served at a higher level of care. This is not always a straightforward or clear clinical judgment. A woman who appears stable prior to transport may become unstable during the transport. Unanticipated birth could occur prior to arrival at the receiving facility. Transfer might also be feasible based on the patient's request.

Whenever maternal transport is an option, the risks and benefits must be thoroughly considered. Several procedures must be completed in order to be compliant with the EMTALA regulations. A conversation between the referring physician and accepting physician at the receiving location should occur prior to transfer. The receiving location should have adequate space and staff to accommodate the woman being transferred and the baby anticipated to be born. A copy of the medical record should accompany the mother on transfer. Prior to the transport, consent is required from the mother regarding the transfer, the destination, and method of transport. It is important to avoid violating the spirit, intent, and rules of the EMTALA law when transferring a pregnant woman. EMTALA violations can result in significant fines and can have negative implications for the reputation of the transferring facility. Common EMTALA violations (Glass, 2004) include:

- Lack of or an inadequate MSE
- Lack of patient stabilization prior to transfer to another facility
- Failure to obtain patient consent for the transfer
- No documented accepting physician
- Transferring with inappropriate equipment and personnel
- Failure to stabilize the patient prior to transfer

TYPES OF MATERNAL–FETAL TRANSPORT

ONE-WAY TRANSPORT

In a one-way transport, the most common type of transport, the referring intuition makes the arrangements for the patient. In this method, usually the local ambulance or helicopter services provides the transportation to the accepting facility. The advantages of one-way transport are that the patient may be transported by the nurse from the referring hospital that patient is familiar with and the actual transport may be faster. The referring facility assumes responsibility and direction of care until a formal hand off is given at the accepting institution. A disadvantage is limited availability of transport vehicles and skilled personnel in emergency obstetric procedures at the originating facility. Often, personnel at level I facilities are not trained in maternal transport in the pre-hospital environment, which could potentially pose an additional safety concern.

TWO-WAY TRANSPORT

In a two-way transport, the receiving facility accepts the patient and then sends a team to transport the patient to their facility. That facility accepts medical and legal responsibility for the patient once the report has been received by the team upon arrival. The advantage of two-way transport is that it allows the receiving institution to bring their highly skilled service directly to the bedside and begin that level of care immediately. The transport team should explain what the patient can expect once they arrive at the receiving intuition. The two-way transport team has been trained in the prehospital management and care of the pregnant patient. A disadvantage may include delay in transfer since travel of the team from the receiving facility to the referring facility adds time to the process.

MODE OF TRANSPORT

FIXED WING (AIRPLANE)

Fixed wing (airplane) can be a viable option for long-distance maternal transports. It also provides a more spacious mode of air transport. Compared to the cost of a rotor wing (helicopter), it may be a less expensive option for air transport. With fixed-wing flights requiring access to a runway and an aircraft, this transport method many times can become a major challenge when time is a factor in moving a patient from one location to another. Finding airplanes that come equipped with personnel ready to deal with obstetrical emergencies can also be a disadvantage for some programs. Potential side effects during flight may include nausea and vomiting, increase in contractions, worsening hypertension or hypotension, decrease in respiratory effort, and unplanned changes in the intravenous (IV) flow rate (O'Brien, 2004).

ROTOR WING (HELICOPTER)

Helicopters are usually used for shorter distances or when the patient has a more urgent need. When speed is important, use of a helicopter offers advantages as a useful tool in accessing timely care for the perinatal patient. (Ohara, 2008). The helicopter is staffed with critical care personnel experienced in airway management and acute condition. Traveling a long distance by ground can affect outcomes for the pregnant patient status, thus making air a more attractive option.

A challenge for helicopters is aircraft availability. Concerns are for appropriate landing zones at either the referring or receiving location. Weather may be problematic for air transport. The cost of helicopter transport may also be a disadvantage for using this as a means for moving the patient from one location to another. The ability to adequately assess the labor status and to continuously monitor the fetus may be of concern due to noise and vibration. A birth during transport is always a concern, especially when the patient is transported in labor. Despite the advantage of air transport, flight teams are often concerned about in-flight birth. However, based on a national survey conducted of 203 flight programs, the incidence of en route birth is rare (Jones, 2001).

GROUND (AMBULANCE)

Ambulances are used for urgent or interfaculty patient transport based on patient condition, distance, and provider request. The major advantage to using ground transport is that it is usually easy to access and there may be different types of units readily available. Ambulances are less affected by weather when compared to air transport. Ground transport is also more economical than other forms of patient transport. Equipment in an ambulance varies depending on whether the ambulance is a basic or a critical care unit. Ambulances are equipped with medical supplies, telemetry monitors, portable oxygen, and personnel such as paramedics and emergency medical technicians (EMTs).

TRANSPORT EQUIPMENT

The transport team requires equipment to adequately monitor the patient during transport and for emergency treatment if necessary. When planning a maternal–fetal transport, it is important to check to make sure everything that is needed is available in the transport vehicle. The following equipment is suggested regardless of the method of transport. Other equipment may be necessary based on the individual clinical situation, including:

- Vital signs monitoring equipment
- Doppler for fetal heart rate (FHR) assessment
- IV administration setup
- Respiratory equipment
- Medications
- Emergency birth equipment
- Infant resuscitation equipment
- Documentation method

TRANSPORT PERSONNEL

Well-trained personnel who can manage obstetrical patients in the prehospital environment are essential for a successful program. The composition of the team may vary depending on resources, regulatory requirements, patient condition, and the vehicle used during transport. When transporting a patient by ground, the team may consist of an EMT or paramedic, respiratory therapist, and/or labor and delivery nurse. For patients requiring air transport, the team may be composed of critical care flight nurses and flight paramedics and/or a labor and delivery nurse. Clinical experience needed to care for the perinatal patient during transport includes annual prehospital safety training, leadership skills, advanced cardiac life support (ACLS) skills, knowledge of how to care for high-risk labor conditions and emergent birth, and neonatal recitation program (NRP) skills. Many programs require that the nurse has labor and delivery extensive experience prior to joining their maternal transport team. It is important that the program has clear guidelines and medical control once they have received the report and assume care of the patient until arriving at the receiving location. During transport, a well-prepared team will be able respond to possible complications or risk in the prehospital environment.

TRANSPORT PLAN AND PATIENT PREPARATION

Once the need for maternal transport has been identified, a discussion with the patient and her family regarding the reason for transfer must occur. The pregnant woman must agree to a transfer to another facility by providing written consent. A copy of the transfer consent should accompany the patient to the receiving location. The referring physician will contact the physician at the accepting location and will review the reason for the referral. Both physicians will decide on the mode of transport based on the distance, weather, patient condition, safety, and cost in most cases (Lupton, 2004). Information should be provided to the family regarding where the patient is being transferred, directions, and contact numbers. All pertinent medical records should accompany the patient to the receiving location.

For the majority of transports, establishing IV access is necessary, supplemental oxygen should be provided as needed, oxygen saturation levels should be monitored, and the patient's bladder should be assessed before departure. Prior to departure, a documented patient assessment should include vital signs, FHR, and uterine activity (Holleran, 1996). When securing the patient to the stretcher, it is important to encourage uterine displacement to promote blood flow during transport. Assessment of maternal–fetal status continues en route based on protocols, orders, and the patient's condition. Care should be taken to maintain physical safety while maintaining respiratory and hemodynamic stability during maternal–fetal transport. Once the woman arrives at the new location, a direct patient hand off from the transport team with the receiving staff is ideal to promote patient safety. Patient hand off information includes any significant events during transport along with the reason for the referral, vital signs, and response to any medication and treatments. (see Fig. 13–1) for a sample documentation form to be used for maternal transport to record these types of data.) This report should include information about emergency contacts and the family that is en route to the hospital. Figures 13–2 and 13–3 provide examples of physician orders that can be used for maternal transport, with Figure 13–3 being specific to a woman in early preterm labor. It is important that the receiving physician keep the primary obstetrician updated on the status of his/her patient and the plan following discharge.

SUMMARY

Maternal transport can enhance access to perinatal care and improve outcomes. A critical systemic interdisciplinary review of referrals can be an effective tool to further identify ways to improve the care provided to perinatal patients. Feedback to the referring hospital from the receiving hospital regarding the patient preparation process can be valuable in promoting quality care, as is feedback from the referring hospital to the receiving hospital when it is focused on how patient needs were met and the timeliness and courteousness of response. Together, the teams can assist each other in providing the best care possible during maternal referral and transport.

MATERNAL TRANSPORT FORM

Please check (✓) the appropriate box (☐) and fill in the blank(s) as needed.

Date: _____ Initiational call time: _____ ☐ Airplane ☐ Helicopter ☐ Ground	RN:		Trip accepted
Miles	Accepting MD	Phone number	
Trip No.	Departed	Arrive Location	Depart	Arrive
Location		Phone		
Referring MD		Phone number		
Patient name		Age	DOB	Weight
Transport Diagnosis				Height

CURRENT LABOR HISTORY

Gravida	Para	Abortion	Living children	Gestational age
Estimated date of confinement	Last menstrual period	Time ☐ Sterile speculum	Time ☐ Vaginal exam	
Dilation ___ cm	Effacement	Station	Membranes ☐ intact	Time PROM

+++ Location of scars

x Location of fetal heart tones

Antenatal testing: ☐ Ultrasound ☐ Amniocentesis ☐ Non stress test

Fetal status / Strip review
Date: _____ Time: _____

PATIENT ASSESSMENT

Allergies/Sensitivities ☐ NKDA ☐ Latex ☐ Other:	Blood Glucose Time _____ Results _____	Circulatory: ☐ WNL ☐ Heart disease ☐ MVP ☐ Chest pain ☐ Blood transfusions
Respiratory ☐ O2 _____ ☐ Asthma ☐ Smoker	Sensory ☐ Visual changes ☐ Glasses ☐ Contacts ☐ Headaches	LOC ☐ Seizure ☐ WNL ☐ Alert	Pain score (1-10)
Reflexes ☐ 4+ ☐ 3+ ☐ 2+ ☐ 1+ ☐ Absent	Urinalysis ☐ Protein ☐ Ketones	Abdomen ☐ Soft ☐ Tender ☐ Rigid	Edema ☐ Face ☐ Hands ☐ Feet

Complications of pregnancy:

| Support person | Contact number |

Status update to referring hospital

Status update to referring hospital

| Date | Time | Call report to RN: _____ |

RN Signature: _____

PATIENT LABEL

FIGURE 13–1. Maternal transport form. (From SSM St. Mary's Health Center, Richmond Heights, MO.)

MATERNAL TRANSPORT FORM

PRE-TRANSPORT NOTES

Date: _____ Time: _____

INTRA-TRANSPORT NOTES

Date: _____ Time: _____

Transfer of care to: Name _____ Date: _____ Time: _____

MEDICATIONS/IV FLUIDS					VITAL SIGNS							
TIME	MEDICATION/FLUID TYPE	DOSE RATE	ROUTE SITE	GIVEN BY REFER HOSP.	TIME	T	HR	RR	BP	SpO2	FHT	CTX

PATIENT LABEL

FIGURE 13–1. *(Continued)*

MATERNAL TRANSPORT PHYSICIAN ORDERS

DRUG MAY BE DISPENSED IN ACCORDANCE WITH THE
HOSPITAL FORMULARY SYSTEM UNLESS CHECKED HERE ⇨ ☐

ALLERGIES: ☐ NO KNOWN ALLERGIES

PATIENT WEIGHT ⇨ _____ ☐ Kgs ☐ Lbs   PATIENT HEIGHT ⇨ _____

IMPORTANT REMINDERS

1. "Daily" instead of "qd"
2. "Units" instead of "u"
3. No trailing zeros (1mg, not 1.0mg)
4. Always use leading zeros (0.1mg, not .1mg)
5. "Morphine" instead of "MSO4"
6. "Magnesium sulfate" instead of "MgSO4"
7. "Every other day" instead of "Q.O.D."
8. "MCG" instead of "µg"
9. "International Units" instead of "IU"

✓	DATE ORDERED	TIME	√	INITIAL HERE TO INDICATE TELEPHONE ORDER READ BACK FOR ACCURACY	ORDERS
					Accepting physician: Dr. _____ Contact #
					IUP:
					Monitoring
					• Vital signs on arrival at referral hospital and review fetal monitor strip before transfer
					• Obtain maternal vital signs and FHR just prior to transport 5-15 minutes prior to departure. Vitals Q 15 minutes during transport. Temperature Q 4 hours, if membranes ruptured then Q 2 hours.
					• EKG monitoring as needed
					• Assess level of consciousness
					• Assess abdominal tenderness and for bladder distention.
					• Position patient to provide for uterine displacement.
					• If indicated to assess cervical dilation, sterile vaginal exam if membranes intact, sterile speculum exam if membranes ruptured
					• Call physician for:
					• Temperature greater than 99.9°F
					• RR greater than 22 or less than 12
					• Pulse greater than 120
					• Systolic BP greater than 160 or less than 80
					• Diastolic BP greater than 100 or less than 40
					• Tetanic contractions and or non reassuring FHT's
					Labs
					☐ GBS culture, bring specimen back to St. Mary's laboratory
					☐ Fern test to rule out ROM
					☐ Fetal fibronectin if no vaginal exam in the past 24 hours
					Intake & Output
					• Foley for bladder distention prn
					• Intake and output prior to departure
					Fluids
					• IV with 18 gauge needle: (not necessary to restart IV if adequate 18 gauge line in place)
					• 1000 ml Lactated Ringers at 125 ml per hour
					Respiratory
					• O2 at 10L/min per non-rebreather mask for fetal intolerance or maternal oxygen saturation level less than 95%
					NPO

PATIENT LABEL

FIGURE 13–2. Maternal transport physician orders. (From SSM St. Mary's Health Center, Richmond Heights, MO.)

MATERNAL TRANSPORT PHYSICIAN ORDERS

DRUG MAY BE DISPENSED IN ACCORDANCE WITH THE
HOSPITAL FORMULARY SYSTEM UNLESS CHECKED HERE ⇨ ☐

ALLERGIES:

PATIENT WEIGHT ⇨ _____   ☐ Kgs ☐ Lbs   PATIENT HEIGHT ⇨ _____

IMPORTANT REMINDERS

1. "Daily" instead of "qd"
2. "Units" instead of "u"
3. No trailing zeros (1mg, not 1.0mg)
4. Always use leading zeros (0.1mg, not .1mg)
5. "Morphine" instead of "MSO4"
6. "Magnesium sulfate" instead of "MgSO4"
7. "Every other day" instead of "Q.O.D."
8. "MCG" instead of "µg"
9. "International Units" instead of "IU"

✓	DATE ORDERED	TIME	✓	ORDERS (INITIAL HERE TO INDICATE TELEPHONE ORDER READ BACK FOR ACCURACY)

Medications:

Antiemetic

☐ Zofran 8 mg IVP one time for nausea

Fetal Lung Maturity

☐ Betamethasone 12 mg IM x 1 if 24 to 34 weeks gestation, for fetal lung maturity

☐ Finger stick per portable blood glucose monitor prior to administration of medication. If blood glucose greater than 200 contact medical control before administration.

GBS Prophylaxis for positive on unknown status

☐ Penicillin 5 million units IVPB x 1

If allergic to Penicillin:

☐ Clindamycin 900 mg IVPB x 1

Additional Orders:

Nurse Signature: _____ Date: _____ Time: _____

Physician Signature: _____ Date: _____ Time: _____

PATIENT LABEL

FIGURE 13–2. *(Continued)*

MATERNAL TRANSPORT PREMATURE LABOR/PROM PHYSICIAN ORDERS

DRUG MAY BE DISPENSED IN ACCORDANCE WITH THE
HOSPITAL FORMULARY SYSTEM UNLESS CHECKED HERE ⇨ ☐

ALLERGIES: ☐ NO KNOWN ALLERGIES

IMPORTANT REMINDERS	
1. "Daily" instead of "qd"	5. "Morphine" instead of "MSO4"
2. "Units" instead of "u"	6. "Magnesium sulfate" instead of "MgSO4"
3. No trailing zeros (1mg, not 1.0mg)	7. "Every other day" instead of "Q.O.D."
4. Always use leading zeros	8. "MCG" instead of "µg"
(0.1mg, not .1mg)	9. "International Units" instead of "IU"

PATIENT WEIGHT ⇨ _____ ☐ Kgs ☐ Lbs   PATIENT HEIGHT ⇨ _____

✓	DATE ORDERED	TIME	▼	INITIAL HERE TO INDICATE TELEPHONE ORDER READ BACK FOR ACCURACY — ORDERS
				Accepting physician: Dr. _____ Contact # _____
				IUP:
				Monitoring
				• Vital signs on arrival at referral hospital and review fetal monitor strip before transfer
				• Obtain maternal vital signs and FHR 5-15 minutes prior to departure. Vitals Q 15 minutes during transport. Temperature Q 4 hours, if membranes ruptured then Q 2 hours.
				• EKG monitoring as needed
				• Assess abdominal tenderness and for bladder distention.
				• Position patient to provide for uterine displacement.
				• Assess level of consciousness
				• Check deep tendon reflexes (DTR) prior to departure and following loading dose of Magnesium Sulfate
				• If indicated to assess cervical dilation, sterile vaginal exam if membranes intact, sterile speculum exam if membranes ruptured
				• Call physician for:
				• Temperature greater than 99.9°F
				• RR greater than 22 or less than 12
				• Pulse greater than 120
				• Systolic BP greater than 160 or less than 80
				• Diastolic BP greater than 100 or less than 40
				• Tetanic contractions and or non reassuring FHT's
				• Active vaginal bleeding
				NPO
				Intake & Output
				• Foley for bladder distention prn
				• Intake and output prior to departure
				Labs
				☐ GBS culture, bring specimen back to St. Mary's laboratory
				☐ Fern test to rule out ROM
				☐ Fetal fibronectin if no vaginal exam in the past 24 hours
				☐ Finger stick blood glucose prior to administration of medication. If blood glucose greater than 200 contact medical control before administration of Terbutaline and/or Betamethasone
				Fluids
				• IV with 18 gauge needle: (not necessary to restart IV if adequate 18 gauge line in place)
				☐ 125mL/hr 1000 ml Lactated Ringers
				☐ 75 mL/hr 1000 ml Lactated Ringers if receiving Magnesium Sulfate IV
				Respiratory
				• O2 at 10L/min per non-rebreather mask for fetal intolerance or maternal oxygen saturation level less than 95%

PATIENT LABEL

FIGURE 13–3. Maternal transport physician orders for premature labor/premature rupture of membranes. (From SSM St. Mary's Health Center, Richmond Heights, MO.)

MATERNAL TRANSPORT PREMATURE LABOR/PROM PHYSICIAN ORDERS

DRUG MAY BE DISPENSED IN ACCORDANCE WITH THE
HOSPITAL FORMULARY SYSTEM UNLESS CHECKED HERE ⇒ ☐

ALLERGIES:

	IMPORTANT REMINDERS	
	1. "Daily" instead of "qd"	5. "Morphine" instead of "MSO4"
	2. "Units" instead of "u"	6. "Magnesium sulfate" instead of "MgSO4"
	3. No trailing zeros (1mg, not 1.0mg)	7. "Every other day" instead of "Q.O.D."
	4. Always use leading zeros	8. "MCG" instead of "μg"
PATIENT WEIGHT ⇒ _____ ☐ Kgs ☐ Lbs PATIENT HEIGHT ⇒ _____	(0.1mg, not .1mg)	9. "International Units" instead of "IU"

✓	DATE ORDERED	TIME	✓	INITIAL HERE TO INDICATE TELEPHONE ORDER READ BACK FOR ACCURACY — **ORDERS**
				Medications
				IV tocolytic medications for preterm labor:
				Choose one: ☐ 2 gm Magnesium Sulfate in 50 mL Sterile Water over 20 minutes
				☐ 4 gm Magnesium Sulfate in 100 mL Sterile Water over 30 minutes
				☐ 6 gm bolus of Magnesium Sulfate (2 gm plus 4 gm dosage noted above)
				☐ Magnesium Sulfate 20 grams in 500 mL Sterile Water run at 2gm/hour (2gm in 50mL) maintenance infusion.
				Increase every 30 minutes by 0.5 grams per hour until contractions less than Q 15 minutes to a maximum dose of
				4 grams per hour.
				• *For absent DTR or change in level of consciousness discontinue Magnesium Sulfate and contact medical control.*
				• *If patient unresponsive and RR less than 8 administer calcium gluconate and contact medical control.*
				Sub-Q or IVP Terbutaline medications in nondiabetic patients
				Choose one: ☐ 0.25 mg Terbutaline IVP every 10 minutes times 2 for non-reassuring fetal heart tones. Hold if
				maternal heart rate over 120 beats per minutes.
				☐ 0.25 mg Terbutaline Sub-Q every 20 minutes times 2 for preterm labor if contractions more frequent
				than Q 15 minutes. Hold if maternal heart rate over 120 beats per minutes
				PO tocolytic medications for preterm labor
				Choose one: ☐ 50 mg Indocin PO times one
				☐ 20 mg Procardia PO times one
				Magnesium Sulfate toxicity
				☐ 10% Calcium gluconate 10 mL IVP over 5 minutes
				Antiemetic
				☐ Zofran 8 mg IVP times 1 for nausea
				Fetal Lung Maturity
				☐ Betamethasone 12 mg IM times 1 if 24 to 34 weeks gestation, for fetal lung maturity
				GBS Prophylaxis for positive on unknown status
				☐ Penicillin 5 million units IVPB x 1
				If allergic to Penicillin:
				☐ Clindamycin 900 mg IVPB x 1
				Additional Orders:
				Nurse Signature: Date: Time:
				Physician Signature: Date: Time:

PATIENT LABEL

FIGURE 13–3. *(Continued)*

REFERENCES

American Academy of Pediatrics & American College of Obstetricians and Gynecologists. (2012). *Guidelines for Perinatal Care* (7th ed.). Elk Grove Village, IL: Authors.

Glass, D. (2004). Emergency Treatment and Labor Act (EMTALA). Avoiding the pitfalls. *The Journal of Perinatal & Neonatal Nursing, 18*(2), 103–114.

Holleran, R. (1996). Obstetric emergencies. In R. Holleran (Ed.), *Flight Nursing* (pp. 596–634). St. Louis, MO: Mosby.

Jones, A. (2001). A national survey of the air medical transport of high-risk obstetric patients. *Air Medical Journal, 20*(2), 17–20.

Lupton, B. (2004). Regionalized neonatal emergency transport. *Seminars in Neonatology, 9*(2), 125–133.

MacDonald, M. A. (1989). *Emergency Transport of the Perinatal Patient.* Boston: Little, Brown and Company.

March of Dimes (1976). *Toward Improving the Outcome of Pregnancy: Recommendations for the Regional Development of Maternal and Perinatal Health Services.* White Plains, NY: March of Dimes Birth Defects Foundation.

March of Dimes (1993). *Toward Improving the Outcome of Pregnancy: The 90s and Beyond* (TIOP II). White Plains, NY: March of Dimes National Foundation.

March of Dimes (2010). *Toward Improving the Outcome of Pregnancy: Enhancing Perinatal Health Through Quality, Safety, and Performance Initiatives* (TIOP III). White Plains, NY: March of Dimes Foundation.

National Quality Forum. (2009). *National Voluntary Consensus Standards for Perinatal Care 2008: A Consensus Report.* Washington, DC: Author.

O'Brien, D. (2004). Long-distance fixed-wing transport of obstetrical patinets. *Southern Medical Association, 97*(9), 816–818.

Ohara, M. (2008). Safety and usefulness of emergency maternal transport using helicopter. *The Journal of Obstetrics and Gynecology Research, 34*(2), 189–194.

The Consolidated Omnibus Budget Reconciliation Act (COBRA). (1985). Pub L No. 9272, § 9121, 100 Stat 82.

U.S. Department of Health and Human Services, Centers for Medicare & Medicaid Services. (2003). *EMTALA: 42 CFR Parts 413, 482, and 489 [CMS-1063-F] RIN 0938-AM34 Medicare Program; Clarifying Policies Related to the Responsibilities of Medicare-Participating Hospitals in Treating Individuals with Emergency Medical Conditions* (Final Rule). Washington, DC: Author.

U.S. Department of Health and Human Services, Centers for Medicare & Medicaid Services. (2009). *Revisions to Appendix V, "Emergency Medical Treatment and Labor Act (EMTALA) Interpretive Guidelines"* (Publication 100-07). Washington, DC: Author.

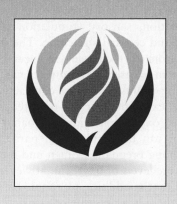

CHAPTER 14

Kathleen Rice Simpson
Nancy O'Brien-Abel

Labor and Birth

Labor and birth are natural processes. Most women do well with support and minimal selected intervention. The minimal intervention philosophy acknowledges that most pregnancies, labors, and births are normal and that intervention creates the potential for iatrogenic maternal–fetal injuries. Interventions should move forward on a continuum from noninvasive to least invasive and from nonpharmacologic to pharmacologic according to the wishes of the woman and the discretion of healthcare providers, based on individual clinical situations. A philosophy of minimal intervention works best in the context of a well-designed safety net, allowing for intervention when necessary, in a clinically timely manner. During the intrapartum period, nurses use knowledge of physiologic and psychosocial aspects of birth and selected pharmacologic therapies to provide comprehensive care for women and families. The focus of this chapter is on nursing interventions that enable the labor and birth process.

OVERVIEW OF LABOR AND BIRTH

ONSET OF LABOR

Multiple theories have been proposed to explain the biophysiologic factors that initiate labor; however, this process is not yet fully understood. A combination of maternal–fetal factors influence labor onset (see Display 14–1). It is likely that a parturition cascade occurs in humans that results in the removal of the mechanisms that maintain uterine quiescence and the initiation of factors that promote uterine activity (Liao, Buhimschi, & Norwitz, 2005). Labor and birth are multifactorial processes that involve interconnected positive feedforward and negative feedback loops that are linked

in a carefully time-regulated fashion (Nathanielsz, 1998; Smith, 2007). These pathways in the fetus, placenta, and mother require sequential initiation and include redundancy that can prevent a single factor from prematurely initiating labor or preventing the initiation of labor (Kilpatrick & Garrison, 2012; Liao et al., 2005). Ongoing research related to preterm birth prevention has suggested that there is a genetic component to the timing of labor (Plunkett et al., 2011), which may help to explain why some women experience preterm birth and others remain pregnant until 41 weeks or more.

A complex series of events must occur during labor and birth that represent a reversal of role for the uterus and cervix during pregnancy. The myometrium, which has remained relatively quiet for many months, has to become active, and the cervix, which has functioned to prevent birth, must lose its resistance. This involves an integrated set of changes within the maternal tissues (myometrium, decidua, and cervix) that occur gradually over a period of days to weeks (Liao et al., 2005; Smith, 2007). Despite extensive research, knowledge of the exact mechanism for spontaneous labor remains incomplete. Most of what is known is from animal studies and in vitro investigations of biopsies obtained from the myometrium and cervix at cesarean birth (Bernal, 2003; Hurd, Gibbs, Ventolini, Horowitz, & Guy, 2005; Liao et al., 2005).

The forces of labor are uterine contractions acting on the resistance of the cervix. The uterine walls are flexible, expanding over time until the onset of labor, when the myometrium converts from a quiet state to a highly active contractile organ. The cervix, composed of connective tissue, remains firmly closed until it is time for labor to begin; then it undergoes rapid, dramatic changes, including ripening, effacement, and dilation (Liao et al., 2005). The conditions and processes that result in term

Possible Causes of the Onset of Labor

Maternal Factor Theories

Uterine muscles are stretched, causing the release of prostaglandin.

Pressure on cervix stimulates nerve plexus, causing the release of oxytocin by the maternal posterior pituitary gland (the Ferguson reflex).

Oxytocin stimulation in circulating blood increases slowly during pregnancy, rises dramatically during labor, and peaks during second stage. Oxytocin and prostaglandin work together to inhibit calcium binding in muscle cells, raising intracellular calcium and activating contractions.

Estrogen/progesterone ratio change: estrogen excites uterine response, and progesterone quiets uterine response. The decrease of progesterone allows estrogen to stimulate the contractile response of the uterus.

Fetal Factor Theories

Placental aging and deterioration triggers initiation of contractions.

Fetal cortisol concentration, produced by the fetal adrenal glands, rises and acts on the placenta to reduce progesterone formation and to increase prostaglandin. Anencephalic fetuses (no adrenal glands) tend to have prolonged gestation.

Prostaglandin, produced by fetal membranes (amnion and chorion) and the decidua, stimulates contractions. When arachidonic acid stored in fetal membranes is released at term, it is converted to prostaglandin.

---

labor are regulated by several compounds and biochemical systems, including progesterone withdrawal and prostaglandin synthesis (Bernal, 2003). Activation of the myometrium requires receptor sites, an increased production of prostaglandin, and the formation of gap junctions. Gap junctions are specialized protein units located within the cell membrane that connect neighboring cells and provide communication channels (Ulmsten, 1997). The number of gap junctions, as well as their permeability and performance, has a direct influence on myometrial function during labor (Bernal, 2003).

It is theorized that after the preparation and activation period, the myometrium is ready to be stimulated for contractions (Liao et al., 2005). Prostaglandin and oxytocin are the most important biochemical factors in stimulating term myometrial activity (Olah & Gee, 1996; Slater, Zervou, & Thornton, 2002). Prostaglandin synthesis during the cervical ripening period also prepares the myometrium to respond to oxytocin (Sheehan, 2006). It is known that oxytocin alone cannot induce the formation of gap junctions. The oxytocin hormone is synthesized by the hypothalamus, then transported to the posterior lobe of the pituitary gland, where it is released into maternal circulation.

The release of oxytocin is caused by stimuli such as breast stimulation, sensory stimulation of the lower genital tract, and cervical stretching. The milk-ejection reflex results from oxytocin released due to breast stimulation. Oxytocin released in response to vaginal and cervical stretching results in uterine contractions through Ferguson's reflex. Differences in reported plasma concentrations of oxytocin during pregnancy and spontaneous labor can be attributed in part to individual variations among pregnant women and methodologies used to measure levels of oxytocin; however, it is generally accepted that in addition to a tonic baseline release of oxytocin, there is a pulsatile release action that may increase in amplitude and frequency during labor (Fuchs et al., 1991).

Two types of oxytocin receptors have been identified and quantified in the human uterus: myometrial and decidual (Liao et al., 2005). Both play an important part in the initiation of spontaneous labor and birth. Oxytocin receptors are present in low concentrations until the later part of the third trimester, during which their numbers increase dramatically. This lack of receptors until late pregnancy probably contributes to the lack of uterine response to oxytocin earlier than during the third trimester (Sultatos, 1997). Oxytocin receptors in the myometrium and decidua reach their peak levels at slightly different times during pregnancy and labor. During pregnancy, as weeks of gestation increase, there is a steady increase in the number of oxytocin receptors in the myometrium (Caldeyro-Barcia & Poseiro, 1960). As pregnancy progresses, the number of oxytocin receptor sites in the myometrium increases by 100-fold at 32 weeks and by 300-fold at the onset of labor (Arias, 2000). This rise in receptor concentration is paralleled by an increase in uterine sensitivity to circulating oxytocin (Kilpatrick & Garrison, 2012). Myometrial receptors are thought to peak in early spontaneous labor and significantly contribute to the initiation of uterine activity (Fuchs, Fuchs, Husslein, & Soloff, 1984). It is likely that the concentration of myometrial receptors play a dominant role in uterine response to endogenous and exogenous oxytocin. Over an approximate 2-week period before the onset of labor, contraction frequency and intensity increase in a pre-labor synchronization of uterine activity. However, these contractions are usually not perceived by the pregnant woman because they are less than 20 mm Hg in intensity (Newman, 2005). As intensity increases beyond 20 to 30 mm Hg, the woman gradually becomes aware of uterine activity, especially via palpation, although these contractions are not noted as painful by most women (Newman, 2005). When contraction intensity is above 30 mm Hg, some women may perceive discomfort. This type of contraction pattern is usually characterized by infrequent contractions and periodic episodes until active labor begins (Newman, 2005). Early labor contractions are concentrated in the lower and middle uterine segments, while active labor contractions originate in the fundal area of the uterus (Newman, 2005).

Oxytocin receptors in the decidua are thought to increase as labor progresses and reach peak levels during birth (Fuchs, Husslein, & Fuchs, 1981). During labor, oxytocin stimulates the production and release of arachidonic acid and prostaglandin F_2 by the decidua that has been sensitized to oxytocin, thus potentiating oxytocin-induced uterine activity (Husslein, Fuchs, & Fuchs, 1981). All oxytocin receptor site interactions do not result in uterine muscle contraction. Although oxytocin does occupy myometrial and decidual receptor sites during labor, the uterus is not in a constant state of contraction. Labor contractions are rhythmic and coordinated, providing evidence that some smooth muscle cells have their oxytocin receptor site occupied without stimulating contraction (Bernal, 2003; Sultatos, 1997).

The exact mechanism of muscle cell coordination during labor remains unknown. One theory is that a signal from pacemaker cells, possibly located in the uterine fundus, is transmitted to other myometrial cells by cell-to-cell communication through gap junctions (Sultatos, 1997). Another theory is that although there is a tonic baseline release of oxytocin from the posterior lobe of the pituitary gland, it is the pulsatile release action that may increase in amplitude and frequency during labor, which could be responsible for the rhythmic nature of uterine contractions (Fuchs et al., 1991). More data are needed to confirm or dispute these theories.

Premonitory signs, such as lightening, urinary frequency, pelvic pressure, changes in vaginal discharge, bloody show, loss of mucous plug, and irregular contractions, are frequently reported several weeks before actual labor begins. Some women also describe changes in sleep patterns and increased energy levels in the final weeks of pregnancy. True labor is characterized by regular uterine contractions resulting in progressive cervical effacement and dilation accompanied by fetal descent into the maternal pelvis (see Display 14–2).

DURATION OF LABOR

There are significant variations in normal labor progress and duration among childbearing women. Classic research by Friedman (1955) described characteristics of normal labor progression in nulliparous women in the 1950s. This research was later expanded to include a series of definitions of labor protraction and arrest (Friedman, 1978). The Friedman (1955, 1978) curve likely represented the ideal labor progression of women during the time these data were collected and analyzed rather than the average labor progression (Zhang, Troendle, & Yancey, 2002). Figures 14–1 A and B provide graphic representations of an expected labor pattern

DISPLAY 14 – 2

Comparison of False and True Labor

False Labor
- Regular contractions
- Decrease in frequency and intensity; longer intervals
- Discomfort in lower abdomen and groin
- Activity has no effect or decreases contractions; disappear with sleep
- No appreciable change in cervix
- Sedation decreases or stops contractions
- Show usually not present

True Labor
- Regular contractions
- Progressive frequency and intensity; closer intervals
- Discomfort begins in back, radiating to the abdomen
- Activity such as walking increases contractions; continue even when sleeping
- Progressive effacement and dilation of cervix
- Sedation does not stop contractions
- Show usually present

and commonly seen deviations based on Friedman's 1955 and 1978 data. Historically, the Friedman labor curve has been widely used in the clinical setting to assess normal labor progression. However, both maternal characteristics and obstetric practices have changed considerably over the past 50 years (Laughon, Branch, Beaver, & Zhang, 2012). Women are older and have higher body mass indices, both of which are associated with progressively longer labors (Hilliard, Chauhan, Zhao, & Rankins, 2012; Kominiarek et al., 2011; Laughon et al., 2012; Treacy, Robson, & O'Herlihy, 2006; Vahratian, Zhang, Troendle, Savitz, & Siega-Riz, 2004). Oxytocin induction and epidural use are also more common and each have been shown to contribute to longer labors (Halpern, Leighton, Ohlsson, Barrett, & Rice, 1998; Harper et al., 2012; Laughon et al., 2012; Osmundson, Ou-Yang, & Grobman, 2010). Figure 14–2 represents data regarding patterns of cervical dilation and fetal descent for nulliparous women in spontaneous labor based on clinical conditions occurring in the present obstetric environment (Zhang, Troendle, et al., 2002). These data are averages; each woman progresses in labor based on individual factors and clinical conditions.

Data from pregnancies at term, in spontaneous active labor, with cephalic, singleton fetuses were compared between the *Collaborative Perinatal Project* (labors during 1959 to 1966) and the *Consortium on Safe Labor* (labors during 2002 to 2008) (Laughon et al., 2012). Based on review of these data, active labor (4 to 10 cm) is longer by a median of 2.6 hours for nulliparous women and active labor (5 to 10 cm) is longer by

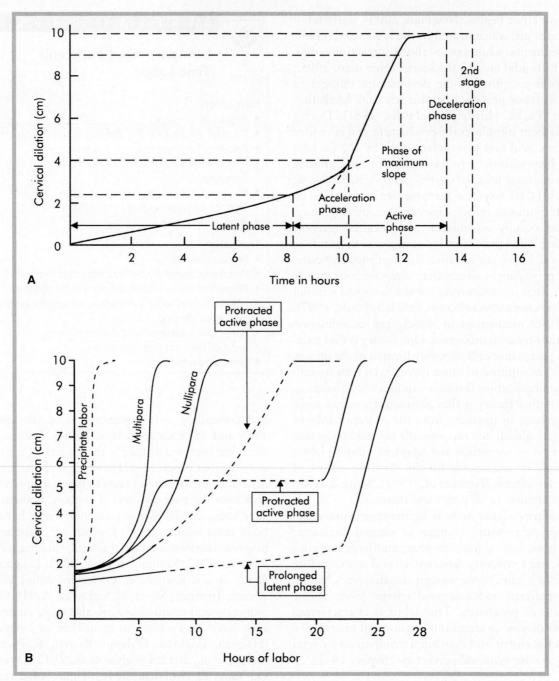

FIGURE 14–1. A, Partogram of normal labor based on Friedman's (1955) labor curve. **B,** Major types of deviation from normal progress of labor based on Friedman's (1978) curve. (From Bobak, I. M., & Jensen, M. D. [1991]. *Essentials of Maternity Nursing* [p. 765]. St. Louis, MO: Mosby–Year Book. Copyright 1991 by Mosby–Year Book. Reprinted with permission.)

median of 2 hours for multiparous women in the modern obstetric cohort when compared to women who labored in the 1950s and 1960s (Laughon et al., 2012). Figures 14–3 A and B represent data comparing active labors of nulliparous and multiparous women from the *Collaborative Perinatal Project* to the *Consortium for Safe Labor*. Due to limited data about cervical dilation before 4 cm in nulliparous women and before 5 cm in multiparous women, the labor curves begin at 4 cm and

5 cm for nulliparous and multiparous women, respectively (Laughon et al., 2012). It is unclear why these differences have developed; however, they likely have been influenced by changes in obstetric practice over the last 50 years, because after adjusting for changes in maternal and pregnancy characteristics, researchers found the increase in length of labor remained significantly longer in the modern cohort compared to the older cohort (Laughon et al., 2012). The modern cohort

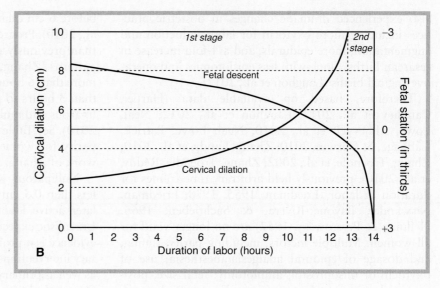

FIGURE 14–2. Patterns of cervical dilation (left) and fetal descent (right) in nulliparous women based on contemporary clinical conditions. (From Zhang, J., Troendle J. F., & Yancey, M. K. [2002]. Reassessing the labor curve in multiparous women. *American Journal of Obstetrics and Gynecology, 187*[4], 824–828.)

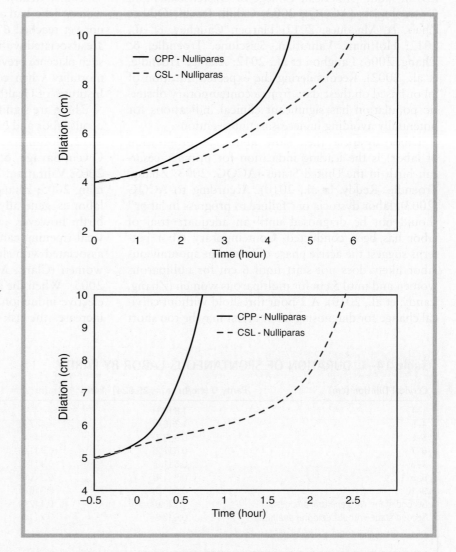

FIGURE 14–3. Comparison of active labor of nulliparous **(A)** and multiparous **(B)** women using data from the Collaborative Perinatal Project (CPP) and the Consortium for Safe Labor (CSL). Due to limited data about cervical dilation before 4 cm in nulliparous women and before 5 cm in multiparous women, the labor curves begin at 4 cm and 5 cm for nulliparous and multiparous women, respectively. (From Laughon, S. K., Branch, D. W., Beaver, J., & Zhang, J. [2012]. Changes in labor patterns over 50 years. *American Journal of Obstetrics and Gynecology, 206*[5], 419.e1–419.e9. doi:10.1016 /j.ajog.2012.03.003)

also experienced dramatic changes in obstetric practices including more oxytocin for labor induction and augmentation, more epidurals, and a 4-fold increase in cesarean births, along with less episiotomies and operative vaginal births (Laughon et al., 2012).

Therefore, based on available data (Harper, Caughey et al., 2012; Laughon et al., 2012; Neal, Lowe, Ahijevych et al., 2010; Neal, Lowe, Patrick, Cabbage, & Corwin, 2010; Zhang, Landy, et al., 2010; Zhang, Troendle, et al., 2002; Zhang, Troendle, Reddy, et al., 2010), previously held arbitrary time frames for duration of labor (Friedman, 1955, 1978; Friedman, Niswander, Bayonet-Rivera, & Sachtleben, 1966; Hellman & Prystowsky, 1952) are no longer valid for all women. Multiple factors, including parity, timing, and dosage of epidural analgesia/anesthesia; use of oxytocin or misoprostol; amniotomy; fetal size, position, and gender; and maternal psyche, age, body mass, labor positions, and pelvic structure influence progress of labor (American College of Obstetricians and Gynecologists [ACOG], 2003; Cahill, Roehl, Odibo, Zhao, & Macones, 2012; Harper, Caughey, et al., 2012; Hoffman, Vahratian, Sciscione, Troendle, & Zhang, 2006; Laughon et al., 2012; Zhang, Troendle, et al., 2002). Reconsidering the expected duration of labor based on these data from a contemporary obstetric population has significant clinical indications for potentially avoiding unnecessary interventions.

Labor dystocia (i.e., slow abnormal progression of labor) is the leading indication for primary cesarean birth in the United States (ACOG, 2003; Zhang, Troendle, Reddy, et al., 2010). According to ACOG (2003), labor dystocia or "failure to progress in labor" should not be diagnosed until an adequate trial of labor has been conducted. Contemporary labor patterns suggest the active phase of first stage spontaneous labor likely does not start until 6 cm for nulliparous women and until 5 cm for multiparous women (Zhang, Landy, et al., 2010). A 2-hour threshold without cervical change for diagnosing labor arrest may be too short before 6 cm dilation (Zhang, Troendle, Mikolajczk, et al., 2010). Progress of labor from 4 to 6 cm is far slower than previously thought based on contemporary labor patterns (Zhang, Landy, et al., 2010). Labor may take more than 6 hours to progress from 4 to 5 cm and more than 3 hours to progress from 5 to 6 cm for both nulliparous and multiparous women (Zhang, Landy, et al., 2010). See Table 14–1 for duration of labor in hours by parity for women in spontaneous labor based on the work of Zhang, Landy, et al. (2010).

Nulliparous women likely have cervical dilation less than 0.5 cm/hr in earlier active labor and faster in later active labor (Neal, Lowe, Patrick, et al., 2010). Unrealistic expectations of faster labor based on outdated evidence is a problem contributing to excessive unnecessary interventions such as labor augmentation techniques as well as primary and repeat cesarean birth in the United States (Neal & Lowe, 2012). Based on data about cesarean birth from the *Consortium for Safe Labor*, Zhang, Troendle, Reddy, et al. (2010) found that one-half of women who had a cesarean birth for labor dystocia had not yet reached 6 cm cervical dilation. Cesarean births are associated with significant risk for future pregnancies such placenta previa, placenta accreta, hysterectomy, and mortality when compared to vaginal births (National Institutes of Health [NIH], 2010).

There are significant differences in length of spontaneous labor and induced labor (Harper, Caughey, et al., 2012; Hoffman et al., 2006; Incerti et al., 2011; Rouse, Owen, Savage, & Hauth, 2001; Simon & Grobman, 2005; Vahratian, Zhang, Troendle, Sciscione, & Hoffman, 2005; Zhang, Landy, et al., 2010). Spontaneous labor is generally shorter with less risk of cesarean birth; however, favorable cervix or preinduction cervical ripening can minimize the risk of cesarean birth associated with electively induced labor for nulliparous women (Clark, Miller, et al., 2009; Vahratian et al., 2005). When the admission Bishop score is less than 6, elective induction for nulliparous women significantly increases the risk of cesarean birth (Frederiks, Lee, &

Table 14–1. DURATION OF SPONTANEOUS LABOR BY PARITY

Cervical Dilation (cm)	Parity 0 (cm/hr; n = 25,624)	Parity 1 (cm/hr; n = 16,755)	Parity 2+ (cm/hr; n = 16,219)
3–4	1.8 (8.1)	–	–
4–5	1.3 (6.4)	1.4 (7.3)	1.4 (7.0)
5–6	0.8 (3.2)	0.8 (3.4)	0.8 (3.4)
6–7	0.6 (2.2)	0.5 (1.9)	0.5 (1.8)
7–8	0.5 (1.6)	0.4 (1.3)	0.4 (1.2)
8–9	0.5 (1.4)	0.3 (1.0)	0.3 (0.9)
9–10	0.5 (1.8)	0.3 (0.9)	0.3 (0.8)
Second stage with epidural analgesia	1.1 (3.6)	0.4 (2.0)	0.3 (1.6)
Second stage without epidural analgesia	0.6 (2.8)	0.2 (1.3)	0.1 (1.1)

Data are median (95th percentile).

From Zhang, J., Landy, H. J., Branch, D. W., Burkman, R., Haberman, S., Gregory, K. D., . . . Reddy, U. M. (2010). Contemporary patterns of spontaneous labor with normal neonatal outcomes. *Obstetrics and Gynecology, 116*(6), 1281–1287. doi:10.1097/AOG.0b013e3181fdef6e

Dekker, 2012; Nielsen, Howard, Crabtree, Batig, & Pates, 2012; Vrouenraets et al., 2005; Zelig, Nichols, Dolinsky, Hecht, & Napolitano, 2012). In a study of 17,794 labors in 2007, Clark, Miller, et al. (2009) found a 50% cesarean birth rate of nulliparous women who were admitted for elective labor induction with cervical dilation of zero centimeters. Figure 14–4 demonstrates rates of cesarean birth after elective labor induction for both nulliparous and multiparous women based on cervical status on admission (Clark, Miller, et al., 2009).

A latent phase as long as 18 hours during labor induction for nulliparous women is not unusual, and most of these women will give birth vaginally if time is allowed to achieve active labor (ACOG, 2009a; Harper, Caughey, et al., 2012; Simon & Grobman, 2005; Zhang, Landy, et al., 2010). Cervical status prior to elective labor induction similarly affects multiparous women's risk of cesarean birth. Clark, Miller, et al. (2009) found a cesarean birth rate of zero for multiparous women admitted for elective induction with a cervical dilation of 5 cm or greater. Regional analgesia/anesthesia lengthens the active phase of labor by approximately 60 to 90 minutes (ACOG, 2002a; Alexander, Sharma, McIntire, & Leveno, 2002). Labor progression for nulliparous and multiparous women appears to be at a similar pace before 6 cm; however, after 6 cm, labor accelerates much faster in multiparous compared to nulliparous women (Zhang, Landy, et al., 2010).

Although multiparous women usually experience faster active labor than nulliparous women, additional childbearing generally has no further effect on labor progression (Vahratian, Hoffman, Troendle, & Zhang, 2006). There also is a relationship between parity and type of labor progression variances. It is known that women in labor with their first child are more likely to experience hypertonic uterine dysfunction, primary inertia, or a prolonged latent phase in early labor (Friedman, 1978). During second and subsequent labors, deviations from the Friedman criteria during active labor, such as hypotonic uterine dysfunction, secondary inertia, and protraction or arrest of the active phase, are more common (Ness, Goldberg, & Berghella, 2005).

Previously, it was thought that limiting the second stage of labor to 2 hours was essential to decrease risks of fetal morbidity and mortality (Hellman & Prystowsky, 1952; Wood, Ng, Hounslow, & Benning, 1973); however, it is now known that waiting beyond 2 hours for the fetus to descend spontaneously is safe for the fetus. The 2-hour recommendation was made before the widespread use of continuous electronic fetal monitoring (EFM) and epidural anesthesia. Based on a substantial body of literature, the arbitrary 2-hour time frame is no longer clinically valid. As long as the fetal heart rate (FHR) is normal and there is evidence of fetal descent, there is no risk to the fetus in waiting a reasonable time for spontaneous birth (Cheng, Hopkins, & Caughey, 2004; Hagelin & Leyon, 1998; Janni et al., 2002; Myles & Santolaya, 2003). Although earlier studies have suggested that the length of the second stage does not influence maternal outcomes (Albers, 1999; Albers, Schiff, & Gorwoda, 1996; Cohen, 1977; Derham, Crowhurst, & Crowther, 1991; Maresh, Choong, & Beard, 1983; Menticoglou, Manning, Harman, & Morrison, 1995; Moon, Smith, & Rayburn, 1990; Paterson, Saunders, & Wadsworth, 1992; Thomson, 1993), later data suggest a prolonged second stage beyond 4 hours may increase maternal risk of operative vaginal birth and perineal trauma (Cheng et al., 2004; Myles & Santolaya, 2003; Sheiner et al., 2006).

Recommendations from ACOG (2000b) include consideration of operative vaginal birth for nulliparous

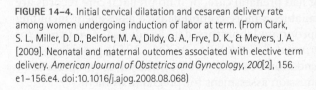

FIGURE 14–4. Initial cervical dilatation and cesarean delivery rate among women undergoing induction of labor at term. (From Clark, S. L., Miller, D. D., Belfort, M. A., Dildy, G. A., Frye, D. K., & Meyers, J. A. [2009]. Neonatal and maternal outcomes associated with elective term delivery. *American Journal of Obstetrics and Gynecology, 200*[2], 156. e1–156.e4. doi:10.1016/j.ajog.2008.08.068)

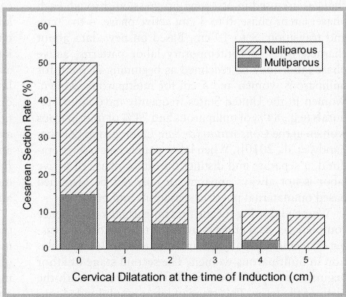

women when there is lack of continuing progress for 3 hours with regional anesthesia or for 2 hours without regional anesthesia. For multiparous women, operative vaginal birth should be considered after lack of continuous progress for 2 hours with regional anesthesia or for 1 hour without regional anesthesia (ACOG, 2000b). These recommendations are for consideration, and are not an absolute necessity for operative vaginal birth. In other words, after these time periods, a complete evaluation of patient progress, maternal–fetal status, and the likelihood that more pushing will safely accomplish vaginal birth should be undertaken.

The recommendations from ACOG (2000b) are based on timing of determination of complete cervical dilation and fetal head engagement. Supportive evidence is based on when patients were noted to be completely dilated via vaginal examination rather than when they were actually 10 cm, so these data are inexact. Frequency of vaginal examinations during labor has a significant effect on accuracy of determination of the beginning of second-stage labor. Other maternal factors, such as length of active pushing and efficacy of maternal pushing efforts, should be considered as well when determining the safest method of birth. Some women may need to individualize pushing efforts based on the fetal response (e.g., pushing with every other or every third contraction or discontinuing pushing temporarily to maintain a normal FHR pattern). Other women may become fatigued after sustained pushing efforts and request a period of rest. Therefore, maternal–fetal status and individual clinical situations provide the best data for labor assessment and management.

STAGES OF LABOR AND BIRTH

Labor and birth have traditionally been divided into four stages. The first stage has been subdivided into the latent, active, and transition phases of labor. Cervical changes are used in assessing progression through each phase: latent phase, 0 to 3 cm; active phase, 4 to 7 cm; and transition, 8 to 10 cm. Based on new data about characteristics of contemporary labor patterns, active phase labor may be redefined as beginning at 6 cm for nulliparous women and 5 cm for multiparous women. Women in the United States frequently have labor epidurals (e.g., 84% of nulliparous and 74% of multiparous women in the *Consortium for Safe Labor* group [Zhang, Landy, et al., 2010]). When labor pain is relieved via epidural, a separate and distinct transition phase of active labor is not always apparent or may not be identified based on maternal physical sensations and behavior.

Women laboring for the first time usually experience complete cervical effacement prior to dilation. Increasing effacement usually occurs simultaneously with dilation in multiparous women. The second stage of labor begins at complete cervical dilation and ends with the birth of the baby. This stage of labor is subdivided into

the initial latent phase (passive fetal descent) and the active pushing phase (Roberts, 2002, 2003). The third stage of labor begins with the birth of the baby and ends with the delivery of the placenta. The fourth stage of labor begins with the delivery of the placenta and lasts until the woman is stable in the immediate postpartum period, usually within the first hour after birth. The immediate postpartum recovery period extends beyond the fourth stage of labor and includes at least the first 2 hours after birth, based on maternal status (American Academy of Pediatrics [AAP] & ACOG, 2012). Table 14–2 summarizes the traditional view of the stages of labor, including cervical changes, uterine activity, maternal activity, and physical sensations. Definitions of stages of labor, including when active labor begins, may change in the future as more data become available regarding characteristics of normal labor in the contemporary obstetric population.

NURSING ASSESSMENTS

Admission Assessment of Maternal–Fetal Status

Major roles of the perinatal nurse caring for laboring women include a thorough admission assessment and ongoing maternal–fetal assessments. In most hospitals, these data are entered electronically into the medical record. Either an electronic or a paper method is appropriate; however, the content should generally be the same. The focus of this assessment is on prior obstetric history, current pregnancy, and labor symptoms. Usually a complete history and physical examination has been conducted by the primary care provider during the prenatal period and is included in the prenatal records that become part of the hospital's medical record. By 36 weeks of gestation, a copy of the prenatal record should be on file in the perinatal unit so pertinent data can easily be accessed when the woman presents in labor. If the woman has received prenatal care and if data regarding a recent history and physical examination confirming normal progress of pregnancy are available for review, the admission evaluation may be limited to an interval history and a physical examination directed at the presenting condition. If the woman has not had prenatal care, or if no prenatal care records are available, a more comprehensive assessment including appropriate laboratory data is advised. *Guidelines for Perinatal Care* (AAP & ACOG, 2012) provide recommendations for the components of a comprehensive admission assessment for pregnant women.

Whereas most pregnant women come to the hospital's labor and birth unit for perinatal care, some women may be seen for an evaluation and treatment of nonobstetric illnesses. Department policies will help determine conditions best treated in the labor and birth unit and those that should be treated in other hospital-care

Table 14–2. STAGES OF LABOR

Stage	Contraction Frequency	Contraction Duration	Contraction Intensity	Physical Sensations	Maternal Behavior
First Stage					
Latent, 0–3 cm	3–30 min; may be irregular	30–40 sec	Mild by palpation; 25–40 mm Hg by intrauterine pressure catheter (IUPC)	Menstrual-like cramps; low, dull backache; light bloody show; diarrhea; possible rupture of membranes	Pain controlled fairly well; able to ambulate and talk through most contractions; range of emotions—excited, talkative, and confident vs. anxious, withdrawn, and apprehensive
Active, 4–7 cm	2–5 min	40–60 sec	Moderate to strong by palpation; 50–70 mm Hg by IUPC	Increasing discomfort; trembling of thighs and legs; pressure on bladder and rectum; persistent backache with occipitoposterior fetal position	Begins to work at maintaining control during contractions; accepts "coaching" efforts of perinatal staff and support persons; quieter
Transition, 8–10 cm	1.5–2 min	60–90 sec	Strong by palpation; 70–90 mm Hg by IUPC	Increased bloody show; urge to push; increased rectal pressure; membranes may rupture if they have not already	Ambulation difficult with uterine contractions; may be irritable and agitated; self-absorbed and may appear to sleep between contractions; need for support increases; verbalizes feelings of discouragement and doubts her ability to cope
Second Stage					
10 cm to birth	2–3 min	40–60 sec	Strong by palpation; 70–100 mm Hg by IUPC	As presenting part descends, urge to push increases; increased rectal and perineal pressure; sensation of burning, tearing, and stretching of vagina and perineum	Excited and eager to push; reluctant, ineffective at pushing
Third Stage					
Birth of the infant to birth of the placenta				Mild uterine contractions; feeling of fullness in vagina as placenta is expelled	Attention is focused on the newborn; feelings of relief

units. Any pregnant woman presenting to a hospital for care should, at a minimum, be assessed for the following: FHR (as appropriate for gestational age), maternal vital signs, and uterine contractions (AAP & ACOG, 2012). The responsible perinatal healthcare provider should be informed promptly if any of the following findings are present or suspected: vaginal bleeding, acute abdominal pain, temperature of 100.4°F or higher, preterm labor, preterm premature rupture of membranes, hypertension, and category II or III (nonreassuring) change throughout FHR pattern (AAP & ACOG, 2012). When a pregnant woman is evaluated for labor, the following factors should be assessed and recorded: blood pressure (BP), pulse, temperature, frequency and duration of uterine contractions, fetal well-being, cervical dilatation and effacement (unless contraindicated [e.g., placenta previa]), preterm rupture of membranes or cervical length as ascertained by transvaginal ultrasound, fetal presentation and station of the presenting part, status of the membranes, date and time of the woman's arrival, and notification of the provider (AAP & ACOG, 2012). The provider should assess and document the maternal pelvic examination and estimated fetal weight (AAP & ACOG, 2012). Previously identified risk factors should be recorded in the prenatal record. If no new risk factors are found, attention may be focused on the following historical factors: time of onset and frequency of contractions; status of the membranes; presence or absence of bleeding; fetal movement; history of allergies; the time, content, and amount of the most recent food or fluid ingestion; and use of any medication (AAP & ACOG, 2012).

At times, pregnant women may come to the hospital before labor is established. They may be experiencing uterine contractions that have not yet resulted in cervical changes or they may be in very early labor.

Onset of labor is established by observing progressive cervical change; thus, differentiation between true and false labor status may require two or more cervical examinations that are separated by an adequate period to observe change (AAP & ACOG, 2012). A policy that allows for the adequate evaluation of labor and prevents unnecessary admissions to the perinatal unit is advisable (AAP & ACOG, 2012). When false or early labor is diagnosed, the woman should be given instructions regarding when to return to the hospital. Fetal status should be determined prior to discharge, ideally using a reactive nonstress test (NST). If a thorough maternal–fetal assessment results in the decision to discharge the woman, it is important to ensure that assessment and discharge processes are consistent with federal regulations as per the Emergency Medical Treatment and Active Labor Act. The leadership teams in some perinatal units have found it helpful to require that two clinicians review fetal data and verify their agreement on fetal status prior to the discharge of a pregnant woman from the hospital.

The initial interaction during the admission process is used to develop rapport with the woman and her family and to get a sense of their expectations for their birth experience. Ideally, the amount of childbirth preparation and type of pain management anticipated during labor is covered during the admission assessment. A review of preferences for childbirth, including a discussion of options that are available at the institution, works best to facilitate a positive experience (Perez, 2005). Although some labor nurses, physicians, and other members of the perinatal team may have negative feelings toward written birth plans, a birth plan can be valuable in helping the nurse meet the couple's expectations and indicates that the woman has given considerable thought to how she would like the labor and birth to proceed (Lothian, 2006). Birth plans that have been discussed previously with the woman's primary healthcare provider can promote her participation in and satisfaction with her care (AAP & ACOG, 2012).

Ongoing Assessment of Maternal–Fetal Status

Limited data are available to support prescribed frequencies of maternal–fetal assessments during labor and birth. No prospective studies have been published concerning how often to assess the mother and fetus during labor. Therefore, a reasonable approach to determining the frequency of assessment is based on individual clinical situations, guidelines, and standards from professional organizations and unit policies. According to AAP and ACOG (2012) maternal temperature, pulse, respirations, and BP should be assessed and recorded at regular intervals during labor or at least every 4 hours. This frequency may be increased, particularly as active labor progresses, according to clinical signs and symptoms.

Frequency of FHR and uterine activity assessment and documentation are guided by professional nursing and medical organizations, unit guidelines, and the clinical situation (ACOG, 2009b, 2010a; Association of Women's Health, Obstetric and Neonatal Nurses [AWHONN], 2008a, 2008b, 2011a; Feinstein, Sprague, & Trepanier, 2009; Simpson & Knox, 2009a; Society of Obstetricians and Gynaecologists of Canada [SOGC], 2007). Generally, the assessment and documentation of fetal status during labor includes FHR baseline, variability, the presence or absence of accelerations and decelerations, and pattern evolution over time. Generally, the assessment and documentation of uterine activity during labor includes contraction frequency, duration, and intensity along with uterine resting tone between contractions. If oxytocin is infusing, the rate in milliunits per minute (mU/min) should be included.

When using EFM, if no risk factors are present at the time of admission or none develop during labor, the FHR should be determined and evaluated at 30-minute intervals during the active phase of the first stage of labor and at 15-minute intervals during the active pushing phase of the second stage of labor, unless fetal risk status or response to labor indicates the need for more frequent assessment (AAP & ACOG, 2012; ACOG, 2009b; AWHONN, 2008a, 2008b; Simpson & Knox, 2009a). If risk factors or complications are present on admission or develop during the course of labor, the FHR should be determined and evaluated every 15 minutes during the active phase of the first stage of labor and every 5 minutes during the active pushing phase of the second stage of labor (AAP & ACOG, 2012; ACOG, 2009b; AWHONN, 2008a, 2008b; Simpson & Knox, 2009a). Continuous EFM is recommended for women with complications (e.g., suspected fetal growth restriction, preeclampsia, type 1 diabetes) (ACOG, 2009b; SOGC, 2007). During oxytocin administration, the FHR should be determined and evaluated every 15 minutes during the active phase of the first stage of labor and every 5 minutes during the active pushing phase of the second stage of labor (AAP & ACOG, 2012; AWHONN, 2008a, 2008b).

When EFM is used to record FHR data permanently, periodic documentation can be used to summarize fetal status during second stage labor maternal pushing efforts, as outlined by unit protocol (AWHONN, 2008a; Simpson & Knox, 2009a). For example, it may be appropriate for a nurse who is at the bedside continually assessing FHR and supporting the woman during the active pushing phase of the second stage of labor to document FHR interpretation in a summary note at intervals of 15 to 30 minutes or more (Simpson & Knox, 2009a).

While most providers in the United States currently choose continuous or intermittent EFM, the institution's policy should include guidelines for intermittent auscultation if electronic monitoring is not the preference of the woman, physician, or certified nurse midwife (CNM). When using intermittent auscultation, if no risk factors or complications are present at the time of admission or none develop during labor, AAP and ACOG (2012) recommend that the FHR should be determined, evaluated, and recorded at least every 30 minutes (preferably before, during, and after a contraction) during the active phase of the first stage of labor and at least every 15 minutes during the active pushing phase of the second stage of labor. If risk factors or complications are present on admission or develop during the course of labor, the FHR should be determined, evaluated, and recorded at least every 15 minutes during the active phase of the first stage of labor and every 5 minutes during the active pushing phase of the second stage of labor (AAP & ACOG, 2012). Frequency ranges of every 15 to 30 minutes during the active phase of the first stage of labor and every 5 to 15 minutes during the active pushing phase of the second stage of labor are recommended by AWHONN based on an evaluation of factors including patient preferences, the phase and stage of labor, maternal response to labor, an assessment of maternal–fetal condition and risk factors, and facility rules and procedures (AWHONN 2008a; Feinstein et al., 2009). Either protocol (AAP & ACOG, 2012; AWHONN, 2008a) is acceptable for intermittent auscultation of the FHR during labor. The AWHONN practice monograph *Fetal Heart Rate Auscultation* (Feinstein et al., 2009) provides a comprehensive discussion about technique, rationale, interpretation, and clinical decision making when using intermittent auscultation during labor.

When auscultation or EFM is used, FHR and uterine activity are documented according to unit protocol. A reasonable approach is to document findings each time they are determined, except when assessing the FHR at 5-minute intervals, due to the difficulty of documenting and concurrently providing labor support to the woman (Simpson & Knox, 2009a). In these cases, summary documentation of fetal status every 15 to 30 minutes, while indicating continuous nursing bedside attendance and evaluation, seems reasonable (Simpson & Knox, 2009a). Generally, assessment data should be documented in the medical record. For example, when a woman is receiving oxytocin for labor induction or augmentation, recommendations are for the assessment of maternal and fetal status every 15 minutes. Nurse staffing of one nurse to one woman receiving oxytocin is recommended (AWHONN, 2010b) and should allow for the ability to document these data in the medical record in a timely manner. When nurse staffing is not as recommended (e.g., the labor nurse is caring for more than one woman receiving oxytocin), the documentation of maternal and fetal status every 15 minutes in real time is a challenge.

Guidelines for ongoing labor assessments are described in AWHONN's practice monographs *Cervical Ripening and Labor* (Simpson, 2013), *Fetal Heart Rate Auscultation* (Feinstein et al., 2009), Evidence-Based Clinical Practice Guidelines *Nursing Care and Management*

of the Second Stage of Labor (AWHONN, 2008b), and *Nursing Care of the Woman Receiving Regional Analgesia/Anesthesia in Labor* (AWHONN, 2011a). *Guidelines for Perinatal Care* (AAP & ACOG, 2012); the ACOG practice bulletins *Intrapartum Fetal Heart Rate Monitoring: Nomenclature, Interpretation, and General Management Principles* (ACOG, 2009b) and *Management of Intrapartum Fetal Heart Rate Tracings* (ACOG, 2010a); the American Society of Anesthesiologists [ASA] publications *Guidelines for Neuraxial Anesthesia in Obstetrics* (ASA, 2010) and *Practice Guidelines for Obstetric Anesthesia* (ASA, 2007); perinatal nursing textbooks; and some state board of health publications are other resources that provide guidelines for initial and ongoing nursing assessments of women in labor. Based on these standards and guidelines, each perinatal center should have expectations for maternal–fetal assessment during labor in the form of clinical policies, protocols, or algorithms. See Display 14–3 and Table 14–3 for suggested guidelines for maternal and fetal assessment during labor, birth, and immediately postpartum.

Maternal–fetal assessment should occur at the bedside by laying hands on the pregnant woman rather than using data obtained from the central monitoring station. Characteristics of FHR patterns may be different when obtained by direct observation of the EFM tracing at the bedside. Direct observation allows for the assessment of maternal anxiety or pain, contractions, and positioning, all of which have the potential to affect vital signs. For example, maternal anxiety or pain can result in increases in BP, pulse, and respirations, while maternal supine positioning can result in hypotension. Repositioning from a semi-Fowler's position to a lateral position may result in a decrease in diastolic BP of up to 10 mm Hg. During second stage pushing, maternal heart rate accelerations have the potential to overlap with FHR decelerations, resulting in signal ambiguity and confusion (Neilson, Freeman, & Mangan, 2008). Maternal pushing efforts that involve the Valsalva maneuver result in an initial increase, then a decrease in BP (Caldeyro-Barcia et al., 1981). Care should be taken to make sure the heart rate that is tracing on the FHR strip as fetal is indeed of fetal origin rather than maternal.

There is insufficient evidence to support a definitive recommendation for the frequency of BP monitoring prior to, during, and after the initiation of epidural analgesia/anesthesia. However, there is evidence that maternal BP can decrease significantly 5 to 15 minutes after initiation or re-bolus of anesthetic/analgesic agents and up to one third of women may develop hypotension within 1 hour of regional anesthetic injection (AWHONN, 2011a). Therefore, a reasonable approach is to assess maternal BP after the initiation or re-bolus of a regional block, including patient-controlled epidural analgesia (PCEA) (AWHONN, 2011a). BP may be assessed every 5 minutes for the first 15 minutes,

Maternal–Fetal–Newborn Assessments During Labor, Birth, and the Immediate Postpartum Period

Maternal Vital Signs

Maternal vital signs should be assessed and recorded at regular intervals, at least every 4 hours. This frequency may be increased, particularly as active labor progresses according to clinical signs and symptoms (AAP & ACOG, 2012).

Intermittent Auscultation of Fetal Heart Rate/Palpation of Uterine Activity

In the absence of risk factors:

- A standard approach is to determine, evaluate and record the fetal heart rate (FHR) every 30 minutes during the active phase of the first stage of labor and at least every 15 minutes during the active pushing phase of the second stage of labor, unless fetal risk status or response to labor indicates the need for more frequent assessment (AAP & ACOG, 2012). Uterine activity is generally assessed at the same frequency as FHR.

When risk factors or complications are present:

- AAP and ACOG (2012) recommend determining, evaluating, and recording the FHR at least every 15 minutes during the active phase of the first stage of labor and at least every 5 minutes during the active pushing phase of the second stage of labor, preferably before, during, and after a uterine contraction. Uterine activity is generally assessed at the same frequency as FHR.
- AWHONN (2008a) suggests auscultation of FHR within the range of every 15–30 minutes during the active phase of the first stage of labor and every 5–15 minutes during the active pushing phase of the second stage of labor (AWHONN, 2008a). Uterine activity is generally assessed at the same frequency as FHR.
- Either protocol is acceptable and should be based on the individual clinical situation.

Electronic Fetal Heart Rate and Uterine Activity Monitoring

Periodic review and documentation of the EFM tracing during active labor should be accomplished based on clinical status and underlying risk factors (ACOG, 2010a).

- A standard approach is to evaluate/review the FHR every 30 minutes during the active phase of the first stage of labor and at least every 15 minutes during the active pushing phase of the second stage of labor, unless fetal risk status or response to labor indicates the need for more frequent assessment (AAP & ACOG, 2012; ACOG, 2009b; AWHONN 2008a, 2008b). Uterine activity is generally assessed at the same frequency as FHR.

When risk factors or complications are present:

- Generally, it is recommended to evaluate/review the FHR every 15 minutes during the active phase of the first stage of labor and every 5 minutes during the active pushing phase of the second stage of labor (AAP & ACOG, 2012; ACOG, 2009b; AWHONN 2008a, 2008b). The exact nature of the risk factor and/or complication will guide the frequency of assessment. Uterine activity is generally assessed at the same frequency as FHR.

Cervical Ripening, Labor Induction, and Labor Augmentation

- Prostaglandin preparations for cervical ripening (e.g., misoprostol, intravaginal PGE$_2$ gel, or vaginal insert) should be administered where FHR and uterine activity can be monitored continuously for an initial observation period. With the dinoprostone vaginal insert (Cervidil [prostaglandin E2]), FHR, and uterine activity should be monitored continuously while in place and for at least 15 minutes after removal. Further monitoring of fetal status and uterine activity during cervical ripening can be governed by individual indications for induction and fetal status (ACOG, 2009a).
- When pharmacologic agents are used for cervical ripening, an assessment of FHR and uterine activity every 30 minutes seems reasonable (AWHONN, 2010b).
- During oxytocin induction or augmentation, FHR monitoring should be as per high-risk patients (AAP & ACOG, 2012). When using EFM, the FHR should be evaluated/reviewed every 15 minutes during the active phase of the first stage of labor and every 5 minutes during the active pushing phase of the second stage of labor (AAP & ACOG, 2012; ACOG, 2009; AWHONN, 2008a, 2008b). Uterine activity is generally assessed at the same frequency as FHR.

Special Considerations for Second Stage Labor

When EFM is used to record FHR data permanently, periodic documentation can be used to summarize an evaluation of fetal status as outlined by unit protocols. Thus, while an evaluation of the FHR may be occurring every 5 minutes or every 15 minutes based on risk status, a summary including findings of fetal status may be documented in the medical record less frequently. It is challenging to simultaneously record FHR and uterine activity data during second stage labor while providing support and encouragement related to maternal pushing efforts. Continuous bedside attendance by the nurse is recommended during second-stage labor maternal pushing efforts (AAP & ACOG, 2012; AWHONN, 2010b). During the active pushing phase of the second stage of labor, summary documentation of fetal status approximately every 30 minutes indicating that there was continuous nursing bedside attendance and evaluation seems reasonable (AWHONN, 2008a; Simpson & Knox, 2009a).

Monitoring and Assessment During Regional Analgesia/Anesthesia

Women who receive epidural analgesia should be monitored in a manner similar to that used for any woman in labor. When regional anesthesia is administered during labor, maternal vital signs should be monitored at regular intervals by a qualified member of the healthcare team (AAP & ACOG, 2012). Neuraxial (regional) anesthesia for labor and/or vaginal birth requires maternal vital signs and FHR be monitored and documented by a qualified individual (ASA, 2010).

- Assess maternal blood pressure (BP) after the initiation or re-bolus of regional block, including patient-controlled epidural anesthesia (PCEA). BP may be assessed every 5 minutes for the first 15 minutes, and then repeated at 30 minutes and at 1 hour after the procedure. More or less frequent monitoring may be indicated based on a consideration of factors (e.g., type of analgesia/anesthesia, route and dose of medication used, maternal–fetal response to medication, maternal–fetal condition, stage of labor, facility protocol) (AWHONN, 2011a).

- Assess pulse and respiratory rates consistent with frequency of BP assessment (AWHONN, 2011a).
- Consider periodic assessment of maternal oxygen saturation for selected women at high risk or those who receive neuraxial opioids as indicated and per institution protocol (AWHONN, 2011a).
- The FHR should be monitored by a qualified individual before and after the administration of neuraxial analgesia for labor. Continuous electronic recording of FHR may not be necessary in every clinical setting and may not be possible during initiation of the block (ASA, 2007).
- Assess the FHR and uterine activity after the initiation or re-bolus of regional block, including PCEA. FHR and uterine activity may be assessed every 5 minutes for the first 15 minutes. More or less frequent monitoring may be indicated based on a consideration of factors (e.g., type of analgesia/anesthesia, route and dose of medication used, maternal–fetal response to medication, maternal–fetal condition, stage of labor, facility protocol) (AWHONN, 2011a).

LABOR PROGRESS

For women who are at no increased risk for complications, an evaluation of the quality of uterine contractions and vaginal examinations should be sufficient to detect abnormalities in the progress of labor (AAP & ACOG, 2012).

- Vaginal examinations include an assessment of dilation and effacement of the cervix and station of the fetal presenting part.
- Generally, uterine activity should be assessed each time the FHR is assessed because uterine activity has implications for fetal status.

ADDITIONAL PARAMETERS DURING LABOR

Assess character and amount of amniotic fluid (e.g., clear, bloody, meconium stained, odorous).

Assess character and amount of bloody show/vaginal bleeding.

Assess maternal and fetal response to labor.

Assess level of maternal discomfort, coping, and effectiveness of pain management/pain relief measures.

Assess labor support person(s) interactions with the woman and contributions to labor support as indicated.

ASSESSMENTS DURING THE IMMEDIATE POSTPARTUM PERIOD (see Chapters 17 and 18 for more detailed information)

Maternal Assessments

- During the period of observation immediately after birth, maternal vital signs and additional signs or events should be monitored and recorded as they occur. Maternal BP and pulse should be assessed and recorded immediately after birth and at least every 15 minutes for 2 hours or more frequently and of longer duration if complications are encountered (AAP & ACOG, 2012; AWHONN, 2011b). The woman's temperature should be taken at least every 4 hours for 8 hours after birth, then at least every 8 hours (AAP & ACOG, 2012).

Newborn Assessments

- Apgar scores should be obtained at 1 minute and 5 minutes after birth. If the 5-minute Apgar score is less than 7, additional scores should be assigned every 5 minutes up to 20 minutes. Temperature, heart and respiratory rates, skin color, adequacy of peripheral circulation, type of respiration, level of consciousness, tone, and activity should be monitored and recorded at least once every 30 minutes until the newborn's condition has remained stable for at least 2 hours (AAP & ACOG, 2012).

SUMMARY

When determining frequency of maternal–fetal assessments during labor, factors such as stage of labor; maternal–fetal risk status; and institutional policies, procedures, and protocols should be taken into consideration. As new standards and guidelines are published from professional organizations, these assessment parameters will need to be reviewed and updated.

---

and then repeated at 30 minutes and at 1 hour after the procedure (AWHONN, 2011a). More or less frequent monitoring may be indicated based on a consideration of factors such as the type of analgesia/anesthesia, route and dose of medication used, the maternal–fetal response to medication, the maternal–fetal condition, the stage of labor, and unit protocol (AWHONN, 2011a). Frequency of subsequent BP assessment while epidural analgesia/anesthesia is in place should be based on a consideration of these variables. Absent evidence from clinical trials to support a specific time frame for the reassessment of BP for this patient population, a reasonable approach is BP assessment approximately every hour.

In many institutions, routine care for healthy women during epidural analgesia/anesthesia includes cardiac monitoring, pulse oximetry, and frequent BP assessment using an automatic BP device. The continuous use of these monitoring devices is not required (AAP & ACOG, 2012; ACOG, 2002a; ASA, 2010; AWHONN, 2011a) and may lead to increased cost and unnecessary technologic interventions for women without identified risk factors. Continuous maternal oxygen saturation (SpO2) monitoring should be discouraged because it often produces inaccurate data due to maternal movement and dislocation of the device. Often, long periods of erroneous recordings of low SpO2 are automatically entered into the electronic medical record and printed on the paper version of the FHR tracing without nursing confirmation that these data accurately reflect maternal condition. Pulse oximeters are designed to measure SpO2 rather than heart rate. Continuous tracing of maternal heart rate on the FHR tracing often obscures the FHR, particularly during second-stage pushing. Spot checks of maternal SpO2 are more appropriate if there is a concern regarding maternal oxygen status. Manual assessment of maternal pulse is more appropriate for differentiating

Table 14–3. MATERNAL–FETAL ASSESSMENT AND DOCUMENTATION GUIDELINES

	Active Labor	Oxytocin	Cervidil/Cytotec	Second-Stage Labor	First hour of Magnesium Sulfate and Any Change in Dose	Magnesium Sulfate Maintenance Dose	All Other Patients
FHR and uterine activity	Every 30 min	Assessment each time rate is increased or at least every 15 min if rate is unchanged	Every 30 min	(Active pushing) Assessment every 5–15 min based on risk status; summary notes every 30 min	Every 15 min	At least every hr	At least every hr
Maternal vital signs	P, R, BP every hr; T every 2 hr unless ROM, then every hr	P, R, BP every hr; T every 2 hr unless ROM, then every hr	P, R, BP every 4 hr; T every 4 hr unless ROM, then every hr	P, R, BP every hr; T every 2 hr unless ROM, then every hr	P, R, BP every 15 min; T every 2 hr unless ROM, then every hr	P, R, BP every hr; T every 2 hr unless ROM, then every hr	T, P, R, BP every 4 hr
Pain status	Every 30 min	Assessment each time rate is increased or at least every 15 min if rate is unchanged	Every 30 min	Assessment every 5–15 min based on risk status; summary notes every 30 min	Every 15 min	At least every hr	At least every hr
Response to labor	Every 30 min	Assessment each time rate is increased or at least every 15 min if rate is unchanged	Every 30 min if applicable	Assessment every 5–15 min based on risk status; summary notes every 30 min	Every 15 min if applicable	At least every hr if applicable	At least every hr if applicable
Comfort measures	Every 30 min if applicable	Assessment each time rate is increased or at least every 15 min if rate is unchanged if applicable	Every 30 min if applicable	Assessment every 5–15 min based on risk status; summary notes every 30 min	Every 15 min if applicable	At least every hr if applicable	At least every hr if applicable
Position	Every 30 min	Assessment each time rate is increased or at least every 15 min if rate is unchanged	Every 30 min	Assessment every 5–15 min based on risk status; summary notes every 30 min	Every 15 min	At least every hr	At least every hr
Oxytocin rate (mU/min)	Assessment each time rate is increased or at least every 15 min if rate is unchanged	Assessment each time rate is increased or at least every 15 min if rate is unchanged					
Vaginal exam/fetal station/progress in descent	As needed	As needed	As needed	As needed, at least every 30 min			
Magnesium sulfate rate (g/hr)					Every 15 min	At least every hr	
Any signs and symptoms of side effects of magnesium sulfate					Every 15 min	At least every hr	
Intake and output	Every 8 hr	Every 8 hr	Every 8 hr	Every 8 hr	Every hour	Every hour	Every 8 hr

BP, blood pressure; FHR, fetal heart rate; P, pulse; R, respirations; ROM, rupture of membrane; T, temperature.
FHR characteristics include baseline rate, variability, and presence or absence of accelerations and decelerations.
Uterine activity includes contraction frequency, duration, intensity, and uterine resting tone.

between maternal heart rate and FHR if there is a concern regarding the origin of heart rate tracing as maternal versus fetal. Unless risk factors have been identified, care for a woman with epidural analgesia/anesthesia may be similar to that of any other woman in labor.

Vaginal Examinations

Nurses should develop proficiency in performing vaginal examinations to assess labor progress and to determine the need for nursing interventions such as position change and timing of medication. They must first be able to identify situations in which a vaginal examination is required and also recognize when a vaginal examination is contraindicated, such as with unexplained vaginal bleeding or with premature rupture of the membranes. Developing clinical proficiency in performing vaginal examinations requires practice and assistance from a knowledgeable preceptor. Because a full assessment may require more time than usual during the period when vaginal examination skills are being acquired, an ideal

patient for nurses to learn the technique has adequate regional analgesia/anesthesia and intact membranes so she can tolerate the potentially longer vaginal examination and there is less risk of infection with the confirmation examination by the preceptor. Usually, patients who are fully informed that the examiner is learning will consent to this type of examination.

Women undergoing a vaginal examination should be minimally exposed and should be advised of the necessity of the examination and the findings. The woman should also be positioned on her back with her head slightly elevated. The vaginal examination should be as quick as possible, but systematic, beginning with an assessment of dilation and effacement, then fetal presentation, station, and position. The normal length of the pregravid cervix is 3.5 to 4 cm. The length of the cervix may vary in women who have had any cervical surgery, such as conization or laser excision procedures. As labor progresses and the fetal presenting part descends, the cervix shortens and dilates changing from long, thick, and closed to thin and 10 cm (Fig. 14–5).

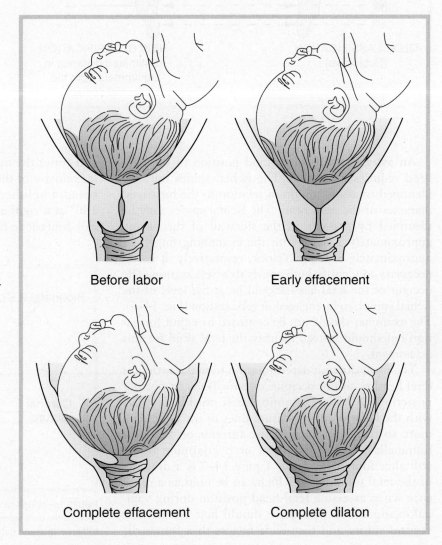

FIGURE 14–5. Cervical dilation and effacement.

Before labor

Early effacement

Complete effacement

Complete dilaton

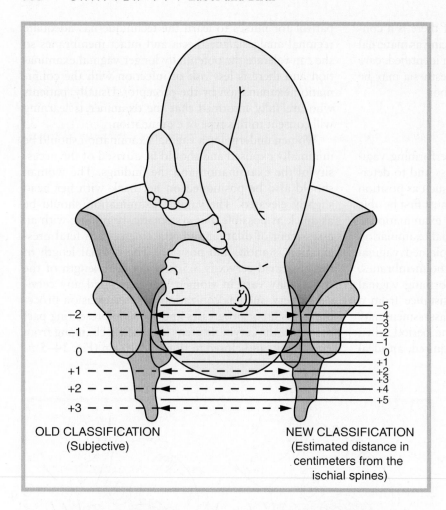

FIGURE 14–6. Fetal station: the relationship of the leading edge of the presenting part of the fetus to the plane of the maternal ischial spines determines the station. Station +1/+3 (old classification) or +2/+5 (new classification) is illustrated. (From Kilpatrick, S., & Garrison, E. [2012]. Normal labor. In S. G. Gabbe, J. R. Niebyl, J. L. Simpson, M. B. Landon, H. L. Galan, E. R. M. Jauniaux, & D. A. Driscoll [Eds.]. *Obstetrics: Normal and Problem Pregnancies*, 5th ed. [pp. 2267–286]. Philadelphia: Elsevier Saunders.)

OLD CLASSIFICATION
(Subjective)

NEW CLASSIFICATION
(Estimated distance in centimeters from the ischial spines)

An assessment of station and position of the fetal head requires more skill. The ischial spines must be identified to assess station in relation to the biparietal diameter of the fetal head. The ischial spines may be identified by pressing in the sidewall of the vagina approximately 1 inch, with the examining fingers at approximately 3 and 9 o'clock, respectively. It is not necessary to identify both spines to assess station. The occiput of the fetal head should be at the level of the ischial spines, to be engaged or zero station (Fig. 14–6). The examiner should not be confused by caput formation but should instead identify the fetal skull for this assessment.

The most difficult determination to make is that of fetal head position: occiput anterior (OA) or occiput posterior (OP). The examining nurse must be familiar with the location of the suture lines in the fetal skull more so than the shape of the anterior or posterior fontanelle because distortion or overlapping bones will alter fontanelle shape. Figure 14–7 is a drawing of the fetal fontanelles, which can be used as a reference when assessing fetal head position during vaginal examination. The nurse should first identify the sagittal suture and then slide fingers to a fontanelle

and count the number of suture lines extending from it exclusive of the sagittal suture (Fig. 14–8). This can be accomplished by sweeping the examining finger 180° at a right angle to the sagittal suture. The anterior fontanelle has three suture lines extending from

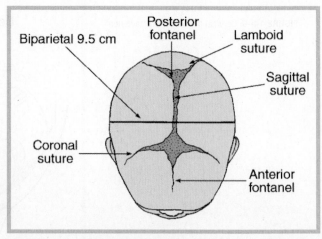

FIGURE 14–7. Fetal fontanelles: fetal presentation, vertex, fetal skull showing the bony segments of the fetal skull important for determining the baby's position and station for birth.

been shown to decrease infections acquired during the intrapartum period, but they may cause local irritation and are absorbed through maternal mucous membranes and fetal skin (AAP & ACOG, 2012). Thus, lubricants containing these agents, and sprays or liquids delivering them directly to the introitus, are not recommended for use during labor (AAP & ACOG, 2012).

Leopold Maneuvers

Leopold maneuvers provide a systematic assessment of fetal position and presentation and should be performed prior to application of EFM, as part of the admission assessment. Information obtained while performing these maneuvers supports assessments made during vaginal examinations and assists in determining the best position to locate the FHR (Fig. 14–9). Leopold maneuvers may be difficult with women who are obese, have tense or guarded abdominal muscles, or have polyhydramnios. In these situations, an ultrasound may be necessary to determine fetal position and presentation.

Fetal Heart Rate Assessment

Systematic assessment of the FHR via EFM includes a determination of the baseline rate, variability, and presence or absence of accelerations and decelerations. Intermittent auscultation of the FHR via stethoscope or handheld ultrasound device includes a determination of the rate and presence or absence of accelerations and decelerations. If decelerations are noted, a further assessment is required to determine the type and duration. Clinical interventions are based on a comprehensive assessment of all of the characteristics of the FHR pattern depicted via EFM or noted during auscultation and the individual clinical situation of the mother and fetus including, but not limited to, gestational age and medications administered to the mother. The FHR can be determined by use of the external ultrasound device of the EFM in most situations. If the clinical situation is such that a continuous external tracing of the FHR is ordered but presents challenges (e.g., a morbidly obese woman at term undergoing a medically indicated labor induction with oxytocin), an internal fetal scalp electrode (FSE) may be applied. See Chapter 15 for a comprehensive discussion about FHR assessment.

Uterine Activity Assessment

A thorough and accurate assessment of the frequency, duration, and intensity of contractions and the uterine resting tone between contractions is an important component of nursing assessments during labor. An assessment of uterine activity begins with direct palpation. Contraction frequency is measured from the beginning

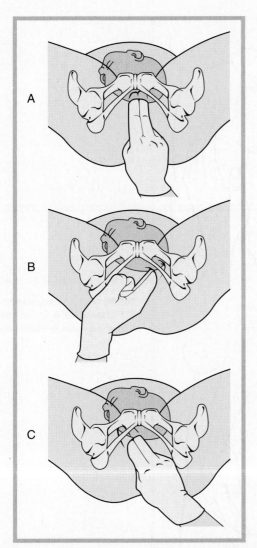

FIGURE 14–8. Vaginal examination. **A,** Determining the station and palpating the sagittal suture. **B,** Identifying the posterior fontanelle. **C,** Identifying the anterior fontanelle. (From Nettina, S. M. [2010]. *Lippincott Manual of Nursing Practice* [9th ed.]. Philadelphia: Lippincott, Williams & Wilkins.)

it, and the posterior fontanelle has two suture lines. It is not necessary to palpate the posterior fontanelle to determine the position of the fetal head. Determination of the position of the fetal head becomes necessary primarily during the second stage when descent is slow. Repositioning the woman to a squatting, side-lying, or hands and knees position to push or using the towel pull technique during pushing may facilitate rotation of the fetal head.

Perineal hygiene is important during periodic vaginal examinations. Attention to clean technique is critical, particularly if membranes are ruptured. Sterile water-soluble lubricants may be used to decrease discomfort during vaginal examinations; however, antiseptics such as povidone-iodine and hexachlorophene should be avoided. These antiseptics have not

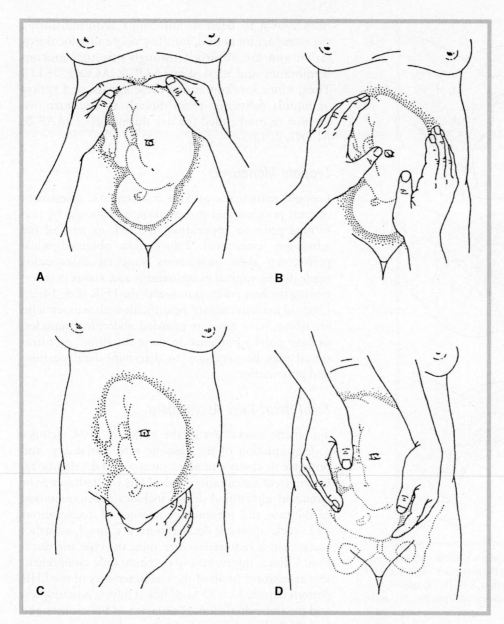

FIGURE 14–9. Leopold maneuvers.
A, First maneuver. B, Second maneuver.
C, Third maneuver. D, Fourth maneuver.

of one contraction to the beginning of the next and is described in minutes. Duration is assessed by the length of the contraction and is described in seconds. Intensity refers to the strength of the contraction and is described as mild, moderate, or strong by palpation, or millimeters of mercury (mm Hg) of intraamniotic pressure with an intrauterine pressure catheter (IUPC). Uterine resting tone is assessed in the absence of contractions or between contractions. By direct palpation, resting tone is described as soft or hard, and by IUPC in terms of mm Hg of intraamniotic pressure.

The external tocodynamometer detects changes in abdominal wall shape during contractions and uterine relaxation. This method provides information about frequency and duration; however, resting tone and intensity must be determined by palpation. Contraction frequency, duration, intensity,

and uterine resting tone can be evaluated by both palpation and an IUPC. The IUPC is more accurate because a direct measurement of intraamniotic pressure is recorded but requires ruptured membranes for insertion. The cervix should be at least 2 to 3 cm dilated before insertion of an IUPC or FSE. As with any procedure, the least invasive approach is preferred unless maternal–fetal status indicates a need for more objective data.

ORAL INTAKE AND INTRAVENOUS FLUIDS DURING LABOR AND BIRTH

Oral Intake

Before the 1940s, women in the United States were encouraged to eat and drink during labor to maintain their stamina for the work of childbirth (American College of Nurse-Midwives [ACNM], 2008). In 1946, Mendelson suggested that maternal aspiration of gastric contents during general anesthesia for cesarean birth was a significant cause of maternal morbidity. This was based on his theory that the delay in gastric emptying during labor contributed to aspiration pneumonitis and that the acidity of the gastric contents determined the severity of maternal complications and risk of death (Mendelson, 1946). For the next 50 years, to prevent aspiration should a cesarean birth be necessary, fasting became the norm for laboring women in most hospitals in the United States. It is now known that regardless of the time of the woman's last meal, the stomach is never completely empty and that fasting does not eliminate stomach contents but rather increases the concentration of hydrochloric acid (ACNM, 2008).

Risks of general anesthesia–related maternal morbidity have decreased significantly since the 1940s but have remained constant over the past 15 years (Hawkins, Chang, Palmer, Gibbs, & Callaghan, 2011). The decreased use of general anesthesia for cesarean birth, published standards for anesthesia care, better anesthesia monitoring, use of cricoid pressure, and routine tracheal intubation with an improved technique have contributed to a decline in maternal mortality (Hawkins et al., 2011). In the cases of anesthesia-related maternal deaths that have been reported in the literature, complications such as advanced maternal age, poor physical status, obesity, emergent procedures, delay in response, high neuraxial block, hypertension, embolism, and hemorrhage appear to be coexisting factors (ACNM, 2008; Davies, Posner, Lee, Cheney, & Domino, 2009; Hawkins et al., 2011). Most women in the United States who have a cesarean birth are given regional anesthesia. The case fatality rate for regional anesthesia between 1997 and 2002 was reported to be 3.8 per million regional anesthetics during cesarean birth (Hawkins et al., 2011). The case fatality rate for general anesthesia during the same period was 6.5 per million general anesthetics for cesarean birth (Hawkins et al., 2011). The leading causes of anesthesia-related pregnancy deaths for 1991 to 2002 were intubation failure or anesthesia induction problems (23%), respiratory failure (20%), and high spinal or epidural block (16%) (Hawkins et al., 2011). Causes of death varied by type of obstetric anesthesia; approximately two thirds of deaths associated with general anesthesia were caused by intubation failure or induction problems, but for women whose deaths were associated with regional anesthesia during cesarean birth, more than one fourth (26%) were caused by high spinal or epidural block, followed by respiratory failure (19%), and drug reaction (19%).

Failed intubation is much more common in obstetrics than in the general population (1 in 280 obstetrics vs. 1 in 2,230 in all other patients); therefore, all members of the perinatal team should be familiar with the ASA (2003) *Difficult Airway Algorithm.*

Physiologic requirements for glucose increase during active labor (Wasserstrum, 1992). Fasting depletes the carbohydrates available; thus, women in labor who are not allowed oral intake may have to metabolize fat for energy (Keppler, 1988). Although there has been limited research about specific nutritional needs during labor, it has been suggested that the energy needs of the laboring woman are similar to those of athletes in competition (ACNM, 2008). Pregnancy and labor are characterized by an exaggerated response to starvation, reflected in part by more rapid development of hypoglycemia and hyperketonemia (Wasserstrum, 1992). Thus, modest amounts of oral intake during labor may be beneficial for women without complications or risks of complications. When women are allowed oral intake during labor, the amount of food and fluids they chose generally decrease as labor progresses (Ludka & Roberts, 1993). Few women choose to eat solid food beyond the latent phase of labor (Parsons, Bidewell, & Nagy, 2006).

In light of the data about the rarity of anesthesia-related maternal mortality and other evidence about nutritional needs of laboring women, in 1999, ASA revised its recommendations for oral intake during labor. These recommendations are supported by ACOG (2009c) and were reaffirmed by ASA in 2007. Examples of clear liquids recommended by ASA (2007) during labor include water, fruit juices without pulp, carbonated beverages, clear tea, black coffee, and sports drinks. Flavored gelatin, fruit ice, popsicles, and broth also are many times offered. The volume of liquid is less important than the type of liquid. ASA (2007) recommends restricting oral fluids on a case-by-case basis for women who are at risk for aspiration (e.g., morbidly obese, diabetic, difficult airway) and for women at risk for operative birth (e.g., indeterminate or abnormal FHR patterns and nonprogression of labor). Although the literature does not quantify modest amounts of fluid, some experts have suggested that the volume of fluid intake may be determined by maternal thirst (O'Sullivan & Hari, 2009).

While there seems to be a consensus that selected oral fluids during labor are generally not harmful in low-risk women, controversy exists regarding solid foods. In a randomized controlled trial of 2,426 nulliparous, nondiabetic women in labor at term, with a cervical dilatation of less than 6 cm, consumption of a light diet was compared to consumption of water (O'Sullivan, Liu, Hart, Seed, & Shennan, 2009). Consumption of a light diet during labor did not influence obstetric or neonatal outcomes nor did it increase the incidence of vomiting. Women who were allowed to eat in labor had similar lengths of labor and operative birth rates as those allowed water only (O'Sullivan et al., 2009). A review of the literature from 1986 to 2009 on oral intake during labor found that foods high in fat slow gastric emptying during labor and that solid food intake is associated with vomiting and increased labor duration, without adverse maternal or neonatal effects (Sharts-Hopko, 2010). A Cochrane Review reports a lack of evidence to support restricting fluids and food during labor in women at low risk for complications (Singata, Tranmer, & Gyte, 2010). Neither benefit nor harm associated with eating during labor was found. Women who ate lightly, compared with those who only consumed water, were no more likely to vomit and had similar lengths of labor and cesarean birth rates (Singata et al., 2010). One randomized controlled trial found no cases of aspiration among women in labor who consumed only liquids and those who consumed low fat, low residue foods during labor (O'Sullivan et al., 2009). The pooled data of the five studies in the Cochrane Review (N = 3,130) were of insufficient power to assess the incidence of aspiration of gastric contents during general anesthesia. Aspiration of gastric contents among women that have cesarean birth is so rare that a randomized clinical trial to determine if oral intake is related to maternal mortality is not feasible (Sharts-Hopko, 2010).

ACOG (2009b), ASA (2007), and the Canadian Anesthesiologists' Society (Merchant et al., 2012) recommend avoiding solid food intake during labor. The risk for aspiration of gastric contents during emergency cesarean birth is the basis for their recommendations. A fasting time for solid food that is predictive of maternal anesthesia complications has not been determined, thus there is insufficient evidence to support safe recommendations for solid intake during labor (ASA, 2007). A fasting time for solid food of at least 6 to 8 hours prior to elective cesarean birth is recommended (ACOG, 2009c; ASA, 2007). A risk assessment of women in labor is the basis of determining whether oral fluid and/or solid intake is appropriate (ACNM, 2008).

Each institution should have a policy for oral nutrition during labor that has been developed in collaboration with anesthesia providers. This policy should not arbitrarily restrict oral and solid intake during labor but rather should be based on what is known about complications that increase the risk of general anesthesia. Women should be informed of the small, but potentially serious, risks of aspiration related to oral intake during labor (ACNM, 2008). It should be made clear that it is the anesthesia that is the risk, not the oral intake, and if labor deviates from the normal, she may be asked to refrain from oral intake (ACNM, 2008).

Intravenous Fluids

Normal healthy women at term have at least 2 L of water stored in their extravascular spaces and have accumulated fat and fluids over the course of the pregnancy. A long labor with the woman fasting may deplete those energy resources. Maternal fluid loss occurs with perspiration, use of various breathing techniques, and vomiting. When fasting during labor became the norm after the 1940s, administration of intravenous (IV) fluids became routine practice. Prophylactic IV access was advocated in anticipation of the administration of rapid volume expanders and blood products in the case of emergencies that can result in maternal hypovolemia and hemorrhage, such as uterine rupture, abruptio placentae, regional anesthesia complications, and immediate postpartum hemorrhage.

IV fluids are thought to increase maternal blood volume, leading to increased blood flow (oxygen) to the placenta and resulting in more oxygen available at the placenta site for maternal–fetal exchange. Therefore, non-glucose-containing IV fluid boluses are often given during an indeterminate or abnormal FHR pattern (Garite & Simpson, 2011). In one study, fetuses of mothers who were given an IV fluid bolus of either 500 mL or 1,000 mL of lactated Ringer's (L/R) solution over 20 minutes had significant increases in fetal SpO_2 that persisted at least 30 minutes after the IV fluid bolus was completed (Simpson & James, 2005b). The greatest increase occurred in the fetuses of mothers who received 1,000 mL. The women in this study were normotensive and adequately hydrated, and their fetuses had normal FHR patterns. Therefore, an IV fluid bolus can result in a transfer of maternal oxygen to the fetus even if the woman is not experiencing hypotension or dehydration (Simpson & James, 2005b). It is likely that the benefits of an IV fluid bolus would be greater if the FHR pattern were indeterminate or abnormal because of the transfer of oxygen through the placenta by passive diffusion from high concentration to low concentration, but more data are needed regarding this common intervention.

The administration of IV solutions containing glucose during labor is controversial. In theory, the administration of glucose averts maternal hypoglycemia and starvation ketosis; however, there is evidence to suggest that maternal IV administration of glucose can have potentially detrimental effects on the fetal status, including increased fetal lactate and decreased fetal pH (ACNM, 2008; Philipson, Kalhan, Riha, & Pimentel, 1987). If the fetus is hypoxic, relatively small elevations in glucose can lead to lactate acidosis (Philipson et al., 1987; Wasserstrum, 1992). IV solutions with glucose can cause fetal hyperglycemia and subsequent reactive hypoglycemia, hyperinsulinism, hyponatremia, acidosis, jaundice, and transient tachypnea in the newborn after birth (ACNM, 2008; Carmen, 1986; Grylack, Chu, & Scanlon, 1984; Mendiola, Grylack, & Scanlon, 1982; Singhi, 1988; Sommer, Norr, & Roberts, 2000). A bolus of IV solution containing glucose can cause marked maternal hyperglycemia (Mendiola et al., 1982; Wasserstrum, 1992). Thus, when the clinical situation is such that a bolus of IV fluids may be necessary to expand plasma volume (e.g., initial treatment for preterm labor, before administration of epidural analgesia/anesthesia, or during hypovolemic maternal emergencies), the IV fluids should not contain glucose (ACNM, 2008; Garite & Simpson, 2011).

Despite the controversy about IV glucose administration during labor, occasionally lactated Ringer's solution with 5% dextrose (D5L/R) may be administered during labor. One liter of D5L/R IV solution provides 180 calories. It is possible that a maintenance rate (125 mL/hr) of glucose-containing IV fluids during labor may be beneficial in shortening labor, although more data are needed before recommendations can be made for the adoption of this type of protocol for routine care. In a double-blinded, randomized controlled trial comparing IV normal saline (NS) with and without dextrose on the course of labor in nulliparous women, patients in active labor were randomized into one of three groups receiving either NS, NS with 5% dextrose, or NS with 10% dextrose at 125 mL/hr (Shrivastava et al., 2009). The administration of a dextrose solution, regardless of concentration, was associated with a shortened labor duration in term vaginally delivered nulliparous women in active labor while there were no significant differences observed in the cesarean section rates between groups or in neonatal outcomes (Shrivastava et al., 2009). Glucose requirements vary depending on weight, use of analgesia/anesthesia, phase of labor, fetal status, and other factors, so it is difficult to determine the optimal rate of glucose infusion during labor.

The most common IV solution used during labor is L/R. An isotonic IV solution should be used to dilute oxytocin during induction and augmentation of labor (ACOG, 2009a). Two randomized controlled trials suggest that the usual amount of IV fluids during labor (125 mL/hr) may be insufficient to meet the needs of women and that inadequate hydration during labor may cause complications of labor (Eslamian, Marsoosi, & Pakneeyat, 2006; Garite, Weeks, Peters-Phair, Pattillo, & Brewster, 2000). These researchers found that women who received 125 mL/hr of L/R solution had longer labors, more oxytocin, and higher rates of cesarean birth when compared with women who received 250 mL/hr of L/R IV fluids. A study of pregnant women comparing different amounts of oral intake considering the same outcome variables would add to what is known about how much and what method of hydration during labor is appropriate.

Individual clinical situations should guide the selection of IV fluids during labor. It is important to avoid boluses of glucose-containing IV solutions during labor, especially in the context of intrauterine resuscitation when the FHR pattern suggests fetal compromise. Thus, if glucose-containing solutions are administered as the main line IV fluids, L/R solution should be available as a piggyback IV solution in case an IV fluid bolus is needed for intrauterine resuscitation or pre-epidural hydration.

More data are needed about the appropriate amount and type of IV fluids during labor. This area of intrapartum care has not been well researched, so practice is based on tradition rather than solid evidence. Current resources for guidelines about IV fluids and oral intake during labor include the Committee Opinion *Oral Intake During Labor* (ACOG, 2009c), *Practice Guidelines for Obstetrical Anesthesia* (ASA, 2007), the Clinical Bulletin *Providing Oral Nutrition to Women in Labor* (ACNM, 2008), and the Evidence Based Clinical Practice Guideline *Nursing Care of the Woman Receiving Regional Analgesia/Anesthesia in Labor* (AWHONN, 2011a).

MATERNAL POSITIONING DURING LABOR AND BIRTH

Unit culture, clinician preferences, and patient cultural background often determine the position women assume during labor and childbirth, such as lying down, squatting, sitting, standing, kneeling, or on all fours. Recumbency, a Western cultural tradition for the convenience of obstetricians, began when more women were hospitalized for childbirth. Early medical research challenging the recumbent position was ignored (Mengert & Murphy, 1933; Vaughn, 1937). Many women today are confined to the bed during the majority of labor as a result of the widespread use of EFM, IVs, oxytocin, and regional analgesia/anesthesia. However, even while in bed, women may be assisted to various positions for labor and birth that may improve maternal and fetal outcomes. Policies that encourage women to walk or change position in labor may result in shorter labors, more efficient contractions, greater comfort, and less need for pain medicine in labor (Shilling, Romano, & DiFranco, 2007).

Ambulation during labor has been shown to decrease the rate of operative birth by 50% (Albers et al., 1997). Women who are encouraged to be mobile during labor report greater comfort and ability to tolerate labor as well as decreased use of analgesia and anesthesia (Bloom et al., 1998). Although the tradition in the United States is to confine women in active labor to the bed, there is no greater risk of adverse maternal–fetal outcomes when women are encouraged to ambulate during labor (Bloom et al., 1998). If continuous EFM has been selected as the method of fetal assessment during labor, use of EFM via telemetry can allow the woman to ambulate while being monitored, even while Cervidil is in place or oxytocin is being administered.

An upright position shortens labor (Chang et al., 2011; DiFranco, Romano, & Keen, 2007; Lawrence, Lewis, Hofmeyr, Dowswell, & Styles, 2009). Duration of both first- and second-stage labor are shorter in women who labor 30° upright as compared to those in a flat recumbent position (Chang et al., 2011; Liu, 1989; Terry, Westcott, O'Shea, & Kelly, 2006). An upright position can also decrease the use of pain medication and the need for oxytocin (Bodner-Adler et al., 2003). In one study, the second stage of labor was decreased when women were in a squatting position, and there was less use of oxytocin, fewer mechanically assisted births, and fewer and less severe lacerations and episiotomies compared to semirecumbent births (Golay, Vedam, & Sorger, 1993). Additional data support these early findings. Evidence suggests that any upright or lateral position during second-stage labor results in less pain, less fatigue, less perineal trauma, fewer episiotomies, fewer operative-assisted births, and fewer FHR abnormalities (Bodner-Adler et al., 2003; Chang et al., 2011; da Silva et al., 2012; de Jong et al., 1997; De Jonge, Van Diem, Scheepers, Buitendijk, & Lagro-Janssen, 2010; Downe, Gerrett, & Renfrew, 2004; Gupta, Hofmeyr, & Shehmar, 2012; Kettle & Tohill, 2011; Ragnar, Altman, Tyden, & Olsson, 2006; Roberts, Algert, Cameron, & Torvaldsen, 2005; Schiessl et al., 2005). Sitting on the toilet may be an acceptable and comfortable alternative to squatting for women who are fatigued (Shermer & Raines, 1997). Perineal edema and pelvic congestion can be prevented when using the toilet for first- or second-stage labor by position changes every 10 to 15 minutes (Shermer & Raines, 1997).

It is important to avoid the supine position during labor because of the relationship between lying flat and maternal hypotension and impedance of uteroplacental blood flow. When the woman in labor is supine, the pressure of the uterus against the spine causes compression of the inferior vena cava, aorta, and iliac arteries (AWHONN, 2008b). If the woman prefers to lie down, a left or right lateral position promotes maternal–fetal exchange at the placental level and enhances fetal well-being (Simpson & James, 2005b). Research has been done to enhance fetal rotation from OP to OA because there is an association between adverse neonatal outcomes and a persistent OP position (Cheng, Shaffer, & Caughey, 2006). A hands-and-knees position for at least 30 minutes during labor may be beneficial in

promoting rotation from OP to OA (Stremler et al., 2005). Other methods that may be beneficial are lateral positioning during labor and using the towel-pull technique during second-stage pushing efforts (AWHONN, 2006). The hands-and-knees position can help to reduce back pain for women in labor and may be useful during both first- and second-stage labor (Stremler et al., 2005). Women are often assisted to hands-and-knees position for certain indeterminate or abnormal FHR patterns but returned to a more standard position for birth. A last minute change of maternal position for birth may be unwarranted because birth may be just as easily accomplished in hands-and-knees position (Bruner, Drummond, Meenan, & Gaskin, 1998; Gannon, 1992). Some women may benefit from the use of a birthing ball for relieving pressure and facilitating a more comfortable position during labor. Figures 14–10 A–V depict positions for labor and birth.

Regional analgesia/anesthesia may limit the use of some positions for labor and birth, particularly if there is significant enough motor blockade to prevent easy repositioning or ambulation. Epidurals that produce less motor block and intrathecal narcotics are becoming more prevalent and are more efficient because they can provide excellent pain management without as much of a limit to mobility (AWHONN, 2011a). Using medication dosages that provide an analgesic

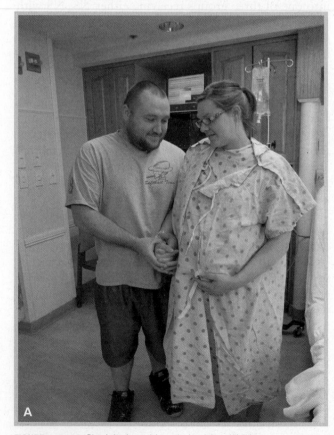

FIGURE 14–10A. Physiologic positions during labor: Walking.

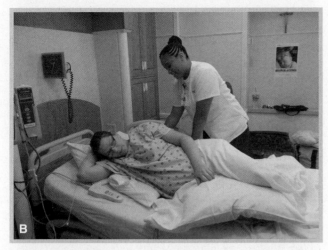

FIGURE 14–10B. Side lying with pillow support.

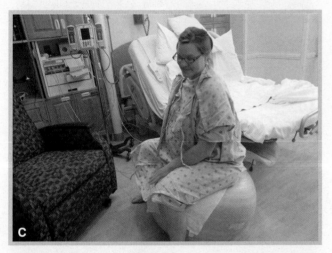

FIGURE 14–10C. Sitting on a birthing ball.

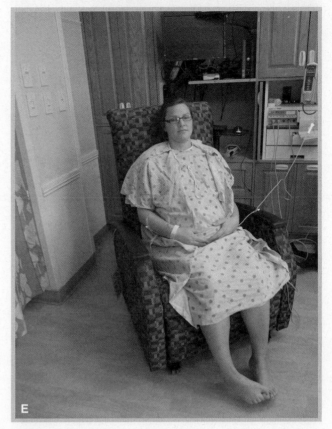

FIGURE 14–10E. Rocking.

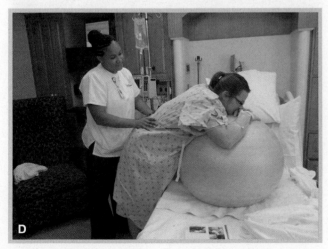

FIGURE 14–10D. Using a birthing ball while standing.

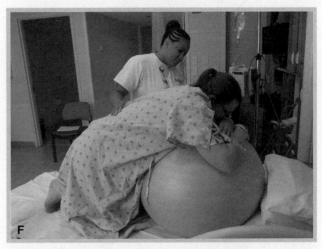

FIGURE 14–10F. Kneeling in bed using a birthing ball.

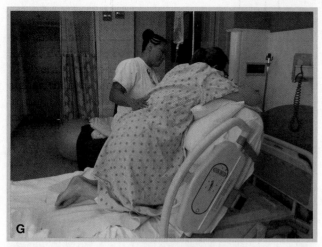

FIGURE 14–10G. Kneeling in bed with head of bed elevated and chest supported.

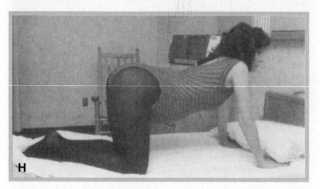

FIGURE 14–10H. Hands and knees.

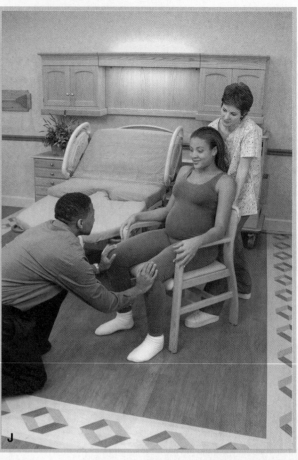

FIGURE 14–10J. Sitting with partner massaging legs. (Courtesy of Hill-Rom.)

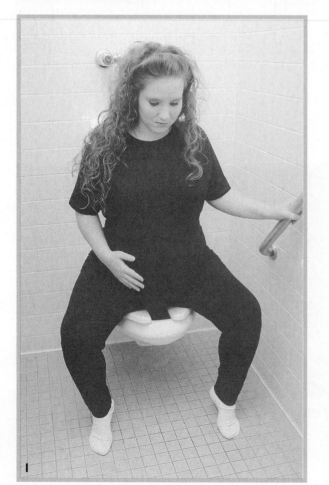

FIGURE 14–10I. Sitting on toilet; also can be used for pushing.

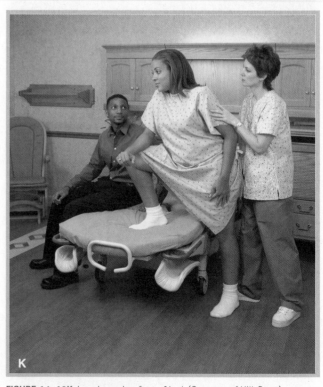

FIGURE 14–10K. Lunging using foot of bed. (Courtesy of Hill-Rom.)

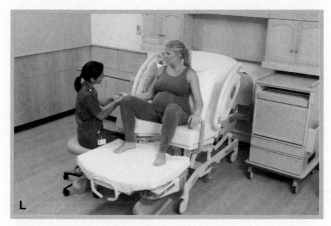

FIGURE 14–10L. Sitting with foot of bed lowered; also can be used for pushing. (Courtesy of Hill-Rom.)

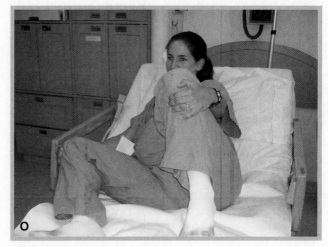

FIGURE 14–10O. Pushing in semi-Fowler's position with right tilt.

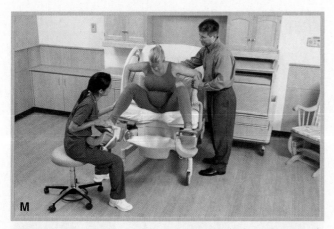

FIGURE 14–10M. Pushing using foot rests as support. (Courtesy of Hill-Rom.)

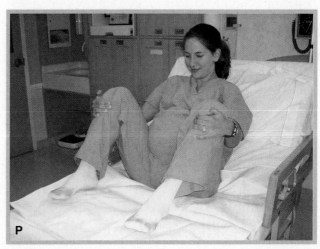

FIGURE 14–10P. Pushing in semi-Fowler's position with mother holding knees back slightly.

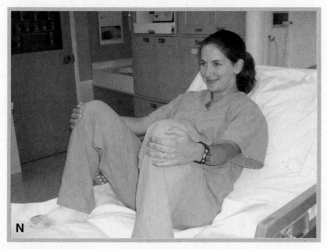

FIGURE 14–10N. Pushing in semi-Fowler's position with feet flat on bed.

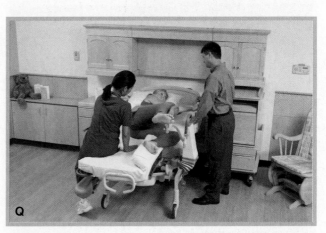

FIGURE 14–10Q. Pushing in side-lying position. (Courtesy of Hill-Rom.)

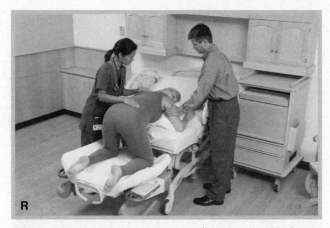

FIGURE 14–10R. Pushing in kneeling position. (Courtesy of Hill-Rom.)

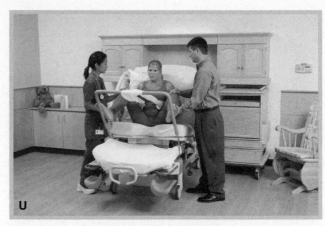

FIGURE 14–10U. Pushing using towel-pull technique with squatting bar and feet supported against bar. (Courtesy of Hill-Rom.)

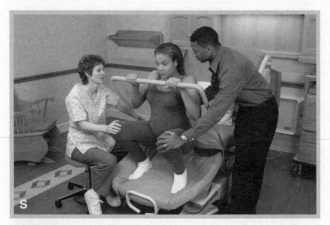

FIGURE 14–10S. Pushing using squatting bar. (Courtesy of Hill-Rom.)

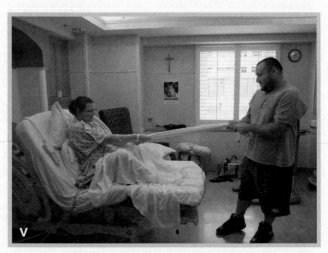

FIGURE 14–10V. Pushing using towel-pull technique with counter-pull of partner.

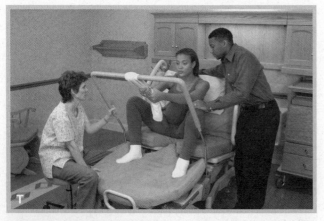

FIGURE 14–10T. Pushing using towel-pull technique with squatting bar and feet flat on bed. (Courtesy of Hill-Rom.)

rather than an anesthetic level of epidural allow the woman to move about more freely and feel pressure as the fetal head descends (AWHONN, 2011a). Feeling pressure will facilitate spontaneous maternal bearing down efforts during the second stage of labor (Roberts, 2002). Nurses should be innovative with the use of positioning techniques for women with epidurals to facilitate birth while maintaining maternal safety. If the mother is confined to the bed, sitting may still be accomplished by adjusting the birthing bed to a more upright position, dropping the lower section, or by helping the mother sit on the side of the bed with a stool for support. When assisting women with epidural analgesia/anesthesia to various positions during labor and/or lowing bed side rails, ensure that the woman is well supported and there are precautions to minimize the risk of patient falls.

Upright positioning during labor is a safe and effective measure that can be encouraged by the perinatal nurse (da Silva et al., 2012; Gupta et al., 2012; Kripke, 2010; Lawrence et al., 2009). Women should be supported in assuming positions of comfort per their choice during labor. Supportive care techniques during labor and interventions to manage the pain most women experience related to labor and birth are covered in detail in Chapter 16.

CARE DURING SECOND-STAGE LABOR

The second stage of labor begins when the cervix is completely dilated. However, women often begin to have an involuntary urge to push prior to complete cervical dilation (Roberts, 2002). This urge to push is triggered by the Ferguson reflex as the presenting fetal part stretches pelvic floor muscles (Ferguson, 1941). Stretch receptors are then activated, releasing endogenous oxytocin, supporting the hypotheses that the urge to push is dependent more on station than dilation (Cosner & deJong, 1993). Women report well-defined urges to push that occur before, during, and after complete dilation (McKay, Barrows, & Roberts, 1990). These findings suggest that "when to push" should be individualized to the maternal response rather than labor routines that dictate pushing at complete dilation (AWHONN, 2006, 2008b; Roberts, 2002). The goals during the second stage of labor should be to support, rather than direct, the woman's involuntary pushing efforts leading to movement of the fetus down and out of the pelvis and to minimize the use of the Valsalva maneuver with its associated negative maternal hemodynamic effects and resultant adverse implications for the fetus (AWHONN, 2006, 2008b; Simpson & James, 2005a). Preparing women who attend childbirth classes to anticipate and actively participate in a physiologic-based second stage of labor may be beneficial in promoting optimal care. Physiologic-based

second stage labor includes delaying pushing until the woman feels the urge to push. Delayed pushing is waiting for fetal descent and or the initiation of the Ferguson reflex before pushing begins in the second stage of labor. Delayed pushing is also referred to as "laboring down," "passive descent," and "rest and descend" (AWHONN, 2008b).

There are generally two approaches to coaching women to push during the second stage of labor: open- and closed-glottis pushing. The traditional approach is to begin pushing and bearing down instructions at complete dilation whether or not the woman feels the urge to push. This technique has been used more frequently since the widespread incidence of epidural analgesia/anesthesia, yet it has no scientific basis and is known to be harmful to maternal–fetal well-being (Aldrich et al., 1995; AWHONN, 2008b; Caldeyro-Barcia, 1979; Langer et al., 1997; Simpson & James, 2005a; Thomson, 1993). Typically, women are coached to take a deep breath and hold it for at least 10 seconds while bearing down three to four times during each contraction. Women are instructed not to make a sound and to bring their knees up toward their abdomen with their elbows outstretched while pushing. Many clinicians will assist by holding the woman's legs back against her abdomen and counting to 10 with each pushing effort. These approaches are outdated and physiologically inappropriate (AWHONN, 2006, 2008b).

When the woman takes a deep breath and holds it (closed glottis), the Valsalva maneuver is instituted. This technique increases intrathoracic pressure, impairs blood return from lower extremities, and initially increases and then decreases BP, resulting in a decrease in uteroplacental blood flow (Barnett & Humenick, 1982; Bassell, Humayun, & Marx, 1980; Caldeyro-Barcia et al., 1981). In the newborn, iatrogenic hypoxemia, acidemia, and lower Apgar scores may result. Sustained pushing of 9 to 15 seconds can result in significant decelerations in the FHR (Caldeyro-Barcia et al., 1981) and decreases in fetal SpO2 (Aldrich et al., 1995; Langer et al., 1997; Simpson & James, 2005a) (Fig. 14–11). Based on results of a randomized clinical trial, when compared to spontaneous pushing, Valsalva pushing can have significant adverse effects including an increase in the length of the second stage of labor, a decrease in Apgar scores at 1 minute and 5 minutes, and a decrease in umbilical cord pH and pO2 (Yildirim & Beji, 2008).

Transient and permanent peroneal nerve damage have been reported following prolonged periods of coached pushing with the woman in the supine lithotomy position. When the woman and/or care provider applies pressure to the peroneal nerve during pushing over a prolonged period, nerve damage resulting in numbness and tingling of the legs, inability to

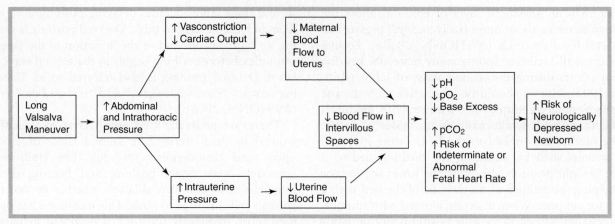

FIGURE 14–11. Coached closed-glottis (Valsalva) pushing during second stage: Effect on maternal hemodynamics and fetal status.

bear weight, and transient loss of feeling may result (Colachis, Pease, & Johnson, 1994; Tubridy & Redmond, 1996; Wong et al., 2003). This type of iatrogenic injury can be prevented by encouraging the woman to keep her feet flat on the bed during second-stage pushing. Healthcare providers should avoid forcibly pushing the woman's legs against her abdomen and placing the woman's legs in stirrups while pushing, as these techniques increase the risk of peroneal nerve damage (Colachis et al., 1994; Tubridy & Redmond, 1996; Wong et al., 2003).

The length and type of pushing, as well as maternal position during pushing, has a direct impact on the fetal response to the second stage of labor and newborn transition to extrauterine life. Avoid sustained closed-glottis pushing if at all possible. The practice of the caregiver counting to 10 with each pushing effort to encourage prolonged breath-holding should be abandoned. There are strategies that can be used to decrease the impact of pushing on fetal well-being. If the fetus is not responding well to maternal pushing efforts, as evidenced by recurrent late and/or variable FHR decelerations, the most appropriate intervention is to modify pushing efforts, which can include pushing with every other or every third contraction and repositioning (Freeman, Garite, Nageotte, & Miller, 2012; Simpson, 2009). If modification of pushing efforts does resolve the FHR pattern, consider stopping pushing temporarily and assisting the woman to a lateral position to allow the fetus to recover (AWHONN, 2006, 2008b). It may be necessary to encourage the woman to push with every other contraction or every third contraction to maintain a normal FHR pattern. A baseline should be able to be identified between contractions. If the fetus does not tolerate pushing and the woman has an epidural, the passive fetal descent approach works best. Discuss concerns

with the physician/CNM if there is pressure or a sense of urgency (unrelated to maternal or fetal status) to get the baby delivered.

At present, there is no reliable method to know which fetuses can tolerate continued physiologic stress of sustained coached closed-glottis pushing. Therefore, the FHR pattern must be used as the indicator as to how well the fetus is responding. It is known that recurrent late and/or variable decelerations during the second stage are associated with respiratory acidemia at birth (Kazandi, Sendag, Akercan, Terek, & Gundem, 2003). Some fetuses may develop metabolic acidemia if this type of pattern continues over a long period (Parer, King, Flanders, Fox, & Kilpatrick, 2006; Shifrin & Ater, 2006). These babies are difficult to resuscitate and may not transition well to extrauterine life. Sustained pushing efforts in the presence of an indeterminate or abnormal FHR pattern during second-stage labor characterized by recurrent late and/or variable decelerations, a rising baseline rate, and decreasing variability increase the risk of fetal harm, such as fetal hypoxic and ischemic injuries (Hamilton, Warrick, Knox, O'Keeffe, & Garite, 2012; Shifrin & Ater, 2006).

In contrast, physiologic second-stage management is based on the principles that the second stage of labor is a normal physiologic event and that women should push spontaneously and give birth with minimal intervention (AWHONN, 2006, 2008b). Second-stage labor has been divided into two phases with the first described as the period from complete dilatation to spontaneous bearing down during which the fetus passively descends until the woman feels the urge to push (Roberts, 2002). The second phase is characterized by vigorous expulsive efforts based on the woman feeling pressure and the urge to push (Roberts & Woolley, 1996). More effective expulsive efforts are associated with delaying pushing until the mother feels the urge to do so (Roberts, 2002). Figure 14–12 provides

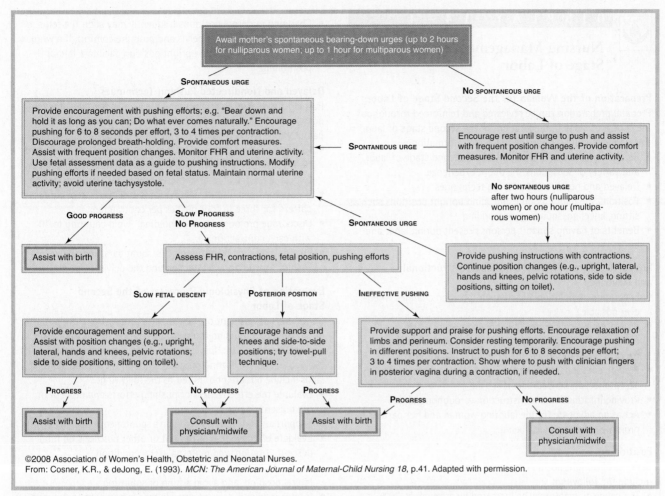

FIGURE 14–12. Suggested algorithm for second stage of labor. (From Association of Women's Health, Obstetric and Neonatal Nurses. [2008b]. *Nursing Care and Management of the Second Stage of Labor: Evidence-Based Clinical Practice Guideline* [2nd ed.].. Washington, DC: Author; Cosner, K. R., & deJong, E. [1993]. Physiologic second-stage labor. *MCN: The American Journal of Maternal Child Nursing, 18*[1], 38–43.)

an algorithm from AWHONN (2008b) for physiologic second-stage management. Display 14–4 lists suggestions from AWHONN (2008b) for optimal second-stage labor care. Appendix 14–A provides an example of a policy for second-stage labor care.

With involuntary pushing, women are observed to hold their breath for 6 seconds while bearing down, and take several breaths in between bearing-down efforts (Roberts, Goldstein, Gruener, Maggio, & Mendez-Bauer, 1987). When pushing spontaneously without instructions, women do not instinctively take a deep breath; they do not start expulsive efforts at the beginning of the contraction, and they use both open- and closed-glottis pushing (Thomson, 1995). This is in contrast to the traditional second-stage coaching instructions that encourage holding breath for 10 seconds while bearing down and allowing only one quick breath between pushes. Open-glottis or gentle pushing avoids fetal stress, has less impact on uteroplacental

blood flow, allows for perineal relaxation, and is more physiologically appropriate (AWHONN, 2006, 2008b; Caldeyro-Barcia et al., 1981; Hanson, 2009; Simpson & James, 2005a). The woman is more in control and responding to her body's own pushing cues, enhancing maternal confidence and satisfaction with the birth experience. Open-glottis pushing as compared to closed-glottis pushing can shorten the length of the second stage of labor (Chang et al., 2011; Parnell, Langhoff-Roos, Iversen, & Damgaard, 1993). Encourage the woman to bear down as long as she can or to do whatever comes naturally (Bloom, Casey, Schaffer, McIntire, & Leveno, 2006). Supporting the woman's voluntary pushing efforts is the best approach (Prins, Boxem, Lucas, & Hutton, 2011). Recent randomized clinical trials have found that women prefer spontaneous voluntary pushing efforts over directed Valsalva pushing (Chang et al., 2011; Prins et al., 2011; Yildirim & Beji, 2008).

DISPLAY 14-4

Nursing Management of the Second Stage of Labor

Preparation of the Woman for the Second Stage of Labor

Prenatal preparation can be reviewed and reinforced throughout the course of labor. In preparation for the second stage of labor, the woman should receive the following information:

- Realistic estimation of duration of the second stage of labor and variety of sensations she might experience
- Delayed and nondirected pushing techniques
- Positions she might assume, including upright positions such as sitting, kneeling, squatting, or standing
- Benefits of having support persons present during labor and birth

Supportive Care: Physical, Emotional, Instructional and Advocacy

- Encourage ambulation and frequent position changes whenever possible.
- Promote physical comfort by applying cool or warm compresses, changing linens, performing vaginal exams only as needed, providing touch and offering fluids as ordered.
- Provide emotional support through reassurance, empathy, acceptance, and encouragement.
- Provide information and instruction throughout labor.
- Act as an advocate for the laboring woman and her partner to promote safety and well-being.

Positioning

Benefits of upright positioning for the second stage of labor include the following:

- The pelvic diameter may be increased by as much as 30%.
- The duration of the second stage of labor may be decreased.
- The intensity of pain and discomfort experienced during the second stage of labor may be minimized.
- Perineal trauma may by decreased, provided the pelvis and perineum are given adequate support.

- Changing maternal positions frequently may align the fetus in a better position in the pelvis and promote comfort. If a woman is unable to maintain an upright position, facilitate lateral positioning.

Delayed and Nondirected Pushing Techniques

Pushing efforts may be delayed until the woman feels the urge to push (up to 2 hours for nulliparous women; up to 1 hour for multiparous women) unless contraindicated by maternal or fetal condition.

- Assess the woman's knowledge of pushing techniques, expectations for pushing, presence of Ferguson's reflex, and readiness to push as well as the fetal presentation, position, and station.
- Encourage open glottis pushing for 6–8 seconds; repeating this pattern for three to four pushes per contraction.
- Discourage prolonged breath-holding. Avoid counting to 10 with each contraction.
- Provide aids such as birthing balls, squat bars, and pillows or cushions to support the woman and the pelvis.

Evaluation of Physiologic Processes of the Second Stage of Labor

Continuous assessment of the woman's progress and evaluation of individualized nursing interventions during the second stage of labor are important. Clinical practice recommendations for evaluating and facilitating progress through the second stage of labor include but are not limited to the following:

- Evaluate the effectiveness of pushing efforts and descent of the presenting part.
- Support and facilitate the woman's spontaneous pushing efforts.
- Evaluate effectiveness of upright or other positions on fetal descent, rotation, and maternal–fetal condition.
- If fetal descent is too rapid, assist the woman to maintain a lateral position, and avoid sitting or squatting.
- If fetal descent is delayed, provide the woman with continuous feedback and encouragement regarding her progress, change maternal position to facilitate rotation and descent, discourage lithotomy or semirecumbent position to facilitate rotation and descent, discourage lithotomy or semirecumbent positions whenever possible, and help the woman maintain an empty bladder.

From Association of Women's Health, Obstetric and Neonatal Nurses. (2008b). *Nursing Care and Management of the Second Stage of Labor: Evidence-Based Clinical Practice Guideline* (2nd ed.). Washington, DC: Author.

Delayed Pushing (Laboring Down/Passive Fetal Descent) for Women with Regional Analgesia/Anesthesia

When women have regional analgesia/anesthesia, they may not feel the urge to push when they are completely dilated. In this situation, an alternative approach to the second stage is to delay pushing while the fetus descends passively. Various researchers have described success with a protocol allowing nulliparous women to wait 2 hours or until the urge to push and allowing multiparous women 1 hour or until the urge to push (Chang et al., 2011; Hansen, Clark, & Foster, 2002; Mayberry, Hammer, Kelly, True-Driver, & De, 1999; Simpson & James, 2005a). A lateral position will facilitate passive fetal descent until the presenting part is low enough to stimulate the Ferguson reflex. There are significantly fewer FHR decelerations when the fetus is allowed to descend spontaneously when compared to coached closed-glottis pushing (Hansen et al., 2002; Simpson & James, 2005a). Maternal fatigue is less when women are allowed a period of passive descent when compared to immediate pushing when there is no urge to push (Chang et al., 2011; Hansen et al., 2002; Lai, Lin, Li, Shey, & Gau, 2009).

Risk of operative vaginal birth is less with delayed pushing until urge to push when compared to pushing immediately at 10 cm (Brancato, Church, & Stone, 2008; Fraser et al., 2000; Roberts, Torvaldsen, Cameron, & Olive, 2004). Injuries to the structure and function of the pelvic floor are less likely when a passive second stage results in a decreased period of maternal expulsive efforts (Devine, Ostergard, & Noblett, 1999). Delaying pushing and avoiding closed-glottis pushing has been shown to decrease the risk of perineal injuries (Albers, Sedler, Bedrick, Teaf, & Peralta, 2006; Sampselle & Hines, 1999; Simpson & James, 2005a). When compared to spontaneous bearing down efforts, coached pushing results in a greater risk of urodynamic stress incontinence, decreased bladder capacity, decreased first urge to void, and detrusor overactivity (Schaffer et al., 2005).

There are no benefits for the mother and fetus to a policy involving immediate and continued pushing when compared to allowing a variable period of rest with spontaneous fetal descent (AWHONN, 2008b; Bloom et al., 2006; Brancato et al., 2008; Handa, Harris, & Ostergard, 1996; Hansen et al., 2002; Maresh et al., 1983; Mayberry et al., 1999; Roberts & Hanson, 2007; Simpson & James, 2005a; Tuuli, Frey, Odibo, Macones, & Cahill, 2012; Vause, Congdon, & Thornton, 1998). The active pushing phase is the most physiologically stressful part of labor for the fetus, so shorting pushing time can promote fetal well-being (Roberts, 2002; Simpson & James, 2005a). Laboring down avoids maternal fatigue and the indeterminate or abnormal FHR patterns associated with sustained coached closed-glottis pushing. Allowing maternal rest and passive fetal descent will not result in a clinically significant increase in the duration of the second stage of labor (Fraser et al., 2000; Hansen et al., 2002). Active pushing time is significantly decreased with delayed pushing (Brancato et al., 2008; Gillesby et al., 2010; Kelly et al., 2010; Simpson & James, 2005b; Tuuli et al., 2012). Throughout passive and active second stage, a periodic assessment of descent of the fetal presenting part via vaginal examination will provide important information about progress and will assist in guiding subsequent care.

Maintaining Adequate Pain Relief While Pushing for Women with Labor Epidurals

In the past, some care providers have discontinued the labor epidural infusion when women are unable to push effectively and/or do not feel an adequate urge to push. The efficacy and ethics of this practice should be questioned (Roberts, 2002). There has been an erroneous assumption by some care providers that the discontinuation of epidural analgesia/anesthesia could speed the second-stage process and avoid an operative vaginal birth or cesarean birth. However, often the opposite occurs. Women who have been receiving adequate regional pain relief and then have discontinuation of the epidural infusion experience significant pain and are at risk for fetal malrotations, dysfunctional uterine activity, a longer second stage,

and forceps- or vacuum-assisted birth (Phillips & Thomas, 1983; Roberts, 2002). The increased catecholamine levels related to severe pain can adversely affect uterine activity and fetal status as well as prolong the second stage (Roberts, 2002). There is no evidence to support the hypothesis that discontinuing epidural analgesia/anesthesia late in labor benefits the mother or baby (Torvaldsen et al., 2004). If women have difficulty feeling the urge to push and effectively working with the pressure as the baby descends, review the level of motor block and type and amount of medications routinely used for regional labor analgesia/anesthesia in the perinatal unit. Consult with anesthesia providers to develop a more appropriate combination of medications that will result in adequate pain relief without an overly dense motor block.

SHOULDER DYSTOCIA

Shoulder dystocia is an uncommon and unpredictable obstetric emergency occurring in 0.2% to 3% of all births (ACOG, 2002b; Bingham, Chauhan, Hayes, Gherman, & Lewis, 2010; Hoffman et al., 2011; Leung et al., 2011; Ouzounian, Gherman, Chauhan, Battista, & Lee, 2012). These data are based on retrospective studies. Data based on prospective studies suggest a higher incidence of 3.3% to 7% of vaginal births (Gurewitsch & Allen, 2011). Recurrent shoulder dystocia occurs in approximately 3.7% to 12% of women who experienced shoulder dystocia during a prior birth (Bingham et al., 2010; Ouzounian et al., 2012). Challenges in determining the actual incidence of shoulder dystocia include: not all are documented as such in the medical record, differences in definitions among providers and in the literature, and shoulder dystocia as a birth complication is not able to be collected from certificates of live births in the United States. Other important data are also often lacking related to shoulder dystocia. The head-to-body interval is not routinely documented in the medical record (Gherman, Chauhan, & Lewis, 2012).

The most common types of injuries to the baby associated with shoulder dystocia include clavicular and humeral fracture, axillary and median nerve injury, transient and permanent brachial plexus injury (Erb's palsy), and fetal/neonatal death (Columbara, Soh, Menacho, Schiff, & Reed, 2011). Shoulder dystocia increases the risk for obstetric brachial plexus injury 100-fold when compared to births without shoulder dystocia (Doumouchtsis & Arulkumaran, 2009). Risk of injury after shoulder dystocia is related to birth weight (>4,000 g), vacuum-assisted vaginal birth, gestational diabetes, maternal obesity, and Hispanic ethnicity (Columbara et al., 2011; Okby & Sheiner, 2012).

Prompt intervention is necessary to decrease the risk of maternal and neonatal complications and long-term

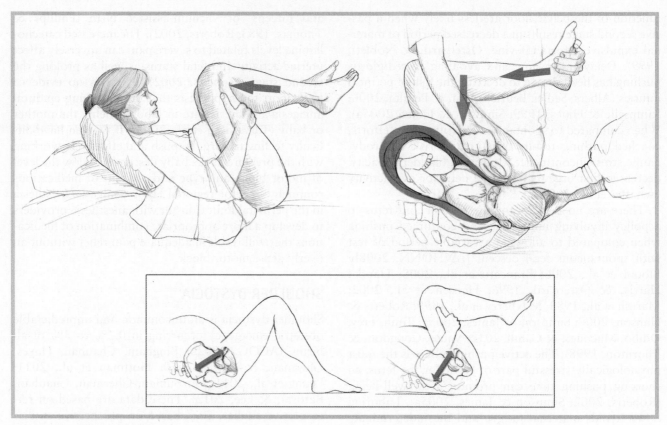

FIGURE 14–13. McRoberts maneuver.

sequelae. While most cases of shoulder dystocia are unpredictable, reasonable steps can be undertaken once shoulder dystocia is identified. A thorough knowledge of what to do should this crisis occur is essential to ensure the best possible outcomes for the mother and baby. Key nursing interventions include calling for additional help; calm, supportive actions; and working in sync with the physician or CNM who is directing the maneuvers to deliver the impacted shoulder.

The Joint Commission's Sentinel Event Alert *Preventing Infant Death and Injury During Delivery* recommended conducting periodic drills for obstetric emergencies such as shoulder dystocia (JCAHO, 2004b). ACOG (2011a) has also recommended drills for obstetric emergencies. Interdisciplinary team training and simulation drills for shoulder dystocia can be beneficial in reducing obstetric brachial plexus injuries. Reported reductions in obstetric brachial plexus injuries related to shoulder dystocia after training include from 30% pretraining to 11% posttraining (Inglis et al., 2011), from 10% pretraining to 4% posttraining (Grobman et al., 2011), and from 9% pretraining to 2% posttraining (Draycott et al., 2008). An evaluation of force applied during simulated shoulder dystocias can be helpful in illustrating the need for changes in practice related to the safe amount of force when an actual shoulder dystocia is encountered (Deering, Weeks, & Benedetti, 2011). The simulation process, including practicing how to

respond effectively to shoulder dystocia, can be useful in introducing and improving concepts of teamwork and interdisciplinary interactions that are necessary for success during an obstetric emergency (Grobman, Hornbogen, Burke, & Costello, 2010).

Interventions described in the literature to relieve the impacted shoulder include the McRoberts maneuver (Fig. 14–13), suprapubic pressure (Fig. 14–14), delivery

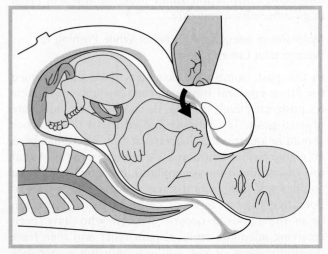

FIGURE 14–14. Suprapubic pressure. (From Penney, D. S., & Perlis, D. W. [1992]. When to use suprapubic or fundal pressure. *MCN: The American Journal of Maternal Child Nursing, 17,* 34–36.)

of the posterior arm, Rubin technique, Woods screw maneuver, Gaskin all-fours maneuver, clavicular fracture, Zavanelli maneuver, and symphysiotomy. While there is no clear evidence-based order of these maneuvers, most clinicians use McRoberts as the initial intervention, followed by suprapubic pressure (ACOG, 2002b; Hoffman et al., 2011). The *Consortium on Safe Labor* (Hoffman et al., 2011) found delivery of the posterior arm following the McRoberts maneuver and suprapubic pressure to be associated with highest rate of vaginal birth when compared to other maneuvers. Although suprapubic pressure and McRoberts are often used prophylactically for women considered to be at high risk for shoulder dystocia, there is no evidence that these interventions reduce the incidence of shoulder dystocia or neonatal adverse outcomes (Beall, Spong, & Ross, 2003). The essential issue during shoulder dystocia is to continue to intervene using an organized expeditious series of steps until the baby has been delivered. If an injury occurs as a result of shoulder dystocia despite the best efforts of the obstetric providers, it is likely that litigation will follow (Gherman, 2002). Birth injuries associated with a shoulder dystocia are the most common reason for obstetric malpractice claims (Colombara, 2011).

Shoulder dystocia is most often diagnosed when attempts at gentle, downward traction on the fetal head fails to result in delivery of the impacted anterior shoulder. The classic "turtle sign," in which the head appears to retract into the perineum, may or may not occur simultaneously. Because the clinical diagnosis of shoulder dystocia is subjectively determined, researchers have used various definitions for shoulder dystocia resulting in studies that are difficult to compare. A definition based on time to birth would be more objective and useful. Spong, Beall, Rodrigues, and Ross (1995) defined shoulder dystocia as a prolonged head-to-body birth interval of ≥60 seconds and/or the use of ancillary obstetric maneuvers. Because the average head-to-body birth interval is approximately 24 seconds for normal vaginal birth, this definition seems reasonable (Gherman et al., 2006). A universally used definition of shoulder dystocia would enhance the ability of researchers to advance science and knowledge about risk factors and appropriate interventions.

Numerous antepartum and pregnancy risk factors associated with shoulder dystocia have been discussed in the literature, including fetal macrosomia (past and/or present pregnancy), preexisting or gestational diabetes mellitus, a previous pregnancy complicated by gestational diabetes, a history of a prior shoulder dystocia, maternal obesity and high gestational weight gain, multiparity, postterm pregnancy, and disproportionate fetal growth with increased abdominal and chest circumference relative to occipitofrontal diameter (ACOG, 2002b; Belfort, White, & Vermeulen, 2012; Gurewitsch & Allen, 2011; Larson & Mandelbaum, 2012; Overland, Vatten, & Eskild, 2012; Tsur, Sergienko, Wiznitzer, Zlotnik, & Sheiner, 2012). Intrapartum risk factors that have been reported include labor induction; abnormal labor progress, including prolonged second-stage labor; and operative vaginal birth (ACOG, 2002b; Gurewitsch & Allen, 2011; Okby & Sheiner, 2012; Tsur et al., 2012). While these factors may increase the risk for shoulder dystocia, most shoulder dystocias are unpredictable and unpreventable (ACOG, 2002b; Okby & Sheiner, 2012; Revicky, Mukhopadhyay, Morris, & Nieto, 2012). Many women have one or more of these risk factors and do not experience shoulder dystocia.

Fetal macrosomia, maternal diabetes, and a history of a prior shoulder dystocia are the risk factors most strongly associated with shoulder dystocia (ACOG, 2002b; Gurewitsch & Allen, 2011). Fetal macrosomia is best defined as an estimated infant weight >4,500 g (9 lb, 15 oz) (ACOG, 2000a); although >4,000 g has been used in some studies. While an estimated fetal weight of >4,000 g may be useful for the identification of increased risks, >4,500 g may be more predictive of neonatal morbidity and >5,000 g may be predictive of increased risk for infant mortality (Boulet, Alexander, Salihu, & Pass, 2003). In the United States, based on natality data from 2009 certificates of live birth, 7.6% of all U.S. infants weigh ≥4,000 g, 1.02% weigh ≥4,500 g, and 0.10% weigh ≥5,000 g (Martin et al., 2011). A clear shift in the birth weight distribution in the United States has occurred over the last two decades. Births at less than 3,500 g have increased, whereas births at higher weights have decreased (Martin et al., 2011). From 1990 to 2009, the percentage of births at 3,500 to 3,999 g declined 10% (from 29.4% to 26.4%), and the percentage of births at ≥4,000 g (≥ 8 lb, 14 oz) dropped 30% (from 10.9% to 7.6%). The decline in birth weight among larger babies was even more pronounced; the percentage of births at 4,500 to 4,999 g declined 42% (from 1.59% to 0.92%), and the percentage of births at ≥5,000 g and greater (≥11 lb) dropped 47% (from 0.19% to 0.10%). The explanations for this shift toward lower birth weights are not fully understood but may be similar to those suggested for the trend toward shorter gestational ages—that is, obstetric intervention earlier in pregnancy and changing maternal demographics and medical risk profiles (Martin et al., 2011).

Risk of shoulder dystocia significantly increases when birth weight is >4,500 g, with reported rates for this weight category ranging from 9.2% to 24% (ACOG, 2002b). Extremely large babies (birth weights >5,000 g [11 lb]) who are born vaginally are reported to have a shoulder dystocia rate of 14% to 20%

(Overland, Spydslaug, Nielsen, & Eskild, 2009; Overland et al., 2012; Vidarsdottir, Geirsson, Hardardottir, Valdimarsdottir, & Dagbjartsson, 2011). In the presence of diabetes, birth weights >4,500 g have been associated with rates of shoulder dystocia from 19.9% to 50% (ACOG, 2002b). However, not all macrosomic fetuses will experience shoulder dystocia and not all cases of shoulder dystocia involve macrosomic fetuses. Approximately 40% to 60% of cases of shoulder dystocia occur in infants weighing less than 4,000 g (Gherman et al., 2006). No birth-weight category is completely free of risk for shoulder dystocia.

Brachial plexus injuries can occur without shoulder dystocia (ACOG, 2002b; Doumouchtsis & Arulkumaran, 2009). Although shoulder dystocia is indeed a major risk factor for obstetric brachial plexus injuries, a significant proportion occur in utero. Propulsive forces of labor, intrauterine maladaptation, and compression of the posterior shoulder against the sacral promontory as well as uterine anomalies are possible intrauterine causes of obstetric brachial plexus injuries (Doumouchtsis & Arulkumaran, 2009).

There have been numerous attempts to develop criteria that would accurately diagnose macrosomia prior to birth, including clinical estimation of fetal weight by abdominal palpation and ultrasonographic parameters. These clinical factors have been statistically associated with shoulder dystocia using retrospective analyses; however, none of these factors or criteria have been shown to have a high positive predictive value for the individual patient when attempting to predict macrosomia or shoulder dystocia, prospectively (ACOG, 2002b; Doumouchtsis & Arulkumaran, 2009). If a fetus is suspected of being >4,500 g, the newborn is more likely (63% to 88%) to weigh <4,500 g (Chauhan et al., 2005). Maternal diabetes is consistently related to the risk of shoulder dystocia (ACOG, 2002b). While it is known that women with diabetes tend to have larger babies, there are also anthropometric differences in babies of diabetic mothers that may explain the propensity for shoulder dystocia in this population (Gherman et al., 2006; Gurewitsch & Allen, 2011). Macrosomic babies of diabetic mothers tend to have larger shoulder and extremity circumferences, a decreased head-to-shoulder ratio, significantly higher body fat, and thicker upper extremity skinfolds when compared to nondiabetic babies of similar birth weight and birth length (Gherman et al., 2006; Gurewitsch & Allen, 2011). The risk of shoulder dystocia for women with diabetes is at least double that of women who do not have diabetes (Gurewitsch & Allen, 2011), with a further increase in risk with the use of vacuum or forceps (Gherman et al., 2006).

Although the diagnosis of fetal macrosomia is imprecise, prophylactic cesarean birth may be considered for suspected fetal macrosomia with estimated fetal weights >5,000 g in women without diabetes and >4,500 g in women with diabetes (ACOG, 2002b). This is a decision made by the CNM or physician in collaboration with the pregnant woman and her family. Individual clinical situations vary, however, and not all women may agree to this course. Macrosomia is relative to maternal pelvic structures and size and fetal presentation and position. Approximately 95% of women that are either at risk for or who actually develop shoulder dystocia have babies that never reach the cutoffs for estimated fetal weights recommended by ACOG (2002b) for consideration of prophylactic cesarean birth. For all practical purposes, shoulder dystocia cannot be predicted with any degree of accuracy (ACOG, 2002b; Chauhan et al., 2005; Gurewitsch & Allen, 2011). The important issue is for perinatal nurses to be aware of maternal–fetal risk factors for individual patients and be prepared if shoulder dystocia should occur.

When shoulder dystocia is suspected, nursing, obstetric, anesthesia, and pediatric staff should be called to attend the birth if not already present. The time of the shoulder dystocia should be documented. The mother is instructed not to push and is positioned with her buttocks at the edge of the bed while preparations and maneuvers to disimpact the shoulder are made under the direction of the physician or CNM. Calmly assisting the woman to the appropriate positions during the maneuvers will help her feel confident that necessary interventions are being done as quickly as possible by competent healthcare providers.

Fundal pressure (see Fig. 14–15) should be avoided during shoulder dystocia because it can further impact the fetal shoulder, resulting in an inability to deliver the fetal body as well as contributing to fetal brachial plexus injuries and fractures of the humerus and clavicle (ACOG, 2002b; Gherman et al., 2006). Gross,

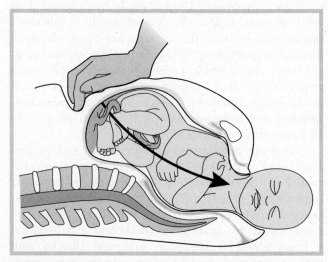

FIGURE 14–15. Fundal pressure. (From Penney, D. S., & Perlis, D. W. [1992]. When to use suprapubic or fundal pressure. *MCN: The: American Journal of Maternal/Child Nursing, 17,* 34–36.)

Shime, and Farine (1987) reported a 77% fetal injury rate when fundal pressure was the only maneuver used to relieve shoulder dystocia. Fundal pressure during shoulder dystocia has been associated with a high rate of permanent brachial plexus injuries (Phelan, Ouzounian, Gherman, Korst, & Goodwin, 1997).

The McRoberts maneuver is usually the first maneuver initiated (Hoffman et al., 2011) and it involves hyperflexion of the woman's thighs against her abdomen (see Fig. 14–13). This position can ease delivery of the shoulder by changing the relationship of the maternal pelvis to the lumbar spine. This maneuver may not actually increase birth canal dimensions, but it does result in flattening of the sacrum relative to the maternal lumbar spine (Gherman, Tramont, Muffley, & Goodwin, 2000). In many cases, the McRoberts maneuver alone or along with suprapubic pressure will result in birth. If the McRoberts maneuver is not immediately successful, the next approach is usually suprapubic pressure (Hoffman et al., 2011).

Firm suprapubic pressure (Fig. 14–14) using the palm of the hand or fist may be used to dislodge the impacted anterior shoulder. The physician or CNM may request the nurse to apply suprapubic pressure posteriorly or laterally to either the right or left side depending on which direction the fetus is facing. Posterior pressure is used to dislodge the anterior shoulder and push it under the symphysis. Lateral pressure to the posterior surface of the anterior shoulder may be used to push the fetal anterior shoulder toward the fetal chest, thereby decreasing shoulder-to-shoulder distance.

If birth does not occur immediately with McRoberts and suprapubic pressure, an appropriate next maneuver is delivery of the posterior arm (Hoffman et al., 2011). Physicians or CNMs gently insert their hand along the curvature of the fetal sacrum and their fingers follow along the humerus to the antecubital fossa. The fetal forearm is flexed and swept across the chest and face and out the vagina. Ideally, the anterior shoulder will slide under the symphysis after the posterior arm is delivered. This technique may result in fracture of the humerus or clavicle.

In the Rubin technique, the fetal shoulders are adducted and displaced into the oblique position, thereby allowing the posterior arm to enter the pelvis. Initially, the Rubin technique described both external and internal maneuvers (Rubin, 1964). During the external maneuver, fetal shoulders are rocked side to side by applying force to the maternal abdomen. If the shoulder dystocia persists, the physician or CNM inserts fingers of one hand vaginally behind the most accessible fetal shoulder and pushes the fetal shoulder toward the anterior surface of the fetal chest in the direction of the fetal face. This most often results in abduction of the shoulders, a smaller shoulder-to-shoulder diameter, and displacement of the anterior shoulder from behind the symphysis pubis.

During shoulder dystocia, the umbilical cord may be partially or completely occluded between the fetal body and maternal pelvis. Compression of the fetal neck, resulting in cerebral venous obstruction, excessive vagal stimulation, and bradycardia, may be combined with reduced arterial oxygen supply to cause clinical deterioration out of proportion to the duration of hypoxia (Kwek & Yeo, 2006). The normally oxygenated fetus can tolerate several minutes of cord compression without significant adverse effects. However, most experts note that a >5-minute head-to-body interval may result in acid–base deterioration in a fetus whose condition was normal prior to the onset of shoulder dystocia (Benedetti, 1995; Leung et al., 2011). Leung et al. (2011) found that pH dropped at a rate of 0.011 per minute of head-to-body interval during birth complicated by shoulder dystocia. When the head-to-body interval exceeds 4 minutes, there is greater risk of neonatal depression (Lerner, Durlacher, Smith, & Hamilton, 2011). If fetal status was not normal prior to the shoulder dystocia, the fetus may have less physiologic reserve (Kwek & Yeo, 2006; Shifrin & Ater, 2006). Constant provider coached pushing efforts for a prolonged period with recurrent late and variable decelerations can result in fetal oxygen desaturation, fetal metabolic acidemia, and risk of fetal hypoxic and ischemic injuries (Hamilton et al., 2012; Parer et al., 2006; Shifrin & Ater, 2006; Simpson & James, 2005a). In this context, the fetus may have less ability to tolerate an additional insult such as shoulder dystocia. In one study using neonatal brain injury as the outcome, brain injury cases were associated with a significantly prolonged head-to-body interval >10 minutes, and ≥7 minutes had a sensitivity of 67% and specificity of 74% in predicting brain injury (Ouzounian, Korst, Ahn, & Phelan, 1998).

If possible, an assessment of fetal status via EFM or handheld ultrasound devices will provide information about how the fetus is tolerating the interventions. However, time should not be lost attempting to locate the FHR if it is not readily identified. It is better to direct attention to dislodging the fetal shoulder by assisting the woman to the appropriate positions and following the direction of the physician or CNM.

The Woods screw maneuver involves placing pressure on the anterior surface of the fetal posterior shoulder and gently rotating the shoulder anteriorly. The concern about this maneuver is that it can result in abduction of the shoulders, resulting in increased shoulder-to-shoulder diameter. As a result, the Rubin technique, which adducts the fetal shoulders and rounds them into a decreased shoulder-to-shoulder diameter, is often preferred.

The Gaskin all-fours maneuver (Fig. 14–16) involves assisting the laboring woman to her hands and knees (not a knee–chest position). In a study of 82 consecutive cases of shoulder dystocia, 83% of the women birthed

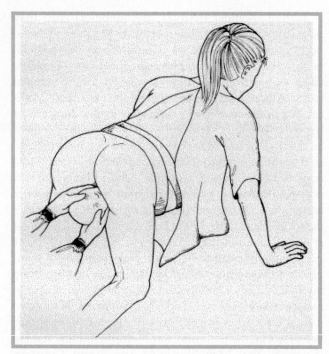

FIGURE 14–16. Gaskin all-fours maneuver. (From Bennett, B. B. [1999]. Shoulder dystocia: an obstetric emergency. *Obstetrics and Gynecology Clinics of North America, 26*[3], 445–458. doi:10.1016/S0889-8545[05]70089-9)

using the Gaskin all-fours maneuver without the need for any additional maneuvers (Bruner et al., 1998). Position change and the effects of gravity appear to provide a rapid, safe, and effective method for reducing shoulder dystocia. The women in the Bruner et al. (1998) study received no anesthesia for labor or birth. For women with epidural analgesia/anesthesia, it may be difficult, but not impossible, to assist the woman to this position.

Episiotomy, as an intervention for shoulder dystocia, is controversial. Because shoulder dystocia is considered a "bony dystocia" and therefore not caused by obstructing soft tissue, its use may not be helpful (ACOG, 2002b). Episiotomy or proctoepisiotomy has been associated with nearly a sevenfold increase in the rate of severe perineal trauma without the benefit of reducing the occurrence of neonatal depression or brachial plexus injury (Gherman et al., 2006). In one large U.S. perinatal service, an analysis of 94,842 births from 1999 to 2009 found the rate of episiotomy during shoulder dystocia decreased from 40% to 4%; however, there was no change in the rate of obstetric brachial plexus injuries (Paris, Greenberg, Ecker, & McElrath, 2011).

While the performance of a symphysiotomy is described in the literature, most practitioners have not had experience with this procedure (Gherman et al., 2006). Risks to the mother include major bladder and urethra damage, long-term pain, and difficulty walking. This procedure is rarely used in the United States (ACOG, 2002b). The deliberate fracture of the clavicles is also described as a method to reduce shoulder

width; however, many practitioners find this procedure technically difficult (Gherman et al., 2006).

In the event that these or other maneuvers do not result in birth, the physician or CNM may attempt to replace the fetal head into the vagina and proceed with cesarean birth. This is known as the Zavanelli maneuver or cephalic replacement. It is important that the head be returned to the occipitoanterior or occipitoposterior position, then flexed, and slowly pushed back into the birth canal. A review of 103 published cases of the Zavanelli maneuver from 1985 to 1997 revealed a 92% success rate, with no reports of fetal injuries in those eventually born via cesarean section (Sandberg, 1999). Others have reported fetal injuries such as Erb's palsy, paresis of the lower extremities, seizures, brain damage, delayed motor development, quadriplegia, cerebral palsy, and death as a result of the Zavanelli maneuver (Gherman et al., 2006). If the Zavanelli maneuver is successful, when possible, an assessment of fetal status via EFM or a handheld ultrasound device is desired while preparing for an emergent cesarean birth. Personnel skilled in neonatal resuscitation should be in attendance at the cesarean birth. The Zavanelli maneuver is not used often. A 2009 survey of obstetricians in the United States revealed that 85% had never used this procedure (Gherman et al., 2012).

Once the shoulder has been disimpacted and birth has occurred, the nurse can direct attention to newborn care and assessment. After the newborn and mother are stabilized, documentation about the events surrounding the birth involving shoulder dystocia is possible. See Display 14–5 for suggestions for medical record documentation following a birth complicated by shoulder dystocia. Use of a standardized checklist in the birth note after a shoulder dystocia can improve documentation of key elements (ACOG, 2012b; Deering, Tobler, & Cypher, 2010; Clark, Belfort, Byrum, Meyers, & Perlin, 2008). Team training and unit protocol implementation can provide similar positive effects on medical record documentation (Grobman et al., 2011; Moragianni, Hacker, & Craparo, 2011; Nguyen, Fox, Friedman, Sandler, & Rebarber, 2011). Ideally, each care provider documents his or her specific actions and interventions. For example, the nurse may record the application of suprapubic pressure and repositioning the woman using the McRoberts maneuver while the physician or CNM will record the techniques and maneuvers they used to disimpact the shoulder and birth the baby. There is no need for duplicate notes by both the nurse and the birth attendant of the same components of the procedure.

Support and communication with the family is important after birth. The woman and her family will likely be concerned about the condition of the baby and will have questions about what occurred. Debriefing with the family soon after the shoulder dystocia can maximize

Suggestions for Medical Record Documentation After a Birth Complicated by Shoulder Dystocia

- Provide emergent nursing care to the woman and baby as a first priority.
- There is no need for duplicate entries of the same data in the medical record. Ideally, the provider documents his or her specific actions and interventions.
- Components of Birth Attendant/Provider Documentation:
  - A brief summary of the series of interventions and clinical events with a focus on a logical step-by-step approach to relieving the impacted shoulder works best in most situations.
  - List the order of each maneuver used in clear and precise terms.
  - Avoid documenting a minute-by-minute account of the emergency unless it is absolutely certain that the times included are accurate.
  - Attempt to approximate the time interval between delivery of the fetal head and body.
  - Review the electronic fetal monitoring strip and talk with other providers in attendance to ensure the most accurate details of clinical circumstances.
  - Note whether an episiotomy was necessary and the condition of the perineum.
  - Include discussion with the woman and her family about the shoulder dystocia and subsequent newborn conditions that occurred after birth; include a note about the content of this conversation and those who were present.
- Components of Nurse Documentation:
  - Include fetal assessment data or attempts to obtain data about the fetal status during the maneuvers.
  - Note the use of the McRoberts maneuver and suprapubic pressure if indicated.
  - Note whether nursing assistance with the maneuvers was under the direction of the physician or certified nurse midwife (CNM).
  - If suprapubic pressure was used, make sure it is noted as such to avoid later allegations of fundal pressure.
  - Include approximate times for calls for assistance and when other providers arrived.
  - Carefully note the condition of the baby at birth and during the immediate newborn period.
  - Describe any resuscitation efforts and those who attended the baby.
  - Make sure that neonatal personnel in attendance understand the difference between suprapubic pressure and fundal pressure to avoid a neonatal note indicating fundal pressure was applied if this is inaccurate.
  - If umbilical blood gases were obtained, make sure they become part of the record.
  - Attempt to document in the medical record within a reasonable time after the mother and newborn are stabilized.
  - Coordinate medical record documentation with the birth attendant/provider.
  - If possible, avoid late entries many hours or days after birth.

communication and provide support. As part of the discussion, the woman should be informed that she is at risk of a recurrent shoulder dystocia in subsequent birth.

THE PERINEUM

Episiotomy

Episiotomy is a median or mediolateral incision into the perineum. According to the latest data based on 2007 hospital procedures, episiotomy is performed during approximately 10% of births in the United States (Martin et al., 2011; Hall, DeFrances, Williams, Golosinskiy, & Schwartzman, 2010). The episiotomy rate has steadily decreased over the past years from 54% in 1992, to 33% in 2000, to 23% in 2004, and 10% in 2007, the latest year for which these data are available (ACOG, 2006b; DeFrances & Podgornik, 2006; Hall et al., 2010; Martin et al., 2011). Although this surgical technique has long been thought to permit the easier passage of the baby and to decrease the risk of perineal trauma, there is little supportive evidence for these beliefs (ACOG, 2006b; Scott, 2005).

Those who consider routine episiotomy to be beneficial cite the following advantages: prevention of perineal tearing; ease of repair when compared to lacerations; reduction in the time and stress of the second stage of labor; decreased compression of fetal head, especially for preterm infants; and allowance of easier manipulation during breech or operative vaginal birth. However, the benefits of routine episiotomy have not been demonstrated by rigorous research (ACOG, 2006b; Carroli & Belizan, 2009; Eason & Feldman, 2000; Eason, Labrecque, Wells, & Feldman, 2000; Hartmann et al., 2005). It appears that personal beliefs, education, and experience of the practitioner, rather than evidence, influence clinical judgment about whether to perform an episiotomy (ACOG, 2006b; Low, Seng, Murtland, & Oakley, 2000).

Based on available data, giving birth over an intact perineum results in less blood loss, less risk of infection, and less perineal pain postpartum (ACOG, 2006b; Eason & Feldman, 2000). Methods to prevent perineal trauma during birth include upright positioning, avoidance of episiotomy, avoidance of forceps or vacuum extractors, passive fetal descent, avoidance of Valsalva pushing, slowing the birth of the fetal head to allow the perineum time to stretch, and birth between contractions (Albers et al., 2006; Andrews, Sultan, Thakar, & Jones, 2006; da Silva et al., 2012; De Jonge et al., 2010; Eason & Feldman, 2000; FitzGerald, Weber, Howden, Cundiff,

& Brown, 2007; Gupta et al., 2012; Hastings-Tolsma, Vincent, Emeis, & Francisco, 2007; Kudish et al., 2006; Mayerhofer et al., 2002; Sampselle & Hines, 1999; Schaffer et al., 2005; Simpson & James, 2005a).

Episiotomy is often performed when the physician or CNM feels that there is a risk of lacerations of the perineum or vagina during birth. The goal is to protect the perineum and to maintain future perineal function and integrity; however, supportive evidence is lacking that these goals can be achieved with routine episiotomy (ACOG, 2006b; Scott, 2005). The use of episiotomy is associated with significant risks such as increased risk of third- and fourth-degree lacerations (Aukee, Sundström, & Kairaluoma, 2006; Hudelist et al., 2005; Ogunyemi, Manigat, Marquis, & Bazargan, 2006), anal sphincter injuries (Andrews et al., 2006; Clemons, Towers, McClure, & O'Boyle, 2005; Dandolu et al., 2005; FitzGerald et al., 2007; Hudelist et al., 2005; Kudish et al., 2006), severe lacerations and injuries in subsequent births (Edwards, Grotegut, Harmanli, Rapkin, & Dandolu, 2006; Peleg, Kennedy, Merrill, & Zlatnik, 1999; Spydslaug, Trogstad, Skrondal, & Eskild, 2005), infection, delayed healing (McGuinness, Norr, & Nacion, 1991), breakdown in repair (Williams & Chames, 2006), increased blood loss (Eason & Feldman, 2000), scarring (Koger, Shatney, Hodge, & McClenathan, 1993), increased pain (Macarthur & Macarthur, 2004), sexual dysfunction (Stamp, Kruzins, & Crowther, 2001), and higher costs secondary to time and suture.

Episiotomy does not protect against problems with perineal muscle function postpartum (Fleming, Newton, & Roberts, 2003). Data from *Mothers' Outcome After Delivery*, a longitudinal cohort study of pelvic floor disorders after childbirth, found that forceps and perineal lacerations, but not episiotomies, were associated with pelvic floor disorders 5 to 10 years after first delivery (Handa, Blomquist, McDermott, Friedman, & Muñoz, 2012). Lacerations of the vagina and perineum are classified according to degree as listed in Display 14–6. Risk factors for third- and fourth-degree lacerations are nulliparity (a 7.2-fold risk), episiotomy (a 2.4-fold risk for nulliparous women and a 4.4-fold risk for multiparous women), increasing gestational age, increasing birth weight, oxytocin, epidural analgesia/anesthesia, operative vaginal birth, and increasing length of the second stage of labor (Landy et al., 2011). In the *Consortium on Safe Labor* database of 228,668 births from 2002 to 2008, third- or fourth-degree lacerations occurred in 2,516 women (2,223 nulliparous [5.8%], 293 [0.6%] multiparous) (Landy et al., 2011).

Nursing interventions during labor can have a direct impact on the use and perceived need for episiotomy. Upright position and open-glottis, gentle pushing that coincide with the woman's natural urges and sensations, aids gradual perineal stretching with less pain, thus

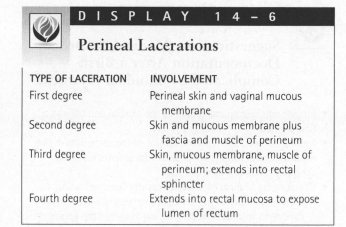

DISPLAY 14 – 6

Perineal Lacerations

TYPE OF LACERATION	INVOLVEMENT
First degree	Perineal skin and vaginal mucous membrane
Second degree	Skin and mucous membrane plus fascia and muscle of perineum
Third degree	Skin, mucous membrane, muscle of perineum; extends into rectal sphincter
Fourth degree	Extends into rectal mucosa to expose lumen of rectum

avoiding the need for episiotomy and resultant perineal trauma (Devine et al., 1999; Eason et al., 2000; Flynn, Franiek, Janssen, Hannah, & Klein, 1997; Sampselle & Hines, 1999; Simpson & James, 2005a). Women who give birth in the lithotomy position are more likely to have an episiotomy than women who give birth in squatting, on hands-and-knees, standing, or in sitting positions (Bodner-Adler et al., 2003; da Silva et al., 2012; de Jong et al., 1997; Gupta & Hofmeyr, 2004; Gupta et al., 2012; Terry et al., 2006). Passive fetal descent and spontaneous bearing down efforts versus directed Valsalva pushing result in fewer episiotomies and perineal lacerations (Albers et al., 2006; Devine et al., 1999; Sampselle & Hines, 1999; Simpson & James, 2005a).

Second-Stage Labor Interventions

Other measures that have been proposed to enhance perineal stretching and decrease perineal trauma are the application of warm compresses, gentle perineal massage and stretching, and warm oil perineal massage during the second stage of labor. There is no evidence from any randomized clinical trial that use of second-stage perineal massage with or without oil decreases the need for episiotomy or the risk of perineal trauma (Albers, Sedler, Bedrick, Teaf, & Peralta, 2005; Eason et al., 2000). One study found that perineal massage during the second stage was associated with a greater risk of perineal trauma (Aikins-Murphy & Feinland, 1998), and another study suggested that some women in labor are uncomfortable with this technique (Albers et al., 2005). There is significant disagreement among providers as to whether second-stage perineal massage should be used (Mayerhofer et al., 2002; Stamp, 1997; Stamp et al., 2001). Perineal massage has not shown to increase the likelihood of an intact perineum or reduce the risk of pain, dyspareunia, or urinary or fecal problems (Albers et al., 2005; Stamp et al., 2001).

According to the latest Cochrane review, warm compresses during second stage may be beneficial in reducing the risk of third- and fourth-degree tears (Aasheim, Nilsen, Lukasse, & Reinar, 2011). Avoiding perineal massage (hands-off approach) during second stage was found to reduce the risk of episiotomy (Aasheim et al., 2011). Absent data to suggest benefit along with limited data to suggest harm, perineal massage during the second stage should be used with caution, if at all, until more evidence is available about risks and benefits.

Antepartum Interventions

Antepartum perineal massage has also been studied as a method to decrease the risk of perineal trauma at birth. Usually, women who choose perineal massage are taught to use the technique daily during the third trimester (Labrecque et al., 1999; Shipman, Boniface, Tefft, & McCloghery, 1997). Very limited data exist to support the role of antepartum perineal massage in reducing the rate of episiotomies and perineal trauma (Eason et al., 2000; Renfrew, Hannah, Albers, & Floyd, 1998). In one study, women who were taught perineal massage reported pain, discomfort, irritation, fatigue, uneasiness with the concept, and negative physician comments (Mynaugh, 1991). The women who practiced perineal massage also experienced more perineal lacerations than those in the control group (Mynaugh, 1991). In another study, perineal massage was effective in reducing the rate of episiotomy for first-time mothers only (Labrecque et al., 1999). In a later study, antenatal perineal massage did not reduce the incidence of episiotomy or abnormal continence scores (Eogan, Daly, & O'Herlihy, 2006). Perineal massage during pregnancy has been shown to neither impair nor substantially protect perineal function at 3 months postpartum (Labrecque, Eason, & Marcoux, 2000). Based on the latest systematic review from the Cochrane Database of Systematic Reviews, antenatal perineal massage may decrease the incidence of episiotomy in women giving birth vaginally for the first time (Beckmann & Garrett, 2009). Perhaps women who practice perineal massage antenatally are more likely to request that episiotomy be avoided unless necessary. More research is needed to determine whether perineal massage performed by the woman in the weeks before labor and birth is effective in avoiding the medical need for episiotomy or reducing the extent of lacerations. If women choose to practice perineal massage during pregnancy, there appears to be no harm in doing so.

EMOTIONAL AND PHYSICAL SUPPORT DURING LABOR AND BIRTH

IMPACT OF THE PSYCHE ON CHILDBIRTH

The psyche plays a major role in the process of labor and birth. A high level of anxiety has been associated with increased catecholamine secretion that can result in ineffective uterine activity and longer and dysfunctional labor (Lederman, Lederman, Work, & McCann, 1985). Anxiety, uncertainty, loss of control, loss of self-confidence, patterns of coping, support systems, fatigue, optimism, fatalism, and aloneness are some of the psychosocial factors to consider when caring for women in labor. Previous birth experiences, present support systems, concerns/questions, anxiety or fear, and cultural considerations further contribute to attitudes and expectations for the current pregnancy experience.

FACILITATING LABOR AND BIRTH

Nursing care during childbirth includes providing information so the woman knows what to expect, interpreting physical sensations, encouraging maternal position changes, reinforcing breathing and other relaxation efforts, support during the second stage, and continued pain management. Women expect that their nurse will provide physical comfort and informational and emotional support as well as technical nursing care and ongoing monitoring of maternal–fetal status during labor (Tumblin & Simkin, 2001). Women appreciate the nurse being there for them (MacKinnon, McIntyre, & Quance, 2005). Some women experience increased anxiety and fear when the labor and birth unit is so busy that they do not have as much nursing contact and support as they had expected (Larkin, Begley, & Devane, 2012). Women value personal control during childbirth and this is an important factor related to the woman's satisfaction with the childbirth experience (Christiaens & Bracke, 2007; Goodman, Mackey, & Tavakoli, 2004). When women have the birth they planned (e.g., vaginal or cesarean), they expressed satisfaction with childbirth, whereas an unplanned cesarean birth is associated with a less favorable view of the experience (Blomquist, Quiroz, Macmillan, McCullough, & Handa, 2011). Helping women to increase their personal control during labor and birth may increase the woman's childbirth satisfaction. Some hospitals offer birth plans for women so they can select options they would like to include as part of their labor and birth. See Display 14–7 for a birth plan that women can complete online, then print and bring to their prenatal visit to discuss with their provider. This birth plan was developed in collaboration with interdisciplinary representatives from the perinatal team. Advantages include the opportunity to consider the anticipated experience well in advance and to discuss expectations with the healthcare provider before arriving at the hospital for labor and birth.

In a systematic review of women's satisfaction with their childbirth experience, women whose experiences were better than expected and women with high expectations were more likely to be satisfied, whereas women with low expectations that were subsequently met had lower levels of satisfaction (Hodnett, 2002).

DISPLAY 14-7

Birth Plan

Expectant Mother's Name _____   Birthdate _____

Expectant Mother's Physician/Nurse Midwife _____

Baby's Physician _____   Baby's Due Date _____

My Labor Support Team • I plan to have the following people with me during my labor and birth:

Partner _____   Relationship _____

Doula _____

Other Support Person _____   Relationship _____

Other Support Person _____   Relationship _____

Other Support Person _____   Relationship _____

Comfort Measures • I plan to try these additional comfort measures (check all that are desired):

☐ Walking, squatting and using a birth ball
☐ Labor in water using a shower or tub
☐ Listening to music (please bring your own)
☐ Massage
☐ Aromatherapy (scented oils, fresh flowers-please bring your own)
☐ Wear my own clothes during labor (hospital gowns are also available)

Monitoring My Contractions and Baby's Heart Rate •
I would prefer (check all that apply):

☐ Checking on the well-being of my baby using intermittent monitoring
☐ Continuous electronic monitoring placed with elastic belts around my abdomen
☐ Using a telemetry unit (when available) so I can be monitored while up and about in my room or hallways
☐ Placement of internal monitors using a fetal scalp electrode and/or intrauterine pressure catheter if medically necessary
☐ Whatever is recommended by my physician/nurse midwife for the safety of myself and baby

Intravenous Access (IV) • I prefer to have IV access using this method:

☐ Saline Lock - access into a vein with short tubing and no fluid attached
☐ Continuous IV - access into a vein with tubing and fluids attached

Pain Management • I plan to:

☐ Labor and give birth with little or no intervention so please don't offer pain medication. I will let you know if I change my mind.
☐ Narcotic pain medication given into my IV if safe for me and my baby
☐ Epidural anesthesia

Bag of Water Breaking • I would prefer to:

☐ Allow my bag of water to break on its own
☐ Have my bag of water artificially broken if medically necessary

Pushing Preferences and Birth • I would like to try (check all that are desired):

☐ Lying on my side to push
☐ Squatting in bed using the squat bar
☐ Sitting upright in bed
☐ On all fours

Episiotomy • I would prefer to:

☐ Not have an episiotomy
☐ Whatever is recommended by my physician/nurse midwife for the safety of myself and baby

Cutting and Umbilical Cord • I plan to:

☐ Have my labor partner cut the umbilical cord
☐ I would prefer that my physician/nurse midwife cut the umbilical cord

Cord Blood Collection and Donation • I plan to:

☐ Donate my baby's cord blood to the public donor blood bank
☐ Arrange for collection of my baby's cord blood for my own private use (Private company I will be using: _____)
☐ I do not plan to have my baby's cord blood collected for private or public use

Immediate Care of My Baby Following Birth • I plan to (check all that are desired):

☐ Have my baby placed skin-to-skin with me on my chest immediately following the birth
☐ Have the nurse clean my baby off first and then placed in my arms for bonding
☐ If possible I would prefer to have little or no separation from my baby

Feeding My Baby • I plan to (check all that are desired):

☐ Initiate breastfeeding shortly after the birth
☐ Exclusively breastfeed my baby on demand
☐ Pump and give my baby breastmilk from a bottle
☐ Bottle feed my baby with infant formula.
  Formula preference:
  ☐ Similac   ☐ Enfamil   ☐ GoodStart

Pacifiers • I would prefer:

☐ Not allow the use of pacifiers or bottles during the hospital stay
☐ Allow pacifiers for my bottle fed baby

Administration of Antibiotic Eye Drops • I would prefer:

☐ Administration of antibiotic eye drops per hospital routine
☐ Delaying the administration of antibiotic eye drops for up to one hour after the birth

Circumcision • I plan to (check all that are desired):

☐ Have my baby boy circumcised
☐ Not have my baby boy circumcised
☐ I would like to arrange for a Bris at the hospital eight days after my baby boy's birth

Rooming In and Bonding With My Baby • I plan to (check all that are desired):

☐ Keep my baby with me as much as possible
☐ Have my formula-fed baby cared for in the newborn nursery at night
☐ Keep my breastfed baby with me at all times including overnight to learn feeding cues
☐ Observe naptime each afternoon and limit visitors during this time
☐ Have my partner spend that night during my hospital stay

Other Things that are Important to Me:

_____

_____

_____

_____

_____

This birth plan serves as a communication tool between you, your physician/nurse midwife and your nursing staff. It helps us know what is most important to you during your baby's birth and hospital stay. The birth process is unique to each woman and can be unpredictable. Expect that you may need to alter your birth plan if health becomes a concern. You can trust our team to honor your wishes while protecting you and your baby. Bring your completed birth plan to one of your prenatal visits. Your physician/nurse midwife will review your plan and answer questions that you may have about what to expect during the labor and birth of your baby.

*Signatures

Expectant Mother _____   Date _____

Physician/Nurse Midwife _____   Date _____

*Signatures serve to acknowledge the expectant mother's birth preference and that her physician/nurse midwife is aware of her wishes.
STL_23573(3/14/12)
_____

From Mercy Hospital – St. Louis. Used with permission.

One-to-one nursing care during labor is a significant patient satisfier, although that type of care is not always feasible in a busy labor unit (Hodnett et al., 2002). Nurse staffing guidelines from AWHONN (2010) delineate types of patients and clinical situations that require one nurse to one woman staffing (see Table 1–3 in Chapter 1 *Perinatal Patient Safety and Professional Liability Issues*). Nursing behaviors that demonstrate valuing and respecting childbearing women are essential in enhancing the quality of the birth experience (Matthews & Callister, 2004).

SUPPORTIVE CARE BY PARTNERS, FAMILY, AND FRIENDS

Attention also should be given to the woman's partner/support person, family members, and friends in attendance. Every effort should be made to support and encourage those in attendance to assist the woman during labor and to allow as many support persons as the woman desires. Arbitrary rules prohibiting more than one support person during labor are contrary to the philosophy that the birth experience belongs to the woman and her family rather to those providing clinical care. Although healthcare providers are sometimes inclined to attempt to control this aspect of the birth process using various arguments for safety and convenience, when examined critically, these arguments have little scientific merit. Women should be able to choose who will be with them during this special and unique life experience. Family-centered care supports the concept that the "family" is defined by the childbearing woman.

In the most recent Cochrane Review, 21 trials involving over 15,000 women were evaluated for effects of labor support on perinatal outcomes (Hodnett, Gates, Hofmeyr, Sakala, & Weston, 2011). Women who have continuous labor support when compared to women who have the usual labor care are more likely to have a spontaneous vaginal birth and are less likely to have a cesarean birth, intrapartum analgesia/anesthesia, operative vaginal birth, a baby with a low 5-minute Apgar score, or to report dissatisfaction with their childbirth experiences (Hodnett et al., 2011; McGrath & Kennell, 2008). Labor was shorter for women with continuous labor support (Hodnett et al., 2011). Continuous labor support is associated with greater benefits when the provider of that support is not a member of the hospital staff (Campbell, Lake, Falk, & Backstrand, 2006; Hodnett et al., 2002; Hodnett et al., 2011). Fewer perinatal complications, fewer newborns with 5-minute Apgar scores less than 7, fewer newborns admitted to the neonatal intensive care unit (NICU), lower rates of analgesia and anesthesia, lower operative birth rates, and shorter labors result when women have a support person as compared to women without support (Campbell et al., 2006; Green, Amis, & Hotelling, 2007; Hodnett et al., 2011; Klaus, Kennell, Robertson, & Sosa, 1986; McGrath & Kennell, 2008; Pascoe, 1993; Sauls, 2002). The presence of a lay support person has also been found to reduce the rate of cesarean births (Klaus, Kennell, McGrath, Robertson, & Hinkley, 1988; McGrath & Kennell, 2008). There is adequate research to validate the significance of promoting support from family members/coaches during the labor and birth experience; thus, all women should have support throughout labor and birth (Hodnett et al., 2011). See Chapter 16 for a more detailed discussion of labor support.

Families should be free to take pictures and make video and/or audio recordings during labor and birth. Policies restricting cameras are in conflict with the philosophy that the birth experience should be what the woman and her family desire within reason. There is no evidence that videos of labor and birth later produced as part of a legal claim increase liability. Videos or pictures showing that the perinatal team provided excellent care in a challenging situation could prove to be beneficial to a situation known to suffer from hindsight bias. Concerns about safety, liability, privacy, and space limitations can be adequately addressed without restrictive policies about visitors and use of cameras during labor and birth if care providers are committed to meeting the needs of childbearing women and their support persons.

SUPPORTING MATERNAL AND FAMILY ATTACHMENT

At birth, skin-to-skin contact between mother and baby has many positive benefits. Although babies were traditionally separated from their mothers immediately after birth for assessment and temperature stabilization and regulation by placing babies in warmers in the delivery room, this practice is not necessary for newborn well-being. Immediate skin-to-skin contact with the baby on the mother's chest after birth and continued contact during the first few days of life can promote normal temperature stabilization and regulation in the newborn and can decrease the risk of neonatal hypothermia and hypoglycemia (Britton, 1980; Bystrova et al., 2003; Fransson, Karlsson, & Nilsson, 2005; Mzurek, Mikieil-Kostyra, Mazur, & Wieczirek, 1999). Duration of breastfeeding and the baby's recognition of the mother's milk odor are enhanced with early skin-to-skin contact immediately after birth (AAP, 2012; ACOG, 2007a; de Chateau & Wiberg, 1984; Mikiel-Kostyra, Boltruszko, Mazur, & Zielenska, 2001; Mikiel-Kostyra, Mazur, & Boltruszko, 2002; Mizuno, Mizuno, Shinohara, & Noda, 2004; Moore, Anderson, Bergman, & Dowswell, 2012; Thukral et al., 2012). Early breastfeeding has similar benefits, so mothers should be encouraged to breast-feed as soon as possible after birth (de Chateau & Wiberg, 1984; Mikiel-Kostyra et al., 2001; Mikiel-Kostyra et al., 2002). Positive long-term effects of early contact include greater communication between mother and baby and encouraging behavior by the mother to the baby (Renfrew, Lang, & Woolbridge, 2000). Most mothers enjoy the experience and would choose skin-to-skin contact for future births (Carfoot, Williamson, & Dickson, 2005).

While some may perceive challenges in providing skin-to-skin contact between the mother and baby immediately after cesarean birth, it can be accomplished by collaboration of the perinatal team including nurses, obstetrics, pediatricians, and anesthesia providers (Fig. 14–17) (Hung & Berg, 2011). In a nurse-led quality improvement project, following the development of a protocol to promote skin-to-skin contact immediately after cesarean birth while in the surgical suite (Fig. 14–18), early skin-to-skin contact increased from 20% to 60% of births in the surgical suite and to 70% within 90 minutes of life. Babies with early skin-to-skin contact in the surgical suite were less likely to have formula supplementation when compared to babies without early skin-to-skin contact. It is important to expend the effort to make skin-to-skin contact a priority immediately after birth for healthy mothers and babies, even for mothers after cesarean birth while they are still in the surgical suite. According to AAP (2012), healthy babies should be placed and remain in direct skin-to-skin contact with their mothers immediately after birth until the first feeding is accomplished. The alert, healthy newborn infant is capable of latching on to a breast without specific assistance within the first hour after birth. The baby should be dried, Apgar scores assigned, and initial

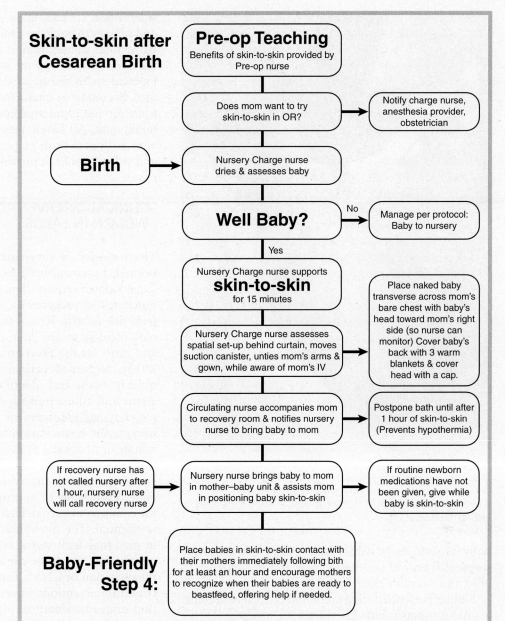

Skin-to-skin after Cesarean Birth

Pre-op Teaching
Benefits of skin-to-skin provided by Pre-op nurse

Does mom want to try skin-to-skin in OR? → Notify charge nurse, anesthesia provider, obstetrician

Birth → Nursery Charge nurse dries & assesses baby

Well Baby? No → Manage per protocol: Baby to nursery

Yes

Nursery Charge nurse supports **skin-to-skin** for 15 minutes → Place naked baby transverse across mom's bare chest with baby's head toward mom's right side (so nurse can monitor) Cover baby's back with 3 warm blankets & cover head with a cap.

Nursery Charge nurse assesses spatial set-up behind curtain, moves suction canister, unties mom's arms & gown, while aware of mom's IV →

Circulating nurse accompanies mom to recovery room & notifies nursery nurse to bring baby to mom → Postpone bath until after 1 hour of skin-to-skin (Prevents hypothermia)

If recovery nurse has not called nursery after 1 hour, nursery nurse will call recovery nurse → Nursery nurse brings baby to mom in mother–baby unit & assists mom in positioning baby skin-to-skin → If routine newborn medications have not been given, give while baby is skin-to-skin

Baby-Friendly Step 4: Place babies in skin-to-skin contact with their mothers immediately following bith for at least an hour and encourage mothers to recognize when their babies are ready to beastfeed, offering help if needed.

FIGURE 14–17. Protocol for providing skin-to-skin contact in the surgical suite during cesarean birth. (Adapted from Hung, K. J., & Berg, O. [2011]. Early skin-to-skin after cesarean to improve breastfeeding. *MCN: The American Journal of Maternal/Child Nursing, 36*[5], 318–324. doi:10.1097/NMC.0b013e3182266314)

physical assessment performed while the baby is with the mother (AAP, 2012). The mother is an optimal heat source for the infant. Weighing, measuring, bathing, needle-sticks, and eye prophylaxis can be delayed until after the first feeding is completed (AAP, 2012). Babies affected by maternal medications may require assistance for effective latch on. Except under unusual circumstances, the newborn should remain with the mother throughout the recovery period (AAP, 2012). Immediate skin-to-skin contact after birth has considerable benefits because it requires minimal financial resources, is not associated with adverse effects among healthy babies, shows an overall positive effect on breastfeeding, and appears to improve newborn stabilization during transition (Hung & Berg, 2011).

Women's expectations and desires regarding who will be present at the birth vary widely. Some women prefer that their partner be the sole participant, while others choose to have more family members and friends share this important event. The desires of the woman should guide this process rather than arbitrarily determined visitor policies. As long as space permits and the safety of the mother and baby are not a consideration, the woman should be able to have as many family members and support persons as she requests. Every effort should be made to have the woman's partner next to her as she is giving birth and to be able to see and touch the baby immediately after birth. If newborn resuscitation is required or unexpected, encourage the partner to be close to the

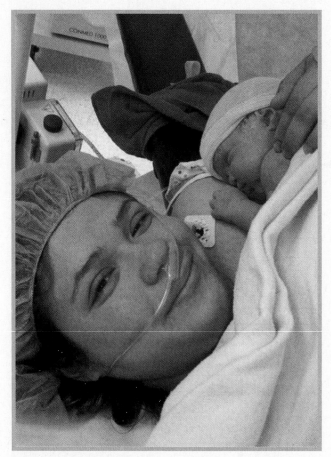

FIGURE 14–18. Skin-to-skin contact of mother and baby in the surgical suite during cesarean birth. (From Hung, K. J., & Berg, O. [2011]. Early skin-to-skin after cesarean to improve breastfeeding. *MCN: The American Journal of Maternal/Child Nursing, 36*[5], 318–324. doi:10.1097/NMC.0b013e3182266314)

baby as soon as possible. As the baby's condition is stabilized, encourage the woman and her partner to hold and examine their baby.

Sibling presence during labor and birth also presents a unique opportunity for nurses to promote family attachment. Parents report that children present during labor and birth show a greater number of mothering and caretaking behaviors than did children not present (DelGiudice, 1986). Sibling classes to prepare children for the birth experience are imperative. These classes should be age related and should include films on childbirth, discussion of maternal behavior and sounds in labor, and reassurance that pain experienced by the mother is temporary. Additionally, each child needs a support person to accompany the child and to be familiar with the child's developmental level, so that both the child's curiosity and concerns for his/her mother and new brother/sister are answered.

As the family is introduced to their newborn immediately at birth, an explanation of umbilical cord clamping/cutting and inspection of the placenta help the family understand the final physiologic separation of the newborn from the mother's life-support system. During skin-to-skin contact, allow the family, support persons, and siblings to be close to the mother to see and touch the baby. After stabilization, if the baby has been wrapped, the nurse can unwrap the newborn and describe normal physical characteristics. Siblings can count fingers and toes. Encouraging interaction with the newborn sets the stage for successful attachment and integration into the family unit. All family members can hold the newborn after birth as desired, and opportunities for photographs and videos should be provided.

CLINICAL INTERVENTIONS FOR WOMEN IN LABOR

The majority of pregnancies, labors, and births are normal, requiring little or no intervention. However, some women require clinical interventions to optimize outcomes in pregnancies with identified maternal or fetal risk factors. Risk status for the woman and fetus may increase at any time during the pregnancy, labor and birth, or the postpartum period (AAP & ACOG, 2012). Nurses in perinatal settings must be able to quickly assess and identify changes in maternal–fetal status and adjust nursing care accordingly. For example, nursing management during labor may require intrauterine resuscitation techniques when an indeterminate or abnormal FHR is noted, or plans for vaginal birth may be quickly changed when an emergent cesarean birth becomes the safest option for the mother and baby. Knowledge of appropriate nursing interventions for common maternal–fetal complications during labor is essential. The nurse must also be aware of changes in maternal–fetal status requiring physician or CNM notification and those requiring bedside evaluation by the physician or CNM. The next section focuses on the clinical interventions of cervical ripening, labor induction and augmentation, operative vaginal birth, and amnioinfusion. Implications for nursing care are presented with key points for assessment and intervention.

CERVICAL RIPENING AND INDUCTION AND AUGMENTATION OF LABOR

Definition of Terms

Cervical ripening is the process of effecting physical softening and distensibility of the cervix in preparation for labor and birth. *Induction of labor* is the stimulation of uterine contractions before the spontaneous onset of labor for the purpose of accomplishing vaginal birth. *Augmentation of labor* is the stimulation of uterine contractions when spontaneous contractions have failed to result in progressive cervical dilation or descent of the fetus. *Tachysystole* is excessive uterine activity, which can be either spontaneous or induced. Tachysystole is defined as more than five contractions in 10 minutes (averaged over 30 minutes) by the National Institute of Child Health and Human Development (NICHD) expert group on EFM that met in 2008 (Macones, Hankins, Spong, Hauth, & Moore, 2008). Additional features of excessive uterine activity include contractions lasting 2 minutes or longer, contractions of normal duration occurring within 1 minute of each other or insufficient return of uterine resting tone between contractions via palpation, or intraamniotic pressure above 25 mm Hg between contractions via IUPC (ACOG, 2003; Simpson, 2013).

Incidence

According to the National Center for Health Statistics (NCHS) (Martin et al., 2011), in 2009 (the most recent year for which natality data on induction are available), the rate of induction of labor in the United States was approximately 23.2% of all births. Data on augmentation are usually similar to the induction rate (Menacker & Martin, 2008); thus based on reported data, approximately one half of women laboring in the United States receive labor stimulation. The 2009 induction rate is 144% higher than the rate in 1990 (9.5%) and represents an all-time high since these data have been recorded from birth certificates (Martin et al., 2011). The latest natality data can be accessed at http://www.cdc.gov/nchs/births.htm. Most clinicians would note that these data seem low when compared to actual clinical practice. The induction rate is calculated based on all women who give birth (Martin et al., 2011). If women who had a planned or repeat cesarean birth are excluded from the denominator and the figures are calculated based on all others who potentially could have had labor induction, the reported rate of induction would be significantly higher (Zhang, Yancey, & Henderson, 2002). It is likely that data regarding induction and augmentation are significantly underreported on birth certificates (Menacker & Martin, 2008).

Indications

Because spontaneous labor is associated with fewer complications than induced labor, induction without a medical indication should be discouraged. According to ACOG (2009a), induction of labor has merit as a therapeutic option when the benefits of expeditious birth outweigh the risks of continuing the pregnancy. Therefore, benefits of labor induction must be weighed against the associated potential maternal and fetal risks (ACOG, 2009a). The various opinions among providers and patients about the exact nature and intensity of some risks and benefits are reflected in clinical practice. Multiple factors influence the decision to induce labor. Not all of the indications are clinical; some are primarily based on convenience (Simpson, 2010). Display 14–8 lists commonly cited convenience issues

DISPLAY 14 – 8

Commonly Cited Convenience Issues for Patients, Physicians, and Institutions Related to Elective Induction of Labor

Patients

Timing of birth to coincide with personal schedules, availability of partners, support persons and family, babysitting issues

Desire for preferred physician to attend the birth rather than a physician partner in the group practice

Wish to "get the pregnancy over with"

Relief from pregnancy discomforts

Avoidance of certain dates such as holidays, preference for certain dates with personal meaning

Income tax deduction enhancement

Physicians

Quality-of-life issues (labor and birth occurs during a weekday, during the day shift, while on call; avoidance of interruptions of office hours, weekends, and evenings; ability to schedule more than one patient on the same day)

Patient satisfaction

Liability concerns

Desire to attend birth of primary patient for reimbursement issues or per patient request

Institutions

Ability to plan for scheduling and staffing

Patient satisfaction

Provider satisfaction

Market share issues

Adapted from Simpson, K. R. (2010). Reconsideration of the costs of convenience: Quality, operational and fiscal strategies to minimize elective labor induction. *Journal of Perinatal and Neonatal Nursing, 24*(1), 42–53. doi:10.1097/JPN.0b013e3181c6abe3

related to elective induction of labor. Display 14–9 lists criteria, indications, and contraindications for cervical ripening and induction and augmentation of labor based on recommendations from ACOG (2003, 2009a). For recommendations from the NICHD expert group (Spong et al., 2011) regarding timing of birth when conditions complicate pregnancy at or after 34 weeks of gestation, see Table 7–1 in Chapter 7 *Preterm Labor and Birth*. These publications can be used to guide unit policy regarding elective births.

According to ACOG (2009a), labor may be induced for logistic reasons, such as a history of rapid labor, distance from the hospital, or "psychosocial indications." The interpretation of psychosocial indications varies widely among providers and is most commonly noted for an elective (i.e., nonmedical indication) induction of labor. When labor is induced for logistic reasons or

DISPLAY 14-9

Criteria, Indications, and Contraindications for Cervical Ripening, Labor Induction, and Labor Augmentation

Criteria for Cervical Ripening and Induction of Labor

- Gestational age, cervical status, pelvic adequacy, fetal size, and fetal presentation should be assessed.
- Any potential risks to the mother and fetus should be considered.
- The medical record should document that a discussion was held between the pregnant woman and her healthcare provider about the indications; the agents and methods of labor induction, including the risks, benefits, and alternative approaches; and the possible need for repeat induction or cesarean birth.
- Nulliparous women undergoing elective induction of labor with an unfavorable cervix should be counseled about a twofold increased risk of cesarean birth.
- Cervical ripening and induction agents should be administered by trained personnel familiar with the effects on mother and fetus.
- Prostaglandin preparations should be administered where uterine activity and fetal heart rate (FHR) can be monitored continuously for an initial observation period. FHR monitoring should be continued if regular uterine contractions persist.
- FHR and uterine contractions should be monitored closely during induction and augmentation as for any high-risk patient in active labor.
- A physician capable of performing a cesarean birth should be readily available.
- For women undergoing trial of labor after a cesarean (TOLAC), induction of labor for maternal or fetal indications remains an option.
- Misoprostol should not be used for third trimester cervical ripening or labor induction in women who have had a cesarean birth or major uterine surgery.

Indications for Cervical Ripening and Induction of Labor

Indications for the induction of labor are not absolute but should take into account maternal and fetal conditions, gestational age, cervical status, and other factors. Following are examples of maternal or fetal conditions that may be indications for the induction of labor:

- Abruptio placentae
- Chorioamnionitis (intraamniotic infection)
- Fetal demise
- Gestational hypertension
- Preeclampsia, eclampsia
- Premature rupture of membranes
- Postterm pregnancy
- Maternal medical conditions (e.g., diabetes mellitus, renal disease, chronic pulmonary disease, chronic hypertension, or antiphospholipid syndrome)

- Fetal compromise (e.g., severe fetal growth restriction, isoimmunization, oligohydramnios)

Labor may also be induced for logistic reasons (e.g., risk of rapid labor, distance from the hospital, or psychosocial indications). In such circumstances, at least one of the following criteria should be met or fetal lung maturity should be established:

- Ultrasound measurement at less than 20 weeks of gestation supports gestational age of 39 weeks or greater.
- Fetal heart tones have been documented as present for 30 weeks by Doppler ultrasonography.
- It has been 36 weeks since a positive serum or urine human chorionic gonadotropin pregnancy test result.
- Testing for fetal lung maturity should not be performed, and is contraindicated, when delivery is mandated for fetal or maternal indications. Conversely, a mature fetal lung maturity test result before 39 weeks of gestation, in the absence of appropriate clinical circumstances, is not an indication for elective labor induction.

Contraindication to Induction of Labor

Generally, the contraindications for labor induction are the same as those for spontaneous labor and vaginal birth. They include, but are not limited to, the following:

- Vasa previa or complete placenta previa
- Transverse fetal lie
- Umbilical cord prolapse
- Previous classical cesarean birth
- Active genital herpes infection
- Previous myomectomy entering the endometrial cavity

Indications for Augmentation of Labor

Augmentation refers to the stimulation of uterine contractions when spontaneous contractions have failed to result in progressive cervical dilation or descent of the fetus. Expectations for labor progress should be based on the most recent data regarding what constitutes normal progress of labor based on parity and other maternal factors. Before augmentation, an assessment of the maternal pelvis and cervix and fetal position, station, and well-being should be performed.

- Augmentation should be considered if the frequency of contractions is less than three contractions per 10 minutes or the intensity of contractions in less than 25 mm Hg above baseline, or both.

Contraindication to Augmentation of Labor

Contraindications to augmentation of labor are similar to those for the induction of labor and may include, but are not limited to, the following:

- Placenta or vasa previa
- Umbilical cord presentation
- Prior classical uterine incision
- Active genital herpes infection
- Pelvic structural deformities
- Invasive cervical cancer

Adapted from American College of Obstetricians and Gynecologists. (2003). *Dystocia and Augmentation of Labor* (Practice Bulletin No. 49). Washington, DC: Author; American College of Obstetricians and Gynecologists. (2008a). *Fetal Lung Maturity* (Practice Bulletin No. 97). Washington, DC: Author. doi:10.1097/AOG.0b013e318188d1c2; American College of Obstetricians and Gynecologists. (2009a). *Induction of Labor* (Practice Bulletin No. 107). Washington, DC: Author. doi:10.1097/AOG.0b013e3181b48ef5; American College of Obstetricians and Gynecologists. (2010c). *Vaginal Birth after Previous Cesarean Delivery* (Practice Bulletin No. 115). Washington, DC: Author. doi:10.1097/AOG.0b013e3181eeb251; Simpson, K. R. (2013). *Cervical Ripening, Labor Induction and Labor Augmentation* [AWHONN Practice Monograph] (4th ed.). Washington, DC: Association of Women's Health, Obstetric and Neonatal Nurses.

psychosocial indications, the pregnant woman should be at least 39 completed weeks of gestation to avoid the risk of iatrogenic prematurity (ACOG, 2009a). Use of checklists for labor induction and planned cesarean birth (ACOG, 2011b, 2011c) can be helpful in ensuring that the appropriate gestational age has been confirmed.

Risk–Benefit Analysis and Informed Consent

Labor induction is not an isolated intervention. The decision for labor induction often results in a cascade of other interventions and activities that have the potential to negatively affect the childbirth process. Labor induction in the United States leads to an IV line, bed rest, and continuous EFM, and often amniotomy, significant discomfort, epidural analgesia/anesthesia, a prolonged stay on the labor unit, and cesarean birth. When considering elective labor induction for a nulliparous woman with an unripe cervix, ACOG (2009a) recommends counseling the patients that they are at twice the risk for cesarean birth when compared to women who are not induced. Nulliparous women should be further informed that electively induced labor may last significantly longer than spontaneous labor, including up to 12 to 18 hours of latent labor (ACOG, 2009a). Based on available data, elective induction for nulliparous women is associated with increased risks of cesarean birth, postpartum hemorrhage, neonatal resuscitation, and a longer hospital length of stay, without improvement in neonatal outcomes (Clark, Miller, et al., 2009; Frederiks, Lee, & Dekker, 2012; Glantz, 2010; Vardo, Thornburg, & Glantz, 2011). Women want to know potential complications of labor induction. In the *Listening to Mothers Survey II,* nearly all first-time mothers surveyed wanted to know every complication (74.7%) or most complications (24%) of labor induction (Declercq, Sakala, Corry, & Applebaum, 2006).

Avoiding associated complications can be accomplished by allowing labor to begin on its own when the mother and baby are healthy (Amis, 2007; AWHONN, 2012). Women can be encouraged by nurses to await spontaneous labor by providing education regarding potential risks of elective induction during prepared childbirth classes and prenatal encounters during the third trimester (AWHONN, 2012; Simpson, Newman, & Chirino, 2010a, 2010b). Although there is some concern that requests by pregnant women to have their labor induced electively are a major reason for the steady increase in elective induction in the United States, in a study of over 3,300 nulliparous women, 70% were offered the option of elective induction by their obstetrician; this discussion occurred in most cases before the estimated date of birth (Simpson et al., 2010a). It is possible that women perceive the offer

of elective induction by their obstetrician as a recommendation. In this study, women who were offered the option of elective induction by their obstetrician were significantly more likely to have an elective induction. However, the education did have a positive effect as 63% of women who chose not to have an elective induction indicated that information about the risks of the procedures presented in prepared childbirth classes was a factor in their choice (Simpson et al., 2010a).

Because of known risks, a risk–benefit analysis is recommended before the procedure as well as a discussion by the provider with the patient of the agents, methods, advantages, disadvantages, and alternative approaches, including the risk of cesarean birth and a repeat induction (ACOG, 2009a; Glantz, 2010; The Joint Commission [TJC], 2012a; Simpson, 2013). Following this discussion, when the woman has enough information to participate in the decision-making process, the provider should obtain informed consent. The medical record should contain documentation that this discussion occurred and that the woman consented to proceed (ACOG, 2009a; TJC, 2012a). It is not the nurse's responsibility to provide the required information to the woman undergoing induction or to obtain informed consent; however, advocating for the woman and fetus includes ensuring that the woman has been fully informed by her primary healthcare provider before beginning the procedure.

The Nurse's Role

The primary role of the labor nurse during cervical ripening, labor induction, or labor augmentation is ongoing maternal and fetal assessment to support safe care. The goal is labor progression without excessive uterine activity or fetal compromise. The nurse providing care for the woman during cervical ripening and induction of labor must be aware of appropriate indications for the use of each mechanical method and pharmacologic agent as well as their actions, expected results, and potential risks. Before any cervical ripening or labor induction agent is used, maternal status and fetal well-being should be established, and cervical status should be assessed and documented in the medical record. Nurses can evaluate cervical status by vaginal examination prior to the induction process. Cervical ripening, labor induction, and labor augmentation are processes that require care by several members of the perinatal team working together to promote patient well-being and successful vaginal birth. An estimation of fetal weight/size and presentation along with an assessment of the maternal pelvis should be determined and documented by the provider (AAP & ACOG, 2007, 2012; ACOG, 2009a). Indications for preinduction cervical ripening and induction of labor also should be documented by the provider. Ongoing maternal–fetal assessments during cervical ripening, labor induction, and labor augmentation are presented in Display 14–3. The absence of fetal well-being necessitates direct bedside evaluation by a physician or CNM, interdisciplinary discussion, and written documentation of further clinical management plans.

Clinical Protocol and Unit Policy Development

Healthcare providers at each institution should develop a policy or protocol for cervical ripening, labor induction, and labor augmentation (AAP & ACOG, 2012; ACOG, 2009a; Simpson, 2013). Suggestions for key concepts to be included are presented in Display 14–10. A sample protocol for labor induction and augmentation is presented in Appendix 14–B. Ideally, physicians, CNMs, and nurses together develop these policies or protocols on the basis of current evidence and published

guidelines from professional organizations such as ACOG, AAP, and AWHONN. The best approach is to develop a single unit policy or protocol rather than allowing each provider to have his or her own protocol with individual variations (Simpson & Knox, 2009b). For example, the group should come to consensus on the IV concentrations, rate of dosage increases, and interval between increases in dosage rate on the basis of available evidence and published guidelines. There should be established processes in place for addressing and preventing elective induction before 39 weeks' gestation. Once the interdisciplinary team agrees on a policy or protocol, it should be expected that all providers will practice within the established unit parameters. Standardization of an oxytocin policy for induction and augmentation of labor among hospitals within a healthcare system can be beneficial in promoting patient safety by selecting appropriate candidates and avoiding

---

DISPLAY 14–10

Suggestions for Key Concepts to Include in Clinical Protocols and Unit Policies for Cervical Ripening, Labor Induction, and Labor Augmentation

Prioritization and Documentation
- Criteria for designating patient priority for cervical ripening and induction based on the nature and intensity of the indication that can be used as a framework for decision making during periods of limited staffing, rooms, or other resources
- Documentation of indication by primary care provider
- Documentation of risk–benefit analysis discussion with the pregnant woman by the primary healthcare provider and informed decision-making process, as recommended by ACOG (2009a), SOGC (2001), and TJC (2012a)
- Specific recommendations for the care of women with a prior history of cesarean birth or uterine scar

Staffing Considerations
- Experience of registered nurse
- Availability of registered nurses to meet recommended nurse-to-patient ratios (one nurse to two women undergoing cervical ripening with pharmacologic agents; one nurse to one woman undergoing labor induction or augmentation with oxytocin)
- Acuity of patient (e.g., medical or obstetric complications)
- Ongoing evaluation of labor status
- Availability and skill level of support personnel
- Contingency plans such as on-call list

Patient Assessment
- Establishment of maternal and fetal well-being
- Establishment of at least 39 completed weeks of gestation if procedure is being performed without a medical indication

- Documentation of cervical status, including Bishop score
- Documentation of pelvic examination and estimated fetal weight
- Method of fetal assessment
- Frequency of maternal–fetal assessments
- Assessment of specific patient needs and requests

Methods and Dosages
- Cervical ripening agents to be used
- Initial oxytocin or misoprostol dosage
- Intervals and amounts for oxytocin dosage increases
- Intervals and amounts for misoprostol dosages
- Orders for oxytocin and documentation in milliunits per minute (mU/min)
- Titration of oxytocin dosage based on progress of labor and maternal–fetal response
- Dosage of misoprostol based on progress of labor and maternal–fetal status
- Maintenance or decrease in oxytocin dosage if labor is progressing

Complications
- Definition of tachysystole
- Interventions for tachysystole
- Interventions for indeterminate or abnormal fetal status
- Criteria for provider notification
- Criteria for bedside evaluation by the provider

Unit Policy
- Algorithm/chain of consultation for addressing clinical disagreements
- Methods for documenting all of the key concepts and interventions outlined in the policy/protocol
- An expectation that the policy will be followed by all members of the healthcare team

Adapted from Simpson, K. R. (2013). *Cervical Ripening, Labor Induction and Labor Augmentation* [AWHONN Practice Monograph] (4th ed.). Washington, DC: Association of Women's Health, Obstetric and Neonatal Nurses.

tachysystole (Krening, Rehling-Anthony, & Garko, 2012; O'Rourke et al., 2011; Simpson, Knox, Martin, George, & Watson, 2011). A systematic review of the potential benefits of establishing an elective induction policy found that their implementation resulted in lower rates of labor induction, cesarean birth, operative/instrumental vaginal births, and maternal/neonatal morbidity in part because women spontaneously gave birth before the scheduled elective induction date after policies were implemented, thereby resulting in lower rates of elective labor induction (Akinsipe, Villalobos, & Ridley, 2012). Each unit should develop processes to periodically evaluate the incidence of oxytocin-induced tachysystole and how the team responds to this clinical situation. A tool to evaluate timely identification and treatment of oxytocin-induced tachysystole during labor is presented in Display 1–7 in Chapter 1 *Perinatal Patient Safety and Professional Liability Issues*.

Staffing Considerations

The number of women who are scheduled for cervical ripening and induction of labor influence nursing staff requirements for labor and birth units. Because inductions of labor are likely to occur during the day, more nurses may be needed during this time than during the late evening or early morning. A record maintained on the unit of women who are scheduled for labor induction is essential to plan staffing and personnel needs based on expected volume. Many units place a limit on the number of scheduled labor inductions that can be performed on any given day to ensure that adequate staff and rooms are available to provide the appropriate level of care. Patient safety is at risk when scheduled procedures such as elective labor induction and cesarean birth are clustered on one or two weekdays for provider convenience without concurrent changes in nurse staffing. This is especially a potential problem in small volume units where there may not be enough nurses to safely handle these artificial peaks in census on busy days and not enough volume on other days to earn productive nursing hours required by the budget while maintaining at least two nurses with obstetric skills in-house at all times.

The development of criteria for designating patient priority for inductions of labor based on the nature and intensity of the indication can provide a useful decision-making framework when conflicts arise. Ideally, these criteria are developed jointly by physician, CNM, and nurse members of a unit practice committee. Requiring documentation of indications and having these data available on the unit may be helpful in designating patient priority when resources are limited. Elective inductions of labor may need to be postponed or rescheduled at times, especially if there are not enough resources available. The establishment of a perinatal nurse on-call system may facilitate securing staffing resources as needed in a timely manner.

The appropriate number of qualified professional registered nurses should be in attendance during cervical ripening and induction or augmentation of labor (AWHONN, 2010b). Current recommendations for the nurse-to-woman ratio for women undergoing cervical ripening with pharmacologic agents is 1:2 (AWHONN, 2010b). Current recommendations for the nurse-to-woman ratio during induction or augmentation of labor with oxytocin is 1:1 (AWHONN, 2010b; SOGC, 2001). If a nurse cannot clinically evaluate the effects of medication at least every 15 minutes or a physician who has privileges to perform a cesarean birth is not readily available, the oxytocin infusion should be discontinued or the initial or subsequent doses of misoprostol should be delayed until this level of maternal–fetal care can be provided (AAP & ACOG, 2012; Simpson, 2013).

Cervical Status

Cervical assessment includes documentation of the Bishop score (Bishop, 1964) and the presence or absence of uterine activity. Cervical status is the most important factor predicting the success of an induction of labor. It is assessed most commonly by using the Bishop pelvic scoring system (Bishop, 1964) (Table 14–4). Perinatal nurses are qualified to assess and document cervical status based on the Bishop scoring system. If the total score is more than 8, the probability of vaginal birth following an induction of labor is similar to that of

Table 14–4. BISHOP SCORE FOR ASSESSING READINESS FOR INDUCTION

Factor	Assigned Value			
	0	1	2	3
Cervical dilation	0	1–2 cm	3–4 cm	5 cm or more
Cervical effacement	0%–30%	40%–50%	60%–70%	80% or more
Fetal station	–3	–2	–1,0	+1,+2
Cervical consistency	Firm	Moderate	Soft	
Cervical position	Posterior	Midposition	Anterior	

From Bishop, E. H. (1964). Pelvic scoring for elective induction. *Obstetrics and Gynecology, 24,* 266.

spontaneous labor (ACOG, 2009a). Despite efforts by many researchers to modify the Bishop score, it remains the most reliable and cost-effective method of predicting the likelihood of successful induction. The risk of cesarean birth after labor induction is inversely related to the Bishop score; a higher rate of cesarean birth is consistently observed in women with a lower Bishop score when compared to women with a more favorable cervix (Caughey et al., 2009). The factor with the strongest association with successful induction seems to be cervical dilation; however, all components collectively can be quite useful in selecting appropriate candidates for labor induction (Baacke & Edwards, 2006). Other factors that have been shown to influence successful labor inductions are maternal age, parity, weight, and height. Younger women, women who are normal weight, women who are tall, and women who are multiparous are more likely to have success with labor induction (Caughey et al., 2009; Crane, 2006; Wing & Farinelli, 2012). Display 14–11 provides information about mechanical methods of cervical ripening and labor induction. Table 14–5 provides information about pharmacologic methods of cervical ripening and induction of labor and augmentation of labor.

Cervical Ripening

Cervical ripening is a complex process that results in physical softening and distensibility of the cervix, eventually leading to beginning cervical effacement

---

DISPLAY 14–11

Mechanical Methods of Cervical Ripening and Labor Induction

Membrane Stripping

- Digital separation of the chorioamniotic membrane from the wall of the cervix and lower uterine segment by inserting the examiner's finger beyond the internal cervical os and then rotating the finger 360° along the lower uterine segment
- Typically performed during an office visit for a pregnant woman ≥39 weeks of gestation with a partially dilated cervix who wants to hasten the onset of spontaneous labor
- Routine membrane stripping is not recommended given no evidence of improved maternal and neonatal outcome.
- The woman should call her physician/certified nurse midwife (CNM) or come to the hospital if the membranes rupture, bleeding occurs, fetal activity decreases, fever develops, regular contractions begin, or discomfort persists between uterine contractions.

Amniotomy

- Artificial rupture of membranes involves the perforation of the chorioamniotic membranes with a plastic hook performed by a qualified physician or CNM.
- Effective method of labor induction for multiparous women with favorable cervices
- Essential to confirm that the fetal vertex, not the umbilical cord or other fetal part, is presenting and well applied to the cervix
- Risks include the possibility of umbilical cord prolapse, cesarean birth, variable decelerations, intraamniotic infection, fetal injury, bleeding from an undiagnosed vasa previa, and commitment to labor with an uncertain outcome.
- Early amniotomy is contraindicated when maternal infection, such as HIV, an active perineal herpes simplex viral infection, and possibly viral hepatitis, is present.
- Medical record documentation should include the indication for amniotomy; amount, color, and odor of amniotic fluid; fetal heart rate (FHR) characteristics before amniotomy; fetal response following the procedure; cervical status; and fetal station.

Transcervical Balloon Catheters

- A deflated Foley catheter, 14–26 French with a 30-mL balloon, is inserted into the extra-amniotic space and then inflated above internal os with 30–80 mL of sterile water.
- The inflated balloon is then retracted to rest against the internal os.
- Appears to be effective for preinduction cervical ripening by causing direct pressure and overstretching of the lower uterine segment and cervix as well as local prostaglandin release
- Balloon catheter usually falls out when cervical dilation occurs
- A double-balloon device has also been utilized (Atad Ripening Device).
- Extra-amniotic saline infusion (EASI): continuous infusion of isotonic fluid into the extra-amniotic space at rates of 20–40 mL/hr. EASI has not been found to improve induction outcomes when compared to balloon catheter alone.

Hygroscopic/Osmotic Dilators

- Natural: Laminaria tents (made from cold water seaweed)
- Synthetic products: *Dilapan-S, Lamicel*
- Absorb fluid from cervical tissue
- Allow for controlled dilation by mechanical pressure and prostaglandin release
- Used primarily during pregnancy termination rather than for cervical ripening in term pregnancies
- Synthetic dilators are more expensive than laminaria; however, they work more quickly.
- Insertion of a large number of small diameter laminaria (2 or 3 mm) preferable to using a few larger ones (6 mm)
- Progressively placed until the cervix is "full"
- The "tails" are allowed to fall into the vagina for ease of identification and removal.
- Laminaria are kept in place with a couple 4 × 4 gauze sponges tucked into the fornix.
- The number of laminaria inserted are documented in medical record.

Advantages of mechanical methods of cervical ripening include low risk of tachysystole, few maternal systemic side effects, low cost, and convenient storage.

Disadvantages of mechanical methods include some maternal discomfort, small increase risk of maternal and neonatal infection, and potential disruption of a low-lying placenta.

Table 14–5. PHARMACOLOGIC AGENTS USED FOR CERVICAL RIPENING/LABOR INDUCTION AND AUGMENTATION

Factor	Pitocin (Oxytocin)	Cervidil (Dinoprostone)	Cytotec (Misoprostol)
Storage and Preparation	Room temperature storage. Available in 20-unit ampules. Several variations in the dilution rate exist. Some protocols suggest adding 10 units of oxytocin to 1,000 mL of an isotonic electrolyte IV solution, resulting in an infusion dosage rate of 1 mU/min = 6 mL/hr. Other commonly reported dilutions are 20 units of oxytocin to 1,000 mL IV fluid (1 mU/min = 3 mL/hr) and 30 units of oxytocin to 500 mL of IV fluid or 60 units of oxytocin to 1,000 mL IV fluid (1 mU/min = 1 mL/hr). One advantage to using 30 units in 500 mL IV fluid or 60 units in 1,000 mL IV fluid is that they result in a 1:1 solution (1 mU/min = 1 mL/hr); therefore, no calculations are needed. The key issue is consistency in practice within each institution.	Keep frozen (−20°C) until immediately before use. No warming required.	Available in 100 micrograms (mcg) & 200 mcg tablets. 100-mcg tablet is not scored; dose should be prepared (cut in four equal pieces) by hospital pharmacy.
Initial Administration	Administered IV in an isotonic electrolyte solution, piggybacked into the main IV line at port most proximal to venous site. Start at 1–2 mU/min.	10 mg dinoprostone in a controlled-release vaginal insert with removable cord is easy to administer and does not require speculum exam.	25 mcg (¼ tablet) placed in the posterior vaginal fornix should be considered for the initial dose. Adverse effects can be minimized by using the lowest dose (25 mcg) no more than every 3–6 hr. Oral administration at equivalent doses to vaginal route is not as efficacious; generally the dose should not exceed 50 mcg.
Patient Considerations	Need not remain in bed during infusion. Intermittent auscultation of the FHR at prescribed intervals or EFM telemetry can be used during ambulation or sitting on a chair or birthing ball. Careful close monitoring for women with history of prior cesarean birth or uterine scar; use lowest dose possible to achieve labor progress.	Remain supine for 2 hr following insertion. Continuous monitoring of FHR and uterine activity is indicated while insert is in place. Ambulation is an option if continuous EFM telemetry is available. Not recommended for use in women with history of prior cesarean birth or uterine scar.	Contraindicated in women with history of prior cesarean birth or uterine scar. Continuous monitoring of FHR and uterine activity is indicated.
Effects	Wide variations in time from initial dose to uterine activity. The biologic half-life is approximately 10–12 min. Three to four half-lives are need to reach physiologic steady state (30–60 min) at which time full effect of dosage on the uterine response can be assessed.	Uterine contractions usually occur within 5–7 hr.	Wide variations exist in time of onset of uterine contractions. Peak action is approximately 1–2 hr when administered intravaginally, but can be up to 4–6 hr for some women.

(continued)

Table 14–5. PHARMACOLOGIC AGENTS USED FOR CERVICAL RIPENING/LABOR INDUCTION AND AUGMENTATION (Continued)

Factor	Pitocin (Oxytocin)	Cervidil (Dinoprostone)	Cytotec (Misoprostol)
Adjusting Dosage	Advance by 1–2 mU/min at intervals no less than every 30–60 min until adequate labor progress is achieved. Titrate dose to maternal–fetal response to labor. Use lowest dose possible to achieve adequate progress of labor (progressive cervical effacement and cervical dilation of approximately 0.5–1.0 cm/hr once active labor has been achieved). Reevaluate clinical situation if oxytocin dosage rate reaches 20 mU/min. Contractions should not be more frequent than every 2 min. Avoid tachysystole. When uterine tachysystole occurs with a normal (category I) FHR tracing, decrease oxytocin. When tachysystole occurs with either an indeterminate or abnormal (category II or III) FHR tracing, decrease or stop oxytocin and initiate intrauterine resuscitative measures.	Remove after 12 hr or at onset of active labor. Remove if uterine tachysystole and/or abnormal (category III) FHR occurs. Removal may be indicated for some types of indeterminate (category II) FHR.	Redosing is permissible if (1) cervical condition remains unfavorable, (2) uterine activity is minimal, (3) FHR is normal (category I), and (4) it has been at least 3 hr since last dose. Consider observation for up to 2 hr after spontaneous rupture of membranes before redosing. Redosing is *withheld* if there are two or more contractions in 10 min, adequate cervical ripening is achieved (Bishop score ≥8, or cervix is 80% effaced and 3 cm dilated), patient enters active labor, or FHR is indeterminate or abnormal (category II or III).
Monitoring	Administer in labor and birth suite, where uterine activity and FHR can be recorded continuously via EFM and evaluated at a minimum every 15 min during the first stage of labor and every 5 min during the second stage of labor. If using intermittent auscultation, determine and record the FHR and palpate uterine contractions at least every 15–30 min during the first stage of labor and every 5–15 min during the second stage of labor based on risk status.	Administer at or near the labor and birth suite, where uterine activity and FHR can be monitored continuously while in place and for at least 15 min after removal. Ambulation is an option if continuous EFM telemetry is available.	Administer at or near labor and birth suite, where uterine activity and FHR can be monitored continuously. Terbutaline, 0.25 mg subcutaneously, also can be used in an attempt to correct indeterminate or abnormal FHR pattern or uterine tachysystole.
Use with Oxytocin, if Needed	N/A	Oxytocin should be delayed for at least 30–60 min after removal of insert. Previous exposure to PGE_2 potentiates contractile response to oxytocin, so careful maternal–fetal monitoring of FHR and uterine activity is warranted.	Oxytocin should be delayed until at least 4 hr after last dose.
Complications	Risk of uterine tachysystole is dose related. Approximately 50% of cases of tachysystole will result in an indeterminate or abnormal (category II or III) FHR.	Rate of uterine tachysystole is about 5%; usually occurs within 1 hr of administration but may occur up to 9.5 hr after administration.	Uterine tachysystole is more common with misoprostol as compared to Prepidil, Cervidil, and oxytocin. Rates of uterine tachysystole are lower with lower dosages (25 mcg) and when dosed less frequently (i.e., less problems when dosed every 6 hr instead of every 3 hr).

EFM, electronic fetal monitoring; FHR, fetal heart rate; IV, intravenous.
Adapted from Simpson, K. R. (2013). *Cervical Ripening and Labor Induction and Augmentation* (4th ed.). (AWHONN Practice Monograph). Washington, DC: Association of Women's Health, Obstetric, and Neonatal Nurses. Used with permission.

and dilation (Wing & Farinelli, 2012). A number of mechanical and pharmacologic methods have been used to induce cervical ripening. The ideal ripening agent or procedure should be simple to use, noninvasive, and effective within a reasonable time period; it should not stimulate or induce labor during the ripening process nor increase maternal, fetal, or neonatal morbidity. Unfortunately, the ideal agent or procedure for cervical ripening has not yet been identified. Mechanical methods are less likely to result in tachysystole and have similar rates of success when compared to pharmacologic agents for cervical ripening (Cromi et al., 2012; Fox et al., 2011; Jozwiak et al., 2012). Based on the most recent Cochrane Review, when compared with oxytocin, mechanical methods for labor induction have less risk of cesarean birth (Jozwiak et al., 2012).

Pharmacologic Methods of Cervical Ripening

Various hormonal preparations are available to induce cervical ripening. These agents include prostaglandin E_1 (PGE_1): misoprostol (Cytotec), and PGE_2 preparations: dinoprostone (Prepidil gel or Cervidil insert). Prepidil, Cervidil, and misoprostol are approved by the U.S. Food and Drug Administration (FDA) for cervical ripening. Nurses caring for women receiving any of these agents should be aware that they may lead to the onset of labor, particularly if the cervix is favorable. When the cervix is unfavorable, cervical softening and thinning are more likely to occur.

Prostaglandin E_2

Dinoprostone (PGE_2) is one of the most frequently prescribed medications for cervical ripening. The mechanism of action is similar to the natural ripening process, and women often go into spontaneous labor following administration. The prostaglandin preparations used successfully for cervical ripening today produce the desired cervical changes, but all tend to increase myometrial contractility. For this reason, prostaglandins for cervical ripening must be viewed as the first step in labor induction. Dinoprostone induces cervical ripening by directly softening the cervix, relaxing the cervical smooth muscle, and producing uterine contractions. An added benefit is the facilitation of postcervical ripening induction by preparing the uterus to produce coordinated contractions with lower doses of oxytocin (Keirse, 2006). Dinoprostone preparations appear to be as efficacious as other methods of cervical ripening (Keirse, 2006). Prepidil is less commonly used among options for cervical ripening. Information about Prepidil can be found at http://www.pfizer.com/files/products/uspi_prepidil.pdf.

Cervidil

The Cervidil vaginal insert is a thin, flat, rectangular-shaped, cross-linked polymer hydrogel that releases dinoprostone from a 10-mg reservoir at a controlled rate of approximately 0.3 mg/hr in vivo (Forest Pharmaceuticals, 2010). The reservoir chip is encased within a pouch of knitted Dacron® polyester with a removal cord. The entire system comes preassembled and prepackaged in sterile foil packets.

Cervidil may be inserted by the perinatal nurse when the nurse has demonstrated competence in insertion and the activity is within the scope of practice as defined by state and provincial regulations. Institutional guidelines should be established for the nurse's role related to the use of Cervidil. Unlike the transcervical preparations, Cervidil does not require visualization of the cervix for insertion. The insert is placed into the posterior fornix of the vagina, with its long axis transverse to the long axis of the vagina. The ribbon end of the retrieval system may be allowed to extrude distally from the vagina or tucked into the vagina. Once placed, Cervidil absorbs moisture, swells, and releases dinoprostone at a controlled rate. The system makes Cervidil relatively simple to insert and requires only a single digital examination.

Cervidil is removed after 12 hours, or when active labor begins (Forest Pharmaceuticals, 2010). Regular contractions (three in 10 minutes lasting 60 seconds or more with moderate patient discomfort) will occur in approximately 25% of women after Cervidil placement (Rayburn, Tassone, & Pearman, 2000). One major advantage of Cervidil is that the system can be easily and quickly removed in the event of uterine tachysystole or other complications. Tachysystole usually occurs within 1 hour after insertion but can occur up to 9.5 hours after the insert has been placed (ACOG, 2009a). If uterine tachysystole occurs, complete reversal of the prostaglandin-induced uterine pattern usually occurs within 15 minutes of removal. If necessary, the woman may be given tocolytic therapy (0.25 mg of terbutaline subcutaneously). Previous exposure to PGE_2 potentiates the contractile response to oxytocin (Forest Pharmaceuticals, 2010; Maul, Macray, & Garfield, 2006), so careful maternal–fetal monitoring is warranted when oxytocin is administered after Cervidil has been used for cervical ripening. Oxytocin administration should be delayed until at least 30 to 60 minutes after removal of the Cervidil insert (ACOG, 2009a). Continuous monitoring of the FHR and uterine activity is indicated while Cervidil is in place (Forest Pharmaceuticals, 2010). Ambulation while Cervidil is in place is an option if continuous EFM via telemetry is available. There have been no studies using methods other than continuous EFM for maternal–fetal assessment. There is risk of initiation of regular contractions progressing to active labor and an approximate 5% rate of tachysystole with Cervidil (ACOG, 2009a; Forest Pharmaceuticals, 2010). Cervidil is not appropriate for outpatient cervical ripening as its use in the outpatient setting has not been studied (ACOG, 2009a).

There is a risk of uterine rupture when prostaglandins are used for women attempting vaginal birth after cesarean birth (VBAC), thus Cervidil is not recommended for these patients (Forest Pharmaceuticals, 2010).

Prostaglandin E_1

Misoprostol (PGE_1) is a synthetic prostaglandin E_1 analogue that has been used for cervical ripening and induction of labor. Misoprostol was originally approved by the FDA for the prevention of peptic ulcers, not for cervical ripening or induction of labor. In April 2002, the FDA removed the contraindication for the use of misoprostol for women during pregnancy because it was widely used for cervical ripening and labor induction and was part of an FDA-approved regime for use with mifepristone to induce abortion in pregnancies of 49 days or less. The FDA (2002) included warnings about potential adverse effects of misoprostol when used for cervical ripening, labor induction, and treatment of serious postpartum hemorrhage in the presence of uterine atony. According to the FDA (2002), a major adverse effect of the obstetric use of misoprostol is uterine tachysystole, which may progress to uterine tetany with marked impairment of uteroplacental blood flow, uterine rupture, or amniotic fluid embolism. The FDA (2002) further noted that pelvic pain, retained placenta, severe genital bleeding, shock, fetal bradycardia, and fetal and maternal death have been reported. As more data are published from ongoing clinical research studies, a clearer understanding of safety and appropriate dosages will emerge.

When used for cervical ripening or induction of labor, 25 micrograms (mcg) placed in the posterior vaginal fornix should be considered for the initial dose (ACOG, 2009a). Higher dosages have been associated with an increased rate of tachysystole (ACOG, 2009a; Wing & Farinelli, 2012). However, it is important to consider that tachysystole and indeterminate or abnormal FHR changes are associated with both the 25- and 50-mcg doses (Crane, Young, Butt, Bennett, & Hutchens, 2001; Keirse, 2006). Tachysystole with and without indeterminate or abnormal FHR changes is significantly higher with the use of misoprostol when compared with Cervidil, Prepidil, and oxytocin (Hofmeyr, Gülmezoglu, & Pileggi, 2010; Wing & Farinelli, 2012). A 4- to 6-hour interval between doses has been associated with less uterine tachysystole than the 3-hour interval (ACOG, 2009a; Wing & Farinelli, 2012).

Uterine rupture is a complication of the use of misoprostol for cervical ripening and labor induction, especially in those who have a uterine scar (Lydon-Rochelle, Holt, Easterling, & Martin, 2001b; Weeks et al., 2007; Wing & Farinelli, 2012). However, it is important to consider that uterine rupture after misoprostol (or oxytocin) can occur in the unscarred uterus, although the risk is lower than for women with a previous uterine scar (Akhan, Iyibozkurt, & Turfanda, 2001; Bennett, 1997; Catanzarite, Cousins, Dowling, & Daneshmand, 2006; Khabbaz et al., 2001). Misoprostol is contraindicated in women with a history of or prior uterine surgery or cesarean birth because of the risk of uterine rupture (ACOG, 2009a, 2010c; Lydon-Rochelle et al., 2001b; Weeks et al., 2007; Wing & Farinelli, 2012).

Because the 100-mcg tablet is unscored, there is no assurance that the PGE_1 is uniformly dispersed throughout the tablet. It is possible that one quarter of a tablet may contain more or less than 25 mcg of PGE_1. The hospital pharmacist should prepare the tablet in four equal parts before administration of a quarter of a tablet intravaginally (Simpson, 2013). Individual providers attempting to break the small tablet into four equal parts increases the risk of inaccurate dose administration.

Advocates of misoprostol for cervical ripening and induction of labor cite the low cost, ease of insertion, and quick action as its main advantages (Wing & Farinelli, 2012). The most commonly reported adverse effects are tachysystole, meconium passage, neonatal umbilical artery pH below 7.16, low 5-minute Apgar scores, admission to the NICU, indeterminate or abnormal FHR patterns, and a higher rate of cesarean birth related to indeterminate or abnormal FHR patterns from tachysystole (Bennett, Butt, Crane, Hutchens, & Young, 1998; Buser, Mora, & Arias, 1997; Farah et al., 1997; Hofmeyr et al., 2010; Sanchez-Ramos & Kaunitz, 2000; Wing & Farinelli, 2012). These adverse effects can be minimized by using the lowest dose (25 mcg) no more than every 3 to 6 hours (ACOG, 2009a). If uterine tachysystole and an indeterminate or abnormal FHR pattern occur with misoprostol and there is no response to routine corrective measures (e.g., maternal repositioning, supplemental oxygen, IV fluid bolus), consider cesarean birth (ACOG, 2009a). Terbutaline, 0.25 mg subcutaneously, also can be used in an attempt to correct the indeterminate or abnormal FHR pattern or the uterine tachysystole (ACOG, 2009a).

If induction or augmentation of labor is required after cervical ripening with misoprostol, some providers opt to use oxytocin. The plasma concentration of misoprostol after vaginal administration of misoprostol rises gradually, reaching peak levels between 1 and 2 hours and declining slowly to an average of 61% of peak level at 4 hours (Arias, 2000; Goldberg, Greenberg, & Darney, 2001; Song, 2000; Zeiman, Fong, Benowitz, Bankster, & Darney, 1997). Some women will have increased plasma concentrations 4 to 6 hours after vaginal administration (Zeiman et al., 1997). Based on these pharmacologic data, the administration of oxytocin should be delayed for at least 4 hours after the last dose of misoprostol (ACOG, 2009a).

Some providers opt to use oral misoprostol, which at equivalent doses to the vaginal route of administration is not as efficacious but is associated with fewer indeterminate or abnormal FHR patterns and episodes of tachysystole when compared to vaginal administration (ACOG, 2009a). Oral administration may offer more patient comfort, satisfaction, and convenience of administration (Wing & Farinelli, 2012). There is a clear, positive dose-response relationship seen between the dosage of oral misoprostol and the rate of tachysystole; 25-mcg and 50-mcg dosages are associated with a lower tachysystole rate, while the tachysystole rate is higher at 200 mcg (Weeks et al., 2007; Wing & Farinelli, 2012). Based on the most recent Cochrane Review, generally, the dose should not exceed 50 mcg orally when administered to a woman with a viable fetus in the third trimester (Alfirevic & Weeks, 2006).

Misoprostol can be administered by perinatal nurses; however, in many institutions, this practice is deferred to physicians or CNMs. If vaginal misoprostol administration is delegated to perinatal nurses, they must have demonstrated competence in insertion and the activity must be within the scope of practice as defined by state and provincial regulations.

Pharmacologic Methods of Induction of Labor

Oxytocin

Oxytocin is the most commonly used induction agent in the United States (ACOG, 2009a). Although oxytocin is an effective means of labor induction in women with a favorable cervix, it is not efficacious as a cervical ripening agent based on multiple randomized trials comparing oxytocin with other methods of cervical ripening (Wing & Farinelli, 2012). Oxytocin following preinduction cervical ripening prostaglandin agents appears to be more efficacious than oxytocin alone as a method of induction (Alfirevic, Kelly, & Dowswell, 2009). An unfavorable cervix generally has been defined as a Bishop score of 6 or less in most randomized trials. If the total score is more than 8, the probability of vaginal delivery after labor induction is similar to that after spontaneous labor. (ACOG, 2009a; Vrouenraets et al., 2005). Therefore, cervical ripening for women with a Bishop score less than 6 is recommended to enhance the likelihood of success.

Oxytocin is a peptide consisting of nine amino acids. Endogenous oxytocin is synthesized by the hypothalamus, then transported to the posterior lobe of the pituitary gland, where it is released into maternal circulation. It is released in response to breast stimulation, sensory stimulation of the lower genital tract, and cervical stretching. Oxytocin released in response to vaginal and cervical stretching results in uterine contractions. Minimal change occurs in myometrial sensitivity to oxytocin from 34 weeks' gestation until term; however, when spontaneous labor is initiated, uterine sensitivity to oxytocin increases rapidly (Wing &

Farinelli, 2012). Therefore, based on this physiologic mechanism, oxytocin is more effective in augmenting labor than in inducing labor (Wing & Farinelli, 2012). Synthetic oxytocin is chemically and physiologically identical to endogenous oxytocin.

Oxytocin circulates in the blood as a free peptide and has a molecular weight of 1,007 d (Zeeman, Khan-Dawood, & Dawood, 1997). Volume of distribution is estimated to be 305 ± 46 mL/kg; thus, oxytocin is distributed into both the intravascular and extravascular compartments (Zeeman et al., 1997). Plasma clearance of oxytocin is through the maternal kidneys and liver by the enzyme oxytocinase, with only a small amount excreted unchanged in the urine. Maternal metabolic clearance rate of oxytocin at term is 19 to 21 mL/kg/min and is unaffected by pregnancy (Zeeman et al., 1997).

During the first stage of spontaneous labor, maternal circulating concentrations of endogenous oxytocin are approximately that which would be achieved with a continuous infusion of exogenous oxytocin at 2 to 4 mU/min (Dawood, Ylikorkala, Trivedi, & Fuchs, 1979). The fetus is thought to secrete oxytocin during labor at a level similar to an infusion of oxytocin at approximately 3 mU/min (Dawood, Wang, Gupta, & Fuchs, 1978). Thus, the combined effects of maternal–fetal contributions to maternal plasma oxytocin concentration is equivalent to a range of about 5 to 7 mU/min (Shyken & Petrie, 1995).

Although there are considerable variations in reports of the biologic half-life of oxytocin, it is now generally agreed that the half-life is between 10 and 12 minutes (Dawood, 1995a; Arias, 2000). Early data based on in vitro studies estimated a plasma half-life of 3 to 4 minutes, but Seitchik, Amico, Robinson, and Castillo (1984) used in vivo methods to study oxytocin pharmacokinetics and found half-life was probably closer to 10 to 15 minutes.

Oxytocin concentration and saturation follow first-order kinetics with a progressive, linear, stepwise increase with each increase in the infusion rate (Arias, 2000). Three to four half-lives of oxytocin are generally needed to reach a steady-state plasma concentration (Stringer, 1996). Uterine response to oxytocin usually occurs within 3 to 5 minutes of IV administration. There is an incremental phase of uterine activity when oxytocin is initiated during which contractions progressively increase in frequency and strength, followed by a stable phase, during which time any further increase in oxytocin will not lead to further normal changes in uterine contractions (Dawood, 1995b; Phaneuf, Rodríguez Liñares, TambyRaja, MacKenzie, & López Bernal, 2000). Instead, abnormal uterine activity such as frequent low-intensity contractions, coupling or tripling of contractions, or uterine tachysystole may be produced with further increases in oxytocin rates. There has long been a myth that these types of abnormal uterine activity patterns are best treated with oxytocin rate increases (i.e., "pit through the pattern"); however, an understanding of their genesis (excessive oxytocin and oxytocin receptor site desensitization) should guide clinicians to reduce the rate or discontinue oxytocin until uterine activity returns to normal. Often, a 30- to 60-minute rest period along with an IV fluid bolus of L/R solution will allow oxytocin receptors to be sensitive to artificial oxytocin and produce uterine contractions that will result in normal uterine activity and labor progress (Dawood, 1995b; Phaneuf et al., 2000; Zeeman et al., 1997).

Continued increases in oxytocin rates over a prolonged period can result in oxytocin receptor desensitization or down-regulation, making oxytocin less effective in producing normal uterine contractions and having the opposite than intended result. Several studies have shown a direct inverse relationship between the duration and dosage of oxytocin and the number of oxytocin receptor sites available for oxytocin uptake during labor (Phaneuf et al., 1998; Phaneuf et al., 2000; Robinson, Schumann, Zhang, & Young, 2003). Prolonged oxytocin infusion at higher than appropriate doses can result in oxytocin side effects such as dysfunctional uterine activity patterns and uterine tachysystole (Dawood, 1995b; Phaneuf et al., 2000). Once active labor is established, oxytocin rates should be discontinued to avoid receptor down-regulation, especially in cases of long labor induction. Prolonged high-dose oxytocin infusions are counterproductive to the augmentation of established labor (Robinson et al., 2003).

Tachysystole is the most concerning side effect of oxytocin. Normal uterine contractions produce intermittent diminution of blood flow to the intervillous space where oxygen exchange occurs. The decreased intervillous blood flow associated with tachysystole ultimately leads to decreased oxygen transfer to the fetus (Simpson & James, 2008). When fetal oxygenation is sufficiently impaired to produce fetal metabolic acidosis from anaerobic glycolysis, direct myocardial depression occurs and the FHR pattern becomes indeterminate or abnormal (ACOG & AAP, 2003). When the intermittent interruption in blood flow caused by excessive uterine activity exceeds a critical level, the fetus responds with evolving hypoxia, acidosis, and ultimately asphyxia if the situation is prolonged (ACOG & AAP, 2003). Therefore, every effort should be made to avoid tachysystole and treat it appropriately when identified (Simpson & Knox, 2009b). Waiting until the FHR is indeterminate or abnormal to treat tachysystole is not consistent with fetal safety (Simpson, 2013). When tachysystole occurs during induced or augmented labor and the FHR pattern is normal, ACOG (2010a) recommends decreasing oxytocin. If there are changes in the FHR pattern, further interventions such as discontinuation of oxytocin, maternal

repositioning, and an IV fluid bolus should be considered (ACOG, 2010a; Simpson, 2013). A simultaneous initiation of maternal repositioning, an IV fluid bolus, and discontinuation of oxytocin will usually resolve oxytocin-induced tachysystole within 6 to 10 minutes (Simpson & James, 2008). See Display 14–12 for a suggested protocol for the treatment of tachysystole.

While oxytocin is the most frequently used medication for labor induction and augmentation, it is also the drug most commonly associated with preventable adverse events during childbirth (Clark, Belfort, Dildy, & Meyers, 2008). The risks of oxytocin are generally dose related and in addition to tachysystole, include fetal compromise, neonatal acidemia, abruptio placentae,

---

DISPLAY 14 – 12

Suggested Clinical Protocol for Oxytocin-Induced Uterine Tachysystole

Oxytocin-Induced Tachysystole (Normal FHR)
- Assist the mother to a lateral position.
- Give intravenous (IV) fluid bolus of at least 500 mL lactated Ringer's (L/R) solution as indicated.
- If uterine activity has not returned to normal after 10–15 minutes, decrease oxytocin rate by at least half; if uterine activity has not returned to normal after 10–15 more minutes, discontinue oxytocin until uterine activity is normal.
- Resume oxytocin after the resolution of tachysystole: If oxytocin has been discontinued for less than 20–30 minutes, the fetal heart rate (FHR) is normal, and contraction frequency, intensity, and duration are normal, resume oxytocin at no more than half the rate that caused the tachysystole and gradually increase the rate as appropriate based on unit protocol and maternal–fetal status. If the oxytocin is discontinued for more than 30–40 minutes, resume oxytocin at the initial dose ordered.

**Oxytocin-Induced Tachysystole
(Indeterminate or Abnormal FHR)**
- Discontinue oxytocin.
- Assist the mother to a lateral position.
- Give IV fluid bolus of at least 500 mL of L/R solution as indicated.
- Consider oxygen at 10 L/min via a nonrebreather face mask (discontinue as soon as possible based on the FHR pattern).
- If no response, consider 0.25 mg terbutaline subcutaneous (SQ).
- Resume oxytocin after the resolution of tachysystole: If oxytocin has been discontinued for less than 20–30 minutes, the FHR is normal, and contraction frequency, intensity, and duration are normal, resume oxytocin at no more than half the rate that caused the tachysystole and gradually increase the rate as appropriate based on unit protocol and maternal-fetal status. If the oxytocin is discontinued for more than 30–40 minutes, resume oxytocin at the initial dose ordered.

and uterine rupture (ACOG, 2009a; Bakker, Kurver, Kuik, & VanGeijin, 2007). Other types of oxytocin errors involve mistaken administration of IV fluids with oxytocin for IV fluid resuscitation during indeterminate or abnormal FHR patterns and/or maternal hypotension and inappropriate elective administration of oxytocin to women who are less than 39 completed weeks of gestation (Simpson & Knox, 2009b). Oxytocin is also often implicated in professional liability claims and thus poses a dual concern for individual clinicians and the organizations in which they practice (Clark, Simpson, Knox, & Garite, 2009). Approximately half of all paid obstetric litigation claims involve allegations of oxytocin misuse (Clark, Belfort, Dildy et al., 2008). Oxytocin administration is a significant source of clinical conflict between nurses and physicians during labor (Simpson, James, & Knox, 2006; Simpson & Lyndon, 2009). Standardized policies for oxytocin are helpful in avoiding conflict as agreed upon dosing for oxytocin and definitions and interventions for oxytocin-induced tachysystole are available for guiding the perinatal team (O'Rourke et al., 2011; Krening et al., 2012; Simpson & Knox, 2009b).

In 2007, oxytocin was added to the Institute for Safe Medication Practices (ISMP, 2007) list of high-alert medications. High-alert medications are defined as those bearing a heightened risk of harm when they are used in error and that may require special safeguards to reduce the risk of error. While oxytocin administered using pharmacologic principles can be therapeutic during labor, inappropriate timing or excessive doses can have a potentially negative effect on the mother and baby (Clark, Simpson, et al., 2009).

DOSAGE AND RATE INCREASE INTERVALS

Based on physiologic and pharmacokinetic principles, Seitchik et al. (1984) recommended at least a 40-minute interval between oxytocin dosage increases because the full effect of oxytocin on the uterine response to increases in dosage cannot be evaluated until steady-state concentration has been achieved. Seitchik et al. (1984) used a sensitive oxytocin radioimmunoassay to show that approximately 40 minutes was required to reach steady-state plasma concentration. Their data suggested that increasing the infusion rate before steady-state concentrations were achieved resulted in laboring women receiving higher doses of oxytocin than necessary. The works of Seitchik and Castillo (1982, 1983) and Seitchik et al. (1984) were the basis of oxytocin protocols with intervals in oxytocin dosage increases between 30 and 60 minutes.

There is no consensus in the literature on the ideal oxytocin dosage regimen, although available data support a lower dosage rate of infusion (Crane & Young, 1998; SOGC, 2001). The most commonly used regime in the United States includes starting at 1 to 2 mU/min with incremental doses of 1 to 2 mU/min every 30 to 40 minutes. Those researchers whose opinions are based on the work of Seitchik et al. (1984) advocate a *physiologic* approach to oxytocin dosage and rate increase intervals. Others support a *pharmacologic* approach based in part on the results from early studies about more aggressive high-dose oxytocin protocols, sometimes referred to as active management of labor (O'Driscoll, Foley, & MacDonald, 1984; O'Driscoll, Jackson, & Gallagher, 1969). It is important to note that high-dose oxytocin is only one component of the active management protocol, which was originally used for augmentation (not induction) among nulliparous women (not multiparous women) in spontaneous active labor.

There have been numerous studies comparing low-dose and high-dose oxytocin dosage protocols as well as 10- to 15-minute versus 30- to 60-minute interval protocols for induction of labor, with varying results (Blakemore, Qin, Petrie, & Paine, 1990; Chua, Arulkumaran, Kurup, Tay, & Ratnam, 1991; Crane & Young, 1998; Goni, Sawhney, & Gopalan, 1995; Hourvitz et al., 1996; Lazor, Philipson, Ingardia, Kobetitsch, & Curry, 1993; Mercer, Pilgrim, & Sibai, 1991; Merrill & Zlatnik, 1999; Muller, Stubbs, & Laurent, 1992; Orhue, 1993a, 1993b, 1994; Satin, Leveno, Sherman, Brewster, & Cunningham, 1992; Satin, Leveno, Sherman, & McIntire, 1994; Wein, 1989). Most researchers noted that higher doses and shorter dose increase intervals led to more uterine tachysystole and indeterminate or abnormal FHR patterns and did not result in a clinically significant decrease in length of labor (Crane & Young, 1998).

A meta-analysis of low-dose versus high-dose oxytocin for labor induction by Crane and Young (1998) found that low-dose protocols resulted in fewer episodes of excessive uterine activity, fewer operative vaginal births, a higher rate of spontaneous vaginal birth, and a trend toward a lower rate of cesarean birth. A cervical dilation rate of 0.5 to 1 cm/hr in the active phase of labor indicates that labor is progressing sufficiently and that oxytocin administration is adequate, especially in nulliparous women (Harper, Caughey, et al., 2012; Rouse et al., 2001; Simon & Grobman, 2005; Vahratian et al., 2005; Zhang, Troendle et al., 2002; Zhang, Landy et al., 2010). Traditional definitions of prolonged latent phase do not apply to induced labor, in which a latent phase exceeding 18 hours is common (ACOG, 2009a; Vahratian et al., 2005). High-dose oxytocin and shorter intervals between rate increases tend to have fewer adverse effects on maternal–fetal status during labor augmentation than during labor induction (Crane & Young, 1998). This result may be due in part to the fact that in spontaneous active labor, the unripe cervix is not a significant factor, and oxytocin receptor sites are thought to be increased in number and sensitivity (Carbillon, Seince, & Uzan, 2001; Dawood, 1995a; Wing & Farinelli, 2012).

Other factors that may influence the dose response to oxytocin include maternal body surface area, parity, week of pregnancy duration, and cervical status (Dawood, 1995a). Although these factors may be significant, to date there are no practical predictive models for determining the required oxytocin dosage for successful labor induction. Until more is known about the pharmacokinetics of oxytocin, each pregnant woman receiving oxytocin will continue to represent an individual bioassay.

Generally, starting doses of 1 to 2 mU/min with increases in 1 to 2 mU/min increments every 30 to 60 minutes are most appropriate and commonly used (see Display 14–12 for a suggested clinical protocol and Appendix 14–B for a sample oxytocin policy). Shorter intervals between dosage increases are associated with a greater risk of tachysystole, somewhat shorter duration of labor, and no reduction in the cesarean birth rate (Crane & Young, 1998). Multiple clinical studies and current data based on physiologic and pharmacologic principles have shown that 90% of pregnant women at term will have labor successfully induced with 6 mU/min or less of oxytocin (Dawood, 1995a, 1995b; Seitchik et al., 1984). There appears to be no advantage to continuing oxytocin once active labor is established. Reducing or discontinuing oxytocin may result in an equal or shorter length of labor compared to labor for women for whom oxytocin is continued or incrementally increased after active labor is achieved (Daniel-Spiegel, Weiner, Ben-Shlomo, & Shalev, 2004).

Although higher doses of oxytocin and short intervals between dosage increments have generally not been found to be beneficial (Crane & Young, 1998), some providers intuitively believe that this approach is better. According to ACOG (2009a), protocols that involve high-dose oxytocin are acceptable; however, ACOG cautions that high-dose oxytocin is associated with more uterine tachysystole. Conversely, SOGC (2001) recommends using the minimum dose to achieve active labor, increasing the dosage no more frequently than every 30 minutes, and reevaluating the clinical situation if the oxytocin dosage rate reaches 20 mU/min.

ADMINISTRATION

Oxytocin is administered intravenously and piggybacked into the mainline solution at the port most proximal to the venous site (see Table 14–5 for a summary of oxytocin administration). There are many variations in the dilution rate. Some protocols suggest adding 10 units of oxytocin to 1,000 mL of an isotonic electrolyte IV solution, resulting in an infusion dosage rate of 1 mU/min = 6 mL/hr. However, other commonly reported dilutions are 20 units of oxytocin to 1,000 mL IV fluid (1 mU/min = 3 mL/hr) and 30 units of oxytocin to 500 mL IV fluid or 60 units of oxytocin to 1,000 mL IV fluid (1 mU/min = 1 mL/hr). One advantage to the dilution rates of 30 units of oxytocin to 500 mL IV fluid or 60 units of oxytocin to 1,000 mL IV fluid is that they result in a 1:1 solution (1 mU/min = 1 mL/hr); therefore, no calculations are needed for the dosage increases, an important consideration for medication safety. The key issues are knowledge of how many mU/min are administered and consistency in clinical practice within each institution. To enhance communication among members of the perinatal healthcare team and to avoid confusion, oxytocin administration rates should always be ordered by the physician or CNM as milliunits per minute and documented in the medical record as milliunits per minute.

Nursing responsibility during oxytocin infusion involves careful titration of the drug to the maternal–fetal response. The titration process includes decreasing the dosage rate or discontinuing the medication when contractions are too frequent, discontinuing the medication when fetal status is indeterminate or abnormal, and increasing the dosage rate when uterine activity and labor progress are inadequate. Often during oxytocin infusion, physicians and nurses are focused on the rate increase section of the protocol while ignoring the clinical criteria for dosage increases. For example, if cervical effacement is occurring or if the woman is progressing in labor as expected based on parity and other individual clinical factors, there is no need to increase the oxytocin rate, even if contractions appear to be mild and infrequent. Labor progress and maternal–fetal response to the medication should be the primary considerations.

When uterine tachysystole occurs or fetal status is such that oxytocin is discontinued, data are limited to guide the decision about the timing and dosage of subsequent IV oxytocin administration. Physiologic and pharmacologic principles may be used to determine the most appropriate dosage. If oxytocin has been discontinued for less than 20 to 30 minutes, the FHR is normal and contraction frequency, intensity, and duration are normal, a suggested protocol may include restarting oxytocin at least at a lower rate of infusion than before the tachysystole occurred. In this clinical situation, many practitioners restart the infusion at half the rate that caused the tachysystole and gradually increase the rate as appropriate based on unit protocol and maternal–fetal status. However, if the oxytocin is discontinued for more than 30 to 40 minutes, most of the exogenous oxytocin is metabolized and plasma levels are similar to that of a woman who has not received IV oxytocin. In this clinical situation, a suggested protocol may include restarting the oxytocin at or near the initial dose ordered. There are individual differences in myometrial sensitivity and the response to oxytocin during labor (Arias, 2000; Ulstem, 1997). It may be necessary to use a lower dose and increase the interval between dosages when there is evidence of the patient's previous sensitivity to the drug. See Display 14–12 for a suggested protocol for managing oxytocin infusion during tachysystole with and without an indeterminate or abnormal FHR pattern.

Misoprostol

Misoprostol is also used for induction of labor. See the section "Cervical Ripening" for a full discussion of misoprostol.

Augmentation of Labor

For some women, labor progresses more slowly than expected. The terms *dystocia* and *failure to progress* are sometimes used to characterize an abnormally long labor. However, this diagnosis is often mistakenly made before the woman has entered the active phase of labor and, therefore, before an adequate trial of labor has been achieved (ACOG, 2003). Often, women have a cesarean birth because of "failure to progress in labor" when, according to ACOG (2003) criteria for the diagnosis of lack of labor progress, active labor has not begun or labor has not been abnormally long (Gifford et al., 2000; Lin & Rouse, 2006; Ness et al., 2005; Zhang, Troendle, et al., 2002; Zhang, Troendle, Reddy, et al., 2010). *Cephalopelvic disproportion* is another common term used when labor has not progressed. This condition can rarely be diagnosed with certainty and is usually related to malposition of the fetal head. According to the latest data, dystocia remains the most common reason for primary cesarean birth in the United States, significantly higher than indeterminate or abnormal fetal status or malpresentation (Zhang, Troendle, Reddy, et al., 2010). ACOG (2003) recommends two practical classifications for labor abnormalities: slower than normal labor (protraction disorders) and complete cessation of contractions (arrest disorders). These disorders require that the woman be in the active phase of labor; thus, a prolonged latent phase is not indicative of dystocia, and this diagnosis cannot be made in the latent phase of labor (ACOG, 2003).

Wide variations in labor progress and duration exist among childbearing women (see previous section on duration of labor). From a physiologic and pharmacologic standpoint, less oxytocin is needed for labor augmentation than for labor induction, but most studies and clinical protocols report higher doses of oxytocin administration during the augmentation of labor. For women in spontaneous active labor, cervical resistance is less than in women who have not yet experienced cervical effacement and dilation. The response to oxytocin seems to depend on preexisting uterine activity and sensitivity rather than the amount given (Arias, 2000).

A systematic review of 10 studies conducted on five different continents between 1987 and 2004 comparing low-dose and high-dose oxytocin for augmentation of labor suggested that high-dose oxytocin (starting range of 4 to 10 mU/min) may be beneficial in shortening labor and decreasing risk of cesarean birth (Wei, Luo, Qi, Xu, & Fraser, 2010). Two of the 10 studies were conducted in Africa with very different clinical conditions than the United States. A significant increase in tachysystole was found with high-dose oxytocin (twice as many women as compared to low dose), but there was no further information about the effects on FHR patterns. There were more babies with Apgar scores less than 7 at 5 minutes of life and more babies with umbilical artery pH less than 7.10 in the high-dose groups (Wei et al., 2010). The authors concluded that 50 women would need to be exposed to high-dose oxytocin during labor augmentation to potentially avoid one cesarean birth (Wei et al., 2010). A retrospective analysis of data from the *Consortium on Safe Labor* (Zhang et al., 2011) compared starting doses of oxytocin for labor augmentation of 1 mU/min, 2 mU/min, and 4 mU/min. Information on intervals between dosage increases was available for only two of the six hospitals included in the study. Length of augmented labor from the start of oxytocin in nulliparous women was 6.9 hours for the 1 mU/min group, 5.3 hours for the 2 mU/min group, and 6.3 hours for the 4 mU/min group (Zhang et al., 2011). Starting at 2 mU/min seemed to be associated with the shortest augmented labor for nulliparous women. There were similar findings for multiparous women although of less clinical significance when considering differences among groups varied from 6 to 24 to 48 minutes. Length of augmented labor from start of oxytocin in multiparous women was 3.8 hours for the 1 mU/min group, 3.1 hours for the 2 mU/min group, and 3.4 hours for the 4 mU/min group (Zhang et al., 2011). There were no differences in the cesarean birth rate among oxytocin dosing groups after controlling for potential confounding variables (Zhang et al., 2011).

Active Management of Labor

Principles of active management of labor (AMOL) were developed by O'Driscoll, Jackson, and Gallagher in 1969. These researchers were faced with limited space in their maternity unit in Dublin, Ireland, and an increasing volume of women in labor. The protocol was initially implemented as a method of shortening labor with a goal of achieving more effective use of space and resources. They discovered that this method of augmentation not only shortened labor for most women but also significantly decreased the cesarean birth rate at their institution (O'Driscoll, Jackson, & Gallagher, 1970). The protocol was designed to be used for *nulliparous women in spontaneous, active labor.* The Dublin active management of labor protocol is precise:

- Candidates include only nulliparous women in spontaneous, active labor with a singleton pregnancy, cephalic presentation, and no evidence of fetal compromise.
- To exclude false and prodromal labor, true labor is specifically defined as contractions with either bloody show, spontaneous rupture of membranes, or complete (100%) cervical effacement.
- Once labor is diagnosed, the woman receives continuous 1:1 labor support from a birth attendant (midwife or labor nurse).
- Amniotomy is performed if membranes have not ruptured spontaneously within 1 hour after labor has been diagnosed.
- If cervical dilation does not progress at least 1 cm/hr, oxytocin augmentation is initiated beginning at 6 mU/min increasing by 6 mU/min every 15 minutes until adequate labor is established, up to a maximum dose of 40 mU/min.
- Tachysystole of uterine activity is defined as more than seven contractions in 15 minutes.

This protocol has been rigorously evaluated in three major randomized controlled studies in the United States (Frigoletto et al., 1995; Lopez-Zeno, Peaceman, Adashek, & Socol, 1992; Rogers et al., 1997). Although all of the studies demonstrated a significant difference in length of labor, none found a significant difference in the cesarean birth rate. All of the studies used protocols very similar to the O'Driscoll et al. (1970) protocol.

The studies that demonstrated this approach was safe for mothers and babies used a nurse-to-woman ratio of 1:1. The principles of active management of labor as a method to decrease cesarean birth rates have not been shown to be successful when applied to labor and birth in the United States. A physiologic dosage regimen for labor induction or augmentation has been suggested as the best approach for most women because of the risks associated with higher doses and increasing the dose at more frequent intervals (such as uterine tachysystole and cesarean birth for indeterminate or abnormal fetal status).

Some practitioners have selected various components of the original AMOL protocol for use in isolation (usually high-dose oxytocin) with varying results. The protocol was found to be safe (although not efficacious in decreasing risk of cesarean birth) when used *in total* for appropriate patients (nulliparous women in spontaneous active labor), with appropriate staffing (one nurse to one woman nursing care), with oxytocin initiated only after cervical changes at less than 1 cm/hr following amniotomy and observation, and with a definition of tachysystole of more than seven contractions

in 15 minutes that did not include an indeterminate or abnormal FHR pattern before intervening. Misapplication of the AMOL protocol using aggressive oxytocin induction regimes as the sole component from the original research is inappropriate (Pates & Satin, 2005). Some have termed this practice the "active mismanagement of labor" (Olah & Gee, 1996), and it is not supported by the original AMOL research team (O'Driscoll, 1996).

Clinical Implications of Labor Induction

Multiple methods of cervical ripening, labor induction, and labor augmentation are currently in use in the United States and Canada. Each method has pros and cons as well as risks and benefits to the mother and fetus. Clearly, the state of the cervix is an important clinical indicator for likelihood of induction success. There is enough evidence to suggest that cervical ripening can increase the chances of success if the indication for induction allows time for cervical ripening. Oxytocin has been used for many years and has proven safe and effective for induction and augmentation. A physiologic dosage regimen for labor induction appears to be the best approach for most women because the risks of higher doses and increasing the doses at more frequent intervals (such as uterine tachysystole and cesarean birth for indeterminate or abnormal fetal status) do not outweigh the benefits (if any) of a slightly shorter labor. Misoprostol is sometimes used for cervical ripening and labor induction. Uterine tachysystole and indeterminate or abnormal FHR patterns related to tachysystole are more common with misoprostol than with oxytocin. Lower doses of misoprostol and increased intervals between doses will decrease the risk to the mother and fetus. Women who are attempting VBAC are at increased risk for uterine rupture with subsequent catastrophic results for both the mother and fetus if pharmacologic agents are used for cervical ripening or labor induction.

The increase in the elective induction rate over the past two decades has profoundly changed the practice of perinatal nursing. Instead of predominately caring for patients who present in spontaneous active labor, many labor nurses spend a significant portion of their time titrating an oxytocin infusion and managing the side effects of oxytocin. Nurses often are pressured by physician colleagues to increase the oxytocin rate to "keep labor on track" and speed the labor process when labor is otherwise proceeding normally at 1 cm/hr and/or there is evidence of excessive uterine activity (Simpson et al., 2006). Although nurses report that they usually resist these types of requests for patient safety reasons, these ongoing clinical conflicts are a source of dissatisfaction for both nurses and physicians (Simpson et al., 2006). Oxytocin mismanagement has become a significant factor in perinatal liability (Clark, Belfort,

Dildy, et al., 2008). The increase in cesarean birth rate, in part the result of widespread elective labor induction of nulliparous women, is changing mother–baby units into surgical units where one third of patients are recovering from major surgery. These shifts in obstetric practice have affected staffing requirements, length of stay, and costs of healthcare for childbearing women and their babies.

There are clinical practices based on the best available evidence that promote the safest care possible for mothers and babies during labor induction. These include, but are not limited to, the following:

- Awaiting spontaneous labor
- If elective, not performing labor induction before 39 completed weeks of gestation
- Cervical readiness before labor induction achieved without pharmacologic agents (if induction is elective)
- Standard physiologic oxytocin protocol including a standard concentration and standard dosing regime
- Agreed upon definition of tachysystole
- Rare cases of uterine tachysystole and, when it occurs, appropriate and timely interventions
- One nurse for each woman undergoing induction of labor
- Common understanding among members of the perinatal team regarding how labor induction will be conducted and an agreement that all team members will participate

Much work lies ahead to provide education to pregnant women so they have enough information to make an informed decision about labor induction. Multiple factors contribute to the steady increase in the rate of induction of labor in the United States. This is a complex issue that involves all participating parties: the pregnant woman, her family, her healthcare provider, the institution, and the intrapartum nurse. More data are needed to fully evaluate the risks and benefits of artificial induction and stimulation of labor. On the basis of what is known, a cautious process that allows for individualization to each clinical situation should be outlined by each institution to ensure the best outcomes for mothers and babies.

OPERATIVE VAGINAL BIRTH

The rate of operative vaginal birth has slowly decreased over recent years from 9% of all births in 1990 (the first year these data were collected from certificates of live births) to 3.7% in 2009 (Martin et al., 2011). Vacuum-assisted births reached a peak at 6.2% in 1997, decreasing to 3.0% in 2009. Forceps-assisted births were at 5.1% in 1990 but were only 0.7% of all births in 2009 (Martin et al., 2011). The 2009 rate for either vacuum- or forceps-assisted births is 61% lower than in 1995 (Martin et al., 2011). However, operative vaginal rates vary widely across the United States, suggesting almost random decision making and the need for outcomes-based data to assist in clinical decision making (Clark, Belfort, Hankins, Meyers, & Houser, 2007). Some predictors of operative vaginal birth are maternal age, parity, previous cesarean birth, diabetes, gestational age, gender, estimated birth weight, induction of labor, oxytocin augmentation, intrapartum fever, prolonged rupture of membranes, meconium-stained amniotic fluid, and epidural anesthesia (Schuit et al., 2012). Nonoperative interventions such as one-to-one labor support, monitoring labor progress, and using oxytocin when labor is not progressing adequately decrease the need for operative vaginal birth (SOGC, 2004). Flexibility in the management of second stage including upright positioning, adequate analgesia/anesthesia, and delaying pushing until the woman has the urge to push also are beneficial in reducing the risk of operative vaginal birth (SOGC, 2004). The rate of operative vaginal birth is reduced when the arbitrary time limit of 2 hours for second stage is abandoned if progress is being made (Fraser et al., 2000; SOGC, 2004).

While no indications are absolute, according to ACOG (2000b) and AAP and ACOG (2012), indications for operative vaginal birth when the fetal head is engaged and the cervix is fully dilated include prolonged second stage, suspicion of immediate or potential fetal compromise, or shortening of the second stage for maternal benefit (e.g., maternal cardiac disease). ACOG (2000b) and AAP and ACOG (2012) define prolonged second stage for nulliparous women as a lack of continuing progress for 3 hours with regional anesthesia or 2 hours without regional analgesia/anesthesia and for multiparous women as a lack of continuing progress for 2 hours with regional anesthesia or 1 hour without regional anesthesia. Multiparous women experiencing a second stage of 3 hours or longer are at increased risk for operative birth, peripartum morbidity, and adverse neonatal outcomes (Cheng, Hopkins, Laros, & Caughey, 2007). Fetal station indicates the level of the leading bony point of the fetal presenting part in centimeters at or below the maternal ischial spines (0 to 5 cm) and is important in the evaluation of fetal progress or descent (see Fig. 14–6) (AAP & ACOG, 2012; ACOG, 2000b). Previously, station was described by dividing the birth canal into thirds (0 to 3+).

According to the *Guidelines for Perinatal Care* (AAP & ACOG, 2012), the following conditions are required for forceps or vacuum-assisted births: a provider with privileges for the procedure, an assessment of maternal pelvis–fetal size relationship including clinical pelvimetry, and estimation of fetal weight, and the position and station of the fetal head, adequate analgesia/anesthesia, willingness to abandon the attempted operative vaginal birth, and a provider in attendance with the ability to perform a cesarean birth.

Although sometimes necessary, operative vaginal birth is not without complications for the woman and baby. Perineal trauma is the main injury risk for women including vaginal and perineal lacerations, extension of the episiotomy, hematoma, and anal sphincter disruption (Aukee et al., 2006; Caughey et al., 2005; Dandolu et al., 2005; FitzGerald et al., 2007; Kudish et al., 2006). Operative vaginal birth significantly increases the risk for all pelvic floor disorders, especially prolapse, 5 to 10 years after a first birth (Handa et al., 2012). Among women with operative vaginal birth, there are significant risks for rehospitalization for postpartum hemorrhage, perineal wound infection complications, and pelvic injuries when compared to women who had spontaneous vaginal birth (Liu et al., 2005; Lydon-Rochelle, Holt, Martin, & Easterling, 2000). The most common reason for rehospitalization for women after operative vaginal birth is perineal wound infection (Lydon-Rochelle et al., 2000). Maternal injuries appear to be more common with forceps as compared to vacuums, whereas fetal injuries are more common with vacuums as compared to forceps (AAP & ACOG, 2012; Johnson, Figueroa, Garry, Elimian, & Maulik, 2004; Mollberg, Hagberg, Bager, Lilja, & Ladfors, 2005). Comparing neonatal outcome between forceps- and vacuum-assisted birth, babies delivered with forceps have more facial nerve palsy, while babies born with vacuums have more cephalohematomas, scalp lacerations, seizures, and 5-minute Apgar scores less than 7 (Werner et al., 2011). Increased risks to the fetus are associated with sequential application of devices (Castro, Hoey, & Towner, 2003; Towner, Castro, Eby-Wilkens, & Gilbert, 1999; Vacca, 2002). Generally, when there is a failed trial of one instrument, use of another is not recommended unless there is a compelling and justifiable reason (ACOG, 2000b; Castro et al., 2003).

Forceps

Forceps are used to assist delivery of the fetal head when birth must be facilitated for the health of the mother or fetus. Piper forceps are sometimes used during vaginal breech births to assist in delivery of the fetal head after the body has been delivered. Maternal conditions that may necessitate use of forceps are medical complications such as cardiac or pulmonary disease, maternal exhaustion, or high level of regional analgesia/anesthesia that diminishes the woman's expulsive efforts. Additional factors associated with use of forceps are birth weight greater than 4,000 g, an OP position, epidural analgesia/anesthesia, maternal age over 35 years, and a prolonged first- or second-stage labor (Mazouni et al., 2006). The fetus may demonstrate signs of compromise via EFM or FHR auscultation during second-stage labor, such as minimal or absent variability associated with bradycardia, tachycardia, or recurrent late or variable decelerations, or prolonged decelerations, suggesting that attempts at assisted birth may be warranted.

A forceps-assisted birth should not be considered unless the cervix is completely dilated, membranes are ruptured, the head is engaged, and the woman has adequate analgesia/anesthesia. The woman's bladder should be emptied prior to application to minimize risks of trauma. If the woman is unable to void, urinary catheterization is usually performed by the birth attendant. The classification of forceps procedures is listed in Table 14–6. All perinatal nurses should be familiar with this classification so that documentation of the procedure is accurate if they are entering these data in the medical record. Consultation with the provider who applied the forceps before medical record documentation is appropriate to ensure accuracy. The number of forceps applications and attempts with traction are usually documented. Ultimately, the responsibility for complete documentation of the operative birth procedure rests with the provider who performed the procedure.

Use of forceps are associated with pain, vaginal and cervical lacerations, extension of the episiotomy, anal sphincter injuries, perineal wound infection, uterine rupture, bladder trauma, fracture of the coccyx, hemorrhage, increased vaginal bleeding, uterine atony, anemia, and pelvic floor disorders (Benavides, Wu, Hundley, Ivester, & Visco, 2005; Caughey et al., 2005; Christianson, Bovbjerg, McDavitt, & Hullfish, 2003; FitzGerald et al., 2007; Handa et al., 2012; Hudelist et al., 2005;

Table 14–6. CRITERIA FOR FORCEPS–ASSISTED BIRTH ACCORDING TO STATION AND ROTATION

Types of Procedure	Criteria
Outlet forceps	1. Scalp is visible at the introitus without separating the labia. 2. Fetal skull has reached the pelvic floor. 3. Sagittal suture is in the anteroposterior diameter or right or left occiput anterior or posterior position. 4. Fetal head is at or on the perineum. 5. Rotation does not exceed 45°.
Low forceps	Leading point of the fetal skull is at station ≥+2 cm and not on the pelvic floor. a. Rotation ≤45° (left or right occiput anterior to occiput anterior, or left or right occiput posterior to occiput posterior) b. Rotation >45°
Midforceps	Station above +2 cm but head engaged
High	Not included in classification.

From American College of Obstetricians and Gynecologists. (2000c). *Operative Vaginal Delivery* (Practice Bulletin No. 17). Washington, DC: Author. Reprinted by permission. Copyright 2000 by American College of Obstetricians and Gynecologists.

Johnson et al., 2004). Babies delivered by forceps are at risk for skin markings, lacerations, bruising, nerve injuries, skull fractures, cephalohematoma, ocular trauma, and intracranial hemorrhage (Doumouchtsis & Arulkumaran, 2006; Dupuis et al., 2005; Towner et al., 1999; Uhing, 2005) and should be observed closely in the immediate newborn period. The incidence of subarachnoid hemorrhage is estimated to be 3.3 per 10,000 forceps-assisted births and subdural hemorrhage 9.8 per 10,000 forceps-assisted births (Doumouchtsis & Arulkumaran, 2006). However, when compared with vacuum-assisted vaginal births or cesarean birth, a forceps-assisted birth is associated with a reduced risk of neonatal seizures and 5-minute Apgar scores less than 7 (Werner et al., 2011). The condition of the mother and newborn at birth should be documented in the medical record. The procedure should be documented by the birth attendant. Neonatal care providers should be made aware of the forceps-assisted vaginal birth (AAP & ACOG, 2012).

Vacuum Extraction

Some physicians and CNMs use vacuum extraction in lieu of forceps, usually dependent on their education, experience, and privileges. A vacuum extractor consists of a soft or rigid cup available in various sizes that has a suction device attached. The cup is placed on the fetal head, and suction is increased gradually until a seal is formed. Gentle traction is then applied to deliver the fetal head. Indications and prerequisites for vacuum extraction or for the use of forceps are generally the same; however, most experts agree that rotation is not appropriate via vacuum extraction (Bofill, Martin, & Morrison, 1998). Proponents of vacuum extraction feel that its advantages include easier application, less force applied to the fetal head, less analgesia/anesthesia needed, less maternal soft tissue injury, fewer fetal injuries, and fewer parental concerns (ACOG, 2000b; Caughey et al., 2005).

Complications from both vacuum- and forceps-assisted births are dependent primarily on skill of the practitioner. The incidence of scalp abrasions and lacerations with vacuum use is approximately 10% (Doumouchtsis & Arulkumaran, 2006). Other common newborn outcomes with vacuum-assisted birth include a chignon, discoloration and bruising of the scalp, blisters and superficial scalp abrasions, and retinal hemorrhage (Vacca, 2002; Uhing, 2005). More serious complications for the baby include extensive or deep scalp lacerations, subgaleal (subaponeurotic) hemorrhage, intracranial hemorrhage, and skull fracture (Vacca, 2002; Uhing, 2005). Approximately 14% to 16% of fetuses delivered with vacuum extractors will develop a cephalohematoma (ACOG, 2000b); however, when the duration of vacuum application at maximum pressure exceeds 5 minutes, this incidence increases to 28% (Bofill et al., 1997). The incidence of subarachnoid hemorrhage after vacuum is estimated to be 2.2 per 10,000 vacuum-assisted births; subdural hemorrhage, 8.0 per 10,000 vacuum-assisted births; and subgaleal hemorrhage, 59 per 10,000 vacuum-assisted births (Doumouchtsis & Arulkumaran, 2006; Towner et al., 1999; Uchil & Arulkumaran, 2003). Avoiding difficult vacuum-assisted births and avoiding the use of forceps to complete a failed vacuum will likely minimize the risk of subgaleal hemorrhages (Uchil & Arulkumaran, 2003). Vacuum devices should not be used to assist births prior to 34 weeks' gestation because of the increased risk of fetal intraventricular hemorrhage (ACOG, 2000b).

There have been reports of neonatal subgaleal hematoma and intracranial hemorrhage after the vacuum extractor has been used. The FDA issued a warning letter to providers in 1998 alerting them to these risks (FDA, 1998). A subgaleal hematoma occurs when emissary veins are damaged and blood accumulates in the potential space between the galea aponeurotica (epicranial aponeurosis) and the periosteum of the skull (pericranium). Because the subaponeurotic space has neither containing membranes nor boundaries, the subgaleal hematoma may extend from the orbital ridges to the nape of the neck. This condition is dangerous because of the large potential space for blood accumulation and the possibility of life-threatening hemorrhage (FDA, 1998). Signs and symptoms of subgaleal hematoma include diffuse swelling of the fetal head and evidence of hypovolemic shock (e.g., pallor, hypotension, tachycardia, and increased respiration rate). These signs and symptoms may be present immediately after birth or may not become clinically apparent until several hours or up to a few days after birth (FDA, 1998). The swelling is usually diffuse, shifts when the newborn's head is repositioned, and indents easily on palpation. In some cases, the swelling is difficult to distinguish from edema of the scalp. On occasion, the hypotension and pallor are the dominant signs while the cranial signs are unremarkable (FDA, 1998). Intracranial hemorrhage includes subdural, subarachnoid, intraventricular, and/or intraparenchymal hemorrhage. Signs and symptoms of intracranial hemorrhage include indications of cerebral irritation such as seizures, lethargy, obtundation, apnea, bulging fontanelle, poor feeding, increased irritability, bradycardia, and/or shock. These signs and symptoms are sometimes delayed until several hours after birth (FDA, 1998). Mortality with subgaleal hemorrhage approaches 25% (Doumouchtsis & Arulkumaran, 2006). A decrease in hematocrit that is greater than 25% of the baseline value at birth in association with significant birth asphyxia is the most important risk factor for newborn mortality (Doumouchtsis & Arulkumaran, 2006).

Maternal complications associated with the use of vacuum devices include pain; vaginal and cervical lacerations; extension of the episiotomy; anal sphincter injuries; perineal wound infection; bladder trauma; hemorrhage; increased vaginal bleeding; uterine atony; and anemia (ACOG, 2000b; Aukee et al., 2006; Caughey et al., 2005; Dandolu et al., 2005; Johnson et al., 2004). A careful assessment following vacuum-assisted birth is necessary to identify maternal complications and to initiate appropriate treatment.

There is a lack of consensus about the number of pulls required to effect birth, the maximum number of cup detachments (pop-offs) that can be tolerated, and the total duration of the procedure (ACOG, 2000b). The concept of the "three pull rule" has become widely accepted as a safety measure for limiting the amount of traction on the fetal head (Vacca, 2002), but what constitutes a safe number of pulls has never been empirically established. Some manufacturers recommend a limit of two pulls. However, there is evidence to suggest that using no more than 600 mm Hg pressure, and abandoning the procedure after three pop-offs and/or 15 to 20 minutes maximum total time of application, is consistent with safe care and a decreased risk of fetal injuries (Bofill, Rust, & Schorr, 1996; Bofill et al., 1998; O'Grady, Gimovsky, & McIlhargie, 1995; Mollberg et al., 2005; Vacca, 2002).

Cup detachment (pop-off) should not be regarded as a normal event or safety feature of using a vacuum (Vacca, 2002). The rapid decompression resulting from a sudden loss of vacuum when the cup detaches completely has been associated with injury to the scalp and its blood vessels (Vacca, 2002). Pop-offs are a warning sign that too much ineffective force is being exerted on the fetal head (Castro et al., 2003; Vacca, 2002). Safety is promoted when the maximum time of application of the vacuum is 15 minutes, and vacuum extraction beyond 20 minutes should be rare (Vacca, 2002, 2006). The recommendations of the manufacturer of the vacuum extractor device being used should be followed. The vacuum pressure should not exceed 500 to 600 mm Hg, the traction force should not exceed 11.5 kg, and the pressure should be released as soon as the contraction ends and the woman stops pushing (Brumfield, Gilstrap, O'Grady, Ross, & Schifrin, 1999; Vacca, 2006). As a general guideline, progress in descent should accompany each traction attempt and no more than three pulls should be attempted (Bofill et al., 1996; Bofill et al., 1998; Brumfield et al., 1999; Vacca, 2006). Traction is used only when the woman is actively pushing.

The vacuum procedure should be timed from the moment of insertion of the cup into the vagina until birth and should not be on the fetal head for longer than 20 to 30 minutes (Bofill et al., 1998; Brumfield et al., 1999). When the cup has been applied at maximum pressure for more than 10 minutes, the rate of fetal injuries increase (Brumfield et al., 1999); thus, while total time of cup application can be 20 minutes, the time of maximum pressure force should not exceed 10 minutes (Paluska, 1997). As with forceps, there should be a willingness to abandon attempts at a vacuum-assisted birth if satisfactory progress is not made (ACOG, 2000b; SOGC, 2004). If the 20-minute time limit is reached, the vacuum cup is removed and the procedure is considered a failed vacuum procedure (Bofill et al., 1998; Vacca, 2002). Three pop-offs, evidence of fetal scalp trauma, and/or no descent with appropriate application and traction should warrant abandoning the vacuum procedure (Bofill et al., 1998). A unit policy about the use of vacuum devices and forceps, including a list of those credentialed in these procedures, facilitates safe maternal–fetal care and avoids clinical controversies at the bedside if there is disagreement between healthcare professionals regarding the amount of pressure, length of application, number of pop-offs and pull attempts, and the need to abandon the procedure. Documentation of fetal station, the duration of application, pressure, number of pulls, and number of pop-offs should be included in the medical record by the provider performing the procedure. Neonatal care providers should be made aware of the vacuum-assisted vaginal birth (AAP & ACOG, 2012).

The Nurse's Role

The birth attendant is responsible for explaining the procedure to the patient and discussing potential risks and benefits. Nurses have a role in educating and reassuring the woman when an assisted vaginal birth is anticipated. Maternal comfort level should be assessed prior to the application of forceps or a vacuum extractor. The urinary bladder may be emptied by the provider or the nurse to decrease the risk of trauma if necessary. If the FHR pattern is the indication for the immediate birth, then the nurse must be prepared for newborn resuscitation ensuring that appropriate equipment, supplies, and personnel are available. Nurses should also be aware of potential complications related to the use of forceps and vacuums and observe both the mother and baby for associated signs and symptoms. Some complications may be life threatening for the mother and baby, so the prompt identification and initiation of appropriate treatment is necessary. Parents should be prepared for and shown any forceps or vacuum extraction marks on their baby and be reassured that they should disappear in a few days.

Complete and accurate medical record documentation of any adverse effects of operative vaginal birth is required. Responsibility for the documentation of station, the position prior to application of the vacuum or forceps, and the complete procedure rests with the provider who performs the operative birth. There is no need for nurses to enter duplicate data in the medical record. The nurse may indicate in the medical record that a forceps- or vacuum-assisted birth was performed and any related nursing interventions.

AMNIOINFUSION

Amnioinfusion is the transcervical instillation of fluid into the amniotic cavity to alleviate umbilical cord compression resulting from decreased amniotic fluid or oligohydramnios (ACOG, 2006a, 2010a). Amnioinfusion is a reasonable and effective measure used to treat recurrent variable FHR decelerations during the first stage of labor that have not been resolved with maternal repositioning. Amnioinfusion has been found to significantly resolve patterns of "moderate" or "severe" variable decelerations but does not affect late decelerations or patterns with absent variability (Hofmeyr & Lawrie, 2012; Miño, Puertas, Miranda, & Herruzo, 1999; Miyazaki & Nevarez, 1985). For women with oligohydramnios and a normal FHR tracing, prophylactic amnioinfusion offers no benefit (Novikova, Hofmeyr, & Essilfie-Appiah, 2010). However, when amnioinfusion is used in women with recurrent variable decelerations, the number of cesarean births performed for FHR abnormalities is reduced (Hofmeyr & Lawrie, 2012). Amnioinfusion is not recommended for treatment of meconium-stained amniotic fluid (AAP & ACOG, 2012). Contraindications may include vaginal bleeding, placenta previa, uterine anomalies, and active infection such as human immunodeficiency virus or herpes virus (Simpson, 2009). An amnioinfusion procedure is presented in Display 14–13.

VAGINAL BIRTH

Although cesarean birth is at an all-time high in the United States, for most (67.1%) women, labor results in vaginal birth (Martin et al., 2011). Routine episiotomy is no longer recommended as a result of the evidence of risks of perineal trauma and its associated sequelae, and its use has greatly decreased over the past decade (ACOG, 2006b; DeFrances & Podgornik, 2006). Healthy women should be allowed and encouraged to give birth in an upright (rather than supine lithotomy) position with minimal intervention. The woman should be allowed and encouraged to have family and support persons at her birth as per her desire in the context of space limitations and clinical conditions (AAP & ACOG, 2012). The birth process should be conducted as a celebration of a natural life event rather than a medical intervention as much as possible based on the clinical situation. At least one registered nurse should be in attendance at every birth to assist the birth attendant and assess maternal–fetal–newborn status. At least one additional person

attending the birth should be solely responsible for the newborn and capable of initiating resuscitation including the administration of positive-pressure ventilation and assisting with chest compressions (AAP & American Heart Association [AHA], 2011). Either this person or an additional person immediately available to the birthing area should have the additional skills required to perform a complete resuscitation, including endotracheal intubation and the administration of medications (AAP & AHA, 2011). Having someone on-call (either at home or in a remote area of the hospital) for newborn resuscitation is not sufficient (AAP & AHA, 2011). When resuscitation is needed, it must be initiated without delay (AAP & AHA, 2011). If the birth is anticipated to be high risk (e.g., meconium staining of the amniotic fluid), at least two persons should be present solely to manage the neonate: one with completed resuscitation skills and one or more to assist (AAP & AHA, 2011). A comprehensive discussion of the newborn's transition to extrauterine life and neonatal resuscitation is presented in Chapter 18.

CESAREAN BIRTH

INCIDENCE

According to the latest data available from the National Center for Health Statistics, after rising for 13 consecutive years, the cesarean birth rate declined slightly from 32.9% in 2009 to 32.8% in 2010 (Hamilton, Martin, & Ventura, 2011). During the mid-1990s, the cesarean rate temporarily decreased due to an upward trend in the number of VBACs (50% increase from 1989 to 1996) (Martin et al., 2011). However, since 1996, the VBAC rate has fallen significantly, while the total cesarean rate has risen 60% (Martin et al., 2011). In 2009, VBAC represented only 1% of all births in the United States (Martin et al., 2011). Once a woman has a cesarean birth, there is more than a 90% chance that subsequent births also will be by cesarean (Martin et al., 2011). Primary cesarean births are also a significant contributor, accounting for 50% of the increasing cesarean rate in one recent study (Barber et al., 2011). These data are consistent with the most recent available U.S. natality data in which 23.8% of all births in 2008 were primary cesarean births (Osterman, Martin, Mathews, & Hamilton, 2011). When compared to 26 other developed countries with cesarean birth rates ranging from 14% (Netherlands) to 40% (Italy), the rate of 32.8% in the United States rate is higher than 22 of the comparison countries (MacDorman, Declercq, & Menacker, 2011).

The most common indications for cesarean birth noted on birth certificates are maternal medical complications and complications of labor such as dystocia, breech/malpresentation, cephalopelvic disproportion,

DISPLAY 14-13

Amnioinfusion

Amnioinfusion is a reasonable therapeutic option when there are recurrent variable decelerations during the first stage of labor that are unresolved with maternal position changes. Ruptured membranes are required.

An institutional protocol may include the following:

- Contraindications (e.g., vaginal bleeding, uterine anomalies, active infections such as HIV or herpes, impending birth)
- Who can perform amnioinfusion
- Who can insert the intrauterine pressure catheter
- What type of fluid may be used (normal saline or lactated Ringer's solution)
- What instillation method may be used (gravity flow or infusion pump)
- What infusion techniques may be used (bolus, continuous, or a combination of both)
- When and why the procedure should be altered (e.g., loss of large amount of fluid resulting from position change or coughing, increased uterine resting tone, reappearance of recurrent variable decelerations, or no fluid return)

General guidelines for the procedure are as follows:

- The amnioinfusion procedure and the indication should be explained to the woman and her support persons prior to initiation.
- During amnioinfusion, room temperature normal saline or lactated Ringer's solution is infused into the uterus transcervically via an intrauterine pressure catheter.
- The initial bolus is usually 250–500 mL given over a 20- to 30-minute period using either an infusion pump or gravity flow. Both methods are appropriate and seem to be equally efficacious.
- Some protocols allow for a continuous infusion of 2–3 mL per minute (120–180 mL/hr) after the bolus until resolution of the variable decelerations (Miller, Miller, & Tucker, 2012). Usually the maximum amount of fluid infused is 1,000 mL (Miller et al., 2012).
- If recurrent variable decelerations have not resolved after the infusion of 800–1,000 mL, the infusion may be discontinued and alternative approaches used (Miller et al., 2012).
- During bolus of the infusion and maintenance rate, the approximate amount of fluid returning should be noted and recorded to avoid iatrogenic polyhydramnios.

- An assessment of fluid return can be accomplished by weighing the underpads (1 mL of fluid equals = 1 g of weight) (Miller et al., 2012).
- As a general consideration, if 250 mL has infused with no return, the amnioinfusion is discontinued until the fluid has returned.
- Overdistention is more likely when the presenting part obstructs flow, thus releasing the fluid by gently elevating the presenting part may be a successful intervention.
- A dual-lumen intrauterine catheter is preferred so that an estimate of uterine resting tone can be assessed during the infusion.
- The uterine resting tone may appear higher than normal during the procedure (from 25 to 40 mm Hg). If there is a concern about an elevated uterine resting tone (>40 mm Hg), temporarily discontinue the infusion to attempt a more accurate assessment. If the uterine resting tone exceeds 25 mm Hg while the infusion is temporarily discontinued for an assessment of uterine resting tone, consider discontinuing the infusion.
- Warming of the solution may not be necessary for full-term fetuses but may be appropriate for preterm or growth-restricted fetuses. Fetal bradycardia may occur if the solution is colder than room temperature and/or is infused too rapidly (Miller et al., 2012). Some providers prefer to warm the solution to body temperature. If the solution is warmed, acceptable temperatures are 93°–96°F (34°–37°C). The safest method to warm the solution is by use of an electronic blood/fluid warmer. Microwaves and other types of warming techniques should not be used to heat the solution.
- Assessment and documentation:
  ○ Contraction intensity and frequency should be continually assessed during the procedure.
  ○ In addition to assessments appropriate for the first stage of labor, additional assessments may include the following:
    ■ Fundal height and leakage of fluids
    ■ Amount, color, and odor of fluid leaking from vagina
    ■ Fetal response such as resolution of the variable decelerations

Documentation may include the maternal and fetal response; uterine resting tone; fluid output; duration of the procedure; and the type, rate, and amount of solution infused.

Adapted from Simpson, K. R. (2009). Physiologic interventions for fetal heart rate patterns. In A. Lyndon & L. U. Ali (Eds.), *AWHONN's Fetal Heart Monitoring Principles and Practices,* (4th ed., pp. 135–155). Dubuque, IA: Kendall Hunt.

---

indeterminate or abnormal fetal status, and placenta previa (Martin et al., 2011). In the *Consortium for Safe Labor* study (Zhang, Troendle, Reddy, et al., 2010), the most common reasons for a cesarean during labor were failure to progress/cephalopelvic disproportion and "nonreassuring" fetal status/fetal distress. The most common reasons for scheduled or planned cesarean birth were prior uterine scar, elective, and fetal malpresentation (Zhang, Troendle, Reddy, et al., 2010). Cesarean birth for indeterminate or abnormal fetal

status increased 1.5- to 5-fold since 1995 (Hendrix & Chauhan, 2005). Cesarean birth is often performed for a lack of progress in labor when the woman is still in the latent phase of labor or when the second stage of labor is not prolonged (Gifford et al., 2000; Harper, Caughey, et al., 2012; Lin & Rouse, 2006; Rouse et al., 2001; Zhang, Landy, et al., 2010). Allowing at least 12 to 18 hours of latent phase labor before a diagnosis of failed induction is made may decrease the risk of cesarean birth (ACOG, 2009a). Compared to women in spontaneous labor, nulliparous women undergoing induction of labor have almost a twofold increased risk of primary cesarean birth; multiparous women a 1.5-fold increased risk (Reisner, Wallin, Zingheim, & Luthy, 2009). The risk of cesarean birth is not increased with the initiation of early neuraxial analgesia when compared to IV opioid analgesia (ACOG, 2006c).

There are significant risks of maternal and newborn complications with cesarean birth (Kolas, Saugstad, Daltveit, Nilsen, & Øian, 2006; MacDorman, Declercq, Menacker, & Malloy, 2006; Sakala & Mayberry, 2006). Babies born via cesarean are at significantly increased risk for respiratory complications and admission to the NICU (Jain & Dudell, 2006; Kolas et al., 2006; Signore, Hemachandra, & Klebanoff, 2006). Approximately 1.1% of babies born via cesarean suffer injuries such as skin lacerations, abrasions, abnormal bruising, subconjunctival hemorrhage, cephalohematoma, clavicular fracture, facial nerve injury, brachial plexus injury, skull fracture, long bone fracture, and intracranial hemorrhage (Alexander et al., 2006). Cesareans following labor are associated with more risk of fetal trauma than cesareans without labor (Baskett, Allen, O'Connell, & Allen, 2007). Duration of the skin incision-to-birth interval, type of incision, and indication for the surgery are influencing factors in fetal injury with cesarean birth (Alexander et al., 2006). Babies born less than 5 minutes after the incision time have a higher injury rate than babies born more than 5 minutes after the incision time (Alexander et al., 2006). Low vertical incisions are associated with the lowest risk of fetal injury while "T" or "J" incisions have a higher risk (Alexander et al., 2006). Cesarean birth after a failed forceps or vacuum attempt as an indication has the highest risk of fetal injury, followed by an indeterminate or abnormal FHR pattern, abnormal presentation, and labor dystocia (Alexander et al., 2006). Because presumed fetal compromise is often a reason for an expedited cesarean with a short interval from incision to birth, risk of injuries are increased with these fetuses.

A cesarean first birth is associated with a higher risk of placenta previa, placental abruption, uterine scar dehiscence, and uterine rupture in the second pregnancy (Getahun, Oyelese, Salihu, & Ananth, 2006; Gilliam, 2006; Lydon-Rochelle et al., 2001a). Maternal morbidity increases with each additional cesarean birth, especially for women with three or more cesarean births, who are at the greatest risk for placenta previa, accreta, and hysterectomy (Marshall, Fu, & Guise, 2011). Women with placenta previa and previous cesarean birth are at a significantly increased risk of placenta accreta, and those women with accreta, regardless of history of previous cesarean, are at a significant increased risk of hysterectomy (Marshall et al., 2011).

There is an approximate 0.5% risk of cesarean hysterectomy related to cesarean birth, with leading indications of placenta accreta (38%) and uterine atony (34%) (Shellhaas et al., 2009). In one study, in the hysterectomy cases with a placenta accreta, 18% occurred with a first cesarean birth while 82% were in women with a prior procedure. In the hysterectomy cases related to uterine atony, 59% were complicated first cesarean births and 41% were in women with a prior cesarean. Major maternal complications of cesarean hysterectomy included transfusion of red blood cells (84%) and other blood products (34%), fever (11%), subsequent laparotomy (4%), ureteral injury (3%), and death (1.6%) (Shellhaas et al., 2009). Accreta hysterectomy cases were more likely than atony hysterectomy cases to require ureteral stents (14% vs. 3%) and to instill sterile milk into the bladder (23% vs. 8%) (Shellhaas et al., 2009).

The incidence of adhesions increases significantly with the number of cesarean births (Marshall et al., 2011; Morales, Gordon, & Bates, 2007). Postsurgical adhesions may result in subfertility, bowel obstruction, pain, injury to the bladder, and increased operative time in subsequent cesarean births (Marshall et al., 2011). Longer operative time increases risks for surgical site infections, greater blood loss, and adverse neonatal outcomes (Marshall et al., 2011; Morales et al., 2007). Women who have a cesarean birth have a significantly increased risk of rehospitalization for uterine infection, surgical wound infection, complications from surgical wound, and cardiopulmonary and thromboembolic complications (Liu et al., 2002; Lydon-Rochelle et al., 2000). They are 30 times more likely to have a surgical wound infection than women who have a vaginal birth (Lydon-Rochelle et al., 2000).

The current rate of surgical site infections in the United States ranges from 1.5% to 3.8% of all cesarean births (Edwards et al., 2009). Risk factors for infection include extremes of age, increased body mass index (BMI), premature rupture of membranes, prolonged duration of surgery, and use of staples for wound closure (Kittur et al., 2012). An Agency for Healthcare Research and Quality review concluded that the impact of repeat cesarean births on perioperative infection is unclear due to inconsistent definitions of infection and the findings that multiple cesarean births do not increase the rate of wound complications beyond the risk of the first cesarean (Guise et al., 2010). Although the rates of excessive bleeding are generally low after cesarean birth, the risk of transfusion increased significantly as the number of previous cesarean births increased (Marshall et al., 2011; Nisenblat et al., 2006). The risk of maternal mortality after cesarean birth from anesthesia complications, puerperal infection, and venous thromboembolism is 3.6 times higher for women who have cesarean birth prior to labor and after failed labor when compared to vaginal birth (Deneux-Tharaux, Carmona, Bouvier-Colle, & Breart, 2006). The average length of inpatient stay for cesarean birth is 3.1 days, as compared to 2.1 days for vaginal birth (Podulka, Stranges, & Steiner, 2011). The average length of stay for cesarean birth with complications is 4.5 days (Podulka et al., 2011). Cesarean birth after labor in the first pregnancy is associated with increased cumulative healthcare costs compared with vaginal birth, regardless of the number or type of subsequent births (Allen, O'Connell, & Baskett, 2006; Druzin & El-Sayed, 2006).

CESAREAN BIRTH BY MATERNAL REQUEST

There are limited data on actual numbers of cesarean deliveries on maternal request (CDMR). Based on birth certificate data, the number of cesarean births without an indicated risk has increased over the past several years. However, these data do not include information regarding whether the mother requested a cesarean birth absent of any risks or whether the decision was made by the provider. Birth certificate data does not include CDMR information (Kirby & Salihu, 2006). There have been attempts to estimate CDMR through the use of diagnostic codes from the *International Classification of Diseases, Ninth Revision, Clinical Modification* (ICD-9-CM). These processes are based on exclusion of codes for cesarean births for other reasons because there is not an ICD-9-CM code for CDMR. Even if there was an associated code, there may be resistance to universal use of a CDMR code by both physicians and patients because of concerns about reimbursement (Gossman, Joesch, & Tanfer, 2006). Based on these issues and with current limitations in natality data collection, the ability to accurately measure the rate of CDMR is not possible at this time and may not be possible for the foreseeable future. Although there is evidence that medical risk factors and complications of labor and delivery are significantly underreported on birth certificates, this limitation alone does not account for the rise in cesarean births without an indicated risk. It is plausible that some of the cesarean births without an indicated risk were as a result of maternal request (NIH, 2006). Estimates of CDMR vary from 0.08% to 2.6% of all births (Declercq et al., 2006; Gossman et al., 2006; NIH, 2006).

At present, limited evidence exists upon which to develop a national policy and clinical practice recommendations related to cesarean birth for nonmedical reasons at term (Lavender, Hofmeyr, Neilson, Kingdon, & Gyte, 2012). However, a review of available evidence is presented based on the findings of the *State of the Science Conference on Cesarean Delivery on Maternal Request*, sponsored by the NIH (2006). Two maternal outcomes are significantly in favor of vaginal birth over cesarean birth. These include a risk of postpartum hemorrhage and an increased maternal hospital length of stay. Other maternal outcomes with weaker

evidence that favor vaginal birth are an increased risk of infections, analgesia/anesthesia complications, subsequent placenta previa, and delayed or impaired breastfeeding. There are no maternal outcomes with strong evidence that favor cesarean birth over vaginal birth. Maternal outcomes with weak evidence to favor cesarean birth are a decreased risk of urinary incontinence and surgical and traumatic complications. For women who have a cesarean birth with future pregnancies after a prior cesarean birth, there is weak evidence of less risk of uterine rupture and cesarean hysterectomy. These women may have decreased fertility after a cesarean birth. Maternal outcomes with equivocal evidence include anorectal function, sexual function, pelvic organ prolapse, subsequent stillbirth, and mortality.

A neonatal outcome with strong evidence that favors vaginal birth over cesarean birth is the decreased risk of respiratory morbidity. Other neonatal outcomes with weak evidence supporting vaginal birth include a risk of iatrogenic prematurity and an increased length of stay. There are no neonatal outcomes with strong evidence that favor cesarean birth over vaginal birth. Neonatal outcomes with weak evidence that favor cesarean birth are fetal mortality, intracranial hemorrhage, neonatal asphyxia, encephalopathy, birth injury, laceration, and neonatal infection.

The following conclusions and recommendations resulted from the NIH (2006) *State of the Science Conference on Cesarean Delivery on Maternal Request*:

- The incidence of cesarean birth without medical or obstetric indication is increasing in the United States, and a component of this increase is CDMR. Given the tools available, the magnitude of this component is difficult to quantify.
- There is insufficient evidence to fully evaluate the benefits and risk of CDMR as compared to planned vaginal birth; more research is needed.
- Until quality evidence becomes available, any decision to perform a CDMR should be carefully individualized and consistent with ethical principles.
- Given that the risks of placenta previa and accreta rise with each cesarean birth, CDMR is not recommended for women desiring more children.
- CDMR should not be performed prior to 39 weeks of gestation or without verification of lung maturity, because of the significant danger of respiratory complications.
- CDMR should not be motivated by an unavailability of effective pain management. Efforts must be made to ensure the availability of pain management services for all women.
- NIH or appropriate federal-level agencies should establish and maintain a Web site to provide up-to-date information on the benefits and risks of all modes of birth.

Although supportive evidence for CDMR is lacking, a number of women may request a cesarean birth absent medical or obstetric indications (Bettes et al., 2007; Pevzner, Preslicka, Bush, & Chan, 2011). The vast majority of women believe vaginal birth is safest for themselves and their baby, but feel that women should be able to choose the route of birth (Pevzner et al., 2011). Most physicians also believe that women have the right to choose a nonmedically indicated cesarean birth; however, not all would agree to perform the procedure (Coleman-Cowger et al., 2010). According to ACOG (2008b), the physician should counsel the woman within the framework of the ethical principles of autonomy, beneficence, nonmaleficence, veracity, and justice using the opportunity to explore the woman's concerns with the goal of reaching a mutually acceptable decision. These same principles apply to nurses caring for women who choose CDMR (Carlton, Callister, & Stoneman, 2005). Beneficence-based clinical judgment favors vaginal birth (Minkoff, Powderly, Chervenak, & McCullough, 2004). Offering or performing CDMR is not consistent with substantive justice–based considerations, and there is no autonomy-based obligation to offer cesarean birth in an ethically and legally appropriate informed consent process (Minkoff et al., 2004). The promotion of CDMR as a standard of care or mandated part of patient counseling is highly questionable in light of finite healthcare resources in the United States (Druzin & El-Sayed, 2006).

Physicians should respond to patient-initiated requests for cesarean birth with a thorough informed consent process (including potential risks and benefits to the mother and fetus in the current pregnancy and implications for risks in future pregnancies) and request that the woman reconsider to ensure her autonomy is meaningfully exercised (ACOG, 2008b; Hankins, 2006; Minkoff et al., 2004). Discussing options, attempting to dissuade women, but ultimately acquiescing to their judgment is not incompatible with obstetric ethics (Minkoff, 2006). If the woman and her physician cannot agree on a route of birth, a referral to another healthcare provider would be appropriate (ACOG, 2008b). With the level of interest in this topic, it is likely that more rigorous research will be conducted and disseminated. As the body of knowledge on CDMR evolves, it is important to develop plans to promulgate this information to healthcare providers, women, and their families so they are able to make an informed decision in their best interests and in the best interests of their baby (Sakala & Mayberry, 2006).

PERIOPERATIVE STANDARDS AND GUIDELINES FOR CESAREAN BIRTH

Perioperative perinatal nursing incorporates the skills of the specialties of obstetrics, surgery, and post-anesthesia care to provide comprehensive care to women who have a cesarean birth. Patients with the same health status and condition should receive a comparable level of quality care regardless of where that care is provided within the hospital (TJC, 2012a). This standard ensures that women having cesarean births with regional or general anesthesia should have perioperative care consistent with those patients who have had general surgical procedures. It is important to distinguish between the concepts of comparable care and equivalent care. Comparable care to that which is provided in the main hospital surgical department is recommended by TJC (2012a); however, equivalent care is not required. The special needs of obstetric patients, their babies, and their families must be considered when planning care and designing protocols and clinical practices. For example, care during cesarean birth should include the woman's support person and family. In the main hospital surgical suite, family members are rarely allowed to be with patients during surgery. However, women having cesarean birth should be allowed to have a support person with them prior to and during the procedure and the recovery period. Some facilities allow more than one support person. Skin-to-skin contact between the healthy mother and baby is recommended after birth while the patient is in the surgical suite. Patient desires and patient safety should guide practice. During the recovery period, the newborn should be allowed to stay with the mother as long as the condition of the mother and baby are stable. Support should be provided so that breastfeeding can be initiated as soon as possible if the woman has chosen to breastfeed.

When unplanned cesarean birth occurs, and the decision is made to proceed, the surgical team should be notified so they can begin preparations. In some facilities, this will involve calling in a surgical team whose members are not in-house, while other facilities maintain a full surgical team around the clock. A full surgical team includes a surgeon, anesthesia provider, surgical first assistant, scrub tech, circulating nurse, and person whose sole responsibility is for potential neonatal resuscitation. All hospitals offering labor and birth services should be equipped to perform an emergency cesarean birth (AAP & ACOG, 2012). In general, the consensus has been that hospitals should have the capacity of beginning a cesarean birth within 30 minutes of the decision to operate (AAP & ACOG, 2012; ACOG & ASA, 2009). However, the scientific evidence to support this threshold is lacking (AAP & ACOG, 2012; ACOG, 2010a). The decision-to-incision interval should be based on the timing that best incorporates maternal and fetal risks and benefits (AAP & ACOG, 2012; ACOG, 2010a). Some high-risk conditions (e.g., morbid obesity, eclampsia, cardiopulmonary compromise, hemorrhage) may require maternal stabilization time before performing emergent cesarean birth (AAP & ACOG, 2012; ACOG, 2010a). On the other hand, some clinical situations require more expeditious birth because they can directly or indirectly cause fetal death or other adverse maternal–fetal outcomes. These include hemorrhage from placenta previa, placental abruption, umbilical cord prolapse, uterine rupture, and an abnormal EFM tracing (AAP & ACOG, 2012; ACOG, 2010a; Silver, 2007).

When the indication for cesarean is an abnormal (Category III) EFM tracing, preparation often requires an assessment of several logistic issues depending on the setting and clinical circumstances (ACOG, 2010a) (see Display 14–14). Sterile materials and supplies needed for emergent cesarean birth are kept sealed but properly arranged and available so that the instrument table can be made ready at once for an obstetric emergency (AAP & ACOG, 2012). Whenever possible, a surgical suite should be kept available for emergent cases. If keeping at least one surgical suite continuously available to handle emergencies is not possible, at a minimum, elective or nonemergent cases should be staggered to allow rapid readiness if an emergency occurs that requires expeditious cesarean birth.

Plans should be in place to call in back-up team members, such as surgeons and anesthesia providers, when those providers primarily responsible for covering the service for obstetric emergencies are not readily available. A list of emergency back-up team members and the quickest method to reach each of them should be available at all times to the labor and delivery charge nurse. Access to direct telephone numbers of those on-call is more likely to result in the fastest communication rather than beepers, which require additional time to send the signal and await response. If the attending physician is notified of an obstetric emergency likely to require emergent cesarean birth while not in-house, including but not limited to, fetal bradycardia, umbilical cord prolapse, significant bleeding, suspected placental abruption, or uterine rupture, and he or she orders preparations for the surgery, hospital policy should allow preparations to begin prior to the arrival of the attending physician. Hospital policies requiring that the physician be in-house to order preparations for emergent cesarean birth can delay the process and potentially contribute to an adverse maternal or fetal outcome.

In July 2004, The Joint Commission, in their Sentinel Event Alert *Preventing Infant Death and Injury During Delivery,* recommended conducting periodic drills for emergent cesarean birth (JCAHO, 2004b). Similar recommendations for drills in emergent situations were offered by ACOG (2011a). Drills for emergent cesarean birth can be helpful in shortening the time from decision to incision. One study found that teamwork training with drills involving all members of the interdisciplinary perinatal team was associated with a shorter decision-to-incision time (21.2 minutes vs. 33.3 minutes) for immediate cesarean birth compared to perinatal teams that had not participated in teamwork training (Nielsen et al., 2007). Use of a contingency team (obstetric and anesthesia attending physicians, chief resident, labor nurse, and surgical scrub nurse), similar to a code team, may have contributed to the improvement. In another study, leaders in a large level III community healthcare center with >5,500 births annually, used a performance improvement process to improve their ability to begin cesarean birth within 30 minutes of the decision to do so (Nageotte & Vander Wal, 2012). While initial baseline data showed that only 25% for cases of fetal intolerance to labor were within the 30 minute time frame, after 3 years of process improvement including collaboration of all caregivers, ongoing data collection and analysis, peer review, and a willingness to change systems, 90% of the cases succeeded in achieving the standard and 100% of cases initiated were initiated within 40 minutes. Specific areas identified that facilitated achieving this goal were complete physician and nursing participation, their understanding of the standard and its importance, and practicing again and again in cases of

---

DISPLAY 14-14

Potential Logistical Considerations in Preparation for Operative Birth in the Context of an Abnormal (Category III) Fetal Heart Rate Tracing

- Obtain informed consent from the woman (verbal or written as feasible).
- Provide information to the woman and her support person/family regarding what is being recommended and the urgency based on maternal and/or fetal status.
- Assemble the surgical team (surgeon, anesthesia personnel, scrub technician, circulating nurse, and baby nurse).
- Assess transit time to the surgical suite and location for operative birth.
- Ensure IV access.
- Review the status of laboratory tests (e.g., complete blood type and screen) and assess the need for availability of blood products.
- Assess the need for preoperative placement of an indwelling Foley catheter and insert if feasible.
- Assemble personnel for neonatal resuscitation, notify members of the neonatal team in-house or on-call, and request their immediate attendance at the birth.

Adapted from American College of Obstetricians and Gynecologists. (2010). *Management of intrapartum fetal heart rate tracings* (Practice Bulletin No. 116). Washington, DC: Author. doi:10.1097/AOG.0b013e3182004fa9

fetal intolerance to labor to decrease their decision-to-incision time (Nageotte & Vander Wal, 2012).

Comprehensive information regarding perioperative care of the woman having a cesarean birth can be found in the evidence-based clinical practice guideline *Perioperative Care of the Pregnant Woman* (AWHONN, 2011b). Recommended practices regarding surgical attire, prevention of retained surgical items, electrosurgery, and maintaining a sterile field are adapted directly from the Association of periOperative Registered Nurses (AORN, 2011) (Table 14–7). Other topics highlighted in the guideline include patient safety and quality improvement, nonobstetric surgery in pregnancy, preoperative education for surgical birth, considerations for an unscheduled surgical birth, care of the obese woman, and postoperative complications (AWHONN, 2011b). A summary of guidelines for perioperative cesarean birth care from AWHONN, ACOG, AAP, ASA, AORN, the

Table 14–7. SUMMARY OF SELECTED AORN PERIOPERATIVE STANDARDS

Surgical Attire
- All individuals who enter the semirestricted and restricted areas of the surgical suite should wear freshly laundered surgical attire or disposable surgical attire intended for use only within the surgical suite.
- Personnel should cover head and facial hair, including sideburns and nape of the neck, when in semirestricted and restricted areas of surgical suite.
- All individuals entering restricted areas of OR suite should wear a mask when open sterile items and equipment are present.
- All personnel entering semirestricted and restricted areas of the surgical suite should confine or remove all jewelry and watches.
- Fingernails should be kept short, clean, natural, and healthy.
- Protective barriers must be made available to reduce the risk of exposure to potentially infectious materials.

Prevention of Retained Surgical Items: Sponge, Sharp, and Instrument Counts
- All counts should include at least one RN.
- Radiopaque surgical soft items (sponges, towels) should be counted on all procedures in which possibility exists that a sponge could be retained.
- Sharps and other miscellaneous items should be counted on all procedures.
- Instruments should be counted for all procedures in which a likelihood exists that an instrument could be retained.
- Additional measures for investigation, reconciliation, documentation, and prevention of retained surgical items should be taken.
- Sponge, sharp, and instrument counts should be documented on the patient's intraoperative record by the RN circulator.

Sponge counts:
- Before the procedure to establish a baseline
- Before closure of a cavity within a cavity
- Before wound closure begins
- At skin closure or the end of the procedure
- At the time of permanent relief of either the scrub or circulator

Instrument counts:
- Before the procedure to establish a baseline
- Before wound closure
- At the time of permanent relief of either the scrub or circulator

Electrosurgery
- Personnel should demonstrate competence in use of ESU and accessories.
- The ESU system should be used in a manner that minimizes the potential for injuries.
- The electrical cord and plugs of the ESU should be handled in a manner that minimizes the potential for damage and subsequent patient injuries.
- The active electrode should be used in a manner that minimizes the potential for injuries.
- When monopolar electrosurgery is used, a dispersive electrode should be used in a manner that minimizes the potential for injuries.
- Potential hazards associated with surgical smoke generated in the practice setting should be identified, and safe practices established.

Maintaining a Sterile Field
- Scrubbed persons should function within a sterile field.
- Sterile drapes should be used to establish a sterile field.
- Items used within sterile field should be sterile.
- All items introduced to a sterile field should be opened, dispensed, and transferred by methods that maintain sterility and integrity.
- A sterile field should be maintained and monitored constantly.
- All personnel moving within or around a sterile field should do so in a manner that maintains the sterile field.

ESU, electrosurgery unit; OR, operating room; RN, registered nurse.
From Association of Women's Health, Obstetric and Neonatal Nurses. (2011b). *Perioperative Care of the Pregnant Woman: Evidence-Based Clinical Practice Guideline.* Washington, DC: Author.
Adapted from the Association of periOperative Registered Nurses. (2011). *Perioperative Standards and Recommended Practices for Inpatient and Ambulatory Settings.* Denver, CO: Author.

American Society of PeriAnesthesia Nurses (ASPAN), and the American Heart Association (AHA) are incorporated into Preoperative Care Intraoperative Care (Display 14–15), Intraoperative Care (Display 14–16), and Post-Anesthesia Recovery Care (Display 14–17).

Advanced cardiac life support (ACLS) competence validation for perinatal nurses who provide post-anesthesia care for obstetric patients is not required (AWHONN, 2010a). However, each hospital must ensure that teams capable of providing ACLS care (e.g., a code team) and the means to provide invasive monitoring or extensive ventilatory support to obstetric patients are available at all times (AWHONN, 2010a). Because the need to implement ACLS skills during the care of obstetric patients is rare, perinatal nurses lack opportunity to use ACLS knowledge and skills and, therefore, to maintain proficiency. Mobilizing the code team when maternal resuscitation requiring ACLS care is needed during the perioperative period may be more appropriate (AWHONN, 2010a). AWHONN (2010a) supports the Joint Commission recommendation that all nurses achieve and maintain competence in basic life support (BLS). Cardiac monitoring of women post-cesarean birth is not required by ASA (2009); however, if similar types of patients in the main

---

DISPLAY 14–15

Perioperative Cesarean Birth Care

PREOPERATIVE CARE

- Obtain an admission assessment comparable to that for all women admitted for labor and birth.
- Provide individualized, family-centered care and a thorough explanation of what to expect in preparation for, during, and after the surgery to the woman and her support person.
- Use an institution-approved safety checklist during preoperative, intraoperative, and postoperative recovery periods according to facility guidelines.
- Obtain a 20- to 30-minute baseline fetal heart rate (FHR) tracing by electronic fetal monitoring (EFM). If the woman is not in active labor and the FHR is normal, EFM may be discontinued after this initial assessment.
- If EFM is being used for a laboring woman, fetal surveillance should continue until the abdominal sterile preparation has begun. If an internal fetal scalp electrode is in use, it should be continued until the abdominal sterile preparation is complete.
- For an emergent cesarean, preparation often requires an assessment of several logistic issues depending on the setting and clinical circumstances, incorporating maternal and fetal risks and benefits. Some maternal conditions (e.g., morbid obesity, eclampsia, cardiopulmonary compromise) may require stabilization time prior to the cesarean.
- Administer preoperative medications according to the healthcare provider order.
- Administer prophylactic antibiotics within 60 minutes before the start of the cesarean birth, according to healthcare provider orders. When this is not possible (e.g., need for emergent cesarean), prophylaxis should be administered as soon as possible after the incision is made.
- In the case of an unplanned cesarean or planned cesarean with rupture of membranes, collaborate with healthcare provider to determine need for intrapartum group B streptococcus (GBS) prophylaxis.
- Document the time of the woman's last solid and liquid oral intake.

- Assess for conditions that may increase her risk for aspiration (e.g., morbid obesity, diabetes, difficult airway, general anesthesia).
- Administer medications (e.g., sodium citrate, sodium bicarbonate, ranitidine, famotidine, metoclopramide) to reduce maternal complications resulting from aspiration according to anesthesia provider orders and facility guidelines.
- Facilitate preoperative blood work according to anesthesia provider orders and facility guidelines. Routine preoperative blood work, including platelet counts, typing, and screening, are generally not indicated in previously healthy women undergoing cesarean birth. The decision to assess preoperative laboratory values should be based on the physical examination, the potential risk for hemorrhage, and facility policies.
- Initiate intravenous (IV) fluids if not already infusing. Consider administering warmed IV fluids and boluses whenever possible.
- Confirm that informed consent is signed.
- Cleanse the lower abdomen to clear the surgical site of soil, debris, and exudate if needed. Consider using preoperative skin cleansing wipes on the abdomen prior to transfer to the surgical suite according to facility guidelines. Do not remove hair unless it will interfere with the surgical incision. If hair needs to be removed, use hair clippers immediately before moving into the surgical suite.
- Insert a Foley catheter; note the amount and color of urine; delay until after anesthesia if possible epidural catheter is placed and dosed, if possible.
- Placement of pneumatic compression devices before cesarean birth is recommended for all women not already receiving thromboprophylaxis. Women undergoing cesarean birth with additional risk factors for thromboembolism, may require thromboprophylaxis with both pneumatic compression devices and anticoagulation therapy. Cesarean birth in the emergency setting should not be delayed because of the timing necessary to implement thromboprophylaxis.
- Implement hypothermia prevention measures (prewarming) 15 minutes prior to the administration of anesthesia and throughout surgery whenever possible (e.g., warmed cotton blankets, forced air warming blanket).
- Transport the woman to the surgical suite.
- Provide hand-off communication according to facility protocol.

For sources, see footnote to Display 14–17.

DISPLAY 14-16

Perioperative Cesarean Birth Care

INTRAOPERATIVE CARE

- Use a facility-approved safety checklist during preoperative, intraoperative, and postoperative recovery periods according to institution guidelines.
- Obtain baseline vital signs prior to the initiation of anesthesia (temperature, pulse, respiration rate, blood pressure, baseline pulse oximeter reading).
- If regional anesthesia is being used, administer preload and/or co-load according to anesthesia provider orders and facility guidelines. Ideally, preload should be administered within approximately 20–30 minutes to ensure optimal prophylactic efficiency. Ideally, co-load should be administered immediately after the initiation of regional anesthesia.
- Conduct a preprocedure verification process according to facility policy and procedure, including relevant documentation (e.g., signed consent form, nursing assessment, preanesthesia assessment), diagnostic test results (e.g., blood work), and any required blood products or special equipment.
- Perform a time-out before the administration of anesthesia and document the completion of the procedure. A second time-out is required prior to the surgery.
- Assist the mother into the appropriate position during the administration of regional anesthesia.
- If general anesthesia is indicated, assist with proper positioning for intubation and cricoid pressure as requested by the anesthesia care provider.
- Position the woman on the surgical table ensuring lateral displacement of the uterus with a hip wedge.
- Insert the urinary catheter according to healthcare provider order and facility guidelines.
- The placement of pneumatic compression devices before a cesarean birth is recommended for all women not already receiving thromboprophylaxis. Women undergoing a cesarean birth with additional risk factors for thromboembolism may require thromboprophylaxis with both pneumatic compression devices and anticoagulation therapy. A cesarean birth in the emergency setting should not be delayed because of the timing necessary to implement thromboprophylaxis.
- If electronic fetal monitoring (EFM) is being used for a laboring woman, fetal surveillance should continue until the abdominal sterile preparation has begun. If an internal fetal scalp electrode is in use, it should be continued until the abdominal sterile preparation is complete.
- Cleanse the lower abdomen and surrounding area using an FDA-approved antiseptic agent for preoperative abdominal preparation according to healthcare provider orders and institution guidelines.
- Dry flammable skin preparation solutions before applying drapes. Place extra absorbing linens on either side of the abdomen prior to the skin preparation and remove as indicated if pooling of antiseptic solution is noted.

- Apply grounding device according to manufacturer's instructions.
- Assist the support person to a position at the head of the surgical table according to the institution protocol.
- Continue warming measures throughout surgery, whenever possible.
- Maintain operating room temperature at 20°–25°C (68°–77°F).
- If prophylactic antibiotics were not administered prior to the incision, prophylaxis should be administered as soon as possible after the incision is made according to healthcare provider orders.
- Confirm equipment and supplies required for normal newborn care and neonatal resuscitation are readily available according to institution guidelines.
- At least two registered nurses (RNs) should attend every cesarean birth. One RN, the circulating nurse, attends to the mother. A second RN attends to the baby. In the case of a multiple birth, one RN should be present for each baby. An additional staff member should be assigned to scrub.
- At least one person should be solely responsible for the newborn and capable of initiating resuscitation, including the administration of positive-pressure ventilation and assisting with chest compressions. Either this person or an additional person immediately available to the birthing area should have the additional skills required to perform a complete resuscitation, including endotracheal intubation and the administration of medications. Having someone on-call (either at home or in a remote area of the hospital) for newborn resuscitation is not sufficient. When resuscitation is needed, it must be initiated without delay.
- If the birth is anticipated to be high risk (e.g., meconium staining of the amniotic fluid), more advanced neonatal resuscitation may be required. In these cases, at least two persons should be present solely to manage the neonate: one with completed resuscitation skills and one or more to assist.
- The newborn should remain in the surgical suite with the mother and support person whenever possible. If mother and baby are in stable condition, facilitate skin-to-skin contact.
- Perform the duties of a circulating nurse according to the facility protocol.
- Ensure that the sponge, needle, and instrument counts are correct according to the facility protocol.
- Assist with the application of abdominal dressing.
- Before leaving the surgical suite, verbally confirm the name of the procedure; the completion of instrument, sponge, and needle counts; specimen labeling; and whether there are any equipment problems.
- Assist in transferring the woman from the surgical table using gentle, smooth movements to decrease her potential for nausea and vomiting.
- For the overweight/obese woman, use an ergonomically safe transfer method.
- Note maternal and newborn status before transport to the post-anesthesia care.
- Assist with transport.
- Provide hand-off communication according to facility protocol.

For sources, see footnote to Display 14–17.

DISPLAY 14–17

Perioperative Cesarean Birth Care

POST–ANESTHESIA RECOVERY CARE

- Use a facility-approved safety checklist during preoperative, intraoperative, and postoperative recovery periods according to facility guidelines
- Confirm the following equipment and supplies are at the bedside as per facility guidelines. These include, but are not limited to:

    Artificial airways

    Oxygen

    Suction

    Equipment to monitor blood pressure, pulse, temperature, oxygen saturation, and blood glucose

- One registered nurse (RN) should be assigned solely to the care of the mother until the critical elements for the mother have been met. Critical elements for the mother are defined as (1) the report has been received from the anesthesia provider, questions answered, and the transfer of care has taken place; (2) the woman is conscious with adequate respiratory status; (3) the initial assessment is completed and documented; and (4) the woman is hemodynamically stable. A second nurse must be available to assist as necessary.
- Use an institution-approved scoring system such as the Aldrete Score (Table 14–8) or Post-Anesthetic Discharge Scoring System (PADSS) to determining the appropriate timing for discharge from phase I and transition to mother–baby care. Discharge from phase I care should be decided in conjunction with the anesthesia care provider.
- Phase I post-anesthesia recovery is a level of care, rather than a location or time frame.
- In post-anesthesia phase I, the nursing roles focus on providing post-anesthesia nursing care in the immediate post-anesthesia period, transitioning to phase II, the inpatient setting, or to an intensive care setting for continued care. Basic life-sustaining needs are of the highest priority. Constant vigilance is required.
- In post-anesthesia phase II, the nursing roles focus on preparation for care in the home or the extended care environment.
- One RN should be assigned solely to the care of the baby until the critical elements for the baby have been met. In the case of multiples, there should be one RN for each baby. Critical elements for the baby's care before the mother's nurse accepts the baby as part of the patient care assignment are defined as (1) the report has been received from the baby nurse, questions answered, and the transfer of care has taken place; (2) the initial assessment and care are completed and documented; (3) identification bracelets have been applied; and (4) the baby's condition is stable.
- Assess the newborn every 30 minutes for the first 2 hours and according to institution guidelines. Assessments include, but may not be limited to, the following:

    Pulse

    Respiratory rate and type

    Skin color

    Level of consciousness

    Tone

    Activity

- After the critical elements have been met, and mother and baby are stable, one RN can assume care for both the mother and the baby, with the second RN available to assist as necessary.
- If the mother has chosen to breast-feed, the baby should be placed at the breast within an hour of birth.
- Assess the maternal status according to facility and professional organization guidelines. Assessments include but may not be limited to the following:

    Level of consciousness (LOC) (orientation to time, place, person, or to pre-op level)

    Blood pressure and pulse (every 15 minutes for 2 hours)

    Color (every 15 minutes)

    Oxygen saturation (every 15 minutes)

    Dressing condition

    Intake and output

    Sensory and motor function

    Temperature (every 15 minutes until normothermic)

- Continue hypothermia prevention (e.g., warmed cotton blankets, forced air warming blanket) as needed.
- Pneumatic compression devices should be left in place until the woman is ambulatory. When reinstitution of anticoagulation therapy is planned postpartum for selected women, pneumatic compression devices should be left in place until the patient is ambulatory and until anticoagulation therapy is restarted according to healthcare provider orders.
- Assess fundal height, tone, and location as well as amount, character, and color of lochia frequently during the initial recovery period and according to facility guidelines.
- Assess for bladder distention. Evaluate the tubing and the catheter for patency.
- Assess for nausea on admission to recovery, on discharge, and more often as indicated. Intravenous (IV) fluid boluses may decrease nausea due to hypotension.
- Administer medications to alleviate or minimize nausea and vomiting (e.g., ondansetron, granisetron, metoclopramide, promethazine, scopolamine) according to healthcare provider orders.
- Assess the woman for pain with each vital sign assessment using a standardized pain scale.
- Provide pharmacologic and nonpharmacologic pain relief measures per obstetric healthcare provider orders and at maternal request.
- Reassess pain at appropriate intervals following both nonpharmacologic and pharmacologic interventions.
- Monitor for side effects related to the administration of IV and intrathecal opioids.
- Assess the woman for pruritus. Administer antipruritic medications (e.g., naloxone, nalbuphine, diphenhydramine, ondansetron, granisetron) according to healthcare provider orders.
- If a woman is breastfeeding, ensure the analgesic medications prescribed for her are considered safe for breastfeeding women.
- Provide support and assistance with infant care and breast-feeding to mothers receiving analgesia after having a surgical birth.

- Provide oral nutrition according to institution guidelines and as tolerated. Offer oral hydration within 2 hours, as indicated. Offer small meals within 8 hours, as indicated.
- Assess for potential postoperative complications relevant to the decision to offer oral nutrition (e.g., abdominal distention, bloating, gassiness, persistent abdominal pain, nausea and/or vomiting, inability to pass flatus, inability to tolerate oral diet).

- Provide hand-off communication according to facility protocol.
- In some perinatal units, discharge from recovery care will not result in the physical transfer of the woman; rather, care will continue in the same room.

Displays 14–15, 14–16, and 14–17 adapted from American Academy of Pediatrics & American College of Obstetricians and Gynecologists. (2012). *Guidelines for Perinatal Care,* (7th ed.). Elk Grove Village, IL: Author; American Academy of Pediatrics & American Heart Association. (2011). *Textbook of Neonatal Resuscitation,* (6th ed.). Elk Grove Village, IL: Author; American College of Obstetricians and Gynecologists. (2007b). *Fetal Monitoring Prior to Scheduled Cesarean Delivery* (Committee Opinion No. 382). Washington, DC: Author; American College of Obstetricians and Gynecologists. (2010a). *Management of Intrapartum Fetal Heart Rate Tracings* (Practice Bulletin No. 116). Washington, DC: Author; American College of Obstetricians and Gynecologists. (2011d). *Thromboembolism in Pregnancy* (Practice Bulletin No. 123). Washington, DC: Author; American College of Obstetricians and Gynecologists. (2011e). *Use of Prophylactic Antibiotics in Labor and Delivery* (Practice Bulletin No. 84). Washington, DC: Author; American College of Obstetricians and Gynecologists. (2012a). *Communication Strategies for Patient Handoffs* (Committee Opinion No. 517). Washington, DC: Author; American Society of Anesthesiologists. (2007). Practice guidelines for obstetrical anesthesia: An updated report by the American Society of Anesthesiologists Task Force on Obstetrical Anesthesia. *Anesthesiology, 106,* 843–863; American Society of PeriAnesthesia Nurses. (2010). *2010–2012 Perianesthesia Nursing Standards and Practice Recommendations.* Cherry Hill, NJ: Author; Association of periOperative Registered Nurses. (2011). *Perioperative Standards and Recommended Practices for Inpatient and Ambulatory Settings.* Denver, CO: Author; Association of Women's Health, Obstetric and Neonatal Nurses. (2010b). *Guidelines for Professional Registered Nurse Staffing for Perinatal Units.* Washington, DC: Author; Association of Women's Health, Obstetric and Neonatal Nurses. (2011b). *Perioperative Care of the Pregnant Woman: Evidence-Based Clinical Practice Guideline.* Washington, DC: Author.

---

hospital post-anesthesia care unit (PACU) are receiving cardiac monitoring, obstetric patients may also. Remote cardiac monitoring is one option that provides a competent individual to assess cardiac data on an ongoing basis without requiring obstetric nurses to do so. Usually the period of cardiac monitoring post-cesarean birth is brief, so this option works well for some facilities. When obstetric nurses are required to interpret findings from cardiac monitoring, adequate education and competence validation processes should be developed.

A method should be in place to ensure that equipment is available for PACU care and maintained according to manufacturer specifications (ASPAN, 2010). The unit should have equipment to administer oxygen, provide constant and intermittent suction, monitor BP, and monitor patient temperature. There should be adjustable lighting and enough space for patient privacy. An electroencephalography (EEG) monitor, bags and masks of the appropriate size, equipment to assess blood glucose, and a pulse oximeter should be readily available. Emergency equipment, including a defibrillator, an emergency communication system, and knowledgeable emergency assistive personnel should be readily available (ASPAN, 2010).

Every effort should be made to avoid hypothermia, beginning in the preoperative phase and continuing into the postoperative phase of perioperative care. Perioperative hypothermia is defined as a core temperature less than 36°C (96.8°F) (ASPAN, 2010; AORN, 2012). Normothermia is a core temperature range of 36°C to 38°C (96.8°F to 100.4°F). Unplanned hypothermia is one of the most common complications of surgery (AORN, 2012). Perioperative hypothermia has been correlated with adverse effects that range from patient discomfort and decreased satisfaction to adverse cardiac

events, altered drug metabolism, increased blood loss, impaired wound healing, and increased surgical wound infections (Hooper et al., 2010). When a woman is anesthetized for cesarean birth, she loses heat intraoperatively and is unable to restore body heat through the normal mechanism of shivering or increased muscle activity (AORN, 2012). The greatest decline temperature occurs during the first hour of surgery and can result in a core temperature drop of approximately 1.6°C (2.7°F) (ASPAN, 2010; AORN, 2012).

Additional factors that have the potential to increase a woman's risk for perioperative hypothermia during a cesarean birth include low ambient room temperature, length of surgical procedure, anesthesia, low BMI, and preoperative systolic BP less than 140 mm Hg (Hooper et al., 2010); however, there is insufficient evidence to support these risk factors as definitive (ASPAN, 2010). Prewarming, defined as warming of peripheral tissues or surface skin before the induction of anesthesia, is recommended to reduce complications associated with perioperative hypothermia and to improve patient satisfaction (Hooper et al., 2010; ASPAN, 2010; AORN, 2012). The perinatal nurse can minimize the risk of hypothermia by prewarming the woman with warm cotton blankets prior to and/or upon arrival in the surgical suite and after sterile drapes are removed, thus limiting the amount of skin surface exposed, limiting time between prepping of the skin and draping, preventing surgical drapes from becoming wet, adjusting the room temperature, warming IV and irrigation fluids, and using forced air warming devices (AORN, 2012). Postoperatively, if the woman's temperature remains normothermic, her temperature should be assessed at least hourly, at discharge from recovery, and as indicated by her condition (ASPAN, 2010; Hopper et al., 2010;

AWHONN, 2011b). If the woman is hypothermic, her temperature should be monitored at least every 15 minutes while providing active warming measures until normothermia is achieved (ASPAN, 2010; Hooper et al., 2010; AWHONN, 2011b).

Phase I post-anesthesia recovery focuses on providing post-anesthesia nursing in the immediate post-anesthesia period, transitioning to phase II in the inpatient setting, or to an intensive care setting for continued care (ASPAN, 2010). Basic life-sustaining needs are of the highest priority; therefore, constant vigilance is required during phase I (ASPAN, 2010). It is important to consider that phase I post-anesthesia recovery is a level of care, rather than a location or time frame. During postoperative recovery, the nurse-to-patient ratio on the perinatal unit should be comparable to that of the main hospital PACU. Phase I recovery for general surgical patients usually occurs in the PACU; however, obstetric patients may be cared for during phase I in a labor and delivery room (LDR) or a labor/delivery/recovery/postpartum room (LDRP) if there is the availability of continuous one nurse–to–one woman care and one nurse for the baby until the critical elements are met when the baby remains with the mother (AWHONN, 2010b).

Critical elements for the mother's post-anesthesia care after cesarean birth before the mother's nurse accepts the baby as part of the patient care assignment are defined as (1) the report has been received from the anesthesia provider, questions answered, and the transfer of care has taken place; (2) the woman is conscious, with adequate respiratory status; (3) the initial assessment is completed and documented; (4) the woman is hemodynamically stable (AWHONN, 2010b). Critical elements for the baby's care before the mother's nurse accepts the baby as part of the patient care assignment are defined as (1) the report has been received from the baby nurse, questions answered, and the transfer of care has taken place; (2) the initial assessment and care are completed and documented; (3) identification bracelets have been applied; and (4) the baby's condition is stable (AWHONN, 2010b). Post-anesthesia recovery care for the mother is as follows: BP levels and maternal pulse should be monitored every 15 minutes for 2 hours and more frequently and of longer duration if complications are encountered; maternal postpartum observation should be designed for the timely identification of excessive blood loss, including hypotension and tachycardia; the amount of vaginal bleeding should be evaluated continuously and the uterine fundus identified, massaged, and assessed for size and degree of contraction; and there should be timely response to changes in maternal vital signs and clinical condition as this is critical to patient safety (AAP & ACOG, 2012; AWHONN, 2010b). Care for the baby at birth is as follows: the baby's airway should be cleared, tactile stimulation provided, and respirations and heart rate evaluated.

An Apgar score should be determined at 1 minute and 5 minutes after birth. If the 5-minute Apgar score is less than 7, additional scores should be assigned every 5 minutes for up to 20 minutes. Temperature, heart rate, and respiratory rates, skin color, adequacy of peripheral circulation, type of respiration, level of consciousness, tone, and activity should be monitored and recorded at least once every 30 minutes until the newborn's condition has remained stable for 2 hours (AAP & ACOG, 2012). If the mother has chosen to breast-feed, the baby should be placed at the breast within the first hour after birth (AAP & ACOG, 2012).

A PACU discharge scoring tool, as shown in Table 14–8, is helpful in conducting a systematic assessment and determining readiness for discharge from post-anesthesia care. Whenever a patient is transferred from one level of care to another level of care requiring a change in caregivers, communicate all pertinent information to

Table 14–8. POST-ANESTHESIA DISCHARGE SCORING

	Criteria	Score
Respiration	Able to breathe deeply and cough freely	2
	Dyspnea/shallow or limited breathing	1
	Apnea	0
Oxygen Saturation	Able to maintain O_2 saturation >92% on room air	2
	Needs O_2 inhalation to maintain O_2 saturation >90%	1
	O_2 saturation <90% even with O_2 supplementation	0
Consciousness	Fully awake	2
	Arousable on calling	1
	Not responding	0
Circulation	BP ± 20 mm Hg pre-anesthetic level	2
	BP ± 20–49 mm Hg of pre-anesthetic level	1
	BP ± 50 mm Hg of pre-anesthetic level	0
Activity	Able to move four extremities	2
	Able to move two extremities	1
	Able to move zero extremities	0
	TOTAL:	——

Example of Aldrete Scoring System, commonly used to determine when patients may be safely discharged from a post-anesthesia care unit phase I level of care to either postsurgical ward or phase II level of care. Individual facilities will determine score (e.g., usually ≥8).
Adapted from Aldrete, J. A. (1995). The post anaesthesia recovery score revisited [Letter]. *Journal of Clinical Anesthesiology, 7*(1), 89–91; Ead, H. (2006). From Aldrete to PADSS: Reviewing discharge criteria after ambulatory surgery. *Journal of PeriAnesthesia Nursing, 21*(4), 259–267; American Society of PeriAnesthesia Nurses. (2010). *Perianesthesia Nursing Standards and Practice Recommendations 2010–2012.* Cherry Hill, NJ: Author; Association of periOperative Registered Nurses. (2012). *Perioperative Standards and Recommended Practices for Inpatient and Ambulatory Settings.* Denver, CO: Author.

the next caregiver. The hand off should be interactive, encouraging questions, with limited interruptions and include a process for verification and an opportunity to review all relevant patient data (ACOG, 2012a). Transfers or patient hand offs present a risk of missing key information with the potential to adversely affect patient status, thus development of a checklist for important clinical content to be included in the hand-off report can be beneficial (Simpson, 2005). Suggested components of a comprehensive transfer report are included in Display 14–18. These components may vary based on the type of care model. In some perinatal

---

DISPLAY 14–18

Suggested Components of Communication (Hand-off) During Transfer from Post-Anesthesia Recovery Care to Postpartum Care for Women After Cesarean Birth

- Vital signs
- Level of consciousness
- Muscular strength and ability to move lower extremities
- Allergies
- Condition of the operative site and dressing
- Fundal height
- Lochia characteristics and amount
- Condition of the perineum if vaginal birth was attempted
- Location and patency of any tubes and/or drains including indwelling urinary catheter
- Intake and output (e.g., intravenous [IV] fluids, oral fluids, estimated blood loss, urinary output)
- Type of analgesia/anesthesia and response
- Medications given and response to those medications (e.g., antibiotics, narcotics)
- Venous thromboembolism (VTE) prophylaxis
- Pain level, interventions for pain, and response to those interventions
- Nausea and vomiting
- Tests ordered with pertinent results, if available
- Initiation of breastfeeding and quality of first breastfeeding experience (e.g., successful latch-on; mother's confidence), if applicable
- Status of the baby (e.g., admitted to special care nursery or neonatal intensive care unit [NICU] and preliminary diagnosis)
- Psychosocial status
- Involvement of the significant other and family
- Plans for immediate care of the baby (e.g., rooming-in if support person will be continuously available to assist the mother)
- If the baby is being relinquished for adoption, the mother's wishes for handling newborn care
- If the mother does not want any publicity or it to be known that she is a patient at the hospital or has given birth
- Discharge orders
- Attending physician
- Attending pediatrician

---

units, discharge from post-anesthesia care will not result in the physical transfer of the patient; rather, care will continue in the same room. Transfer of care from one caregiver to another may or may not occur at this time. In other units, discharge from post-anesthesia care will result in a physical transfer of the patient from the obstetric PACU to the mother–baby unit, and care will be transferred to another nurse.

Perioperative Patient Safety

Patient safety goals from The Joint Commission (2012b) include strategies to decrease the risk of potentially preventable surgical errors and perioperative harm. A recent closed-claims review of 444 surgical errors revealed that most errors (75%) occur during the intraoperative period, 25% during preoperative care, 35% during postoperative care, with approximately 33% occurring during multiple phases of care and approximately 66% involving more than one clinician (Rogers et al., 2006). Patients having a cesarean birth are particularly susceptible to two types of adverse surgical events: retained foreign bodies such as instruments, sponges, or needles and anesthesia awareness.

Risk of a retained instrument or sponge is significantly increased with emergency surgery, unplanned changes in procedure, not counting sponges or instruments, and higher body mass (Gawande, Studdert, Orav, Brennan, & Zinner, 2003). Cesarean birth is often emergent, at times proceeding without a complete count. A cesarean birth can develop into a significant postpartum hemorrhage and/or a cesarean hysterectomy. In some institutions, a cesarean hysterectomy may involve the addition of other experts to the original surgical team to assist with the procedure. Pregnant women have a higher body mass than the general population. Obesity and a higher BMI predispose obstetric patients to an increased risk of retained foreign bodies and anesthesia-related adverse events (Gawande et al., 2003). Every effort should be made to obtain a complete count of instruments, sponges, and needles prior to beginning a cesarean birth (AORN, 2012). However, if a count is not possible due to emergent conditions, an X-ray following the surgery while the patient is still on the surgical table is a reasonable option to decrease the likelihood of a retained instrument, sponge, or needle (Gawande et al., 2003). This option has merit for selected high-risk cases even when the counts are believed to be correct because in the overwhelming majority of cases of retained instruments, sponges, or needles, the final count is recorded as correct (Gawande et al., 2003). A unit policy should be in place to guide practice for surgical situations involving a high risk of retained foreign bodies.

Anesthesia awareness occurs under general anesthesia when a patient becomes cognizant of some or all of the events during surgery and has direct recall of those events (JCAHO, 2004a). Because of the routine use of neuromuscular blocking agents (also known as paralytics) during general anesthesia, the patient is often unable to communicate with the surgical team when this occurs (JCAHO, 2004a). Women having cesarean birth are at risk for anesthesia awareness because anesthesia providers usually give the mother light anesthesia to avoid causing depression in the newborn (Spitellie, Holmes, & Domino, 2002; Ghoneim, Block, Haffarnan, & Mathews, 2009). The most common patient perceptions of awareness are sounds and conversations, sensation of paralysis, anxiety and panic, helplessness and powerlessness, and pain. The least common are visual perceptions, feeling the intubation or tube, and feeling the operation without pain, although some patients do feel significant pain (Spitellie et al., 2002). The exact incidence of anesthesia awareness with recall in the United States is unknown but is estimated to be approximately 0.24%, or 26,000 cases per year based on 20 million general anesthetics per year (Sebel et al., 2004). Many patients who experience anesthesia awareness are adversely affected long after the surgery (Bischoff & Rundshagen, 2011; JCAHO, 2004a; Radovanovic & Radovanovic, 2011; Spitellie et al., 2002). The psychological sequelae of anesthesia awareness includes sleep disturbances, nightmares, anxiety and panic attacks, flashbacks, avoidance of medical care, and post-traumatic stress disorder (PTSD) (Bruchas, Kent, Wilson, & Domino, 2011; JCAHO, 2004a; Spitellie et al., 2002). Most patients who develop PTSD recover in a few months to a few years; however, it is estimated that 10% to 25% of patients who experience PTSD as a result of anesthesia awareness suffer from chronic PTSD. Implementing the JCAHO (2004a) recommendations for preventing and managing anesthesia awareness may decrease the risk to the woman having a cesarean birth.

The term "wrong-site surgery" is used to refer to any surgical procedure performed on the wrong patient, wrong body part, wrong side of the body, or at the wrong level of the correctly identified anatomic site (TJC, 2012b). The following definitions are useful to describe potential surgical errors (ACOG, 2010b). Wrong-side surgery indicates a surgical procedure performed on the wrong extremity or side of the patient's body (e.g., the left ovary rather than the right ovary). Wrong-patient surgery describes a surgical procedure performed on a different person than the one intended to receive the operation (e.g., circumcision of a baby whose parents did not intend or consent to circumcise or a tubal ligation performed during cesarean birth of a woman who did not consent to tubal ligation). Wrong-level surgery and wrong-part surgery are used to indicate surgical procedures that are performed at the correct operative site but at the wrong level or part of the operative field or patient's anatomy.

The following are factors that may contribute to an increased risk of surgical errors (ACOG, 2010b; TJC, 2012b; Rogers et al., 2006): emergent cases, multiple surgeons involved in the case, multiple procedures during a single surgical visit, changes in members of the surgical team during the procedure, unusual time pressures to start or complete the procedure, and unusual physical characteristics, including morbid obesity or physical deformity. Some of these factors apply to obstetric patients having a cesarean birth. A common theme in cases of surgical errors involves failed communication between the surgeon or surgeons, nurses, other members of the healthcare team, and the patient (ACOG, 2010b; Rogers et al., 2006). Communication is crucial throughout the surgical process, particularly during the preoperative assessment of the patient and the procedures used to verify the planned procedure. Effective preoperative patient assessment includes a review of the medical record or imaging studies immediately before starting surgery. To facilitate this step, all relevant information sources, verified by a predetermined checklist, should be available in the operating room and rechecked by the entire surgical team before the operation begins (ACOG, 2010b). A formal procedure for final confirmation of the correct patient and surgical procedure (a "time-out") that requires the participation of all members of the surgical team is helpful (TJC, 2012b). It is inappropriate to place total reliance on the surgeon or to assume that the surgeon should never be questioned (ACOG, 2010b). The risk of error may be reduced by involving the entire surgical team in the verification process and encouraging any member of that team to point out a possible error without fear of ridicule or reprimand (ACOG, 2010b).

Beepers, radios, telephone calls, and other potential distractions in the surgical environment should be kept to a minimum, if allowed at all, especially during critical stages of the operation such as the birth and during surgical counts (ACOG, 2010b). Nonessential conversation should be postponed until surgery is finished (ACOG, 2010b). Appropriate nurse staffing during a cesarean birth is essential for patient safety. A circulating nurse and another person whose sole responsibility is the baby in case neonatal resuscitation is necessary are minimally required in addition to the other members of the surgical team (AORN, 2012; AAP & AHA, 2011).

Because of the potential for serious harm from surgical errors, vigorous efforts are required to eliminate or reduce their frequency (ACOG, 2010b). Preventing these types of errors requires a team effort by all individuals participating in the surgical process. Although all members of the surgical team share in this responsibility, according to ACOG (2010b), the primary surgeon should oversee these efforts. The circulating nurse partners with the surgeon in ensuring that the process is as safe as it can be for mothers and babies during a cesarean birth. This may present a challenge to the circulating nurse if all members of the surgical team do not value or actively participate in perioperative safety procedures. Often, there is pressure to proceed with the case prior to completing all of the components of the perioperative safety protocol, including reviewing the preoperative checklist, the patient history, the reason for surgery, and time-out. While these pressures may occur in the face of an emergency, often they are the result of the desire by some members of the surgical team to complete the case as soon as possible for their convenience. Support from the perinatal leadership team is essential to promote universal active participation by all members of the surgical team with appropriate actionable follow-up for those who do not comply. Rarely is there an emergency during which the time-out process and all surgical counts cannot be safely implemented. In nearly all cases, there is time to conduct the surgical counting process; make sure it is the right patient, the right procedure, and the right site; and that documented consent has been procured.

In 2003, JCAHO published the *Universal Protocol for Preventing Wrong Site, Wrong Procedure, and Wrong Person Surgery*. The universal protocol is based on three levels of activity before initiation of any surgical procedure:

1. *Preoperative verification process*
   The healthcare team ensures that all relevant documents and studies are available before the procedure starts and that the documents have been reviewed and are consistent with each other, with the patient's expectations, and with the team's understanding of the intended patient, procedure, site, and as applicable, any implants. The team must address missing information or discrepancies before starting the procedure.

2. *Marking of the operative site*
   The healthcare team, including the patient (if possible), unambiguously identifies the intended site of incision or insertion by marking all operative sites involving laterality, multiple structures, or multiple levels. The site for cesarean birth is not included as part of this process.

3. *"Time-out" before starting the procedure*
   The operative team conducts a final verification of the correct patient, procedure, site, and as applicable, implants. A relatively new but essential element of this overall process is the formal enlistment of active involvement by the patient to avert errors in the operative arena. Involving the patient in this manner requires personal effort by the surgeon to educate the patient during the preoperative evaluation process. The patient, who has the greatest stake in avoiding errors, thus becomes integrally involved in helping ensure that errors are avoided.

SUPPORTING MOTHER–BABY ATTACHMENT AFTER CESAREAN BIRTH

Whether anticipated or unexpected, the need for surgical birth increases the family's anxiety, places additional strain on the maternal–newborn relationship, makes postpartum recovery more difficult for the woman and family, and creates a need for accepting the altered birth experience. Women who give birth via cesarean have special needs for information, the presence of the partner throughout cesarean birth, and sustained contact with their newborn (Fig. 14–19). An unplanned emergent cesarean birth can result in significant stress for the new mother. Continuity in caregivers, choice where possible, and control over specific aspects of care can reduce stress. In order to facilitate a positive birth experience and attachment to the newborn, consideration should be given to the ongoing attention of the family's understanding of cesarean birth, ways to maintain the father or support person's presence throughout the birth experience, and early and sustained contact with the newborn (Fig. 14–20). Support and encouragement in the surgical suite and immediately postpartum are key indicators of breastfeeding success after a cesarean birth (Zanardo et al., 2010). Encouraging sibling interaction promotes the attachment and integration of the baby into the family (Fig. 14–21).

If the mother who has had a cesarean birth requests rooming-in with her newborn in the immediate postoperative period, it is important that a support person be available to assist her with newborn care. Women in the immediate postoperative period are likely receiving parental or regional pain medications and may inadvertently fall asleep while holding their baby, thus increasing the risk of injuries to the baby. Women recovering from cesarean birth have limited mobility and may be unsteady on their feet the first

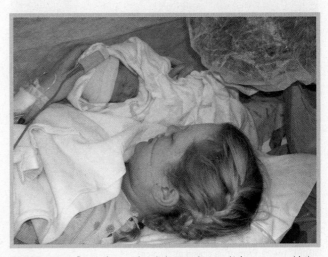

FIGURE 14–19. Promoting mother–baby attachment during cesarean birth.

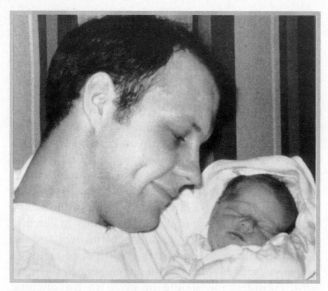

FIGURE 14–20. Promoting father involvement.

few times getting out of bed after surgery. They are at risk of falling when ambulating unassisted to care for their baby in the early recovery period. A policy requiring rooming-in for post-cesarean birth mothers is not appropriate for safety reasons; unit policies and practice should be based on the individual patient's condition and availability of a support person for assistance.

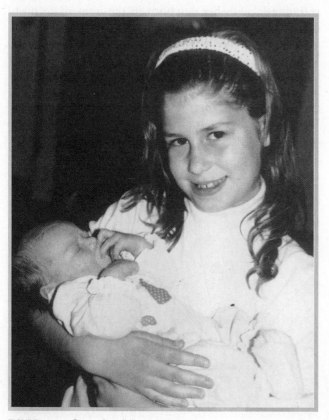

FIGURE 14–21. Promoting sibling attachment.

VAGINAL BIRTH AFTER PREVIOUS CESAREAN

A trial of labor after previous cesarean (TOLAC) offers these women the opportunity of achieving a VBAC. The VBAC rate (VBACs per 100 women with a prior cesarean birth) increased from approximately 5% in 1985 to a high of 28.3% by 1996, at which time the total cesarean birth rate dipped to 20.7%. Over the next 10 years, the VBAC rate fell dramatically to 8.5% in 2006, while the overall cesarean birth rate increased to 32.8% (Hamilton et al., 2011). The steep decline in the VBAC rate corresponds with an increasing repeat cesarean birth rate. Based on current data, once a woman has a cesarean birth, there is approximately a 92% chance that her next birth will be a cesarean (Martin et al., 2011). The continuing decrease in the VBAC rate, and subsequent increase in the repeat cesarean rate, may be related to reports of associate risks, physician or maternal preference, more conservative practice guidelines such as the requirement for immediate availability of a surgical team during a TOLAC, legal pressures, as well as the continuing debate regarding the potential risks and benefits of vaginal birth compared to cesarean birth (Martin et al., 2011).

In March 2010, the Eunice Kennedy Shriver National Institute of Child Health and Human Development and Office of Medical Application of NIH convened a Consensus Development Conference on VBAC to evaluate evidence regarding the safety and outcome of TOLAC and VBAC. The NIH panel recognized TOLAC as a reasonable option for many pregnant women with one prior low transverse uterine incision (NIH, 2010). Overall benefits of TOLAC are directly related to having a VBAC, which provides women the lowest morbidity (ACOG, 2010c; NIH, 2010). Women who successfully achieve VBAC avoid major abdominal surgery, resulting in lower rates of hemorrhage and infection, and have a shorter recovery compared with elective repeat cesareans (ACOG, 2010c). For women considering future pregnancies, VBAC may avoid consequences of multiple cesarean births including hysterectomy, bowel or bladder injury, transfusion, infection, placenta previa, and placenta accreta (ACOG, 2010c). Most maternal morbidity that occurs during TOLAC happens when a repeat cesarean birth becomes necessary (ACOG, 2010c; NIH, 2010). Therefore, VBAC is associated with the fewest complications than elective repeat cesareans; however, a failed TOLAC is associated with more complications than an elective repeat cesarean (ACOG, 2010c). In some cases, benefits for the mother may come as a price for the fetus, or vice versa, posing an ethical dilemma for the woman and her caregiver (NIH, 2010). When TOLAC and an elective repeat cesarean are medically equivalent options, the woman's preferences should be honored in a shared decision-making process (NIH, 2010).

Multiple studies of women attempting TOLAC have shown that 60% to 80% will result in successful vaginal births (ACOG, 2010c; Guise et al., 2010). However, an individual woman's chance for VBAC success varies depending on her demographic and obstetric characteristics (ACOG, 2010c). Display 14–19 lists factors to consider when deciding on TOLAC. Highly favorable influences for a successful VBAC are a previous vaginal delivery and spontaneous labor (ACOG, 2010c; Scott, 2011).

Uterine Rupture

Uterine rupture is the most serious complication of TOLAC, and can be life-threatening to both the mother and the neonate. The risk of clinically determined uterine rupture during TOLAC in women with low transverse uterine incision is approximately 0.5% to 0.9% (ACOG, 2010c), although absolute risk varies based on the type of previous uterine scar, the number of prior cesarean births, whether the mother had a prior vaginal birth, whether labor was spontaneous or induced, the cervical ripening/induction agent, a history of postpartum fever after a previous cesarean birth, a previous preterm cesarean birth, a single-layer uterine closure, an interval between pregnancies of less than 24 months, BMI, race, and maternal age over 30 years (ACOG, 2010c; Cahill et al., 2007; Cahill et al., 2008; Cahill, Tuuli, Odibo, Stamilio, & Macones, 2010; Hibbard et al., 2006; Landon et al., 2006; Scifres, Rohn, Odibo, Stamilio, & Macones, 2011; Shanks & Cahill, 2011). Labor dystocia after 7 cm for women having TOLAC may be associated with uterine rupture (Harper, Cahill, et al., 2012).

In general, labor should progress during TOLAC based on what would be expected related to clinical history. Labor curves and rates of cervical change for women having TOLAC and women without a previous cesarean birth are similar (Graseck et al., 2012). There does not appear to be an increased risk of uterine rupture during TOLAC for women with a history of multiple cesareans when compared to women with a history of a single cesarean (Landon et al., 2006). Women with three or more prior cesareans have similar rates of success and risks of morbidity during TOLAC when compared to women with one prior cesarean and women that give birth via repeat cesarean (Cahill, Tuuli, et al., 2010). Clinical suspicion for uterine rupture should be high for women during TOLAC who require frequent epidural dosing (Cahill, Odibo, Allsworth, & Macones, 2010). In some studies, the reported incidence of uterine rupture has varied due to true, catastrophic uterine ruptures being counted together with asymptomatic scar dehiscence (ACOG, 2010c).

Waiting for spontaneous labor, thus avoiding cervical ripening agents and oxytocin, appears to significantly decrease the risk of uterine rupture for women

---

DISPLAY 14–19

Trial of Labor After Cesarean (TOLAC): Clinical Factors to Consider

STRONGEST PREDICTORS OF SUCCESSFUL TOLAC
- Prior vaginal birth
- Spontaneous labor

ADDITIONAL FACTORS ASSOCIATED WITH SUCCESS
- Prior incision low transverse
- Clinically adequate pelvis and normal fetal size
- No other uterine scars, anomalies, or previous rupture
- Patient enthusiasm and informed consent
- Physician available capable of monitoring labor and fetus and performing cesarean
- Anesthesia, blood bank, and staff available and simulation training for emergency cesarean birth

DECREASED PROBABILITY OF SUCCESS
- Recurrent indication for initial cesarean (e.g., labor dystocia)
- Increased maternal age
- Non-white ethnicity
- Gestational age >40 weeks
- Maternal obesity
- Preeclampsia
- Short interpregnancy interval
- Increased neonatal birth weight

CAUTION AND POTENTIAL CONTRAINDICATIONS
- Prior classical or T-shaped incision or previous fundal surgery
- Contracted pelvis, macrosomia, or both
- Recurrent indication for initial cesarean
- Medical or obstetric condition precluding vaginal birth
- Patient refusal
- Induction with unfavorable cervix
- Augmentation of labor
- Inability to preform emergency cesarean birth

Adapted from American College of Obstetricians and Gynecologists. (2010c). *Vaginal Birth After Previous Cesarean Delivery* (Practice Bulletin No. 115). Washington, DC: Author. doi:10.1097/AOG.0b013e3181eeb251; Scott, J. R. (2011). Vaginal birth after cesarean delivery. *Obstetrics and Gynecology, 118*(2), 342–350. doi:10.1097/AOG.0b013e3182245b39

---

attempting VBAC (ACOG, 2010c; Shanks & Cahill, 2011). There are enough data to suggest that prostaglandins and high rates of oxytocin infusion increase the risk for rupture (ACOG, 2010c; Cahill et al., 2007). Uterine ruptures at the scar site and sites remote from the previous scar site have been reported with high doses of oxytocin. It has been theorized that prostaglandins induce local biochemical modifications that weaken the prior uterine scar, thus predisposing it to rupture. Misoprostol should not be used for third trimester cervical ripening or labor induction in women who have had a cesarean birth or major uterine surgery

(ACOG, 2010c). Women undergoing a trial of labor require comprehensive care by an interdisciplinary perinatal team. The patient and family need additional reassurance and support. Women attempting TOLAC require close surveillance and continuous EFM of FHR and uterine activity (ACOG, 2010c; Cahill et al., 2007). There are no data to suggest FSEs or IUPCs are superior to external monitoring (ACOG, 2010c; Bakker et al., 2010). The IUPC does not assist in the diagnosis of uterine rupture (ACOG, 2010c). IV access is a reasonable precaution because of the risk of uterine rupture, which would require the administration of rapid volume expanders and blood products. Rate of cervical dilation and fetal descent should be assessed frequently and abnormal labor progress reported to the primary care provider. Epidural analgesia/anesthesia for labor may be used for TOLAC as no high quality evidence suggests that epidural analgesia/anesthesia contributes to an unsuccessful TOLAC (ACOG, 2010c).

The most common presenting sign associated with uterine rupture is FHR abnormality, which has been found in 70% of the cases of uterine ruptures (ACOG, 2010c; Leung, Farmer, Leung, Medearis, & Paul, 1993). Acute signs of uterine rupture are variable and may include fetal bradycardia, changes in uterine contraction patterns, vaginal bleeding, loss of station, or new onset of intense uterine pain (ACOG, 2010c; Leung, Farmer, et al., 1993; Ridgeway, Weyrich, & Benedetti, 2004; Scott, 2011; Yap, Kim, & Laros, 2001). Uterine or abdominal pain in the area of the previous incision may be described as mild to "tearing" in nature (Scott, 2011). Bleeding, either vaginal or intraabdominal, may produce anxiety, restlessness, weakness, dizziness, gross hematuria, shoulder pain, and shock (Scott, 2011). Because uterine rupture is often sudden and may be catastrophic, any of these findings warrant rapid laparotomy (Scott, 2011). If complete cord compression occurs or the fetus is extruded from the uterus, the outcome may be poor. In a classic study, Leung, Leung, and Paul (1993) evaluated 78 cases of uterine rupture in a large tertiary medical center and reported significant neonatal morbidity when 18 minutes or more elapsed between the onset of prolonged deceleration and birth. When the prolonged deceleration was preceded by "severe" late or variable decelerations, fetal asphyxia occurred as early as 10 minutes from the onset of prolonged deceleration. An evaluation of 36 cases of uterine rupture by Holmgrem, Scott, Porter, Esplin, and Bardsley (2012) found that babies born within 18 minutes after uterine rupture had normal umbilical pH levels or 5-minute Apgar scores greater than 7, whereas a longer time frame was associated with adverse outcomes. Prompt intervention does not always prevent severe, fetal metabolic acidosis or neonatal death. Even in facilities with immediate access to cesarean birth, uterine rupture can result in catastrophic outcome.

Although the actual numbers of adverse fetal or neonatal outcomes are low with VBAC, risks to the baby associated with uterine rupture are significant and can be catastrophic. They include hypoxemia, neurologic depression, pathologic fetal acidosis, seizures, asphyxia, hypoxic ischemic encephalopathy, cerebral palsy, and death (Chauhan, Martin, Hendricks, & Morrison, 2003; Guise et al., 2004; Holmgren et al., 2012; Landon et al., 2004; Smith, Pell, Cameron, & Dobbie, 2002; Yap et al., 2001).

Common sequelae associated with uterine rupture include excessive hemorrhage requiring surgical exploration; the need for hysterectomy; the need for blood product transfusion; hypovolemia; hypovolemic shock; injury to the bladder or ureters; bowel laceration; extrusion of any part of the fetus, cord, or placenta through the disruption; emergent cesarean birth for suspected rupture; emergent cesarean birth for indeterminate or abnormal fetal status; and general anesthesia (Guise et al., 2004; Hibbard et al., 2001; Kirkendall, Jauregui, Kim, & Phelan, 2000; Landon et al., 2004; Pare, Quinones, & Macones, 2006). Many women with uterine rupture experience more than one of these complications (Landon et al., 2004).

Because of the risks associated with TOLAC and the unpredictable nature of uterine rupture and other complications, ACOG (2010c) has made recommendations for healthcare providers and facilities offering TOLAC:

1. A TOLAC should be undertaken at facilities capable of emergency surgery.
2. A TOLAC may be undertaken in facilities with staff immediately available to provide emergency care.
3. When resources for immediate cesarean birth are not available, healthcare providers and patients considering TOLAC should discuss the hospital's resources and availability of obstetric, pediatric, anesthetic, and operating room staffs.
4. The decision to offer and pursue TOLAC in a setting in which the option of immediate cesarean birth is more limited should be carefully considered by patients and their healthcare providers. In such situations, the best alternative may be to refer patients to a facility with available resources.
5. Healthcare providers and insurance carriers should do all they can to facilitate transfer of care or comanagement in support of a desired TOLAC, and such plans should be initiated early in the course of antenatal care.
6. Respect for patient autonomy supports that patients should be allowed to accept increased levels of risk; however, patients should be clearly informed of such a potential increase in risk and management alternatives.

7. After counseling, the ultimate decision to undergo TOLAC or repeat cesarean birth should be made by the patient in consultation with her healthcare provider. The potential risks and benefits of both TOLAC and elective repeat cesarean birth should be discussed. Documentation of counseling and the management plan should be included in the medical record.

Rupture of the uterus is an obstetric emergency. Maternal–fetal survival depends on prompt identification and surgical intervention. Rapid volume expanders, blood, and blood products should be readily available. Policies, procedures, and protocols should be written and evaluated to ensure optimum care for women who are having a trial of labor after a previous cesarean birth. If the primary care provider is a family practitioner or CNM without privileges or the ability to perform an emergent cesarean birth, clear policies and protocols should be in place to ensure appropriate and timely surgical coverage in case of maternal complications.

Safe care during a trial of labor to attempt VBAC is resource intensive. Many obstetric units do not have the financial and personnel resources to provide in-house anesthesia and a surgical team for the course of VBAC labor. Approximately 37% of U.S. hospitals providing perinatal services have fewer than 500 births per year; 8% have less than 100 births per year (Simpson, 2011). These hospitals and others without around the clock anesthesia and surgical team support may find it challenging to supply the resources to meet the full scope of the ACOG (2010c) recommendations during VBAC labor. Not all obstetricians have the desire or the ability to devote the time to remain in-house during VBAC labor. The decision to offer a trial of labor for women attempting VBAC should be based on a commitment of resources and an agreement of providers to be in-house during the course of labor. If this commitment cannot be made for whatever reason, the hospital should not offer planned VBAC care. Alternatives are repeat cesarean birth or patient referral to another hospital with resources consistent with the ACOG (2010c) recommendations.

SUMMARY

Nurses who care for women during the intrapartum period require knowledge of the labor process and a thorough understanding of techniques and interventions that enhance safe labor and birth. The woman's desires about her labor and birth experience should guide care. We should consider ourselves supportive guests at the woman's momentous life event rather than routine interventionists. A philosophy that labor and birth are normal processes will enable appropriate care and avoid unnecessary interventions that can lead to iatrogenic maternal–fetal injuries.

Some of the age-old nursing traditions surrounding birth have not been found to be based on sound scientific evidence. Positioning for labor and birth has evolved from supine lithotomy to positions that are more woman and fetus oriented. For most women, fasting during labor is not necessary to avoid adverse outcomes. Aggressive coached closed-glottis, second-stage pushing techniques should be abandoned in favor of second-stage care practices that are more mother and baby friendly. Routine episiotomy should become a thing of the past. Nurses can influence changes related to routine childbirth practices by keeping abreast of current research in perinatal nursing and using this knowledge when caring for laboring women. There are many opportunities for nursing research to evaluate efficacy and effects of routine interventions during labor and birth.

Cervical ripening procedures, labor induction/augmentation, and operative births are necessary interventions for some women to promote optimal maternal and fetal outcome, but the least invasive approach should be the first considered. Ideally, women and their babies are exposed to the risks of cervical ripening, labor induction, and/or labor augmentation in the context of medically indicated conditions only. Babies should not be born electively before their time for convenience. Nurses must also have expertise in perioperative standards for women experiencing cesarean births. This chapter has presented an overview of nursing considerations for clinical practice during childbirth. Perinatal care based on national standards, current research, and principles of patient safety will enhance quality outcomes for women and newborns. The nurse has an important role in supporting a positive childbirth experience (Fig. 14–22). Attending the birth of a healthy baby and sharing the joy with the new mother is one of the most rewarding experiences in perinatal nursing practice.

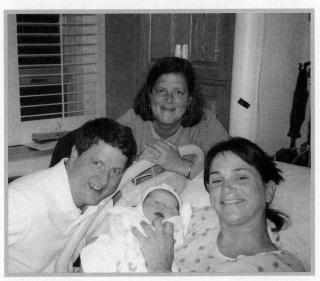

FIGURE 14–22. The nurse and the new family.

REFERENCES

Aasheim, V., Nilsen, A. B., Lukasse, M., & Reinar, L. M. (2011). Perineal techniques during the second stage of labour for reducing perineal trauma. *Cochrane Database of Systematic Reviews*, (12), CD006672. doi:10.1002/14651858.CD006672.pub2

Aikins-Murphy, P., & Feinland, J. B. (1998). Perineal outcomes in a home birth setting. *Birth: Issues in Perinatal Care and Education, 25*(4), 226–234.

Akhan, S. E., Iyibozkurt, A. C., & Turfanda, A. (2001). Unscarred uterine rupture after induction of labor with misoprostol: A case report. *Clinical and Experimental Obstetrics and Gynecology, 28*(2), 118–120.

Akinsipe, D. C., Villalobos, L. E., & Ridley, R. T. (2012). A systematic review of implementing an elective labor induction policy. *Journal of Obstetric, Gynecologic and Neonatal Nursing, 41*(1), 5–16. doi:10.1111/j.1552-6909.2011.01320.x

Albers, L. L. (1999). The duration of labor in healthy women. *Journal of Perinatology, 19*(2), 114–119

Albers, L. L., Anderson, D., Cragin, L., Daniels, S. M., Hunter, C., Sedler, K. D., & Teaf, D. (1997). The relationship of ambulation in labor to operative delivery. *Journal of Nurse Midwifery, 42*(1), 4–8.

Albers, L. L., Schiff, M., & Gorwoda, J. G. (1996). The length of active labor in normal pregnancies. *Obstetrics and Gynecology, 87*(3), 355–359.

Albers, L. L., Sedler, K. D., Bedrick, E. J., Teaf, D., & Peralta, P. (2005). Midwifery care measures in the second stage of labor and reduction of genital tract trauma at birth: A randomized trial. *Journal of Midwifery and Women's Health, 50*(5), 365–372. doi:10.1016/j.jmwh.2005.05.012

Albers, L. L., Sedler, K. D., Bedrick, E. J., Teaf, D., & Peralta, P. (2006). Factors related to genital tract trauma in normal spontaneous vaginal births. *Birth, 33*(2), 94–100. doi:10.1111/j.0730-7659.2006.00085

Aldrete, J. A. (1995). The post anaesthesia recovery score revisited (Letter). *Journal of Clinical Anesthesiology, 7*(1), 89–91.

Aldrich, C. J., D'Antona, D., Spencer, J. A. D., Wyatt, J. S., Peebles, D. M., Delpy, D. T., & Reynolds, E. O. (1995). The effect of maternal pushing on cerebral oxygenation and blood volume during the second stage of labour. *British Journal of Obstetrics and Gynecology, 102*(6), 448–453.

Alexander, J. M., Leveno, K. J., Hauth, J., Landon, M. B., Thom, E., Spong, C. Y., . . . Gabbe, S. G. (2006). Fetal injury associated with cesarean delivery. *Obstetrics and Gynecology, 108*(4), 885–890. doi:10.1097/01.AOG.0000237116.72011.f3

Alexander, J. M., Sharma, S. K., McIntire, D. D., & Leveno, K. J. (2002). Epidural anesthesia lengthens the Friedman active phase of labor. *Obstetrics and Gynecology, 100*(1), 46–50.

Alfirevic, Z., Kelly, A. J., & Dowswell, T. (2009). Intravenous oxytocin alone for cervical ripening and induction of labour. *Cochrane Database of Systematic Reviews, 7*(4), CD003246. doi:10.1002/14651858.CD003246.pub2

Alfirevic, Z., & Weeks, A. (2006). Oral misoprostol for induction of labour. *Cochrane Database of Systematic Reviews, 19*(2), CD001338. doi:10.1002/14651858.CD001338.pub2

Allen, V. M., O'Connell, C. M., & Baskett, T. F. (2006). Maternal morbidity associated with cesarean delivery without labor compared with induction of labor at term. *Obstetrics and Gynecology, 108*(2), 286–294. doi:10.1097/01.AOG.0000215988.23224.e4

American Academy of Pediatrics. (2012). Breastfeeding and the use of human milk (Policy Statement). *Pediatrics, 1129*(3), e827–e841. doi:10.1542/peds.2011-3552

American Academy of Pediatrics & American College of Obstetricians and Gynecologists. (2012). *Guidelines for Perinatal Care* (7th ed.). Elk Grove Village, IL: Author.

American Academy of Pediatrics & American Heart Association. (2011). *Textbook of Neonatal Resuscitation* (6th ed.). Elk Grove Village, IL: Author.

American College of Nurse-Midwives. (2008). *Providing Oral Nutrition to Women in Labor* (ACNM Clinical Bulletin No. 10). Silver Spring, MD: Author. doi:10.1016/j.jmwh.2008.03.006

American College of Obstetricians and Gynecologists. (2000a). *Fetal Macrosomia* (Practice Bulletin No. 22; Reaffirmed, 2010). Washington, DC: Author.

American College of Obstetricians and Gynecologists. (2000b). *Operative Vaginal Delivery* (Practice Bulletin No. 17; Reaffirmed, 2012). Washington, DC: Author.

American College of Obstetricians and Gynecologists. (2002a). *Obstetric Analgesia and Anesthesia* (Practice Bulletin No. 36; Reaffirmed, 2012). Washington, DC: Author.

American College of Obstetricians and Gynecologists. (2002b). *Shoulder Dystocia* (Practice Bulletin No. 40; Reaffirmed, 2010). Washington, DC: Author.

American College of Obstetricians and Gynecologists. (2003). *Dystocia and Augmentation of Labor* (Practice Bulletin No. 49; Reaffirmed, 2011). Washington, DC: Author.

American College of Obstetricians and Gynecologists. (2006a). *Amnioinfusion Does Not Prevent Meconium Aspiration Syndrome* (Committee Opinion No. 346; Reaffirmed, 2010). Washington, DC: Author.

American College of Obstetricians and Gynecologists. (2006b). *Episiotomy* (Practice Bulletin No. 71; Reaffirmed, 2011). Washington, DC: Author.

American College of Obstetricians and Gynecologists. (2006c). *Analgesia and Cesarean Delivery Rates* (Committee Opinion No. 339; Reaffirmed, 2010). Washington, DC: Author.

American College of Obstetricians and Gynecologists. (2007a). Breastfeeding: Maternal and infant aspects. *ACOG Clinical Review, 12*(1, Suppl.), 1–16.

American College of Obstetricians and Gynecologists. (2007b). *Fetal Monitoring Prior to Scheduled Cesarean Delivery* (Committee Opinion No. 382). Washington, DC: Author. doi:10.1097/01.AOG.0000263933.13135.43

American College of Obstetricians and Gynecologists. (2008a). *Fetal Lung Maturity* (Practice Bulletin No. 97). Washington, DC: Author. doi:10.1097/AOG.0b013e318188d1c2

American College of Obstetricians and Gynecologists. (2008b). *Surgery and Patient Choice* (Committee Opinion No. 395). Washington, DC: Author. doi:10.1097/01.AOG.0000291581.16747.24

American College of Obstetricians and Gynecologists. (2009a). *Induction of Labor* (Practice Bulletin No. 107). Washington, DC: Author. doi:10.1097/AOG.0b013e3181b48ef5

American College of Obstetricians and Gynecologists. (2009b). *Intrapartum Fetal Heart Rate Monitoring: Nomenclature, Interpretation, and General Management Principles* (Practice Bulletin No. 106). Washington, DC: Author. doi:10.1097/AOG.0b013e3181aef106

American College of Obstetricians and Gynecologists. (2009c). *Oral Intake during Labor* (Committee Opinion No. 441; Reaffirmed, 2011). Washington, DC: Author. doi:10.1097/AOG.0b013e3181ba0649

American College of Obstetricians and Gynecologists. (2010a). *Management of Intrapartum Fetal Heart Rate Tracings* (Practice Bulletin No. 116). Washington, DC: Author. doi:10.1097/AOG.0b013e3182004fa9

American College of Obstetricians and Gynecologists. (2010b). *Patient Safety in the Surgical Environment* (Committee Opinion No. 464). Washington, DC: Author. doi:10.1097/AOG.0b013e3181f69b22

American College of Obstetricians and Gynecologists. (2010c). *Vaginal Birth after Previous Cesarean Delivery* (Practice Bulletin No. 115). Washington, DC: Author. doi:10.1097/AOG.0b013e3181eeb251

American College of Obstetricians and Gynecologists. (2011a). *Preparing for Clinical Emergencies in Obstetrics and Gynecology* (Committee Opinion No. 487). Washington, DC: Author. doi:10.1097/AOG.0b013e31821922eb

American College of Obstetricians and Gynecologists. (2011b). *Scheduling Induction of Labor* (Patient Safety Checklist No. 5). Washington, DC: Author. doi:10.1097/AOG.0b013e318240d429

American College of Obstetricians and Gynecologists. (2011c). *Scheduling Planned Cesarean Delivery* (Patient Safety Checklist No. 3). Washington, DC: Author. doi:10.1097/AOG.0b013e31823ed20d

American College of Obstetricians and Gynecologists. (2011d). *Thromboembolism in Pregnancy* (Practice Bulletin No. 123). Washington, DC: Author. doi:10.1097/AOG.0b013e3182310c4c

American College of Obstetricians and Gynecologists. (2011e). *Use of Prophylactic Antibiotics in Labor and Delivery* (Practice Bulletin No. 84). Washington, DC: Author. doi:10.1097/AOG.0b013e3182238c31

American College of Obstetricians and Gynecologists. (2012a). *Communication Strategies for Patient Handoffs* (Committee Opinion No. 517). Washington, DC: Author. doi:10.1097/AOG.0b013e318249ff4f

American College of Obstetricians and Gynecologists. (2012b). *Documenting Shoulder Dystocia* (Patient Safety Checklist No. 6). Washington, DC: Author. doi:10.1097/AOG.0b013e318268053c

American College of Obstetricians and Gynecologists & American Academy of Pediatrics. (2003). *Neonatal Encephalopathy and Cerebral Palsy: Defining the Pathogenesis and Pathophysiology.* Washington, DC: Author.

American College of Obstetricians and Gynecologists & American Society of Anesthesiologists. (2009). *Optimal Goals for Anesthesia Care in Obstetrics* (Committee Opinion No. 433). Washington, DC: Author. doi:10.1097/AOG.0b013e3181a6d04f

American Society of Anesthesiologists. (2003). Practice guidelines for management of the difficult airway: An updated report from the American Society of Anesthesiologists Task Force on management of the difficult airway. *Anesthesiology, 98*(5), 1269–1277.

American Society of Anesthesiologists. (2007). Practice guidelines for obstetrical anesthesia: An updated report by the American Society of Anesthesiologists Task Force on Obstetrical Anesthesia. *Anesthesiology, 106,* 843–863. doi:10.1097/01.anes.0000264744.63275.10

American Society of Anesthesiologists. (2009). *Standards for Postanesthesia Care.* Park Ridge, IL: Author.

American Society of Anesthesiologists. (2010). *Guidelines for Neuraxial Anesthesia in Obstetrics.* Park Ridge, IL: Author.

American Society of PeriAnesthesia Nurses. (2010). *Perianesthesia Nursing Standards and Practice Recommendations 2010–2012.* Cherry Hill, NJ: Author.

Amis, D. (2007). Labor begins on its own. *Journal of Perinatal Education, 16*(3), 16–20. doi:10.1624/105812407X217093

Andrews, V., Sultan, A. H., Thakar, R., & Jones, P. W. (2006). Risk factors for obstetric anal sphincter injury: A prospective study. *Birth, 33*(2), 117–122. doi:10.1111/j.0730-7659.2006.00088.x

Arias, F. (2000). Pharmacology of oxytocin and prostaglandins. *Clinical Obstetrics and Gynecology, 43*(3), 455–468.

Association of periOperative Registered Nurses. (2011). *Perioperative Standards and Recommended Practices for Inpatient and Ambulatory Settings.* Denver, CO: Author.

Association of periOperative Registered Nurses. (2012). *Perioperative Standards and Recommended Practices for Inpatient and Ambulatory Settings.* Denver, CO: Author.

Association of Women's Health, Obstetric and Neonatal Nurses. (2006). *Second Stage Labor Support.* (High Touch Nursing Care During Labor: Video Series). Longmont, CO: Injoy Birth and Parenting Videos.

Association of Women's Health, Obstetric and Neonatal Nurses. (2008a). *Fetal Heart Monitoring* (Position Statement). Washington, DC: Author.

Association of Women's Health, Obstetric and Neonatal Nurses. (2008b). *Nursing Care and Management of the Second Stage of Labor: Evidence-Based Clinical Practice Guideline* (2nd ed.). Washington, DC: Author.

Association of Women's Health, Obstetric and Neonatal Nurses. (2010a). *Advanced Cardiac Life Support in Obstetric Settings* (Position Statement). Washington, DC: Author. doi:10.1111/j.1552-6909.2010.01176

Association of Women's Health, Obstetric and Neonatal Nurses. (2010b). *Guidelines for Professional Registered Nurse Staffing for Perinatal Units.* Washington, DC: Author.

Association of Women's Health, Obstetric and Neonatal Nurses. (2011a). *Nursing Care of the Woman Receiving Regional Analgesia/Anesthesia in Labor: Evidence-Based Clinical Practice Guideline* (2nd ed.). Washington, DC: Author.

Association of Women's Health, Obstetric and Neonatal Nurses. (2011b). *Perioperative Care of the Pregnant Woman: Evidence-Based Clinical Practice Guideline.* Washington, DC: Author.

Association of Women's Health, Obstetric and Neonatal Nurses. (2012). *40 reasons to go the full 40 weeks.* Washington, DC: Author. Retrieved from http://www.health4mom.org/a/40_reasons_121611

Aukee, P., Sundström, H., & Kairaluoma, M. V. (2006). The role of mediolateral episiotomy during labour: Analysis of risk factors for obstetric anal sphincter tears. *Acta Obstetricia et Gynecologica Scandinavica, 85*(7), 856–860. doi:10.1080/00016340500408283

Baacke, K. A., & Edwards, R. K. (2006). Preinduction cervical assessment. *Clinical Obstetrics and Gynecology, 49*(3), 564–572.

Bakker, P. C. A. M., Kurver, P. H. J., Kuik, D. J., & Van Geijn, H. P. (2007). Elevated uterine activity increases the risk of fetal acidosis at birth. *American Journal of Obstetrics and Gynecology, 196,* 313.e1–313.e6.

Bakker, J. J. H., Verhoeven, C. J. M., Janssen, P. F., van Lith, J. M., van Oudgaarden, E. D., Bloemenkamp, K. W. M., . . .van der Post, J. A. M. (2010. Outcomes after internal versus external tocodynamometry for monitoring labor. *New England Journal of Medicine, 362*(4), 306–313. doi:10.1056/NEJMoa0902748

Barber, E. L., Lundsberg, L. S., Belanger, K., Pettker, C. M., Funai, E. F., & Illuzzi, J. L. (2011). Indications contributing to the increasing cesarean delivery rate. *Obstetrics and Gynecology, 118*(1), 29–38. doi:10.1097/AOG.0b013e31821e5f65

Barnett, M. M., & Humenick, S. S. (1982). Infant outcome in relation to second stage labor pushing method. *Birth and the Family Journal, 9*(4), 221–229.

Baskett, T. F., Allen, V. M., O'Connell, C. M., & Allen, A. C. (2007). Fetal trauma in term pregnancy. *American Journal of Obstetrics and Gynecology, 197*(5), 499.e1–499.e7. doi:10.1016/j.ajog.2007.03.065

Bassell, G. M., Humayun, S. G., & Marx, G. F. (1980). Maternal bearing down efforts: Another fetal risk. *Obstetrics and Gynecology, 56*(1), 39–41.

Beall, M. H., Spong, C. Y., & Ross, M. G. (2003). A randomized controlled trial of prophylactic maneuvers to reduce head-to-body delivery time in patients at risk for shoulder dystocia. *Obstetrics and Gynecology, 102*(1), 31–35.

Beckmann, M. M., & Garrett, A. J. (2009). Antenatal perineal massage for reducing perineal trauma. *Cochrane Database of Systematic Reviews,* (1), CD005126. doi:10.1002/14651858.CD005123.pub2

Belfort, M. A., White, G. L., & Vermeulen, F. M. (2012). Association of fetal cranial shape with shoulder dystocia. *Ultrasound Obstetrics and Gynecology, 39*(3), 304–309. doi:10.1002/uog.9066

Benavides, L., Wu, J. M., Hundley, A. F., Ivester, T. S., & Visco, A. G. (2005). The impact of occiput posterior fetal head position on the risk of anal sphincter injury in forceps-assisted vaginal deliveries. *American Journal of Obstetrics and Gynecology, 192*(5), 1702–1706. doi:10.1016/j.ajog.2004.11.047

Benedetti, T. J. (1995). Shoulder dystocia. *Contemporary OB/GYN, 40*(3), 39–43.

Bennett, B. B. (1997). Uterine rupture during induction of labor at term with intravaginal misoprostol. *Obstetrics and Gynecology, 89*(5, Pt. 1), 832–833.

Bennett, K. A., Butt, K., Crane, J. M. G., Hutchens, D., & Young, D. C. (1998). A masked randomized comparison of oral and vaginal misoprostol for labor induction. *Obstetrics and Gynecology, 92*(4, Pt. 1), 481–486.

Bernal, A. L. (2003). Mechanisms of labour: Biochemical aspects. *British Journal of Obstetrics and Gynaecology, 110*(Suppl. 20), 39–45.

Bettes, B. A., Coleman, V. H., Zinberg, S., Spong, C. Y., Portnoy, B., DeVoto, E., & Schulkin, J. (2007). Cesarean delivery on maternal request: Obstetrician-gynecologists' knowledge, perception, and practice patterns. *Obstetrics and Gynecology, 109*(1), 57–66. doi:10.1097/01.AOG.0000249608.11864.b6

Bingham, J., Chauhan, S. P., Hayes, E., Gherman, R., & Lewis, D. (2010). Recurrent shoulder dystocia: A review. *Obstetrical and Gynecological Survey, 65*(3), 183–188. doi:10.1097/OGX.0b013e3181cb8fbc

Bischoff, P., & Rundshagen, I. (2011). Awareness under general anesthesia. *Deutsches Arzteblatt International, 108*(1–2): 1–7. doi:10.3238/arztebl.2011.0001

Bishop, E. H. (1964). Pelvic scoring for elective induction. *Obstetrics and Gynecology, 24*, 266–268.

Blakemore, K. J., Qin, N. G., Petrie, R. H., & Paine, L. L. (1990). A prospective comparison of hourly and quarter-hourly oxytocin dose increase intervals for the induction of labor at term. *Obstetrics and Gynecology, 75*(5), 757–761.

Blomquist, J. L., Quiroz, L. H., Macmillan, D., McCullough, A., & Handa, V. L. (2011). Mothers' satisfaction with planned vaginal and planned cesarean birth. *American Journal of Perinatology, 28*(5), 383–388. doi:10.1055/s-0031-1274508

Bloom, S. L., Casey, B. M., Schaffer, J. I., McIntire, D. D., & Leveno, K. J. (2006). A randomized trial of coached versus uncoached maternal pushing during the second stage of labor. *American Journal of Obstetrics and Gynecology, 194*(1), 10–13. doi:10.1016/j.ajog.2005.06.022

Bloom, S. L., McIntire, D. D., Kelly, M. A., Beimer, H. L., Burpo, R. H., Garcia, M. A., & Leveno, K. J. (1998). Lack of effect of walking on labor and delivery. *New England Journal of Medicine, 339*(2), 76–79.

Bodner-Adler, B., Bodner, K., Kimberger, O., Lozanov, P., Hussiein, P., & Mayerhofer, K. (2003). Women's position during labour: Influence on maternal and neonatal outcome. *Wiener Klinische Wochenschrift, 115*(19–20), 720–723.

Bofill, J. A., Martin, J. N. Jr., & Morrison, J. C. (1998). The Mississippi operative vaginal delivery trial: Lessons learned. *Contemporary OB/GYN, 48*(10), 60–79.

Bofill, J. A., Rust, O. A., Devidas, M., Roberts, W. E., Morrison, J. C., & Martin, J. N. Jr. (1997). Neonatal cephalohematoma from vacuum extraction. *Journal of Reproductive Medicine, 42*(9), 565–569.

Bofill, J. A., Rust, O. A., & Schorr, S. J. (1996). A randomized prospective trial of the obstetric forceps versus the M-cup vacuum extractor. *American Journal of Obstetrics and Gynecology, 175*(5), 1325–1330.

Boulet, S. L., Alexander, G. R., Salihu, H. M., & Pass, M. (2003). Macrosomic births in the United States: Determinants, outcomes, and proposed grades of risk. *American Journal of Obstetrics and Gynecology, 188*(5), 1372–1378. doi:10.1067/mob.2003.302

Brancato, R. M., Church, S., & Stone, P. W. (2008). A meta-analysis of passive descent versus immediate pushing in nulliparous women with epidural analgesia in the second stage of labor. *Journal of Obstetric, Gynecologic and Neonatal Nursing, 37*(1), 4–12. doi:10.1111/j.1552-6909.2007.00205.x

Britton, G. R. (1980). Early mother-infant contact and infant temperature stabilization. *Journal of Obstetric, Gynecologic and Neonatal Nursing, 9*(2), 84–86.

Bruchas, R. R., Kent, C. D., Wilson, H. D., & Domino, K. B. (2011). Anesthesia awareness: Narrative review of psychological sequelae, treatment, and incidence. *Journal of Clinical Psychology in Medical Settings, 18*(3), 257–267. doi:10.1007/s10880-011-9233

Brumfield, C., Gilstrap, L. C., O'Grady, J. P., Ross, M. G., & Schifrin, B. S. (1999). Cutting your legal risks with vacuum-assisted deliveries. *OBG Management, 3*, 2–6.

Bruner, J. P., Drummond, S. B., Meenan, A. L., & Gaskin, I. M. (1998). All-fours maneuver for reducing shoulder dystocia during labor. *Journal of Reproductive Medicine, 43*(5), 439–443.

Buser, D., Mora, G., & Arias, F. (1997). A randomized comparison between misoprostol and dinoprostone for cervical ripening and labor induction in patients with unfavorable cervices. *Obstetrics and Gynecology, 89*(4), 581–585.

Bystrova, K., Widstrom, A. M., Matthiesen, A. S., Ransjo-Arvidson, A. B., Welles-Nystrom, B., Wassberg, C., . . . Uvnäs-Moberg K. (2003). Skin-to-skin contact may reduce negative consequences of "the stress of being born": A study on temperature in newborn infants subjected to different ward routines in St. Petersberg. *Acta Paediatrica, 92*(3), 320–326. doi:10.1111/j.1651-2227.2003.tb00553.x

Cahill, A. G., Odibo, A. O., Allsworth, J. E., & Macones, G. A. (2010). Frequent epidural dosing as a marker for impending uterine rupture in patients who attempt vaginal birth after cesarean delivery. *American Journal of Obstetrics and Gynecology, 202*(4), 355.e1–335.e5. doi:10.1016/j.ajog.2010.01.041

Cahill, A. G., Roehl, K. A., Odibo, A. O., Zhao, Q., & Macones, G. A. (2012). Impact of fetal gender on the labor curve. *American Journal of Obstetrics and Gynecology, 206*(4), 335.e1–335.e5. doi:10.1016/j.ajog.2012.01.021

Cahill, A. G., Stamilio, D. M., Odibo, A. O., Peipert, J. F., Stevens, E. J., & Macones, G. A. (2007). Does a maximum dose of oxytocin affect risk for uterine rupture in candidates for vaginal birth after cesarean delivery? *American Journal of Obstetrics and Gynecology, 197*(5), 495.e1–495.e5. doi:10.1016/j.ajog.2007.04.005

Cahill, A. G., Stamilio, D. M., Odibo, A. O., Peipert, J., Stevens, E., & Macones, G. A. (2008). Racial disparity in the success and complications of vaginal birth after cesarean delivery. *Obstetrics and Gynecology, 111*(3), 654–658. doi:10.1097/AOG.0b013e318163be22

Cahill, A. G., Tuuli, M., Odibo, A. O., Stamilio, D. M., & Macones, G. A. (2010). Vaginal birth after caesarean for women with three or more prior caesareans: Assessing safety and success. *BJOG, An International Journal of Obstetrics & Gynaecology, 117*(4), 422–427. doi:10.1111/j.1471-0528.2010.02498.x

Caldeyro-Barcia, R. (1979). The influence of maternal bearing-down efforts during second stage on fetal wellbeing. *Birth and the Family Journal, 6*, 17–21.

Caldeyro-Barcia, R., Giussi, G., Storch, E., Poseiro, J. J., Kettenhuber, K., & Ballejo, G. (1981). The bearing down efforts and their effects on fetal heart rate, oxygenation, and acid-base balance. *Journal of Perinatal Medicine, 9*(Suppl. 1), 63–67.

Caldeyro-Barcia, R., & Poseiro, J. J. (1960). Physiology of the uterine contraction. *Clinical Obstetrics and Gynecology, 3*, 386–408.

Campbell, D. A., Lake, M. F., Falk, M., & Backstrand, J. R. (2006). A randomized control trial of continuous support in labor by a lay doula. *Journal of Obstetric, Gynecologic and Neonatal Nursing, 35*(4), 456–464. doi:10.1111/j.1552-6909.2006.00067.x

Carbillon, L., Seince, N., & Uzan, M. (2001). Myometrial maturation and labour. *Annals of Medicine, 33*, 571–578.

Carfoot, S., Williamson, P., & Dickson, R. (2005). A randomised controlled trial in the north of England examining the effects of skin-to-skin care on breast feeding. *Midwifery, 21*(1), 71–79.

Carlton, T., Callister, L. C., & Stoneman, E. (2005). Decision making in laboring women: Ethical issues for perinatal nurses. *Journal of Perinatal and Neonatal Nursing, 19*(2), 145–154.

Carmen, S. (1986). Neonatal hypoglycemia in response to maternal glucose infusion before delivery. *Journal of Obstetric, Gynecologic and Neonatal Nursing, 15*(4), 319–322.

Carroli, G., & Belizan, J. (2009). Episiotomy for vaginal birth. *Cochrane Database of Systematic Reviews*, (1), CD000081. doi:10.1002/14651858.CD000081.pub2

Castro, M. A., Hoey, S. D., & Towner, D. (2003). Controversies in the use of the vacuum extractor. *Seminars in Perinatology, 27*(1), 46–53.

Catanzarite, V., Cousins, L., Dowling, D., & Daneshmand, S. (2006). Oxytocin-associated rupture of an unscarred uterus in a primagravida. *Obstetrics and Gynecology, 108*(3, Pt. 2), 723–725. doi:10.1097/01.AOG.0000215559.21051.dc

Caughey, A. B., Sandberg, P. L., Zlatnik, M. G., Thiet, M., Parer, J. T., & Laros, R. K. (2005). Forceps compared with vacuum: Rates of neonatal and maternal morbidity. *Obstetrics and Gynecology, 106*(5, Pt. 1), 908–912. doi:10.1097/01.AOG.0000182616.39503.b2

Caughey, A. B., Sundaram, V., Kaimal, A. J., Cheng, Y. W., Gienger, A., Little, S. E., . . . Bravata, D. M. (2009). *Maternal and Neonatal Outcomes of Elective Induction of Labor* (Evidence Reports/Technology Assessments, No. 176). Rockville, MD: Agency for Healthcare Research and Quality. Retrieved from http://www.ahrq.gov/clinic/tp/eiltp.htm

Chang S. C., Chou, M. M., Lin, K. C., Lin, L. C., Lin, Y. L., & Kuo, S. C. (2011). Effects of a pushing intervention on pain, fatigue and birthing experiences among Taiwanese women during the second stage of labour. *Midwifery, 27*(6), 825–831. doi:10.1016/j.midw.2010.08.009

Chauhan, S. P., Grobman, W. A., Gherman, R. A., Chauhan, V. B., Chang, G., Magann, E. F., & Hendrix, N. W. (2005). Suspicion and treatment of the macrosomic fetus: A review. *American Journal of Obstetrics and Gynecology, 193*(2), 332–346. doi:10.1016/j.ajog.2004.12.020

Chauhan, S. P., Martin, J. N. Jr., Hendricks, C. E., & Morrison, J. C. (2003). Maternal and perinatal complications with uterine rupture in 142,075 patients who attempted vaginal birth after cesarean delivery: A review of the literature. *American Journal of Obstetrics and Gynecology, 189*(2), 408–417. doi:10.1067/S0002-9378(03)00675-6

Cheng, Y. W., Hopkins, L. M., & Caughey, A. B. (2004). How long is too long: Does a prolonged second stage of labor in nulliparous women affect maternal and neonatal outcomes? *American Journal of Obstetrics and Gynecology, 191*(3), 933–938. doi:10.1016/j.ajog.2004.05.044

Cheng, Y. W., Hopkins, L. M., Laros, R. K. Jr., & Caughey, A. B. (2007). Duration of the second stage of labor in multiparous women: Maternal and neonatal outcomes. *American Journal of Obstetrics and Gynecology, 196*(6), 585.e1–585.e6. doi:10.1016/j.ajog.2007.03.021

Cheng, Y. W., Shaffer, B. L., & Caughey, A. B. (2006). The association between persistent occiput posterior position and neonatal outcomes. *Obstetrics and Gynecology, 107*(4), 837–844. doi:10.1097/01.AOG.0000206217.07883.a2

Christiaens, W., & Bracke, P. (2007). Assessment of social psychological determinants of satisfaction with childbirth in a cross-national perspective. *BMC Pregnancy Childbirth, 7*, 26. doi:10.1186/1471-2393-7-26

Christianson, L. M., Bovbjerg, V. E., McDavitt, E. C., & Hullfish, K. L. (2003). Risk factors for perineal injury during delivery. *American Journal of Obstetrics and Gynecologists, 189*(1), 255–260. doi:10.1067/mob.2003.547

Chua, S., Arulkumaran, S., Kurup, A., Tay, D., & Ratnam, S. S. (1991). Oxytocin titration for induction of labour: A prospective randomized study of 15 versus 30-minute dose increment schedules. *Australian New Zealand Journal of Obstetrics and Gynaecology, 31*(2), 134–137.

Clark, S. L., Belfort, M. A., Byrum, S. L., Meyers, J. A., & Perlin, J. B. (2008). Improved outcomes, fewer cesarean deliveries, and reduced litigation: Results of a new paradigm in patient safety. *American Journal of Obstetrics and Gynecology, 199*(2), 105.e1–105.e7. doi:10.1016/j.ajog.2008.02.031

Clark, S. L., Belfort, M. A., Dildy, G. A., & Meyers, J. A. (2008). Reducing obstetric litigation through alterations in practice

patterns. *Obstetrics and Gynecology, 112*(6), 1279–1283. doi:10.1097/AOG.0b013e31818da2c7

Clark, S. L., Belfort, M. A., Hankins, G. D. V., Meyers, J. A., & Houser, F. M. (2007). Variation in the rates of operative delivery in the United States. *American Journal of Obstetrics and Gynecology, 196*(6), 526.e1–526.e5. doi:10.1016/j.ajog.2007.01.024

Clark, S. L., Miller, D. D., Belfort, M. A., Dildy, G. A., Frye, D. K., & Meyers, J. A. (2009). Neonatal and maternal outcomes associated with elective term delivery. *American Journal of Obstetrics and Gynecology, 200*(2), 156.e1–156.e4. doi:10.1016/j.ajog.2008.08.068

Clark, S. L., Simpson, K. R., Knox, G. E., & Garite, T. J. (2009). Oxytocin: New perspectives on an old drug. *American Journal of Obstetrics and Gynecology, 200*(1), 35.e1–35.e6. doi:10.1016/j.ajog.2008.06.010

Clemons, J. L., Towers, G. D., McClure, G. B., & O'Boyle, A. L. (2005). Decreased anal sphincter lacerations associated with restrictive episiotomy use. *American Journal of Obstetrics and Gynecologists, 192*(5), 1620–1625. doi:10.1016/j.ajog.2004.11.017

Cohen, W. R. (1977). Influence of the duration of second stage labor on perinatal outcome and puerperal morbidity. *Obstetrics and Gynecology, 49*(3), 266–269.

Colachis, S. C., Pease, W. S., & Johnson, E. W. (1994). A preventable cause of foot drop during childbirth. *American Journal of Obstetrics and Gynecology, 171*(1), 270–272.

Coleman-Cowger, V. H., Erickson, K., Spong, C. Y., Portnoy, B., Croswell, J., & Schulkin, J. (2010). Current practice of cesarean delivery on maternal request following the 2006 state-of-the-science conference. *Journal of Reproductive Medicine, 55*(1–2), 25–30.

Colombara, D. V., Soh, J. D., Menacho, L. A., Schiff, M. A., & Reed, S. D. (2011). Birth injury in a subsequent vaginal delivery among women with a history of shoulder dystocia. *Journal of Perinatal Medicine, 39*(6), 709–715. doi:10.1515/JPM.2011.074

Cosner, K. R., & deJong, E. (1993). Physiologic second-stage labor. *MCN: The American Journal of Maternal Child Nursing, 18*(1), 38–43.

Crane, J. M. (2006). Factors predicting labor induction success: A critical analysis. *Clinical Obstetrics and Gynecology, 49*(3), 573–584.

Crane, J. M., & Young, D. C. (1998). Meta-analysis of low-dose versus high-dose oxytocin for labour induction. *Journal of the Society of Obstetricians and Gynaecologists of Canada, 20*(13), 1215–1223.

Crane, J. M., Young, D. C., Butt, K. D., Bennett, K. A., & Hutchens, D. (2001). Excessive uterine activity accompanying induced labor. *American Journal of Obstetrics and Gynecology, 97*(6), 926–931.

Cromi A., Ghezzi, F., Uccella, S., Agosti, M., Serati, M., Marchitelli, G., & Bolis, P. (2012). A randomized trial of preinduction cervical ripening: Dinoprostone vaginal insert versus double-balloon catheter. *American Journal of Obstetrics and Gynecology, 207*(2), 125.e1–125.e7. doi:10.1016/j.ajog.2012.05.020

Dandolu, V., Chatwani, A., Harmanli, O., Floro, C., Gaaughan, J. P., & Hernandez, E. (2005). Risk factors for obstetrical anal sphincter lacerations. *International Urogynecology Journal and Pelvic Floor Dysfunction, 16*(4), 304–307.

Daniel-Spiegel, E., Weiner, Z., Ben-Shlomo, I., & Shalev, E. (2004). For how long should oxytocin be continued during induction of labour? *British Journal of Obstetrics and Gynaecology, 111*(4), 331–334. doi:10.1111/j.1471-0528.2004.00096.x

da Silva, F. M., de Oliveira, S. M., Bick, D., Osava, R. H., Tuesta, E. F., & Riesco, M. L. (2012). Risk factors for birth-related perineal trauma: A cross-sectional study in a birth centre. *Journal of Clinical Nursing, 21*(15–16), 2209–2218. doi:10.1111/j.1365-2702.2012.04133.x

Davies, J. M., Posner, K. L., Lee, L. A., Cheney, F. W., & Domino, K. B. (2009). Liability associated with obstetric anesthesia: A closed claims analysis. *Anesthesiology, 110*(1), 131–139. doi:10.1097/ALN.0b013e318190e16a

Dawood, M. Y. (1995a). Novel approach to oxytocin induction-augmentation of labor: Application of oxytocin physiology during pregnancy. *Advances in Experimental Medicine and Biology, 395*, 585–594.

Dawood, M. Y. (1995b). Pharmacologic stimulation of uterine contractions. *Seminars in Perinatology, 19*(1), 73–83.

Dawood, M. Y., Wang, C. F., Gupta, R., & Fuchs, F. (1978). Fetal contribution to oxytocin in human labor. *Obstetrics and Gynecology, 52*(2), 205–209.

Dawood, M. Y., Ylikorkala, O., Trivedi, D., & Fuchs, F. (1979). Oxytocin in maternal circulation and amniotic fluid during pregnancy. *Journal of Clinical Endocrinology and Metabolism, 49*(3), 429–434.

de Chateau, P., & Wiberg, B. (1984). Long-term effect on mother-infant behavior of extra contact during the first hour post partum. III: Follow-up at one year. *Scandinavian Journal of Social Medicine, 12*(2), 91–103.

Declercq, E. R., Sakala, C., Corry, M. P., & Applebaum, S. (2006). *Listening to Mothers II: Report of the Second National US Survey of Women's Childbearing Experiences.* New York: Childbirth Connection.

Deering, S. H., Tobler, K., & Cypher, R. (2010). Improvement in documentation using an electronic checklist for shoulder dystocia deliveries. *Obstetrics and Gynecology, 116*(1), 63–66. doi:10.1097/AOG.0b013e3181e42220

Deering, S. H., Weeks, L., & Benedetti, T. (2011). Evaluation of force applied during deliveries complicated by shoulder dystocia using simulation. *American Journal of Obstetrics and Gynecology, 204*(3), 234.e1–234.e5. doi:10.1016/j.ajog.2010.10.904

DeFrances, C. J., & Podgornik, M. N. (2006). *2004 National Hospital Discharge Survey* (Advance data from Vital and Health Statistics No. 371). Hyattsville, MD: National Center for Health Statistics.

de Jong, P. R., Johanson, R. B., Baxen, P., Adrians, V. D., van der Westhuisen, S., & Jones, P. W. (1997). Randomised trial comparing the upright and supine positions for the second stage of labour. *British Journal of Obstetrics and Gynaecology, 104*(5), 567–571.

De Jonge, A., Van Diem, M. T., Scheepers, P. L., Buitendijk, S. E., Lagro-Janssen, A. L. (2010). Risk of perineal damage is not a reason to discourage a sitting birthing position: A secondary analysis. *International Journal of Clinical Practice, 64*(5), 611–618. doi:10.1111/j.1742-1241.2009.02316.x

DelGiudice, G. T. (1986). The relationship between sibling jealousy and presence at a sibling's birth. *Birth, 13*(4), 250–254.

Deneux-Tharaux, C., Carmona, E., Bouvier-Colle, M. H., & Breart, G. (2006). Postpartum maternal mortality and cesarean delivery. *Obstetrics and Gynecology, 108*(3), 541–548. doi:10.1097/01.AOG.0000233154.62729.24

Derham, R. J., Crowhurst, J., & Crowther, C. (1991). The second stage of labor: Durational dilemmas. *Australian New Zealand Journal of Obstetrics and Gynaecology, 31*(1), 31–36.

Devine, J. B., Ostergard, D. R., & Noblett, K. L. (1999). Long-term complications of the second stage of labor. *Contemporary OB/GYN, 49*(6), 119–126.

DiFranco, J. T., Romano, A. M., & Keen, R. (2007). Spontaneous pushing in upright or gravity-neutral positions. *Journal of Perinatal Education, 16*(3), 35–38. doi:10.1624/105812407X217138

Doumouchtsis, S. K., & Arulkumaran, S. (2006). Head injuries after instrumental vaginal deliveries. *Current Opinion in Obstetrics and Gynecology, 18*(2), 129–134. doi:10.1097/01.gco.0000192983.76976.68

Doumouchtsis, S. K., & Arulkumaran, S. (2009). Are all brachial plexus injuries caused by shoulder dystocia? *Obstetrical and Gynecological Survey, 64*(9), 615–623. doi:10.1097/OGX.0b013e3181b27a3a

Downe, S., Gerrett, D., & Renfrew, M. J. (2004). A prospective randomised trial on the effect of position in the passive second stage of labour on birth outcome in nulliparous women using epidural analgesia. *Midwifery, 20*(2), 157–168.

Draycott, T. J., Crofts, J. F., Ash, J. P., Wilson, L. V., Yard, E., Sibanda, T., & Whitelaw, A. (2008). Improving neonatal outcome through practical shoulder dystocia training. *Obstetrics and Gynecology, 112*(1), 14–20. doi:10.1097/AOG.0b013e31817bbc61

Druzin, M. L., & El-Sayed, Y. Y. (2006). Cesarean delivery on maternal request: Wise use of finite resources? A view from the trenches. *Seminars in Perinatology, 30*(5), 305–308. doi:10.1053/j.semperi.2006.07.012

Dupuis, O., Silveira, R., Dupong, C., Mottolese, C., Kahn, P., Dittmar, A., & Rudigoz, R. C. (2005). Comparison of "instrumented-associated" and "spontaneous" obstetric depressed skull fractures in a cohort of 68 neonates. *American Journal of Obstetrics and Gynecology, 192*(1), 165–170. doi:10.1016/j.ajog.2004.06.035

Ead, H. (2006). From Aldrete to PADSS: Reviewing discharge criteria after ambulatory surgery. *Journal of PeriAnesthesia Nursing, 21*(4), 259–267.

Eason, E., & Feldman, P. (2000). Much ado about a little cut: Is episiotomy worthwhile? *Obstetrics and Gynecology, 95*(4), 616–618.

Eason, E., Labrecque, M., Wells, G., & Feldman, P. (2000). Preventing perineal trauma during childbirth: A systematic review. *Obstetrics and Gynecology, 95*(3), 464–471.

Edwards, H., Grotegut, C., Harmanli, O. H., Rapkin, D., & Dandolu, V. (2006). Is severe perineal damage increased in women with prior anal sphincter injury? *Journal of Maternal-Fetal and Neonatal Medicine, 19*(11), 723–737. doi:10.1080/14767050600921307

Edwards, J. R., Peterson, K. D., Mu, Y., Banerjee, S., Allen-Bridson, K., Morrell, G., . . . Horan, T. C. (2009). National Healthcare Safety Network (NHSN) report: Data summary for 2006 through 2008, issued December 2009. *AJIC: American Journal of Infection Control, 37*(10),783–805. doi:10.1016/j.ajic.2009.10.001

Eogan, M., Daly, L., & O'Herlihy, C. (2006). The effect of regular antenatal perineal massage on postnatal pain and anal sphincter injury: A prospective observational study. *Journal of Maternal-Fetal and Neonatal Medicine, 19*(4), 225–229. doi:10.1080/14767050600593155

Eslaman, L., Marsoosi, V., & Pakneeyat, Y. (2006). Increased intravenous fluid intake and the course of labor in nulliparous women. *European Journal of Obstetrics and Gynecology, 93*(2), 102–105. doi:10.1016/j.ijgo.2006.01.023

Farah, L. A., Sanchez-Ramos, L., Del Valle, G. O., Gaudier, F. L., Delke, I., & Kaunitz, A. M. (1997). Randomized trial of two doses of the prostaglandin E1 analog misoprostol for labor induction. *American Journal of Obstetrics and Gynecology, 177*(2), 364–369.

Feinstein, N. F., Sprague, A., & Trepanier, M. J. (2009). *Fetal Heart Rate Auscultation* (2nd ed.) (Practice Monograph). Washington, DC: Association of Women's Health, Obstetric, and Neonatal Nurses.

Ferguson, J. K. W. (1941). Study of motility of intact uterus at term. *Surgery, Gynecology and Obstetrics, 73*, 359–366.

FitzGerald, M. P., Weber, A. M., Howden, N., Cundiff, G. W., & Brown, M. B. (2007). Risk factors for anal sphincter tear during vaginal delivery. *Obstetrics and Gynecology, 109*(1), 29–34. doi:10.1097/01.AOG.0000242616.56617.ff

Fleming, N., Newton, E. R., & Roberts, J. (2003). Changes in postpartum perineal muscle function in women with and without episiotomies. *Journal of Midwifery and Women's Health, 48*(1), 53–59.

Flynn, P., Franiek, J., Janssen, P., Hannah, W. J., & Klein, M. C. (1997). How can second stage management prevent perineal trauma? *Canadian Journal of Family Practice, 43*(1), 73–84.

Food and Drug Administration. (1998). *Need for Caution When Using Vacuum Assisted Delivery Devices* (FDA Public Health Advisory). Washington, DC: Author.

Food and Drug Administration. (2002). *FDA approves new labeling information for Cytotec (misoprostol)*. Retrieved from http://www.fda.gov/cder.

Forest Pharmaceuticals, Inc. (2010). *Cervidil Prescribing Information*. St. Louis, MO: Author. Retrieved from http://frx.com/pi/cervidil_pi.pdf

Fox, N. S., Saltzman, D. H., Roman, A. S., Klauser, C. K., Moshier, E., & Rebarber, A. (2011). Intravaginal misoprostol versus Foley catheter for labour induction: A meta-analysis. *BJOG, An International Journal of Obstetrics and Gynaecology, 118*(6), 647–654. doi:10.1111/j.1471-0528.2011.02905.x

Fransson, A. L., Karlsson, H., & Nilsson, K. (2005). Temperature variation in newborn babies: Importance of physical contact with the mother. *Archives of Disease in Childhood. Fetal and Neonatal Edition, 90*(6), F500–F504. doi:10.1136/adc.2004.066589

Fraser, W. D., Marcoux, S., Krauss, I., Douglas, J., Goulet, C., & Boulvain, M. (2000). Multicenter randomized controlled trial of delayed pushing for nulliparous women in the second stage of labor with continuous epidural analgesia. *American Journal of Obstetrics and Gynecology, 182*(5), 1165–1172.

Frederiks, F., Lee, S., & Dekker, G. (2012). Risk factors for failed induction in nulliparous women. *Journal of Maternal-Fetal and Neonatal Medicine, 283*(6), 1239–1243.

Freeman, R. K., Garite, T. J., Nageotte, M. P., & Miller, L. A. (2012). *Fetal Heart Rate Monitoring* (4th ed.). Philadelphia: Lippincott Williams & Wilkins.

Friedman, E. A. (1955). Primigravid labor: A graphicostatistical analysis. *Obstetrics and Gynecology, 6*, 567–589.

Friedman, E. A. (1978). *Labor: Clinical Evaluation of Management* (2nd ed.). New York: Appleton-Century-Crofts.

Friedman, E. A., Niswander, K. R., Bayonet-Rivera, N. P., & Sachtleben, M. R. (1966). Relationship of prelabor evaluation to inducibility and the course of labor. *Obstetrics and Gynecology, 28*, 495–501.

Frigoletto, F. D. Jr., Lieberman, E., Lang, J. M., Cohen, A., Barss, V., Ringer, S., & Datta, S. (1995). A clinical trial of active management of labor. *New England Journal of Medicine, 333*(12), 745–750.

Fuchs, A. R., Fuchs, F., Husslein, P., & Soloff, M. S. (1984). Oxytocin receptors in the human uterus during pregnancy and parturition. *American Journal of Obstetrics and Gynecology, 150*(12), 734–741.

Fuchs, A. R., Husslein, P., & Fuchs, F. (1981). Oxytocin and the initiation of human parturition. II: Stimulation of prostaglandin production in the human decidua by oxytocin. *American Journal of Obstetrics and Gynecology, 141*(6), 694–699.

Fuchs, A. R., Romero, R., Keefe, D., Parra, M., Oyarzun, E., & Behnke, E. (1991). *American Journal of Obstetrics and Gynecology, 165*(5, Pt. 1), 1515–1523.

Gannon, J. M. (1992). Delivery on the hands and knees: A case study approach. *Journal of Nurse-Midwifery, 37*(1), 48–52.

Garite, T. J., & Simpson, K. R. (2011). Intrauterine resuscitation during labor. *Clinical Obstetrics and Gynecology, 54*(1), 28–39. doi:10.1097/GRF.0b013e31820a062b

Garite, T. J., Weeks, J., Peters-Phair, K., Pattillo, C., & Brewster, W. R. (2000). A randomized controlled trial of the effect of increased intravenous hydration on the course of labor in nulliparous women. *American Journal of Obstetrics and Gynecology, 183*(6), 1544–1548.

Gawande, A. A., Studdert, D. M., Orav, E. J., Brennan, T. A., & Zinner, M. J. (2003). Risk factors for retained instruments and sponges after surgery. *New England Journal of Medicine, 348*(3), 229–235.

Getahun, D., Oyelese, Y., Salihu, H. M., & Ananth, C. V. (2006). Previous cesarean delivery and risks of placenta previa and placental abruption. *Obstetrics and Gynecology, 107*(4), 771–778.

Gherman, R. B. (2002). Shoulder dystocia: An evidence-based evaluation of the obstetric nightmare. *Clinical Obstetrics and Gynecology, 45*(2), 345–362.

Gherman, R. B., Chauhan, S. P., & Lewis, D. F. (2012). A survey of central association members about the definition, management, and complications of shoulder dystocia. *Obstetrics and Gynecology, 119*(4), 830–837. doi:10.1097/AOG.0b013e31824be910

Gherman, R. B., Chauhan, S., Ouzounian, J. G., Lerner, H., Gonik, B., & Goodwin, M. (2006). Shoulder dystocia: The unpreventable obstetric emergency with empiric management guidelines. *American Journal of Obstetrics and Gynecology, 195*(3), 657–672. doi:10.1016/j.ajog.2005.09.007

Gherman, R. B., Tramont, J., Muffley, P., & Goodwin, T. M. (2000). Analysis of McRoberts' maneuver by x-ray pelvimetry. *Obstetrics and Gynecology, 95*(1), 43–47.

Ghoneim, M. M., Block, R. I., Haffarnan, M., & Mathews, M. J. (2009). Awareness during anesthesia: Risk factors, causes and sequelae: A review of reported cases in the literature. *Anesthesia and Analgesia, 108*(2), 527–535. doi:10.1213/ane.0b013e318193c634

Gifford, D. S., Morton, S. C., Fiske, M., Keesey, J., Keeler, E., & Kahn, K. L. (2000). Lack of progress as a reason for cesarean. *Obstetrics and Gynecology, 95*(4), 589–595.

Gillesby, E., Burns, S., Dempsey, A., Kirby, S., Mogensen, K., Naylor, K., . . . Whelan, B. (2010). Comparison of delayed versus immediate pushing during second stage of labor for nulliparous women with epidural anesthesia. *Journal of Obstetric, Gynecologic, and Neonatal Nursing, 39*(6), 635–644. doi:10.1111/j.1552-6909.2010.01195.x

Gilliam, M. (2006). Cesarean delivery on request: Reproductive consequences. *Seminars in Perinatology, 30*(5), 257–260. doi:10.1053/j.semperi.2006.07.005

Glantz, J. C. (2010). Term labor induction compared with expectant management. *Obstetrics and Gynecology, 115*(1), 70–76. doi:10.1097/AOG.0b013e3181c4ef96

Golay, J., Vedam, S., & Sorger, L. (1993). The squatting position for the second stage of labor: Effects on labor and on maternal and fetal well being. *Birth: Issues in Perinatal Care and Education 20*(2), 73–78.

Goldberg, A. B., Greenberg, M. B., & Darney, P. D. (2001). Misoprostol and pregnancy. *New England Journal of Medicine, 344*(1), 38–47.

Goni, S., Sawhney, H., & Gopalan, S. (1995). Oxytocin induction of labor: A comparison of 20- and 60-min dose increment levels. *International Journal of Gynaecology and Obstetrics, 48*(1), 31–36.

Goodman, P., Mackey, M. C., & Tavakoli, A. S. (2004). Factors related to childbirth satisfaction. *Journal of Advanced Nursing, 46*(2), 212–219. doi:10.1111/j.1365-2648.2003.02981.x

Gossman, G. L., Joesch, J. M., & Tanfer, K. (2006). Trends in maternal request cesarean delivery from 1991 to 2004. *Obstetrics and Gynecology, 108*(6), 1506–1516. doi:10.1097/01.AOG.0000242564.79349.b7

Graseck, A. S., Odibo, A. O., Tuuli, M., Roehl, K. A., Macones, G. A., & Cahill, A. G. (2012). Normal first stage of labor in women undergoing trial of labor after cesarean delivery. *Obstetrics and Gynecology, 119*(4), 732–736. doi:10.1097/AOG.0b013e31824c096c

Green, J., Amis, D., & Hotelling, B. A. (2007). Continuous labor support. *Journal of Perinatal Education, 16*(3), 25–28. doi:10.1624/105812407X217110

Grobman, W. A., Hornbogen, A., Burke, C., & Costello, R. (2010). Development and implementation of a team-centered shoulder dystocia protocol. *Simulation in Healthcare, 5*(4), 199–203. doi:10.1097/SIH.0b013e3181da5caa

Grobman, W. A., Miller, D., Burke, C., Hornbogen, A., Tam, K., & Costello, R. (2011). Outcomes associated with introduction of a shoulder dystocia protocol. *American Journal of Obstetrics and Gynecology, 205*(6), 513–517. doi:10.1016/j.ajog.2011.05.002

Gross, S. J., Shime, J., & Farine, D. (1987). Shoulder dystocia: Predictors and outcome. A five year review. *American Journal of Obstetrics and Gynecology, 156*(2), 334–336.

Grylack, L. J., Chu, S. S., & Scanlon, J. W. (1984). Use of intravenous fluids before cesarean section: Effects on perinatal glucose, insulin, and sodium homeostasis. *Obstetrics and Gynecology, 63*(5), 654–658.

Guise, J. M., Berlin, M., McDonagh, M., Osterwell, P., Chan, B., & Helfand, M. (2004). Safety of vaginal birth after cesarean: A systematic review. *Obstetrics and Gynecology, 103*(3), 420–429.

Guise, J. M., Eden, K., Emeis, C., Denman, M. A., Marshall, N., Fu, R., . . . McDonagh, M. (2010). *Vaginal birth after cesarean: New insights* (Evidence Report/Technology Assessment No. 191; Agency for Healthcare Research and Quality Publication No. 10-E001). Rockville, MD: Agency for Healthcare Research and Quality.

Gupta, J. K., Hofmeyr, G. J., & Shehmar, M. (2012). Position in the second stage of labour for women without epidural anaesthesia. *Cochrane Database of Systematic Reviews,* (5), CD002006. doi:10.1002/14651858.CD002006.pub3

Gurewitsch, E. D., & Allen, R. H. (2011). *Obstetrics and Gynecology Clinics of North America, 38*(2), 247–269. doi:10.1016/j.ogc.2011.02.015

Hagelin, A., & Leyon, J. (1998). The effect of labor on the acid-base status of the newborn. *Acta Obstetricia et Gynecologica Scandinavica, 77*(8), 841–844.

Hall, M. J., DeFrances, C. J., Williams, S. N., Golosinskiy, A., & Schwartzman, A. (2010). National hospital discharge survey: 2007 Summary. *National Health Statistics Reports, 29,* 1–24.

Halpern, S. H., Leighton, B. L., Ohlsson, A., Barrett, J. F., & Rice, A. (1998). Effect of epidural vs opioid analgesia on the progress of labor: A meta-analysis. *Journal of the American Medical Association, 280*(24), 2105–2110.

Hamilton, B. E., Martin, J. A., & Ventura, S. J. (2011). Births: Preliminary data for 2010. *National Vital Statistics Reports, 60*(2), 1–36. Hyattsville, MD: National Center for Health Statistics. Retrieved from http://www.cdc.gov/nchs/nvss/new_births.htm

Hamilton, E., Warrick, P., Knox, E., O'Keeffe, D., & Garite, T. (2012). High uterine contraction rates in births with normal and abnormal umbilical artery gases. *Journal of Maternal-Fetal and Neonatal Medicine, 25*(11), 2302–2307.

Handa, V. L., Blomquist, J. L., McDermott, K. C., Friedman, S., & Muñoz, A. (2012). Pelvic floor disorders after vaginal birth: Effect of episiotomy, perineal laceration, and operative birth. *Obstetrics and Gynecology, 119*(2, Pt. 1), 233–239. doi:10.1097/AOG.0b013e318240df4f

Handa, V. L., Harris, T. A., & Ostergard, D. R. (1996). Protecting the pelvic floor: Obstetric management to prevent incontinence and pelvic organ prolapse. *Obstetrics and Gynecology, 88*(3), 470–478.

Hankins, G. D. V. (2006). Cesarean section on request at 39 weeks: Impact on shoulder dystocia, fetal trauma, neonatal encephalopathy, and intrauterine fetal demise. *Seminars in Perinatology, 30*(5), 276–287. doi:10.1053/j.semperi.2006.07.009

Hansen, S. L., Clark, S. L., & Foster, J. C. (2002). Active pushing versus passive fetal descent in the second stage of labor: A randomized controlled trial. *Obstetrics and Gynecology, 99*(1), 29–34.

Hanson, L. (2009). Second-stage labor care: Challenges in spontaneous bearing down. *Journal of Perinatal and Neonatal Nursing, 23*(1), 31–39. doi:10.1097/JPN.0b013e318196526b

Harper, L. M., Cahill, A. G., Roehl, K. A., Odibo, A. O., Stamilio, D. M., & Macones, G. A. (2012). The pattern of labor preceding uterine rupture. *American Journal of Obstetrics and Gynecology, 207*(3), 210.e1–210.e6.

Harper, L. M., Caughey, A. B., Odibo, A. O., Roehl, K. A., Zhao, Q., & Cahill, A. G. (2012). Normal progress of induced labor. *Obstetrics and Gynecology, 119*(6), 1113–1118. doi:10.1097/AOG.0b013e318253d7aa

Hartmann, K., Viswanathan, M., Palmieri, R., Gartiehner, G., Thorp, J. Jr., & Lohr, K. N. (2005). Outcomes of routine episiotomy. *Journal of the American Medical Association, 293*(17), 2141–2148. doi:10.1001/jama.295.12.1361

Hastings-Tolsma, M., Vincent, D., Emeis, C., & Francisco, T. (2007). Getting through birth in one piece: Protecting the perineum.

MCN: The American Journal of Maternal/Child Nursing, 32(3), 158–164. doi:10.1097/01.NMC.0000269565.20111.92

Hawkins, J. L., Chang, J., Palmer, S. K., Gibbs, C. P., & Callaghan, W. M. (2011). Anesthesia-related maternal mortality in the United States: 1979–2002. *Obstetrics and Gynecology, 117*(1), 69–74. doi:10.1097/AOG.0b013e31820093a9

Hellman, L. M., & Prystowsky, H. (1952). The duration of the second stage of labor. *American Journal of Obstetrics and Gynecology, 63*(6), 1223–1233.

Hendrix, N. W., & Chauhan, S. P. (2005). Cesarean delivery for nonreassuring fetal heart rate tracing. *Obstetrics and Gynecology Clinics of North America, 32*(4), 273–286. doi:10.1016/j.ogc.2005.01.003

Hibbard, J. U., Gilbert, S., Landon, M. B., Hauth, J. C., Leveno, K. J., Spong, C. Y., . . . Gabbe, S. G. (2006). Trial of labor or repeat cesarean delivery in women with morbid obesity and previous cesarean delivery. *Obstetrics and Gynecology, 108*(1), 125–133. doi:10.1097/01.AOG.0000223871.69852.31

Hibbard, J. U., Ismail, M. A., Wang, Y., Te, C., Karrison, T., & Ismail, M. A. (2001). Failed vaginal birth after cesarean section: How risky is it? I. Maternal morbidity. *American Journal of Obstetrics and Gynecology, 184*(7), 1365–1371.

Hilliard, A. M., Chauhan, S. P., Zhao, Y., & Rankins, N. C. (2012). Effect of obesity on length of labor in nulliparous women. *American Journal of Perinatology, 29*(2), 127–132. doi:10.1055/s-0031-1295653

Hodnett, E. D. (2002). Pain and women's satisfaction with the experience of childbirth: A systematic review. *American Journal of Obstetrics and Gynecology, 186*(5, Suppl.), S160–S172.

Hodnett, E. D., Gates, S., Hofmeyr, G. J., Sakala, C., & Weston, J. (2011). Continuous support for women during childbirth. *Cochrane Database of Systematic Reviews, 16*(2), CD003766. doi:10.1002/14651858.CD003766.pub3

Hodnett, E. D., Lowe, N. K., Hannah, M. E., Willan, A. R., Stevens, B., Weston, J. A., . . . Stremler, R. (2002). Effectiveness of nurse providers of birth labor support in North American hospitals: A randomized controlled trial. *Journal of the American Medical Association, 288*(11), 1373–1381. doi:10.1001/jama.2012.4796

Hoffman, M. K., Bailit, J. L., Branch, D. W., Burkman, R. T., Van Veldhusien, P., Lu, L., . . . Zhang, J. (2011). A comparison of obstetric maneuvers for the acute management of shoulder dystocia. *Obstetrics and Gynecology, 117*(6), 1272–1278. doi:10.1097/AOG.0b013e31821a12c9

Hoffman, M. K., Vahratian, A., Sciscione, A. C., Troendle, J. F., & Zhang, J. (2006). Comparison of labor progression between induced and noninduced multiparous women. *Obstetrics and Gynecology, 107*(5), 1029–1034. doi:10.1097/01.AOG.0000210528.32940.c6

Hofmeyr, G. J., Gülmezoglu, A. M., & Pileggi, C. (2010). Vaginal misoprostol for cervical ripening and induction of labour. *Cochrane Database of Systematic Reviews,* (10), CD000941. doi:10.1002/14651858.CD000941.pub2

Hofmeyr, G. J., & Lawrie, T. A. (2012). Amnioinfusion for potential of suspected umbilical cord compression in labour. *Cochrane Database of Systematic Reviews,* (2), CD000013. doi:10.1002/14651858.CD000013.pub2

Holmgren, C., Scott, J. R., Porter, T. F., Esplin, M. S., & Bardsley, T. (2012). Uterine rupture with attempted vaginal birth after cesarean delivery: Decision-to-delivery time and neonatal outcome. *Obstetrics and Gynecology, 119*(4), 725–731. doi:10.1097/AOG.0b013e318249a1d7

Hooper, V. D., Chard, R., Clifford, T., Fetzer, S., Fossum, S., Godden, B., . . . Wilson, L. (2010). ASPAN's evidence based clinical practice guideline for the promotion of perioperative normothermia: Second edition. *Journal of PeriAnesthesia Nursing, 25*(6), 346–365. doi:10.1016/j.jopan.2010.10.006

Hourvitz, A., Alcalay, M., Korach, J., Lusky, A., Barkai, G., & Seidman, D. S. (1996). A prospective study of high- versus low-dose oxytocin for induction of labor. *Acta Obstetricia et Gynecologica Scandinavica, 75*(7), 636–641.

Hudelist, G., Gelle'n, J., Singer, C., Ruecklinger, E., Czerwenka, K., Kandolf, O., & Keckstein, J. (2005). Factors predicting severe perineal trauma during childbirth: Role of forceps delivery routinely combined with mediolateral episiotomy. *American Journal of Obstetrics and Gynecology, 192*(3), 875–881. doi:10.1016/j.ajog.2004.09.035

Hung, K. J., & Berg, O. (2011). Early skin-to-skin after cesarean to improve breastfeeding. *MCN: The American Journal of Maternal Child Nursing, 36*(5), 318–324. doi:10.1097/NMC.0b013e3182266314

Hurd, W. W., Gibbs, S. G., Ventolini, G., Horowitz, G. M., & Guy, S. R. (2005). Shortening increases spontaneous contractility in myometrium from pregnant women at term. *American Journal of Obstetrics and Gynecology, 192*(4), 1295–1301. doi:10.1016/j.ajog.2005.01.030

Husslein, P., Fuchs, A. R., & Fuchs, F. (1981). Oxytocin and the initiation of human parturition 1, prostaglandin release during induction of labor by oxytocin. *American Journal of Obstetrics and Gynecology, 141*(6), 688–693.

Incerti, M., Locatelli, A., Ghidini, A., Ciriello, E., Consonni, S., & Pezzullo, J. C. (2011). Variability in rate of cervical dilation in nulliparous women at term. *Birth, 38*(1), 30–35. doi:10.1111/j.1523-536X.2010.00443.x

Inglis, S. R., Feier, N., Chetiyaar, J. B., Naylor, M. H., Sumersille, M., Cervellione, K. L., & Predanic, M. (2011). Effects of shoulder dystocia training on the incidence of brachial plexus injury. *American Journal of Obstetrics and Gynecology, 204*(4), 322.e1–322.e6. doi:10.1016/j.ajog.2011.01.027

Institute for Safe Medication Practices. (2007). *High-Alert Medications.* Huntingdon Valley, PA: Author.

Jain, L., & Dudell, G. G. (2006). Respiratory transition in infants delivered by cesarean section. *Seminars in Perinatology, 30*(5), 296–304. doi:10.1053/j.semperi.2006.07.011

Janni, W., Schiessl, B., Peschers, U., Huber, S., Strobl, B., Hantschmann, P., . . . Kainer, F. (2002). The prognostic impact of a prolonged second stage of labor on maternal and fetal outcome. *Acta Obstetricia et Gynecologica Scandinavica, 81*(3), 214–221. doi:10.1034/j.1600-0412.2002.810305.x

Johnson, J. H., Figueroa, R., Garry, D., Elimian, A., & Maulik, D. (2004). Immediate maternal and neonatal effects of forceps and vacuum-assisted deliveries. *Obstetrics and Gynecology, 103*(3), 513–518.

Joint Commission on Accreditation of Healthcare Organizations. (2003). *Universal Protocol for Preventing Wrong Site, Wrong Procedure, and Wrong Persons Surgery.* Oakbrook Terrace, IL: Author.

Joint Commission on Accreditation of Healthcare Organizations. (2004a). *Preventing and Managing the Impact of Anesthesia Awareness* (Sentinel Alert No. 32). Oakbrook Terrace, IL: Author.

Joint Commission on Accreditation of Healthcare Organizations. (2004b). *Preventing Infant Death and Injury during Delivery* (Sentinel Event Alert No. 30). Oakbrook Terrace, IL: Author.

Joint Commission on Accreditation of Healthcare Organizations. (2010). *Preventing Maternal Death* (Sentinel Event Alert No. 44). Oakbrook Terrace, IL: Author.

Joint Commission on Accreditation of Healthcare Organizations. (2012a). *Comprehensive Accreditation Manual for Hospitals.* Oakbrook Terrace, IL: Author.

Joint Commission on Accreditation of Healthcare Organizations. (2012b). *Patient Safety Goals for Hospitals 2012.* Oakbrook Terrace, IL: Author.

Jozwiak, M., Bloemenkamp, K. W., Kelly, A. J., Mol, B. W., Irion, O., & Boulvain, M. (2012). Mechanical methods for induction of labour. *Cochrane Database of Systematic Reviews,* (3), CD001233. doi:10.1002/14651858.CD001233.pub2

Kazandi, M., Sendag, R., Akercan, F., Terek, M. C., & Gundem, G. (2003). Different type of variable decelerations and their effects to neonatal outcomes. *Singapore Medical Journal, 44*(5), 243–247.

Keirse, M. J. (2006). Natural prostaglandins for induction of labor and preinduction cervical ripening. *Clinical Obstetrics and Gynecology, 49*(3), 609–626.

Kelly, M., Johnson, E., Lee, V., Massey, L., Purser, D., Ring, K., . . . Wood, D. (2010). Delayed versus immediate pushing in second stage of labor. *MCN: The American Journal of Maternal Child Nursing, 35*(2), 81–88. doi:10.1097/NMC.0b013e3181cae7ad

Keppler, A. B. (1988). The use of intravenous fluids during labor. *Birth, 15*(2), 75–79.

Kettle, C., & Tohill, S. (2011). Perinatal care. *Clinical Evidence Online,* pii: 1401. Retrieved from http://www.ncbi.nlm.nih.gov/pmc/articles/PMC2907946/pdf/2008-1401.pdf

Khabbaz, A. Y., Usta, I. M., El-Hajj, M. I., Abu-Musa, A., Seoud, M., & Nassar, A. H. (2001). Rupture of an unscarred uterus with misoprostol induction: Case report and review of the literature. *Journal of Maternal-Fetal and Neonatal Medicine, 10*(2), 141–145.

Kilpatrick, S., & Garrison, E. (2012). Normal labor. In S. G. Gabbe, J. R. Niebyl, J. L. Simpson, M. B. Landon, H. L. Galan, E. R. M. Jauniaux, & D. A Driscoll (Eds.), *Obstetrics: Normal and Problem Pregnancies* (5th ed., pp. 2267–2286). Philadelphia, PA: Elsevier Saunders.

Kirby, R. S., & Salihu, H. M. (2006). Back to the future? A critical commentary on the 2003 U.S. national standard certificate of live birth. *Birth, 33*(3), 238–244. doi:10.1111/j.1523-536X.2006.00109.x

Kirkendall, C., Jauregui, I., Kim, J. O., & Phelan, J. (2000). Catastrophic uterine rupture: Maternal and fetal characteristics. *Obstetrics and Gynecology, 95*(4 Suppl.), S74.

Kittur, N. D., McMullen, K. M., Russo, A. J., Ruhl, L., Kay, H. H., & Warren, D. K. (2012). Long-term effect of infection prevention practices and case mix on cesarean surgical site infections. *Obstetrics and Gynecology, 120*(2, Pt. 1), 246–251. doi:10.1097/AOG.0b013e31825f032a

Klaus, M. H., Kennell, J. H., McGrath, S., Robertson, S. S., & Hinkley, C. (1988). Medical intervention: The effect of social support during labor (Part 2 abstract). *Pediatric Research, 23*(4), 211A.

Klaus, M. H., Kennell, J. H., Robertson, S. S., & Sosa, R. (1986). Effects of social support during parturition and maternal and infant morbidity. *British Medical Journal, 293*(6547), 585–587.

Koger, K. E., Shatney, C. H., Hodge, K., & McClenathan, J. H. (1993). Surgical scar endometrioma. *Surgery, Gynecology, and Obstetrics, 177*(3), 243–246.

Kolas, T., Saugstad, O. D., Daltveit, A. K., Nilsen, S. T., & Øian, P. (2006). Planned cesarean versus planned vaginal delivery at term: Comparison of newborn infant outcomes. *American Journal of Obstetrics and Gynecology, 195*(6), 1538–1543. doi:10.1016/j.ajog.2006.05.005

Kominiarek, M. A., Zhang, J., Vanveldhuisen, P., Troendle, J., Beaver, J., & Hibbard, J. U. (2011). Contemporary labor patterns: The impact of maternal body mass index. *American Journal of Obstetrics and Gynecology, 205*(3), 244.e1–244.e8. doi:10.1016/j.ajog.2011.06.014

Krening, C. F., Rehling-Anthony, K., & Garko, C. (2012). Oxytocin administration: The transition to a safer model of care. *Journal of Perinatal and Neonatal Nursing, 26*(1), 15–24. doi:10.1097/JPN.0b013e318240c7d4

Kripke, C. (2010). Upright vs. recumbent maternal position during first stage of labor. *American Family Physician, 81*(3), 285.

Kudish, B., Blackwell, S., Mcneely, S. G., Bujold, E., Kruger, M., Hendrix, S. L., & Sokol, R. (2006). Operative vaginal delivery and midline episiotomy: A bad combination for the perineum.

American Journal of Obstetrics and Gynecology, 195(3), 749–754. doi:10.1016/j.ajog.2006.06.078

Kwek, K., & Yeo, G. S. H. (2006). Shoulder dystocia and injuries: Prevention and management. *Current Opinion in Obstetrics and Gynecology, 18*(2), 123–128. doi:10.1097/01.gco.0000192976.38858.90

Labrecque, M., Eason, E., & Marcoux, S. (2000). Randomized trial of perineal massage during pregnancy: Perineal symptoms three months after delivery. *American Journal of Obstetrics and Gynecology, 182*(1, Pt. 1), 76–80.

Labrecque, M., Eason, E., Marcoux, S., Lemieux, F., Pinault, J. J., Feldman, P., & Laperriere, L. (1999). Randomized controlled trial of prevention of perineal trauma by perineal massage during pregnancy. *American Journal of Obstetrics and Gynecology, 180*(3, Pt. 1), 593–600.

Lai, M. L., Lin, K. C., Li, H. Y., Shey, K. S., & Gau, M. L. (2009). Effects of delayed pushing during the second stage of labour on postpartum fatigue and birth outcomes in nulliparous women. *Journal of Nursing Research, 17*(1), 62–72. doi:10.1097/JNR.0b013e3181999e78

Landon, M. B., Hauth, J. C., Leveno, K. J., Spong, C. Y., Leindecker, S., Varner, M. W., . . . Gabbe, S. G. (2004). Maternal and perinatal outcomes associated with a trial of labor after prior cesarean delivery. *New England Journal of Medicine, 351*(25), 2581–2589.

Landon, M. B., Spong, C. Y., Thom, E., Hauth, J. C., Bloom, S. L. Varner, M. W., . . . Gabbe, S. G. (2006). Risk of uterine rupture with a trial of labor in women with multiple and single prior cesarean delivery. *Obstetrics and Gynecology, 108*(1), 12–20. doi:10.1097/01.AOG.0000224694.32531.f3

Landy, H. J., Laughon, S. K., Bailit, J. L., Kominiarek, M. A., Gonzalez-Quintero, V. H., Ramirez, M., . . . Zhang, J. (2011). Characteristics associated with severe perineal and cervical lacerations during vaginal delivery. *Obstetrics and Gynecology, 117*(3), 627–635. doi:10.1097/AOG.0b013e31820afaf2

Langer, B., Carbonne, B., Goffinet, F., Le Goueff, F., Berkane, N., & Laville, M. (1997). Fetal pulse oximetry and fetal heart rate monitoring during stage II of labour. *European Journal of Obstetrics and Gynecology, 72*(Suppl. 1), S57–S61.

Larkin, P., Begley, C. M., & Devane, D. (2012). 'Not enough people to look after you': An exploration of women's experiences of childbirth in the Republic of Ireland. *Midwifery, 28*(1), 98–105. doi:10.1016/j.midw.2010.11.007

Larson, A., & Mandelbaum, D. E. (2012). Association of head circumference and shoulder dystocia in macrosomic neonates. *Maternal and Child Health Journal.* Advance online publication. doi:10.1007/s10995-012-1013-z

Laughon, S. K., Branch, D. W., Beaver, J., & Zhang, J. (2012). Changes in labor patterns over 50 years. *American Journal of Obstetrics and Gynecology, 206*(5), 419.e1–419.e9. doi:10.1016/j.ajog.2012.03.003

Lavender, T., Hofmeyr, G. J., Neilson, J. P., Kingdon, C., & Gyte, G. M. (2012). Caesarean section for non-medical reasons at term. *Cochrane Database of Systematic Reviews,* (3), CD004660. doi:10.1002/14651858.CD004660.pub3

Lawrence, A., Lewis, L., Hofmeyr, G. J., Dowswell, T., & Styles, C. (2009). Maternal positions and mobility during first stage labour. *Cochrane Database of Systematic Reviews,* (2), CD003934. doi:10.1002/14651858.CD003934.pub2

Lazor, L. Z., Philipson, E. H., Ingardia, C. J., Kobetitsch, E. S., & Curry, S. L. (1993). A randomized comparison of 15- and 40-minute dosing protocols for labor augmentation and induction. *Obstetrics and Gynecology, 82*(6), 1009–1012.

Lederman, R. P., Lederman, E., Work, B., & McCann, D. S. (1985). Anxiety and epinephrine in multiparous women in labor: Relationship to duration of labor and fetal heart rate pattern. *American Journal of Obstetrics and Gynecology, 153*(8), 870–877.

Lerner, H., Durlacher, K., Smith, S., & Hamilton, E. (2011). Relationship between head-to-body delivery interval in shoulder dystocia and neonatal depression. *Obstetrics and Gynecology, 118*(2, Pt. 1), 318–322. doi:10.1097/AOG.0b013e31822467e9

Leung, A., Farmer, R. M., Leung, E. K., Medearis, A. L., & Paul, R. H. (1993). Risk factors associated with uterine rupture during trial of labor after cesarean birth: A case control study. *American Journal of Obstetrics and Gynecology, 168*(5), 1358–1363.

Leung, A., Leung, E., & Paul, R. (1993). Uterine rupture after previous cesarean delivery: Maternal and fetal consequences. *American Journal of Obstetrics and Gynecology, 169*(4), 945–950.

Leung, T. Y., Stuart, O., Sahota, D. S., Suen, S. S., Lau, T. K., & Lao, T. T. (2011). Head-to-body delivery interval and risk of fetal acidosis and hypoxic ischaemic encephalopathy in shoulder dystocia: A retrospective review. *BJOG: An International Journal of Obstetrics and Gynaecology, 118*(4), 474–479. doi:10.1111/j.1471-0528.2010.02834.x

Liao, J. B., Buhimschi, C. S., & Norwitz, E. R. (2005). Normal labor: Mechanism and duration. *Obstetrics and Gynecology Clinics of North America, 32*(2), 145–164. doi:10.1016/j.ogc.2005.01.001

Lin, M. G., & Rouse, D. J. (2006). What is a failed labor induction? *Clinical Obstetrics and Gynecology, 49*(3), 585–593.

Liu, S., Heaman, M., Joseph, K. S., Liston, R. M., Huang, L., Sauve, R., & Kramer, M. S. (2005). Risk of maternal postpartum readmission associated with mode of delivery. *Obstetrics and Gynecology, 105*(4), 836–842. doi:10.1097/01.AOG.0000154153.31193.2c

Liu, S., Heaman, M., Kramer, M. S., Demissie, K., Wen, S. W., & Marcoux, S. (2002). Length of hospital stay, obstetric conditions at childbirth, and maternal readmission: A population-based cohort study. *American Journal of Obstetrics and Gynecology, 187*(3), 681–687. doi:10.1067/mob.2002.125765

Liu, Y. C. (1989). The effects of the upright position during childbirth. *Image, The Journal of Nursing Scholarship, 21*(1), 14–18.

Lopez-Zeno, J. A., Peaceman, A. M., Adashek, J. A., & Socol, M. L. (1992). A controlled trial of a program for the active management of labor. *New England Journal of Medicine, 326*(7), 450–454.

Lothian, J. (2006). Birth plans: The good, the bad, and the future. *Journal of Obstetric, Gynecologic and Neonatal Nursing, 35*(2), 295–303. doi:10.1111/j.1552-6909.2006.00042.x

Low, L, K., Seng, J. S., Murtland, T. L., & Oakley, D. (2000). Clinician-specific episiotomy rates: Impacts on perineal outcomes. *Journal of Nurse Midwifery and Women's Health, 43*(2), 87–93.

Ludka, L., & Roberts, C. (1993). Eating and drinking in labor: A literature review. *Journal of Nurse Midwifery, 38*(4), 199–207.

Lydon-Rochelle, M., Holt, V. L., Easterling, T. R., & Martin, D. P. (2001a). Risk of uterine rupture during labor among women with a prior cesarean delivery. *New England Journal of Medicine, 345*(1), 3–8.

Lydon-Rochelle, M., Holt, V. L., Easterling, T. R., & Martin, D. P. (2001b). First-birth cesarean and placental abruption or previa at second birth. *Obstetrics and Gynecology, 97*(5, Pt. 1), 765–769.

Lydon-Rochelle, M., Holt, V. L., Martin, D. P., & Easterling, T. R. (2000). Association between method of delivery and maternal rehospitalization. *Journal of the American Medical Association, 283*(18), 2411–2416.

Macarthur, A. J., & Macarthur, C. (2004). Incidence, severity, and determinants of perineal pain after vaginal delivery: A prospective cohort study. *American Journal of Obstetrics and Gynecology, 191*(4), 1199–1204. doi:10.1016/j.ajog.2004.02.064

MacDorman, M., Declercq, E., & Menacker, F. (2011). Recent trends and patterns in cesarean and vaginal birth after cesarean (VBAC) deliveries in the United States. *Clinics in Perinatology, 38*(2), 179–192. doi:10.1016/j.clp.2011.03.007

MacDorman, M. F., Declercq, E., Menacker, F., & Malloy, M. H. (2006). Infant and neonatal mortality for primary cesarean and vaginal births to women with "no indicated risk", United States, 1998–2001 birth cohorts. *Birth, 33*(3), 175–182. doi:10.1111/j.1523-536X.2006.00102.x

MacKinnon, K., McIntyre, M., & Quance, M. (2005). The meaning of the nurse's presence during childbirth. *Journal of Obstetric, Gynecologic and Neonatal Nursing, 34*(1), 28–36. doi:10.1177/0884217504272808

Macones, G. A., Hankins, G. D. V., Spong, C. Y., Hauth, J., & Moore, T. (2008). The 2008 National Institute of Child Health and Human Development workshop report on electronic fetal monitoring. *Obstetrics and Gynecology, 112*(3), 661–666. doi:10.1097/AOG.0b013e3181841395

Maresh, M., Choong, K. H., & Beard, R. W. (1983). Delayed pushing with lumbar epidural analgesia in labour. *British Journal of Obstetrics and Gynaecology, 90*(7), 623–627.

Marshall, N. E., Fu, R., & Guise, J.-M. (2011). Impact of multiple cesarean deliveries on maternal morbidity: A systematic review. *American Journal of Obstetrics and Gynecololology, 205*(3), 262. e1–262.e8. doi:10.1016/j.ajog.2011.06.035

Martin, J. A., Hamilton, B. E., Ventura, S. J., Osterman, M. J. K., Kirmeyer, S., Mathews, T. J., & Wilson, E. C. (2011). Births: Final data for 2009. *National Vital Statistics Reports, 60*(1), 1–72.

Matthews, R., & Callister, L. C. (2004). Childbearing women's perceptions of nursing care that promotes dignity. *Journal of Obstetric, Gynecologic and Neonatal Nursing, 33*(4), 498–507. doi:10.1177/0884217504266896

Maul, H., Macray, L., & Garfield, R. E. (2006). Cervical ripening: Biochemical, molecular, and clinical considerations. *Clinical Obstetrics and Gynecology, 49*(3), 551–563.

Mayberry, L. J., Hammer, R., Kelly, C., True-Driver, B., & De, A. (1999). Use of delayed pushing with epidural anesthesia: Findings from a randomized controlled trial. *Journal of Perinatology, 19*(1), 26–30.

Mayberry, L. J., Strange, L. B., Suplee, P. D., & Gennaro, S. (2003). Use of upright positioning with epidural analgesia: Findings from an observational study. *MCN: The American Journal of Maternal Child Nursing, 28*(3), 152–159.

Mayerhofer, K., Bodner-Adler, B., Bodner, K., Rabl, M., Kaider, A., Wagenbichler, P., . . . Husslein, P. (2002). Traditional care of the perineum during birth: A prospective, randomized, multicenter study of 1,076 women. *Journal of Reproductive Medicine, 47*(6), 477–482.

Mazouni, C., Porcu, G., Bretell, F., Loundou, A., Heckenroth, H., & Gamerre, M. (2006). Risk factors for forceps delivery in nulliparous patients. *Acta Obstetricia et Gynecologica Scandinavica, 85*(3), 298–301. doi:10.1080/00016340500500782

McGrath, S. K., & Kennell, J. H. (2008). A randomized controlled trial of continuous labor support for middle-class couples: Effect on cesarean delivery rates. *Birth, 35*(2), 92–97. doi:10.1111/j.1523-536X.2008.00221.x

McGuinness, M., Norr, K., & Nacion, K. (1991). Comparison between different perineal outcomes on tissue healing. *Journal of Nurse-Midwifery, 36*(3), 192–198.

McKay, S., Barrows, T., & Roberts J. (1990). Women's views of second-stage labor as assessed by interviews and videotapes. *Birth, 17*(4), 192–198.

Menacker, F., & Martin, J. A. (2008). Expanded health data from the new birth certificate, 2005. *National Vital Statistics Report, 56*(3), 1–24.

Mendelson, C. L. (1946). The aspiration of stomach contents into the lungs during obstetric anesthesia. *American Journal of Obstetrics and Gynecology, 52*, 191–205.

Mendiola, J., Grylack, L. J., & Scanlon, J. W., (1982). Effects of intrapartum maternal glucose infusion on the normal fetus and newborn. *Anesthesia and Analgesia, 61*(1), 32–35.

Mengert, W., & Murphy, D. (1933). Intra-abdominal pressures created by voluntary muscular effort. *Surgery and Gynecologic Obstetrics, 57*, 745–751.

Menticoglou, S. M., Manning, F., Harman, C., & Morrison, I. (1995). Perinatal outcome in relation to second-stage duration. *American Journal of Obstetrics and Gynecology, 173*(3), 906–912.

Mercer, B., Pilgrim, P., & Sibai, B. (1991). Labor induction with continuous low-dose oxytocin infusion: A randomized trial. *Obstetrics and Gynecology, 77*(5), 659–663.

Merchant, R., Chartrand, D., Dain, S., Dobson, J., Kurrek, M., LeDez, K., . . . Shukla, R. (2012). Guidelines to the practice of anesthesia revised edition 2012. *Canadian Journal of Anesthesia, 59*(1), 1–14. doi:10.1007/s12630-011-9609-0

Merrill, D. C., & Zlatnik, F. J. (1999). Randomized, double-masked comparison of oxytocin dosage in induction and augmentation of labor. *Obstetrics and Gynecology, 94*(3), 455–463.

Mikiel-Kostyra, K., Boltruszko, I., Mazur, J., & Zielenska, M. (2001). Skin-to-skin contact after birth as a factor determining breastfeeding duration. *Medycyna Wieku Rozwojowego, 5*(2), 179–189.

Mikiel-Kostyra, K., Mazur, J., & Boltruszko, I. (2002). Effect of early skin-to-skin contact after delivery on duration of breastfeeding: A prospective cohort study. *Acta Paediatrica, 91*(12), 1301–1306.

Miller, L. A., Miller, D., & Tucker, S. M. (2012). *Pocket Guide to Fetal Monitoring: A Multidisciplinary Approach*. St. Louis: Mosby.

Minkoff, H. (2006). The ethics of cesarean section by choice. *Seminars in Perinatology, 30*(5), 309–312. doi:10.1053/j.semperi.2006.07.013

Minkoff, H., Powderly, K. R., Chervenak, F., & McCullough, L. B. (2004). Ethical dimensions of elective primary cesarean delivery. *Obstetrics and Gynecology, 103*(2), 387–392.

Miño, M., Puertas, A., Miranda, J. A., & Herruzo, A. J. (1999). Amnioinfusion in term labor with low amniotic fluid due to rupture of membranes: A new indication. *European Journal of Obstetrics, Gynecology, and Reproductive Biology, 82*(1), 29–34.

Miyazaki, F. S., & Nevarez, F. (1985). Saline amnioinfusion for relief of repetitive variable decelerations: A prospective randomized study. *American Journal of Obstetrics and Gynecology, 153*(3), 301–306.

Mizuno, K., Mizuno, N., Shinohara, T., & Noda, M. (2004). Mother-infant skin-to-skin contact after delivery results in early recognition of own mother's mild odor. *Acta Paediatrica, 93*(12), 1640–1645.

Mollberg, M., Hagberg, H., Bager, B., Lilja, H., & Ladfors, L. (2005). Risk factors for obstetric brachial palsy among neonates delivered by vacuum extraction. *Obstetrics and Gynecology, 106*(5, Pt. 1), 913–918. doi:10.1097/01.AOG.0000183595.32077.83

Moon, J. M., Smith, C. V., & Rayburn, W. F. (1990). Perinatal outcome after a prolonged second stage of labor. *Journal of Reproductive Medicine, 35*(3), 229–231.

Moore, E. R., Anderson, G. C., Bergman, N., & Dowswell, T. (2012). T. Early skin-to-skin contact for mothers and their healthy newborn infants. *Cochrane Database of Systematic Reviews,* (5), CD003519. doi:10.1002/14651858.CD003519.pub3

Moore, L. E., & Rayburn, W. F. (2006). Elective induction of labor. *Clinical Obstetrics and Gynecology, 49*(3), 698–704.

Moragianni, V. A., Hacker, M. R., & Craparo, F. J. (2011). Improved overall delivery documentation following implementation of a standardized shoulder dystocia delivery form. *Journal of Perinatal Medicine, 40*(1), 97–100. doi:10.1515/JPM.2011.112

Morales, K. J., Gordon, M. C., & Bates, G. W. Jr. (2007). Postcesarean delivery adhesions associated with delayed delivery of infant. *American Journal of Obstetrics and Gynecology, 201*(5), 56.e1–56.e6. doi:10.1016/j.ajog.2006.12.017

Muller, P. R., Stubbs, T. M., & Laurent, S. L. (1992). A prospective randomized clinical trial comparing two oxytocin induction protocols. *American Journal of Obstetrics and Gynecology, 167*(2), 373–380.

Myles, T. D., & Santolaya, J. (2003). Maternal and neonatal outcomes in patients with a prolonged second stage labor. *Obstetrics and Gynecology, 102*(1), 52–58.

Mynaugh, P. A. (1991). A randomized study of two methods of teaching perineal massage: Effects on practice rates, episiotomy rates, and lacerations. *Birth: Issues in Perinatal Care and Education, 18*(3), 153–159.

Mzurek, T., Mikieil-Kostyra, K., Mazur, J., & Wieczorek, P. (1999). Influence of immediate newborn care on infant adaptation to the environment. *Medycyna Wieku Rozwojowego, 3*(2), 215–224.

Nageotte, M. P., & Vander Wal, B. (2012). Achievement of the 30-minute standard in obstetrics-can it be done? *American Journal of Obstetrics and Gynecology, 206*(2), 104–107. doi:10.1016/j.ajog.2011.09.008

Nathanielsz, P. W. (1998). Comparison studies on the initiation of labor. *European Journal of Obstetrics, Gynecology and Reproductive Biology, 78*(2), 127–132.

National Institutes of Health. (2006). Cesarean delivery on maternal request. *NIH Consensus and State of the Science Statements, 23*(1), 1–36. Bethesda, MD: Author. Retrieved from http://consensus.nih.gov/2006/cesareanstatement.pdf

National Institutes of Health. (2010). Vaginal birth after cesarean: New insights. *NIH Consensus and State of the Science Statements, 27*(3), 1–48. Bethesda, MD: Author. Retrieved from http://consensus.nih.gov/2010/vbacstatement.htm

Neal, J. L., & Lowe, N. K. (2012). Physiologic partograph to improve birth safety and outcomes among low-risk, nulliparous women with spontaneous labor onset. *Medical Hypotheses, 78*(2), 319–326. doi:10.1016/j.mehy.2011.11.012

Neal, J. L., Lowe, N. K., Ahijevych, K. L., Patrick, T. E., Cabbage, L. A., & Corwin, E. J. (2010). "Active labor" duration and dilation rates among low-risk, nulliparous women with spontaneous labor onset: A systematic review. *Journal of Midwifery and Women's Health, 55*(4), 308–318. doi:10.1016/j.jmwh.2009.08.004

Neal, J. L., Lowe, N. K., Patrick, T. E., Cabbage, L. A., & Corwin, E. J. (2010). What is the slowest-yet-normal cervical dilation rate among nulliparous women with spontaneous labor onset? *Journal of Obstetric, Gynecologic, and Neonatal Nursing, 39*(4), 361–369. doi:10.1111/j.1552-6909.2010.01154.x

Neilson, D. R., Freeman, R. K., & Mangan, S. (2008). Signal ambiguity resulting in unexpected outcome with external fetal heart rate monitoring. *American Journal of Obstetrics and Gynecology, 198*(6), 717–724. doi:10.1016/j.ajog.2008.02.030

Ness, A., Goldberg, J., & Berghella, V. (2005). Abnormalities of the first and second stages of labor. *Obstetrics and Gynecology Clinics of North America, 32*(2), 201–220.

Newman, R. B. (2005). Uterine contraction assessment. *Obstetrics and Gynecology Clinics of North America, 32*(3), 341–367.

Nguyen, T., Fox, N. S., Friedman, F. Jr., Sandler, R., & Rebarber, A. (2011). The sequential effect of computerized delivery charting and simulation training on shoulder dystocia documentation. *Journal of Maternal-Fetal and Neonatal Medicine, 24*(11), 1357–1361. doi:10.3109/14767058.2010.551151

Nielsen, P. E., Goldman, M. B., Mann, S., Shapiro, D. E., Marcus, R. G., Pratt, S. D., . . . Sachs, B. P. (2007). Effects of teamwork training on adverse outcomes and process of care in labor and delivery: A randomized controlled trial. *Obstetrics and Gynecology, 109*(1), 48–55. doi:10.1097/01.AOG.0000250900.53126.c2

Nielsen, P. E., Howard, B. C., Crabtree, T., Batig, A. L., & Pates, J. A. (2012). The distribution and predictive value of Bishop scores in nulliparas between 37 and 42 weeks gestation. *Journal of Maternal-Fetal and Neonatal Medicine, 25*(3), 281–285. doi:10.3109/14767058.2011.573831

Nisenblat, V., Barak, S., Grness, O. B., Degani, S., Ohel, G., & Gonen, R. (2006). Maternal complications associated with multiple cesarean deliveries. *Obstetrics and Gynecology, 108*(1), 21–26. doi:10.1097/01.AOG.0000222380.11069.11

Novikova, N., Hofmeyr, G. J., & Essilfie-Appiah, G. (2010). Prophylactic versus therapeutic amnioinfusion for oligohydramnios in labour. *Cochrane Database of Systematic Reviews,* (2), CD000176. doi:10.1002/14651858.CD000176

O'Driscoll, K. (1996). Active management of labor: True purpose has been misunderstood. *British Medical Journal, 309*(6960), 1015.

O'Driscoll, K., Foley, M., & MacDonald, D. (1984). Active management of labor as an alternative to cesarean section for dystocia. *Obstetrics and Gynecology, 63*(4), 485–490.

O'Driscoll, K., Jackson, R. J., & Gallagher, J. T. (1969). Prevention of prolonged labour. *British Medical Journal, 2*(655), 477–480.

O'Driscoll, K., Jackson, R. J., & Gallagher, J. T. (1970). Active management of labour and cephalopelvic disproportion. *Journal of Obstetrics and Gynaecology of the British Commonwealth, 77*(5), 385–389.

O'Grady, J. P., Gimovsky, M. L., & McIlhargie, C. J. (1995). *Vacuum Extraction in Modern Obstetric Practice.* New York: The Parthenon Publishing Group.

Ogunyemi, G., Manigat, B., Marquis, J., & Bazargan, M. (2006). Demographic variations and clinical associations of episiotomy and severe perineal lacerations in vaginal delivery. *Journal of the National Medical Association, 98*(11), 1874–1881.

Okby, R., & Sheiner, E. (2012). Risk factors for neonatal brachial plexus paralysis. *Archives of Gynecology and Obstetrics, 286*(2), 333–336. doi:10.1007/s00404-012-2272-z

Olah, K. S., & Gee, H. (1996). The active mismanagement of labour. *British Journal of Obstetrics and Gynaecology, 103*(8), 729–731.

Orhue, A. A. (1993a). A randomized trial of 30-min and 15 min oxytocin infusion regime for induction of labor at term for women of low parity. *International Journal of Gynaecology and Obstetrics, 40*(3), 219–225.

Orhue, A. A. (1993b). A randomized trial of 45-minutes and 15 minutes incremental oxytocin infusion regimes for the induction of labour in women of high parity. *British Journal of Obstetrics and Gynaecology, 100*(1), 126–129.

Orhue, A. A. (1994). Incremental increases in oxytocin infusion regimens for induction of labor at term in primigravidas: A randomized controlled trial. *Obstetrics and Gynecology, 83*(2), 229–233.

O'Rourke, T. P., Girardi, G. J., Balaskas, T. N., Havlisch, R. A., Landstrom, G., Kirby, B., . . . Simpson, K. R. (2011). Implementation of a system-wide policy for labor induction. *MCN: The American Journal of Maternal Child Nursing, 36*(5), 305–311. doi:10.1097/NMC.0b013e3182069e12

Osmundson, S., Ou-Yang, R. J., & Grobman, W. A. (2010). Elective induction compared with expectant management in nulliparous women with a favorable cervix. *Obstetrics and Gynecology, 116*(3), 601–605. doi:10.1097/AOG.0b013e3181eb6e9b

Osterman, M. J. K., Martin, J. A., Mathews, T. J., & Hamilton, B. E. (2011). Expanded data from the new birth certificate, 2008. *National Vital Statistics Reports, 59*(7), 1–29.

O'Sullivan, G., & Hari, M. S. (2009). Aspiration: Risk, prophylaxis, and treatment. In D. H. Chestnut, L. S. Polley, L. C. Tsen, & C. A. Wong (Eds.), *Chestnut's Obstetric Anesthesia: Principles and Practice* (4th ed., pp. 711–717). Philadelphia: Mosby Elsevier.

O'Sullivan, G., Liu, B., Hart, D., Seed, P., & Shennan, A. (2009). Effect of food intake during labour on obstetric outcome: Randomized controlled trial. *British Medical Journal, 338,* b784. doi:10.1136/bmj. b784

Ouzounian, J. G., Gherman, R. B., Chauhan, S., Battista, L. R, & Lee, R. H. (2012). Recurrent shoulder dystocia: Analysis of incidence and risk factors. *American Journal of Perinatology, 29*(7), 515–528. doi:10.1055/s-0032-1310522

Ouzounian, J. G., Korst, L. M., Ahn, M. O., & Phelan, J. P. (1998). Shoulder dystocia and neonatal brain injury: Significance of the head–shoulder interval. *American Journal of Obstetrics and Gynecology, 178*(Suppl. 1), S76.

Overland, E. A., Spydslaug, A., Nielsen, C. S., & Eskild, A. (2009). Risk of shoulder dystocia in second delivery: Does a history of shoulder dystocia matter? *American Journal of Obstetrics and Gynecology, 200*(5), 506.e1–506.e6. doi:10.1016/j.ajog.2008.12.038

Overland, E. A., Vatten, L. J., & Eskild, A. (2012). Risk of shoulder dystocia: Associations with parity and offspring birthweight. A population study of 1 914 544 deliveries. *Archives of Gynecology and Obstetrics, 285*(5), 1225–1229. doi:10.1111/j.1600-0412.2012.01354.x

Paluska, S. A. (1997). Vacuum-assisted vaginal delivery. *American Family Physician, 55*(6), 2197–2203.

Pare, E., Quinones, J. N., & Macones, G. A. (2006). Vaginal birth after cesarean section versus elective repeat cesarean section: Assessment of maternal downstream health outcomes. *British Journal of Obstetrics and Gynaecology, 113*(1), 75–85. doi:10.1111/j.1471-0528.2005.00793.x

Parer, J. T., King, T., Flanders, S., Fox, M., & Kilpatrick, S. J. (2006). Fetal acidemia and electronic fetal heart rate patterns: Is there evidence of an association? *Journal of Maternal-Fetal and Neonatal Medicine, 19*(5), 289–294. doi:10.1080/14767050500526172

Paris, A. E., Greenberg, J. A., Ecker, J. L., & McElrath, T. F. (2011). Is an episiotomy necessary with a shoulder dystocia? *American Journal of Obstetrics and Gynecology, 205*(3), 217.e1–217.e3. doi:10.1016/j.ajog.2011.04.006

Parnell, C., Langhoff-Roos, J., Iversen, R., & Damgaard, P. (1993). Pushing method in the explusive phase of labor: A randomized trial. *Acta Obstetricia et Gynecologica Scandinavica, 72*(1), 31–35.

Parsons, M., Bidewell, J., & Nagy, S. (2006). Natural eating behavior in latent labor and its effect on outcomes in active labor. *Journal of Midwifery and Women's Health, 51*(1), e1–e6. doi:10.1016/j.jmwh.2005.08.015

Pascoe, J. M. (1993). Social support during labor and duration of labor: A community based study. *Public Health Nursing, 10*(2), 97–99.

Paterson, C. M., Saunders, N. S., & Wadsworth, J. (1992). The characteristics of the second stage of labor in 25,069 singleton deliveries in the North West Thames Health Region, 1988. *British Journal of Obstetrics and Gynaecology, 99*(5), 377–380.

Pates, J. A., & Satin, A. J. (2005). Active management of labor. *Obstetrics and Gynecology Clinics of North America, 32*(2), 221–230.

Peleg, D., Kennedy, C. M., Merrill, D., & Zlatnik, F. J. (1999). Risk of repetition of a severe perineal laceration. *Obstetrics and Gynecology, 93*(6), 1021–1024.

Perez, P. G. (2005). Birth plans: Are they really necessary? *MCN: The American Journal of Maternal Child Nursing, 30*(5), 288.

Pevzner, L., Preslicka, C., Bush, M. C., & Chan, K. (2011). Women's attitudes regarding mode of delivery and cesarean delivery on maternal request. *Journal of Maternal-Fetal and Neonatal Medicine, 24*(7), 894–899. doi:10.3109/14767058.2010.531797

Phaneuf, S., Asboth, G., Carrasco, M. P., Rodriguez Linares, B., Kimura, T., Harris, A., & Lopez-Bernal, A. (1998). Desensitization of oxytocin receptors in human myometrium. *Human Reproduction Update, 4*(5), 625–633.

Phaneuf, S., Rodríguez Liñares, B., TambyRaja, R. L., MacKenzie, I. Z., & López Bernal, A. (2000). Loss of myometrial oxytocin receptors during oxytocin-induced and oxytocin-augmented labour. *Journal of Reproduction and Fertility, 120*(1), 91–97.

Phelan, J. P., Ouzounian, J. G., Gherman, R. B., Korst, L. M., & Goodwin, M. (1997). Shoulder dystocia and permanent Erb's palsy: The role of fundal pressure. *American Journal of Obstetrics and Gynecology, 176*(Suppl. 1), S138.

Philipson, E. H., Kalhan, S. C., Riha, M. M., & Pimental, R. (1987). Effects of maternal glucose infusion on fetal acid-base status in human pregnancy. *American Journal of Obstetrics and Gynecology, 157*(4, Pt. 1), 866–873.

Phillips, K. C., & Thomas, T. A. (1983). Second stage of labour with or without extradural analgesia. *Anaesthesia, 38*(10), 972–976.

Plunkett, J., Doniger, S., Orabona, G., Morgan, T., Haataja, R., Hallman, M., . . . Muglia, L. (2011). An evolutionary genomic approach to identify genes involved in human birth timing. *PLoS Genetics, 7*(4), e1001365. doi:10.1371/journal.pgen.1001365

Podulka, J., Stranges, E., & Steiner, C. (2011) *Hospitalizations Related to Childbirth, 2008.* (HCUP Statistical Brief No. 110). Rockville, MD: Agency for Healthcare Research and Quality.

Prins, M., Boxem, J., Lucas, C., & Hutton, E. (2011). Effect of spontaneous pushing versus Valsalva pushing in the second stage of labour on mother and fetus: A systematic review of randomised trials. *BJOG, An International Journal of Obstetrics and Gynaecology, 118*(6), 662–670. doi:10.1111/j.1471-0528.2011.02910.x

Radovanovic, D., & Radovanovic, Z. (2011). Awareness during general anaesthesia—implications of explicit intraoperative recall. *European Review for Medical and Pharmacological Sciences, 15*(9), 1085–1089.

Ragnar, I., Altman, D., Tyden, T., & Olsson, S. E. (2006). Comparison of the maternal experience and duration of labour in two upright delivery positions: A randomised controlled trial. *British Journal of Obstetrics and Gynaecology, 113*(2), 165–170. doi:10.1111/j.1471-0528.2005.00824.x

Rayburn, W. F., Tassone, S., & Pearman, C. (2000). Is Cervidil appropriate for outpatient cervical ripening? *Obstetrics and Gynecology, 95*(Suppl. 4), S63.

Reisner, D. P., Wallin, T. K., Zingheim, R. W., & Luthy, D. A. (2009). Rediction of elective inductions in a large community hospital. *American Journal of Obstetrics and Gynecology, 200*(6), 674.e1–674.e7. doi:10.1016/j.ajog.2009.02.021

Renfrew, M. J., Hannah, W., Albers, L., & Floyd, E. (1998). Practices that minimize trauma to the genital tract in childbirth: A systematic review of the literature. *Birth: Issues in Perinatal Care and Education, 25*(3), 143–160.

Renfrew, M. J., Lang, S., & Woolbridge, M. W. (2000). Early versus delayed initiation of breastfeeding. *Cochrane Database of Systematic Reviews, (2),* CD000043.

Revicky, V., Mukhopadhyay, S., Morris, E. P., & Nieto, J. J. (2012). Can we predict shoulder dystocia? *Archives of Gynecology and Obstetrics, 285*(2), 291–295. doi:10.1007/s00404-011-1953

Ridgeway, J. J., Weyrich, D. L., & Benedetti, T. J. (2004). Fetal heart rate changes associated with uterine rupture. *Obstetrics and Gynecology, 103*(3), 506–512.

Roberts, C. L., Algert, C. S., Cameron, C. A., & Torvaldsen, S. (2005). A meta-analysis of upright positions in the second stage of labor to reduce instrumental deliveries in women with epidural anesthesia. *Acta Obstetricia et Gynecologica Scandinavica, 84*(8), 794–798. doi:10.1111/j.0001-6349.2005.00786.x

Roberts, C. L., Torvaldsen, S., Cameron, C. A., & Olive, E. (2004). Delayed versus early pushing in women with epidural analgesia: A systematic review and meta-analysis. *British Journal of Obstetrics and Gynaecology, 111*(12), 1333–1340. doi:10.1111/j.1471-0528.2004.00282.x

Roberts, J. E. (2002). The "push" for evidence: Management of the second stage. *Journal of Midwifery and Women's Health, 47*(1), 2–15.

Roberts, J. E. (2003). A new understanding of the second stage of labor: Implications for nursing care. *Journal of Obstetric, Gynecologic, and Neonatal Nursing, 32*(6), 794–801. doi:10.1177/0884217503258497

Roberts, J. E., Goldstein, S. A., Gruener, J. S., Maggio, M., & Mendez-Bauer, C. (1987). A descriptive analysis of involuntary bearing-down efforts during the expulsive phase of labor. *Journal of Obstetric, Gynecologic, and Neonatal Nursing, 16*(1), 48–55.

Roberts, J., & Hanson, L. (2007). Best practices in second stage labor care: Maternal bearing down and positioning. *Journal of Midwifery and Women's Health, 52*(3), 238–245. doi:10.1016/j.jmwh.2006.12.011

Roberts, J., & Woolley, D. (1996). A second look at the second stage of labor. *Journal of Obstetric, Gynecologic, and Neonatal Nursing, 25*(5), 415–423.

Robinson, C., Schumann, R., Zhang, P., & Young, R. C. (2003). Oxytocin-induced desensitization of the oxytocin receptor.

American Journal of Obstetrics and Gynecology, 188(2), 497–502. doi:10.1067/mob.2003.22

Rogers, R., Gilson, G. J., Miller, A. C., Izquierdo, L. E., Curet, L. B., & Qualls, C. R. (1997). Active management of labor: Does it make a difference? *American Journal of Obstetrics and Gynecology, 177*(3), 599–605.

Rogers, S. O. Jr., Gawande, A. A., Kwaan, M., Puopolo, A. L., Yoon, C., Brennan, T. A., . . . Studdert, D. M. (2006). Analysis of surgical errors in closed malpractice claims at 4 liability insurers. *Surgery, 140*(1), 26–33. doi:10.1016/j.surg.2006.01.008

Rouse, D. J., Owen, J., Savage, K. G., & Hauth, J. C. (2001). Active phase labor arrest: Revisiting the 2-hour minimum. *Obstetrics and Gynecology, 98*(4), 550–554.

Rubin, A. (1964). Management of shoulder dystocia. *Journal of American Medical Association, 139*, 835–838.

Sakala, C., & Mayberry, L. J. (2006). Vaginal or cesarean birth: Application of an advocacy organization-driven research translational model. *Nursing Research, 55*(2, Suppl.), S68–S74.

Sampselle, C. M., & Hines, S. (1999). Spontaneous pushing during birth: Relationship to perineal outcomes. *Journal of Nurse Midwifery, 44*(1), 36–39.

Sanchez-Ramos, L., & Kaunitz, A. M. (2000). Misoprostol for cervical ripening and labor induction: A systematic review of the literature. *Clinical Obstetrics and Gynecology, 43*(3), 475–488.

Sandberg, E. C. (1999). The Zavanelli maneuver: 12 years of recorded experience. *Obstetrics and Gynecology, 93*(2), 312–317.

Satin, A. J., Leveno, K. J., Sherman, M. L., Brewster, D. S., & Cunningham, F. G. (1992). High-versus low-dose oxytocin for labor stimulation. *Obstetrics and Gynecology, 80*(1), 111–116.

Satin, A. J., Leveno, K. J., Sherman, M. L., & McIntire, D. (1994). High-dose oxytocin: 20- versus 40-minute dosage interval. *Obstetrics and Gynecology, 83*(2), 234–238.

Sauls, D. J. (2002). Effects of labor support on mothers, babies, and birth outcomes. *Journal of Obstetric, Gynecologic and Neonatal Nursing, 31*(6), 733–741. doi:10.1177/0884217502239209

Schaffer, J. I., Bloom, S. L., Casey, B. M., McIntire, D. D., Nihira, M. A., & Leveno, K. J. (2005). A randomized trial of the effects of coached vs uncoached maternal pushing during the second stage of labor on postpartum pelvic floor structure and function. *American Journal of Obstetrics and Gynecology, 192*(5), 1692–1696. doi:10.1016/j.ajog.2004.11.043

Schiessl, B., Janni, W., Jundt, K., Rammel, G., Peschers, U., & Kainer, F. (2005). Obstetrical procedures influencing the duration of the second stage of labor. *European Journal of Obstetrics, Gynecology, and Reproductive Biology, 118*(1), 17–20.

Schuit, E., Kwee, A., Westerhuis, M., Van Dessel, H., Graziosi, G., Van Lith, J., . . . Groenwold, R. (2012). A clinical prediction model to assess the risk of operative delivery. *BJOG, An International Journal of Obstetrics & Gynaecology, 119*(8), 915–923. doi:10.1111/j.1471-0528.2012.03334.x

Scifres, C. M., Rohn, A., Odibo, A., Stamilio, D., & Macones, G. A. (2011). Predicting significant maternal morbidity in women attempting vaginal birth after cesarean section. *American Journal of Perinatology, 28*(3), 181–186. doi:10.1055/s-0030-1266159

Scott, J. R. (2005). Episiotomy and vaginal trauma. *Obstetrics and Gynecology Clinics of North America, 32*(2), 307–321.

Scott, J. R. (2011). Vaginal birth after cesarean delivery: A common sense approach. *Obstetrics and Gynecology, 118*(2), 342–350. doi:10.1097/AOG.0b013e3182245b39

Sebel, P. S., Bowdle, T. A., Ghoneim, M. M., Rampil, I. J., Padilla, R. E., Gan, T. J., . . . Domino, K. B. (2004). The incidence of awareness during anesthesia: A multicenter United States study. *Anesthesia and Analgesia, 99*(3), 833–839. doi:10.1213/01.ANE.0000130261.90896.6C

Seitchik, J., Amico, J., Robinson, A. G., & Castillo, M. (1984). Oxytocin augmentation of dysfunctional labor: IV. Oxytocin pharmacokinetics. *American Journal of Obstetrics and Gynecology, 150*(3), 225–228.

Seitchik, J., & Castillo, M. (1982). Oxytocin augmentation of dysfunctional labor: I. Clinical data. *American Journal of Obstetrics and Gynecology, 144*(8), 899–905.

Seitchik, J., & Castillo, M. (1983). Oxytocin augmentation of dysfunctional labor: III. Multiparous patients. *American Journal of Obstetrics and Gynecology, 145*(7), 777–780.

Shanks, A. L., & Cahill, A. G. (2011). Delivery after prior cesarean: Success rate and factors. *Clinics in Perinatology, 38*(2), 233–245. doi:10.1016/j.clp.2011.03.011

Sharts-Hopko, N. C. (2010). Oral intake in labor: A review of the evidence. *MCN: The American Journal of Maternal/Child Nursing, 35*(4), 197–203. doi:10.1097/NMC.0b013e3181db48f5

Sheehan, P. M. (2006). A possible role for progesterone metabolites in human parturition. *Australian and New Zealand Journal of Obstetrics and Gynaecology, 46*(2), 159–163.

Sheiner, E., Walfisch, A., Hallak, M., Marley, S., Mazor, M., & Shoham-Vardi, I. (2006). Length of second stage labor as a predictor of perineal outcome after vaginal delivery. *Journal of Reproductive Medicine, 51*(2), 115–119.

Shellhaas, C. S., Gilbert, S., Landon, M. B., Varner, M. W., Leveno, K. J., Hauth, J. C., . . . Gabbe, S. G. (2009). The frequency and complication rates of hysterectomy accompanying cesarean delivery. *Obstetrics and Gynecology, 114*(2, Pt. 1), 224–229. doi:10.1097/AOG.0b013e3181ad9442

Shermer, R. H., & Raines, D. A. (1997). Positioning during the second stage of labor: Moving back to the basics. *Journal of Obstetric, Gynecologic, and Neonatal Nursing, 26*(6), 727–734.

Shifrin, B. S., & Ater, S. (2006). Fetal hypoxic and ischemic injuries. *Current Opinion in Obstetrics and Gynecology, 18*(2), 112–122. doi:10.1097/01.gco.0000192984.15095.7c

Shilling, T., Romano, A. M., & DiFranco, J. T. (2007). Freedom of movement throughout labor. *Journal of Perinatal Education, 16*(3), 21–24. doi:10.1624/105812407X217101

Shipman, M. K., Boniface, D. R., Tefft, M. E., & McCloghery, F. (1997). Antenatal perineal massage and subsequent perineal outcomes: A randomized controlled trial. *British Journal of Obstetrics and Gynaecology, 104*(7), 787–791.

Shrivastava, V. K., Garite, T. J., Jenkins, S. M., Saul, L., Rumney, P., Preslicka, C., & Chan, K. (2009). A randomized, double-blinded, controlled trial comparing parenteral normal saline with and without dextrose on the course of labor in nulliparas. *American Journal of Obstetrics and Gynecology, 200*(4), 379.e1–379.e6. doi:10.1016/j.ajog.2008.11.030

Shyken, J. M., & Petrie, R. H. (1995). Oxytocin to induce labor. *Clinical Obstetrics and Gynecology, 38*(2), 232–245.

Signore, C., Hemachandra, A., & Klebanoff, M. (2006). Neonatal morbidity and morbidity after elective cesarean delivery versus routine expectant management: A decision analysis. *Seminars in Perinatology, 30*(5), 288–295. doi:10.1053/j.semperi.2006.07.010

Silver, R. M. (2007). Fetal death. *Obstetrics and Gynecology, 109*(1), 153–167. doi:10.1097/01.AOG.0000248537.89739.96

Simon, C. E., & Grobman, W. A. (2005). When has an induction failed? *Obstetrics and Gynecology, 105*(4), 705–709. doi:10.1097/01.AOG.0000157437.10998.e7

Simpson, K. R. (2005). Handling handoffs safely. *MCN: The American Journal of Maternal Child Nursing, 30*(2), 76.

Simpson, K. R. (2009). Physiologic interventions for fetal heart rate patterns. In A. Lyndon & L. U. Ali (Eds.), *AWHONN's Fetal Heart Monitoring Principles and Practices* (4th ed., pp. 135–155). Dubuque, IA: Kendall Hunt.

Simpson, K. R. (2010). Reconsideration of the costs of convenience: Quality, operational and fiscal strategies to minimize elective labor induction. *Journal of Perinatal and Neonatal Nursing, 24*(1), 42–53. doi:10.1097/JPN.0b013e3181c6abe3

Simpson, K. R. (2011). An overview of distribution of births in United States hospitals in 2008 with implications for small volume perinatal units in rural hospitals. *Journal of Obstetric, Gynecologic and Neonatal Nursing, 40*(4), 432–439. doi:10.1111/j.1552-6909.2011.01262.x

Simpson, K. R. (2013). *Cervical Ripening, Labor Induction and Labor Augmentation* [AWHONN Practice Monograph] (4th ed.). Washington, DC: Association of Women's Health, Obstetric and Neonatal Nurses.

Simpson, K. R., & James, D. C. (2005a). Effects of immediate versus delayed pushing during second stage labor on fetal wellbeing. *Nursing Research, 54*(3), 149–157.

Simpson, K. R., & James, D. C. (2005b). Efficacy of intrauterine resuscitation techniques in improving fetal oxygen status during labor. *Obstetrics and Gynecology, 105*(6), 1362–1368. doi:10.1097/01.AOG.0000164474.03350.7c

Simpson, K. R., & James, D. C. (2008). Effects of oxytocin-induced uterine hyperstimulation during labor on fetal oxygen status and fetal heart rate patterns. *American Journal of Obstetrics and Gynecology, 199*(1), 34.e1–34.e5. doi:10.1016/j.ajog.2007.12.015

Simpson, K. R., James, D. C., & Knox, G. E. (2006). Nurse-physician communication during labor and birth: Implications for patient safety. *Journal of Obstetric, Gynecologic and Neonatal Nursing, 35*(4), 547–556. doi:10.1111/j.1552-6909.2006.00075.x

Simpson, K. R., & Knox, G. E. (2009a). Communication of fetal heart monitoring information. In A. Lyndon & L. U. Ali (Eds.), *AWHONN's Fetal Heart Monitoring Principles and Practice* (4th ed., pp. 177–209). Dubuque, IA: Kendall Hunt.

Simpson, K. R., & Knox, G. E. (2009b). Oxytocin as a high alert medication: Implications for perinatal patient safety. *MCN: The American Journal of Maternal Child Nursing, 34*(1), 8–15. doi:10.1097/01.NMC.0000343859.62828.ee

Simpson, K. R., Knox, G. E., Martin, M. George, C., & Watson, S. R. (2011). MHA Keystone Obstetrics: A statewide collaborative for perinatal patient safety in Michigan. *Joint Commission Journal on Quality and Patient Safety, 37*(12), 544–552.

Simpson, K. R., & Lyndon, A. (2009). Clinical disagreements during labor and birth: How does real life compare to best practice? *MCN: The American Journal of Maternal Child Nursing, 34*(1), 31–39. doi:10.1097/01.NMC.0000343863.72237.2b

Simpson, K. R., Newman, G., & Chirino, O. R. (2010a). Patient education to reduce elective inductions. *MCN: The American Journal of Maternal Child Nursing, 35*(4), 188–194. doi:10.1097/NMC.0b013e3181d9c6d6

Simpson, K. R., Newman, G., & Chirino, O. R. (2010b). Patients' perspectives on the role of prepared childbirth education in decision-making regarding elective labor induction. *Journal of Perinatal Education, 19*(3), 21–32. doi:10.1624/105812410X514396

Singata, M., Tranmer, J., & Gyte, G. M. L. (2010). Restricting oral fluid and food intake during labour. *Cochrane Database of Systematic Reviews*, (1), CD003930. doi:10.1002/14651858.CD003932.pub2

Singhi, S. (1988). Effect of maternal intrapartum glucose therapy on neonatal blood glucose levels and neurobehavioral status of hypoglycemic term infants. *Journal of Perinatal Medicine, 16*(3), 217–224.

Slater, D. M., Zervou, S., & Thornton, S. (2002). Prostaglandins and prostanoid receptors in human pregnancy and parturition. *Journal of the Society for Gynecologic Investigation, 9*(3), 118–124.

Smith, G. C. S., Pell, J. P., Cameron, A. D., & Dobbie, R. (2002). Risk of perinatal death associated with labor after previous cesarean delivery in uncomplicated term pregnancies. *Journal of the American Medial Association, 287*(20), 2684–2690.

Smith, R. (2007). Parturition. *New England Journal of Medicine, 356*(3), 271–283.

Society of Obstetricians and Gynaecologists of Canada. (2001). *Induction of Labour at Term* (Clinical Practice Guideline No. 107). Ottawa, Canada: Author.

Society of Obstetricians and Gynaecologists of Canada. (2004). *Guidelines for Operative Vaginal Birth* (Clinical Practice Guideline No. 148). Ottawa, Canada: Author.

Society of Obstetricians and Gynaecologists of Canada. (2007). Fetal health surveillance: Antepartum and intrapartum consensus guideline. *Journal of Obstetric and Gynaecology Canada, 29*(9, Suppl. 4), S1–S56.

Sommer, P. A., Norr, K., & Roberts, J. (2000). Clinical decision-making regarding intravenous hydration in normal labor in a birth center setting. *Journal of Midwifery and Women's Health, 45*(2), 114–121.

Song, J. (2000). Use of misoprostol in obstetrics and gynecology. *Obstetrical and Gynecological Survey, 55*(8), 503–510.

Spitellie, P. H., Holmes, M. A., & Domino, K. B. (2002). Awareness during anesthesia. *Anesthesiology Clinics of North America, 20*(3), 555–570.

Spong, C. Y., Beall, M., Rodrigues, D., & Ross, M. G. (1995). An objective definition of shoulder dystocia: Prolonged head-to-body delivery intervals and/or the use of ancillary obstetric maneuvers. *Obstetrics and Gynecology, 86*(3), 433–436.

Spong, C. Y., Mercer, B. M., D'Alton, M., Kilpatrick, S., Blackwell, S., & Saade, G. (2011). Timing of indicated late-preterm and early-term birth. *Obstetrics and Gynecology, 118*(2, Pt. 1), 323–333. doi:10.1097/AOG.0b013e3182255999

Spydslaug, A., Trogstad, L. I., Skrondal, A., & Eskild, A. (2005). Recurrent risk of anal sphincter laceration among women with vaginal deliveries. *Obstetrics and Gynecology, 105*(2), 307–313. doi:10.1097/01.AOG.0000151114.35498.e9

Stamp, G. E. (1997). Care of the perineum in the second stage of labour: A study of the views and practices of Australian midwives. *Midwifery, 13*(2), 100–104.

Stamp, G., Kruzins, G., & Crowther, C. (2001). Perineal massage in labour and prevention of perineal trauma: Randomised controlled trial. *British Medical Journal, 322*(7297), 1277–1280.

Stremler, R., Hodnett, E., Petryshen, P., Stevens, B., Weston, J., & Willan, A. R. (2005). Randomized controlled trial of hands-and-knees positioning for occipitoposterior position in labor. *Birth, 32*(4), 243–251. doi:10.1111/j.0730-7659.2005.00382.x

Stringer, J. L. (1996). *Basic Concepts in Pharmacology*. St. Louis: McGraw-Hill.

Sultatos, L. G. (1997). Mechanisms of drugs that affect uterine motility. *Journal of Nurse Midwifery, 42*(2), 367–370.

Terry, R. R., Westcott, J., O'Shea, L., & Kelly, F. (2006). Postpartum outcomes in supine delivery by physicians vs nonsupine delivery by midwives. *Journal of the American Osteopathic Association, 106*(4), 199–202.

Thomson, A. M. (1993). Pushing techniques in the second stage of labour. *Journal of Advanced Nursing, 18*(2), 171–177.

Thomson, A. M. (1995). Maternal behaviour during spontaneous and directed pushing in the second stage of labour. *Journal of Advanced Nursing, 22*(6), 1027–1034.

Thukral, A., Sankar, M. J., Agarwal, R., Gupta, N., Deorari, A. K., & Paul, V. K. (2012). Early skin-to-skin contact and breast-feeding behavior in term neonates: A randomized controlled trial. *Neonatology, 102*(2), 114–119. doi:10.1159/000337839

Torvaldsen, S., Roberts, C. L., Bell, J. C., & Raynes-Greenow, C. H. (2004). Discontinuation of epidural analgesia late in labour for reducing the adverse delivery outcomes associated with epidural analgesia. *Cochrane Database of Systematic Reviews*, (4), CD004457. doi:10.1002/14651858.CD004457.pub2

Towner, D., Castro, M. A., Eby-Wilkens, E., & Gilbert W. M. (1999). Effect of mode of delivery in nulliparous women on neonatal intracranial injury. *New England Journal of Medicine, 341*(23), 1709–1704.

Treacy, A., Robson, M., & O'Herlihy, C. (2006). Dystocia increases with advancing maternal age. *American Journal of Obstetrics and Gynecology, 195*(3), 760–763. doi:10.1016/j.ajog.2006.05.052

Tsur, A., Sergienko, R., Wiznitzer, A., Zlotnik, A., & Sheiner, E (2012). Critical analysis of risk factors for shoulder dystocia. *Archives of Gynecology and Obstetrics, 285*(5), 1225–1229. doi:10.1007/s00404-011-2139-8

Tubridy, N., & Redmond, J. M. T. (1996). Neurological symptoms attributed to epidural analgesia in labour: An observational study of seven cases. *British Journal of Obstetrics and Gynaecology, 103*(8), 832–833.

Tumblin, A., & Simkin, P. (2001). Pregnant women's perceptions of their nurse's role during labor and delivery. *Birth, 28*(1), 52–56.

Tuuli, M. G., Frey, H. A., Odibo, A. O., Macones, G. A., & Cahill, A. G. (2012). Immediate compared with delayed pushing in the second stage of labor: A systematic review and meta-analysis. *Obstetrics and Gynecology, 120*(3), 660–668. doi:10.1097/AOG.0b013e3182639fae

Uchil, D., & Arulkumaran, S. (2003). Neonatal subgaleal hemorrhage and its relationship to delivery by vacuum extraction. *Obstetrical and Gynecological Survey, 58*(10), 687–693.

Uhing, M. R. (2005). Management of birth injuries. *Clinics in Perinatology, 32*(1), 19–38. doi:10.1016/j.clp.2004.11.007

Ulmsten, U. (1997). Onset and forces of term labor. *Acta Obstetricia et Gynecologica Scandinavica, 76*(6), 499–514.

Vacca, A. (2002). Vacuum-assisted delivery. *Best Practice & Research: Clinical Obstetrics and Gynaecology, 16*(1), 17–30.

Vacca, A. (2006). Vacuum-assisted delivery: An analysis of traction forces and maternal and neonatal outcomes. *Australian and New Zealand Journal of Obstetrics and Gynaecology, 46*(2), 124–127. doi:10.1111/j.1479-828X.2006.00540.x

Vahratian, A., Hoffman, M. K., Troendle, J. F., & Zhang, J. (2006). The impact of parity on course of labor in a contemporary population. *Birth, 33*(1), 12–17. doi:10.1111/j.0730-7659.2006.00069.x

Vahratian, A., Zhang, J., Troendle, J. F., Savitz, D. A., & Siega-Riz, A. M. (2004). Maternal prepregnancy overweight and obesity and the pattern of labor progression in term nulliparous women. *Obstetrics and Gynecology, 104*(5, Pt. 1), 943–951. doi:10.1097/01.AOG.0000142713.53197.91

Vahratian, A., Zhang, J., Troendle, J. F., Sciscione, A. C., & Hoffman, M. K. (2005). Labor progression and risk of cesarean delivery in electively induced nulliparas. *Obstetrics and Gynecology, 105*(4), 698–704. doi:10.1097/01.AOG.0000157436.68847.3b

Vardo, J. H., Thornburg, L. L., & Glantz, J. C. (2011). Maternal and neonatal morbidity among nulliparous women undergoing elective induction of labor. *Journal of Reproductive Medicine, 56*(1–2), 25–30.

Vaughn, K. O. (1937). *Safe Childbirth: The Three Essentials.* London, United Kingdom: Ballière, Tindall, and Cox.

Vause, S., Congdon, H. M., & Thornton, J. G. (1998). Immediate and delayed pushing in the second stage of labour for nulliparous women with epidural analgesia: A randomized controlled trial. *British Journal of Obstetrics and Gynaecology, 105*(2), 186–188.

Vidarsdottir, H., Geirsson, R. T., Hardardottir, H., Valdimarsdottir, U., & Dagbjartsson, A. (2011). Obstetric and neonatal risks among extremely macrosomic babies and their mothers. *American Journal of Obstetrics and Gynecology, 204*(5), 423.e1–423.e6. doi:10.1016/j.ajog.2010.12.036

Vrouenraets, F. P. J. M., Roumen, F. J. M. E., Dehing, C. J. G., van den Akker, E. S. A., Aarts, M. J. B., & Scheve, E. J. T. (2005). Bishop score and risk of cesarean delivery after induction of labor in nulliparous women. *Obstetrics and Gynecology, 105*(4), 690–697. doi:10.1097/01.AOG.0000152338.76759.38

Wasserstrum, N. (1992). Issues in fluid management during labor: General considerations. *Clinics in Obstetrics and Gynecology, 35*(3), 505–513.

Weeks, A., Alfirevic, Z., Faúndes, A., Hofmeyr, G. J., Safar, P., & Wing, D. (2007). Misoprostol for induction of labor with a live fetus. *International Journal of Gynaecology and Obstetrics, 99*(Suppl. 2), S194–S197. doi:10.1016/j.ijgo.2007.09.011

Wei, S. Q., Luo, Z. C., Qi, H. P., Xu, H., & Fraser, W. D. (2010). High-dose vs low-dose oxytocin for labor augmentation: A systematic review. *American Journal of Obstetrics and Gynecology, 203*(4), 296–304. doi:10.1016/j.ajog.2010.03.007

Wein, P. (1989). Efficacy of different starting doses of oxytocin for induction of labor. *Obstetrics and Gynecology, 74*(6), 863–868.

Werner, E. F., Janevic, T. M., Illuzzi, J., Funai, E. F., Savitz, D. A., & Lipkind, H. S. (2011). Mode of delivery in nulliparous women and neonatal intracranial injury. *Obstetrics and Gynecology, 118*(6), 1239–1246. doi:10.1097/AOG.0b013e31823835d3

Williams, M. K., & Chames, M. C. (2006). Risk factors for the breakdown of perineal laceration repair after vaginal delivery. *American Journal of Obstetrics and Gynecology, 195*(3), 755–759. doi:10.1016/j.ajog.2006.06.085

Wing, D. A., & Farinelli, C. K. (2012). Abnormal labor and induction of labor. In S. G. Gabbe, J. R. Niebyl, J. L. Simpson, M. B. Landon, H. L. Galan, E. R. M. Jauniaux, & D. A. Driscoll (Eds.). *Obstetrics: Normal and Problem Pregnancies* (5th ed., pp. 287–311). Philadelphia: Elsevier Saunders.

Wong, C. A., Scavone, B. M., Dugan, S., Smith, J. C., Prather, H., Ganchiff, J. N., & McCarthy, R. J. (2003). Incidence of postpartum lumbosacral spine and lower extremity nerve injuries. *Obstetrics and Gynecology, 101*(2), 279–288.

Wood, C., Ng, K., Hounslow, D., & Benning, H. (1973). The influences of different birth times upon fetal condition in normal deliveries. *Journal of Obstetrics and Gynaecology of the British Commonwealth, 80*(4), 289–294.

Yap, O. W., Kim, E. S., & Laros, R. K. Jr. (2001). Maternal and neonatal outcomes after uterine rupture in labor. *American Journal of Obstetrics and Gynecology, 184*(7), 1576–1581.

Yildirim, G., & Beji, N. K. (2008). Effects of pushing techniques in birth on mother and fetus: A randomized study. *Birth, 35*(1), 25–30 doi:10.1111/j.1523-536X.2007.00208.x

Zanardo, V., Svegliado, G., Cavallin, F., Giustardi A., Cosmi, E., Litta, P., & Trevisanuto, D. (2010). Elective cesarean delivery: Does it have a negative effect on breastfeeding? *Birth, 37*(4), 275–279. doi:10.1111/j.1523-536X.2010.00421.x

Zeeman, G. G., Khan-Dawood, F. S., & Dawood, M. Y. (1997). Oxytocin and its receptor in pregnancy and parturition: Current concepts and clinical implications. *Obstetrics and Gynecology, 89*(5, Pt. 2), 873–883.

Zeiman, M., Fong, S. K., Benowitz, N. L., Banskter, D., & Darney, P. D. (1997). Absorption kinetics of misoprostol with oral and vaginal administration. *Obstetrics and Gynecology, 90*(1), 88–92.

Zelig, C. M., Nichols, S. F., Dolinsky, B. M., Hecht, M. W., & Napolitano, P. G. (2012). Interaction between maternal obesity and Bishop score in predicting successful induction of labor in term, nulliparous patients. *American Journal of Perinatology.* Advance online publication. doi:10.1055/s-0032-1322510

Zhang, J., Branch, D. W., Ramirez, M. M., Laughon, S. K., Reddy, U., Hoffman, M., . . . Hibbard, J. U. (2011). Oxytocin regimen for labor augmentation, labor progression, and perinatal outcomes. *Obstetrics and Gynecology, 188*(2, Pt. 1), 249–256. doi:10.1097/AOG.0b013e3182220192

Zhang, J., Landy, H. J., Branch, D. W., Burkman, R., Haberman, S., Gregory, K. D, . . . Reddy, U. M. (2010). Contemporary patterns of spontaneous labor with normal neonatal outcomes. *Obstetrics and Gynecology, 116*(6), 1281–1287. doi:10.1097/AOG.0b013e3181fdef6e

Zhang, J., Troendle, J., Mikolajczyk, R., Sundaram, R., Beaver, J., & Fraser, W. (2010). The natural history of the normal first stage of labor. *Obstetrics and Gynecology, 115*(4), 705–710. doi:10.1097/AOG.0b013e3181d55925

Zhang, J., Troendle, J., Reddy, U. M., Laughon, S. K., Branch, D. W., Burkman, R., . . . van Veldhuisen, P. (2010). Contemporary cesarean delivery practice in the United States. *American Journal of Obstetrics and Gynecology, 203*(4), 326.e1–326.e10. doi:10.1016/j.ajog.2010.06.058

Zhang, J., Troendle, J. F., & Yancey, M. K. (2002). Reassessing the labor curve in multiparous women. *American Journal of Obstetrics and Gynecology, 187*(4), 824–828.

Zhang, J., Yancey, M. K., & Henderson, C. E. (2002). U. S. National trends in labor induction, 1989–1998. *Journal of Reproductive Medicine, 47*(2), 120–124.

APPENDIX 14–A

Second-Stage Labor Care

PURPOSE

To promote safe and effective care during second stage labor.

These clinical guidelines apply to all women in labor, with an emphasis on women with regional analgesia/anesthesia.

SUGGESTED CLINICAL GUIDELINES

WHEN TO BEGIN MATERNAL PUSHING EFFORTS

Delay pushing until the woman has the urge to push (up to 2 hours for nulliparous women with regional analgesia/anesthesia; up to 1 hour for multiparous women with regional analgesia/anesthesia) to shorten the active pushing phase.

HOW TO ENCOURAGE MATERNAL PUSHING EFFORTS

Discourage prolonged breath holding. Instead, instruct the woman to bear down and allow her to choose whether or not to hold her breath while pushing.

Discourage more than three to four pushing efforts with each contraction and more than 6 to 8 seconds of each pushing effort.

Take steps to maintain a normal fetal heart rate (FHR) pattern while pushing. Modify maternal pushing efforts based on fetal status. Push with every other or every third contraction if necessary to avoid recurrent FHR decelerations. In some situations, it may be necessary to stop pushing temporarily to allow the fetus to recover.

MATERNAL POSITIONING

Encourage repositioning often based on maternal comfort and fetal status.
Use semi-Fowlers with the mother's feet flat on the bed.
Use lateral positioning as an alternative.
Avoid hyperflexing the mother's knees against her abdomen.

Consider the towel-pull technique for maternal fatigue and/or promotion of fetal rotation.
Avoid supine positioning.
Avoid the use of stirrups during pushing.

UTERINE ACTIVITY

If oxytocin is infusing, consider decreasing or discontinuing oxytocin to approximate physiologic second-stage labor contraction patterns.

Avoid uterine tachysystole in the second stage of labor; treat in a timely manner before the FHR pattern becomes indeterminate or abnormal.

MATERNAL–FETAL ASSESSMENT

Assess characteristics of the FHR pattern and uterine activity:

Physiologic conditions during passive fetal descent are similar to late first-stage labor. Therefore, maternal–fetal assessment frequencies during first-stage labor, based on risk status, can be used during passive fetal descent.
During the passive decent phase: every 30 minutes if no maternal–fetal risk factors have been identified; every 15 minutes if maternal–fetal risk factors have been identified and/or if oxytocin is infusing.
During the active pushing phase: every 15 minutes if no maternal–fetal risk factors have been identified; every 5 minutes if maternal–fetal risk factors have been identified and/or if oxytocin is infusing.

MEDICAL RECORD DOCUMENTATION

Each time maternal–fetal status is documented during second-stage labor, the following aspects are included:

FHR characteristics (baseline rate, variability, presence or absence of accelerations, and presence or absence of decelerations)
Uterine activity characteristics (frequency, duration, intensity, and resting tone as appropriate to monitoring method)
Maternal position

Oxytocin rate, if infusing

How the woman is tolerating/responding to push-ing (during the active pushing phase)

Pain perception

Summary documentation every 15 to 30 minutes during the active pushing phase including these aspects is appropriate, noting continuous bedside attendance and assessment.

MATERNAL COMFORT/PAIN RELIEF

Maintain pain relief measures; avoid decreasing or dis-continuing the epidural infusion.

Reposition as necessary.

URINARY BLADDER STATUS

Avoid use of Foley catheters during labor.

Encourage the mother to void on the bedpan; if she is unable, consider use of an in-and-out catheter if bladder needs to be emptied.

If Foley catheter has been in use during labor, dis-continue during pushing.

PHYSICIAN/NURSE MIDWIFE COMMUNICATION

Notify physician/nurse midwife when birth is immi-nent and/or maternal–fetal condition is such that bed-side evaluation/attendance is requested.

REFERENCES

American Academy of Pediatrics and American College of Obstetri-cians and Gynecologists. (2012). *Guidelines for Perinatal Care.* Elk Grove Village, IL: Author.

American College of Obstetricians and Gynecologists. (2000). *Oper-ative Vaginal Delivery* (Practice Bulletin No. 17). Washington, DC: Author.

American College of Obstetricians and Gynecologists. (2003). *Dys-tocia and Augmentation of Labor* (Practice Bulletin No. 49). Washington, DC: Author.

Association of Women's Health, Obstetric and Neonatal Nurses. (2008). *Nursing Management of the Second Stage of Labor: Evidence-Based Clinical Practice Guideline* (2nd ed.). Washington, DC: Author.

APPENDIX   1 4 – B

Induction/Augmentation of Labor with Oxytocin

PURPOSE

To promote safe and effective use of oxytocin for induction and augmentation of labor.

POLICY

PHYSICIAN/NURSE MIDWIFE/NURSE RESPONSIBILITIES:

Responsibility for the decision to use oxytocin for labor induction or augmentation rests with the attending obstetrician and/or certified nurse midwife (CNM).

Labor nurses may refuse to administer oxytocin if in their best judgment it is contraindicated, or if the needs of the service make it difficult or impossible to adequately monitor maternal–fetal status. The attend-ing physician and/or CNM will be notified.

GUIDELINES FOR PRACTICE:

BEFORE OXYTOCIN ADMINISTRATION

Verify that the physician and/or CNM has discussed the indications and the potential risks and benefits of induction or augmentation of labor with the pregnant

woman and that maternal consent is documented in the medical record.

Verify that the indication for induction is document-ed in the medical record. If indication is elective, verify gestational age of ≥39 completed weeks of gestation.

Follow routine admission procedure and perform vaginal examination to evaluate cervical status and fetal station and presentation. Document the Bishop score in the medical record (see the following). The labor nurse, CNM, attending physician, or resident physician in training may determine cervical status based on the Bishop score. The labor nurse may per-form the initial vaginal examination and subsequent vaginal examinations during labor.

Assist the woman to a position of comfort, preferably the left or right lateral position or an upright position.

Apply an electronic fetal monitor (EFM) and record the fetal heart rate (FHR) for at least 30 minutes prior to the initiation of oxytocin infusion. Before oxytocin is administered, the FHR should be normal. Notify physician and/or CNM if the FHR is indeterminate/abnormal.

OXYTOCIN DOSAGE AND ADMINISTRATION

Pre-mixed solution of 30 units in 500 mL of lactated Ringer's (L/R) solution (1 milliunit per minute [mU/min] = 1 milliliter per hour [mL/hr])

BISHOP SCORING SYSTEM

Score	Dilatation (cm)	Effacement (%)	Station	Consistency	Position of Cervix
0	Closed	0–30	–3	Firm	Posterior
1	1–2	40–50	–2	Medium	Midposition
2	3–4	60–70	–1, 0	Soft	Anterior
3	≥5	≥80	+1, +2		

From Bishop, E. H. (1964). Pelvic scoring for elective induction. *Obstetrics and Gynecology, 24,* 266.

Start oxytocin at 1 to 2 mU/min and gradually increase by 1 to 2 mU/min every 30 to 40 minutes until adequate progress of labor is established and/or contractions are every 2 to 3 minutes.

Once adequate labor is established, maintain or decrease oxytocin to baseline rate necessary for continued labor progress.

Decrease or discontinue oxytocin infusion during the second stage of labor to approximate physiologic second-stage contraction patterns.

The oxytocin infusion may be increased to 20 mU/min per this protocol at the discretion of the nurse. A bedside evaluation of the attending physician and/or CNM is needed to increase beyond 20 mU/min. This should be considered only in unusual clinical situations.

MATERNAL–FETAL ASSESSMENT AND DOCUMENTATION

An assessment of maternal–fetal status, described in the following, should occur every 15 minutes during the first stage of labor and every 5 minutes during the active pushing phase of the second stage of labor while oxytocin is being administered. Summary documentation may occur at 30-minute intervals during the active pushing phase of second-stage labor with a note that the nurse is in continuous bedside attendance assessing maternal–fetal status. The following documentation in the medical record is required each time oxytocin dosage rate is increased or decreased (or at least every 15 minutes if the dosage is unchanged):

Fetal Heart Rate: baseline rate, baseline variability, presence or absence of FHR accelerations, presence or absence of FHR decelerations, and interventions as appropriate

Uterine Activity: contraction frequency, duration, intensity, and uterine resting tone by palpation or intrauterine pressure catheter (IUPC)

Maternal Response to Labor: the woman's response to the contractions (i.e., not feeling contractions, using breathing techniques with contractions, requires intense labor coaching with contractions, comfortable with contractions with epidural analgesia)

Oxytocin Dose: in milliunits per minute

If a registered nurse is not available to clinically evaluate the effects of the oxytocin infusion at least every 15 minutes, the infusion should be discontinued until that level of nursing care is available (Simpson, 2013). The attending physician will be notified. A registered nurse may provide care for two women undergoing cervical ripening with pharmacologic agents or one woman undergoing labor induction or augmentation with oxytocin.

MATERNAL ACTIVITY

Encourage the woman to try alternatives to bed rest such as ambulating in the labor and delivery room (LDR) or hall or using the rocking chair. Other labor support techniques for women who wish to be out of bed include use of the birthing ball and a warm shower. When the woman is out of bed during oxytocin infusion, use EFM telemetry unit to monitor FHR and uterine activity.

TACHYSYSTOLE

Tachysystole is defined as (ACOG, 2003, 2009; Simpson, 2013; Macones et al., 2008):

more than five contractions in 10 minutes (averaged over 30 minutes),
contractions lasting 2 minutes or more,
contractions of normal duration occurring within 1 minute of each other, or
insufficient return of uterine resting tone between contractions via palpation or intraamniotic pressure above 25 mm Hg between contractions via IUPC

SUGGESTED CLINICAL PROTOCOL FOR OXYTOCIN-INDUCED UTERINE TACHYSYSTOLE

Oxytocin-Induced Tachysystole (Normal FHR)

- Maternal repositioning (either left or right)
- Intravenous (IV) fluid bolus of L/R solution
- If uterine activity has not returned to normal after 10 minutes, decrease oxytocin rate by at least half; if uterine activity has not returned to normal after 10 more minutes, discontinue oxytocin until uterine activity is less than five contractions in 10 minutes.

Oxytocin-Induced Tachysystole (Indeterminate/Abnormal FHR)

- Discontinue oxytocin.
- Maternal repositioning (either left or right).
- IV fluid bolus of L/R solution.
- Consider oxygen at 10 L/min via nonrebreather facemask if the first interventions listed previously do not resolve the indeterminate/abnormal FHR pattern and/or variability is minimal or absent. Discontinue as soon as possible.
- If no response, consider 0.25 mg terbutaline SQ.
- Notify primary provider of actions taken and maternal–fetal response.

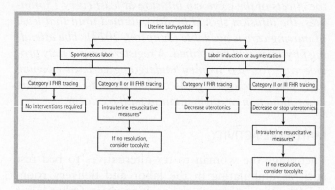

Resumption of Oxytocin After Resolution of Tachysystole:

- If oxytocin has been discontinued for less than 20 to 30 minutes, the FHR is normal and contraction frequency, intensity, and duration are normal, resume oxytocin at no more than half the rate that caused the tachysystole and gradually increase the rate as appropriate based on unit protocol and maternal–fetal status. If the oxytocin is discontinued for more than 30 to 40 minutes, resume oxytocin at the initial dose ordered.

INDETERMINATE/ABNORMAL FETAL STATUS

Identification of indeterminate/abnormal fetal status requires notification of the physician and/or CNM after interventions to resolve the clinical situation, documentation in the medical record of the interventions to resolve the clinical situation, the maternal–fetal response, and the content of the conversation between the nurse and the provider.

EPIDURAL ANALGESIA/ANESTHESIA

Women receiving oxytocin who have epidural analgesia/anesthesia should have pelvic examinations periodically as clinically indicated to assess labor progress.

INTERNAL MONITORING

Internal monitoring may be appropriate based on the individual clinical situation. If unable to record an interpretable FHR tracing and/or uterine activity tracing, women receiving oxytocin may have fetal scalp electrode (FSE) and/or IUPC placed, if indicated. Membranes must be ruptured and the cervix must be at least 2 to 3 cm dilated before the nurse can insert a FSE or IUPC.

Insertion of a FSE or IUPC requires a physician or CNM order. Oxytocin is not in itself an indication for internal monitoring if external monitoring produces an interpretable tracing and there is not a clinical need for more accurate data about intrauterine pressure.

If unable to insert internal monitors and/or the FHR and/or uterine activity continues to be unable to be recorded, the oxytocin infusion should be discontinued until an interpretable FHR pattern and uterine activity pattern can be recorded. The physician and/or the CNM who ordered the oxytocin should be notified.

CARE OF WOMEN ATTEMPTING VAGINAL BIRTH AFTER CESAREAN

Oxytocin may be used to induce or augment labor of women attempting vaginal birth after cesarean birth (VBAC). Verify that the consent for VBAC labor has been obtained and included in the medical record. Continuous EFM is recommended with insertion of an IPUC as soon as clinically possible. The lowest dose of oxytocin required to achieve adequate labor progress should be used. Oxytocin rates beyond 20 mU/min are not recommended.

REFERENCES

American Academy of Pediatrics and American College of Obstetricians and Gynecologists. (2012). *Guidelines for Perinatal Care.* Elk Grove Village, IL: Author.

American College of Obstetricians and Gynecologists. (2003). *Dystocia and Augmentation of Labor* (Practice Bulletin No. 49). Washington, DC: Author.

American College of Obstetricians and Gynecologists. (2009). *Intrapartum Fetal Heart Rate Monitoring: Nomenclature, Interpretation and General Management Principles* (Practice Bulletin No. 106). Washington, DC: Author.

American College of Obstetricians and Gynecologists. (2010). *Management of Intrapartum Fetal Heart Rate Tracings* (Practice Bulletin No. 116). Washington, DC: Author.

Simpson, K. R. (2013). *Cervical Ripening, Labor Induction and Labor Augmentation* (AWHONN Practice Monograph). Washington, DC: Association of Women's Health, Obstetric and Neonatal Nurses.

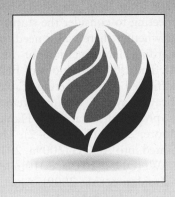

Audrey Lyndon
Nancy O'Brien-Abel
Kathleen Rice Simpson

Fetal Assessment during Labor

INTRODUCTION

The introduction of electronic fetal monitoring (EFM) in the late 1960s has had a far-reaching impact on perinatal care and the practice of nursing, midwifery, and medicine. Despite debate about advantages and limitations, effects on perinatal morbidity and mortality, and role in healthcare costs and malpractice litigation, EFM is used in the majority of labor and birth units in the United States and Canada today. This chapter discusses the physiologic basis for fetal heart rate (FHR) monitoring, defines FHR patterns, and reviews intrapartum management of FHR patterns.

HISTORICAL PERSPECTIVES

Publication of the discovery of fetal heart tones in 1822 marked the beginning of modern obstetric practice (Sureau, 1996; Goodlin, 1979). Jean Alexandre Le Jumeau, Vicomte de Kergaradec used a stethoscope hoping to hear the noise of the water in the uterus. Although M. Maior of Geneva was the first person credited with identifying fetal heart tones, Kergaradec was the first person astute enough to suggest in print potential clinical uses for FHR auscultation (Kennedy, 1843; Goodlin, 1979). In the early 1800s, researchers working independently in Switzerland, Ireland, Germany, France, and the United States described fetal heart tones, and in 1833, the British obstetrician William Kennedy described fetal heart sounds as a "quick double pulsation" with a usual rate of 130 to 140 beats per minute (bpm). Kennedy (1843) noted the rate was sometimes slower and sometimes much faster, depending on "inherent vital causes" (p. 107). He documented fetal heart variation in labor, including rates as high as 180 to 200 bpm in ill mothers

and slowing and cessation of the FHR prior to stillbirth. In 1858, Schwartz of Germany suggested that the FHR be counted often during labor, both between and during contractions, to promote improved outcomes. Schwartz described the association between fetal bradycardia and decreased uteroplacental blood flow during contractions. In 1849, Killian proposed forceps-assisted birth for an FHR of fewer than 100 bpm or greater than 180 bpm (Goodlin, 1979). Soon after, Winckel described specific FHR criteria to be used for the diagnosis of fetal distress via auscultation (Goodlin, 1979). After the invention of the fetoscope in the early 1900s, fetal heart sounds were commonly assessed in order to document fetal viability during the prenatal period. Winckel's criteria were used in clinical practice until the 1950s when Hon raised concern about the subjectivity of counting heartbeats during labor.

Although interest in continuous recording of fetal heart tones by various methods dates to the later years of the 19th century, the major development of modern clinical EFM occurred during the 1960s. In 1906, Cramer produced the first electrocardiographic (ECG) recording of the fetal heartbeat. Research using abdominal leads to obtain the fetal ECG continued but remained impractical for clinical use until the mid-1960s, when techniques capable of excluding the maternal ECG from the recording became available. By the 1950s, research on electronic methods of FHR monitoring escalated. In 1958, Hon published the first report of continuous fetal ECG monitoring using a device placed on the maternal abdomen. By the 1960s, Hon, Caldeyro-Barcia, and Hammacher were reporting successful attempts at developing an electronic FHR monitor that could continuously record FHR data (Caldeyro-Barcia et al., 1966; Hammacher, 1969; Hon, 1963). Although many others have contributed to what is known about fetal assessment during labor, EFM, as it is used today, is largely the result of the work of these three investigators working independently on separate continents. In 1968, the first commercially available EFMs were introduced.

Coinciding with the development of EFM technology was the emergence of data that refuted the effectiveness of intermittent auscultation (IA) with Delee or Pinard fetoscopes. The Benson, Shubeck, Deutschberger, Weiss, and Berendes (1968) study of more than 24,000 births, called the Collaborative Perinatal Project, concluded that FHR auscultation during labor was unreliable in determining fetal distress except in extreme cases of terminal bradycardias. Based on this report and rapid technologic advances, IA of the FHR between contractions was rapidly replaced with continuous EFM during the 1970s. Over the next three decades, EFM became the preferred method of fetal surveillance during the intrapartum period in the United States and Canada.

During the 1980s and 1990s, several randomized trials that compared IA to continuous EFM were conducted (MacDonald, Grant, Sheridan-Pereira, Boylan, & Chalmers, 1985; Thacker, Stroup, & Peterson, 1995; Vintzileos et al., 1993). Disappointingly, EFM did not decrease perinatal mortality or prevent cerebral palsy. Equally important, the women in EFM groups experienced a fourfold increase in operative birth (Thacker et al., 1995). The potential reasons why EFM did not demonstrate efficacy in the randomized trials include methodological flaws, inconsistent criteria and terminology to describe fetal status, and the use of outcome variables for which there were insufficient sample sizes to determine a significant difference between IA and continuous EFM.

The demonstrated increase in cesarean birth rates fueled reexamination of all aspects of EFM use. In 1997, the National Institute of Child Health and Human Development (NICHD) of the National Institutes of Health convened a panel of FHR monitoring experts. This group proposed quantitative definitions of FHR characteristics to serve as a basis for standardizing research that uses FHR data (NICHD, 1997). Between 1997 and 2004, there was gradual but sporadic adoption of the proposed standardized FHR definitions in clinical practice in the United States. In July 2004, the Joint Commission on Accreditation of Healthcare Organizations (JCAHO; now known as The Joint Commission [TJC]) recommended use of a standard language for communication and documentation of FHR patterns. In May 2005, the Association of Women's Health, Obstetric and Neonatal Nurses (AWHONN) and the American College of Obstetricians and Gynecologists (ACOG) formally supported adoption of the NICHD definitions for FHR patterns as the standardized language for communicating fetal status (ACOG, 2005a;

AWHONN, 2005). In 2008, the NICHD held an interdisciplinary meeting to consider the status of FHR terminology and whether there was a need for additional guidance regarding interpretation of FHR patterns (Spong, 2008). The 1997 definitions of FHR characteristics were reaffirmed at this meeting (Table 15–1), and a new classification system for interpretation of FHR patterns was proposed (Macones, Hankins, Spong, Hauth, & Moore, 2008) (Table 15–2). These changes were incorporated into ACOG (2009a, 2010b) practice bulletins, the AWHONN (2010a, 2010b) fetal monitoring program (Lyndon & Ali, 2009), American College of Nurse-Midwives (ACNM; 2010a, 2010b) documents, and National Certification Corporation (NCC) certification examinations.

Currently, clinical reliance on EFM remains high despite the lack of positive results from published research. To date, EFM is the primary screening technique for the clinical determination of the adequacy of fetal oxygenation during labor. This paradox is better understood following a review of the physiology of the fetal heart and its adaptations during labor. The feelings of many clinicians about EFM versus IA were summarized by Cibils in 1996 (p. 1383): "It is difficult to understand the premise that the intermittent recording (by a crude method) of a given biologic variable [the FHR] will be better to make a clinical decision affecting the mother and fetus than the continuous, precise recording of the same variable." Chen, Chauhan, Ananth, Vintzileos, and Abuhamad (2011) conducted retrospective cohort study of over 4 million U.S. births occurring between 24 and 44 weeks' gestation in 2004, using linked birth certificate and infant death certificate data. They found that EFM was used in 89% of births, and EFM use was associated with a substantially decreased risk of low Apgar scores (<4), low Apgar score with seizures, and early neonatal death. However, as pointed out by Devoe (2011a), the design of the Chen et al. study cannot address causality or the nature of the relationship between the use of EFM and the observed outcomes. Moreover, the study did not examine EFM tracings, the labor process, or other myriad circumstances surrounding each birth, and the birth certificate–recorded rate of EFM use was substantially lower than that reported by mothers who have given birth (Declercq, Sakala, Corry & Appelbaum, 2006). Hence, although the study provides some support for the use of EFM, true confirmatory data about improved outcomes when EFM is used during labor are still lacking. Nevertheless, most clinicians prefer EFM as the intrapartum method of fetal assessment, and it is recommended by ACOG (2009a) and the Society of Obstetricians and Gynaecologists of Canada (SOGC) (2007) for high-risk maternal–fetal conditions during labor.

Table 15–1. FETAL HEART RATE CHARACTERISTICS

Term	Definition
Baseline rate	Approximate mean FHR rounded to increments of 5 bpm during a 10-min window excluding accelerations and decelerations and periods of marked variability. There must be ≥2 min of identifiable baseline segments (not necessarily contiguous) in any 10-min window, or the baseline for that period is indeterminate. In such cases, one may need to refer to the previous 10-min window for determination of the baseline.
Bradycardia	Baseline rate of <110 bpm.
Tachycardia	Baseline rate of >160 bpm.
Baseline variability	Determined in a 10-min window, excluding accelerations and decelerations. Fluctuations in the baseline FHR that are irregular in amplitude and frequency and are visually quantified as the amplitude of the peak-to-trough in bpm.
- Absent variability	Amplitude range undetectable.
- Minimal variability	Amplitude range visually detectable but ≤5 bpm. (Greater than undetectable but ≤5 bpm.)
- Moderate variability	Amplitude range 6–25 bpm.
- Marked variability	Amplitude range >25 bpm.
Acceleration	Visually apparent **abrupt** increase in FHR. *Abrupt* increase is defined as an increase from onset of acceleration to peak is <30 sec. Peak must be ≥15 bpm and must last ≥15 sec from the onset to return. Acceleration lasting ≥10 min is defined as a baseline change. Before 32 weeks of gestation, accelerations are defined as having a peak ≥10 bpm and duration of ≥10 sec.
Prolonged acceleration	Acceleration ≥ 2 min but <10 min in duration.
Early deceleration	Visually apparent, usually symmetrical, **gradual** decrease and return of FHR associated with a uterine contraction. The *gradual* FHR decrease is defined as one from the onset to FHR nadir of ≥30 sec. The decrease in FHR is calculated from onset to nadir of deceleration. The nadir of the deceleration occurs at the same time as the peak of the contraction. In most cases, the onset, nadir, and recovery of the deceleration are coincident with the beginning, peak, and ending of the contraction, respectively.
Late deceleration	Visually apparent, usually symmetrical, **gradual** decrease and return of FHR associated with a uterine contraction. The *gradual* FHR decrease is defined as from the onset to FHR nadir of ≥30 sec. The decrease in FHR is calculated from onset to the nadir of deceleration. The deceleration is delayed in timing, with nadir of the deceleration occurring after the peak of the contraction. In most cases, the onset, nadir, and recovery of the deceleration occur after the beginning, peak, and ending of the contraction, respectively.
Variable deceleration	Visually apparent **abrupt** decrease in FHR. An *abrupt* FHR decrease is defined as from the onset of the deceleration to beginning of FHR nadir of <30 sec. The decrease in FHR is calculated from the onset to the nadir of deceleration. The decrease in FHR is ≥15 bpm, lasting ≥15 sec, and <2 min in duration. When variable decelerations are associated with uterine contractions, their onset, depth, and duration commonly vary with successive uterine contractions.
Prolonged deceleration	Visually apparent decrease in FHR from baseline that is ≥15 bpm, lasting ≥2 min, but <10 min. A deceleration that lasts ≥10 min is baseline change.
Recurrent	Occurring with ≥50% of contractions in any 20-min window.
Intermittent	Occurring with <50% of contractions in any 20-min window.
Sinusoidal pattern	Visually apparent, smooth, sine wave–like undulating pattern in FHR baseline with cycle frequency of 3–5/min that persists for ≥20 min.

FHR, fetal heart rate.
Adapted from Lyndon, A., O'Brien-Abel, N., & Simpson, K. R. (2009). Fetal heart rate interpretation. In A. Lyndon & L. U. Ali (Eds.), *Fetal Heart Monitoring Principles and Practices* (4th ed., p. 105). Washington, DC: Association of Women's Health, Obstetric and Neonatal Nurses/Kendall Hunt; Macones, G. A., Hankins, G. D., Spong, C. Y., Hauth, J. D., & Moore, T. (2008). The 2008 National Institute of Child Health Human Development workshop report on electronic fetal monitoring: Update on definitions, interpretations, and research guidelines. *Obstetrics & Gynecology, 112*, 661–666, and *Journal of Obstetric, Gynecologic and Neonatal Nursing, 37*, 510–515.

DEFINITIONS AND APPROPRIATE USE OF TERMS DESCRIBING FETAL HEART RATE PATTERNS

Appropriate clinical management of variant FHR patterns and effective clinical communication are both enhanced by use of standardized definitions that convey agreed upon meanings among the members of the healthcare team. Adoption of a common language for FHR characteristics and pattern definitions, as well as medical record documentation that is mutually agreed upon and routinely used by all providers, enhances interdisciplinary communication and, therefore, maternal–fetal safety (JCAHO, 2004). Both oral communication and written documentation must accurately convey the clinician's level of concern and/or record the presumed diagnosis. The chances of miscommunication between care providers, especially during telephone

Table 15–2. THREE-TIERED SYSTEM FOR FETAL HEART RATE INTERPRETATION

Classification	Definition	Interpretation
Category I	Includes **all** of the following characteristics: Baseline rate 110–160 bpm Moderate baseline variability Accelerations present or absent Late or variable decelerations absent Early decelerations present or absent	Normal: Predictive of normal fetal acid–base balance at the time of observation
Category II	All tracings that do not meet criteria for category I or category III Represents an "appreciable fraction" of tracings encountered in clinical care	Indeterminate: Not predictive of abnormal fetal acid–base status but cannot be classified as category I or III
Category III	Either: Absent baseline variability and any of the following: Recurrent late deceleration Recurrent variable decelerations Bradycardia OR Sinusoidal pattern	Abnormal: Associated with abnormal fetal acid–base status at the time of observation

Adapted from Macones, G. A., Hankins, G. D., Spong, C. Y., Hauth, J., & Moore, T. (2008). The 2008 National Institute of Child Health and Human Development workshop report on electronic fetal monitoring: Update on definitions, interpretation, and research guidelines. *Obstetrics and Gynecology, 112*(3), 661–666, and *Journal of Obstetric, Gynecologic, and Neonatal Nursing, 37*(5), 510–515.

conversations about fetal status, are decreased when everyone is speaking the same language (Simpson & Knox, 2006, 2009). Timely intervention is dependent on clear communication between providers sharing care of an individual patient (Fox, Kilpatrick, King, & Parer, 2000; Miller, 2005; Simpson & Knox, 2009). The NICHD (Macones et al., 2008) nomenclature is the basis for the pattern descriptions in this chapter.

The three-tiered classification system for FHR pattern interpretation put forth by the NICHD reflects both the presence and absence of scientific consensus on FHR interpretation (Macones et al., 2008) (see Table 15–2). There is little controversy concerning what constitutes a normal FHR pattern. Most clinicians agree on the definition of a normal (category I) FHR tracing (i.e., baseline rate within 110 to 160 bpm, moderate FHR variability, and absence of late or variable decelerations; accelerations and early decelerations may both be present or absent in a normal tracing). There is good evidence that this type of FHR tracing confers an extremely high predictability of a normally oxygenated fetus when it is obtained (ACOG, 2009a; Macones et al., 2008). Of note, while the presence of spontaneous or induced accelerations is predictive of normal fetal acid–base status at the time of observation, the absence of accelerations is not a reliable predictor of fetal acidemia (Macones et al., 2008).

At the other end of the spectrum from normality, several patterns are likely predictive of current or impending fetal asphyxia so severe that the fetus is at risk for neurologic and other fetal damage or death (Macones et al., 2008). These patterns are classified as abnormal (category III) and include absent baseline FHR variability with recurrent late or variable decelerations or bradycardia, or a sinusoidal FHR pattern. Patterns at this end of the spectrum are considered predictive of abnormal fetal acid–base status and require prompt evaluation and intervention (Macones et al., 2008).

Many fetuses have FHR tracings that are intermediate between these two extremes, and there is no consensus on their presumed condition or clinical management because there is inconsistent evidence in the literature regarding their predictive value in relation to fetal acid–base status. These tracings are classified as indeterminate (category II). Category II tracings include all tracings that are not categorized as category I or category III. This includes tracings demonstrating alterations in baseline (e.g., bradycardia with minimal or moderate variability) and tracings with recurrent late or variable decelerations and minimal or moderate variability, among others. Category II tracings are not considered predictive of abnormal acid–base status at the time they are observed, but they also cannot reliably be placed in category I on the basis of current evidence (Macones et al., 2008). These tracings can be conceptualized as representing some level of fetal physiologic stress. Thus evaluation, attempts to ameliorate or reduce any identified stressors, reevaluation, and close surveillance of these tracings are appropriate (ACOG, 2010b); most clinicians do not wait until the FHR pattern is at the extreme end of abnormality before intervening to attempt to improve fetal status via one or more intrauterine resuscitation techniques (Garite & Simpson, 2011; Simpson, 2007).

A review of the literature on the association between FHR patterns and fetal acidemia found moderate FHR variability was strongly associated with an umbilical cord pH >7.15 or newborn vigor (5-minute Apgar score ≥7). Absent or minimal FHR variability with late or variable decelerations was the strongest predictor of newborn acidemia. The correlation between diminished variability and acidemia was 23%, which the investigators suggest was low because studies reviewed did not always differentiate between decreased and absent variability, and the association with absent variability is likely stronger. The investigators found increasing depth of decelerations was correlated with low pH (<7.15). Acidemia took time to develop except in situations of sudden profound bradycardia. In the context of decreasing variability with recurrent decelerations, newborn acidemia developed over a period of time approaching 1 hour (Parer, King, Flanders, Fox, & Kilpatrick, 2006).

Further data suggest normal fetal status (category I) is associated with normal short-term neonatal outcomes. Based on an analysis of 48,444 EFM tracings of women in term labor in 10 hospitals, babies whose tracings during the last 2 hours prior to birth were exclusively normal (category I) did well, with only 0.6% having Apgar scores <7 at 5 minutes of life and 0.2% having low Apgar scores with neonatal intensive care unit (NICU) admission. However, when more than 75% of the EFM tracing in last 2 hours prior to birth was indeterminate (category II), low Apgar scores at 5 minutes increased to 1.3% of babies and low Apgar score at 5 minutes with NICU admission increased to 0.7% (Jackson, Holmgren, Esplin, Henry, & Varner, 2011).

Analysis of this large database of women in term labor allowed estimation of the frequency of types of EFM tracings based on the NICHD-defined FHR categories (Macones et al., 2008). When all of labor was included, most tracings (77.9%) were normal (category I), 22.1% were indeterminate (category II), and 0.004% were abnormal (category III). During the last 2 hours of labor prior to birth, normal (category I) decreased to 60.9% of the duration, indeterminate (category II) increased to 39.1%, and abnormal (category III) increased to 0.006%. These last 2 hours included women in second-stage labor that had a vaginal or cesarean birth and women that had a cesarean birth without second-stage labor (Jackson et al., 2011). The strength of the association between time in an indeterminate (category II) tracing and the risk of Apgar score less than 7 with a NICU admission in this study did not increase until more than 50% of the last 2 hours of labor were spent in category II. This is consistent with the findings of Parer et al. (2006) that, in the absence of catastrophic events, acidemia develops over a period of time approximating an hour. Thus, there is supportive evidence for the classification

system developed by NICHD in relation to presumed fetal acid–base status across a continuum of FHR findings. Ideally, members of the perinatal team have a shared method of interpreting FHR patterns and an agreed upon management guideline for specific FHR patterns (Fox et al., 2000; Knox & Simpson, 2011).

Terms such as *stress* and *distress* lack the precise meaning needed to discriminate levels of concern. In 1998, ACOG recommended that *nonreassuring fetal status* replace the term *fetal distress* in its committee opinion *Inappropriate Use of the Terms Fetal Distress and Birth Asphyxia*. This committee opinion was reaffirmed in 2005 (ACOG, 2005b). The three-tiered interpretation system developed by the NICHD EFM expert group was introduced in 2008 (Macones et al., 2008). The term *fetal distress* has a low positive predictive value, even in high-risk populations, and is often associated with an infant who is in good condition at birth as determined by the Apgar score or umbilical cord blood gas analysis or both. Communication between clinicians caring for the woman and those caring for her baby is best served by categorization of the FHR as normal, indeterminate, or abnormal, followed by a further description of findings when the tracing is indeterminate (category II) or abnormal (category III). Further description should include baseline variability, recurrent variable or late decelerations, prolonged decelerations, fetal tachycardia or bradycardia, maternal risk factors, proximity to birth, and identification of the level of urgency for intervention. It is important that team members explicitly reach and confirm agreement on the necessity of intervention or the parameters for continued close surveillance (Lyndon, Zlatnik, & Wachter, 2011).

Whereas in the past, the term *fetal distress* generally referred to an ill fetus, categorization of the FHR pattern describes the clinician's interpretation of data regarding fetal status (i.e., the presumptive relationship between the FHR pattern and fetal acid–base status). The three-tiered categorization scheme acknowledges the imprecision inherent in the interpretation of the data as well as the dynamic nature of the fetal response to labor (Macones et al., 2008). Therefore, the diagnosis of category II or III tracing can be consistent with the birth of a vigorous baby as the predictive value of even category III tracings for neurologic outcome in infants is poor despite indication of increased risk for fetal acidemia (ACOG, 2010b).

Another problematic issue is use of *asphyxia* and or *acidosis* when making a presumptive diagnosis of intrapartum hypoxia. *Asphyxia* means insufficiency or absence of exchange of respiratory gases. The pathologic consequence of asphyxia is injury to the fetal tissues, primarily the brain, with subsequent neurologic impairment. However, asphyxia is a continuum of oxygen deficit that moves from hypoxemia (decreased oxygen content in blood) to acidemia (increased hydrogen ion concentration in blood), then acidosis (increased hydrogen ion concentration in the tissue) (King & Parer, 2000). Hypoxemia and acidemia are detectable via pH measurements of fetal scalp blood or umbilical cord blood at birth. These values reveal the acid–base balance within blood but not within tissue and therefore cannot directly reveal the extent or duration of metabolic acidosis or level of asphyxia in tissue. Thus, the use of terms like *asphyxia* and *acidosis* in communication and medical record documentation about characteristics of the FHR and fetal and/or newborn status is both inappropriate and confusing (Fahey & King, 2005) and should be avoided.

TECHNIQUES OF FETAL HEART RATE MONITORING

ASSESSMENT OF UTERINE ACTIVITY

During the intrapartum period, the FHR is interpreted relative to uterine activity. Therefore, interpretation of FHR patterns includes a complete assessment of four components of the uterine contractions: (1) frequency, (2) duration, (3) intensity, and (4) the uterine resting tone between contractions. These assessments can be made by either palpation, external tocodynamometer (*tokos* is Greek for *childbirth*), or the use of an intrauterine pressure catheter (IUPC).

Assessment of uterine activity begins with palpation. Contraction frequency is measured from the beginning of one contraction to the beginning of the next and is described in minutes. Duration is the length of the contraction and is described in seconds. Intensity refers to the strength of the contraction and is described as mild, moderate, or strong by palpation, or in millimeters of mercury (mm Hg) or Montevideo units (MVUs) if an IUPC is used. Uterine resting tone is assessed in the absence of contractions or between contractions. By direct palpation, resting tone is described as soft or hard and via IUPC in terms of mm Hg or MVUs. As with any procedure, the least invasive approach is preferred unless maternal–fetal status indicates a need for more precise data.

Each technique has some limitations. Intensity cannot be determined with a tocodynamometer. The tocodynamometer detects pressure changes from the tightening of the fundus during contractions through the maternal abdomen. This technique gives a relatively accurate reading of the duration and frequency of contractions but is unable to assess intensity or resting tone. Thus, manual palpation is an essential component of external uterine activity monitoring (Harmon, 2009). With an IUPC, the peak of the contraction as indicated on the fetal monitor tracing depicts the actual strength of the contraction measured in mm Hg pressure within the

amniotic fluid. The IUPC is most accurate because direct measurement of intraamniotic pressure is recorded, but it requires ruptured membranes for insertion, and technical difficulties requiring troubleshooting are not uncommon (Harmon, 2009).

Normal contraction characteristics in the active phase of labor include frequency every 2 to 3 minutes, duration of 80 to 90 seconds, and strong to palpation (Clark, Simpson, Knox, & Garite, 2009). Both contraction characteristics and labor progress are evaluated to determine the adequacy of uterine activity. Some uterine activity patterns are dysfunctional or inadequate for generating progress in labor (Fig. 15–1 A–C). Normal uterine activity is defined as less than or equal to five contractions in 10 minutes averaged over 30 minutes; tachysystole is defined as more than five contractions in 10 minutes averaged over 30 minutes (Macones et al., 2008). Clarke et al. (2009) propose consistent achievement of 200 to 220 MVUs as an indication of adequate labor forces in women receiving oxytocin; however, excessive uterine activity should be avoided to minimize risk of fetal harm. There is an association between higher MVUs and risk of neonatal acidemia at birth. In a study of 1,433 FHR and uterine activity patterns, babies of women with MVUs averaging 236 during first-stage labor were not acidemic at birth, whereas babies of mothers with MVUs averaging 261 had an umbilical artery pH of 7.11 or less (Bakker, Kurver, Kuik, & Van Geijn, 2007). Tachysystole can be spontaneous as a result of endogenous maternal oxytocin or prostaglandins; however, it is more often seen during exogenous stimulation with agents used in cervical ripening and induction and augmentation of labor (Simpson, 2009a).

Coupling or *tripling* refers to a pattern of two or three contractions with little or no interval followed by a regular interval of approximately 2 to 5 minutes. This pattern may be indicative of a dysfunctional labor process and saturation or down-regulation of uterine oxytocin receptor sites (Dawood, 1995; Phaneuf, Rodriguez Linares, TambyRaja, MacKenzie, & Lopez Bernal, 2000; Zeeman, Khan-Dawood, & Dawood, 1997). If coupling or tripling occurs, a suggested intervention to promote normal uterine activity is temporary discontinuation of oxytocin, maternal repositioning, and an intravenous (IV) fluid bolus of lactated Ringer's solution with resumption of oxytocin after 30 to 60 minutes.

EXTERNAL DOPPLER VERSUS FETAL SCALP ELECTRODE

The FHR can be detected via a Doppler ultrasound transducer or fetal electrode. Leopold's maneuvers are used to determine the fetal position prior to applying the Doppler transducer (see Chapter 14). The Doppler transducer is

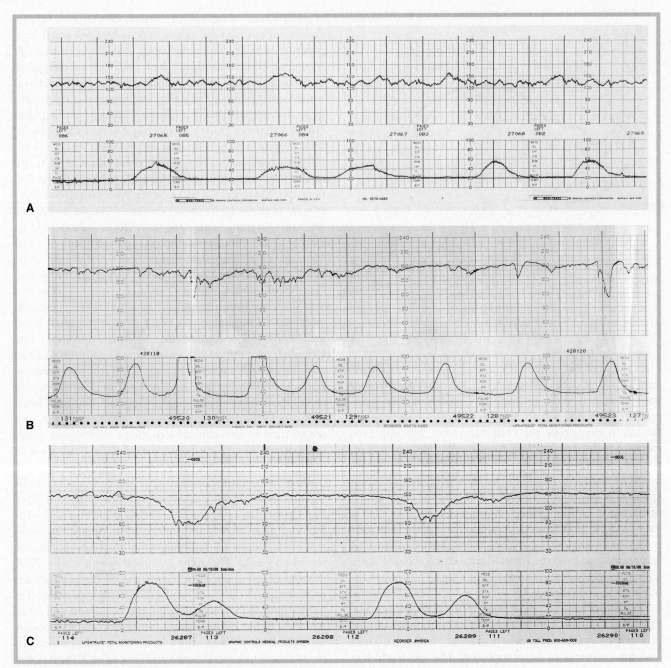

FIGURE 15–1. Three types of uterine contractions. **A,** Normal contraction frequency, duration, and intensity and uterine resting tone. **B,** Tachysystole. **C,** Coupling of contractions.

applied to the maternal abdomen over the fetal back or chest and transmits a high frequency ultrasound. The transducer detects the ultrasound wave that is bounced back off the fetal heart and then counts the FHR by measuring the shift in ultrasound wave frequency between the generated wave and the returning wave reflected off the moving heart (Fig. 15–2). The resulting "Doppler shift" waveform goes through "autocorrelation," where it is digitized, smoothed, compared with adjacent wave forms, and averaged over three consecutive heartbeats to produce the FHR. This signal is amplified and converted by the monitor to both visual and auditory output of the FHR (Harmon, 2009). The ultrasound wave will not conduct to the fetus if there is air between the emission of the wave and the object it is reflecting off. Gel applied to the transducer helps eliminate air between the transducer and maternal abdomen.

In the United States, the monitor plots the calculated FHR on paper that is moving at 3 cm/min, or on a graphic computer representation of monitor paper moving at the same speed. Because there is variability in the time interval between heartbeats in a normally oxygenated

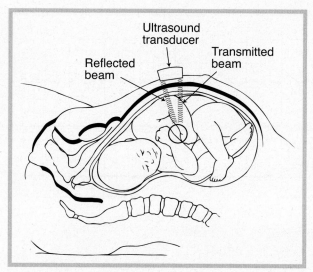

FIGURE 15–2. The Doppler ultrasound device for detecting cardiac activity. The frequency of the reflected beam is changed when it is reflected from a moving structure. (Adapted from Parer, J. T. [1997]. *Handbook of Fetal Heart Rate Monitoring* [2nd ed., p. 104]. Philadelphia: W.B. Saunders. Used with permission.)

fetus, the line produced over time has a jagged, irregular appearance resulting from the different rates of consecutive recorded heartbeats. Early Doppler technology tended to exaggerate the FHR variability, but improvements in technology have resulted in a Doppler recording that sufficiently reflects the true variability in the FHR under observation. In some other countries, the recording speed may be set at 1 cm/min, changing the appearance of the FHR patterns observed. Although the Doppler is easy to apply, maternal or fetal movement, uterine contractions, or maternal positions can interrupt a continuous recording. In cases where the mother is significantly overweight, a continuous recording via external monitoring may be challenging.

The direct fetal scalp electrode (FSE) is the most accurate way to assess the FHR but is invasive and should not be used unless the cervix is at least 2 to 3 cm dilated and the membranes have ruptured. The electrode has three leads, which detect the PQRST complex. The filter within the electronics of the machine removes all components except the R wave. The R wave then triggers the machine to count; it waits for a second complex, filters all but the R wave, and then calculates how much time elapsed from the first to the second R wave in a fashion similar to the technique used with Doppler ultrasound. The elapsed time between R intervals is converted into bpm, and the pen records that rate on the paper. Both Doppler ultrasound and FSE are appropriate methods for electronic detection and interpretation of FHR patterns (Macones et al., 2008).

It is important to avoid confusing the maternal heart rate with the FHR. Clinical conditions that increase risk of confusion include low FHR baseline, maternal pushing efforts during second-stage labor, maternal

repositioning, maternal obesity, and maternal tachycardia, which may be associated with an elevated temperature, anxiety, or medications (Neilson, Freeman, & Mangan, 2008; Simpson, 2011). An abrupt change in the characteristics of the FHR tracing or FHR accelerations consistently coincident with uterine contractions or with maternal pushing efforts should be evaluated to confirm that the tracing is of fetal origin. In the case of fetal demise, a recording may be produced of the maternal heart rate either via the external ultrasound transducer detecting maternal aortic pulsations or via the FSE detecting the maternal ECG. When there are two sources of data (e.g., maternal heart rate via pulse oximetry and fetal or maternal heart rate via external ultrasound or via FSE), the fetal monitor may display coincident alerts to suggest that both data sources are detecting the same heart rate. When these alerts are displayed, confirmation of two distinct heart rates, one from the fetus and one from the mother, should be undertaken. Potential strategies to minimize risk of confusing maternal heart rate with FHR include confirming maternal heart rate by palpation of maternal pulse during initiation of EFM and comparing it with FHR, repeating this confirmation periodically during first- and second-stage labor, paying close attention to distinguishing between maternal heart rate and FHR during second-stage pushing efforts, and recognizing other clinical situations that could result in maternal heart rate being recorded as FHR such as extremes of maternal weight (Simpson, 2011).

Both Doppler ultrasound and FSEs can produce FHR recordings that are inadequate for interpretation. Use of EFM during labor requires knowledge of sources of artifact and solutions for resolution. Many times, the problem is secondary to equipment malfunction and can be remedied easily. The most common reasons why FHR tracings do not record accurately, the FHR tracing that is produced, and the solutions to the problems are listed in Table 15–3. In November 2009, the U.S. Food and Drug Administration (FDA) issued a recall of specific models of fetal monitors and sent a letter to healthcare providers outlining potential problems. The FDA (2009) noted that the following technical issues had been reported: switching between the FHR and maternal heart rate, halving of the FHR, a mismatch between the audible and printed FHR, false decelerations, and noisy or erratic signals. The concern was that clinical decisions based on unrecognized inaccuracies in the FHR tracing could lead healthcare professionals to perform unnecessary interventions such as cesarean birth, could fail to identify the need for interventions, and/or could fail to identify and treat fetal compromise (FDA, 2009).

Application of an FSE is invasive and increases risk of maternal–fetal infection. Therefore, it should be used only when continuous recordings are indicated and are unable to be obtained with external monitoring. If the recording obtained via external EFM is continuous, there is no need for an FSE as there is

Table 15–3. SOURCES OF ARTIFACT OR ERROR IN FETAL HEART RATE RECORDINGS

	Recording Produced	Solution
Signal errors		
Faulty leg plate, electrode, or monitor	No recording.	Replace equipment.
Transducer does not detect fetal heart	Intermittent recording consistently.	Move transducer.
• Maternal muscle movements		
• Uterine contractions		
• Maternal positioning		
• Maternal obesity		
Interference by maternal signal	Recording will be maternal heart rate.	Recognize maternal heart beat and use alternative method or adjust placement of transducer.
Limitation of machinery		
Counting process omits FHR that is >30 bpm different from preceding beat	Arrhythmia will be audible but does not appear on record.	Use fetal ECG if improved recording needed. Arrhythmias tend to be regular, and artifact tends to be irregular.
Halving or doubling of audible FHR	Very slow rates may be doubled and very fast rates (>240 bpm) may be halved.	Auscultate to determine correct rate.
Interpretive errors		
Maternal heart rate recorded	Rate recorded will equal maternal pulse EFM may provide electronic cues that recording is maternal in nature.	Compare with maternal pulse. Palpate maternal pulse.
• Fetal death		
• Electrode on cervix		
Scaling error	Two paper speeds are possible on some machines (1 and 3 cm/min). FHR pattern will change at slower speed, exaggerating variability.	Ensure paper speed of 3 cm/min prior to applying transducers

ECG, electrocardiogram; EFM, electronic fetal monitoring; FHR, fetal heart rate.
Adapted from Parer, J. T. (1997). *Handbook of Fetal Heart Rate Monitoring* (2nd ed.). Philadelphia: W. B. Saunders.

no clinical difference in data interpretation. There is evidence to suggest that application of a direct electrode could enhance maternal–fetal transmission of HIV when used in women who are HIV seropositive (Maiques, Garcia-Tejedor, Perales, & Navarro, 1999); therefore, use of an FSE is contraindicated in women who are known to be HIV seropositive (American Academy of Pediatrics [AAP] & ACOG, 2012). Other relative contraindications to the application of a direct fetal lead include women who have active or chronic hepatitis, group B streptococcus, and herpes simplex virus (HSV) or other known and nontreated sexually transmitted diseases (Phillips, n.d.). While the indicted use of an FSE may be reasonable in the setting of HSV without active lesions (AAP & ACOG, 2012), current recommendations are to avoid techniques that result in a break in the skin when these infectious agents are known to be present (AAP & ACOG, 2012; Maiques et al., 1999). Application of a direct fetal lead also may be deferred for women who are known hemophilia carriers and fetal carrier status is either confirmed or unknown (Phillips, n.d.).

INTERMITTENT AUSCULTATION

Prior to the introduction of Doppler technology, IA of the FHR was accomplished with a Pinard or DeLee stethoscope. A baseline FHR can be obtained, and the presence

or absence of decelerations can be noted without determination of variability or the type of deceleration with this technique. Auscultation with a non-Doppler stethoscope is no longer common practice in the United States. Today, when the FHR is assessed during labor via an IA protocol, a handheld Doppler unit is typically used (Display 15–1). There is limited evidence to suggest improved outcomes for fetuses of women assessed via EFM as compared to IA; thus, IA is an appropriate

DISPLAY 15–1

Capabilities of Auscultation Devices

FETOSCOPE
- Detect FHR baseline
- Detect FHR rhythm
- Verify the presence of an arrhythmia
- Detect increases and decreases from FHR baseline
- Clarify double or half counting by EFM

DOPPLER
- Detect FHR baseline
- Detect FHR rhythm
- Detect increases and decreases from FHR baseline

EFM, electronic fetal monitoring; FHR, fetal heart rate.
From Feinstein, N. F., Sprague, A., & Trepanier, M. J. (2008). *Fetal Heart Rate Auscultation* (2nd ed.). Washington, D. C.: Association of Women's Health, Obstetric and Neonatal Nurses.

(ACOG, 2010b) and, in some cases, preferred (SOGC, 2007) method of FHR monitoring. SOGC (2007) recommends IA as the primary method of FHR monitoring for women with uncomplicated pregnancy and labor. However, ACOG (2010a), ACNM (2010a), and SOGC recommend that continuous EFM be used for high-risk women, and ACOG suggests women receiving oxytocin be monitored as for high-risk conditions (AAP & ACOG, 2012; ACOG, 2009b). SOGC recommends EFM for augmentation of labor and suggests EFM may be appropriate for labor induction.

Current recommendations for using auscultation during the intrapartum period are outlined by AWHONN (Feinstein, Sprague, & Trepanier, 2008), ACNM (2010a), ACOG (2009a), SOCG (2007), and in the *Guidelines for Perinatal Care* (AAP & ACOG, 2012). However, there are inconsistencies in the recommendations from AAP, ACOG, AWHONN, ACNM, and SOGC regarding patients for whom IA is appropriate and the frequency of assessment when using IA. Because protocols in clinical trials varied, AWHONN suggests auscultation of the FHR every 15 to 30 minutes in the active phase of the first stage of labor and every 5 to 15 minutes in the active phase of the second stage of labor (AWHONN, 2009; Feinstein et al., 2008). ACOG suggests an assessment frequency for IA of every 30 minutes in the active phase of the first stage of labor and every 15 minutes in the second stage of labor for women without identified risk factors (AAP & ACOG, 2012); and at least every 15 minutes in the active phase of first-stage labor and at least every 5 minutes during second-stage labor for women with identified risk factors (ACOG, 2009a). SOGC (2007) recommends assessment hourly in latent labor, every 15 to 30 minutes in the active phase of first-stage labor, and every 5 minutes during second-stage labor. ACNM recommends auscultation every 15

to 30 minutes in the active phase of the first stage of labor, every 15 minutes in second stage prior to pushing, and every 5 minutes while pushing (ACNM, 2010a). No clinical trials have examined methods of fetal assessment during the latent phase of labor. The variation in recommendations among professional societies reflects the variation in protocols used for clinical trials and the mix of both low- and high-risk patients in most trials. Therefore, clinical judgment and unit policy should guide decisions when deciding the method and frequency of fetal assessment. When auscultation is used as the primary method of fetal surveillance during labor, a 1:1 nurse–fetus ratio is required (ACNM, 2010a; AWHONN, 2009). Categories for interpretation of IA findings are listed in Table 15–4.

The decision to use IA or EFM is made in collaboration with the laboring woman, as there remains a lack of consistent, high-quality evidence to definitively recommend one approach over the other (Devoe, 2011a). The decision is based on many factors, including patient history, fetal condition, risk classification, and hospital policies and procedures. As with EFM, there are benefits and limitations to the use of IA (Display 15–2). Both IA and EFM are effective in fetal evaluation when used appropriately (AAP & ACOG, 2012; ACNM, 2010a; ACOG, 2010b; AWHONN, 2009; SOGC, 2007).

PHYSIOLOGIC BASIS FOR FETAL HEART RATE MONITORING

EFM is a technique for assessing the adequacy of fetal oxygenation. As previously noted, while a normal FHR tracing (category I) is a good predictor of a normoxic fetus, the reverse is not true. Because the high rate of false-positive indeterminate and abnormal FHR

Table 15–4. CLASSIFICATION & INTERPRETATION OF AUSCULTATED FHR

	Characteristics	Interpretation
Category I	**All** of the following: Normal FHR baseline between 110 and 160 bpm Regular rhythm Presence of FHR increases or accelerations from the baseline Absence of FHR decreases of decelerations from the baseline	Normal: Normal auscultated FHR characteristics are predictive of fetal well-being at the time of observation.
Category II	**Any** of the following: Irregular rhythm Presence of FHR decreases or decelerations from the baseline Tachycardia (baseline >160 bpm >10 min in duration) Bradycardia (baseline <110 bpm >10 min in duration)	Indeterminate: Findings cannot be classified as abnormal, as variability cannot be determined by auscultation. These findings require evaluation, ongoing surveillance, and reevaluation consistent with overall clinical circumstances. In emergent situation (e.g., bradycardia), preparations to expedite birth should occur simultaneously with efforts to ameliorate and verify the nature of the FHR findings.

FHR, fetal heart rate.
Adapted from Lyndon, A., O'Brien-Abel, N., & Simpson, K. R. (2009). Fetal heart rate interpretation. In A. Lyndon & L. U. Ali (Eds.), *Fetal Heart Monitoring Principles and Practices* (4th ed., pp. 101–133). Washington, DC: Association of Women's Health, Obstetric and Neonatal Nurses/Kendall Hunt.

tracings has many origins and several clinical implications, a working knowledge of FHR physiology can aid clinical interpretation of FHR patterns during labor. The following section reviews the importance of maternal oxygenation, uteroplacental exchange, umbilical blood flow, and factors influencing FHR regulation. Subsequently, we review the characteristics of the normal FHR, interventions for managing alterations in FHR, and FHR pattern evolution.

MATERNAL OXYGEN STATUS

Fetal oxygenation depends on well-oxygenated maternal blood flow to the placenta. Adequate maternal hemoglobin levels, adequate maternal oxygen saturation (SaO_2), and adequate oxygen tension in maternal arterial blood P_aO_2 are needed to for fetal oxygenation. While most pregnant women are healthy and well-oxygenated, maternal conditions that may impair oxygen delivery to the fetus include severe anemia, asthma, congenital cardiac defects, congestive heart failure, lung disease, or seizures.

UTERINE, PLACENTAL, AND UMBILICAL BLOOD FLOW

Adequate uterine blood flow is required for the passage of respiratory gases and substances across the placenta. Uterine blood flow increases throughout pregnancy and in a singleton pregnancy at term is approximately 700 mL/min or 10% to 15% of maternal cardiac output (Blackburn, 2007; Parer, 1997). While uterine blood also supplies the myometrium and endometrium, the intervillous space within the placenta receives 70% to 90% of the total uterine blood flow near term (Parer, 1997). In the intervillous space, well-oxygenated maternal blood propelled by maternal arterial blood pressure surrounds the fetal chorionic villi, allowing exchange of oxygen, carbon dioxide, and other substances between the maternal and fetal circulations (Fig. 15–3). The newly oxygenated fetal blood within the fetal villi flows into veins that converge into a single umbilical vein, which carries the oxygenated blood and nutrients to the fetus. Deoxygenated blood and waste products return from the fetus to the placenta via two umbilical arteries, which divide successively into smaller vessels, eventually creating an arteriovenous system within each chorionic villus (Blackburn, 2007).

Maternal–fetal exchange of oxygen, carbon dioxide, nutrients, waste products, water, and other substances is facilitated by the large surface area of the placental membrane separating the maternal and fetal blood (Fig. 15–4). Mechanisms by which these substances transfer across the placental membrane include passive diffusion, facilitated diffusion, active transport, hydrostatic pressure, breaks or leaks, and pinocytosis. Oxygen and carbon dioxide are exchanged rapidly by passive diffusion. Passive diffusion allows movement down the concentration gradient from an area of high concentration, across a membrane, to an area of lower concentration. The concentration gradients and characteristics of fetal hemoglobin favor transfer of oxygen from mother to fetus and transfer of carbon dioxide from fetus to mother.

Clinical factors that can potentially decrease uteroplacental perfusion and fetal oxygenation include excessive uterine contractions or hypertonus; maternal hypotension or hypertension; placental changes due to decreased surface area, degenerative changes, infarcts, calcification, infection, or edema; and vasoconstriction. In addition, umbilical cord entanglement, compression, or occlusion may impede fetal oxygenation. Therefore, a primary goal in intrapartum care is to maximize uterine blood flow, uteroplacental exchange, and umbilical blood flow, thereby minimizing risk to the fetus.

FETAL HEART RATE REGULATION

The cardioregulatory center in the medulla oblongata interacts with the parasympathetic and sympathetic branches of the autonomic nervous systems, baroreceptors, chemoreceptors, fetal hormones, sleep/wake cycles,

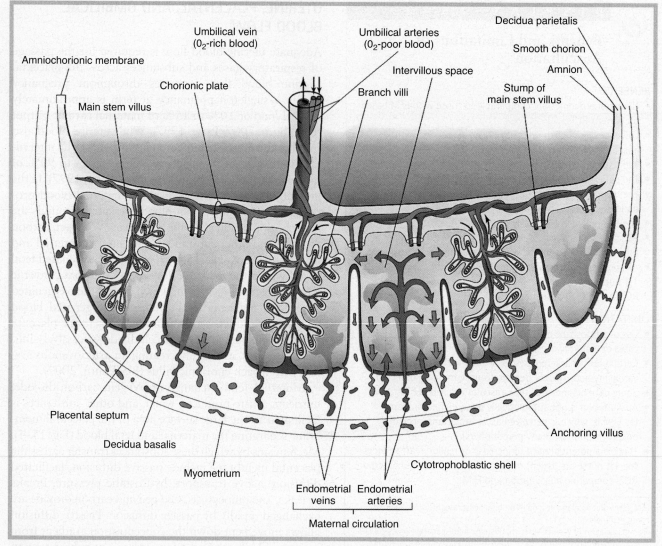

FIGURE 15–3. Schematic drawing of a transverse section through a full-term placenta showing maternal uteroplacental circulation and fetal–placental circulation. (From Moore, K. L., & Persaud, T. V. N. [2003]. *The Developing Human: Clinically Oriented Embryology* [7th ed., p. 126]. Philadelphia: Saunders. Used with permission from Elsevier.)

breathing movements, painful stimuli, sound vibrations, and temperature to influence FHR (O'Brien-Abel, 2009). Major factors believed to influence the integration of FHR control are outlined in Table 15–5. Interplay between the two components of the autonomic nervous system (sympathetic and parasympathetic), higher cortical functions in the brain, and chemoreceptors and baroreceptors are all reflected in the baseline rate and, in part, make up the FHR variability seen on the recording from an FHR monitor.

Sympathetic nervous system fibers are widely distributed throughout the fetal myocardium at term. Stimulation of these nerve fibers releases norepinephrine, causing increased heart rate, strength of cardiac contractions, and cardiac output (Parer, 1997; Nageotte & Gilstrap, 2009). The average baseline FHR in the normal fetus at 20 weeks' gestation is 155 bpm; at 30 weeks, 144 bpm; and at term before labor, 140 bpm

(Nageotte & Gilstrap, 2009). This slow, gradual decrease in FHR seen with advancing gestational age is due to an increased dominance of the parasympathetic over the sympathetic branch of the autonomic nervous system. While the sympathetic branch is dominant in an extremely premature fetus, a baseline FHR greater than 160 bpm should be further evaluated to rule out fetal compromise, rather than assuming the tachycardia is secondary to prematurity (Freeman, Garite, & Nageotte, 2003).

The parasympathetic nervous system influences the fetal heart via the vagus nerve, which innervates the sinoatrial (SA) and atrioventricular nodes within the heart. Stimulation of the vagus nerve releases acetylcholine, which decreases firing of the SA node, resulting in a slower heart rate in a normal fetus (Dalton, Phill, Dawes, & Patrick, 1983; Parer & Nageotte, 2004). With advancing gestational age,

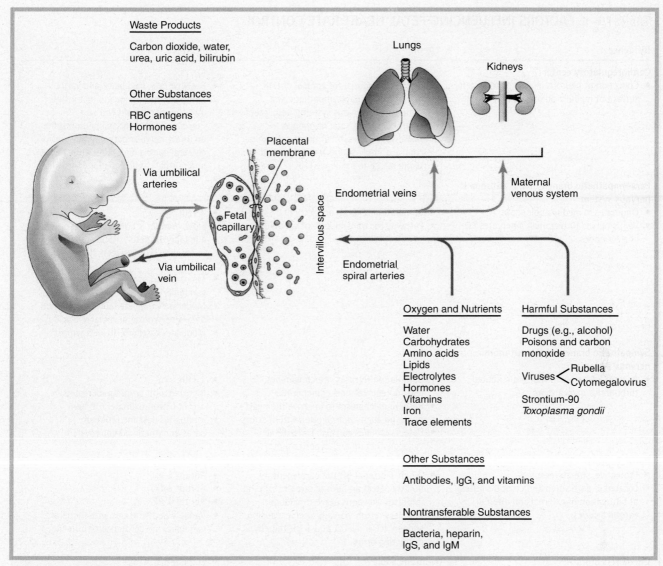

Waste Products

Carbon dioxide, water,
urea, uric acid, bilirubin

Other Substances

RBC antigens
Hormones

Via umbilical
arteries

Placental
membrane

Fetal
capillary

Via umbilical
vein

Intervillous space

Lungs

Kidneys

Endometrial veins

Maternal
venous system

Endometrial
spiral arteries

Oxygen and Nutrients

Water
Carbohydrates
Amino acids
Lipids
Electrolytes
Hormones
Vitamins
Iron
Trace elements

Harmful Substances

Drugs (e.g., alcohol)
Poisons and carbon
monoxide

Viruses ⟨ Rubella
Cytomegalovirus

Strontium-90
Toxoplasma gondii

Other Substances

Antibodies, IgG, and vitamins

Nontransferable Substances

Bacteria, heparin,
IgS, and IgM

FIGURE 15–4. Transfer of substances between the mother and the fetus across the placental membrane. Ig, immuno-globulin; RBC, red blood cell. (From Moore, K. L., & Persaud, T. V. N. [2003]. *The Developing Human: Clinically Oriented Embryology* [7th ed., p. 128]. Philadelphia: Saunders. Used with permission from Elsevier.)

this vagal influence results in approximately 10 bpm difference in baseline FHR between 28 and 30 weeks' gestation and term. The second important function of the parasympathetic system is the transmission of FHR variability. Vagal stimulation of the SA node is the primary influence in the transmission of impulses causing FHR variability. Because severe hypoxia and metabolic acidosis will decrease central nervous system (CNS) function, the presence of moderate FHR variability reliably indicates a well-oxygenated, nonacidemic fetus (ACOG, 2010b; Garite, 2007; Macones et al., 2008).

Chemoreceptors, located centrally in the medulla oblongata and peripherally in the aortic arch and carotid sinuses, have their greatest effect on the regulation of respiration and in the control of circulation (Nageotte & Gilstrap, 2009; Parer, 1997). When uteroplacental

blood flow falls below the threshold needed for normal respiratory gas exchange, increased carbon dioxide tension (PCO_2) in fetal vessels stimulates the chemoreceptors to fire, resulting in slowing of the FHR (Freeman et al., 2003). The influence of chemoreceptors may be seen in the mechanism of late decelerations and in variable decelerations with hypoxemia.

Baroreceptors, located in the aortic arch and carotid sinuses, are small stretch receptors that quickly detect increases in fetal arterial blood pressure (Nageotte & Gilstrap, 2009; Parer, 1997). When umbilical blood flow is occluded, fetal arterial blood pressure quickly increases, triggering the baroreceptors to send impulses via the vagus nerve to the midbrain to abruptly decrease the FHR, cardiac output, and blood pressure, thereby protecting the fetus. The influence of baroreceptors may be seen in the mechanism of variable decelerations.

Table 15-5. FACTORS INFLUENCING FETAL HEART RATE CONTROL

Influence	Action	FHR Effect
Cardioregulatory center • Collection of neurons in ventral and lateral surface of medulla oblongata	• Integrating source for control of FHR • Interacts with parasympathetic and sympathetic nervous systems, baroreceptors, chemoreceptors, fetal hormones, sleep/wake cycles, breathing movements, painful stimuli, sound, vibrations, and temperature to influence FHR	• Baseline rate, variability, and various FHR patterns provide indirect insights into functioning of CNS • Presence of FHR variability represents an intact nervous pathway through cerebral cortex, midbrain, vagus nerve, and normal cardiac conduction system
Parasympathetic branch of the autonomic nervous system • Originates in medulla oblongata • Vagus nerve (10th cranial) innervates SA and AV nodes	• Stimulation releases acetylcholine • Pathway for transmission of variability	• ↓ FHR • Slow, gradual ↓ FHR with ↑ gestational age (approximately 10 bpm difference in baseline FHR between 28 wk and term) • Maintains transmission of beat-to-beat variability • Moderate variability indicates absence of severe hypoxia or metabolic acidosis • Modulates baseline FHR with sympathetic
Sympathetic branch of the autonomic nervous system • At term, nerve fibers widely distributed throughout myocardium	• Stimulation releases catecholamines (e.g., norepinephrine, epinephrine) • Reserve mechanism to improve the heart's pumping ability during intermittent stress • Catecholamines can also cause fetal vasoconstriction and hypertension	• ↑ FHR • Blocking with propranolol results in ↓ FHR of approximately 10 bpm • Modulates baseline FHR with parasympathetic nervous system
Baroreceptors • Protective, stretch receptors • Located in aortic arch and carotid sinuses at bifurcation of external and internal carotid arteries	• When ↑ arterial BP, the baroreceptors quickly detect amount of stretch, sending impulses via vagus nerve to midbrain • Impulses return via vagus nerve, causing sudden ↓ FHR, ↓ CO, and ↓ BP, thereby protecting fetus	• Abrupt ↓ FHR • Abrupt ↓ CO • Abrupt ↓ BP • Variable decelerations with moderate variability are baroreceptor influenced

Chemoreceptors
• Central—located in medulla oblongata
• Peripheral—in aortic arch and carotid sinuses
	In the adult
	• When arterial blood perfusing chemoreceptors contains ↑ PCO_2 or ↓ PO_2:
	  ○ Central chemoreceptors respond with reflex tachycardia and hypertension, most likely in an attempt to circulate blood and ↓ the PCO_2
	  ○ Peripheral chemoreceptors respond with bradycardia
		In the fetus:
		• Interaction of central and peripheral chemoreceptors poorly understood
		• Combined effect is slowing of FHR
		• Described in mechanism of late decelerations and in variable decelerations resulting from umbilical arterial occlusion coupled with hypoxemia
		• When blood flow is below threshold for normal respiratory gas exchange, ↑ PCO_2 stimulates chemoreceptors to slow FHR

Hormonal regulation • Epinephrine and norepinephrine secreted from the adrenal medulla • Arginine vasopressin secreted from posterior pituitary • Renin-angiotensin-aldosterone secreted from kidneys	• In response to stressful situations, compensatory response shunts blood away from less vital organs and toward brain, heart, and adrenal glands • In adult, responds to ↓ plasma volume, ↑ plasma osmolarity • In fetal sheep, hypoxemia most potent stimulus; distributes blood flow • Responds to ↓ plasma volume or ↓ BP; protects fetus from hemorrhagic stress by stimulating vasoconstriction	• ↓ FHR, ↑ strength of cardiac contractions, ↑ CO, ↑ arterial BP • ↑ FHR, ↑ CO, ↑ arterial BP • Sinusoidal heart rate pattern in experimental studies • ↑ FHR, ↑ CO, ↑ arterial BP

(continued)

Table 15–5. FACTORS INFLUENCING FETAL HEART RATE CONTROL *(Continued)*

Influence	Action	FHR Effect
Frank-Starling mechanism • In the adult, CO = HR × SV • SV is influenced by Frank-Starling mechanism, which states that ↑ inflow of blood into heart stretches cardiac muscle, thereby resulting in ↑ force of contraction and ↑ SV	• In the fetus, this mechanism has not been found to apply on the basis of studies involving fetal and adult lambs • Compared with adult, fetal SV does not fluctuate significantly	• Fetal CO ≈ HR • Modest variations in baseline FHR probably have little effect on fetal CO • However, during FHR >240 bpm or FHR <60 bpm, fetal CO is substantially decreased

AV, atrioventricular; BP, blood pressure; CNS, central nervous system; CO, cardiac output; FHR, fetal heart rate; HR, heart rate; PCO_2, partial pressure of carbon dioxide; PO_2, partial pressure of oxygen; SA, sinoatrial; SV, stroke volume.
From O'Brien-Abel, N. (2009). Physiologic basis for fetal monitoring. In A. Lyndon & L. U. Ali (Eds.), *Fetal Heart Monitoring Principles and Practices* (4th ed., pp. 35–36). Washington, DC: Association of Women's Health, Obstetric and Neonatal Nurses/Kendall Hunt. Used with permission.

Fetal monitoring is an ongoing indirect assessment of physiologic factors affecting fetal oxygenation and thereby fetal acid–base status. Uteroplacental blood flow, intervillous space perfusion, umbilical blood flow, and intrinsic influences of parasympathetic and sympathetic nervous system, baroreceptors, and chemoreceptors are reflected in the characteristics of the observed FHR. Ongoing assessment and interpretation of FHR characteristics are used to determine fetal oxygenation and rule out fetal acidemia.

CHARACTERISTICS OF THE NORMAL FETAL HEART RATE

FHR pattern interpretation involves assessment of five components of the FHR as well as the relationship of FHR characteristics to both uterine activity and the overall clinical situation. Characteristics of the FHR to be evaluated include (1) baseline rate, (2) FHR variability, (3) presence or absence of accelerations, (4) other periodic and/or episodic changes, and (5) evolution over time (Macones et al., 2008). Periodic and episodic changes refer to accelerations and decelerations. Periodic changes in FHR occur in response to uterine activity. Episodic changes are not associated with uterine activity and may occur randomly. This section reviews the characteristics of the normal FHR (category I tracings), and the next section will review the etiology and management of the most common periodic and episodic changes seen in category II and III tracings, as well as some other less common alterations in FHR.

BASELINE RATE

The baseline FHR is the approximate mean FHR rounded to increments of 5 bpm during a 10-minute segment, excluding periodic or episodic changes, periods of marked FHR variability, and segments of the baseline that differ by >25 bpm (Macones et al., 2008). In determining the baseline rate, at least 2 minutes of identifiable

baseline are required, although they do not need to be contiguous. If, during a 10-minute segment, there are not at least 2 minutes of identifiable baseline, the baseline for that period is indeterminate. In this case, one may need to refer to the previous 10-minute segment(s) for determination of the baseline. The normal baseline FHR range is 110 to 160 bpm (Macones et al., 2008). Bradycardia is a baseline FHR <110 bpm; tachycardia is a baseline FHR >160 bpm (Macones et al., 2008). Since the baseline is determined over a 10-minute period, a baseline change has occurred once the change in FHR has been sustained for at least 10 minutes. Periodic and episodic changes are quantified relative to the most recently determined adjacent baseline FHR.

VARIABILITY

Variability is a characteristic of the FHR baseline defined as fluctuations in the baseline FHR that occur with irregular amplitude and frequency (Macones et al., 2008). The FHR of the healthy fetus is displayed as an irregular line on the monitor tracing. These irregularities demonstrate the FHR variability, which reflects the slight difference in time interval between successive heartbeats (short-term component), and cyclic fluctuations over time (long-term component). The irregular fluctuations of the FHR are visually quantitated as the amplitude of the peak-to-trough in beats per minute as follows:

Absent variability has an amplitude range that is undetectable.
Minimal variability has an amplitude range that is detectable, but less than or equal to 5 bpm.
Moderate variability has an amplitude range of 6 to 25 bpm.
Marked variability has an amplitude range greater than 25 bpm.

Clinically, variability is visually determined as a unit without separating short- and long-term components (Macones et al., 2008; NICHD, 1997). As a characteristic of the baseline, variability is assessed during the baseline and not during periodic changes such as decelerations.

ACCELERATIONS

Accelerations may be present or absent in a normal (category I) FHR tracing. Accelerations are visually apparent abrupt increases (defined as onset of acceleration to peak in <30 seconds) in FHR above the baseline (Fig. 15–5). The acme is at least 15 bpm above the baseline, and the acceleration lasts at least 15 seconds but less than 2 minutes from the onset to return to baseline (Macones et al., 2008). The FHR only needs to reach a peak ≥15 bpm above baseline with onset-return criteria as described previously; it does not need to be sustained at ≥15 bpm above baseline. Before 32 weeks of gestation, accelerations are defined as having an acme of at least 10 bpm above the baseline and duration of at least 10 seconds (Macones et al., 2008). Like moderate variability, the presence of accelerations indicates central oxygenation and predicts the absence of fetal metabolic acidemia (ACOG, 2009a; Clark, Gimovsky, & Miller, 1984; Macones et al., 2008). Accelerations can occur as periodic or episodic changes in the FHR. The absence of accelerations is not a reliable predictor of fetal acidemia (Macones et al., 2008).

EARLY DECELERATIONS

Early decelerations may or may not be present in a normal (category I) FHR tracing (Macones et al., 2008). Early decelerations are characterized by a visually apparent *gradual* (defined as onset of deceleration to nadir ≥30 seconds) decrease and return to baseline FHR associated with a uterine contraction. Early decelerations are typically symmetrical and coincident in timing with the uterine contraction; in most cases, the onset, nadir, and recovery of the deceleration are coincident with the beginning, peak, and ending of the contraction, respectively (Macones et al., 2008).

Early decelerations are presumed to be a response to fetal head compression. Altered cerebral blood flow causes the decrease in heart rate through a vagal reflex. When the contraction occurs, pressure on the fetal head stimulates the vagus nerve. The heart rate begins to drop at the onset of the contraction when the head compression begins and returns to the baseline rate at the end of the contraction when the head is no longer compressed (Freeman et al., 2003). Early decelerations are benign, requiring no intervention or treatment and are not associated with fetal hypoxia or low Apgar scores. The key to assessment of early decelerations is to make sure one distinguishes them from late decelerations. The presence of variability is a key clinical factor. Vagal stimulation occurs as a result of head compression, not secondary to hypoxemia, and will not result in a decrease in variability.

UTERINE ACTIVITY

Uterine activity is a key characteristic for interpretation of the overall clinical picture and the FHR pattern. Uterine activity is quantified by determining the number of contractions present in a 10-minute segment averaged over 30 minutes (Macones et al., 2008). Uterine activity should be further characterized in terms of contraction duration and intensity and the quality and duration of resting tone (Lyndon, O'Brien-Abel, & Simpson, 2009; Macones et al., 2008). The frequency of uterine activity is classified as either normal or tachysystole (Macones et al., 2008):

Normal uterine activity is ≤5 or fewer contractions in 10 minutes, averaged over 30 minutes.
Tachysystole occurs when there are >5 contractions in 10 minutes, averaged over 30 minutes.
Tachysystole is further characterized by the presence or absence of FHR decelerations.

Although the definition for tachysystole includes an averaging of contractions over a 30-minute period, this is not meant to imply that 30 minutes is required before tachysystole can be determined or that interventions

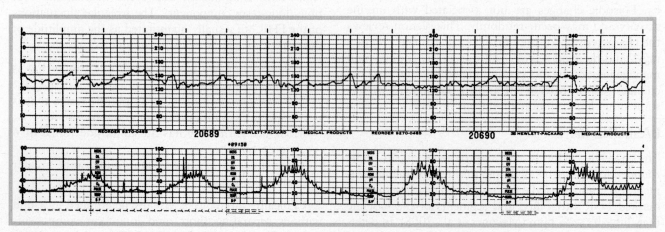

FIGURE 15–5. Accelerations of the fetal heart rate.

to decrease uterine activity should be delayed until tachysystole has been occurring for 30 minutes. One or two 10-minute segments of more than five contractions is sufficient to identify excessive uterine activity and initiate appropriate interventions.

INTERVENTIONS FOR INDETERMINATE OR ABNORMAL FETAL HEART RATE PATTERNS

Before discussing the etiology and individual management of periodic or episodic changes in the FHR, a general review of the initial assessment and interventions used to maximize fetal oxygenation in the presence of variant FHR patterns is warranted. When an indeterminate (category II) or abnormal (category III) FHR pattern is identified, initial assessment may include a cervical exam to rule out umbilical cord prolapse, rapid cervical dilation, or rapid descent of the fetal head; a review of uterine activity to rule out tachysystole; and an evaluation of maternal vital signs, in particular temperature and blood pressure, to rule out maternal fever or maternal hypotension (ACOG, 2010b). These assessment data can guide appropriate treatment to attempt to resolve the pattern. *Intrauterine resuscitation* refers to a series of interventions to promote fetal well-being that include a change in maternal position, a decrease in uterine activity or uterine contraction frequency, administration of IV fluids, and administration of oxygen, and sometimes administration of terbutaline sulfate or amnioinfusion (ACOG, 2010b; Garite & Simpson, 2011; Simpson, 2009b). Other resuscitative techniques include correction of maternal hypotension and modification of

second-stage labor maternal pushing efforts (Garite & Simpson, 2011; Simpson, 2009b). The type of resuscitative technique is based on the specific characteristics of the observed FHR pattern and maternal condition. In some cases, a combination of techniques will be required. A summary of the goals and techniques for intrauterine resuscitation are presented in Table 15–6. These interventions are directed at improving maternal blood flow to the placenta and oxygen delivery to the fetus. Data suggest that these techniques can improve fetal oxygen status, but there is no evidence that these techniques will reverse asphyxia. If the clinical characteristics of the FHR patterns are thought to represent a serious risk for acidemia, these measures should be initiated only if doing so does not delay the move toward expeditious birth (Lyndon et al., 2009; Simpson, 2007, 2009b).

POSITION CHANGE

Changing maternal position alters the relationship between the umbilical cord and fetal parts or the uterine wall and alters maternal cardiac output. It is usually done to minimize or correct cord compression and to improve uterine blood flow (increased uterine blood flow may also decrease the frequency of uterine contractions) (Simpson, 2009b). Position change can resolve or decrease the severity of prolonged decelerations and/or variable decelerations. Position change may also modify late decelerations if the etiology of this pattern is decreased uterine blood flow (usually secondary to supine positioning and inferior vena caval compression), as venous return and cardiac output are increased in the lateral position (Clark et al., 1991).

Table 15–6. INTRAUTERINE RESUSCITATION

Goal	Techniques/Methods
Promote fetal oxygenation	Lateral positioning (either left or right)
	Oxygen administration at 10 L/min via nonrebreather face mask
	IV fluid bolus of at least 500 mL of lactated Ringer's solution
	Discontinuation of oxytocin/removal of Cervidil/withholding next dose of Cytotec
	Stopping pushing temporarily or pushing with every other, or every third, contraction (during second-stage labor)
Reduce uterine activity	Discontinuation of oxytocin/removal of Cervidil/withhold next dose of Cytotec
	IV fluid bolus of at least 500 mL of lactated Ringer's solution
	Lateral positioning (either left or right)
	If no response, consider terbutaline 0.25 mg subcutaneously
Alleviate umbilical cord compression	Repositioning
	Amnioinfusion (during first-stage labor)
	Stopping pushing temporarily or pushing with every other, or every third, contraction (during second-stage labor)
Correct maternal hypotension	Lateral positioning (either left or right)
	IV fluid bolus of at least 500 mL of lactated Ringer's solution
	If no response, consider ephedrine 5–10 mg IV push

IV, intravenous.

Generally, it is best to avoid supine positioning to prevent compression of the vena cava, reduced cardiac output, and supine hypotensive syndrome. Several studies comparing the effects of right lateral, left lateral, and supine maternal positions on fetal oxygen status suggest that lateral positioning on either the left or the right is more favorable for enhancing fetus oxygenation when compared to a supine position (Aldrich et al., 1995; Carbonne, Benachi, Leveque, Cabrol, & Papiernik, 1996; Simpson & James, 2005b).

REDUCTION OF UTERINE ACTIVITY

When uterine contractions are too frequent, there may be insufficient time for blood flow through the intervillous space to normalize gas exchange, because at intrauterine pressures over 35 mm Hg, all uterine contractions result in stasis of blood flow at their peak. If FHR decelerations occur with tachysystole, reduction of contraction activity will improve fetal oxygenation (Simpson, 2009a). Reduction of uterine activity can occur by reducing oxytocin dosage or discontinuing oxytocin administration, if in use. Lateral positioning of the mother and a crystalloid IV fluid bolus may also reduce uterine activity. If oxytocin is in use, tachysystole is present, and the FHR is abnormal (category III), oxytocin should be discontinued (Simpson, 2009a). Oxytocin should be decreased when tachysystole occurs in the context of a normal (category I) FHR tracing (Simpson, 2009a). Clinical judgment is required to determine whether to decrease versus discontinue oxytocin for category II tracing depending on their specific presentation

(ACOG, 2010b). For example, oxytocin may need to be discontinued in the context of category II tracings with minimal variability and recurrent decelerations, but it may be appropriate to continue oxytocin at a decreased rate in a tracing with moderate variability and intermittent variable decelerations. A suggested protocol for management of oxytocin-induced tachysystole is presented in Table 15–7. Similarly, the next dose of pharmacologic agents used to ripen the cervix or stimulate contractions should be delayed until uterine activity returns to normal and the FHR improves. Administration of tocolytics is another option occasionally used as a temporary measure to provide intrauterine resuscitation for a prolonged deceleration or other variant FHR patterns secondary to tachysystole, by reducing uterine activity. A subcutaneous dose of terbutaline 0.25 mg is often used for this purpose.

INTRAVENOUS FLUID ADMINISTRATION

IV fluid administration is thought to improve uteroplacental perfusion through expansion of maternal intravascular volume. Reductions in uterine blood flow may occur as a result of hypovolemia, hypotension, and sympathetic nervous system blockade following regional analgesia/anesthesia and other conditions. Data suggest that increasing IV fluids will positively affect uterine blood flow and, thus, fetal oxygenation, even in women who are normotensive and well hydrated. Fetal oxygen saturation (FSpO2) was significantly increased after at least a 500-mL bolus of lactated Ringer's solution over 20 minutes in normotensive women who were otherwise

---

Table 15–7. SUGGESTED CLINICAL PROTOCOL FOR OXYTOCIN-INDUCED TACHYSYSTOLE

Oxytocin-Induced Tachysystole (Normal FHR)

- Assist the mother to a lateral position.
- Give IV fluid bolus of at least 500 mL lactated Ringer's solution as indicated.
- If uterine activity has not returned to normal after 10–15 min, decrease oxytocin rate by at least half; if uterine activity has not returned to normal after 10–15 more minutes, discontinue oxytocin until uterine activity less than five contractions in 10 min.
- Resume oxytocin after resolution of tachysystole: If oxytocin has been discontinued for less than 20–30 min, the FHR is normal, and contraction frequency, intensity, and duration are normal, resume oxytocin at no more than half the rate that caused the tachysystole and gradually increase the rate as appropriate based on unit protocol and maternal–fetal status. If the oxytocin is discontinued for more than 30–40 min, resume oxytocin at the initial dose ordered.

Oxytocin-Induced Tachysystole (Indeterminate or Abnormal FHR)

- Discontinue oxytocin.
- Assist the mother to a lateral position.
- Give IV fluid bolus of at least 500 mL of lactated Ringer's solution as indicated.
- Consider oxygen at 10 L/min via nonrebreather face mask (discontinue as soon as possible based on the FHR pattern).
- If no response, consider 0.25 mg terbutaline SQ.
- To resume oxytocin after resolution of tachysystole: If oxytocin has been discontinued for less than 20–30 min, the FHR is normal, and contraction frequency, intensity, and duration are normal, resume oxytocin at no more than half the rate that caused the tachysystole and gradually increase the rate as appropriate based on unit protocol and maternal–fetal status. If the oxytocin is discontinued for more than 30–40 min, resume oxytocin at the initial dose ordered.

FHR, fetal heart rate; IV, intravenous; SQ, subcutaneous.

receiving lactated Ringer's solution at 125 mL/hr (Simpson & James, 2005b). The increase in FSpO2 was greatest with a 1,000-mL IV fluid bolus. The positive effects on fetal oxygen status continued for more than 30 minutes after the IV fluid bolus (Simpson & James, 2005b). Thus, an IV fluid bolus of 500 to 1,000 mL may be useful as an intrauterine resuscitation technique. However, caution is indicated when increasing IV fluids or giving repeated IV fluid boluses. Some clinical situations, such as preeclampsia, preterm labor treated with magnesium sulfate, or preterm labor treated with corticosteroids and beta-sympathomimetic medications, carry an increased risk for pulmonary edema that might necessitate fluid restriction. Oxytocin has an antidiuretic effect, so prolonged use of oxytocin can also lead to fluid overload if IV fluids are used too liberally. An extreme effect of fluid overload related to excessive use of oxytocin is water intoxication. Glucose-containing IV fluids should not be used for volume expansion or intrauterine resuscitation (Simpson, 2009b).

OXYGEN ADMINISTRATION

Intrauterine resuscitation frequently includes maternal oxygen administration. Although this therapy appears to be beneficial in improving fetal oxygen status during labor, recent concern for potential adverse effects of oxygen therapy suggests adoption of a judicious approach to the use of oxygen in laboring women. In a classic study about the effects of maternal oxygen administration on the fetus, 100% oxygen via face mask corrected "nonreassuring" FHR patterns by decreasing the baseline FHR during fetal tachycardia and reducing or eliminating late decelerations (Althabe, Schwarcz, Pose, Escarcena, & Caldeyro-Barcia, 1967). There is evidence that FSpO2 will increase as a result of maternal oxygen administration of at least 10 L/min via nonrebreather face mask (Haydon et al., 2006; McNamara, Johnson, & Lilford, 1993; Simpson & James, 2005b), and some evidence that maternal oxygen administration increases fetal cerebral oxygenation (Aldrich, Wyatt, Spencer, Reynolds, & Delpy, 1994). Fetuses with lower oxygen saturation appear to benefit most from maternal oxygen administration (Haydon et al., 2006; Simpson & James, 2005b).

Even though healthy women in labor have nearly 100% SpO2 (usually between 96% and 99%), increasing inspired oxygen increases blood oxygen tension and results in more oxygen delivered to the fetus and the fetal cerebral tissues (Aldrich et al., 1994; McNamara et al., 1993). There is a more rapid increase in FSpO2 when oxygen is given as compared to the decrease in FSpO2 when it is discontinued, suggesting that the fetus responds to the change in oxygen concentration gradient by accepting oxygen more rapidly than it releases it (McNamara et al., 1993). In one study, increased FSpO2 persisted 30 minutes after discontinuation of maternal oxygen (Simpson & James, 2005b). Fetal hemoglobin has a higher affinity for oxygen than adult hemoglobin, and fetal hematocrit is higher than adults. These physiologic factors allow for a steeper increase in fetal oxygen concentration and FSpO2 during maternal oxygen therapy.

When administering oxygen to the mother, the nonrebreather face mask works best because the fraction of inspired oxygen (FIO_2) at 10 L/min is approximately 80% to 100%, as compared to a simple face mask (FIO_2 27% to 40%) or nasal cannula (FIO_2 31%) (Simpson & James, 2005b). There is inconsistent evidence concerning how long maternal oxygen therapy should be continued and its effects on fetal acid–base status. One study found a deterioration in umbilical cord blood values when maternal oxygen was administered for more than 10 minutes during second-stage labor (Thorp, Trobough, Evans, Hedrick, & Yeast, 1995), while others found no change in acid–base status as measured by umbilical cord gases when maternal oxygen was administered from 15 to 60 minutes during second-stage labor or prior to cesarean birth (Haruta, Funato, Sumida, & Shinkai, 1984; Jozwik et al., 2000). Of note, much of the research on maternal oxygen administration was conducted with very small samples of women, the interventions were not randomized, and there was often no control group. A 2008 Cochrane review, using only studies that were randomized controlled trials (RCTs), concluded that there is not enough evidence to support prophylactic oxygen administration and that there were no randomized trials of oxygen administration for "fetal distress" (Fawole & Hofmeyr, 2003/2008). Questions have also been raised regarding the potentially deleterious production of oxygen free radicals in both the mother and fetus under conditions of increased oxygen tension (Simpson, 2008). However, fetal hypoxia also produces oxygen free radicals. Thus, based on the available evidence, maternal oxygen therapy as an intrauterine resuscitation technique for 15 to 30 minutes appears to be reasonable based on the fetal response as noted by the FHR pattern (Haydon et al., 2006; Jozwik et al., 2000; Simpson, 2008). Prolonged oxygen administration should be avoided as there is not enough data on beneficial versus potentially negative effects of prolonged administration.

TREATMENT FOR ANESTHESIA–RELATED HYPOTENSION

Conduction anesthetics/analgesics produce a sympathetic blockade, increasing the risk of decreased placental blood flow with or without overt maternal hypotension (Dado, 2011). This may result in late or prolonged decelerations or bradycardia and is the rationale for prehydration with IV fluid prior to administration of conduction analgesia/anesthesia.

If decelerations or bradycardia occur and maternal repositioning and IV fluid bolus are not successful in resolving them, ephedrine may be given to increase maternal blood pressure. Ephedrine and phenylephrine are the recommended agents because they are least likely to reduce uterine blood flow, and phenylephrine may be preferred in situations where there is a fetal bradycardia (ACOG, 2009a; American Society of Anesthesiologists [ASA], 2007). Bradycardias may also be due to increased uterine tone with intrathecal opioid administration. This problem may be treated with nitroglycerine (Dado, 2011).

AMNIOINFUSION

Amnioinfusion may be helpful in the treatment of recurrent variable decelerations during first-stage labor that have not resolved with maternal position changes (ACOG, 2010b). During amnioinfusion, normal saline or lactated Ringer's solution is introduced transcervically via a double lumen IUPC into the uterus either by gravity flow or through an infusion pump. Amnioinfusion may significantly resolve patterns of "moderate to severe" variable decelerations but does not affect late decelerations or patterns with absent variability (Mino, Puertas, Miranda, & Herruzo, 1999; Miyazaki & Nevarez, 1985). Amnioinfusion is no longer recommended as a treatment for meconium-stained fluid (ACOG, 2006a) because it did not reduce the risk of moderate or severe meconium aspiration syndrome or perinatal death in a multinational study of 1,998 women in labor at term (Fraser et al., 2005). Thus, amnioinfusion should be limited to the treatment of recurrent variable decelerations during first-stage labor that have not resolved with maternal position changes.

Amnioinfusion does not seem to affect the length of labor (Strong, 1997) and appears to be safe for women who are attempting a vaginal birth after a previous cesarean birth (Ouzounian, Miller, & Paul, 1996). Careful monitoring and documentation of fluid infused is important to avoid iatrogenic polyhydramnios. See Chapter 14 for a comprehensive discussion of the technique for amnioinfusion.

MODIFICATION OF MATERNAL PUSHING EFFORTS

When the FHR demonstrates recurrent decelerations during second-stage pushing, stopping pushing temporarily or pushing with every other or every third contraction based on the fetal response can be effective at allowing the fetus to recover and maintain adequate reserves (AWHONN, 2008). As a potential preventive measure, delaying active pushing until the woman feels the urge to push can minimize fetal stress (AWHONN, 2008; Simpson & James, 2005a). See Chapter 14 for a comprehensive discussion of nursing care during second-stage labor.

FETAL HEART RATE PATTERNS

ALTERATIONS IN BASELINE RATE

Changes in baseline rate that can occur are (1) tachycardia (a rate greater than 160 bpm) and (2) bradycardia (a rate below 110 bpm) (Macones et al., 2008).

Tachycardia

A baseline tachycardia (FHR >160 bpm for 10 minutes or more) may be caused by fetal conditions such as infection, hypoxemia, anemia, prematurity (<26 to 28 weeks' gestation), supraventricular tachycardia, and congenital anomalies; maternal conditions such as fever, dehydration, and infection; or medical problems such as hyperthyroidism. Beta-sympathomimetic drugs such as terbutaline and ritodrine may also cause both maternal and fetal tachycardia. Tachycardia represents increased sympathetic and/or decreased parasympathetic autonomic tone. There are a number of causes of tachycardia that do not reflect a risk of acidemia. The most common of these is an elevation in maternal temperature, although medications administered to the mother and extreme prematurity are other potential factors.

Fetal tachycardia in the presence of chorioamnionitis may be secondary to the maternal fever, an indication of fetal infection, or both. Thus, the determination of risk for acidemia in a fetus with tachycardia is especially difficult, and baseline variability is especially important in evaluating fetal tachycardia. Tachycardia with moderate variability in the absence of FHR decelerations rarely represents fetal acidemia (Krebs, Petres, Dunn, Jordaan, & Segreti, 1979; Low, Victory, & Derrick, 1999). In the presence of normal FHR variability and no periodic changes, the tachycardia is assumed to be due to some cause other than fetal oxygen deficit. Tachycardia sometimes occurs during recovery from oxygen deprivation and probably represents catecholamine activity following sympathetic nervous or adrenal medullary activity in response to acute nonrepetitive hypoxemic stress. There is some controversy in the literature about whether concern for tachycardia should be heightened in the presence of thick meconium staining (Cahill, Parks, Harper, Heitmann, & O'Neill, 2009; Xu, Mas-Calvet, Wei, Luo, & Fraser, 2009). Fetal tachycardia without FHR variability signifies a significant risk for fetal acidemia. Acidemia cannot be reliably excluded in the context of fetal tachycardia with minimal variability or absent accelerations (ACOG, 2010b).

Nursing interventions for tachycardia include assessment of maternal temperature and hydration. Elevated maternal temperature is the most common etiology of fetal tachycardia in the intrapartum period. Nursing interventions include notification of the physician or midwife, assisting the woman to a lateral position, an infusion of IV fluids, and, if variability is minimal or absent, administration of oxygen at 10 L/min via nonrebreather face mask. If the fetal tachycardia is associated with absent variability or recurrent late or variable decelerations, bedside evaluation by a physician is necessary. If maternal fever is ruled out as the etiology of the tachycardia, oxytocin infusion should be decreased or discontinued if infusing, or the next dose of Cervidil, Prepidil, or misoprostol should be delayed until fetal status improves.

Bradycardia

A baseline bradycardia (FHR <110 bpm for 10 minutes or more) may be caused by fetal conditions such as hypoxemia secondary to an acute decrease in oxygen flow to the fetus, vagal stimulation, and rarely, cardiac anomalies such as complete heart block (CHB) or hypothermia. Bradycardias may cause hypoxemia or may be the result of hypoxemia. The depth, duration, and presence or absence of variability are critical components in making a clinical association between the bradycardia seen and the presence or absence of fetal hypoxemia. In addition, in the context of a drop in heart rate that is not returning to previous baseline, intervention is needed before a definitive distinction can be made between a true baseline change and a prolonged deceleration (ACOG, 2010b).

A sudden, profound bradycardia is an obstetric emergency that may signal uterine rupture, prolapsed umbilical cord, rupture of a vasa previa, or placental abruption (Fig. 15–6). This pattern, sometimes called "terminal" bradycardia, may precede death in utero if birth does not occur rapidly. The onset of a recurrent decelerations or fetal bradycardia when a woman is laboring after a prior cesarean birth should cause concern for the onset of uterine rupture, initiation of bedside evaluation by the provider, and preparation for an emergent cesarean birth. FHR abnormalities are the most common sign of uterine rupture, occurring in 70% of cases (ACOG, 2010a). While variable, late, or prolonged decelerations may be seen initially, bradycardia is the FHR pattern most associated with uterine rupture (Leung, Leung, & Paul, 1993; Menihan, 1998; Ridgeway, Weyrich, & Benedetti, 2004). Leung et al. (1993) evaluated the fetal consequences of catastrophic uterine rupture when the diagnosis was made at the onset of a fetal bradycardia. All babies with a previously normal FHR pattern born within 17 minutes following the onset of a prolonged deceleration survived without significant perinatal morbidity (Leung et al., 1993). However, if "severe" late or variable decelerations are present prior to the onset of bradycardia, the fetus tolerated a shorter period of prolonged FHR deceleration, and there was significantly increased risk for metabolic acidosis (Leung et al., 1993). When "severe" late and variable decelerations precede the onset of a prolonged deceleration associated with uterine rupture, perinatal asphyxia can occur as early as 10 minutes after the onset of a prolonged deceleration (Leung et al., 1993). Similarly, Kamoshita et al. (2010) reviewed a retrospective case series of 19 women with "reassuring" tracings followed by serious causes (e.g., abruption, cord prolapse, uterine rupture) of sudden, sustained bradycardia under 100 bpm that occurred

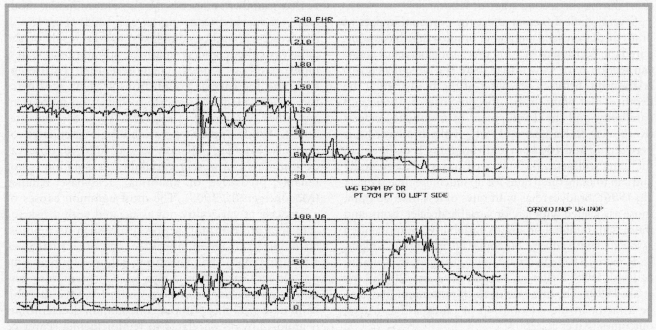

FIGURE 15–6. Terminal bradycardia.

over a 1-year period. This group observed normal neurologic outcomes in babies at 2 years when cesarean birth occurred in less than 25 minutes from the onset of bradycardia and three deaths that occurred in the context of longer event to birth times due to cord prolapse outside the delivery setting. See Chapter 14 for a discussion of uterine rupture associated with women attempting a trial of labor after a previous cesarean birth.

Bradycardias that occur during the second stage of labor following a previously normal FHR pattern may be less concerning. These may be due to increased vagal tone from head compression (Parer & Nageotte, 2004), or occasionally umbilical cord occlusion. If the variability remains moderate or minimal and the FHR does not fall below 80 to 90 bpm, expediting birth is not warranted (Gull et al., 1996). However, efforts should be made to modify maternal pushing efforts to allow the fetus to recover.

During a second-stage bradycardia, the woman should be encouraged to push while in either right or left lateral position, avoiding the supine position. She should be encouraged to push with every other or every third contraction to allow the fetus to gain a few added minutes of improved blood flow (AWHONN, 2008). Coaching a laboring woman to push with every other contraction may be difficult if she has no anesthesia, so this strategy may only be possible with regional anesthesia in place. However, Valsalva pushing (prolonged breath holding) is likely to worsen the situation and should be avoided (AWHONN, 2008). If the woman has a regional anesthetic, another option is to allow the fetus to descend passively with the uterine contractions if the contractions are of sufficient strength. See Chapter 14 for a discussion about nursing interventions during the second stage of labor.

Several clinical factors affect the potential impact of bradycardia on fetal outcome. Studies that have compared the decision to incision times for emergency cesarean section have shown that there is a time-dependent relationship between the onset of the bradycardia, the depth of the bradycardia, the presence or absence of variability, and the development of metabolic acidosis (Korhonen & Kariniemi, 1994). If the bradycardia is between 80 and 100 bpm and variability is maintained, the fetus will generally stay well oxygenated centrally and can tolerate these rates for an indefinite time (Gull et al., 1996). Bradycardias with rates of less than 60 bpm, those associated with late or variable decelerations, and those with minimal or absent variability are most often associated with adverse outcome (Beard, Filshie, Knight, & Roberts, 1971; Berkus, Langer, Samueloff, Xenakis, & Field, 1999; Dellinger, Boehm, & Crane, 2000; Low et al., 1999). The presence of thick meconium may also be a factor in the relationship of bradycardia to fetal outcomes (Xu et al., 2009).

In the case of a fetal demise, both the external ultrasound transducer and the direct fetal electrode can record maternal heart rate, which will appear the same as a bradycardic FHR. The external transducer can record maternal heart rate from the aorta, and the direct lead will record maternal heart rate conducted through the dead fetal tissue. Likewise, the external transducer can record maternal heart rate with a live fetus if incorrectly positioned. Thus, a fetal bradycardia can be missed if clinicians assume that a low rate is maternal. Therefore, evaluation of maternal pulse in order to differentiate it from FHR should be one of the initial nursing assessments when bradycardia is observed. This assessment is accomplished by palpating the maternal pulse. When the monitor is recording the maternal heart rate, maternal pulse is synchronous with the monitor signal. As previously mentioned, some fetal monitors provide cues or alerts that the heart rate being detected may be maternal rather than fetal. If these cues are displayed, confirmation that FHR is the source of the tracing is warranted.

Nursing interventions for bradycardia include notifying the physician or midwife with a request for bedside evaluation, a vaginal exam to rule out a prolapsed umbilical cord, assisting the woman to a lateral position, administering an infusion of IV fluids, oxygen at 10 L/min via a nonrebreather face mask, and discontinuing oxytocin if infusing. If the bradycardia persists, preparations for an operative birth, including moving the patient to the location where birth can be accomplished most expeditiously, may be warranted.

ALTERATIONS IN VARIABILITY

FHR variability is described as absent, minimal, moderate, or marked (Macones et al., 2008) (Fig. 15–7). Moderate variability complexes are the result of the parasympathetic and sympathetic stimuli, fetal states, higher cortical centers, chemoreceptors, baroreceptors, and the cardiac conductions system, and therefore reflect adequate cerebral oxygenation more than any other component of the FHR (Parer & Nageotte, 2004). While moderate variability is predictive of normal acid–base balance at the time of observation, minimal or absent variability in isolation is not reliably predictive of abnormal acid–base balance (Macones et al., 2008). The most common causes of a decrease in variability not associated with a risk for acidemia are centrally acting drugs such as opioids, tranquilizers, magnesium sulfate, and other analgesics administered to women during labor. Minimal (but not absent) variability is also seen in premature gestations and during fetal sleep cycles (ACOG, 2010b). Minimal variability without concomitant decelerations is almost always unrelated to fetal acidemia (Parer &

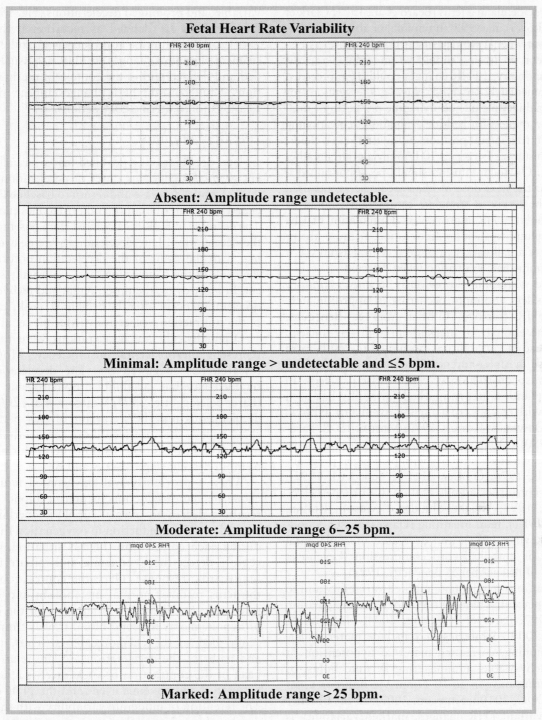

FIGURE 15–7. Fetal heart rate variability.

Livingston, 1990). However, ACOG (2010b) recommends considering a tracing with persistent minimal variability without accelerations and no response to scalp or vibroacoustic stimulation (VAS) as possibly associated with fetal acidemia unless normal scalp pH can be confirmed. A fetus with a defective cardiac conduction system, anencephaly, or congenital neurologic deficit may present with minimal or absent variability; and in the case of congenital neurologic impairment,

this FHR pattern may actually represent an asphyxial insult that occurred during the antepartum period (MacLennan, 1999).

Conversely, absent variability is seen in cases where the fetus has cerebral asphyxia and therefore experiences loss of either fine-tuning within the cardioregulatory center in the brain or direct myocardial depression. Loss of variability especially in the presence of other periodic patterns during labor is the most sensitive indicator of metabolic acidemia in a fetus (Beard et al., 1971; Clark et al., 1984; Low et al., 1999). If minimal or absent variability is present when a woman first arrives for care, assessment of fetal well-being should be undertaken rapidly, as other unobserved FHR changes could have preceded what is immediately observed. Nursing interventions for absent variability include notifying the physician or midwife with a request for bedside evaluation, repositioning the woman to a lateral position, administering IV fluids, and administering oxygen at 10 L/min via nonrebreather face mask. Oxytocin infusion should be discontinued if infusing or the next dose of pharmacologic agents used to ripen the cervix or stimulate contractions should be delayed until the FHR improves. Fetal stimulation may be used to attempt to elicit an acceleration. Because absent variability is a hallmark sign of deep central asphyxia, it warrants immediate evaluation when detected.

Marked variability (previously termed *saltatory pattern*) is less common, occurring in approximately 2% of FHR tracings (O'Brien-Abel & Benedetti, 1992). The etiology of marked variability is unclear. The increase in variability is presumed to result from an increase in alpha-adrenergic activity, which causes selective vasoconstriction of certain vascular beds. In fetal sheep and monkeys, marked variability has been observed with episodes of acute hypoxemia or hypoxia (Dalton, Dawes, & Patrick, 1977; Martin, 1978; Parer et al., 1980). Other studies of human fetuses have associated marked variability with prolonged pregnancies (Cibils, 1976; O'Brien-Abel & Benedetti, 1992), maternal ephedrine administration (O'Brien-Abel & Benedetti, 1992; Wright, Shnider, Levinson, Rolbin, & Parer, 1981), fetal breathing (Dawes, Visser, Goodman, & Levine, 1981), and decreased uteroplacental perfusion or umbilical cord compression (Leveno et al., 1984; O'Brien-Abel & Benedetti, 1992).

Interventions to eliminate marked variability aim to promote placental blood flow and fetal oxygenation (Parer, 1997; Parer & Nageotte, 2004; Nagoette & Gilstrap, 2009). Strategies may include maternal lateral positioning, correcting maternal hypotension or uterine tachysystole, administering IV fluid bolus, or administering oxygen at 10 L/min via nonrebreather mask (ACOG, 2010b; Simpson, 2007). In the absence of other variant FHR changes, marked variability is not associated with fetal acidemia (O'Brien-Abel & Benedetti, 1992; Wright, Shnider et al., 1981).

PERIODIC AND EPISODIC CHANGES IN FETAL HEART RATE

Periodic changes in heart rate are transient and last anywhere from a few seconds to 1 or 2 minutes or more, as compared to baseline changes in the heart rate, which must last a minimum of 10 minutes. The four types of FHR decelerations are early, late,

variable, and prolonged decelerations (Fig. 15–8 A–D). Decelerations are defined as recurrent if they occur with ≥50% of uterine contractions in any 20-minute segment. Periodic changes in FHR are usually identified and defined within the context of uterine contractions, while episodic FHR changes appear to have no relationship to uterine contractions.

Late Decelerations

A late deceleration is defined as a visually apparent *gradual* (defined as onset of deceleration to nadir ≥30 seconds) decrease and return to baseline FHR associated with a uterine contraction (Macones et al., 2008). The decrease in FHR is calculated from onset to nadir of the deceleration. Late decelerations are delayed in timing, with the nadir of the deceleration occurring after the peak of the contraction, and are usually symmetrical. In most cases, the onset, nadir, and recovery of the deceleration occur after the beginning, peak, and ending of the contraction, respectively (Macones et al., 2008).

Originally, all late decelerations were thought to represent uteroplacental insufficiency. More recent research has suggested that late decelerations with retained baseline variability are neurogenic in origin (Parer & Nageotte, 2004; Westgate et al., 2007). Early decelerations may be a variant of this pattern, and some believe they are seen more frequently in fetuses in an occiput posterior position and/or during periods of rapid descent (Fig. 15–9 A and B).

When a previously well-oxygenated fetus experiences an acute reduction in uterine blood flow, the resulting decreased oxygen supply is overlaid on the normal transient reduction in oxygenation that occurs during each contraction. In this situation, chemoreceptors detect the hypoxemia and initiate the vagal bradycardic response. Once the contraction recedes, the fetus resumes normal metabolism and the heart rate recovers. There is a brief delay in the detection of hypoxemia as the fetal blood travels from the placental bed to the chemoreceptors. Thus, the onset and nadir of the deceleration are late relative to the peak of the contraction because there is a lag in time between the hypoxemic event and the FHR response. The retention of moderate variability with this type of deceleration suggests the fetus is not significantly acidemic at the time such a pattern is observed (ACOG, 2009a; Parer et al., 2006); however, close surveillance is warranted and intrauterine resuscitation measures are appropriate (ACOG, 2010b).

Late decelerations with concomitant minimal or absent variability are possibly secondary to fetal hypoxia and acidemia (Beard et al., 1971; Berkus et al., 1999; Clark et al., 1984). This type of periodic change occurs when there is insufficient oxygen for myocardial metabolism and/or normal cerebral function. These FHR patterns are likely to occur when there is chronic placental

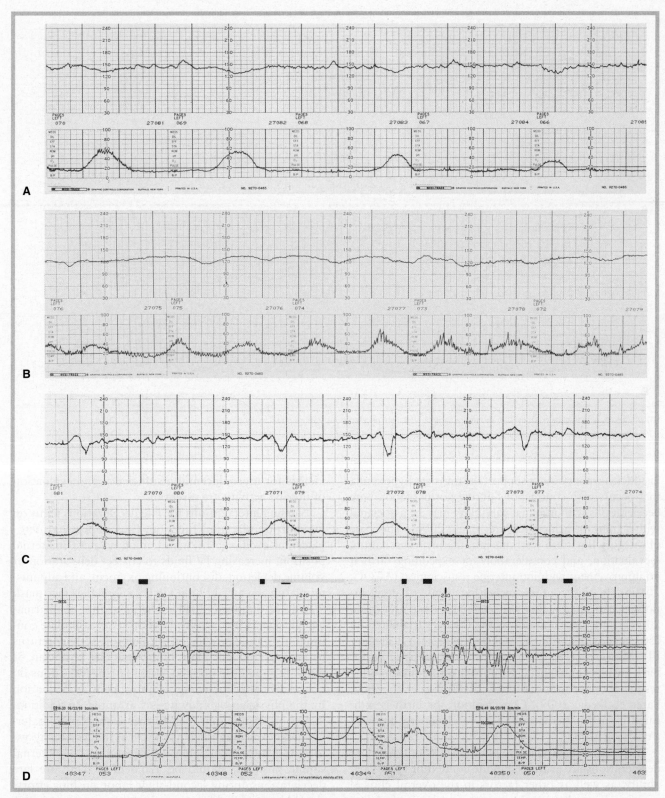

FIGURE 15–8. Four types of fetal heart rate decelerations. **A**, Early. **B**, Late. **C**, Variable. **D**, Prolonged.

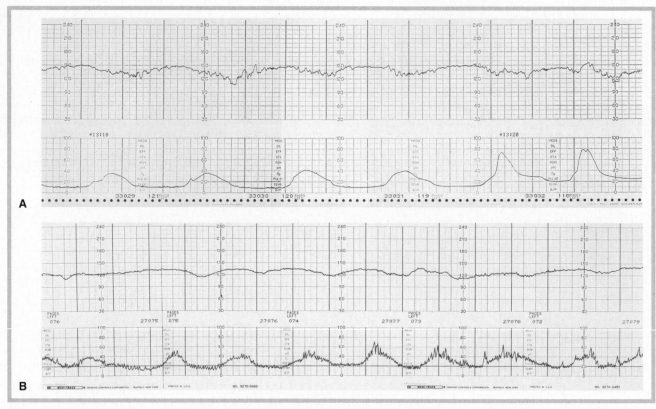

FIGURE 15–9. **A,** Late decelerations with moderate variability. **B,** Late decelerations with minimal variability.

insufficiency that cannot support the transient hypoxemia that occurs with contractions during normal labor. Late decelerations with minimal variability may be associated with significant acidemia (Parer et al., 2006). This type of category II pattern warrants intrauterine resuscitation, reevaluation, and consideration for expediting birth if no improvement with intrauterine resuscitation (ACOG, 2010b). In this context, increasing depth of decelerations is associated with lower fetal pH levels (Parer et al., 2006). Late decelerations with absent variability are associated with abnormal fetal acid–base status (category III) (Macones et al., 2008) and warrant preparation for birth while simultaneously implementing intrauterine resuscitation measures (ACOG, 2010b; Fox et al., 2000; Parer & Ikeda, 2007). Consideration for birth is indicated if such patterns cannot be resolved expeditiously (ACOG, 2010b).

It follows from the previous discussion that late decelerations are evaluated in the context of FHR variability, as well as other factors in the overall clinical picture. Late decelerations with moderate baseline variability and a stable rate with accelerations warrant less concern than late decelerations in the presence of an abnormal baseline rate, minimal variability, and absence of accelerations. If the FHR pattern was normal prior to the onset of decelerations, an iatrogenic cause, such as maternal hypotension, frequently can be determined. Evaluation of maternal history for risk factors for uteroplacental insufficiency and evaluation of uterine activity are essential.

Nursing interventions for late decelerations focus on maximizing placental function, thus improving uteroplacental exchange by maintaining a lateral maternal position, increasing IV fluids to correct dehydration or volume depletion, discontinuing oxytocin, and administering oxygen at 10 L/min via nonrebreather face mask (Garite & Simpson, 2011). The next dose of pharmacologic agents used to ripen the cervix or stimulate contractions should be delayed until uterine activity returns to normal and the FHR improves. The physician or midwife should be notified. If the late decelerations do not resolve after these interventions, bedside evaluation by the physician or midwife is warranted. In addition, iatrogenic insults that may further compromise maternal–fetal exchange, such as oxytocin-induced tachysystole or maternal hypotension secondary to maternal supine position, should be avoided. If there are late decelerations during second-stage labor, pushing efforts should be modified based on the fetal response.

Variable Decelerations

A variable deceleration is defined as a visually apparent *abrupt* (defined as onset of deceleration to beginning of nadir <30 seconds) decrease in FHR below the baseline (Macones et al., 2008). The decrease is calculated from the onset to the nadir of the contraction and is ≥15 bpm, lasting ≥15 seconds, and <2 minutes from onset to return to baseline. Variable decelerations typically vary in their onset, depth, and duration relative to uterine contractions.

Variable decelerations are the most frequently seen FHR deceleration pattern in labor (ACOG, 2010b). The initial rapid deceleration of the FHR is a response to vagal stimulation resulting from umbilical cord compression. When the umbilical arteries are occluded, the low-resistance placental circuit is abruptly withdrawn, resulting in increased peripheral vascular resistance and sudden fetal hypertension. Hypertension immediately stimulates fetal baroreceptors, producing a vagal reflex response and rapid slowing of the FHR. When the umbilical cord is released, the FHR typically returns rapidly to predeceleration values (Freeman et al., 2003; Lee, Di Loreto, & O'Lane, 1975). When variable decelerations occur during the second stage of labor, they may also be caused by the marked head compression and resultant intense vagal stimulation that occurs during rapid descent. When there is oligohydramnios, the cord is more vulnerable to compression because of the lack of cushioning provided by the amniotic fluid (Galvan, Van Mullem, & Broekhuizen, 1989). In this case, the variable decelerations may occur in response to fetal movement or uterine contractions, and they may be frequent or occasional. Variable decelerations have multiple appearances in all aspects except one: The initial FHR drop is abrupt.

Nursing interventions to correct variable decelerations focus on determining the likely source of cord compression and alleviating it if possible (Garite & Simpson, 2011). In most cases, alleviating the cord compression begins with assisting the woman to a lateral or modified Sims' position to release the cord from where it is entrapped. A vaginal examination is appropriate to palpate for an umbilical cord prolapse.

If there are recurrent variable decelerations during second-stage labor, maternal pushing efforts should be modified based on the fetal response. Pushing with every other, or every third, contraction may allow more blood flow to the fetus and the fetus to recover between contractions (AWHONN, 2008; Freeman et al., 2003). When variable decelerations continue despite modified pushing efforts, it may be necessary to stop pushing temporarily. Women without regional analgesia/anesthesia may have difficulty controlling their urge to push and may need significant encouragement to not push while the fetus recovers. Discontinue oxytocin until fetal status improves and uterine activity returns to normal. Oxygen may be given at 10 L/min via a nonrebreather face mask, and IV fluids may be increased. If position changes do not result in resolution of the variable decelerations, notification of the physician or midwife is warranted, and a request for bedside evaluation may be indicated based on the clinical situation.

When variable decelerations occur during first-stage labor and maternal position changes do not result in resolution, amnioinfusion may be considered (ACOG, 2010b; Garite & Simpson, 2011). Recurrent variable decelerations in the context of absent variability are associated with abnormal acid–base status (Macones et al., 2008). In this situation, prompt birth should be considered if intrauterine resuscitation measures do not result in improved fetal status (ACOG, 2010b).

Prolonged Decelerations

A prolonged deceleration of the FHR is a visually apparent decrease in FHR below the baseline that is ≥15 bpm, lasting ≥2 minutes, but <10 minutes from onset to return to baseline (Macones et al., 2008). The decrease is calculated from the adjacent baseline. During a prolonged deceleration, the heart rate usually drops abruptly, and stays down for several minutes. Prolonged decelerations may occur in the presence or absence of contractions and may have either an abrupt or slow return to the baseline rate. Prolonged decelerations may be the result of a longer episode of cord compression, maternal hypotension, excessive uterine activity, vagal stimulation, uterine rupture, vasa previa rupture, or rarely, maternal seizures or maternal respiratory or cardiac arrest.

This type of deceleration may also be seen when there is a transient decrease in uteroplacental blood flow in a previously well-functioning maternal–fetal unit. This occasionally occurs during the administration of regional anesthesia and/or when the patient is in a supine position (Freeman et al., 2003). Nonrecurrent prolonged decelerations that are preceded and followed by an FHR that has a normal baseline and moderate variability are not associated with fetal hypoxemia of clinical significance. ACOG (2010b) recommends prompt birth in cases of prolonged decelerations with minimal or absent variability.

Nursing interventions for prolonged decelerations include discontinuing oxytocin if infusing, increasing IV fluids, administering oxygen at 10 L/min via nonrebreather face mask, a vaginal exam to rule out prolapsed cord, and repositioning the woman to remove pressure from the umbilical cord. Delay the next dose of pharmacologic agents used to ripen the cervix or stimulate contractions until uterine activity returns to normal and the FHR improves. The physician or midwife should be notified and a bedside evaluation requested. A tocolytic agent may also be administered to decrease uterine activity (ACOG, 2010b). If there are prolonged decelerations during second-stage labor, modify pushing efforts based on the fetal response (AWHONN, 2008). When a prolonged deceleration occurs during antepartum testing, an ultrasound measurement of amniotic fluid volume is indicated. A decision tree with suggested general guidelines for the management of selected FHR tracings is provided in Figure 15–10.

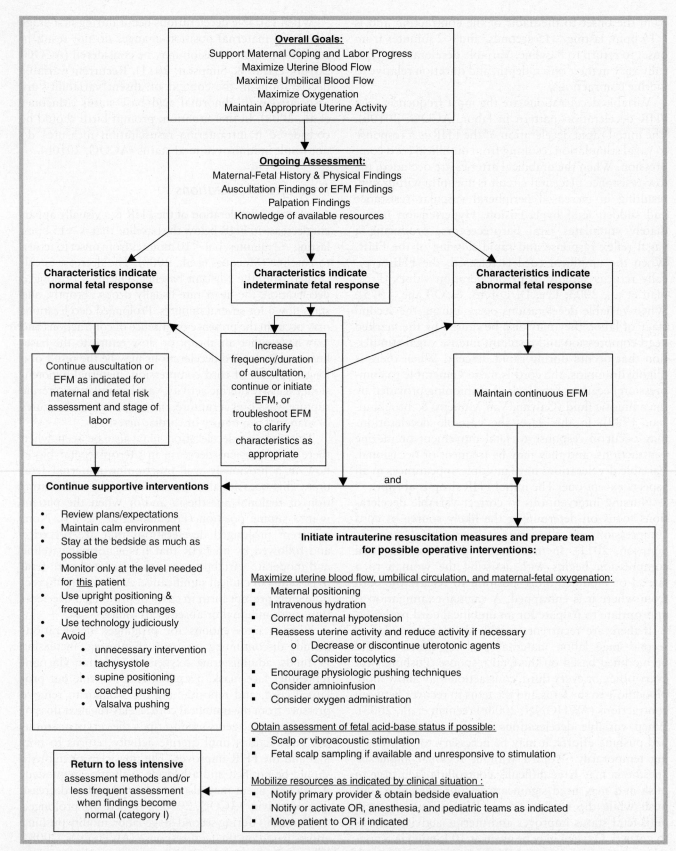

FIGURE 15–10. Fetal monitoring decision tree. EFM, electronic fetal monitoring. (From Lyndon, A., O'Brien-Abel, N., & Simpson, K. R. [2009]. Fetal heart rate interpretation. In A. Lyndon & L. U. Ali [Eds.], *Fetal Heart Monitoring Principles and Practices* [4th ed., p. 128]. Washington, DC: Association of Women's Health, Obstetric and Neonatal Nurses/ Kendall Hunt. Used with permission.)

UNUSUAL FETAL HEART RATE PATTERNS

As a general caveat, whenever an unusual tracing is observed from the beginning of electronic monitoring, consider the possibility of a fetus with a congenital anomaly. An initial tracing with minimal or absent variability without accelerations or with other unusual characteristics should prompt an urgent assessment of fetal well-being. This may include fetal stimulation, an ultrasound evaluation, or other assessments as indicated by the overall clinical picture. Although most fetuses with congenital anomalies have normal FHR tracings (Nageotte & Gilstrap, 2009), hydrocephalic and anencephalic fetuses may present with unusual FHR patterns that do not fit any category or definition (Freeman et al., 2003). If possible, an ultrasound examination may be performed to rule out gross anomalies as the cause of the pattern, even though the results of the ultrasound examination may be inconclusive. An anomaly that affects the fetal CNS most likely will have an impact on the variability and/or the fetal cardiac system's ability to accelerate and decelerate. Unusual decelerations with a flat, fixed rate may be seen.

Sinusoidal Heart Rate Pattern

The sinusoidal FHR pattern is a visually apparent undulating smooth sine wavelike pattern in FHR baseline with a cycle frequency of three to five per minute, which persists for *at least* 20 minutes (Macones et al., 2008) (Fig. 15–11). First identified in 1972, the sinusoidal FHR pattern was associated with severely affected, Rh-sensitized, and dying fetuses (Manseau, Vaquier, Chavinie, & Sureau, 1972). The FHR pattern was named "sinusoidal" due to its sine waveform.

A true sinusoidal FHR pattern is a rare occurrence. When identified, it has been associated with severe fetal anemia as a result of Rh isoimmunization, massive fetomaternal hemorrhage, twin-to-twin transfusion syndrome, ruptured vasa previa, traumatic fetal bleeding with severe anemia, fetal intracranial hemorrhage, and severe fetal asphyxia (Modanlou & Murata, 2004). Other conditions associated with a true sinusoidal FHR include fetal infection, fetal cardiac anomalies, neonatal hypoxia, congenital hydrocephalus, gastroschisis, and maternal cardiopulmonary bypass (Modanlou & Murata, 2004). Whatever the pathogenesis, a true sinusoidal FHR pattern is an ominous finding that implies fetal jeopardy and requires immediate fetal evaluation.

A sinusoidal-appearing FHR pattern has been noted to follow the maternal administration of some opioid medications (especially butorphanol and fentanyl), fetal sleep cycles, thumb-sucking, or rhythmic movements of the fetal mouth (Modanlou & Murata, 2004). As the medication is excreted, the fetus awakens or the fetus stops sucking, and the sinusoidal-appearing

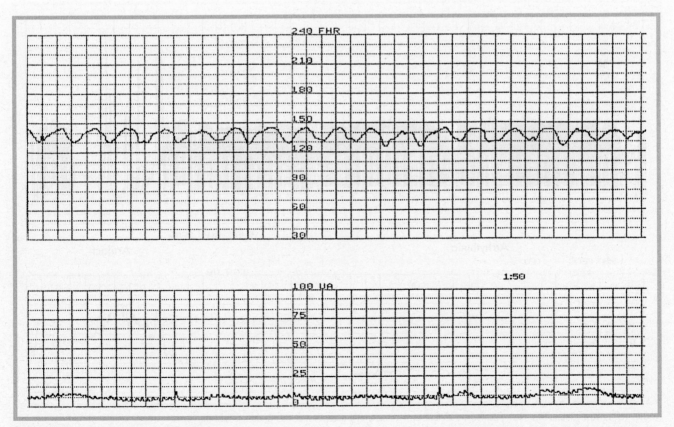

FIGURE 15–11. Sinusoidal fetal heart rate pattern.

pattern resolves, thus giving it the name of "pseudosinusoidal" or "drug-induced sinusoidal." In contrast to the true sinusoidal FHR pattern, this undulating pattern is of short duration and both preceded and followed by a normal FHR (Modanlou & Murata, 2004). No treatment is indicated.

Fetal Arrhythmias

Fetal cardiac arrhythmias occur in approximately 1% to 2% of all pregnancies and are usually benign (Kleinman, Nehgme, Copel, 2004). Of those, approximately 90% are due to irregular rhythm, and less than 10% are due to sustained bradyarrhythmias or tachyarrhythmias with clinical significance to the fetus (Kleinman & Nehgme, 2004).

Arrhythmias due to irregular rhythm have been recognized with increasing frequency at routine prenatal visits (Fig. 15–12). Most of these arrhythmias are ectopic premature atrial contractions (PACs) detected by listening to the fetal heart. The most common finding is the impression that the fetal heart is intermittently "skipping" beats. In most cases, the skipping actually represents either a pause following an extrasystole that has not reset the sinus node pacemaker or an extrasystole occurring early in the cardiac cycle with a stroke volume that is inadequate to produce a detectable Doppler signal (Kleinman & Nehgme, 2004). PACs may be exacerbated by maternal caffeine ingestion, decongestant medications, or tobacco (Sklansky, 2009). While the extrasystoles may be a source of anxiety for the parents, the extrasystoles usually resolve spontaneously, and affected fetuses only rarely develop persistent tachyarrhythmias requiring further evaluation.

Sustained fetal tachyarrhythmias or bradyarrhythmias are rare. However, when detected during routine prenatal visits, they require multidisciplinary evaluation. Supraventricular tachycardia (SVT) is the most common arrhythmia that has potentially significant clinical consequences. SVT typically occurs at 240 to 260 bpm with minimal or absent FHR variability. While most commonly diagnosed in fetuses with structurally normal hearts, SVT frequently is a result of electrical reentry arising from a circus movement of electrical energy between the atrial and ventricular myocardium (Kleinman & Nehgme, 2004). SVT typically manifests as an intermittent tachyarrhythmia; however, sustained SVT may occur. Decisions about treatment of sustained SVT with antiarrhythmic agents (e.g., digoxin, propranolol, flecainide, sotalol, amiodarone) requires a careful risk/benefit analysis. Considerations include development of hydrops fetalis, gestational age, lung maturity, provider experience with cardioconversion, neonatal intensive care

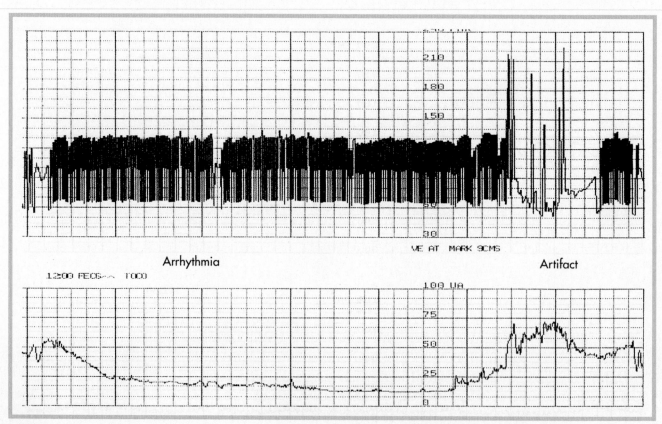

FIGURE 15–12 Arrhythmia. This tracing demonstrates fetal arrhythmia and artifact. Notice the randomness of the artifactual information compared with the organization of the arrhythmia.

experience with varying gestational ages for fetuses with and without hydrops, and parental wishes (Kleinman & Nehgme, 2004).

In CHB, the atrial electrical impulses are unable to pass through the conduction system to activate the ventricles. This results in the ventricles depolarizing at their own intrinsic rate of 40 to 80 bpm. Approximately 50% of fetuses with CHB have structurally normal hearts; however, transplacental passage of maternal antibodies (anti-Ro and anti-La) can damage the cardiac conduction system typically after 18 to 20 weeks gestation (Sklansky, 2009; Copel, Friedman, & Kleinman, 1997). Often, mothers of these fetuses have symptoms consistent with Sjögren's syndrome, systemic lupus erythematosus, or related connective tissue disorders (Sklansky, 2009). These fetuses generally tolerate the arrhythmia well if they are able to maintain a ventricular rate greater than 55 bpm (Kleinman & Nehgme, 2004). The other half of fetuses with CHB have underlying congenital heart disease, often appearing as a complex lesion in the central portion of the heart involving the atrioventricular junction. Unfortunately, the prognosis for fetuses with structural cardiac defects or hydrops fetalis is quite poor (Kleinman & Nehgme, 2004).

Assessment of the FHR with external ultrasound component of the EFM may be difficult in the presence of extrasystoles due to the inability to see a consistent baseline or to evaluate variability. These arrhythmias may be verified by auscultating the FHR for irregular rhythm or, if appropriate, applying the FSE to accurately record the extrasystoles as brief upward or downward excursions. Tachyarrhythmias and bradyarrhythmias may appear as halved or doubled the actual heart rate when monitored electronically. Auscultating and counting the actual FHR or ultrasound imaging may verify the arrhythmia. If the heart rate is regular to auscultation, yet there are unusual excursions on the EFM tracing, the most likely explanation is that it is artifactual information. An artifact may be caused by the FSE having a poor attachment to the fetal presenting part or equipment problems. Attempts to correct the problem include changing the cable or fetal monitor and/or replacing the direct electrode (see Table 15–3).

CLINICAL IMPLICATIONS FOR MONITORING THE FETUS LESS THAN 32 WEEKS' GESTATION DURING LABOR

While the principles of EFM are the same for the preterm fetus as for the term fetus, there are differences in FHR patterns of preterm fetuses when compared to those in term labor, and there are unique clinical implications for obtaining and interpreting EFM

data during preterm labor. Perinatal complications such as preeclampsia, intraamniotic infection, oligohydramnios, umbilical cord compression, placental abruption, intrauterine growth restriction, uteroplacental insufficiency, and multiple gestation are more common during preterm labor. These complications are often associated with indeterminate or abnormal FHR patterns. There is evidence to suggest that these FHR patterns have greater significance for outcomes for the preterm fetus (Matsuda, Maeda, & Kouno, 2003).

The preterm fetus is more susceptible to hypoxic insults and more likely to develop and die from complications of prematurity if born depressed, hypoxemic, or acidemic (Freeman et al., 2003). An abnormal FHR pattern and some types of indeterminate FHR patterns (e.g., minimal to absent variability, late decelerations, recurrent variable decelerations, tachycardia) may be predictive of perinatal asphyxia and long-term neurologic outcome for the preterm fetus (Braithwaite, Milligan, & Shennan, 1986; Douvas, Meeks, Graves, Walsh, & Morrison, 1984; Low et al., 1992; Matsuda et al., 2003; Shy et al., 1990; Westgren, Malcus, & Svenningsen, 1986).

In fetuses less than 28 weeks' gestation, approximately 60% will have an indeterminate or abnormal FHR tracing during the 24 hours prior to birth (Ayoubi et al., 2002). Decelerations (five or more per hour, in which FHR amplitude decreased at least 60 bpm for greater than 30 seconds) and "bradycardia" (less than 120 bpm for greater than 10 minutes) were most common (56%), followed by tachycardia (greater than 160 bpm) (25%) and minimal or absent variability (20%). Of these findings, minimal or absent variability was most significantly correlated with neonatal death at 2 months of age, with only 38% of these infants surviving. Neither decelerations or bradycardia nor fetal tachycardia appeared to affect neonatal mortality rates, with 65% and 74%, respectively, surviving. Compared to the term fetus, the progression from a normal to an indeterminate or abnormal FHR tracing occurs more often and more quickly in the premature fetus (Freeman et al., 2003). Thus, timeliness of identification and initiation of interventions for variant FHR patterns may be more critical and of more lasting consequences when the fetus is preterm.

BASELINE RATE

With advancing gestational age, average baseline FHR at term decreases to approximately 140 bpm before labor. In the preterm fetus, baseline FHR is often in the upper end of the normal range, closer to 160 bpm. In one study, 78% of fetuses less than 33 weeks' gestation had periods of tachycardia (greater than 160 bpm), as compared to only 20% of fetuses greater than 33 weeks' gestation (Westgren et al., 1986). An FHR greater than 160 bpm may indicate evolving fetal hypoxemia, maternal fever, intraamniotic infection, or the side effects of terbutaline administration. The presence of fetal tachycardia is more predictive of acidemia, low Apgar scores, and adverse neonatal outcomes in the preterm fetus compared to the term fetus (Burrus, O'Shea, Veille, & Mueller-Heubach, 1994; Westgren, Holmquist, Svenningsen, & Ingemarsson, 1982). Therefore, baseline rate, as well as other features of the FHR, merits special attention by the nurse responsible for monitoring the labor of a woman with a preterm pregnancy.

VARIABILITY

Minimal variability may be seen more often in the preterm fetus than in the term fetus (Freeman et al., 2003; To & Leung, 1998; Westgren et al., 1982). Loss of variability in the preterm fetus is more predictive of low Apgar scores and acidemia compared to the fetus at term (Douvas et al., 1984; Freeman et al., 2003; Westgren, Hormquist, Ingemarsson, & Svenningsen, 1984). When compared with FHR decelerations, bradycardia, or tachycardia, the finding of minimal or absent variability is most strongly associated with neonatal death in fetuses less than 28 weeks' gestation (Ayoubi et al., 2002). The combination of loss of variability and fetal tachycardia is more often associated with low Apgar scores and acidemia in the preterm fetus (Freeman et al., 2003).

Medications may also influence FHR variability in the preterm fetus. IV magnesium sulfate may be given to women in preterm labor for neuroprotection or to inhibit uterine contractions, or for seizure prophylaxis in laboring women diagnosed with preeclampsia. While studies vary regarding the effect of magnesium sulfate on FHR variability, decreased variability should always be assessed with caution taking into consideration of additional factors (e.g., early gestational age, preeclampsia) that may be causing the decreased variability (ACOG, 2009a; Wright, Ridgway, Wright, Covington, & Bobitt, 1996). Antenatal corticosteroids may be given to the women in preterm labor to enhance fetal lung maturity. Both betamethasone and dexamethasone may cause a transient increase in baseline variability for about 24 hours, followed by decreased variability, which returns to pretreatment variability by the fourth to the seventh day; however, these changes are not indicative of deterioration in fetal status (ACOG, 2009a; Lunshof et al., 2005; Senat et al., 1998; Subtil et al., 2003). IV or intramuscular (IM) opioids may result in minimal variability. It is important to know the duration of the effects of any pain medication given to be able to accurately distinguish between expected FHR side effects and evolving fetal hypoxemia.

ACCELERATIONS

Accelerations of the preterm FHR are generally lower in amplitude and less frequent than those of the term fetus, although most preterm fetuses, even at 24 to 26 weeks' gestation and beyond, will have accelerations of at least 15 bpm lasting 15 seconds (Freeman et al., 2003). The number and amplitude of accelerations increase over the course of gestation as the fetus matures (Kisilevsky, Hains, & Low, 2001). Before 32 weeks of gestation, accelerations are defined as having an acme of at least 10 bpm above baseline with a duration of at least 10 seconds above the baseline (ACOG, 2009a, 2010b; Macones et al., 2008). Similar to moderate variability, the presence of FHR accelerations is highly predictive of normal acid–base status at the time of assessment (ACOG, 2010b).

Antenatal corticosteroid administration may cause a transient increase in fetal movement and FHR accelerations within 12 hours of the first injection and within 6 hours of a second dose (Lunshof et al., 2005; Subtil et al., 2003). The increase in fetal movement and FHR accelerations may be more common in 29 to 33 weeks' gestation fetuses compared to 25 to 28 weeks' gestation fetuses (Lunshof et al., 2005). As with variability, IV or IM opioid medication may temporarily depress the fetal neurologic system, resulting in fewer FHR accelerations and/or FHR accelerations of lower amplitude.

DECELERATIONS

During labor, variable decelerations are more common in the preterm fetus, occurring 55% (34 to 36 weeks' gestation) and 70% (28 to 33 weeks' gestation) of the time compared with 30% to 50% in the fetus at term (Freeman et al., 2003; Westgren et al., 1982). Variable decelerations during preterm labor are associated with a higher rate of hypoxemia, acidemia, neurologic abnormalities, and adverse long-term outcomes (Holmes, Oppenheimer, Gravelle, Walker, & Blayney, 2001; Westgren et al., 1984). There is evidence to suggest that variable decelerations in the premature fetus may also be associated with intraventricular hemorrhage in a manner unrelated to fetal acidemia (Holmes et al., 2001).

Although there does not appear to be an increased incidence of late decelerations during preterm labor, conditions that are more likely to result in late decelerations are more common (Freeman et al., 2003). These include uteroplacental insufficiency, intraamniotic infection, preeclampsia, intrauterine growth restriction, and placental abruption. Late decelerations have more significance for the preterm fetus because there is an association between late decelerations during preterm labor and adverse outcomes such as hypoxemia, academia, and long-term neurologic abnormalities

(Westgren et al., 1984; Zanini, Paul, & Huey, 1980). Prolonged decelerations occur at a similar frequency for the preterm and term fetus (Freeman et al., 2003).

MONITORING PRETERM MULTIPLE GESTATIONS

When monitoring more than one fetus, it is important to maintain two distinct FHRs. Some newer generation monitors designed to accommodate multiple gestations have features to distinguish the two fetuses being monitored. Independent volume controls aid transducer placement by allowing both FHRs to be heard simultaneously. FHRs recorded on the tracing may be offset to facilitate interpretation. Some monitors even provide visual and audible indications when synchronous fetal or maternal heart rate signals are detected. These system cues can be helpful but do not replace a careful nursing assessment of each FHR pattern. The mother may be able to provide assistance in determining the position of each baby by indicating where she feels fetal movement, or ultrasound guidance may be needed to accurately locate and identify individual FHRs for placement of transducers. Despite attempts to continuously monitor multiples for prolonged periods of time, an interpretable tracing may be difficult to obtain. In a study of monoamniotic twins, successful monitoring occurred in only half of the fetuses at 27 to 30 weeks' gestation. At earlier gestations (<27 weeks), successful monitoring of both fetuses was accomplished only 37% of the time (Quinn, Cao, Lacoursiere, & Schrimmer, 2011).

Although some fetal twin pairs may have synchronous FHR patterns at times, most fetuses in multiple gestations will not have completely synchronous FHR patterns during labor (Fig. 15–13 A and B). Tactile communication occurs between twins in utero, and these movements often result in simultaneous accelerations of the FHR during nonstress testing (Sherer, Nawrocki, Peco, Metlay, & Woods, 1990). Periods of reactivity and nonreactivity of the FHR also are similar during nonstress testing (Sherer, D'Amico, Cox, Metlay, & Woods, 1994). The assumption can be made that these conditions and FHR reactions would apply to the intrapartum period, but there have been no confirmatory studies. The published data are limited to FHR patterns of twins during antepartum testing, although authors mentioned incidental data. Some twin fetuses will have asynchronous FHR patterns over the course of labor, especially if there are differences in fetal well-being. Accelerations and decelerations usually occur within the same time frame but will not be identical in duration or excursion from the baseline (Gallagher, Costigan, & Johnson, 1992). There were no studies found about intrapartum FHR patterns of triplets and higher order

multiples, presumably because these pregnancies almost always result in cesarean birth without labor. However, in selected cases when fetal status is normal and fetal presentation is favorable, women with triplets can labor and give birth vaginally.

ASSESSMENT OF PATTERN EVOLUTION

In clinical practice, interpretation of the FHR is an ongoing assessment that includes multiple perinatal factors, specific FHR characteristics, and most importantly, the evolution of the FHR pattern as labor progresses (Fig. 15–14). An abnormal FHR can suddenly develop spontaneously, but usually, the evolution from normal follows a typical pattern over time. FHR patterns that result from an acute event such as umbilical cord prolapse, uterine rupture, or placental abruption are typically noted immediately and acted on quickly by the perinatal team. However, when fetal deterioration occurs progressively over a long period, the clinical symptoms may not be fully appreciated by all members of the perinatal team. A loss of situational awareness can occur and, as a result, timely interventions may be delayed. When the FHR evolves from a baseline within normal limits, moderate variability, and accelerations to variant patterns with minimal to absent variability and recurrent late, variable, or prolonged decelerations, the risk of fetal deterioration toward metabolic acidemia is significant despite the low predictive value of abnormal (category III) tracings for abnormal neurologic outcomes in the neonate (ACOG, 2010b; Freeman et al., 2003). Oxytocin-induced tachysystole can exacerbate the situation, so it is essential to carefully titrate the oxytocin infusion based on contraction frequency and the fetal response (Simpson, 2009a). If the usual intrauterine resuscitation techniques do not result in pattern resolution, consider expeditious birth. A request for bedside evaluation by the primary provider is warranted so that plans can be made and implemented for fetal rescue in a timely manner (Simpson, 2005b).

Evolving FHR patterns that occur during the second stage of labor can be problematic as providers may at times be more oriented to the imminence of birth than to the evolution of the FHR tracing. Yet the active pushing phase of the second stage presents increased physiologic fetal stress with maternal bearing down efforts (Roberts, 2002), and care should be taken to avoid iatrogenic stress and to allow recovery between uterine contractions. One way to minimize fetal risk during the second stage is to allow the fetus to descend passively and to delay pushing until the woman feels the urge to push. Shortening the active pushing phase by allowing passive fetal descent can minimize the decrease in fetal oxygen status that is associated with maternal pushing efforts (Simpson & James, 2005a).

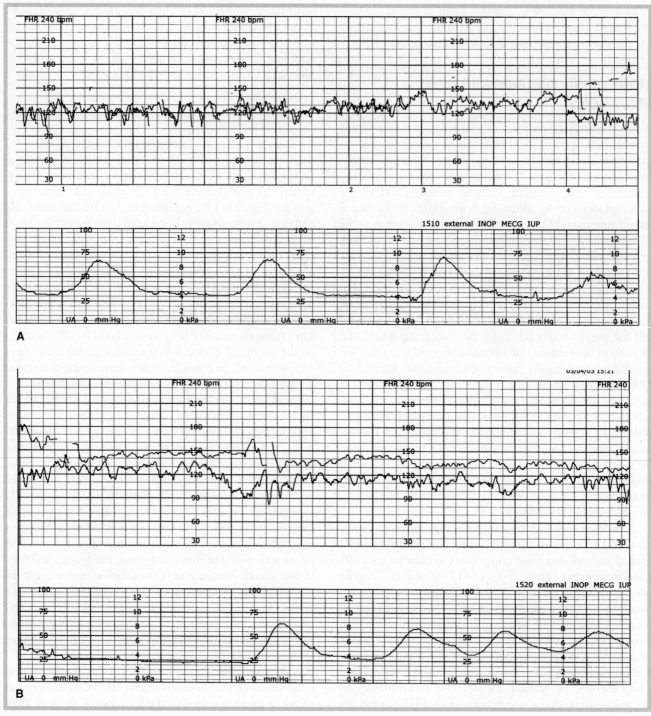

FIGURE 15–13. A, Synchronous fetal heart rate patterns of twins. B, Asynchronous fetal heart rate patterns of twins.

It is common during the second stage of labor for the FHR to develop variable decelerations that become progressively more severe as the woman pushes with contractions and the fetus descends. In this scenario, if the contractions are of normal frequency with adequate resting tone and the pattern is secondary to vagal stimulation during head compression, the FHR will maintain variability because the decelerations are not caused by hypoxia (Parer & Nageotte, 2004). These decelerations can resolve intermittently as the vertex adjusts to pelvic diameters and may resolve completely when the vertex crowns. If the etiology of this pattern is cord occlusion that is worsening as the fetus descends, the decelerations may become more severe and develop a concomitant loss of variability as the fetus develops hypoxemia.

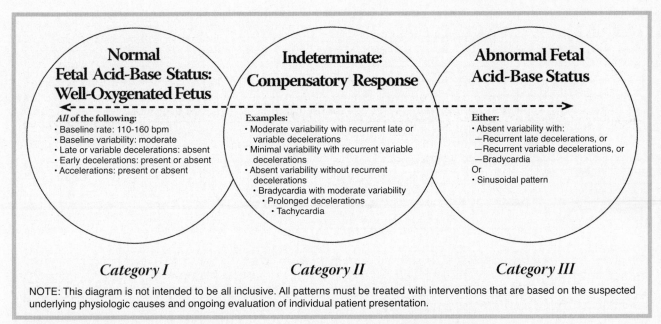

FIGURE 15–14. Dynamic physiologic response model. (From Lyndon, A., O'Brien-Abel, N., & Simpson, K. R. [2009]. Fetal heart rate interpretation. In A. Lyndon & L. U. Ali [Eds.], *Fetal Heart Monitoring Principles and Practices* [4th ed., p. 116]. Washington, DC: Association of Women's Health, Obstetric and Neonatal Nurses/Kendall Hunt. Used with permission.)

When oxytocin is continued during second-stage pushing, it is especially important to avoid tachysystole. Normally during the second stage, contractions tend to become slightly less frequent, which may allow the fetus to tolerate the stress of maternal pushing efforts, umbilical cord compression, and vagal stimulation. When contractions are too frequent over a prolonged period, the fetus may not be able to tolerate this physiologic stress (Bakker et al., 2007).

Interventions for variable decelerations during the second stage should also include assessment of the pushing technique used. When recurrent variable decelerations during the second stage are associated with closed glottis pushing, the most appropriate approach is to encourage the woman to push with every other, or every third, contraction and to discourage prolonged breath holding (AWHONN, 2008). In some cases, it is best to temporarily discontinue pushing to allow the fetus to recover. These techniques can be attempted for all women but are most effective for women who have regional analgesia/anesthesia. Open glottis pushing with the woman bearing down for no more than 6 to 8 seconds per pushing effort will have a less negative effect on fetal status than repetitive closed glottis pushing (AWHONN, 2008; Simpson & James, 2005a) (Fig. 15–15 A and B). Encouraging the woman to bear down as long as she can is more favorable for fetal well-being than telling the woman to take a deep breath and hold it for 10 seconds without making a sound (Simpson & James, 2005a). Counting to 10 with each pushing effort to encourage pushing efforts lasting 10 seconds or more is no longer considered the

most appropriate method of second-stage labor coaching (AWHONN, 2008; Roberts, 2002). Three to four pushing efforts per contraction will minimize risk of fetal compromise and promote adequate fetal descent (AWHONN, 2008). The provider should assess variable decelerations that evolve into longer or deeper decelerations or are associated with tachycardia or decreasing variability and intervene to minimize additional stress via intrauterine resuscitation, discontinuation of oxytocin, and potentially emergent birth (ACOG, 2009a, 2010b). Appropriate care during the second stage of labor can prevent iatrogenic fetal stress and the birth of a depressed baby.

The end-stage bradycardia that retains mild-to-moderate variability is another expression of head compression during rapid descent. If moderate variability is retained and the rate remains above 80 to 90 bpm, this pattern should be watched but considered a benign variant. Conversely, a bradycardia that slopes down over several minutes and loses variability within the first 4 minutes of descent is a pattern evolution that signals fetal decompensation and warrants rapid intervention (Gull et al., 1996).

It is extremely important to recognize an FHR pattern that precedes death. In any stage of labor, bradycardias that are preceded by a period of late or variable decelerations or minimal variability and bradycardias that are associated with absent variability are associated with metabolic acidosis in the fetus (Beard et al., 1971; Berkus et al., 1999; Clark et al., 1984; Dellinger et al., 2000; Low et al., 1999; Macones et al., 2008), and birth is recommended if the pattern cannot be

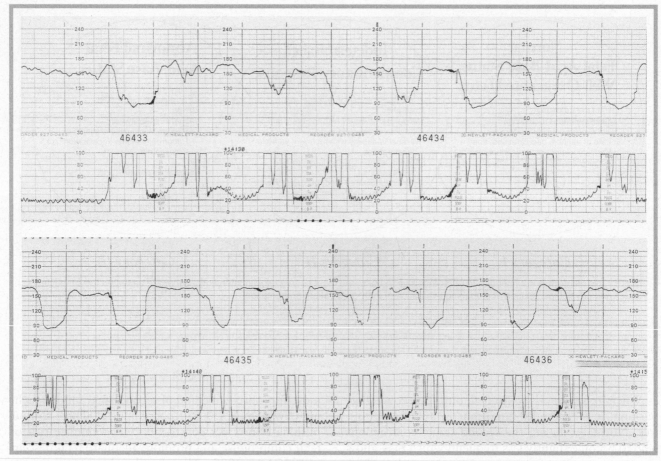

FIGURE 15–15. Iatrogenic category III fetal heart rate pattern as a result of coached closed glottis pushing during the second stage of labor.

resolved (ACOG, 2010b) (see Fig. 15–6). In either situation, if the problem causing fetal hypoxia is not corrected, the FHR eventually becomes a flat, fixed pattern with absent variability prior to death. Scalp stimulation elicits no response. Multiple authors have reviewed the relationship between FHR patterns and neonatal outcomes. The presence of accelerations most reliably indicates adequate oxygenation to the brain, and moderate baseline variability is highly suggestive of the same. A normal baseline rate with moderate variability, with or without accelerations, conveys a high level of security that the fetus is well oxygenated at the time of observation (ACOG, 2009a, 2010b; Macones et al., 2008). Many FHR tracings obtained during labor include some type of variant pattern, and the majority of these fetuses are also well oxygenated. In a study examining the frequency of categories of FHR patterns during term labor, most tracings (77.9%) were normal (category I), 22.1% were indeterminate (category II), and 0.004% were abnormal (category III) (Jackson, Holmgren, Esplin, Henry, & Varner, 2011). Because the range of tracings in category II is quite wide, clinical judgment and knowledge of the underlying physiology are required to determine the appropriate level of concern and level of intervention needed. Nurses caring for women during

labor should be able to promptly recognize abnormal (category III) patterns and request immediate medical consultation, as these abnormal tracings do convey a risk for fetal metabolic acidemia.

ANCILLARY METHODS FOR ASSESSING FETAL ACID–BASE STATUS

Because most variant FHR tracings are not associated with an underlying fetal hypoxemia, it is occasionally helpful to use ancillary testing that can discriminate between the fetus with hypoxemia and the fetus that is centrally well oxygenated. This discrimination can potentially avoid unnecessary interventions if the results of the test are normal. Preferred ancillary methods for evaluating fetal status are fetal scalp stimulation and VAS as they are less invasive than fetal scalp sampling and are readily available. Umbilical cord blood gas and pH values are used to determine fetal acid–base status at the time of birth.

FETAL SCALP AND ACOUSTIC STIMULATION

An acceleration of the FHR of at least 15 bpm above the baseline with a duration of at least 15 seconds highly correlates with a fetal blood pH >7.19, whether the acceleration is spontaneous or in response to fetal stimulation (Clark et al., 1984). Thus, eliciting accelerations through fetal stimulation can be a useful way to rule out fetal acidemia. Stimulation tests include fetal scalp stimulation and fetal acoustic stimulation. Stimulation tests should be performed while the FHR is at baseline, not during a deceleration (Clark et al., 1984; Freeman et al., 2003; Garite, 2007). Likewise, accelerations elicited by VAS have a similar correlation with fetal normoxia (Lin, Vassallo, & Mittendorf, 2001; Porter & Clark, 1999; Skupski, Rosenberg, & Eglinton, 2002). The absence of an acceleration response to digital or acoustic stimulation is not diagnostic of fetal acidemia; rather, it is an indeterminate finding (Macones et al., 2008; Porter & Clark, 1999; Skupski et al., 2002) and should be managed accordingly (ACOG, 2010b).

Digital scalp stimulation is performed by placing firm, digital pressure on the fetal scalp during a vaginal examination. To perform VAS, a commercially distributed vibroacoustic stimulator or a battery-powered artificial larynx is positioned over the fetal vertex or breech and a stimulus of 1 to 2 seconds is applied (ACOG, 1999). This may be repeated up to three times for progressively longer durations up to 3 seconds to elicit FHR accelerations (ACOG, 1999; Druzin, Smith, Gabbe & Reed, 2007). While some evidence supports the use of VAS during labor (ACOG, 2010b), no RCTs to date have addressed the safety and efficacy of VAS in the context of labor (East et al., 2005). Because digital scalp stimulation and VAS are less invasive and easier to perform than fetal scalp sampling while providing similar information about the likelihood of fetal acidemia, scalp pH is used rarely in the United States (ACOG, 2009a). ACOG (2010b) recommends that when an FHR tracing has minimal or absent variability and no accelerations and does not respond to intrauterine resuscitation measures, additional assessment such as digital scalp stimulation or VAS should be done.

UMBILICAL CORD BLOOD GAS AND ACID–BASE ANALYSIS

Umbilical Cord Blood Analysis

Umbilical cord blood gas and pH determinations provide an objective method of determining fetal acid–base status immediately before birth (Blickstein & Green, 2007). Risk of moderate and severe newborn encephalopathy and respiratory and other complications occur in 10% of neonates with umbilical arterial base deficit of 12 to 16 mmol/L (or base excess of −12 to −16 mmol/L, increasing to 40% in neonates with an umbilical arterial base deficit greater than 16 mmol/L [base excess less than −16 mmol/L]) (ACOG, 2006b).

Umbilical cord blood sampling is often performed when an event during labor or birth may have the potential to be associated with an adverse neonatal outcome. Situations in which the obstetric care provider may wish to obtain venous and arterial blood samples include low 5-minute Apgar score, expedited birth for fetal compromise (e.g., umbilical cord prolapse, uterine rupture, placental abruption), abnormal and some indeterminate FHR tracings, severe intrauterine growth restriction, maternal thyroid disease, acute chorioamnionitis, multifetal gestation, thick meconium, and premature or postterm births (ACOG, 2006b; Blickstein & Green, 2007; Gibbs, Rosenberg, Warren, Galan, & Rumack, 2004; Nageotte & Gilstrap, 2009).

A suggested procedure for having cord blood available for determining gases and pH if needed is to place a double-clamped segment of the umbilical cord on the delivery table immediately after birth. If the newborn appears vigorous and the 5-minute Apgar score is satisfactory, the umbilical cord segment may be discarded. However, if problems with the neonate's condition persist, blood samples from the artery and vein of the umbilical cord segment are drawn separately and sent to the laboratory for blood gas analysis (ACOG, 2006b). Clamped segments of the umbilical cord and cord blood samples in heparinized syringes are both stable at room temperature for up to 60 minutes (ACOG, 2006b; Blickstein & Green, 2007; Gibbs et al., 2004).

The umbilical artery provides the most accurate information for determining neonatal acid–base status at birth. Drawing a separate sample from the umbilical vein will help verify that a true arterial specimen was obtained. While normal cord blood values are usually described in ranges, Table 15–8 provides single-digit values to serve as an initial reference of normal and abnormal umbilical artery cord blood acid–base values. Table 15–9 provides a quick reference for each type of acidemia (respiratory, metabolic, mixed) and corresponding increases or decreases in acid–base measurements (pH, PCO_2, bicarbonate [HCO_3], base deficit, base excess). Respiratory acidemia may occur when the flow of gases in the umbilical cord is interrupted, resulting in an elevated fetal PCO_2. Metabolic acidemia may occur with prolonged disruption of fetal oxygenation, resulting in anaerobic metabolism and the buildup of lactic acid in excess of fetal capacity to buffer acids. Decreased bicarbonate and increased base deficit or decreased base excess are reflective of this process. While metabolic acidemia is more serious than respiratory acidemia, most infants born with metabolic acidemia will develop normally (ACOG, 2006b).

Table 15–8. SINGLE-DIGIT VALUE GUIDELINE FOR INITIAL ASSESSMENT OF NORMAL AND ABNORMAL UMBILICAL ARTERY CORD BLOOD ACID–BASE VALUES

	Normal Values	Respiratory Acidemia	Metabolic Acidemia
pH	≥ 7.10	<7.10	<7.10
PO_2 (mm Hg)	>20	Variable	<20
PCO_2 (mm Hg)	<60	>60	<60
Bicarbonate (mEq/L)	>22	≥ 22	<22
Base deficit (mEq/L)	≤ 12	<12	>12
Base excess (mEq/L)	≥ -12	>-12	<-12

The values presented are suggested as a guide for evaluating acid–base status. All umbilical cord blood values should be evaluated in relation to the specific clinical findings and situation for a given patient. Note that greater absolute values of base deficit or excess are associated with acidemia.
Data from Andres, R. L., Saade, G., Gilstrap, L. C., Wilkins, I., Witlin, A., Zlatnik, F., & Hankins, G. V. (1999). Association between umbilical blood gas parameters and neonatal morbidity and death in neonates with pathologic fetal acidemia. *American Journal of Obstetrics and Gynecology, 181*(4), 867–871; Nageotte, M. P. & Gilstrap, L. C. (2009). Intrapartum fetal surveillance. In R. K. Creasy & R. Resnick (Eds.), *Maternal-Fetal Medicine* (6th ed., pp. 397–417). Philadelphia: Saunders; Low, J. A., Lindsay, B. G., & Derrick, E. J. (1997). Threshold of metabolic acidosis associated with newborn complications. *American Journal of Obstetrics and Gynecology, 177*(6), 1391–1394.

ST Segment Analysis

Ongoing efforts to improve the predictive value of FHR data for differentiating the compromised fetus from the uncompromised fetus when variant FHR patterns are present have included fetal pulse oximetry and ST segment analysis (STAN). While fetal pulse oximetry initially appeared promising, it did not gain widespread clinical use in the United States because it did not reduce the overall cesarean rate in a large multicenter trial (Garite et al., 2000), and it was eventually withdrawn from the market in the United States, although still is in use in Europe. STAN is still under active investigation in Europe and the United States. STAN uses select components of the fetal ECG signal to determine whether fetal myocardial ischemia is present. The system includes a fetal ECG electrode, a maternal skin reference electrode, and a microprocessor-based fetal monitor that continuously identifies the fetal ST segment and T-wave changes from the fetal cardiac cycle (Belfort & Saade, 2011b). When the STAN monitor detects significant changes in the ST interval compared to the baseline T/QRS ratio, it flags an ST event on the monitor and in the event log (Devoe, 2011b). The fetal STAN™ system is manufactured by Neoventa Medical in Mölndal, Sweden.

While fetal STAN has been used and studied in Europe, enthusiasm for this practice in the United States has been somewhat lacking. Study results in Europe are difficult to extrapolate to the U.S. population due to differences in obstetric practice and patient case mix as well as differences in definitions of key terms such as metabolic acidosis and neonatal encephalopathy (Belfort & Saade, 2011b). Additionally, as STAN is not a stand-alone component that can be used with current fetal monitors, the cost of replacing fetal monitors with those that can provide STAN data is a concern and a significant barrier to widespread adoption in the United States. A meta-analysis of five RCTs published between 1993 and 2010 that included 15,352 patients in which ST analysis was compared with conventional EFM found that the addition of ST analysis for intrapartum fetal monitoring resulted in reduction of fetal blood sampling and operative vaginal births. Although individual studies of ST analysis tended to show a decrease in metabolic acidosis at birth, there was no significant reduction in metabolic acidosis when these studies were pooled in the meta-analysis (Becker et al., 2012). More data are needed regarding this method of adjunct fetal assessment. The Maternal Fetal Medicine Units Networks of the NICHD has initiated an RCT of the STAN technology as an adjunct to EFM versus FHR monitoring alone. Approximately 11,000 women in labor with singleton cephalic pregnancy at ≥ 36 weeks' gestation are being enrolled at multiple sites in the United States. Primary outcome measures include intrapartum fetal death, neonatal death, Apgar score ≤ 3 at 5 minutes, neonatal seizure, cord artery pH ≤ 7.05 and base deficit ≥ 12 mmol/L, intubation for ventilation at delivery, or presence of neonatal encephalopathy. Results of this RCT are expected in 2013 (Belfort & Saade, 2011a).

Table 15–9. SIGNIFICANCE OF DEVIATION FROM NORMAL VALUES

Type of Acidemia	pH	PO_2	PCO_2	HCO_3	Base Deficit	Base Excess
Respiratory	Decreased	Variable	Increased	Normal	Normal	Normal
Metabolic	Decreased	Decreased	Normal	Decreased	Increased	Decreased
Mixed	Decreased	Decreased	Increased	Decreased	Increased	Decreased

NURSING ASSESSMENT AND MANAGEMENT STRATEGIES

PATIENT EDUCATION ABOUT FETAL HEART RATE MONITORING

Preparation for fetal monitoring includes a discussion of risks and benefits of methods of fetal assessment in the context of the woman's values, preferences, obstetric history, and treatment plan so that the woman may make an informed decision about monitoring (Carter et al., 2010). In a national survey about childbirth, 76% of women said they should make decisions for themselves about labor interventions after consulting with their care team, 23% thought decision making was best shared between mother and care team, and 3% wanted the team to make decisions after consulting with the mother. Respondents also wanted to know about most or all potential complications in order to inform their decision making (Declercq et al., 2006). While continuous EFM may be recommended for many women (e.g., those with obstetric risk factors and those receiving induction or augmentation of labor), EFM is not without risk and may often be used simply out of routine and convenience (Wood, 2003). Indeed, 96% of women surveyed reported receiving EFM all or most of the time during labor and only 3% of women receiving only IA during labor (Declercq et al., 2006), yet these numbers are out of proportion to induction rates and risk factor rates.

An assessment of the woman's preferences, knowledge, and prior discussions with providers regarding monitoring methods is a good starting point for discussion. Monitoring methods appropriate to the woman's individual situation should be described and offered, with adequate time provided for answering the woman's questions. Ideally, concerns regarding fetal assessment and monitoring during labor will have been discussed between the woman and her perinatal healthcare provider prior to admission. It is important to keep in mind that options for ongoing fetal assessment may include intermittent EFM and IA for many women in addition to continuous EFM (AAP & ACOG, 2012; ACOG, 2009a, 2010b; Feinstein et al., 2008).

NURSING ASSESSMENT OF THE FETAL HEART RATE

A systematic, organized approach to interpreting FHR patterns prevents misinterpretation and confusion. The deceleration in the middle of the tracing is eye catching and anxiety producing, but it may not be the most important aspect of the tracing. Assessment of the entire FHR tracing, including previous fetal status, uterine contractions, and all procedures that transpired prior to the deceleration, is required. Integration of maternal obstetric and medical history is of critical importance for appropriate interpretation of FHR findings. Assessments should include, but are not limited to, the following: (1) maternal–fetal risk for uteroplacental insufficiency, (2) administration of regional analgesia/anesthesia, (3) administration of medications or maternal substance use, (4) pharmacologic agents used for cervical ripening and labor induction/augmentation, and (5) trends or changes in FHR characteristics over time.

Physical assessment should include maternal vital signs, hydration status, and position, as these factors can have an influence on fetal status. For example, maternal fever can cause fetal tachycardia, whereas supine positioning or hypotension can cause fetal bradycardia.

Experienced perinatal nurses assess FHR patterns for evidence of fetal well-being very quickly. They use a mental checklist that includes the following questions (Lyndon et al., 2009; Simpson, 2009b):

- What is the baseline FHR?
- Is it within normal limits for this fetus?
- If not, what clinical factors could be contributing to this baseline rate?
- Is there evidence of moderate baseline variability?
- Are accelerations present?
- If accelerations are not present and variability is minimal or absent, does external or fetal scalp stimulation elicit an acceleration of the FHR appropriate for gestational age?
- What clinical factors could be contributing to this baseline variability?
- Are there periodic or episodic FHR patterns?
- If so, what are they and what are the appropriate interventions (if any)?
- Does the FHR pattern suggest a chronic or acute maternal–fetal condition?
- Is uterine activity normal in frequency, duration, intensity, and resting tone?
- What is the relationship between the FHR and uterine activity?
- How has the FHR changed over time?
- If the FHR pattern is indeterminate (category II) or abnormal (category III), do the appropriate interventions resolve the situation?
- If not, are further interventions needed based on the overall clinical picture?
- Is the FHR pattern such that notification of the physician or midwife is warranted?
- How close or how far is the woman from birth?
- What team members need to be aware of current maternal–fetal status?
- Are there complications team members should prepare for?

Nurses who are learning the principles of EFM may require more time to complete an assessment of fetal status; however, the essential components of a comprehensive assessment remain the same. It is helpful to devise a systematic method for FHR assessment and related appropriate interventions and consistently use that method in clinical practice to enhance optimal maternal–fetal outcomes.

After collecting all pertinent data, the following characteristics of the FHR tracing are interpreted and documented in the medical record: (1) uterine activity: frequency, duration, intensity, and resting tone; (2) baseline FHR and variability; (3) presence or absence of accelerations; and (4) presence or absence of decelerations (Display 15–3). There is no need to provide detailed descriptions of FHR decelerations in medical record documentation: Simply identify them by name. In the past, some clinicians were taught to descriptively document decelerations by depth, duration, and return to baseline rate (i.e., deceleration down to 60 bpm for 90 seconds with a slow return to baseline). However, this advice was based on concern for loss of the tracing in systems where paper tracings were microfilmed separately from the rest of the medical record. In the current environment, this type of description is time consuming and unnecessary when the electronic tracing is recorded and integrated in the labor record, as it is with most obstetric surveillance systems. Additional detailed descriptions of the tracing diminishes time available for nursing care and may increase professional liability if the case should be reviewed after an adverse outcome and the medical record documentation concerning the decelerations does not match exactly with the decelerations as noted on the FHR tracing. Identification of the deceleration as early, late, variable, or prolonged implies that the deceleration meets criteria for these types of decelerations as defined by NICHD (Macones et al., 2008), and

this is sufficient for the medical record. During interdisciplinary communication regarding FHR patterns, detailed descriptions may be necessary and appropriate for clarification and appreciation of the need for immediacy of intervention.

If the FHR pattern is indeterminate or abnormal, nursing intervention is based first on identification of the precipitating event, when possible, and then prioritized based on the level of concern. Eliminating the cause (e.g., uterine tachysystole or maternal hypotension) and/or instituting interventions that provide intrauterine resuscitation may be all that is necessary for the resumption of a normal FHR pattern (see Table 15–6). Conversely, the presence of any category III tracing and some category II tracings warrants immediate bedside evaluation by a physician who can initiate a cesarean birth. A decision tree for FHR management is presented in Figure 15–10. Depending on the clinical situation, there may be a decision for operative birth.

INTERDISCIPLINARY COMMUNICATION

It is not unusual for disagreements in the interpretation of FHR patterns to exist between different members of the perinatal healthcare team (ACOG, 2009a; Beckmann, Van Mullem, Beckmann, & Broekhuizen, 1997; Lyndon et al., 2011; Simpson, James, & Knox, 2006; Simpson & Lyndon, 2009). Intrapartum fetal assessment is one of the most important clinical situations in which nurses, physicians, and midwives need to work together and trust each other's judgment (Clark et al., 2009; Fox et al., 2000; Simpson et al., 2006; Simpson & Knox, 2009). Much of the communication about ongoing maternal–fetal status during labor occurs while the nurse is at the bedside and the provider is in the office or at home (Simpson, 2005a; Simpson et al., 2006). If the nurse determines that the FHR pattern is indeterminate or abnormal, the physician or midwife should be notified. Effective clinical communication is timely, direct, respectful, and explicitly identifies the level of concern and urgency (Lyndon et al., 2011). Nurses should describe their concerns and observations so that a clear plan of management can collaboratively be determined. Requests for orders for interventions and a bedside evaluation, if necessary, should be clearly stated. "Please come in to review the FHR pattern" is more effective in obtaining a bedside evaluation than "I'm worried about the fetus." If the situation is acute, "I need you to come now" is a clear, concise request for immediate action. Communication regarding indeterminate or abnormal FHR patterns should include characteristics of the pattern (baseline rate, variability, and presence or absence of accelerations and decelerations), pattern evolution (i.e., how long this FHR pattern has been developing and changing over time), the clinical context (e.g., bleeding, tachysystole, hypotension), intrauterine resuscitation

---

D I S P L A Y   1 5 - 3

Essential Components of Documentation of Fetal Heart Rate Patterns

1. Baseline rate
2. Baseline variability
3. Presence or absence of accelerations
4. Periodic or episodic decelerations
5. Changes of trends of FHR patterns over time

FHR, fetal heart rate.
Adapted from National Institute of Child Health and Human Development Research Planning Workshop. (1997). Electronic fetal heart rate monitoring: Research guidelines for interpretation. *American Journal of Obstetrics and Gynecology, 177*(6), 1385–1390, and *Journal of Obstetric Gynecology and Neonatal Nursing, 26*(6), 635–640.

techniques implemented and the fetal response, and request for further interventions and evaluation (e.g., amnioinfusion, ephedrine or phenylephrine, terbutaline, bedside evaluation as soon as possible, immediate bedside evaluation, preparations for emergent cesarean birth) (Fox et al., 2000; Simpson & Knox, 2009). The general content of this conversation, including the provider's response, should be documented in the medical record. If the discussion results in a clinical disagreement that cannot be resolved by the direct care providers, nurses should follow institutional policy about resolution of clinical disagreements. This type of policy is usually known as the chain of consultation or chain of authority. See Chapter 1 for a discussion of the chain of consultation.

Physicians, midwives, and nurses are responsible for maintaining competence in FHR pattern interpretation and appropriate use of interventions. One way to both maintain competence and promote interdisciplinary collaboration is participation in EFM education programs that include physicians, midwives, and nurses. A group process can be used to review EFM strips, expected responses, appropriate interpretations, and related interventions. Interdisciplinary team discussions can lead to an increased knowledge of EFM principles for everyone involved and can be a mechanism for decreasing hierarchy and improving interdisciplinary understanding and teamwork. Developing case studies containing clinical ambiguity is an ideal avenue for clarifying ongoing clinical issues where interpretation and expectations of all provider groups are not in sync (Miller, 2005). Educational collaboration between nurses, midwives, and physicians who are jointly responsible for FHR pattern interpretation and clinical interventions enhances collaboration in everyday clinical interactions and thus promotes maternal–fetal safety (JCAHO, 2004).

Certification in EFM is another option to promote interdisciplinary knowledge related to fetal assessment. When all members of the team hold certification in EFM, there is recognition that everyone has the same level of EFM knowledge and skill and that this knowledge and these skills are not discipline specific. Preparing for the certification exam as a group can enhance interdisciplinary team collegiality and effective communication when there is a question concerning fetal status based on the FHR pattern.

ISSUES IN THE USE OF FETAL HEART RATE MONITORING DURING LABOR

EFFICACY OF ELECTRONIC FETAL HEART RATE MONITORING

When EFM was developed and introduced into clinical practice, the hope was that this technique for fetal assessment would lead to a reduction in the overall incidence of cerebral palsy and intrapartum stillbirth (AAP & ACOG, 2012; ACOG, 2009a). This expectation was due in part to the opinion of experts in the 1960s and 1970s that most cases of cerebral palsy and other neurologic morbidity were the result of asphyxia during labor and birth. The randomized trials conducted during the 1980s failed to show a decrease in the incidence of cerebral palsy among infants who were monitored during labor (Shy et al., 1990). Yet the incidence of cesarean birth and assisted operative birth in the cohorts monitored increased fourfold (Thacker et al.,1995). These results have led many to the conclusion that EFM is not efficacious (Freeman, 1990). More recent reviews of the methodology used in the randomized trials in combination with newer information on the genesis of cerebral palsy have brought to light some of the reasons why FHR monitoring did poorly in the randomized trials that were conducted (ACOG, 2005c; Parer & King, 2000). Because this controversy remains unresolved, it is worth reviewing in the context of this text.

FETAL HEART RATE MONITORING AND CEREBRAL PALSY

EFM has been in wide use for more than 30 years with no change in the incidence of cerebral palsy (2 per 1,000 live births) (ACOG, 2009a; Penning & Garite, 1999). Thus, the original hope that EFM would predict and therefore prevent fetal asphyxia, which would in turn prevent cerebral palsy, has not come to pass. The majority of cases of infant and childhood cerebral palsy are related to prenatal events rather than the labor and birth process. Most cases of cerebral palsy are associated with prematurity, disorders of coagulation, and intrauterine exposure to maternal infections (Grether & Nelson, 1997). Interruption of the oxygen supply to the fetus contributes to approximately 6% of cases of cerebral palsy (Nelson & Grether, 1999), and most experts believe that no more than 2% to 20% of cases of cerebral palsy are due to intrapartum events of any cause (MacDonald, 1996; Nelson, 1988). These wide-ranging estimates are the result of imprecise interpretation of EFM data during labor as well as variations in diagnostic classification of the severity and type of cerebral palsy (Lent, 1999). ACOG estimates that no more than 4% of encephalopathy cases can be attributed to intrapartum events in isolation (ACOG, 2009a). In addition, the dramatically improved survival rates of extremely preterm infants have the potential to actually increase the incidence of cerebral palsy, and advances in neonatal care may also improve the survival rate of asphyxiated infants of any gestational age. These factors may obscure any effect that EFM has had on the incidence of cerebral palsy. In 1999, an international panel composed of specialists and researchers in perinatology, neonatology,

---

DISPLAY 15–4

Criteria to Define an Acute Intrapartum Hypoxic Event as Sufficient to Cause Cerebral Palsy

1.1: Essential criteria (must meet all four)

1. Evidence of a metabolic acidosis in fetal umbilical cord arterial blood obtained at birth (pH <7 and base deficit ≥12 mmol/L)
2. Early onset of severe or moderate neonatal encephalopathy in infants born at 34 or more weeks of gestation
3. Cerebral palsy of the spastic quadriplegic or dyskinetic type*
4. Exclusion of other identifiable etiologies such as trauma, coagulation disorders, infectious conditions, or genetic disorders

1.2: Criteria that collectively suggest an intrapartum timing (within close proximity to labor and birth [e.g., 0–48 hours]) but are nonspecific to asphyxial insults

1. A sentinel (signal) hypoxic event occurring immediately before or during labor
2. A sudden and sustained fetal bradycardia or the absence of fetal heart rate variability in the presence of recurrent, late, or variable decelerations, usually after a hypoxic sentinel event when the pattern was previously normal
3. Apgar scores of 0–3 beyond 5 minutes
4. Onset of multisystem involvement within 72 hours of birth
5. Early imaging study showing evidence of acute nonfocal cerebral abnormality

---

* Spastic quadriplegia and, less commonly, dyskinetic cerebral palsy are the only types of cerebral palsy associated with acute hypoxic intrapartum events. Spastic quadriplegia is not specific to intrapartum hypoxia. Hemiparetic cerebral palsy, hemiplegic cerebral palsy, spastic diplegia, and ataxia are unlikely to result from acute intrapartum hypoxia.
Data from American College of Obstetricians and Gynecologists & American Academy of Pediatrics. (2003). *Neonatal Encephalopathy and Cerebral Palsy: Defining the Pathogenesis and Pathophysiology.* Washington, DC: Author; MacLennan, A. (1999). A template for defining a causal relation between acute intrapartum events and cerebral palsy: International consensus statement. *British Medical Journal, 319*(7216), 1054–1059; Nelson, K. B., & Grether, J. K. (1998). Potentially asphyxiating conditions and spastic cerebral palsy in infants of normal birth weight. *American Journal of Obstetricians and Gynecologists, 179*(2), 507–513.

---

midwifery, science, and epidemiology reviewed the literature on the causation of cerebral palsy (MacLennan, 1999). The *International Consensus Statement* published by this group lists clinical and biochemical factors that define the criteria that would implicate an acute intrapartum event as the etiology of cerebral palsy (Display 15–4).

SENSITIVITY, SPECIFICITY, AND RELIABILITY OF ELECTRONIC FETAL MONITORING

EFM sensitivity (the ability to detect a healthy fetus when it is indeed healthy) is high, while specificity (the ability to detect a compromised fetus when it is compromised and not include healthy fetuses in the criteria) is low (Simpson & Knox, 2000). When the FHR is normal, there is a very high probability that the fetus is adequately oxygenated and not acidemic at the time of observation (Macones et al., 2008). Thus, EFM is a sensitive screening tool: It is very good at ruling out fetal compromise. Conversely, it is estimated that even the most ominous FHR patterns are associated with, at most, a 50% to 65% incidence of neonatal depression (Martin, 1998). Overall, EFM can have up to a 99.8% false-positive rate for term fetuses (Nelson, Dambrosia, Ting, & Grether, 1996). Therefore, EFM is not very specific: It is not highly accurate for definitively identifying fetal compromise. The sensitivity and specificity limitations of EFM are related to its inability to directly evaluate fetal oxygen status.

Further complicating the issue is the fact that both interobserver and intraobserver reliability in interpreting EFM data is inconsistent (Martin, 1998; Paneth, Bommarito, & Stricker, 1993). Not only do experienced clinicians continue to differ in interpretations when evaluating a specific FHR pattern (Wolfberg et al., 2008), they also disagree with their own interpretation when asked to review the same FHR tracing, and their interpretations of the tracing may be influenced by knowledge of the outcome (Di Lieto et al., 2003; Figueras et al., 2005). This phenomenon particularly affects interpretations suggesting fetal compromise (Simpson & Knox, 2000). By contrast, diagnosis of fetal well-being (adequate fetal oxygenation) has much higher interobserver and intraobserver reliability: Agreement is highest on identification of normal baseline, "normal" variability, and presence of accelerations (Di Lieto et al., 2003; Figueras et al., 2005; Wolfberg et al., 2008). Therefore, communication issues and professional disagreements regarding EFM interpretation are much more likely to occur when attempting to assign a diagnosis of fetal compromise than that of fetal well-being.

The differential predictability between sensitivity and specificity and the lack of reliability between different providers is the basis of the fundamental issue confounding the use of EFM (Simpson & Knox, 2000). The lack of common understanding by all involved professionals about how FHR monitoring can be relied upon when determining fetal status undermines the ability of this technique to guide clinical management (Fox et al., 2000). If the FHR pattern has a normal baseline rate, moderate variability, and no late, variable, or prolonged decelerations (i.e., is a category I tracing), there is little disagreement about the prediction of fetal well-being. Similarly, category III patterns, those with absent variability and either bradycardia, variable, or late decelerations, or a sinusoidal FHR, generate significant agreement. These patterns clearly suggest that the fetus is at risk for acidemia. However, many FHR patterns are between these two extremes, falling into category II. When different members of the care team simultaneously make different assumptions concerning EFM data, communication between the involved professionals is compromised (Fox et al., 2000). Therefore, interdisciplinary processes that promote common understanding of EFM principles are highly recommended to promote the safest care possible for the mother and fetus (JCAHO, 2004).

SUMMARY

Monitoring and interpreting the FHR are critical elements of intrapartum care (see Fig. 15–10). Standardized terms and definitions must be routinely used by all members of the perinatal healthcare team (ACNM, 2010b; ACOG, 2005c; AWHONN, 2005; JCAHO, 2004). Knowledge of the physiology underlying specific FHR patterns has increased over time. Nurses, midwives, and physicians must keep abreast of evolving knowledge in order to provide the best care for mothers and babies during labor. An appreciation of FHR pattern evolution and the use of variability in determining the risk for fetal acidemia is critical. Clinicians caring for women in labor should be able to rapidly identify FHR patterns that truly reflect the absence of fetal acidemia and those that consistently indicate a significant risk for fetal acidemia (Parer et al., 2006). Finally, an interdisciplinary team approach in which there exists mutual respect and true collaboration between nurses, midwives, and physicians will create a clinical environment that enhances safe and effective intrapartum care.

REFERENCES

Aldrich, C. J., D'Antona, D., Spencer, J. A., Wyatt, J. S., Peebles, D. M., Delpy, D. T., & Reynolds, E. O. (1995). The effect of maternal posture on fetal cerebral oxygenation during labour. *British Journal of Obstetrics and Gynaecology, 102*(1), 14–19.

Aldrich, C. J., Wyatt, J. S., Spencer, J. A., Reynolds, E. O., & Delpy, D. T. (1994). The effect of maternal oxygen administration on human fetal cerebral oxygenation measured during labour by near infrared spectroscopy. *British Journal of Obstetrics and Gynaecology, 101*(6), 509–513.

Althabe, O., Jr., Schwarcz, R. L., Pose, S. V., Escarcena, L., & Caldeyro-Barcia, R. (1967). Effects on fetal heart rate and fetal pO2 of oxygen administration to the mother. *American Journal of Obstetrics and Gynecology, 98*(6), 858–870.

Andres, R. L., Saade, G., Gilstrap, L. C., Wilkins, I., Witlin, A., Zlatnik, F., & Hankins, G. V. (1999). Association between umbilical blood gas parameters and neonatal morbidity and death in neonates with pathologic fetal acidemia. *American Journal of Obstetrics and Gynecology, 181*(4), 867–871.

American Academy of Pediatrics & American College of Obstetricians and Gynecologists. (2012). *Guidelines for Perinatal Care* (7th ed.). Elk Grove Village, IL: Author.

American College of Nurse-Midwives. (2010a). *Intermittent Auscultation for Intrapartum Fetal Heart Rate Surveillance.* Silver Spring, MD: Author. doi:10.1016/j.jmwh.2010.05.007

American College of Nurse-Midwives. (2010b). *Standardized Nomenclature for Electronic Fetal Monitoring* (Position Statement). Silver Spring, MD: Author. Retrieved from http://www.midwife.org/siteFiles/position/Standardized_Nomenclature_for_Electronic_Fetal_Monitoring_03_2010_001.pdf

American College of Obstetricians and Gynecologists. (1999). *Antepartum Fetal Surveillance* (Practice Bulletin No. 9). Washington, DC: Author.

American College of Obstetricians and Gynecologists. (2005a). *Intrapartum Fetal Heart Rate Monitoring* (Practice Bulletin No. 70). Washington, DC: Author.

American College of Obstetricians and Gynecologists. (2005b). *Inappropriate Use of the Terms Fetal Distress and Birth Asphyxia* (Committee Opinion No. 326). Washington, DC: Author.

American College of Obstetricians and Gynecologists. (2005c). *Intrapartum Fetal Heart Rate Monitoring* (Practice Bulletin No. 62). Washington, DC: Author.

American College of Obstetricians and Gynecologists. (2006a). *Amnioinfusion Does Not Prevent Meconium Aspiration Syndrome* (Committee Opinion No. 346). Washington, DC: Author.

American College of Obstetricians and Gynecologists. (2006b). *Umbilical Cord Blood Gas and Acid-Base Analysis* (Committee Opinion No. 348). Washington, DC: Author.

American College of Obstetricians and Gynecologists. (2009a). *Intrapartum Fetal Heart Rate Monitoring: Nomenclature, Interpretation, and General Management Principles* (Practice Bulletin No. 106). Washington, DC: Author. doi:10.1097/AOG.0b013e3181aef106

American College of Obstetricians and Gynecologists. (2009b). *Induction of Labor* (Practice Bulletin No. 107). Washington, DC: Author. doi:10.1097/AOG.0b013e3181b48ef5

American College of Obstetricians and Gynecologists. (2010a). *Vaginal Birth After Previous Cesarean Delivery* (Practice Bulletin No. 115). Washington, DC: Author. doi:10.1097/AOG.0b013e3181eeb251

American College of Obstetricians and Gynecologists. (2010b). *Management of Intrapartum Fetal Heart Rate Tracings* (Practice Bulletin No. 116). Washington, DC: Author. doi:10.1097/AOG.0b013e3182004fa9

American College of Obstetricians and Gynecologists & American Academy of Pediatrics. (2003). *Neonatal Encephalopathy and Cerebral Palsy: Defining the Pathogenesis and Pathophysiology.* Washington, DC: Author.

American Society of Anesthesiologists. (2007). Practice guidelines for obstetric anesthesia: An updated report by the American Society of Anesthesiologists Task Force on Obstetric Anesthesia. *Anesthesiology, 106,* 843–863.

Association of Women's Health, Obstetric and Neonatal Nurses. (2000). *Symposium Fetal Heart Rate Auscultation.* Washington, DC: Author.

Association of Women's Health, Obstetric and Neonatal Nurses. (2005). *NICHD Transitional Teaching Guide.* Washington, DC: Author.

Association of Women's Health, Obstetric and Neonatal Nurses. (2008). *Nursing Care and Management of the Second Stage of Labor: Evidence-Based Practice Guideline* (2nd ed.). Washington, DC: Author.

Association of Women's Health, Obstetric and Neonatal Nurses. (2009). *Position Statement: Fetal Heart Monitoring.* Washington, DC: Author.

Association of Women's Health, Obstetric and Neonatal Nurses. (2010a). *Advanced Fetal Monitoring Course.* Washington, DC: Author.

Association of Women's Health, Obstetric and Neonatal Nurses. (2010b). *AWHONN Intermediate Fetal Heart Monitoring Course Instructor Teaching Materials.* Washington, DC: Kendall Hunt.

Ayoubi, J. M., Audibert, F., Vial, M., Pons, J. C., Taylor, S., & Frydman, R. (2002). Fetal heart rate and survival of the very premature newborn. *American Journal of Obstetrics and Gynecology, 187*(4), 1026–1030.

Bakker, P. C., Kurver, P. H., Kuik, D. J., & Van Geijn, H. P. (2007). Elevated uterine activity increases the risk of fetal acidosis at birth. *American Journal of Obstetrics and Gynecology, 196*(4), 313.e1–313.e6. doi:10.1016/j.ajog.2006.11.035

Beard, R. W., Filshie, G. M., Knight, C. A., & Roberts, G. M. (1971). The significance of the changes in the continuous fetal heart rate in the first stage of labour. *Journal of Obstetrics and Gynaecology of the British Commonwealth, 78*(10), 865–881.

Becker, J. H., Bax, L., Amer-Wahlin, I., Ojala, K., Vayssiere, C., Westerhuis, M. E. M. H., . . . Moons, K. G. M. (2012). ST analysis of the fetal electrocardiogram in intrapartum fetal monitoring: A meta-analysis. *Obstetrics and Gynecology, 119*(1), 145–154. doi:10.1097/AOG.0b013e31823d8230

Beckmann, C. A., Van Mullem, C., Beckmann, C. R., & Broekhuizen, F. F. (1997). Interpreting fetal heart rate tracings. Is there a difference between labor and delivery nurses and obstetricians? *Journal of Reproductive Medicine, 42*(10), 647–650.

Belfort, M. A., & Saade, G. R. (2011a). ST segment analysis as an adjunct to electronic fetal monitoring, Part I: Background, physiology, and interpretation. *Clinics in Perinatology, 38*(1), 143–157, vii. doi:10.1016/j.clp.2010.12.009

Belfort, M. A., & Saade, G. R. (2011b). ST segment analysis (STAN) as an adjunct to electronic fetal monitoring, Part II: Clinical studies and future directions. *Clinics in Perinatology, 38*(1), 159–167, vii. doi:10.1016/j.clp.2010.12.010

Benson, R. C., Shubeck, F., Deutschberger, J., Weiss, W., & Berendes, H. (1968). Fetal heart rate as a predictor of fetal distress. A report from the collaborative project. *Obstetrics and Gynecology, 32*(2), 259–266.

Berkus, M. D., Langer, O., Samueloff, A., Xenakis, E. M., & Field, N. T. (1999). Electronic fetal monitoring: What's reassuring? *Acta Obstetricia et Gynecologica Scandinavica, 78*(1), 15–21.

Blackburn, S. T. (2007). *Maternal, Fetal, and Neonatal Physiology: A Clinical Perspective* (3rd ed.). St. Louis, MO: Saunders.

Blickstein, I., & Green, T. (2007). Umbilical cord blood gases. *Clinics in Perinatology, 34*(3), 451–459. doi:10.1016/j.clp.2007.05.001

Braithwaite, N. D., Milligan, J. E., & Shennan, A. T. (1986). Fetal heart rate monitoring and neonatal mortality in the very preterm infant. *American Journal of Obstetrics and Gynecology, 154*(2), 250–254.

Burrus, D. R., O'Shea, T. M., Jr., Veille, J. C., & Mueller-Heubach, E. (1994). The predictive value of intrapartum fetal heart rate abnormalities in the extremely premature infant. *American Journal of Obstetrics and Gynecology, 171*(4), 1128–1132.

Cahill, A. G., Parks, L., Harper, L., Heitmann, E., & O'Neill, K. (2009). Abnormal fetal heart rate tracings in patients with thick meconium staining of the amniotic fluid: Xu et al. *American Journal of Obstetrics and Gynecology, 200*(3), 342–343; discussion e341–344. doi:10.1016/j.ajog.2008.12.054

Caldeyro-Barcia, R., Mendez-Bauer, C., Poseiro, J. J., Escarcena, B. S., Pose, S. V., Bieniarz, J., . . . Althabe, O. (1966). Control of human fetal heart rate during labor. In D. E. Cassels (Ed.), *The Heart and Circulation in the Newborn and Infant* (pp. 7–36). New York: The Chicago Heart Association/Grune & Stratton.

Carbonne, B., Benachi, A., Leveque, M. L., Cabrol, D., & Papiernik, E. (1996). Maternal position during labor: Effects on fetal oxygen saturation measured by pulse oximetry. *Obstetrics & Gynecology, 88*(5), 797–800. doi:10.1016/0029-7844(96)00298-0

Carter, M. C., Corry, M., Delbanco, S., Foster, T. C., Friedland, R., Gabel, R., . . . Simpson, K. R. (2010). 2020 Vision for a high-quality, high-value maternity care system. *Women's Health Issues, 20*(1, Suppl.), S7–S17. doi:10.1016/j.whi.2009.11.006

Chen, H. Y., Chauhan, S. P., Ananth, C. V., Vintzileos, A. M., & Abuhamad, A. Z. (2011). Electronic fetal heart rate monitoring and its relationship to neonatal and infant mortality in the United States. *American Journal of Obstetrics and Gynecology, 204*(6), 491.e1–491.e10. doi:10.1016/j.ajog.2011.04.024

Cibils, L. A. (1976). Clinical significance of fetal heart rate patterns during labor. I. Baseline patterns. *American Journal of Obstetrics and Gynecology, 125*(3), 290–305.

Cibils, L. A. (1996). On intrapartum fetal monitoring. *American Journal of Obstetrics and Gynecology, 174*(4), 1382–1389.

Clark, S. L., Cotton, D. B., Pivarnik, J. M., Lee, W., Hankins, G. D., Benedetti, T. J., & Phelan, J. P. (1991). Position change and central hemodynamic profile during normal third-trimester pregnancy and post partum. *American Journal of Obstetrics and Gynecology, 164*(3), 883–887.

Clark, S. L., Gimovsky, M. L., & Miller, F. C. (1984). The scalp stimulation test: A clinical alternative to fetal scalp blood sampling. *American Journal of Obstetrics and Gynecology, 148*(3), 274–277.

Clark, S. L., Simpson, K. R., Knox, G. E., & Garite, T. J. (2009). Oxytocin: New perspectives on an old drug. *American Journal of Obstetrics and Gynecology, 200*(1), 35.e1–35.e6. doi:10.1016/j.ajog.2008.06.010

Copel, J. A., Friedman, A. H., & Kleinman, C. S. (1997). Management of fetal cardiac arrhythmias. *Fetal Diagnosis and Therapy, 24*(1), 201–221.

Cramer, M. V. (1906). Ueber die dierkte ableitung der akionsstrome des menschlchen hersens vom oesophagus und uber das elektrokardiogramm des fotus. *Muenchener Medizinische Wochenschrift, 53*, 811–813.

Dado, L. A. (2011). Anesthesia for the complicated obstetric patient. In M. L. Foley, T. H. Strong, Jr., & T. J. Garite (Eds.), *Obstetric Intensive Care Manual* (3rd ed., pp. 231–246). New York: McGraw-Hill.

Dalton, K. J., Dawes, G. S., & Patrick, J. E. (1977). Diurnal, respiratory, and other rhythms of fetal heart rate in lambs. *American Journal of Obstetrics and Gynecology, 127*(4), 414–424.

Dalton, K. J., Phill, D., Dawes, G. S., & Patrick, J. E. (1983). The autonomic nervous system and fetal heart rate variability. *American Journal of Obstetrics and Gynecology, 146*(4), 456–462.

Dawes, G. S., Visser, G. H., Goodman, J. D., & Levine, D. H. (1981). Numerical analysis of the human fetal heart rate: Modulation by breathing and movement. *American Journal of Obstetrics and Gynecology, 140*(5), 535–544.

Dawood, M. Y. (1995). Pharmacologic stimulation of uterine contraction. *Seminars in Perinatology, 19*(1), 73–83.

Declercq, E. R., Sakala, C., Corry, M., & Applebaum, S. (2006). *Listening to Mothers II: Report of the Second National U.S. Survey of Women's Childbearing Experiences.* New York: Childbirth Connection.

Dellinger, E. H., Boehm, F. H., & Crane, M. M. (2000). Electronic fetal heart rate monitoring: Early neonatal outcomes associated with normal rate, fetal stress, and fetal distress. *American Journal of Obstetrics and Gynecology, 182*(1, Pt. 1), 214–220.

Devoe, L. D. (2011a). Electronic fetal monitoring: Does it really lead to better outcomes? *American Journal of Obstetrics and Gynecology, 204*(6), 455–456. doi:10.1016/j.ajog.2011.04.023

Devoe, L. D. (2011b). Fetal ECG analysis for intrapartum electronic fetal monitoring: A review. *Clinical Obstetrics and Gynecology, 54*(1), 56–65. doi:10.1097/GRF.0b013e31820a0ee7

Di Lieto, A., Giani, U., Campanile, M., De Falco, M., Scaramellino, M., & Papa, R. (2003). Conventional and computerized antepartum telecardiotocography. Experienced and inexperienced observers versus computerized analysis. *Gynecologic and Obstetric Investigation, 55*(1), 37–40. doi:10.1159/000068955

Douvas, S. G., Meeks, G. R., Graves, G., Walsh, D. A., & Morrison, J. C. (1984). Intrapartum fetal heart rate monitoring as a predictor of fetal distress and immediate neonatal condition in low-birth weight (less than or equal to 1,800 grams) infants. *American Journal of Obstetrics and Gynecology, 148*(3), 300–302.

Druzin, M. L., Smith, J. F., Gabbe, S. G., & Reed, K. L. (2007). Antepartum fetal evaluation. In S. G. Gabbe, J. R. Niebyl, & J. L. Simpson (Eds.), *Obstetrics: Normal and Problem Pregnancies* (5th ed., pp. 267–300). Philadelphia: Churchill Livingstone.

East, C. E., Smyth, R., Leader, L. R., Henshall, N. E., Colditz, P. B., & Tan, K. H. (2005). Vibroacoustic stimulation for fetal assessment in labour in the presence of a nonreassuring fetal heart rate trace. *Cochrane Database of Systematic Reviews*, (2), CD004664. doi:10.1002/14651858.CD004664.pub2

Fahey, J., & King, T. L. (2005). Intrauterine asphyxia: Clinical implications for providers of intrapartum care. *Journal of Midwifery & Womens Health, 50*(6), 498–506. doi:10.1016/j.jmwh.2005.08.007

Fawole, B., & Hofmeyr, G. J. (2003/2008). Maternal oxygen administration for fetal distress. *Cochrane Database of Systematic Reviews, 4.* doi:10.1002/14651858.CD000136

Feinstein, N. F., Sprague, A., & Trepanier, M. J. (2008). *Fetal Heart Rate Auscultation* (2nd ed.). Washington, DC: Association of Women's Health, Obstetric and Neonatal Nurses.

Figueras, F., Albela, S., Bonino, S., Palacio, M., Barrau, E., Hernandez, S., . . . Cararach, V. (2005). Visual analysis of antepartum fetal heart rate tracings: Inter- and intra-observer agreement and impact of knowledge of neonatal outcome. *Journal of Perinatal Medicine, 33*(3), 241–245. doi:10.1515/JPM.2005.044

Fox, M., Kilpatrick, S., King, T., & Parer, J. T. (2000). Fetal heart rate monitoring: Interpretation and collaborative management. *Journal of Midwifery & Womens Health, 45*(6), 498–507.

Fraser, W. D., Hofmeyr, J., Lede, R., Faron, G., Alexander, S., Goffinet, F., . . . Wei, B. (2005). Amnioinfusion for the prevention of the meconium aspiration syndrome. *New England Journal of Medicine, 353*(9), 909–917. doi:10.1056/NEJMoa050223

Freeman, R. (1990). Intrapartum fetal monitoring: A disappointing story. *New England Journal of Medicine, 322*(9), 624–626.

Freeman, R. K., Garite, T. J., & Nageotte, M. P. (2003). *Fetal Heart Monitoring* (3rd ed.). Philadelphia: Lippincott.

Gallagher, M. W., Costigan, K., & Johnson, T. R. (1992). Fetal heart rate accelerations, fetal movement, and fetal behavior patterns in twin gestations. *American Journal of Obstetrics and Gynecology, 167*(4, Pt. 1), 1140–1144.

Galvan, B. J., Van Mullem, C., & Broekhuizen, F. F. (1989). Using amnioinfusion for the relief of repetitive variable decelerations during labor. *Journal of Obstetric, Gynecologic and Neonatal Nursing, 18*(3), 222–229.

Garite, T. J. (2007). Intrapartum fetal evaluation. In S. G. Gabbe, J. R. Niebyl, & J. L. Simpson (Eds.), *Obstetrics: Normal and Problem Pregnancies* (5th ed., pp. 364–395). Philadelphia: Churchill Livingstone Elsevier.

Garite, T. J., Dildy, G. A., McNamara, H., Nageotte, M. P., Boehm, F. H., Dellinger, E. H., . . . Swedlow, D. B. (2000). A multicenter controlled trial of fetal pulse oximetry in the intrapartum management of nonreassuring fetal heart rate patterns. *American Journal of Obstetrics and Gynecology, 183*(5), 1049–1058. doi:10.1067/mob.2000.110632

Garite, T. J., & Simpson, K. R. (2011). Intrauterine resuscitation during labor. *Clinical Obstetrics and Gynecology, 54*(1), 28–39. doi:10.1097/GRF.0b013e31820a062b

Gibbs, R. S., Rosenberg, A. R., Warren, C. J., Galan, H. L., & Rumack, C. M. (2004). Suggestions for practice to accompany neonatal encephalopathy and cerebral palsy. *Obstetrics and Gynecology, 103*(4), 778–779. doi:10.1097/01.AOG.0000119227.67228.34

Goodlin, R. C. (1979). History of fetal monitoring. *American Journal of Obstetrics and Gynecology, 133*(3), 323–352.

Grether, J. K., & Nelson, K. B. (1997). Maternal infection and cerebral palsy in infants of normal birth weight. *Journal of the American Medical Association, 278*(3), 207–211.

Gull, I., Jaffa, A. J., Oren, M., Grisaru, D., Peyser, M. R., & Lessing, J. B. (1996). Acid accumulation during end-stage bradycardia in term fetuses: How long is too long? *British Journal of Obstetrics and Gynaecology, 103*(11), 1096–1101.

Hammacher, K. (1969). The clinical significance of cardiotocography. In P. Huntingford, K. Huter, & E. Salez (Eds.), *Perinatal Medicine,* 1st European Congress, Berlin (p. 81). New York: Academic Press.

Harmon, K. M. (2009). Techniques for fetal heart assessment. In A. Lyndon & L. U. Ali (Eds.), *Fetal Heart Monitoring Principles and Practices* (4th ed.). Washington, DC: Association of Womens Health, Obstetric and Neonatal Nurses/Kendall Hunt.

Haruta, M., Funato, T., Sumida, T., & Shinkai, T. (1984). [The influence of maternal oxygen inhalation for 30 to 60 minutes on fetal oxygenation]. *Nippon Sanka Fujinka Gakkai Zasshi. Acta Obstetrica et Gynaecologica Japonica, 36*(10), 1921–1929.

Haydon, M. L., Gorenberg, D. M., Nageotte, M. P., Ghamsary, M., Rumney, P. J., Patillo, C., & Garite, T. J. (2006). The effect of maternal oxygen administration on fetal pulse oximetry during labor in fetuses with nonreassuring fetal heart rate patterns. *American Journal of Obstetrics and Gynecology, 195*(3), 735–738. doi:10.1016/j.ajog.2006.06.084

Holmes, P., Oppenheimer, L. W., Gravelle, A., Walker, M., & Blayney, M. (2001). The effect of variable heart rate decelerations on intraventricular hemorrhage and other perinatal outcomes in preterm infants. *Journal of Maternal-Fetal Medicine, 10*(4), 264–268.

Hon, E. H. (1958). The electronic evaluation of the fetal heart rate: Preliminary report. *American Journal of Obstetrics and Gynecology, 75*(6), 1215–1230.

Hon, E. (1963). The classification of fetal heart rate I: A revised working classification. *Obstetrics and Gynecology, 22*(2), 137–146.

Jackson, M., Holmgren, C. M., Esplin, M. S., Henry, E., & Varner, M. W. (2011). Frequency of fetal heart rate categories and short-term neonatal outcome. *Obstetrics and Gynecology, 118*(4), 803–808. doi:10.1097/AOG.0b013e31822f1b50

Joint Commission on Accreditation of Healthcare Organizations. (2004). *Preventing Infant Death and Injury During Delivery* (Sentinel Event Alert No. 30). Oakbrook Terrace, IL: Author.

Jozwik, M., Sledziewski, A., Klubowicz, Z., Zak, J., Sajewska, G., & Pietrzycki, B. (2000). [Use of oxygen therapy during labour and acid-base status in the newborn]. *Medycyna Wieku Rozwojowego (Developmental Period Medicine), 4*(4), 403–411.

Kamoshita, E., Amano, K., Kanai, Y., Mochizuki, J., Ikeda, Y., Kikuchi, S., . . . Unno, N. (2010). Effect of the interval between onset of sustained fetal bradycardia and cesarean delivery on long-term neonatal neurologic prognosis. *International Journal of Gynecology & Obstetrics, 111*(1), 23–27. doi:10.1016/j.ijgo.2010.05.022

Kennedy, E. (1843). Audible evidences of pregnancy. In *Observations on Obstetric Auscultation: With an Analysis of the Evidences of Pregnancy; and an Inquiry Into the Proofs of the Life and Death of the Foetus in Utero* (pp. 71–146). New York: J. & H. G. Langley. (Original work published 1833)

King, T., & Parer, J. (2000). The physiology of fetal heart rate patterns and perinatal asphyxia. *Journal of Perinatal & Neonatal Nursing, 14*(3), 19–39.

Kisilevsky, B. S., Hains, S. M., & Low, J. A. (2001). Maturation of fetal heart rate and body movement in 24-33-week-old fetuses threatening to deliver prematurely. *Developmental Psychobiology, 38*(1), 78–86. doi:10.1002/1098-2302(2001)38:1<78::AID-DEV7>3.0.CO

Kleinman, C. S., & Nehgme, R. A. (2004). Cardiac arrhythmias in the human fetus. *Pediatric Cardiology, 25*(3), 234–251. doi:10.1007/s00246-003-0589-x

Kleinman, C. S., Nehgme, R., & Copel, J. A. (2004). Fetal cardiac arrhythmias. In R. K. Creasy & R. Resnick (Eds.), *Maternal-Fetal Medicine* (5th ed., pp. 465–482). Philadelphia: W. B. Saunders.

Knox, G. E., & Simpson, K. R. (2011). Perinatal high reliability. *American Journal of Obstetrics and Gynecology, 204*(5), 373–377. doi: 10.1016/j.ajog.2010.10.900

Korhonen, J., & Kariniemi, V. (1994). Emergency cesarean section: The effect of delay on umbilical arterial gas balance and Apgar scores. *Acta Obstetricia et Gynecologica Scandinavica, 73*(10), 782–786.

Krebs, H. B., Petres, R. E., Dunn, L. J., Jordaan, H. V., & Segreti, A. (1979). Intrapartum fetal heart rate monitoring. I. Classification and prognosis of fetal heart rate patterns. *American Journal of Obstetrics and Gynecology, 133*(7), 762–772.

Lee, C. Y., Di Loreto, P. C., & O'Lane, J. M. (1975). A study of fetal heart rate acceleration patterns. *Obstetrics & Gynecology, 45*(2), 142–146.

Lent, M. (1999). The medical and legal risks of the electronic fetal monitor. *Stanford Law Review, 51*(4), 807–837.

Leung, A. S., Leung, E. K., & Paul, R. H. (1993). Uterine rupture after previous cesarean delivery: Maternal and fetal consequences. *American Journal of Obstetrics and Gynecology, 169*(4), 945–950.

Leveno, K. J., Quirk, J. G., Jr., Cunningham, F. G., Nelson, S. D., Santos-Ramos, R., Toofanian, A., & DePalma, R. T. (1984). Prolonged pregnancy. I. Observations concerning the causes of fetal distress. *American Journal of Obstetrics and Gynecology, 150*(5), 465–473.

Lin, C. C., Vassallo, B., & Mittendorf, R. (2001). Is intrapartum vibroacoustic stimulation an effective predictor of fetal acidosis? *Journal of Perinatal Medicine, 29*(6), 506–512. doi:10.1515/JPM.2001.070

Low, J. A., Galbraith, R. S., Muir, D. W., Killen, H. L., Pater, E. A., & Karchmar, E. J. (1992). Mortality and morbidity after intrapartum asphyxia in the preterm fetus. *Obstetrics and Gynecology, 80*(1), 57–61.

Low, J. A., Lindsay, B. G., & Derrick, E. J. (1997). Threshold of metabolic acidosis associated with newborn complications. *American Journal of Obstetrics and Gynecology, 177*(6), 1391–1394.

Low, J. A., Victory, R., & Derrick, E. J. (1999). Predictive value of electronic fetal monitoring for intrapartum fetal asphyxia with metabolic acidosis. *Obstetrics and Gynecology, 93*(2), 285–291.

Lunshof, M. S., Boer, K., Wolf, H., Koppen, S., Velderman, J. K., & Mulder, E. J. (2005). Short-term (0–48 h) effects of maternal betamethasone administration on fetal heart rate and its variability. *Pediatric Research, 57*(4), 545–549. doi:10.1203/01.PDR.0000155948.83570.EB

Lyndon, A., & Ali, L. U. (Eds.). (2009). *Fetal Heart Monitoring Principles and Practices* (4th ed.). Washington, DC: Association of Women's Health, Obstetric and Neonatal Nursing/Kendall Hunt.

Lyndon, A., O'Brien-Abel, N., & Simpson, K. R. (2009). Fetal heart rate interpretation. In A. Lyndon & L. U. Ali (Eds.), *Fetal Heart Monitoring Principles and Practices* (4th ed., pp. 101–133). Washington, DC: Association of Women's Health, Obstetric and Neonatal Nurses/Kendall Hunt.

Lyndon, A., Zlatnik, M. G., & Wachter, R. M. (2011). Effective physician-nurse communication: A patient safety essential for labor and delivery. *American Journal of Obstetrics and Gynecology, 205*(2), 91–96. doi:10.1016/j.ajog.2011.04.021

MacDonald, D. (1996). Cerebral palsy and intrapartum fetal monitoring. *New England Journal of Medicine, 334*(10), 659–660. doi:10.1056/NEJM199603073341011

MacDonald, D., Grant, A., Sheridan-Pereira, M., Boylan, P., & Chalmers, I. (1985). The Dublin randomized controlled trial of intrapartum fetal heart rate monitoring. *American Journal of Obstetrics and Gynecology, 152*(5), 524–539.

MacLennan, A. (1999). A template for defining a causal relation between acute intrapartum events and cerebral palsy: International consensus statement. *BMJ (Clinical Research Ed.), 319*(7216), 1054–1059.

Macones, G. A., Hankins, G. D., Spong, C. Y., Hauth, J., & Moore, T. (2008). The 2008 National Institute of Child Health and Human Development workshop report on electronic fetal monitoring: Update on definitions, interpretation, and research guidelines. *Journal of Obstetric, Gynecologic, and Neonatal Nursing, 37*(5), 510–515. doi:10.1111/j.1552-6909.2008.00284.x

Maiques, V., Garcia-Tejedor, A., Perales, A., & Navarro, C. (1999). Intrapartum fetal invasive procedures and perinatal transmission of HIV. *European Journal of Obstetrics, Gynecology, and Reproductive Biology, 87*(1), 63–67.

Manseau, P., Vaquier, J., Chavinie, J., & Sureau, C. (1972). [Sinusoidal fetal cardiac rhythm. An aspect evocative of fetal distress during pregnancy]. *Journal de Gynecologie, Obstetrique et Biologie de la Reproduction, 1*(4), 343–352.

Martin, C. B., Jr. (1978). Regulation of the fetal heart rate and genesis of FHR patterns. *Seminars in Perinatology, 2*(2), 131–146.

Martin, C. B., Jr. (1998). Electronic fetal monitoring: A brief summary of its development, problems and prospects. *European Journal of Obstetrics, Gynecology, and Reproductive Biology, 78*(2), 133–140.

Matsuda, Y., Maeda, T., & Kouno, S. (2003). The critical period of non-reassuring fetal heart rate patterns in preterm gestation. *European Journal of Obstetrics, Gynecology, and Reproductive Biology, 106*(1), 36–39.

McNamara, H., Johnson, N., & Lilford, R. (1993). The effect on fetal arteriolar oxygen saturation resulting from giving oxygen to the mother measured by pulse oximetry. *British Journal of Obstetrics and Gynaecology, 100*(5), 446–449.

Menihan, C. A. (1998). Uterine rupture in women attempting a vaginal birth following prior cesarean birth. *Journal of Perinatology, 18*(6, Pt. 1), 440–443.

Miller, L. A. (2005). System errors in intrapartum electronic fetal monitoring: A case review. *Journal of Midwifery & Womens Health, 50*(6), 507–516. doi:10.1016/j.jmwh.2004.09.012

Mino, M., Puertas, A., Miranda, J. A., & Herruzo, A. J. (1999). Amnioinfusion in term labor with low amniotic fluid due to rupture of membranes: A new indication. *European Journal of Obstetrics, Gynecology, and Reproductive Biology, 82*(1), 29–34.

Miyazaki, F. S., & Nevarez, F. (1985). Saline amnioinfusion for relief of repetitive variable decelerations: A prospective randomized study. *American Journal of Obstetrics and Gynecology, 153*(3), 301–306.

Modanlou, H. D., & Murata, Y. (2004). Sinusoidal heart rate pattern: Reappraisal of its definition and clinical significance. *Journal of Obstetrics and Gynaecology Research, 30*(3), 169–180. doi:10.1111/j.1447-0756.2004.00186.x

Moore, K. L., & Persaud, T. V. N. (2003). *The Developing Human: Clinically Oriented Embryology*, 7th ed. Philadelphia: Saunders.

Nageotte, M. P., & Gilstrap, L. C. (2009). Intrapartum fetal surveillance. In R. K. Creasy & R. Resnick (Eds.), *Maternal-Fetal Medicine* (6th ed., pp. 397–417). Philadelphia: Saunders.

National Institute of Child Health and Human Development Research Planning Workshop. (1997). Electronic fetal heart rate monitoring: Research guidelines for interpretation. *American Journal of Obstetrics and Gynecology, 177*(6), 1385–1390.

Neilson, D. R., Jr., Freeman, R. K., & Mangan, S. (2008). Signal ambiguity resulting in unexpected outcome with external fetal heart rate monitoring. *American Journal of Obstetrics and Gynecology, 198*(6), 717–724. doi:10.1016/j.ajog.2008.02.030

Nelson, K. B. (1988). What proportion of cerebral palsy is related to birth asphyxia? *Journal of Pediatrics, 112*(4), 572–574.

Nelson, K. B., Dambrosia, J. M., Ting, T. Y., & Grether, J. K. (1996). Uncertain value of electronic fetal monitoring in predicting cerebral palsy. *New England Journal of Medicine, 334*(10), 613–618. doi:10.1056/NEJM199603073341001

Nelson, K. B., & Grether, J. K. (1998). Potentially asphyxiating conditions and spastic cerebral palsy in infants of normal birth weight. *American Journal of Obstetrics and Gynecology, 179*(2), 507–513.

Nelson, K. B., & Grether, J. K. (1999). Causes of cerebral palsy. *Current Opinion in Pediatrics, 11*(6), 487–491.

O'Brien-Abel, N. (2009). Physiologic basis for fetal monitoring. In A. Lyndon & L. U. Ali (Eds.), *Fetal Heart Monitoring: Principles and Practice* (4th ed., pp. 21–42). Washington, DC: Association of Women's Health, Obstetric and Neonatal Nurses/Kendall Hunt.

O'Brien-Abel, N. E., & Benedetti, T. J. (1992). Saltatory fetal heart rate pattern. *Journal of Perinatology, 12*(1), 13–17.

Ouzounian, J. G., Miller, D. A., & Paul, R. H. (1996). Amnioinfusion in women with previous cesarean births: A preliminary report. *American Journal of Obstetrics and Gynecology, 174*(2), 783–786.

Paneth, N., Bommarito, M., & Stricker, J. (1993). Electronic fetal monitoring and later outcome. *Clinical and Investigative Medicine. Medecine Clinique et Experimentale, 16*(2), 159–165.

Parer, J. T. (1997). *Handbook of Fetal Heart Rate Monitoring* (2nd ed.). Philadelphia: W. B. Saunders.

Parer, J. T., Dijkstra, H. R., Vredebregt, P. P., Harris, J. L., Krueger, T. R., & Reuss, M. L. (1980). Increased fetal heart rate variability with acute hypoxia in chronically instrumented sheep. *European Journal of Obstetrics, Gynecology, and Reproductive Biology, 10*(6), 393–399.

Parer, J. T., & Ikeda, T. (2007). A framework for standardized management of intrapartum fetal heart rate patterns. *American Journal of Obstetrics and Gynecology, 197*(1), 26.e1–26.e6. doi:10.1016/j.ajog.2007.03.037

Parer, J. T., & King, T. (2000). Fetal heart rate monitoring: Is it salvageable? *American Journal of Obstetrics and Gynecology, 182*(4), 982–987.

Parer, J. T., King, T., Flanders, S., Fox, M., & Kilpatrick, S. J. (2006). Fetal acidemia and electronic fetal heart rate patterns: Is there evidence of an association? *Journal of Maternal Fetal and Neonatal Medicine, 19*(5), 289–294. doi:10.1080/14767050500526172

Parer, J. T., & Livingston, E. G. (1990). What is fetal distress? *American Journal of Obstetrics and Gynecology, 162*(6), 1421–1425; discussion 1425–1427.

Parer, J. T., & Nageotte, M. P. (2004). Intrapartum fetal surveillance. In R. K. Creasy & R. Resnick (Eds.), *Maternal-Fetal Medicine* (5th ed., pp. 403–427). Philadelphia: W. B. Saunders.

Penning, S., & Garite, T. J. (1999). Management of fetal distress. *Obstetrics and Gynecology Clinics of North America, 26*(2), 259–274.

Phaneuf, S., Rodriguez Linares, B., TambyRaja, R. L., MacKenzie, I. Z., & Lopez Bernal, A. (2000). Loss of myometrial oxytocin receptors during oxytocin-induced and oxytocin-augmented labour. *Journal of Reproduction and Fertility, 120*(1), 91–97.

Phillips. (n.d.). *Fetal spiral electrode package insert*. In P. M. Systems (Ed.), (Vol. 9898 031 37631, pp. A-989803137631 Rev B;989803137054–989803130040 Rev B).

Porter, T. F., & Clark, S. L. (1999). Vibroacoustic and scalp stimulation. *Obstetrics and Gynecology Clinics of North America, 26*(4), 657–669.

Quinn, K. H., Cao, C. T., Lacoursiere, D. Y., & Schrimmer, D. (2011). Monoamniotic twin pregnancy: Continuous inpatient electronic fetal monitoring—an impossible goal? *American Journal of Obstetrics and Gynecology, 204*(2), 161.e1–161.e6. doi:10.1016/j.ajog.2010.08.044

Ridgeway, J. J., Weyrich, D. L., & Benedetti, T. J. (2004). Fetal heart rate changes associated with uterine rupture. *Obstetrics and Gynecology, 103*(3), 506–512. doi:10.1097/01.AOG.0000113619.67704.99

Roberts, J. E. (2002). The "push" for evidence: Management of the second stage. *Journal of Midwifery and Women's Health, 47*(1), 2–15.

Senat, M. V., Minoui, S., Multon, O., Fernandez, H., Frydman, R., & Ville, Y. (1998). Effect of dexamethasone and betamethasone on fetal heart rate variability in preterm labour: A randomised study. *British Journal of Obstetrics and Gynaecology, 105*(7), 749–755.

Sherer, D. M., D'Amico, M. L., Cox, C., Metlay, L. A., & Woods, J. R., Jr. (1994). Association of in utero behavioral patterns of twins with each other as indicated by fetal heart rate reactivity and nonreactivity. *American Journal of Perinatology, 11*(3), 208–212. doi:10.1055/s-2008-1040747

Sherer, D. M., Nawrocki, M. N., Peco, N. E., Metlay, L. A., & Woods, J. R., Jr. (1990). The occurrence of simultaneous fetal heart rate accelerations in twins during nonstress testing. *Obstetrics and Gynecology, 76*(5, Pt. 1), 817–821.

Shy, K. K., Luthy, D. A., Bennett, F. C., Whitfield, M., Larson, E. B., van Belle, G., . . . Stenchever, M. A. (1990). Effects of electronic fetal-heart-rate monitoring, as compared with periodic auscultation, on the neurologic development of premature infants. *New England Journal of Medicine, 322*(9), 588–593. doi:10.1056/NEJM199003013220904

Simpson, K. R. (2005a). The context and clinical evidence for common nursing practices during labor. *MCN: American Journal of Maternal Child Nursing, 30*(6), 356–363.

Simpson, K. R. (2005b). Failure to rescue: Implications for evaluating quality of care during labor and birth. *Journal of Perinatal and Neonatal Nursing, 19*(1), 24–34.

Simpson, K. R. (2007). Intrauterine resuscitation during labor: Review of current methods and supportive evidence. *Journal of Midwifery & Women's Health, 52*(3), 229–237. doi:10.1016/j.jmwh.2006.12.010

Simpson, K. R. (2008). Intrauterine resuscitation during labor: Should maternal oxygen administration be a first-line measure? *Seminars in Fetal and Neonatal Medicine, 13*(6), 362–367. doi:10.1016/j.siny.2008.04.016

Simpson, K. R. (2009a). *Cervical Ripening and Induction and Augmentation of Labor* (3rd ed.). Washington, DC: Association of Women's Health, Obstetric and Neonatal Nurses.

Simpson, K. R. (2009b). Physiologic interventions for fetal heart rate patterns. In A. Lyndon & L. U. Ali (Eds.), *Fetal Heart Monitoring Principles and Oractices* (pp. 135–155). Washington, DC: Association of Women's Health, Obstetric and Neonatal Nurses/Kendall Hunt.

Simpson, K. R. (2011). Avoiding confusion of maternal heart rate with fetal heart rate during labor. *MCN: The American Journal of Maternal Child Nursing, 36*(4), 272. doi:10.1097/NMC.0b013e318217a61a

Simpson, K. R., & James, D. C. (2005a). Effects of immediate versus delayed pushing during second-stage labor on fetal well-being: A randomized clinical trial. *Nursing Research, 54*(3), 149–157.

Simpson, K. R., & James, D. C. (2005b). Efficacy of intrauterine resuscitation techniques in improving fetal oxygen status during labor. *Obstetrics and Gynecology, 105*(6), 1362–1368. doi:10.1097/01.AOG.0000164474.03350.7c

Simpson, K. R., James, D. C., & Knox, G. E. (2006). Nurse-physician communication during labor and birth: Implications for patient safety. *Journal of Obstetric, Gynecologic, and Neonatal Nursing, 35*(4), 547–556. doi:10.1111/j.1552-6909.2006.00075.x

Simpson, K. R., & Knox, G. E. (2000). Risk management and electronic fetal monitoring: Decreasing risk of adverse outcomes and liability exposure. *Journal of Perinatal and Neonatal Nursing, 14*(3), 40–52.

Simpson, K. R., & Knox, G. E. (2006). Essential criteria to promote safe care during labor and birth. *AWHONN Lifelines, 9*(6), 478–483.

Simpson, K. R., & Knox, G. E. (2009). Communication of fetal heart monitoring information. In A. Lyndon & L. U. Ali (Eds.), *Fetal Heart Monitoring Principles and Practices* (4th ed., pp. 177–209). Washington, DC: Association of Women's Health, Obstetric and Neonatal Nurses/Kendall Hunt.

Simpson, K. R., & Lyndon, A. (2009). Clinical disagreements during labor and birth: How does real life compare to best practice? *MCN: The American Journal of Maternal Child Nursing, 34*(1), 31–39. doi:10.1097/01.NMC.0000343863.72237.2b

Sklansky, M. (2009). Fetal cardiac malformations and arrhythmias. In R. K. Creasy & R. Resnick (Eds.), *Maternal-Fetal Medicine* (6th ed., pp. 305–345). Philadelphia: Saunders.

Skupski, D. W., Rosenberg, C. R., & Eglinton, G. S. (2002). Intrapartum fetal stimulation tests: A meta-analysis. *Obstetrics and Gynecology, 99*(1), 129–134.

Society of Obstetricians and Gynaecologists of Canada. (2007). Fetal health surveillance: Antepartum and intrapartum consensus guideline. *Journal of Obstetrics and Gynaecology Canada, 29*(9, Suppl. 4), S1–S56.

Spong, C. Y. (2008). Electronic fetal heart rate monitoring: Another look. *Obstetrics and Gynecology, 112*(3), 506–507. doi:10.1097/AOG.0b013e318185f872

Strong, T. H., Jr. (1997). The effect of amnioinfusion on the duration of labor. *Obstetrics and Gynecology, 89*(6), 1044–1046.

Subtil, D., Tiberghien, P., Devos, P., Therby, D., Leclerc, G., Vaast, P., & Puech, F. (2003). Immediate and delayed effects of antenatal corticosteroids on fetal heart rate: A randomized trial that compares betamethasone acetate and phosphate, betamethasone phosphate, and dexamethasone. *American Journal of Obstetrics and Gynecology, 188*(2), 524–531.

Sureau, C. (1996). Historical perspectives: Forgotten past, unpredictable future. *Baillieres Clinical Obstetrics and Gynaecology, 10*(2), 167–184.

Thacker, S. B., Stroup, D. F., & Peterson, H. B. (1995). Efficacy and safety of intrapartum electronic fetal monitoring: An update. *Obstetrics and Gynecology, 86*(4, Pt. 1), 613–620.

Thorp, J. A., Trobough, T., Evans, R., Hedrick, J., & Yeast, J. D. (1995). The effect of maternal oxygen administration during the second stage of labor on umbilical cord blood gas values: A randomized controlled prospective trial. *American Journal of Obstetrics and Gynecology, 172*(2, Pt. 1), 465–474.

To, W. W., & Leung, W. C. (1998). The incidence of abnormal findings from intrapartum cardiotocogram monitoring in term and preterm labours. *Australian and New Zealand Journal of Obstetrics and Gynaecology, 38*(3), 258–261.

United States Food and Drug Administration. (2009). *Safety alert: Phillips avalon fetal monitors (Safety alerts for human medical products)*. MedWatch: The FDA Safety Information and Adverse Event Reporting Program. Retrieved from http://www.fda.gov/Safety/MedWatch/SafetyInformation/SafetyAlertsforHumanMedicalProducts/ucm181505.htm

Vintzileos, A. M., Antsaklis, A., Varvarigos, I., Papas, C., Sofatzis, I., & Montgomery, J. T. (1993). A randomized trial of intrapartum electronic fetal heart rate monitoring versus intermittent auscultation. *Obstetrics and Gynecology, 81*(6), 899–907.

Westgate, J. A., Wibbens, B., Bennet, L., Wassink, G., Parer, J. T., & Gunn, A. J. (2007). The intrapartum deceleration in center stage: A physiologic approach to the interpretation of fetal heart rate changes in labor. *American Journal of Obstetrics and Gynecology, 197*(3), 236.e1–236.e11. doi:10.1016/j.ajog.2007.03.063

Westgren, M., Holmquist, P., Svenningsen, N. W., & Ingemarsson, I. (1982). Intrapartum fetal monitoring in preterm deliveries: Prospective study. *Obstetrics and Gynecology, 60*(1), 99–106.

Westgren, M., Hormquist, P., Ingemarsson, I., & Svenningsen, N. (1984). Intrapartum fetal acidosis in preterm infants: Fetal monitoring and long-term morbidity. *Obstetrics and Gynecology, 63*(3), 355–359.

Westgren, M., Malcus, P., & Svenningsen, N. W. (1986). Intrauterine asphyxia and long-term outcome in preterm fetuses. *Obstetrics and Gynecology, 67*(4), 512–516.

Wolfberg, A. J., Derosier, D. J., Roberts, T., Syed, Z., Clifford, G. D., Acker, D., & Plessis, A. D. (2008). A comparison of subjective and mathematical estimations of fetal heart rate variability. *Journal of Maternal Fetal and Neonatal Medicine, 21*(2), 101–104. doi:10.1080/14767050701836792

Wood, S. H. (2003). Should women be given a choice about fetal assessment in labor? *MCN: American Journal of Maternal Child Nursing, 28*(5), 292–298.

Wright, J. W., Ridgway, L. E., Wright, B. D., Covington, D. L., & Bobitt, J. R. (1996). Effect of MgSO4 on heart rate monitoring in the preterm fetus. *Journal of Reproductive Medicine, 41*(8), 605–608.

Wright, R. G., Shnider, S. M., Levinson, G., Rolbin, S. H., & Parer, J. T. (1981). The effect of maternal administration of ephedrine on fetal heart rate and variability. *Obstetrics and Gynecology, 57*(6), 734–738.

Xu, H., Mas-Calvet, M., Wei, S. Q., Luo, Z. C., & Fraser, W. D. (2009). Abnormal fetal heart rate tracing patterns in patients with thick meconium staining of the amniotic fluid: Association with perinatal outcomes. *American Journal of Obstetrics and Gynecology, 200*(3), 283.e1–283.e7. doi:10.1016/j.ajog.2008.08.043

Zanini, B., Paul, R. H., & Huey, J. R. (1980). Intrapartum fetal heart rate: Correlation with scalp pH in the preterm fetus. *American Journal of Obstetrics and Gynecology, 136*(1), 43–47.

Zeeman, G. G., Khan-Dawood, F. S., & Dawood, M. Y. (1997). Oxytocin and its receptor in pregnancy and parturition: Current concepts and clinical implications. *Obstetrics and Gynecology, 89*(5, Pt. 2), 873–883.

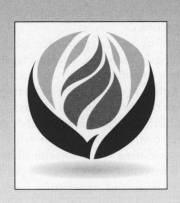

CHAPTER 16

Carol Burke

Pain in Labor: Nonpharmacologic and Pharmacologic Management

A woman's experience of pain in labor is complex, multidimensional, unique to the individual, and may vary from labor to labor. Unlike an acute or chronic insult, pain during labor is usually not associated with a pathologic process. Labor is a normal, physiologic process that causes severe pain for most women. An appreciation of each woman's unique experience of pain is possible when the perinatal nurse understands the physiologic and psychosocial factors influencing pain perception. This chapter will present the physiologic basis for pain, psychosocial factors influencing pain perception, pain management options, and nursing care for nonpharmacologic and pharmacologic methods during labor. For the majority of women in all societies and cultures, natural childbirth is likely to be one of the most painful events in their lifetime (Lowe, 2002). Pain in labor is not easily defined or simple to assess (Roberts, Gulliver, Fisher, & Cloyes, 2010).

During labor, responsibility for managing pain and providing comfort is shared by the laboring woman, nurses, physicians, certified nurse midwives (CNMs), and labor-support persons. Interventions exist along a continuum, from nonpharmacologic to pharmacologic. As healthcare professionals move along this continuum, the potential for complications and side effects increase. The goal of pain management during labor is to assist the woman in managing her pain without interrupting labor or doing harm to the woman or her fetus or newborn. Approaches to pain management in childbirth have addressed the sensory, affective, cognitive, and behavioral dimensions of pain, while more recently a multidimensional approach has been advocated, addressing all dimensions of labor pain (Lowe, 2002; Wesselmann, 2008). A study of low-risk women in labor concluded that four factors were critical to women's experience of childbirth: (1) personal expectations, (2) the amount of support from caregivers, (3) the quality of the caregiver–patient relationship, and (4) the involvement in decision making (Hodnett et al., 2002).

PHYSIOLOGIC BASIS FOR PAIN

Most pain during childbirth results from normal physiologic events. During the first stage of labor, visceral pain results from uterine contractions leading to uterine muscle hypoxia; lactic acid accumulation; cervical and lower uterine segment stretching; traction on ovaries, fallopian tubes, and uterine ligaments; and pressure on the bony pelvis. Afferent pain impulses are carried along sympathetic nerve fibers entering the neuraxis between the 10th and 12th thoracic and first lumbar spinal segments. An additional somatic component arises from perineal stretching and pressure on the urethra, bladder, and rectum causing afferent pain impulses to fire late in the first stage and persist throughout the second stage. This pain is transmitted along the pudendal nerve carried along sympathetic nerve fibers entering the neuraxis between the second and fourth sacral spinal segments (El-Wahab & Robinson, 2011). Some women in labor experience continuous low-back pain that is distinct from uterine contractions. This pain may be related to pressure from the fetal occipital bone on the neural plexus and bony structures of the maternal spine and pelvis. The third stage is usually not particularly painful in comparison.

PHYSIOLOGIC RESPONSES TO PAIN

Pain during labor may result in anxiety and a stress response. Pain induces a physiologic stress response, which can precipitate widespread physiologic and potentially adverse effects on the progress of labor and the well-being of the mother and fetus. Unrelieved anxiety and stress cause increased production of cortisol, glucagon, and catecholamines, which increase metabolism and oxygen consumption (Hawkins, 2010; Reynolds, 2011). Increased levels of catecholamines have been shown to cause uterine hypoperfusion and decreased blood flow to the placenta, resulting in uterine irritability, preterm labor, dystocia, and fetal asphyxia (Wesselmann, 2008). Increased adrenaline levels may prolong labor through beta-receptor-mediated uterine relaxation (Wesselmann, 2008). Due to the release of catecholamines, maternal tachycardia, hypertension, and a rise in cardiac output all increase myocardial workload and, hence, oxygen demand. Respiratory effects include hyperventilation leading to maternal hypocarbia and respiratory alkalosis. While these responses may be innocuous during the course of an uncomplicated labor, they can precipitate heart failure and even ischemia in women with poor cardiorespiratory reserve (El-Wahab & Robinson, 2011). Additionally, it has been suggested that postnatal depression may be less common among women who receive effective analgesia in labor (Flink, Mroczek, Sullivan, & Linton, 2009).

THE EXPERIENCE OF PAIN

Unique circumstances of every labor influence the experience of pain. Responsiveness of the cervix to uterine contractions is influenced by prior surgical or diagnostic procedures that compromise the integrity of the cervix. Prior surgical procedures may result in an incompetent cervix and shorter labor or cause scarring and adhesions, resulting in failure to dilate and protract labor. Many medical and nursing procedures are uncomfortable. Interventions such as pharmacologic agents used for cervical ripening, induction and augmentation of labor, vaginal examinations performed in the supine position, bed rest, amniotomy, tight external electronic fetal monitor (EFM) belts, and enemas may change the character of labor contractions and increase discomfort. Length of labor does not necessarily correlate directly with a woman's perception of pain. Women with short labors may experience very intense pain due to frequent uterine contractions. Women with a fetus in a persistent posterior position report severe pain during and between uterine contractions.

As duration of intense pain increases, discouragement and fatigue increase, decreasing the woman's ability to cope effectively with contractions. Fatigue may occur with a prolonged latent phase, as reported by the woman on admission that she has not slept well for days. Cultural differences with labor pain, acceptance, and personal control in pain relief render pain medication use during labor variable. The use of pain medication is lowest if women have a positive attitude toward labor pain and experience control over the reception of pain medication (Christiaens, Verhaeghe, & Bracke, 2010). Catastrophizing (where a person may think only in terms of negative thoughts about the pain and outcome) is associated with increased pain reports, even when coping strategies are being used (Escott, Slade, & Spiby, 2009).

Labor pain is an example of acute pain. It has a high degree of variability among individuals and at different points in labor. In a study of primiparous women during the first stage of labor, 60% described the pain during first stage of labor as unbearable, intolerable, extremely severe, and excruciating (Melzack, 1984). Descriptions of pain during the first and second stage of labor vary (Table 16–1). Some women describe a decrease in intensity during the second stage, perhaps because of maternal focus on pushing. Others experience more painful sensations, possibly because of the position of the fetus descending through the birth canal.

Many women experience intense pain in labor, which may increase in severity and duration over time. Childbirth pain is one of the most severe types of pain a woman will experience in her lifetime (Camann, 2005). When the McGill Pain Questionnaire was used to compare reports of intensity of pain for a variety of clinical experiences (e.g., chronic back pain, nonterminal cancer pain, phantom limb pain, sprains, fractures), only the pain associated with accidental amputation of a digit and causalgia pain caused more pain than labor (Niven & Gijsbers, 1989). It is clear that a woman's expectation of her labor helps shape her experience, and the level of pain for many women is different from anticipated (Lally, Murtagh, Jacphail, & Thomson, 2008).

Table 16–1. DESCRIPTIONS OF PAIN EXPERIENCE DURING LABOR AND BIRTH

Stage	Sensory	Affective
Stage 1	Cramping, pulling, aching, heavy, sharp, stabbing, cutting, intermittent, localized, global, sore, heavy, throbbing	Exciting, intense, tiring, exhausting, scary, frightening, bearable or unbearable, distressing, horrible, agonizing, indescribable, overwhelming, engulfing
Stage 2	Painful pressure, burning, ripping, tearing, piercing, explosive, localized	Exhausting, overwhelming, out-of-body feeling, inner focused or tunnel vision, exciting, horrible, excruciating, terrifying, less intense

PSYCHOSOCIAL FACTORS INFLUENCING PAIN PERCEPTION

In addition to the physiologic factors that influence the perception of pain, psychosocial factors influence an individual's experience. These factors include labor support, childbirth preparation, and the healthcare environment.

LABOR SUPPORT

Women identify labor support as a continuous presence by another, emotional support (reassurance, encouragement, and guidance), physical comforting, providing information, and guidance for the woman and her partner regarding decision making, facilitation of communication, anticipatory guidance, and explanations of procedures (Simkin & Bolding, 2004; Roberts et al., 2010). Providing for physical comfort includes offering a variety of nonpharmacologic and pharmacologic interventions. Emotional support includes behaviors such as giving praise, encouragement, and reassurance; being positive; appearing calm and confident; assisting with breathing and relaxation; providing explanations about labor progress; identifying ways to include family members in the experience; and treating women with respect (Bryanton, Fraser-Davey, & Sullivan, 1994; Sleutel, 2000). Methods of labor support are found in Display 16–1.

REGISTERED NURSE

It is the position of the Association of Women's Health, Obstetric and Neonatal Nurses (AWHONN) that supporting and caring for women during labor is best performed by a registered nurse (Display 16–2). Comprehensive nursing education, clinical patient-management skills, and previous experience make the registered nurse uniquely qualified to provide the professional care and complex emotional care women and families need during labor and birth (AWHONN, 2000). The perinatal nurse must be able to support the laboring woman and assist her in maximizing the potential of the woman's birth plan. Multiple strategies may be necessary during the course of labor. Perinatal nurses should develop expertise in a variety of pain-management strategies.

Nurses may spend anywhere from 12.4% (Gale, Fothergill-Bourbonnais, & Chamberlain, 2001) to 58% (Miltner, 2002) of their time providing supportive care to patients, usually doing so in conjunction with some technical activity. Factors that have contributed to individual nurses spending less time with women include increased technology associated with giving birth, increased requests for epidural anesthesia, and institutional staffing patterns. As use of technology has expanded in obstetrics, the perinatal nurse has moved

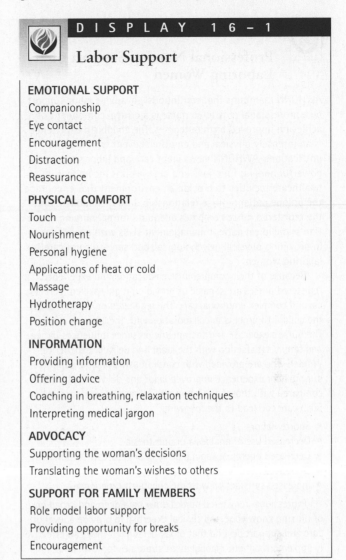

DISPLAY 16–1

Labor Support

EMOTIONAL SUPPORT
Companionship
Eye contact
Encouragement
Distraction
Reassurance

PHYSICAL COMFORT
Touch
Nourishment
Personal hygiene
Applications of heat or cold
Massage
Hydrotherapy
Position change

INFORMATION
Providing information
Offering advice
Coaching in breathing, relaxation techniques
Interpreting medical jargon

ADVOCACY
Supporting the woman's decisions
Translating the woman's wishes to others

SUPPORT FOR FAMILY MEMBERS
Role model labor support
Providing opportunity for breaks
Encouragement

from providing hands-on comfort to monitoring the equipment, imputing data into the electronic medical record and relying on pharmacologic interventions. Technology, especially when coupled with epidural analgesia, requires the nurse to divide her focus between the woman and machines. If pharmacologic methods have been used, the woman's pain may be lessened and the nurse may feel that her presence is no longer needed. The nurse may perceive that caring for a woman with an epidural is less physically and emotionally draining for the nurse than caring for a woman who is planning non-pharmacologic management. If the culture of the perinatal unit allows ease of access to neuraxial analgesia, nurses new to the specialty will have limited opportunity to learn about or use nonpharmacologic measures.

It is important that the nurse recognizes the value of her presence and not be distracted by the technology. The registered nurse who understands the physiologic events of labor and has been educated about supportive care in labor should take the lead in providing

D I S P L A Y 1 6 – 2

Professional Nursing Support of Laboring Women

AWHONN maintains that continuously available labor support by a professional registered nurse is a critical component of achieving improved birth outcomes. The childbirth experience is an intensely physical and emotional event with lifelong implications. AWHONN views labor care and labor support as powerful nursing functions and believes it is incumbent on healthcare facilities to provide an environment that encourages the unique patient–nurse relationship during childbirth. Only the registered nurse combines adequate formal nursing education and clinical patient management skills with experience in providing physical, psychological, and sociocultural care to laboring women.

Because of their comprehensive education and experience, registered nurses are capable of providing highly skilled technical and complex emotional care. The registered nurse facilitates the childbirth process in collaboration with the laboring woman. The nurse's expertise and therapeutic presence influences patient and family satisfaction with the labor and delivery experience. Women who are provided with continuously available support during labor experience improved labor and delivery outcomes compared with those who labor without a skilled support person. Such care can lead to the following:

- Shorter labors
- Decreased use of analgesia or anesthesia
- Decreased operative vaginal delivery or cesarean section
- Decreased need for oxytocin
- Increased satisfaction with the childbirth experience

Professional registered nurses draw on a deep and broad base of nursing knowledge and clinical expertise to provide a level of care and support beyond that of lay personnel. They can effectively implement patient management strategies for low- and high-risk patients. The registered nurse can assess, plan, implement, and evaluate an individualized plan of care based on each woman's physical, psychological, and sociocultural needs, including desires and expectations of the laboring process. The support provided by the professional registered nurse should include the following:

- Assessment and management of the physiologic and psychologic processes of labor
- Provision of emotional support and physical comfort measures
- Evaluation of fetal well-being during labor
- Instruction regarding the labor process
- Patient advocacy—the clinical assessment and evaluation that results from collaboration among professional members of the healthcare team
- Role modeling to facilitate family participation during labor and birth
- Direct collaboration with other members of the healthcare team to coordinate patient care

In today's healthcare environment, numerous factors may influence the nurse's ability to provide bedside labor care:

- A limited number of available experienced registered nurses
- Limited financial resources
- Rigid organizational processes and structures
- Cumbersome documentation requirements
- Decreasing reimbursement by third-party payers in the United States

AWHONN challenges healthcare facilities to continuously evaluate the impact of patient–nurse ratios on resource use, overall operating expenses, patient outcomes, and patient satisfaction. AWHONN also supports evaluation models that can measure the impact a registered professional nurse has on indirect cost savings, such as savings resulting from lower cesarean section rates, shorter labors, and fewer technologic interventions.

AWHONN encourages women and families to request labor support from a professional registered nurse or advanced practice nurse (e.g., clinical nurse specialist, CNM, or nurse practitioner) for labor and birth.

Studies on professional nursing care for laboring women are in progress. AWHONN supports continued research efforts to document the essential role of professional nursing labor support on maternal–newborn outcomes and the potential financial benefits of such support for the healthcare system.

CNM, certified nurse midwife.
From Association of Women's Health, Obstetric and Neonatal Nurses. (2000). *Professional nursing support of laboring women*. Washington, DC: Author.

---

labor support and role model labor support behaviors for others present during labor and birth. Perinatal nurses should remain at the bedside when women are experiencing severe pain. This allows the nurse to provide support to the laboring woman and her partner. According to Chapman (2000), nurses who remained at the bedside, explained what was occurring with the labor, and included the expectant father were viewed by those fathers as providing the most support.

HUSBAND OR SIGNIFICANT OTHER

Labor support ideally is provided by a variety of individuals (Table 16–2). Qualitative research has demonstrated that one of the most significant aspects of the experience of labor for women is the presence of one or more support persons (Lavender, Walkinshaw, & Walton, 1999). Postpartum women report that one of the things contributing to a positive labor experience was the presence of a family member or friend in the room even if "they just sit there" (Lavender et al., 1999). At the time of admission, the laboring woman should identify family members or friends who will act as labor-support persons.

Fathers have an important role in providing physical and emotional support during childbirth. Chapman (1992) described three roles assumed by expectant fathers during labor without epidural analgesia or anesthesia:

- Coaches actively assisted their partners during and after labor contractions with breathing and relaxation techniques. Coaches led or directed their

Table 16–2. PROVIDING LABOR SUPPORT

Clinical Practice	Referenced Rationale
1. Labor support ideally is continuous and provided by a variety of individuals.	A Cochrane review has addressed the effect of continuous support in 15 trials involving 12,791 women in 11 countries and concluded that women who had continuous 1:1 support were (1) more likely to have a spontaneous vaginal birth, (2) less likely to require analgesia, and (3) less likely to report dissatisfaction with their childbirth experience (Hodnett, Gates, Hafmeyr, & Sakala, 2003).
2. Trained lay doulas are effective at providing labor support.	Pain was reduced by continuous labor support, particularly those in which laypersons trained as doulas provided the support (Simkin & Bolding, 2004).
3. Labor support should begin in early labor and continued through delivery.	Support in early labor seems to have provided greater benefit than when begun in active labor (Simkin & Bolding, 2004).
4. Fathers and other support persons may require assistance and suggestions with support measures.	As pain intensifies, women become frustrated, irritable, exhausted, and panicky. These personality changes may be totally unfamiliar qualities that the men had never seen their partners demonstrate or demonstrated to the degree manifested in labor.
5. Content related to changing emotions should be presented in prenatal classes.	It is important that childbirth educators present content related to coping and not coping, discuss the transition, and teach men in their classes about the emotions they can expect to witness and experience themselves during labor.

partners through labor and birth and viewed themselves as managers or directors of the experience.

- Teammates assisted their partners throughout the experience of labor and birth by responding to requests for physical or emotional support or both. They sometimes led their partners, but their usual role was that of follower or helper.
- Witnesses viewed themselves primarily as companions who were there to provide emotional and moral support. They were present during labor and birth to observe the process and to witness the birth of their child.

These roles were identified by organizing behaviors that partners were observed performing during labor or behaviors women described in interviews after birth. Most men in the study adopted the role of witness rather than teammate or coach (Chapman, 1992).

Chandler and Field (1997) report that witnessing their partners in severe pain caused men to feel helpless and fearful. They became discouraged when the comfort measures they tried did not help their partners. Ultimately, they felt they had failed in their role. These results contrast with the intentions of childbirth educators, who perceive themselves as preparing coaches and teammates for laboring women, and with perinatal nurses, who expect fathers and other family members to take a more active role in labor support.

The theoretical experience of expectant fathers when their partners received epidural analgesia or anesthesia is outlined in Display 16–3 (Chapman, 2000). During labor, critical experiences for men occurred at two points. In the holding-out phase of labor, before making the decision to receive an epidural, men experienced a sense of "losing her." As pain became more severe, women underwent personality changes, becoming frustrated, irritable, exhausted, and panicky. These personality changes may be totally unfamiliar qualities

that the men had never seen their partners demonstrate or demonstrate to the degree that they do while in labor. Women also gradually turn inward as they attempt to cope with the pain. Withdrawing into themselves causes women to be unable to communicate their needs and to become unresponsive to their partners' attempts at labor support. Men feel increased levels of anxiety, helplessness, frustration, and emotional pain (Chapman, 2000). These findings are consistent with the work of Somers-Smith (1999), who found that fathers experience childbirth as a stressful event.

DISPLAY 16 – 3

Grounded Theory of the Expectant Father's Epidural Labor Experience

Holding-Out Phase: During labor, when couples are planning to avoid an epidural or seeing how far they can get in labor without needing an epidural.

Surrendering Phase: The point at which the decision is made to receive an epidural, which is described as yielding to the need for an epidural, giving up, and feeling they have experienced all the pain they can handle and done everything they can to avoid an epidural.

Waiting Phase: Period of time after making the decision to receive an epidural until the anesthesia care provider arrives.

Getting Phase: Period of time when the anesthesia provider is present, making assessments, preparing equipment, and placing the epidural.

Cruising Phase: The time after the epidural has provided pain relief. Couples' focus changes to rest and relaxation. Labor has gone from a stressful process to a calm experience. Both may fall asleep, due to exhaustion from the stress of coping with the pain of labor.

Chapman, L. L. (2000). Expectant fathers and labor epidurals. *MCN: The American Journal of Maternal Child Nursing, 25*(3), 133–139.

The second and most dramatic phase for men sharing the experience of labor is during the cruising phase. After the epidural has provided relief from the pain of labor, men describe a sensation of "she's back." The laboring woman again is aware of her surroundings and is interacting with those around her. From a man's perspective, labor has gone from a stressful event to a calm experience. Rather than describing their experience in terms of the role they assumed during labor and the frustration and disconnected feelings they had as labor intensified and women's behavior changed (Chapman, 1991, 1992), these men described their experience by the degree of frustration they felt before the epidural and the degree of enjoyment after the epidural (Chapman, 2000). It is important that childbirth educators present this content, discuss this process, and teach men in their classes about the emotions they can expect to witness and experience during labor.

DOULA

There is increased interest in the role of the professional or lay labor-support person (doula), who is present during labor in addition to the perinatal nurse. The movement toward professional or lay labor support is a result of the inability of perinatal nurses to provide women with the support they want during labor and the recognition that husbands or significant others do not always make the best coaches during labor. Being in a hospital and seeing one's wife in labor may be very stressful for some fathers (Klaus, Kennell, & Klaus, 2002). Childbirth education programs have traditionally provided training labor-support persons. However, the assumption that the husband or significant other makes the best coach may not be accurate (Chapman, 1992). It is important for the father of the baby to be present during the labor and birth, but the presence of a doula may be what the laboring woman needs.

Labor-support persons, or doulas, with a variety of credentials and levels of education, assist women and their partners during pregnancy, birth, and the postpartum period. "A doula is a supportive companion (other than a friend or loved one) who is professionally trained to provide labor support" (Gilliland, 2002, p. 762). Most often seen during labor, their main goal is to ensure that the woman feels safe and confident (Ballen & Fulcher, 2006). A doula remains continuously at the side of the woman to provide emotional support and physical comfort (Klaus et al., 2002). While not provided by all programs, a unique aspect of the doula role occurs postpartum, usually after discharge from the hospital. During a home visit, the doula is able to make time to review with the new mother her labor and birth experience with the goal of creating a satisfying birth experience. "The doula allows the woman to reflect on her experience, fills in gaps in her memory, praises her, and sometimes helps reframe upsetting or difficult aspects of the birth" (Ballen & Fulcher, 2006, p. 305). Table 16–3 contrasts the role of a doula with that of the perinatal nurse.

Table 16–3. DIFFERENTIATING THE ROLES OF THE NURSE AND THE DOULA

Registered Nurse	Doula
Professional education and license to practice nursing. Follows evidence-based standards and guidelines from professional organizations.	Often trained, though this is not required. May be prepared through a formal education program; may be certified.
Meets the woman for the first time during labor.	Usually meets and begins to form a relationship with the woman during her pregnancy to try to understand her expectations, needs, fears, and concerns.
Performs clinical tasks within the scope of practice of the registered nurse.	Supportive role; performs no clinical tasks.
Consults with the obstetrical care provider.	Has no direct communication responsibility to the obstetrical care provider.
Provides intermittent labor support; presence in the LDR/LDRP is not continuous; may be caring for more than one patient; depending on the length of labor, more than one nurse may care for the woman.	Provides continuous labor support; leaves the LDR/LDRP only for bathroom breaks; stays with the woman throughout her labor and birth and into the early postpartum period.
Keeps patient informed of labor progress: what is normal and what to expect.	Keeps patient informed of labor progress in lay terms: what is normal and what to expect.
Advocates for the patient by communicating her needs and desires to the obstetrical care provider.	Assists the patient to formulate and articulate her questions and concerns to the nurse and the obstetrical care provider.
Responsible for documenting assessments in medical record.	May document events of the labor and birth to share and review with the woman later to ensure positive memories.
Has a legal accountability and responsibility for his/her actions.	Responsibilities decided between doula and the family.
May have minimal or no contact with the patient after the birth.	Some type of follow-up visit(s) is usually part of the program.

LDR, labor and delivery room; LDRP, labor, delivery, recovery, and postpartum room.

In a meta-analysis of 11 clinical trials in which continuous support by a doula was compared with traditional intermittent support of a labor and delivery nurse, continuous support was associated with significantly shorter labors; decreased use of analgesia, oxytocin, and forceps; and decreased cesarean births (Scott, Berkowitz, & Klaus, 1999). In a culture in which women experience traditional labor without their husbands, those accompanied by a female support person had significantly shorter labors, less use of analgesia and oxytocin, and fewer admissions to the neonatal intensive care unit (NICU) (Mosallam, Rizk, Thomas, & Ezimokhai, 2004). Women who had the benefit of a doula during labor expressed significantly less emotional distress and had higher self-esteem at 4 months postpartum than women who had attended a traditional Lamaze class (Manning-Orenstein, 1998). When low-income pregnant women were randomized to be accompanied in labor by their family and a trained doula or just family members, those in the experimental group had significantly shorter labors and greater cervical dilation at the time of epidural anesthesia (Campbell, Lake, Falk, & Backstrand, 2006).

Doulas (also known as labor assistants, birth companions, labor support specialists, professional labor assistants, and monitrices) may be volunteers or paid and are available through a variety of programs, either hospital based, community based, or as a private, contracted service. Hospital- and community-based programs are often available to underserved populations, women who may be newly emigrating, or women who might be alone during childbirth (e.g., adolescents, incarcerated women). Individual hospitals or community-based healthcare agencies may be involved in training doulas, or there are national organizations where training and certification are available (Display 16–4). Services of a doula are generally arranged by the expectant couple or presented as an available option by a healthcare agency before labor.

The husband or significant other, family members and friends, and/or a doula should be welcomed and encouraged to provide labor support. The presence of one or all of these additional individuals does not decrease the ultimate responsibility of the perinatal nurse but instead adds to a positive birth experience. Labor support, when provided by nursing personnel, a partner, family members, or friends, affects a woman's perception of labor (Lowe, 2002; Wright, McCrea, Stringer, & Murphy-Black, 2000). In a meta-analysis of 15 clinical trials, continuous support from a nurse, CNM, or lay person resulted in decreased operative vaginal birth, cesarean birth, 5-minute Apgar scores less than 7, and use of medication for pain relief (Hodnett, Gates, Hafmeyr, & Sakala, 2003). In a systematic review of the literature, Hodnett (2000) found the attitudes and behaviors of caregivers are a stronger

DISPLAY 16 – 4

Associations That Train and Certify Doulas

ALACE (Association of Labor Assistants & Childbirth Educators) http://www.alace.org

CHILDBIRTH EDUCATION SPECIALISTS http://www.childbirth education.net

DONA (Doulas of North America International) http://www.dona.org

CHILDBIRTH INTERNATIONAL http://www.childbirthinternational.com

INTUITIVE DOULA http://www.intuitivedoula.com

ICEA (International Childbirth Education Association) http://www.icea.org

Adapted from Ballen, L. E., & Fulcher, A. J. (2006). Nurses and doulas: Complementary roles to provide optimal maternity care. *Journal of Obstetric, Gynecologic, and Neonatal Nursing, 35*(2), 304–311.

influence on satisfaction with childbirth than many other factors. Women who received continuous support during labor are less likely to request intrapartum analgesia, require an operative birth, or report dissatisfaction with their childbirth experience (Hodnett et al., 2003).

CHILDBIRTH PREPARATION

An awareness of the childbirth preparation and skills that the woman and her partner are prepared to use are helpful when planning nursing support strategies during labor. The desire for pain relief during labor varies in women with a spectrum from natural childbirth to the most invasive technique (e.g., neuraxial analgesia). Prenatal education should provide information on an assortment of pain management and coping skills to hopefully meet the expectations of the woman. Most pregnant women have concerns about labor process and their ability to handle painful contractions. Childbirth classes provide an opportunity to help women understand and let go of fears about labor and birth and begin to develop confidence in their ability to give birth. Antenatal education in preparation for childbirth is available in a number of formats including in a classroom, online, and through video display. Content and bias varies depending on the author and presenter of the material. Both pharmacologic and nonpharmacologic pain relief methods may be presented as alternatives or complimentary to each other, which may influence the woman's coping ability and choice. The common goal of all birthing classes is to provide the knowledge and confidence to give birth and to make informed decisions. Anxiety-reducing strategies and a variety of coping techniques integrated into the physiology of the birth process will provide an aid to pain management. Guidelines from 2008 from the National

Institute for Clinical Excellence (NICE; 2008) reviewed studies from the United States, the United Kingdom, and Australia and recommend preparation for labor and birth to include information about coping with pain in labor and the birth plan. Knowledge regarding pregnancy, birth, and parenting issues is increased following attendance at antenatal classes, and the wish to receive this information is a strong motivator for attending classes. Classes need to include information about decision making, including both informed consent and the women's right to an informed refusal. For the woman, it takes courage and confidence to communicate effectively with the healthcare team and her provider in making clear her expectations of labor and birth (Lothian, 2005).

A broad range of nonpharmacologic behavioral strategies including controlled breathing, relaxation, positioning, and massage are usually presented in both the Lamaze and Bradley courses (Table 16–4). The Lamaze® philosophy, also known as psychoprophylaxis, teaches that birth is a normal, natural, and healthy process. The goal of Lamaze® is to explore all the ways women can find strength and comfort during labor and birth. It is based on the Pavlovian concept of conditioned reflex training. Classes focus on relaxation techniques, but they also encourage the mother to condition her response to pain through training and preparation. This conditioning is meant to teach expectant mothers constructive responses to the pain and stress of labor as opposed to tensing muscles in response to pain. The basis of Lamaze® childbirth preparation is the belief that pain during childbirth leads to fear and tension, which increases the experience of pain. As fear and anxiety heighten, muscle tension increases, inhibiting the effectiveness of contractions, increasing discomfort, and further heightening fear and anxiety. Other techniques are also used to decrease a woman's perception of pain such as distraction (a woman might be encouraged, for example, to focus on a special object from home or a photo) or massage by a supportive coach. Lamaze® courses are neutral regarding the use of drugs and routine medical interventions during labor and delivery and educate mothers about their options so informed decisions can be made. Nonpharmacologic and pharmacologic pain-management strategies provide women with specific techniques they can use to cope with the discomfort of labor, thereby increasing their feelings of control.

The Bradley Method® (also called "Husband-Coached Birth") places an emphasis on a natural approach to birth and on the active participation and teamwork with the baby's father as the birth coach. A major goal of this method is the avoidance of medications unless absolutely necessary. Other topics include the importance of good nutrition and exercise during pregnancy, relaxation techniques (such as deep breathing and concentration on body signals) as a method of coping with labor, and the empowerment of parents to

Table 16–4. COMPARISON OF PRENATAL EDUCATION CLASSES

Type	Objective	Class Content
Lamaze® International http://www.lamaze.org	Supports birth as normal, natural, and healthy and empowers expectant women and their partners to make informed decisions about interventions.	4–6 wk class Labor rehearsals Normal labor, birth, and early postpartum Positioning for labor and birth Relaxation and massage techniques to ease pain Labor support Communication skills Information about medical procedures Breastfeeding Healthy lifestyle
The Bradley Method®: http://www.bradleybirth.com	Helps the woman and her husband prepare for a natural labor and birth without the use of medication.	12-wk class Importance of nutrition and exercise Relaxation techniques to manage pain Labor rehearsals How to avoid a cesarean birth Postpartum care Breastfeeding Guidance for coach/doula about supporting and advocating for the mother
Hospital based	Provides information about procedures available at the particular hospital. Usually taught by registered nurse from the hospital.	1- or 2-day class May include elements of Lamaze® and Bradley® Physical/emotional changes in pregnancy Information on cesarean birth, induction, augmentation, common labor and delivery interventions, and medication options May include postpartum and newborn care

trust their instincts to become active, informed participants in the birth process. The course is traditionally offered in 12 sessions. Although Bradley® emphasizes a birth experience without pain medication, the classes do prepare parents for unexpected complications or situations, including emergency cesarean birth. After the birth, immediate breastfeeding and constant contact between parents and baby are stressed.

Hospital-based classes are offered in the third trimester and welcome the involvement of a birth companion during classes. The hospital-based prenatal class presents content seemingly biased to that particular institution and may focus primarily on the medical model. Usually a tour of the facility is included in the classes. Carlton et al. (2005) question whether some hospital-based education serves to socialize women about the "appropriate" ways of giving birth rather than educating them.

There is a relationship between women's expectation of labor and their actual experience of labor (Green, 1993). Women who expect breathing and relaxation techniques to work are more likely to find them helpful. Women who wish to avoid medications can be successful with the help of educational preparation, their support system, and perinatal nurses who respect that plan. The labor admission assessment should include questions related to the type and amount of childbirth preparation (e.g., classes, reading, video tape viewing). As part of the admission assessment, the nurse should ask about the couple's plans for pain management during labor and whether this subject was discussed with her obstetric provider. Asking about their plans and goals validates their efforts to prepare for labor and birth. Nurses should assure the woman and her support persons that the couple's goals are understood and that achievement is a shared objective. Nurses have a responsibility whenever possible to facilitate an experience for each couple that matches their expectations (Carlton, Callister, & Stoneman, 2005). Knowledge and skills learned in childbirth-preparation classes are enhanced when the nurse present during labor and birth believes in and actively supports the couple as they apply these principles.

HEALTHCARE ENVIRONMENT

Every perinatal unit takes a unique approach to caring for laboring women. A culture develops over time and is accepted by most of those working within the department as a reflection of their values and beliefs. Cultural differences may be as significant as the availability of labor, delivery, recovery, and postpartum rooms (LDRPs) or as subtle as the routine initiation of intravenous fluids on admission. These practices reflect the evolution of intrapartum care within a particular institution. Unit culture extends to treatment of pain and influences the woman's perception of pain. Nurses who value nonpharmacologic approaches to pain management use these techniques in clinical practice.

PAIN TOLERANCE

Pain is a culturally bound phenomenon. When a patient expresses pain, the form that expression takes is related to what her culture has taught her is appropriate. Pain tolerance may be defined as the level of stimuli at which the laboring woman asks to have the stimulation stopped. In labor, it is the point at which a woman requests pharmacologic pain relief or increased comfort measures. Descriptive words such as mild, moderate, and severe do not provide a measure of pain tolerance because laboring women may describe pain as severe but may not request pain medication. A woman's pain tolerance or the length of time she is able to go without medication may be increased by the use of nonpharmacologic pain management techniques (O'Sullivan, 2009).

The Joint Commission (TJC; 2011), in 2001, established pain management standards for healthcare organizations, which require that patients (1) have appropriate assessment and management of pain, (2) are screened for pain during the initial assessment and reassessed periodically, and (3) are educated about pain management. Many hospitals use a rating scale to quantify the pain from 0 to 10, with a response of 4 or greater requiring intervention and 10 being excruciating pain. TJC does not mandate this particular rating scale but rather that their standards are followed.

Most hospitals have adapted one of the many available standardized pain assessment tools. Those used in adult populations, for the most part, require that the patient rate the intensity of pain she is experiencing. They are useful because there is some objectivity added to assessing and documenting phenomena that are very subjective. What these simplistic tools cannot tell the nurse is how the pain is being interpreted or translated by the woman in labor. What is her perception of the pain and how much is she suffering during labor? Only by being present and really listening, observing, and empathizing with a woman during labor can the nurse begin to understand what the experience of pain is for her and what interventions might be helpful to provide some relief (King & McCool, 2004). There is still a need for research to find a suitable assessment instrument for the evaluation of labor pain (Bergh, Stener-Victorin, Wallin, & Martensson, 2011).

Roberts et al. (2010) developed and implemented an alternative tool to the 0 to 10 rating scale, called The Coping with Labor Algorithm, which qualifies the woman's ability and internal consciousness as coping or not coping with her labor. Signs of coping include rhythmic motion, breathing patterns, and stating she is coping. Noncoping cues include lack of concentration, crying, and stating she is no longer coping. Both pathways incorporate nursing and supportive actions. The coping algorithm was found to be useful in the hospital setting and is being evaluated in other hospitals for ease of use and applicability. The Coping with Labor Algorithm has passed a Joint Commission survey.

Although pain may be quantified, it is only one component of a woman's overall experience of labor and delivery. Personal satisfaction is not always correlated with the level of pain and should be included in the evaluation of pain (Tournaire & Theau-Yonneau, 2007). Research has shown that alternative coping techniques may improve a women's sense of control and satisfaction with childbirth (Kimber, McNabb, McCourt, Haines, & Brocklehurst, 2008). Helping women cope with labor through methods to impact the affective component and decrease the sensory component may be viewed as ineffective by clinicians supportive of the pharmacologic model (Lowe, 2002).

THE NONPHARMACOLOGIC MODEL

The nonpharmacologic model views childbirth as a unique individual experience and a normal physiologic process that involves pain. The goal is to eliminate the suffering, helplessness, distress, and loss of control. This model will not provide complete pain relief, but allows techniques that allow a woman to cope with her labor pain; therefore, it is inaccurate to use terms such as *pain relief* when referring to these interventions. Alternatively, the complete removal of pain does not always convert to a more satisfying experience. A woman's ability to actively participate in her labor can transform the experience from suffering to active participation and confidence in her ability to cope with the aid of her support system. The nonpharmacologic model is appealing

to women and caregivers who are interested in reducing labor pain without creating potentially serious side effects and high costs. It includes a wide variety of techniques to address both physical sensations of pain and to prevent suffering by addressing the emotional and spiritual components of care (Simkin & Bolding, 2004). Ultimately, it is a nurse's role to support the laboring woman to make informed choices that achieve a woman's vision of birth, while ensuring the safety of both the mother and infant. Few randomized, controlled clinical trials exist validating all these techniques. Some interventions, such as positioning, counter-pressure, heat and cold, touch, massage, and injections of sterile water, may decrease pain. Other interventions, such as relaxation, imagery, focusing, breathing techniques, and music, more likely benefit a woman by decreasing anxiety, improving overall mood, and increasing the individual's sense of control in a painful situation (McCaffery & Pasero, 1999).

Women choose pain-management strategies based on their previous experience with pain, what they learned in prenatal classes and from primary healthcare providers' recommendations, and listening to what worked for family members and friends. The advantage of nonpharmacologic pain management strategies is their simplicity and relative ease to initiate, the sense of control women receive when they actively manage their pain, the lack of serious side effects, and the fact that they do not generally add additional costs to the birth process (Simkin & O'Hara, 2002). Also, nonpharmacologic interventions do not require additional medical interventions and provide the opportunity for the woman's significant others to be involved in the birth experience. The 2006 "Listening to Mothers II Survey" noted that 69% of the mothers used some type of nonpharmacologic intervention during labor (Declercq, Sakala, Corry, & Applebaum, 2007) (Fig. 16–1).

FIGURE 16–1. Frequency of nonpharmacologic use during labor. (Adapted from Declercq, E. R., Sakala, C., Corry, M. P., & Applebaum, S. [2007]. Listening to mothers II: Report of the second national U. S. survey of women's childbearing experiences. *Journal of Perinatal Education, 16*(4), 15–17.)

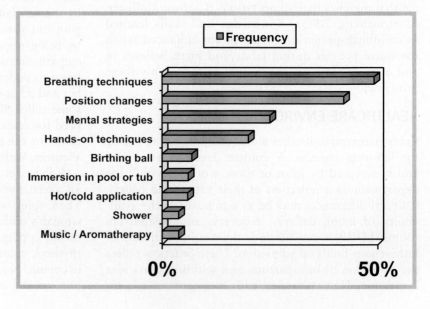

There are three classifications of nonpharmacologic methods or comfort measures that can be used to decrease or alter painful sensations associated with labor and birth: (1) measures to reduce painful stimuli, (2) methods that activate peripheral sensory receptors to block transmission of painful stimuli, and (3) cognitive techniques that enhance inhibitory neural pathways, thereby reducing a woman's negative psychologic reaction to pain (Table 16–5).

The effectiveness of nonpharmacologic pain-management strategies can be explained by Melzack and Wall's (1965) early work on the gate control and the processes responsible for the transmission of pain. The first process is explained by the structure of the central nervous system, which is composed of large and small sensory nerve fibers. Impulses are carried by the spinal cord from the site of the stimuli to the cerebral cortex, where impulses are interpreted. Small, thinly myelinated, or unmyelinated fibers transport impulses such as pressure and pain from the uterus, cervix, and pelvic joints. Large myelinated fibers transport impulses from the skin. Because passage along large fibers occurs more quickly, it is possible for cutaneous stimulation to block or alter painful impulses. Based on this premise, tactile stimulation in the form of touch or massage is often used effectively during labor. The second process is stimulation of the reticular activating system in the brain stem. The reticular activating system interprets auditory, visual, and painful sensory stimuli. When the cerebral cortex focuses on auditory or visual stimulation, painful stimulation is less able to pass through the "gate." Many forms of distraction are used during labor to decrease pain perception.

Melzack (1999) has reevaluated the Gate Control Theory, adding to it the possibility of multiple influences within the brain, a neuromatrix that is ultimately responsible for how each individual perceives pain. These other influences include past experiences, cultural conditioning, emotional state, level of anxiety, understanding of the labor process, and the meaning that the current situation has for the individual are used by the cerebral cortex to interpret a sensation as painful. Just as thoughts and emotions can increase pain, they can also increase feelings of confidence and control, decreasing painful sensations. Prenatal education and labor support are effective pain-management strategies because they enhance maternal confidence and a sense of control.

CUTANEOUS PAIN RELIEF TECHNIQUES

Maternal Position and Movement

Women naturally choose positions of comfort and are more likely to change position during early labor. Modern technology (e.g., EFM, intravenous tubing and catheters, automatic blood pressure monitors, fetal scalp electrodes) and pharmacologic use may interfere with a woman's ability to find a comfortable position and frequently restricts her to bed. Many nurses and physicians encourage bed rest for labor because it helps them feel more in control of the situation, and they believe it may be safer for the woman and fetus. However, it is possible to use most of the technology available in obstetrics without maintaining continuous bed rest. An upright position can be accomplished in a recliner, rocking chair, or birthing bed adjusted to a chair position. EFM telemetry units, transducers that can be submerged in water, or intermittent auscultation of the fetal heart rate (FHR) can be used to evaluate fetal response to labor while the woman is ambulating or using hydrotherapy. Women should be encouraged to change their position frequently during labor. Changing position alters the relationship between the fetus and pelvis and the efficiency of uterine contractions (Zwelling, 2010). Table 16–6 lists a variety of positions available to women in labor along with the benefits of each. Maintaining a horizontal position during labor is associated with decreased blood flow and may increase uterine muscle hypoxia, resulting in the increased perception of pain associated with uterine contractions (Mayberry et al., 2000). Molina, Sola, Lopez, and Pires (1997) noted decreased pain in vertical as compared with horizontal positions before 6 cm of dilation.

Women report less pain in an upright position during the second stage of labor than women in a semi-Fowler's or semi-recumbent position (AWHONN, 2008). Upright positions during labor cause more intense and frequent contractions and more rapid cervical dilation. Changing position in labor and including some upright positions

Table 16–5. NONPHARMACOLOGIC METHODS TO CONTROL PAIN

Technique	Examples
Cutaneous measures to reduce painful stimuli	Massage
	Touch
	Back rub
	Counter-pressure
	Movement and positioning
	Application of heat or cold
	Acupuncture
	Hydrotherapy
Auditory or visual techniques to block the transmission of painful stimuli	Focal point
	Breathing techniques
	Attention focusing
	Distraction
	Hypnosis
	Music
Cognitive processes to control the degree to which a sensation is interpreted as painful	Prenatal education
	Relaxation
	Labor support
	Imagery

Table 16–6. LABOR POSITIONS

Positions	Effect of Positions
Standing or any upright position	Takes advantage of gravity during and between contractions Contractions less painful and more productive Fetus well aligned with angle of pelvis May speed labor if woman has been recumbent May increase urge to push in second stage
Walking	Movement causes changes in pelvic joints, encouraging rotation and descent
Standing and leaning forward on person or object (e.g., partner, bed, birth ball)	May relieve backache; good position for back rub More restful than standing Can maintain continuous electronic fetal monitor
Slow dancing (mother embraces partner around neck, rests head on his/her chest or shoulder; with partner's arms around mother's trunk, interlocking fingers at her low back, she can drop her arms and rests against her partner to increase relaxation)	Swaying movements to music may causes changes in pelvic joints, encouraging rotation and descent Rhythm and music add comfort Being embraced by loved one increases sense of well-being Position permits partner to give back pressure to relieve back pain
Sitting upright	Resting position More gravity advantage than supine
Rocking in chair	Rocking movement is relaxing and increases comfort Using foot stool decreases tension in lower extremities
Sitting on toilet or commode	May help relax perineum for effective bearing down
Hands and knees (can achieve this position by kneeling on bed with head raised, kneeling on floor while leaning on a chair or birthing ball)	Helps relieve backache from occipitoposterior Assists rotation of baby from occipitoposterior Allows freedom of movement for pelvic rocking Vaginal examinations possible Takes pressure off hemorrhoids
Side lying	Helps lower elevated blood pressure; increases perfusion of blood to the placenta and fetus Takes pressure off hemorrhoids Easier to relax between pushing efforts Effective position for pushing during second stage
Squatting while supporting herself on object like side of the bed or chair	Takes advantage of gravity Widens pelvic outlet; may enhance rotation and descent of the fetus
Supported squat: mother leans with back against standing partner who holds her under the arms and takes all her weight during contraction	Makes bearing down efforts more spontaneous Helpful if mother does not feel an urge to push
Supported squat: partner sits on high bed or counter with feet supported on chairs or foot stool; with thighs spread, mother backs between legs and places flexed arms over thighs; partner grips woman's sides with his thighs; she lowers herself, allowing partner to support her full weight	Mechanical advantage during second stage as upper trunk presses on uterine fundus Lengthens mother's trunk, allowing more room for asynclitic fetus to maneuver into position Eliminates restriction of pelvic joint mobility that can be caused by external pressure from bed or chair

Adapted from Simkin, P. (1995). Reducing pain and enhancing progress in labor: A guide to nonpharmacologic methods for maternity caregivers. *Birth*, *22*(3), 161–171.

may result in more efficient labors (Cluett & Burns, 2009). Women may initially resist suggestions to change position or may find new positions uncomfortable. When encouraging a woman to change position, the nurse should provide extra support and encouragement and suggest that she remain in the new position through several contractions before deciding whether it is comfortable. In the absence of any staff instructions, women moved about in bed, but only a small percentage chose upright positions or ambulation during either the first or second stage (Cluett & Burns, 2009).

Pillows should be used generously to maintain positions and to support extremities. When a side-lying position is used, pillows can be placed behind the back and between the knees. In a semi-Fowler's position, pillows can be placed under knees or arms. Shorter women sitting in a chair may find that a pillow or stool under their feet decreases stretching of leg muscles. Women who labor with the baby's head in an occipital-posterior position report significantly less back pain when using hands-and-knees positioning (Zwelling, 2010). Positioning and movements in labor are recommended for other purposes than comfort, such as rotating an asynclitic fetus and correcting slow progress in dilation or descent.

Birthing Ball

Standard physiotherapy balls routinely used in physical therapy and exercise programs have permeated the labor setting. The woman can maintain an upright position by sitting on the ball or kneeling on the bed with her arms and chest draped over the ball. The rotation of the ball helps the mother to sway her hips side to side or in a circle. This movement helps to stretch her body and align a fetus from an asynclitic position. The birthing ball can facilitate position changes and be used as a comfort tool for women in labor. A woman can sit on it and rock or lightly bounce to decrease perineal pressure. She can also lean over the ball, decreasing back pain with an occiput posterior position. Birthing balls are one of the best tools for facilitating an upright position and can be used with an epidural only with assistance and support.

Touch and Massage

Touch in the form of hand holding, stroking, embracing, or patting communicates caring and reassurance. Cultural influences and personal factors may affect individual responses to touch; however, touch is universal and may soothe and reassure the laboring woman.

In hospitals, nurses have varying comfort levels with touch and may be more likely to advise support persons to provide the intervention. Usual touch by the nurse (only as necessary to perform clinical procedures) is different than comforting (nonclinical) touch. Perinatal nurses and others who provide support during labor use touch consciously and unconsciously throughout labor to communicate their support and presence, to relieve muscle tension, and to decrease the pain of labor. The interventions of touch and massage have not undergone sufficient scientific study to provide clear conclusions regarding benefits and risks. Some women appreciate touch and massage in labor, and these simple interventions may relieve pain and anxiety. The reaction of each woman should guide the nurse in the acceptability and value of these soothing measures (Declercq et al., 2007).

Interventions can be used by the perinatal nurse or other labor-support person to relieve back labor. These techniques include counter-pressure, bilateral hip pressure (e.g., double-hip squeeze), and the knee press (Simkin, 1995). These maneuvers are performed by applying localized pressure to reduce sacroiliac pain resulting from strain on sacroiliac ligaments caused by mechanisms of labor. Counter-pressure requires application of enough force to meet the intensity of

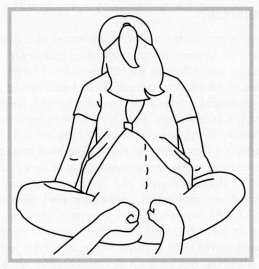

FIGURE 16–2. Firm counter-pressure of the fists on the lower back.

pressure from the fetal occipital bone against the sacrum (Fig. 16–2). Steady pressure from the heel of a support person's hand or another firm object counteracts the strain against the sacroiliac ligaments caused by the fetal occiput (Simkin, 1995).

Massage is the manipulation of the soft tissues of the body to enhance health and healing. Massage has been used to decrease fatigue, tension, emotional distress, and chronic and acute pain. Purposeful use of massage is employed during labor as a relaxation and stress-reduction technique. This technique is effective at reducing pain because it functions as a distraction, may stimulate cutaneous nerve fibers that block painful impulses, and stimulates the local release of endorphins (Gentz, 2001; Huntley, Coon, & Ernst, 2004). In two randomized controlled trials, where the experimental group received several massages during labor, self-reports of anxiety levels were the same in both groups, while nurses reported observing significantly less behavioral manifestations of pain (Chang, Wang, & Chen, 2002) and pain scores were significantly less during early and active labor (Chang, Chen, & Huang, 2006).

All forms of massage are accomplished with moderate pressure, activating large myelinated nerve fibers. Because habituation can occur, decreasing the beneficial effects of massage, the type of stroke and location should vary during labor. In a randomized controlled trial during which partners provided massage during labor, women reported significantly less pain and anxiety (Field, Hemandez-Reif, Taylor, Quintino, & Burman, 1997). Relaxation and massage have been shown to be factors in promoting labor progress, decreasing pain perception, and increasing the woman's ability to cope with labor (Zwelling, Johnson, & Allen, 2006).

Hydrotherapy

Hydrotherapy, or the use of warm water as a complimentary nonpharmacologic pain relief technique, may be desired and effective for the woman in labor. It is capable of promoting relaxation and decreasing pain without the risks caused by other treatments. Benfield, Herman, Katz, Wilson, and Davis (2001) published a small study of laboring women at 4-cm cervical dilation noting a therapeutic effect of decreased anxiety at 15 minutes of warm water immersion with an added benefit of decreased pain and anxiety at 60 minutes compared to nonbathers. A randomized controlled study of 108 women found the pain index scores among women who used the immersion bath were significantly lower than in those women without immersion (daSilva, deOliveira, & Nobre, 2009). Kiani (2009) concluded that a warm water pool can be an effective way to decrease labor pain and alleviate suffering especially during the first and second stages of labor. Numerous positive benefits have been shown by use of hydrotherapy (Cluett & Burns, 2009) and are listed in Display 16–5.

Positive benefits of water immersion include ease of positioning, buoyancy, hydrostatic pressure, and thermal relaxation. Hydrotherapy allows freedom of movement and helps facilitate maternal participation leading to a more normal labor process. Buoyancy in the tub allows for an almost weightless feeling, and women may have more opportunity to move during labor, which enhances progress due to the ease of movement. Using water immersion and covering the abdomen with warm water, the hydrostatic pressure of the water provides stability and relieves some of the pain associated with uterine contractions. In addition, hydrostatic pressure moves fluid from the extravascular to the intravascular spaces reducing blood pressure and edema and promoting diuresis (Florence & Palmer, 2003). Warm water provides soothing stimulation of nerves in the skin, promoting vasodilatation,

reversal of sympathetic nervous system response, and a reduction in catecholamine production (Florence & Palmer, 2003). Hydrotherapy is postulated to provide pain relief through the perception of warmth by the nerve receptors in skin. These nerve impulses travel to the cerebral cortex and initiate the gate mechanism, thereby decreasing pain perception. The potential combined effects of these changes are postulated to result in increased intravascular volume, improved uterine perfusion, decreased pain, decreased blood pressure due to vasodilatation, increased relaxation, and shortened labor (Simkin & O'Hara, 2002). The water temperature should be maintained between 36°C and 37°C (96.8°F and 98.6°F) to promote relaxation and maintain warmth. Warmer water may raise both maternal and fetal temperature and may lead to fetal tachycardia and elevated neonatal temperature (Simkin & O'Hara, 2002). Maternal effects of hydrotherapy include weakness, dizziness, nausea, tachycardia, or hypotension. These are usually related to an increase in body temperature or dehydration. Cool liquids should be provided to the mother to maintain her comfort, and hourly monitoring of the water temperature will help to maintain optimal temperature.

A repeated concern regarding the safety to the fetus is whether hydrotherapy can be used with ruptured membranes. Water does not enter the vagina during tub bathing. This topic has been studied with no increase in the incidence of chorioamnionitis, postpartum endometritis, neonatal infections, or need for antibiotics (Zwelling et al., 2006; Eriksson, Mattsson, & Ladfors, 1997).

Safety considerations including rapid draining of the water and movement to the birthing bed must be planned when immersion is used. A safety huddle including the woman and her support person, nurses, and provider staff should occur prior to entry to the tub, which includes expectations of duration of hydrotherapy, need for emergent exit, and avoidance of injury from falls. Tubs may be ordinary bathtubs, water-saving reclining tubs, or portable tubs. The manufacturer's recommendations and the hospital's infection control department are sources for appropriate cleaning and safety requirements.

If water immersion is not an option, hydrotherapy may be achieved in the form of a warm shower spray using a flexible hand-held unit guided by the mother, her support person, or the nurse. Aiming at the lower uterine segment, the warm stream of water may help to relieve the stretching sensations of the ligaments and promote local vasodilatation that facilitates muscle relaxation and reduces pain of tense muscles (Mackey, 2001). Significant others supporting the woman in labor can assist her by holding the shower wand and adjusting the temperature as needed. The mother may stand or sit in the shower on a supportive bench or chair as tolerated and desired, even for long periods of

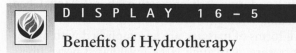

DISPLAY 16–5

Benefits of Hydrotherapy

- Pain and anxiety relief
- Increased diuresis
- Decreased edema
- Decreased blood pressure
- Enhanced fetal rotation due to increased buoyancy
- Faster cervical dilation
- Less use of intramuscular and intravenous medication
- Less use of epidural anesthesia
- Fewer operative births (vacuum and forceps)
- Less perineal trauma
- Fewer episiotomies

time. Whether in a tub or a shower, hydrotherapy is a proven means of relaxation and provides temporary pain relief in labor (Simkin & O'Hara, 2002).

Hospital resources may not accommodate immersion tubs or allow women to bring inflatable devices for use in labor or provide the opportunity to shower during labor. An alternative source of heat may be provided by the use of a hot water bottle, warm moist towel, heating pad, and chemical warm packs. Caution must be used when using external devices so that scalding of the skin does not occur. Hospital-established protocols may prohibit the use of external heating devices.

Cold compresses may be an option for the mother if heat is not preferable. An ice pack, frozen gel pack, cold towels, or chemical cool pack applied to the lower back may provide pain relief for the laboring woman. A cool cloth to the forehead, neck, or wrist areas may provide comfort. Cold may provide relief of musculoskeletal pain and may be an appropriate intervention to suggest if heat is not an option or desired.

The advantages of using thermal interventions as a nonpharmacologic method of pain relief may include a reduction and/or delay in the use of drugs, allowing the laboring woman to have a more active role in the labor process (Table 16–7). Hospital policies and culture may influence the use of hydrotherapy and other alternative methods of pain relief (Stark, Rudell, & Haus, 2008).

Hypnosis

Hypnosis is the induction of a deeply relaxed state based on the power of suggestion to encourage changes in behavior or relief of symptoms. Positive affirmations, suggestions, and visualizations to relax the body, guide thoughts, and control breathing are techniques used with hypnosis. A tape is often played to help the woman enter a calm state of self-hypnosis. Common hypnotic pain relief techniques are "glove anesthesia" in which the woman imagines that her hand is numb and that it can spread numbness to other areas by placing her hand on painful areas. Other techniques interpret the contractions as acceptable and powerful surges of energy that cause only a light pressure sensation (Ketterhagen, VandeVusse, & Berner, 2002). A systematic review of hypnosis for pain relief in labor including randomized control trials found that the need for analgesics was reduced; however, bias was found in many studies (Cyna, McAuliffe, & Andrew, 2004). Hypnosis as a means of reducing pain relief in labor cannot be recommended until further studies have been performed.

Music

Music can be used during labor as a distraction and to provide a focus. Evidence suggests that the perception

and response to pain and music travel through the same neural pathways in the limbic system and that use of particular types of music perceived as relaxing may decrease anxiety associated with the perception of pain (Browning, 2000). Familiar music associated with restful or pleasant recollections may be an adjunct to relaxation and imagery to manage the pain of labor.

Music creates an atmosphere in the birthing room that also may change the approach of healthcare professionals to laboring women. Perinatal nurses and physicians become more relaxed, slow their activities, and respond with increased respect for the unique personal event in progress (DiFranco, 2000). When women use earphones or headsets to listen to music, the music provides a distraction and the woman is in constant control of the volume. Ultimately, choosing music that helps her relax or improve her mood will give the woman a greater sense of control.

Music can be effective at increasing pain tolerance or cue to woman to move or breathe rhythmically. Most studies, however, lack significance or validate benefits (DiFranco, 2000).

Yoga

Yoga, a method of India origin, proposes control of the body and mind. Energy yoga uses special training of breathing, achieves changes in levels of consciousness, relaxation, and inner peace. Supporters claim that yoga shortens the duration of labor, decreases pain, and reduces the need of analgesic medication (Tournaire & Theau-Yonneau, 2007).

Intradermal Injections of Sterile Water

Intradermal injections of sterile water (IISW) to control the pain of labor was first introduced in obstetric literature in the late 1980s and uses counter-irritation to offset localized pain in the same dermatome distribution. Four small intradermal injections of 0.05 to 0.1 mL of sterile water are done with a 1-mL syringe and a 25-gauge needle to form four small blebs. These subdermal injections are placed over the sacrum of a woman's back, one over each posterior superior iliac spine and two others 3 cm below and 1 cm medial to each of the first sites (Fig. 16–3). Exact locations of the injections do not appear to be critical to its success (Simkin & Bolding, 2004). Although it is not totally understood how this technique relieves the lower back pain associated with the first stage of labor, the Gate Control Theory is a plausible explanation. Sterile water causes distension of the skin, which irritates nerve endings, blocking other painful sensations (Huntley et al., 2004).

One hour after women with lower back pain were given IISW, they reported less pain (Martensson & Wallin, 1999) or no pain (Lytzen, Cederberg,

Table 16–7. HYDROTHERAPY IN LABOR

Clinical Practice	Referenced Rationale
1. Warm water immersion using a tub may be considered as a complimentary therapy for pain relief of the laboring women meeting the following eligibility criteria: • 37 weeks' or greater gestation • Cephalic presentation, singleton • 30-minute Category I FHR tracing prior to tub entry • Active labor	The use of hydrotherapy during labor, whether in a shower or a tub, is a proven means of relaxation and pain relief (Cluett & Burns, 2009; Royal College of Obstetricians and Gynaecologists [RCOG], 2006). The warm water stimulates the release of endorphins, relaxes muscles to decrease tension, stimulates large-diameter nerve fibers to close the gate on pain, and promotes better circulation and oxygenation (Garland & Jones, 1997).
2. If baseline FHR >160 or maternal temp >100.4°F develops during water immersion, the water should be cooled or the mother assisted out of the tub to cool. If fetal tachycardia or elevated temperature persists despite these measures, the mother should not return to the tub, and the MD/CNM notified.	Fetal tachycardia may be a result of maternal hyperthermia since there were no differences for Apgar score less than 7 at 5 min, neonatal unit admissions, or neonatal infection rates when immersion was used. (Cluett & Burns, 2009).
3. FHR may be auscultated or telemetry used according to the institution's fetal monitoring protocol while in the tub or shower.	Changes in water temperature by as little as 2°F have been noted to be associated with impact on maternal heart rate, cardiac output, diastolic blood pressure, and core body temperature. Recommended temperature to avoid potentially harmful effects is 96.0°–98.6°F/36°–37°C (Florence & Palmer, 2003; Eriksson, Ladfors, Mattsson, & Fall, 1996)
4. Water temperature should remain between 96.0° and 98.6°F (36°–37°C). The water temperature is documented every hour while the patient is in the tub. Water in the tub should cover the maternal abdomen.	With relaxation and comfort, stress hormone production may decrease. Increased comfort with submersion and decreased stress hormone production may improve uterine contractility. In a study of nulliparas with dystocia, immersion in water reduced the rate of labor augmentation without resulting in longer labors (Cluett, Pickering, Getliffe, St. James, & Saunders, 2004).
5. Vital signs are checked and documented according to hospital protocol.	Cervical dilation at the onset of the bath may indirectly influence the duration of labor. Use of the tub early in labor may result in a longer duration of the bath and suppression of the posterior gland's production of oxytocin (Cluett & Burns, 2009; Nikodem, 2004).
6. Ambulation and other nonpharmacologic measures are recommended until cervical dilation is 4–5 cm and contraction pattern is well established. Earlier entry into the tub may slow the progress of labor.	Frequency of fetal monitoring should be consistent with recognized standards of care and institutional policies and based on the stage of labor. When cervical dilation was 5 cm or greater upon entry to the tub, a decreased used of oxytocin, epidural analgesia, and shorter labor resulted (Eriksson et al., 1996).
7. Provide hydration for the mother with cold/cool drinks (e.g., water, juice, sport drinks, any clear liquid).	Several physiologic changes occur with immersion in warm water. Buoyancy allows for support of extremities, while hydrostatic pressure gives equal resistance to all muscle groups, providing stability. This support and stability allow for freedom of movement and a sense of weightlessness that may encourage movement (Simkin & O'Hara, 2002). Women with a normal, uncomplicated labor may drink modest amounts of clear liquids such as water, fruit juice without pulp, carbonated beverages, clear tea, black coffee, and sports drinks (ACOG, 2009c).
8. If an IV is started, protect the site with plastic covering.	The data on IV fluids type and infusion rate are insufficient for a strong recommendation (Berghella, Baxter, & Chauhan, 2008).
9. Water is changed or the patient is removed from the tub if excessive feces or debris accumulates during labor that cannot be easily removed with a tropical fish net.	Contraindications include thick meconium, oxytocin infusion, bleeding or large bloody show, epidural analgesia or anesthesia, and nonreassuring fetal status.
10. Use of water immersion for labor is documented in the medical record.	Documentation and record keeping is a fundamental part of clinical practice (Williams, Davies, & Ross, 2009). Warm water may cause dizziness, and a decrease in catecholamine release will decrease blood pressure.
11. Support person or member of the nursing staff should be present at all times. Shower seat should be available in the shower for the laboring woman as well as a seat outside of the shower or tub for their support person.	Labor support is essential, especially for the woman with an unmedicated labor.

CNM, certified nurse midwife; FHR, fetal heart rate; IV, intravenous; MD, medical doctor.

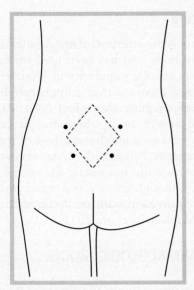

FIGURE 16–3. Location of injection sites in relation to the Michaelis rhomboid for intradermal injections of sterile water. (From Martensson, L. & Wallin, G. [1999]. Labor pain treated with cutaneous injections of sterile water: A randomized controlled trial. *British Journal of Obstetrics and Gynecology, 106*[7], 634.)

& Moller-Nielsen, 1989). In randomized controlled clinical trials, when the effect of IISW was compared with injections of normal saline, women receiving the sterile water reported less pain at 45 minutes (Bahasadri, Ahmadi-Abhari, Dehghani-Nik, & Habibi, 2006), 1 hour (Trolle, Moller, Kronborg, & Thomsen, 1991), and 2 hours after the injections were given (Wiruchpongsanon, 2006). When IISW was compared with transcutaneous electrical nerve stimulation (TENS) or standard care such as back massage, whirlpool bath, or position change, women receiving IISW reported less pain than those using TENS or receiving standard care (Labrecque, Nouwen, Bergeron, & Rancourt, 1999). Although the studies included random assignment of participants to a treatment or control group, a major limitation of all studies of TENS and IISW was inadequate sample size to detect significant differences.

The advantages of IISW include the following:

- Can be performed by a registered nurse
- Is not a technically difficult procedure
- Provides one more strategy for pain control
- Can be repeated as often as needed

The only side effect associated with the procedure is intense stinging pain at the time of injection that lasts about 30 seconds and a hyperemic zone around the papule that lasts for several hours after injection (Lytzen et al., 1989). This method may be an alternative for women with lower back pain but who wish to avoid epidural analgesia. Pain relief is noted for 45 to 120 minutes.

COGNITIVE TECHNIQUES ALTERING PAIN PERCEPTION

Relaxation

Achieving a state of relaxation is the basis of all nonpharmacologic interventions during labor. Women benefit from a state of relaxation because it conserves energy rather than creating fatigue from the prolonged tension of voluntary muscles. Relaxation enhances the effectiveness of nonpharmacologic and pharmacologic pain-management strategies. Relaxation is a skill and a physical state. The degree of relaxation a woman can achieve will influence the amount of anxiety she feels. Many women are first introduced to these skills during childbirth classes. How well they learn and are able to use these skills depends on quality of instruction, the amount of time they practice, and their belief that this technique can be beneficial. Relaxation is as contagious as panic, tension, and feelings of being overwhelmed. Relaxation skills cannot be taught during active labor, but an environment that promotes relaxation can be created by the perinatal nurse (Display 16–6). When actually faced with the forces of labor, women who learned relaxation techniques during childbirth classes will need the presence of an informed perinatal nurse to reinforce and encourage the use of these techniques during labor.

Guided Imagery

Guided imagery is a relaxation technique using visualization to purposely direct thoughts to relieve stress and provide a sense of relief. Childbirth educators teach imagery as a skill, encouraging expectant women

---

D I S P L A Y   1 6 – 6

Creating a Relaxed Environment During Labor

- Control the amount of light, noise, and interruptions.
- Maintain an unhurried demeanor.
- Use a calm, soft, slow voice.
- Recognize the signs of tension:
  - Changes in voice
  - Frowning
  - Clenched fists
  - Stiff, straight posture
  - Tense arms or legs
  - Stiff, raised shoulders
- Maintain eye contact.
- Use touch or massage if this is acceptable to the woman.
- Sit, rather than stand, next to the woman.
- Introduce caregivers to the woman and her support partner.
- Respect the birth plan.

to focus on pleasant scenes or experiences to increase their level of relaxation. Nurses encourage women to use imagery by making statements such as "think of the baby moving through the birth canal," "think of the baby moving down and out," and "think about the cervix gently opening like a flower one petal at a time." Imagery is used to keep women focused and to encourage the use of the contraction as a stimulus for strength and power.

Attention Focusing and Distraction

During early labor, distraction is an effective strategy. Distraction is the process by which stimuli from the environment draw a woman's attention away from her pain. Walking in the hallway, sitting in a chair, talking with visitors, watching television, playing cards, and using the telephone keep laboring women occupied. Most women reach a point during labor when they no longer are able to talk comfortably through contractions. Labor is hard work that requires intense concentration to maintain a sense of control. Women are helped to concentrate by focusing on an object in the room or a support person's face or eyes. Attention focusing involves deliberate, intentional activities on the part of the laboring woman. These activities include patterned breathing and visualization or imagery.

Patterned Breathing

Breathing techniques are usually taught in prenatal classes and are used as a distraction during labor to decrease pain and promote relaxation. On admission, the perinatal nurse reviews with the woman and her support person the specific techniques they were taught in prenatal class. If a woman has not attended class, early labor is the time to discuss and practice a slow, controlled breathing pattern.

Most women are taught to take a deep breath at the beginning of a contraction. This breath ensures oxygen to the mother and baby, signals to people in the room that a contraction is beginning, and stretches and tenses respiratory muscles. Exhaling this breath relaxes respiratory muscles and voluntary muscles. At some point during labor, perinatal nurses may find it necessary to breathe synchronously with a couple through several contractions. Women are encouraged to breathe slowly. However, as labor pain increases, women may need to use a lighter, more accelerated breathing (i.e., no more than two times their normal rate). Alternatively, a pant–blow method of breathing, in which a woman takes three to four light panting breaths followed by an exhale (i.e., blow), may be used. When attempting to control the urge to push, a rapid and shallow breathing pattern may be helpful.

Acupuncture

Acupuncture is the insertion of fine needles into specific areas of the body and has been used for centuries in China and is gaining popularity in Western countries. One proposed theory is that acupuncture blocks pain stimuli from reaching the spinal cord. Acupuncture might have benefit as an alternative or complement to patients who seek another method of pain relief in labor (Florence & Palmer, 2003). Another study found that acupuncture did not reduce the need for epidural anesthesia, although there was a trend toward lower analgesic requirement with no detrimental impact on outcome (MacKenzie et al., 2011).

THE PHARMACOLOGIC MODEL

The pharmacologic model of care views pain as pathologic and seeks to reduce pain to an acceptable patient threshold. Pain generally signals a potential threat, which should be eased or eliminated. Labor pain, however, does not usually indicate pathology, but rather a signal that normal labor is progressing. Alleviation and control of pain are of major importance in medicine. The American College of Obstetricians and Gynecologists (ACOG) and the American Society of Anesthesiologists (ASA) agree that pain management should be offered to the laboring woman (ASA, 2009b). The decision for pain management should be based on the patient's preference in collaboration with her obstetric provider. ACOG and ASA published a joint statement in which both organizations supported a woman's right to adequate pain relief in labor:

> Labor causes severe pain for many women. There is no other circumstance where it is considered acceptable to an individual to experience untreated severe pain, amenable to safe intervention, while under a physician's care. In the absence of a medical contraindication, maternal request is a sufficient medical indication for pain relief during labor. Pain management should be provided whenever medically indicated. (ASA, 2009b; ACOG, 2002)

The ASA has conducted series of surveys over the past 20 years revealing an overall increase in the use of regional analgesia and a decrease in the percentage of women receiving either parenteral or no analgesia during labor in all hospitals regardless of volume of births (Bucklin, Hawkins, Anderson, & Ullrich, 2005). The reported use of neuraxial anesthesia is more than 70% in women who give birth in U.S. hospitals with a delivery volume greater than 1,500 deliveries per year, perhaps because parenteral analgesia has limited effectiveness and a greater potential for neonatal toxicity (Briggs & Wan, 2006). The use of pain-relieving drugs during labor is now part of standard care in many countries throughout the world (Ullman, Smith, Burns, Mori, & Dowswell, 2010). The patterns of pain may vary during the day, with peak and trough times reported at different times of the day. Therapeutic effects of opioids and local anesthetics also demonstrate circadian variations (Touitou, Dispersyn, & Pain, 2010).

The woman should clearly understand the benefits and potential maternal–fetal side effects of pharmacologic methods. This information is best discussed during the prenatal period with her obstetric provider. During labor, the woman may be exhausted, distressed, and not coping. She may feel remorseful following the birth if pharmacologic methods were not in her birth plan, or may suffer from posttraumatic stress disorder if the pain was unrelenting (Flink et al., 2009). Postpartum depression may be more common when analgesia is not used (Hawkins, 2010). The neuraxial procedure and potential complications must be discussed between the anesthesiologist, obstetric care provider, and the woman with sufficient time for her questions to be answered. Some institutions provide the opportunity for women to meet with an anesthesia provider before admission. Without this type of preparation, obtaining true informed consent from a woman in active labor is practically impossible. The perinatal nurse assesses preferences for pain management on admission and conducts ongoing assessments of factors influencing pain perception throughout labor.

Pharmacologic pain management strategies used during labor include sedatives and hypnotics, parenteral opioids, local anesthesia, and neuraxial analgesia. Using pain medications during labor brings with it unique concerns that are not faced in other clinical areas. These include concerns about the effects medications may have on the course and outcome of labor and the fetus or newborn. Women experiencing prolonged latent labor may benefit from the brief period of therapeutic rest or sleep.

SEDATIVES AND HYPNOTICS

The term *sedative–hypnotic* describes the effect this group of medications has on the individual; it is not a classification of drug. The effects of these drugs are dose related. In low doses, they cause sedation, and higher doses cause a hypnotic effect. Two classifications of drugs used in labor to provide sedative–hypnotic effects are barbiturates and H_1-receptor antagonists (i.e., antihistamines).

Historically, women experiencing prolonged latent labor were thought to benefit from the brief period of therapeutic rest or sleep following administration of barbiturates. Barbiturates such as secobarbital sodium (Seconal) and pentobarbital (Nembutal) given orally or as an intramuscular injection have little analgesic action, depress the central nervous system, decrease anxiety, and can potentiate respiratory depression (Faucher & Brucker, 2000). Barbiturates are lipid soluble, easily cross the placenta, and have a long

half-life. Seconal has been found in maternal and fetal blood samples for up to 40 hours after administration and therefore is rarely used in modern-day obstetrics (Florence & Palmer, 2003).

Zolpidem tartrate (Ambien) is unrelated to barbiturates but possesses the sedative and hypnotic properties of benzodiazepines. The usual dosage of 5 to 10 mg has a mean peak blood concentration of 1.6 hours and half-life of 1.4 to 4.5 hours. This drug may enable the exhausted woman to rest and recover from hypertonic uterine dysfunction or prolonged latent phase so that she is better able to cope with active labor (Florence & Palmer, 2003).

H_1-receptor antagonists include promethazine hydrochloride (Phenergan), hydroxyzine hydrochloride (Vistaril), and propiomazine (Largon). These medications may be administered with narcotics during labor to relieve anxiety, increase sedation, and decrease nausea and vomiting. Promethazine hydrochloride can cause respiratory depression and, if combined with an opioid, may cause hypotension and sedation leading to a fall risk should the woman ambulate (Poole, 2003). H_1-receptor antagonists traditionally have been thought to potentiate the effects of narcotics; however, there is no objective evidence to support this belief (Wakefield, 1999). Although all H_1-receptor antagonists have a sedative effect on the woman in labor, they do cross the placenta, but do not appear to increase neonatal depression (Althaus & Wax, 2005).

Inhalational Analgesia

Inhalational analgesia is provided by breathing in subanesthetic concentrations of volatile agents, the aim being that the mother should remain conscious with preservation of her laryngeal reflexes (O'Sullivan, 2010). Nitrous oxide administered as Entonox (a 50:50 oxygen:nitrous oxide mixture) is given via a demand valve connected to a facemask or mouthpiece. This form of analgesia is widely used in the United Kingdom, Australia, Finland, and Canada; however, it is used very little in the United States. The efficacy and safety of nitrous oxide for labor analgesia has not been recently evaluated. Rosen (2002) concluded in a review of 11 randomized controlled trials that current published work does not provide clear quantitative objective evidence of the analgesic efficacy of nitrous oxide. The peak analgesic effect of nitrous oxide lags behind the start of its administration by 50 seconds, out of synchronization with typical peak and duration of a uterine contraction. Uterine contractions usually peak at 30 seconds and, with the disproportionate delay of nitrous onset, the opportune time for analgesic effects is missed. Studies designed to determine the best techniques for its intermittent administration to attain the highest concentrations at the time of peak pain during a contraction are indicated (Rosen, 2002). Maternal satisfaction has been reported in about half of cases, and there is no clear qualitative evidence of the efficacy in relieving labor pain (Tournaire & Theau-Yonneau, 2007).

The effects on human fetuses exposed to nitrous oxide or other anesthetic agents in utero are unknown (Rosen, 2002). Nitrous oxide administration does not affect uterine activity and thus would not be expected to affect the course of the first and second stage of labor or rate of cesarean birth. Nitrous oxide readily passes across the placenta; however, there is little apparent effect on Apgar scores, acid–base balance, and neurologic and adaptive capacity scores (Reynolds, 2010).

Environmental pollution occurs frequently during inhaled administration, and healthcare workers are often exposed to levels of nitrous oxide in excess of occupational exposure limits (Sanders, Weimann, & Maze, 2008). Although the long-term effects on the health of workers are unclear, there may be an increased risk of adverse reproductive outcomes in healthcare workers due to occupational exposure. This may pose health risks to exposed healthcare workers and other participants in the mother's care, and may contribute significantly to global warming. Nitrous oxide is a greenhouse gas and because it is inert in the body, all used gas will ultimately escape into the atmosphere. The impact of the medical use of nitrous oxide on the greenhouse effect is less than 0.05% and produces less than 1% of the entire nitrous oxide in the atmosphere (Volmanen, Palomaki, & Ahonen, 2011).

Although nitrous oxide has a long history of safe use, the resulting maternal hypoxemia may put an "at-risk" fetus in jeopardy. Opportunities for continued research on nitrous oxide to include techniques to improve the timing of administration to better coincide with the pain of uterine contraction, safety of administration by nonanesthesia personnel, the efficacy of additional coadministered methods to improve analgesia, and the development of methods to better measure the degree of maternal pain relief when nitrous oxide is used during labor (Rosen, 2002).

PARENTERAL OPIOIDS

The use of opiates in labor is approximately 40% to 56% both in the United States and the United Kingdom (Ullman et al., 2010). Women not willing or not able to utilize the neuraxial technique may choose parenteral opioids. Advantages include cost, ease of availability, and administration. The greatest risk of harm is to the fetus related to placental transfer and longer half-life due to reduced neonatal metabolism. Any drug present in maternal blood and transferred to the central nervous system must readily cross the blood–brain barrier and therefore also the placenta (Reynolds, 2010; Florence & Palmer, 2003). Opioids provide less effective pain relief than neuraxial analgesia and have direct pharmacologic effects on the fetus and newborn. Opioids have been shown to cause neonatal respiratory depression with lower Apgar and neurobehavioral scores. The greatest risk occurs if it is administered 2 to 3 hours prior to delivery.

There are three types of drugs that may be parenterally administered during labor: opioids (morphine and meperidine), synthetic opioids (fentanyl and remifentanil), and opioid agonist-antagonists (butorphanol and nalbuphine). These drugs bind to one of four receptor sites (mu, kappa, sigma, or delta) on nerve cells located in the brain and spinal cord. Table 16–8 highlights

Table 16–8. PARENTERAL OPIOID AGENTS USED IN LABOR AND THEIR RECEPTOR-BINDING RELATIONSHIPS

Receptor	Receptor Properties	Medication
Mu	Supraspinal analgesia Respiratory depression Euphoria Physical dependence	Morphine Meperidine Butorphanol (weak) Fentanyl Sufentanil Remifentanil Alfentanil
Kappa	Spinal analgesia Miosis Sedation Slight respiratory depression	Morphine (weak) Butorphanol Nalbuphine
Sigma	Dysphoria Hallucinations Respiratory and vasomotor stimulation May not mediate analgesia	Butorphanol (partial) Nalbuphine Fentanyl (partial)
Delta	Spinal analgesia and smooth muscle relaxation	Morphine (weak) Codeine (weak)

Adapted from Faucher, M. A., & Brucker, M. C. (2000). Intrapartum pain: Pharmacologic management. *Journal of Obstetric, Gynecologic, and Neonatal Nursing, 29*(2), 169–180.

the most commonly used opioids and their receptor-binding patterns. Individual drugs have an affinity for one or more receptor sites, which accounts for differences in pharmacodynamics and side effects. Depending on the dose, route of administration, and stage of labor, parenteral analgesia does not eliminate pain, but instead causes a blunting effect, inducing somnolence and decreasing the perception of pain, allowing women to relax and rest between contractions. Table 16–9 lists parenteral opioid analgesics used in labor including dose, route of administration, onset of action, time of peak effect, and duration of action. After administration of these medications, the frequency and duration of contractions may decrease (Althaus & Wax, 2005). For this reason, parenteral analgesia is usually not administered until a labor pattern is well established. Following administration, some women experience a short period of decreased uterine activity followed by an increase in uterine activity. Both effects may be the result of decreased anxiety and serum concentrations of catecholamines (Mussell, 1998). When given during labor, these medications often cause women to doze between contractions. If medication administration does result in dozing, coaching by a support person or nurse is important to help the woman anticipate and recognize the beginning of a contraction rather than have her startled awake at the peak of a contraction. Opioids readily cross the placenta by passive diffusion leading to minimal variability on the FHR baseline. These drugs have consequences for the infant with resulting respiratory depression, inhibited suckling at the breast, and decreased alertness (Ullman et al., 2010). The opioid choice for analgesia in labor is dependent on what is available and customary in each hospital. There is insufficient evidence to support the choice of one opioid over another (Ullman et al., 2010).

Morphine and meperidine have a strong affinity for mu receptors, resulting in effective analgesia and dose-dependent respiratory depression. Opioids readily cross the placenta and can have a cumulative effect, increasing the potential for maternal and neonatal respiratory depression as the woman receives more medication. Morphine sulfate may cause allergic reactions in sulfite-sensitive people, which is more common in women with asthma. Morphine may be used during a prolonged period of early labor to rest prior to active labor. Neonatal side effects are related to dosage and timing of administration. Because of the potential for neonatal respiratory depression, the timing of administration relative to birth of the newborn is important. Ideally, birth should occur within 1 hour or after 4 hours following administration (Althaus & Wax, 2005). Many clinical sites have abandoned the use of meperidine during labor because of untoward effects. In the fetus, breathing movements, muscular activity, oxygen saturation, and variability are all reduced following administration of meperidine. Neonatal effects may be apparent for the first few hours and include reduced oxygen saturation, increased CO_2 levels, acidosis, decreased suckling leading to impaired breastfeeding, and diminished thermoregulation (Reynolds, 2010). In addition, the metabolite normeperidine has a prolonged half-life, up to 60 hours in the neonate, and may affect neonatal behavior regardless of the timing of administration to the mother (Reynolds, 2010).

Naloxone hydrochloride (Narcan), a narcotic antagonist, reverses the respiratory depression caused by parenteral narcotics received by the mother within the past 4 hours. It is administered to the newborn who continues to experience respiratory depression after positive pressure ventilation has restored a normal heart rate (American Heart Association & American Academy of Pediatrics [AAP], 2010). In a randomized controlled trial comparing neonatal outcomes using meperidine and fentanyl during labor, significantly fewer neonates required resuscitation and naloxone hydrochloride in

Table 16–9. PARENTERAL OPIOID DOSING

Drug	Dose	Route	Onset of Action (min)	Peak Effect (min)	Duration of Action (hr)
Meperidine (Demerol)	50–100 mg	IM	50	40–50	2–4
	25–50 mg	IV	10	5–10	2–4
Morphine	5–10 mg	IM	10–20	60–90	4–6
	1–2 mg	IV	3–5	20	4–6
Butorphanol (Stadol)	2–4 mg	IM	10–30	30–60	3–4
	1–2 mg	IV	1–2	2–3	3–4
Nalbuphine (Nubain)	0.2 mg/kg	IM	15	60	3–6
	0.1–0.2 mg/kg	IV	2–3	30	3–6
Fentanyl (Sublimaze)	50–100 mg	IM	7–15	20–30	1–2
	25–50 mg	V	2–3	3–5	0.5–1
Remifentanil	20 mcg	V (PCA)	1	1	15 min

IM, intramuscular; IV, intravascular; PCA, patient-controlled analgesia; V, vascular.

the group whose mothers received fentanyl (Rayburn, Smith, Parriott, & Woods, 1989). Naloxone should not be given to infants of mothers who are addicted or who are suspected of being addicted to narcotics or who are in a methadone treatment program. In these infants, naloxone can cause neonatal seizures.

The synthetic opioids, fentanyl and remifentanil, have advantages of short duration of action, intravenous pharmacologic action, and are suited for systemic labor analgesia. Remifentanil rapidly transfers across the placenta and is metabolized rapidly in the fetus; therefore, neonatal depression is avoided. These synthetic opioids do not cause as much sedation, nausea, and emesis as in patients who are experienced with opioids (Reynolds, 2010). The time to peak effect of fentanyl is 3 to 4 minutes, it is well tolerated, and is administered using a patient-controlled analgesia (PCA) pump. Remifentanil is a more expensive, novel μ-receptor agonist that has been used in obstetric anesthesia and analgesia for almost 10 years. It is preferred for the rapid onset of effect (approximately 1 minute), rapid degradation, and elimination in the fetus. It does not accumulate even after prolonged administration. Efficacy and safety in labor are well established; however, fetal and maternal monitoring are required with this drug (Evron & Ezri, 2007; Hinova & Fernando, 2009; Volmanen et al., 2011). Remifentanil regimen requires close maternal monitoring (suggested 1:1 nursing ratio), continuous oxygen saturation monitoring, and a dedicated intravenous cannula for this particular drug administration (Hinova & Fernando, 2009; Volmanen et al., 2011). No study has identified an increased incidence of indeterminate or abnormal FHR recording after remifentanil has been used for labor analgesia, and no neonate has required naloxone after delivery (D'Onofrio, Novelli, Mecacci, & Scarselli, 2009; Hinova & Fernando, 2009). There is evidence supporting the analgesic effects and suitability of synthetic opioids for first-stage labor analgesia, especially for laboring women who refuse or cannot receive neuraxial analgesia.

Neuraxial analgesia has progressed significantly since first introduced for labor, and the quality of research methodology continues to improve over time resulting in safe patient outcomes (Hong, 2010). Butorphanol (Stadol) and Nalbuphine (Nubain), with affinity for the kappa and sigma receptors, provide effective analgesia with less respiratory depression. Agonist–antagonists have limited effect on maternal respiratory depression, regardless of the number of doses (Althaus & Wax, 2005). The advantage of the agonist–antagonists is the "ceiling effect" related to maternal respiratory depression. Intravenous butorphanol and nalbuphine during labor have been associated with transient sinusoidal-like FHR patterns during labor (ACOG, 2009a). This nonpathologic sinusoidal pattern may be noted for 10 to 90 minutes but without any adverse neonatal outcomes

(Florence & Palmer, 2003). Because it can increase blood pressure, butorphanol should be avoided if the woman has hypertension or preeclampsia (ACOG, 2009b). Nalbuphine, if administered to an opioid-dependent person, can precipitate drug withdrawal symptoms because of its strong antagonist effect at the mu receptor site.

NEURAXIAL ANALGESIA

Neuraxial analgesia has progressed significantly since first introduced for labor, and the quality of research methodology continues to improve over time resulting in safe patient outcomes (Hong, 2010). Neuraxial analgesia in labor can be initiated with an epidural, spinal, or a combined spinal epidural (CSE) technique, which combines a local anesthetic and opioid analgesic introduced into the lumbar epidural space. The goal of neuraxial analgesia techniques during labor is to provide sufficient analgesia effect with as little motor block as possible. With the discovery of spinal cord opioid receptors in the late 1970s and the use of spinal and epidural opioids, pain management in labor was transformed from anesthesia to analgesia. Lower concentrations of local anesthetic, in combination with narcotics such as fentanyl (Sublimaze), sufentanil (Sufenta), alfentanil (Alfenta), and remifentanil (Ultiva), result in increased pain relief without significant motor block (ASA, 2007b). Of the various pharmacologic methods available for use during labor, neuraxial analgesia techniques are the most flexible and effective, and they result in the least central nervous system depression of the mother and neonate (ACOG, 2004). Because parenteral analgesia has limited effectiveness and a greater potential for neonatal toxicity, many women in labor today receive neuraxial analgesia (Briggs & Wan, 2006). The ACOG Committee on Obstetrical Practice and the ASA Committee on Obstetric Anesthesia collaborated to update a position statement on the optimal goals for anesthesia care in obstetrics (Display 16–7).

When randomized controlled clinical trials were conducted to evaluate the effects of patient-controlled epidural analgesia (PCEA) with patient-controlled intravenous opioid analgesia (PCIA), the group using PCIA required more antiemetics, reported more sedation, and newborns required more resuscitation, received naloxone more often (Halpern et al., 2004), and had lower 1-minute Apgar scores (Wong et al., 2005), while the PCEA group had lower pain scores (Halpern et al., 2004; Wong et al., 2005) and higher patient satisfaction scores (Halpern et al., 2004). In addition, studies have demonstrated that there was no difference in the rate of cesarean birth rate or operative vaginal birth between women receiving PCEA or PCIA (Halpern et al., 2004; Wong et al., 2005). When the length of labor was compared for women receiving PCEA and PCIA, labor for the PCEA group was longer,

DISPLAY 16-7

Optimal Goals for Anesthesia Care in Obstetrics

I. Availability of a licensed practitioner who is credentialed to administer an appropriate anesthetic whenever necessary. For many women, regional anesthesia (epidural, spinal, or combined spinal epidural) will be the most appropriate anesthetic.

II. Availability of a licensed practitioner who is credentialed to maintain support of vital functions during any obstetric emergency.

III. Availability of anesthesia and surgical personnel to permit the start of a cesarean delivery within 30 minutes of the decision to perform the procedure; in cases of vaginal birth after cesarean (VBAC), appropriate facilities and personnel, including obstetric anesthesia, nursing personnel, and a physician capable of monitoring labor and performing cesarean delivery, immediately available during active labor to perform emergency cesarean delivery. The definition of immediate availability of personnel and facilities remains a local decision, based on each institution's available resources and geographic location.

IV. Appointment of a qualified anesthesiologist to be responsible for all anesthetics administered. There are obstetric units where obstetricians or obstetrician-supervised nurse anesthetists administer anesthetics. The administration of general or regional anesthesia requires both medical judgment and technical skills. Thus, a physician with privileges in anesthesiology should be readily available.

Persons administering or supervising obstetric anesthesia should be qualified to manage the infrequent but occasionally life-threatening complications of major regional anesthesia such as respiratory and cardiovascular failure, toxic local anesthetic convulsions, or vomiting and aspiration. Mastering and retaining the skills and knowledge necessary to manage these complications require adequate training and frequent application.

To ensure the safest and most effective anesthesia for obstetric patients, the director of anesthesia services, with the approval of the medical staff, should develop and enforce written policies regarding provision of obstetric anesthesia such as the following:

I. Availability of a qualified physician with obstetrical privileges to perform operative vaginal or cesarean delivery during administration of anesthesia. Regional and/or general anesthesia should not be administered until the patient has been examined and the fetal status and progress of labor evaluated by a qualified individual. A physician with obstetrical privileges who has knowledge of the maternal and fetal status and the progress of labor, and who approves the initiation of labor anesthesia, should be readily available to deal with any obstetric complications that may arise.

II. Availability of equipment, facilities, and support personnel equal to that provided in the surgical suite. This should include the availability of a properly equipped and staffed recovery room capable of receiving and caring for all patients recovering from major regional or general anesthesia. Birthing facilities, when used for analgesia or anesthesia, must be appropriately equipped to provide safe anesthetic care during labor and delivery or post-anesthesia recovery care.

III. Personnel other than the surgical team should be immediately available to assume responsibility for resuscitation of

a depressed newborn. The surgeon and anesthesiologist are responsible for the mother and may not be able to leave her care for the newborn, even when a regional anesthetic is functioning adequately. Individuals qualified to perform neonatal resuscitation should demonstrate the following:

A. Proficiency in rapid and accurate evaluation of the newborn condition, including Apgar scoring.

B. Knowledge of the pathogenesis of a depressed newborn (acidosis, drugs, hypovolemia, trauma, anomalies, and infection), as well as specific indications for resuscitation.

C. Proficiency in newborn airway management, laryngoscopy, endotracheal intubations, suctioning of airways, artificial ventilation, cardiac massage, and maintenance of thermal stability.

In larger maternity units and those functioning as high-risk centers, 24-hour in-house anesthesia, obstetric, and neonatal specialists are usually necessary. Preferably, the obstetric anesthesia services should be directed by an anesthesiologist with special training or experience in obstetric anesthesia. These units will also frequently require the availability of more sophisticated monitoring equipment and specially trained nursing personnel.

A survey jointly sponsored by the ASA and ACOG found that many hospitals in the United States have not yet achieved the previous goals. Deficiencies were most evident in smaller delivery units, which are typical in some geographic locations. Currently, approximately 50% of hospitals providing obstetric care have fewer than 500 deliveries per year. Providing comprehensive care for obstetric patients in these small units is extremely inefficient, not cost-effective, and frequently impossible. Thus, the following recommendations are made:

1. Whenever possible, consolidate small units.
2. When geographic factors require the existence of smaller units, these units should be part of a well-established regional perinatal system.

The availability of the appropriate personnel to assist in the management of a variety of obstetric problems is a necessary feature of good obstetric care. The presence of a pediatrician or other trained physician at a high-risk cesarean delivery to care for the newborn or the availability of an anesthesiologist during active labor and delivery when VBAC is attempted, and at a breech or twin delivery are examples. Frequently, these professionals spend a considerable amount of time standing by for the possibility that their services may be needed emergently but may ultimately not be required to perform the tasks for which they are present. Reasonable compensation for these standby services is justifiable and necessary.

A variety of other mechanisms have been suggested to increase the availability and quality of anesthesia services in obstetrics. Improved hospital design to place labor and delivery suites closer to the operating rooms would allow for more efficient supervision of nurse anesthetists. Anesthesia equipment in the labor and delivery area must be comparable to that in the operating room.

Finally, good interpersonal relations between obstetricians and anesthesiologists are important. Encourage joint meetings between the two departments. Anesthesiologists should recognize the special needs and concerns of the obstetrician, and obstetricians should recognize the anesthesiologist as a consultant in the management of pain and life-support measures. Both should recognize the need to provide high-quality care for all patients.

American College of Obstetricians and Gynecologists. (2009). *Optimal Goals for Anesthesia Care in Obstetrics* (Committee Opinion No. 433). Washington, DC: Author.

Table 16–10. COMPARISON OF NEURAXIAL TO OPIOID ANALGESIA

Neuraxial Analgesia (PCEA)	Patient-Controlled IV Opioid Analgesia
Higher patient satisfaction scores	Higher level of patient control and choice
Maternal hypotension, some nausea	More nausea
Maternal pain relief	Maternal sedation
Can be given early in labor	Not recommended until labor well established
Labor duration longer and second stage longer	May prolong latent phase
Potential increase need for oxytocin administration	
Increased operative vaginal delivery (vacuum and forceps)	
Maternal fever, which may lead to fetal tachycardia and neonatal septic workup	Newborn required more resuscitation, required naloxone and lower 1-minute Apgar score
Larger doses of fentanyl may be associated with slightly impaired breastfeeding	Meperidine may decrease sucking reflex.
Rare, life-threatening complications	Maternal respiratory depression
No difference in cesarean birth rate	

IV, intravenous; PCEA, patient-controlled epidural analgesia.

reaching statistical significance, but the increased length of time is not thought to have any clinical significance (Halpern et al., 2004; Liu & Sia, 2004). A randomized control trial found nulliparous women with epidural analgesia had a significantly shorter active pushing time when passive descent (laboring down) occurred (Gillesby et al., 2010). The timing of neuraxial analgesia, given before or after cervical dilatation reaches 5 cm, does not have an effect on cesarean birth rate (Wong et al., 2005). The current recommendation by ACOG is that use of neuraxial analgesia techniques and the timing of catheter placement does not influence cesarean birth rate and "should not influence the method of pain relief that women can choose during labor" (ACOG, 2006). Table 16–10 compares patient-controlled neuraxial analgesia to parenteral analgesia. There is no evidence that discontinuing the epidural infusion during the second stage of labor may improve the woman's ability to push. Efforts to sustain adequate epidural analgesia in the second stage should always be made (Abenhaim & Fraser, 2008).

The anesthesiologist or certified registered nurse anesthetist (CRNA) is responsible for identifying women with contraindications to the procedure (Display 16–8). Use of neuraxial analgesia techniques is not contraindicated in the presence of an indeterminate or abnormal FHR pattern (Vincent & Chestnut, 1998). However, it should be used judiciously when nonreassuring FHR or conditions associated with uteroplacental insufficiency exist (Thorp, 1999). The advantages of spinal or epidural analgesia or anesthesia are outlined in Display 16–9. However, an obstetric concern such as twin gestation, maternal hypertension, difficult airway, or obesity validates the practice of prophylactic placement of an epidural catheter early in labor. This access catheter permits rapid administration

DISPLAY 16–8

Contraindications to Neuraxial Analgesia

- Coagulation disorders
- Local infection at the site of injection
- Maternal hypotension and shock
- Nonreassuring FHR pattern requiring immediate birth
- Maternal inability to cooperate
- Allergy to local anesthetics
- Last dose of low-molecular-weight heparin within 12 hours

FHR, fetal heart rate.

DISPLAY 16–9

Advantages of Neuraxial Analgesia

- It generally provides superior pain relief, and position changes are less uncomfortable.
- The method usually provides sufficient anesthesia for episiotomy and/or repair of lacerations.
- Placement of an epidural catheter in labor means that an emergency cesarean section can occur more quickly, should this become necessary.
- Patient for whom general anesthesia is a risk (e.g., marked obesity; history of difficult/failed intubation; abnormalities of face, neck, spine; severe medical complications such as cardiac, pulmonary, or neurologic disease) may benefit from having an epidural catheter placed and functioning in early labor.

and/or extension of the block for emergent cesarean birth and lessens the risks associated with urgent use of general anesthesia (ASA, 2007b).

Obese patients present unique challenges for the anesthesia care provider in terms of positioning, identification of anatomic landmarks, and the midline and location of the epidural space (Saravanakumar, Rao, & Cooper, 2006; Roofthooft, 2009). Obesity in pregnancy is defined as a body mass index (BMI) of 30 kg/m^2 or greater (Roofthooft, 2009). Significant physiologic changes with the obese patient include the airway and respiratory systems and cardiovascular systems, which lead to increased anesthetic and obstetric risk. Difficult or failed tracheal intubation rate is higher in women whose BMI is 33 kg/m^2 or greater (Roofthooft, 2009). The obese laboring woman experiences increased work of breathing due to chest wall weight and higher ventilatory requirements, making the woman susceptible to rapid desaturation. Obesity increases cardiac output because every extra 100 g of adipose tissue increases the cardiac output by up to 50 mL/min (Roofthooft, 2009). Obesity also increases the need for cesarean birth due to fetal macrosomia and labor dystocia. Therefore, having a functional epidural catheter in place is advantageous should a need arise suddenly. Placing the catheter during early labor, when the woman is still comfortable, may make the process easier and more controlled due to her ability to cooperate. Not only are the obstetric risks increased with obesity, but the anesthetic complications are more frequent. Therefore, careful anticipatory planning and consults with the anesthesia provider is paramount to coordinate care for the obese woman.

STANDARD EPIDURAL

Epidural anesthesia is noted as "the gold standard" pain relief in labor and delivery (Hawkins, 2010; O'Sullivan, 2009). It involves the injection of a local anesthetic agent (e.g., lidocaine or bupivacaine) and an opioid analgesic agent (e.g., morphine or fentanyl) into the lumbar epidural space (Fig. 16–4). The injected agent gradually diffuses across the dura into the subarachnoid space, where it acts primarily on the spinal nerve roots and to a lesser degree on the spinal cord and paravertebral nerves. For many years, epidural anesthesia was limited to local anesthetics such as lidocaine (Xylocaine) and chloroprocaine (Nesacaine). These drugs act on nerve fibers as they cross the epidural space, causing sensory blockade. To obtain a therapeutic level of pain relief, the dose of local anesthetic resulted in loss of motor function. With the introduction of bupivacaine (Marcaine), practitioners found a longer duration of action, minimal motor blockade, and lack of neonatal neurobehavioral effects (Cohen, 1997). Ropivacaine (Naropin) has properties similar to those of bupivacaine, but this local anesthetic causes less motor block (Merson, 2001) and less cardiotoxic effects (Althaus & Wax, 2005).

Epidural narcotics act by diffusion of epidural medications across the dura mater membrane into the cerebrospinal fluid and binding to opiate receptors in the dorsal horn of the spinal cord. In contrast, a spinal block requires a needle puncture of the dura mater and

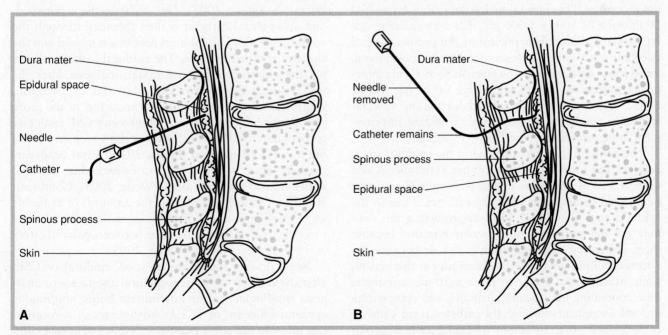

FIGURE 16–4. A, A needle is inserted into the epidural space. **B**, A catheter is threaded into the epidural space; the needle is then removed. The catheter allows medication to be administered intermittently or continuously to relieve pain during labor and childbirth.

direct injection of medications into the cerebrospinal fluid. The epidural block requires more medication than a spinal block for similar clinical effects. Adding a narcotic to the local anesthetic lessens the risk of toxicity by decreasing the amount of local anesthetic needed, reducing the motor blockade, increasing the duration of pain relief, and improving the quality of pain relief (ASA, 2007b). There was no difference in incidence of side effects (e.g., nausea and hypotension), increased duration of labor, or adverse neonatal outcomes when epidural local anesthetics with opioids were compared with epidural local anesthetics without opioids (ASA, 2007b). Opioid in the epidural infusion may cause pruritus, which for most women will last approximately 45 to 60 minutes after the initial loading dose (Wong, 2009). Adding a small amount of epinephrine decreases the amount of narcotic needed to obtain satisfactory pain relief (Armstrong et al., 2002; Polley, Columb, Naughton, Wagner, & van de Ven, 2002). Medications commonly used for neuraxial analgesia as well as their side effects are described in Table 16–11.

Successful epidural analgesia produces a segmental sympathetic and sensory nerve block and a decrease in endogenous catecholamines with the onset of pain relief. The sympathetic nerve blockade and the decrease in circulating catecholamines may lead to hypotension and a decrease in uteroplacental blood flow due to vasodilatation. Hypotension, defined as a systolic reading less than 100 mm Hg or a 20% decrease, may result in a reduction in venous return and cardiac output (Poole, 2003). Hypotension may occur in up to 80% of women (El-Wahab & Robinson, 2011) and therefore requires close monitoring of blood pressure by the nurse during the procedure. Pre-epidural hydration with a crystalloid IV infusion of 500 to 1,000 mL increases vascular volume and may blunt the hypotension. If it persists, despite adequate intravenous hydration and lateral positioning, intravenous ephedrine can be given in 5- to 10-mg incremental injections for a total dosage of 30 mg (Poole, 2003). For some women, the reduction in vascular resistance results in a statistically significant improvement in uteroplacental blood flow (Hong, 2010).

The epidural catheter is placed in the epidural space between the fourth and fifth lumbar vertebrae. A test dose of a local anesthetic mixed with epinephrine may be injected to determine that the catheter is not in the epidural vein (Fig. 16–3). In some women, a test dose may not determine an intravascular injection because there is existing maternal tachycardia or because the effects occur too quickly to be observed. For this reason, some practitioners prefer to place a 10-mL anesthetic dose combining bupivacaine, fentanyl, and epinephrine in 5-mL increments through the catheter. If the catheter is positioned correctly, onset of analgesia is approximately 5 minutes, and decreased sensation in lower extremities occurs within 20 minutes (Wong, 2009).

When the anesthesiologist or CRNA is satisfied that the catheter is properly placed, a bolus of anesthetic medication is injected. Depending on the specific medications used, women begin to feel relief in 5 to 10 minutes. A complete block usually occurs in 15 to 20 minutes. A small group of women experience what is called "windows," areas or even whole sides of their body where pain relief is not obtained. In circumstances where the patient is not satisfied with her pain relief, a bolus might be given or the catheter removed and replaced. The failure to obtain complete pain relief despite proper placement of the catheter may be due to the presence of connective tissue bands in the epidural space that limit areas that can be reached by the medication infused into the epidural space (Althaus & Wax, 2005).

COMBINED SPINAL EPIDURAL

CSE offers the advantages of both the epidural and spinal techniques as it provides rapid-onset pain relief and minimal motor blockade to the laboring woman. It is performed by first placing a 17- or 18-gauge Tuohy needle in the epidural space using the loss-of-resistance technique. After the needle is positioned in the epidural space, the smaller gauge spinal needle is placed through the epidural needle into the adjacent dural sac ("needle-through-needle" technique) (Hong, 2010). Within the dural sac are the contents of the intrathecal space including cerebrospinal fluid, the spinal cord, and the spinal nerve roots. Intrathecal analgesia is achieved faster and with a very low dose of local and opioid analgesia (combination of bupivacaine and fentanyl) necessary to produce epidural analgesia (Atienzar, Palanca, Torres, Borras, & Esteve, 2008). The spinal needle is removed, and an epidural catheter is then threaded through the epidural needle. The epidural needle is removed and the catheter is taped in place. The epidural catheter allows for the continuation of neuraxial analgesia after the initial spinal dose wears off. Maternal hypotension, pruritus, and motor nerve block are a few of the more prevalent problems. Women who receive CSE analgesia report significantly more pruritus than women receiving a standard epidural (Hong, 2010). Fetal bradycardia can occur with reported rates exceeding the risk with epidural analgesia alone (Wong, 2009). Continued anesthesia studies will explore the amounts of available local anesthetic and opiate drugs in intrathecal mixtures to strike a better balance between patient safety and therapeutic efficacy (Wong, 2009).

Regardless of the technique used, epidural or CSE, after the catheter is in place, epidural anesthesia or analgesia is administered by intermittent bolus, continuous epidural infusion, or PCEA. Advantages of a continuous infusion include a consistent level of pain relief and prevention of hemodynamic changes associated with the repeated occurrence of pain. Continuous flow through

Table 16–11. MEDICATIONS COMMONLY USED FOR REGIONAL ANALGESIA/ANESTHESIA DURING LABOR

Anesthesia Agents

Drug	Route	Concentration (%)	Volume (mL)	Dose (mg)	Side Effects/Adverse Reactions[†]	Nursing Implications
Bupivacaine	Epidural block	0.25	10–20	25–50	Hypotension*	Monitor maternal vital signs
		0.50	10–20	50–100	FHR changes*	Monitor FHR
	Intermittent infusion	0.125–0.375	5–10		Dysrhythmias[†]	Ensure resuscitation equipment available
	Continuous infusion	0.0625–0.25	8–15		Bronchospasm[†]	
	Caudal block	0.25	15–30	37.5–75	Seizures[†]	
		0.5	15–30	75–150	Respiratory arrest[†]	
	Surgical spinal	0.75 in 8.25% dextrose			Cardiovascular collapse[†]	
Lidocaine	Epidural block	1	25–30	250–300	Hypotension*	Monitor maternal vital signs
		1.5	15–20	225–300	FHR changes*	Monitor FHR
		2	10–15	200–300	Muscular twitching[†]	Ensure resuscitation equipment available
	Intermittent injection	0.75–1.5	5–10		Light-headedness[†]	
	Continuous infusion	0.5–1.0	8–15		Edema[†]	
	Caudal block	1	20–30	200–300	CNS depression[†]	
	Spinal surgical	5.0 in 7.5% dextrose	1.5–2.0	75–100	Tinnitus[†]	
					Coma[†]	
					Seizures[†]	
					Respiratory arrest[†]	
					Cardiovascular collapse[†]	
Ropivacaine	Intermittent injection	0.125–0.25	5–10	20–30	Hypotension*	Monitor maternal vital signs
	Continuous infusion	0.125–0.25	6–12	12–28	FHR changes*	Monitor FHR
					Neonatal jaundice*	Ensure resuscitation equipment available

Narcotic Agents

Drug	Route	Concentration (mcg/mL)	Rate (mL/hr)	Side Effects/Adverse Reactions[†]	Nursing Implications
Fentanyl	PCEA	1–3	8–20	FHR changes*	Prolonged administration may ↑ risk of maternal/fetal/neonatal respiratory/CNS depression
	CSE	10–25		Hypotension*	Crosses placenta rapidly
				Nausea*	Monitor for maternal/neonatal respiratory depression
				Pruritus*	Determine allergy status
				Sedation*	Ensure naloxone and resuscitation equipment available
				Vomiting*	
				Urinary retention*	
				Dysrhythmias[†]	
				Respiratory depression[†]	
Sufentanil	PCEA	0.75–1	5–15	FHR changes*	May improve and prolong anesthesia
	CSE	5.0–11.5		Hypotension*	Monitor for maternal/neonatal respiratory depression
				Nausea*	Ensure naloxone and resuscitation equipment available
				Vomiting*	
				Pruritus*	
				Sedation*	
				Respiratory depression[†]	

CNS, central nervous system; CSE, combined spinal epidural; FHR, fetal heart rate; PCEA, patient-controlled epidural analgesia.
*Potential side effect. [†]Potential adverse reaction. [†]Adverse reactions are rare.

the catheter also stabilizes the catheter, decreasing the risk of migration into an epidural vein or through the dura into the subarachnoid space. The continuous infusion may be a local anesthetic alone (bupivacaine, lidocaine, or ropivacaine) or a combination of a local and a narcotic (fentanyl or sufentanil). Women who receive local anesthetic alone need more medication to obtain satisfactory pain relief than women who receive a combination of local and opioid (Hong, 2010; Wong, McCarthy, & Hewlett, 2011). When a local anesthetic is combined with an opioid, there is less motor blockade, no difference in rate of spontaneous versus operative vaginal delivery or perineal pain during second-stage labor, and increased maternal satisfaction with pain management (Russell & Reynolds, 1996). As cervical dilatation progresses, some women require an increase in the rate of the continuous infusion or a second bolus with a higher concentration of local anesthetic or narcotic.

ADVERSE EVENTS

Adverse events are known to occur with neuraxial analgesia. Rare, life-threatening, and life-altering major complications include high spinal block, accidental intravascular injection, epidural hematoma, and meningitis. Other, more common adverse effects are reported with varying degrees of frequency and include maternal hypotension, FHR changes, reduced success in breastfeeding initiation, headache, and maternal fever.

Major Complications

Inadvertent placement of the catheter and infusion into the intrathecal space can cause a high spinal block resulting in immediate upper thoracic sensory loss and severe lower extremity motor blockade. The anesthetic agent may ascend intrathecally to the brain stem leading to respiratory paralysis, total autonomic blockage, and loss of consciousness.

An accidental intravenous injection of epinephrine and a local anesthetic agent into an epidural vein may lead to systemic toxicity causing almost immediate increased maternal heart rate, palpitations, increased blood pressure, numbness of the tongue or around the mouth, metallic taste, tinnitus, slurred speech, jitteriness, or agitation, which may culminate in seizures and cardiac arrest. The nurse must be prepared to always have emergency equipment immediately available, recognize these complications, and anticipate the need for cardiopulmonary support. Intravenous lipid emulsion has emerged as an effective therapy for cardiotoxic effects of lipid soluble local anesthetics such as bupivacaine or ropivacaine (Hawkins, 2010).

Bleeding within the spinal neuraxis can lead to a very rare spinal or epidural hematoma (Ruppen, Derry, McQuay, and Moore, 2006; Horlocker et al., 2010). Coagulopathy (pathologic or therapeutic),

thrombocytopenia (usual threshold $<80 \times 10^9$/L with no decreasing trend), or spinal deformities leading to a difficult catheter placement may contribute to the development of a hematoma. Early signs of a hematoma include severe back pain, progressive sensory or motor blockade following initial signs of regression, and deteriorating function of the lower extremities and the bowel and bladder (Horlocker et al., 2010). If the woman develops an unusually prolonged motor block with suspicion of hematoma, immediate evaluation utilizing spinal imaging followed by emergent laminectomy and decompression is required to preserve neurologic integrity (Beilin & Abramovitz, 2007).

One study determined that the risk of meningitis was 9 cases in 1.2 million (Ruppen et al., 2006). Potential causes include movement of the laboring woman in bed with possible contamination with streptococci, inadequate skin preparation prior to needle insertion, and droplet contamination from the anesthesia provider not wearing a mask during placement. The American Society of Regional Anesthesia and Pain Medicine (ASRA) recommends an alcohol-based chlorhexidine solution (2% chlorhexidine in 70% alcohol) as skin prep for neuraxial anesthesia/analgesia (Hebl, 2006). Signs and symptoms of meningitis may occur within 12 hours to a few days following birth and include fever, severe unrelenting headache, neck stiffness, sensitivity to light, nausea, and vomiting. Drowsiness, confusion, and seizure are advanced signs. Bacterial meningitis is serious and requires prompt antibiotic treatment to improve the chances of a recovery without serious complications. Meningitis can lead to serious long-term consequences such as deafness, epilepsy, hydrocephalus, and cognitive deficits, especially if not treated quickly. Cerebrospinal fluid obtained through a lumbar puncture will reveal an increased leukocyte and protein level and a lowered glucose level. Vancomycin and third-generation cephalosporin are the recommended first-line antibiotic therapy (Horlocker et al., 2010).

Common Complications

As stated earlier, maternal hypotension is thought to be due to an anesthetic-induced sympathectomy and vasodilatation. While neuraxial analgesia does not depend on maternal blood levels for its effect, opioids used in both CSE and epidural anesthesia do pass into maternal blood, cross the placenta, and produce fetal and neonatal depression when given in large doses (Reynolds, 2010). Low dose local anesthetic and opioid solutions may cause minimal variability of the FHR (O'Sullivan, 2009). Late and prolonged decelerations and fetal bradycardia are more common with CSE but are not associated with an increased cesarean birth rate (Reynolds, 2010). More studies are needed to determine the long-term effects of labor analgesia or delivery anesthesia on infant development (Sun, 2011). In a small study, larger doses of epidural fentanyl (>150 μg) given during the course of labor was suggested to interfere with early breastfeeding success (Beilin et al., 2005).

Headache may occur after unintentional dural puncture with a 17- or 18-gauge epidural needle, also known as a wet tap. The incidence of a wet tap is about 1:100, with approximately 70% of patients complaining of a severe headache (Hawkins, 2010; El-Wahab & Robinson, 2011). An epidural blood patch, using 15 to 25 mL of the patient's own blood into the epidural space will provide immediate relief to 65% to 90% of patients (Hawkins, 2010).

The precise etiology of the maternal hyperthermia related to epidural analgesia remains unknown. It is likely that the rise is due to an alteration in maternal thermoregulatory physiology due to an imbalance between heat production and heat loss. However, an infectious etiology can never be completely discounted. Women with intrapartum fever are more likely to deliver by cesarean birth or operative vaginal delivery and the infant is more likely to undergo an evaluation for neonatal sepsis including antibiotic therapy while culture results are pending (Verani, McGee, Schrag, 2010; Yancey, Zhang, Schwatz, Dietrick, & Klebanoff, 2001; Osborne et al., 2008). Epidurals associated with maternal hyperthermia occur more so in nulliparous women and the risk appears to increase with duration of labor (El-Wahab & Robinson, 2011; Kuczkowski & Reisner, 2003; Yancey et al., 2001). The maternal–fetal temperature affects uteroplacental blood flow and fetal oxygen delivery due to higher maternal oxygen consumption (Kuczkowski & Reisner, 2003). Fetal temperature is approximately 0.5°C higher than maternal temperature. Fetal hyperthermia is associated with an increased risk of neonatal encephalopathy; therefore, prevention of fetal exposure to intrauterine hyperthermia is paramount.

NURSING CARE

In 2011, AWHONN published the second edition of the evidence-based guideline for nursing care of the woman receiving regional analgesia/anesthesia in labor. The clinical position statement providing guidelines for practice for nurses caring for pregnant women receiving anesthesia/anesthesia by catheter techniques (e.g., epidural, intrathecal, spinal, PCEA catheters) follows.

Only qualified, credentialed, licensed anesthesia care providers, as described by the ASA and the American Association of Nurse Anesthetists and/or as authorized by state law, should perform the following procedures:

- Insertion, initial injection, bolus injection, rebolus injection or initiation of a continuous infusion of catheters for analgesia/anesthesia
- Verification of correct catheter placement

- Increasing or decreasing the rate of the continuous infusion

Following stabilization of vital signs after either initial insertion, initial injection, bolus injection, rebolus injection, or initiation of continuous infusion by a licensed, credentialed anesthesia care provider, nonanesthetist registered nurses, in communication with the obstetric and anesthesia care providers, may:

- Monitor the patient's vital signs, mobility, level of consciousness, and perception of pain.
- Monitor the status of the fetus.
- Replace empty infusion syringes or infusion bags with new, pre-prepared solutions containing the same medication and concentration, according to standing orders provided by the anesthesia care provider.
- Stop the continuous infusion if there is a safety concern or if the woman has given birth.
- Remove the catheter, if educational criteria have been met and institutional policy and law allow. Removal of the catheter by a registered nurse is contingent upon receipt of a specific order from a qualified anesthesia or physician provider.
- Initiate emergency therapeutic measures according to institutional policy and/or protocol if complications arise.

Nonanesthetist registered nurses should **not**:

- Rebolus an epidural either by injecting medication into the catheter or increasing the rate of a continuous infusion
- Increase/decrease the rate of a continuous infusion
- Reinitiate an infusion once it has been stopped
- Manipulate PCEA doses or dosage intervals
- Be responsible for obtaining informed consent for analgesia/anesthesia procedures; however, the nurse may witness the patient signature for informed consent prior to analgesia/anesthesia administration (AWHONN, 2007)

Perinatal nurses must be comfortable with the operation of additional technology, familiar with nursing care during all phases of the procedure, and able to recognize potential complications. Continuous epidural anesthesia is always delivered through an infusion pump, and continuous EFM is the most frequently used method of fetal assessment. Depending on institutional practice, women may also be monitored using a cardiac monitor, pulse oximeter, and automatic blood pressure devices. *Guidelines for Perinatal Care* (AAP & ACOG, 2007) suggest a 1:1 nurse–patient ratio for initiating epidural anesthesia.

Published statements from professional organizations and individual state nursing practice acts are inconsistent regarding the role of the nurse in caring for women in labor who receive anesthesia or analgesia and do not provide specific guidelines for how often and what type of monitoring will lead to optimal maternal–fetal outcomes. Controversy exists in the literature and in clinical practice about the frequency of maternal–fetal assessments during epidural anesthesia or analgesia for laboring women. Many perinatal units have policies that require completion of specific aspects of maternal–fetal assessment every 15 to 30 minutes for women with epidurals. There are, however, no published standards of care or practice guidelines from the ASA, American Association of Nurse Anesthetists, ACOG, or AWHONN that prescribe what the maternal–fetal assessment includes or the specific frequencies for making assessments during epidural infusion for labor and delivery. Existing published standards are general and outlined in Display 16–10. Nursing

and medical textbooks may contain suggested protocols and valuable clinical information, but they alone do not define standards of care. There are no research-based data to demonstrate optimal time intervals for maternal–fetal assessments during epidural infusion. The type and amount of medication used, the level of the block given, and the maternal–fetal status should be considered when determining intensity of monitoring. Perinatal nurses, in collaboration with obstetric and anesthesia providers in each institution, must develop protocols that delineate responsibilities and care for women receiving epidural anesthesia or analgesia during labor and delivery. Table 16–12 presents an overview of the nursing care to consider as policies and procedures are developed for care of the intrapartum patient receiving neuraxial analgesia.

DISPLAY 16–10

Professional Organizations' Guidelines for Maternal–Fetal Assessment Frequency During Neuraxial Analgesia

	AWHONN	ASA	ACOG
MATERNAL ASSESSMENTS	BP after the initiation or rebolus of a regional block, including PCEA. BP, P, and R assessed every 5 minutes for the first 15 minutes. More or less frequent monitoring may be indicated based on consideration of factors such as the type of analgesia/anesthesia, route and dose of medication used, the maternal–fetal response to medication, maternal–fetal condition, the stage of labor, or facility protocol.	Requires that the parturient's vital signs and the FHR be monitored and documented by a qualified individual. Additional monitoring appropriate to the clinical condition of the parturient and the fetus should be employed when indicated.	When regional anesthesia is administered during labor, the patient's vital signs should be monitored at regular intervals by a qualified member of the healthcare team.
FETAL ASSESSMENTS	Assess the FHR tracing before initiating regional analgesia, ideally, to identify a reassuring pattern. If a nonreassuring FHR pattern is identified, initiate corrective measures as needed and notify the anesthesia/obstetric care provider. Assess FHR after the initiation or rebolus of a regional block, including PCEA. FHR may be assessed every 5 minutes for the first 15 minutes. More or less frequent monitoring may be indicated based on consideration of factors such as the type of analgesia/anesthesia, route and dose of medication used, the maternal–fetal response to medication, maternal–fetal condition, the stage of labor, or facility protocol. The frequency of subsequent assessment should be based on consideration of the variables listed previously.	FHR should be monitored by a qualified individual before and after administration of regional analgesia for labor. Continuous electronic recording of the FHR may not be necessary in every clinical setting and may not be possible during initiation of neuraxial anesthesia.	

ACOG, American College of Obstetricians and Gynecologists; ASA, American Society of Anesthesiologists; AWHONN, Association of Women's Health, Obstetric and Neonatal Nurses; BP, blood pressure; FHR, fetal heart rate; P, pulse; PCEA, patient-controlled epidural analgesia; R, respiration.
From American Academy of Pediatrics & American College of Obstetricians and Gynecologists. (2007). *Guidelines for Perinatal Care* (6th ed.). Elk Grove Village, IL: Author; American Society of Anesthesiologists. (2007a). *Guidelines for Regional Anesthesia in Obstetrics*. Park Ridge, IL: Author; Association of Women's Health, Obstetric and Neonatal Nurses. (2007). Role of the registered nurse (RN) in the care of the pregnant woman receiving analgesia/anesthesia by catheter techniques (epidural, intrathecal, spinal, PCEA catheters) (Position Statement). Washington, DC: Author.

Table 16–12. CARE OF PATIENTS RECEIVING NEURAXIAL ANALGESIA

Nursing Care	Referenced Rationale
1. Review understanding of neuraxial analgesia and clarify concerns and information as needed. Include support systems as available.	Women are increasingly encouraged to take an active role in decision making regarding pregnancy, labor, and delivery (Lally et al., 2008).
2. Notify the obstetric and anesthesia care providers of the woman's request for neuraxial analgesia.	The woman has a right to request pain relief during labor. A focused history and physical shall be completed prior to the initiation of anesthesia/analgesia. Labor progress and fetal status must be evaluated prior to initiation of neuraxial analgesia by a qualified obstetric care provider (ASA, 2009b).
3. Assess for any contraindications to the procedure prior to initiation, including: • Coagulopathy and/or thrombocytopenia • Local or systemic infection • Inadequate staffing	A specific platelet count predictive of neuraxial anesthetic complications has not been determined. A platelet count is clinically useful for laboring women with suspected preeclampsia or HELLP syndrome and for other disorders associated with coagulopathy (ASA, 2007a). The recommendation from ASA (2007a) is that a blood type and screen or cross-match should be based on maternal history, anticipated hemorrhage complications, and hospital policies. Continuous bedside nursing attendance should be provided during the initiation of regional anesthesia until the woman's condition is stable (at least for the first 30 min following the initial dose of medication) (AWHONN, 2010).
4. The FHR should be monitored 20–30 min before and continuously after administration of neuraxial analgesia. Continuous EFM may not be possible during placement of the epidural catheter.	Anesthetic and analgesia agents may influence the FHR pattern. Recording the FHR reduces fetal and neonatal complications (ASA, 2009a). Administration of regional analgesia during labor has resulted in decreased uteroplacental blood flow, and alterations in the FHR such as late decelerations, variable decelerations, bradycardia, tachycardia, and increased and decreased variability have been reported (Wong, 2009)
5. Initiate large-bore IV access and provide a bolus of 500–1,000 mL Hartmann's solution (Ringer's lactate) 15–30 min before the procedure.	Avoid rapidly infusing IV fluids into women with cardiac disease or severe preeclampsia without direct measurement of hemodynamic status.
6. Conduct a preprocedure verification process (time out) prior to initiation of the neuraxial procedure and document completion of this verification.	The purpose of the time out is to conduct a final validation that the correct patient, site, and procedure are identified (ACOG, 2009d; TJC, 2011).
7. Emergency preparedness: Verify the immediate availability of emergency response and equipment. Advise colleagues that the procedure will soon begin. An emergency cesarean birth may become necessary due to a prolonged deceleration or bradycardia that does not respond to the intrauterine resuscitation techniques.	Regional anesthesia should be initiated and maintained only in areas in which resuscitation equipment and drugs are immediately available (ASA, 2008; AWHONN, 2009).
8. Assist the woman to maintain a sitting or side-lying position with feet supported on a chair or stool and head flexed forward supported by herself with elbows resting on knees or leaning against the shoulder of a support person. Stress the importance of remaining still during insertion of the catheter. Encourage the use of breathing and relaxation techniques during the procedure.	Avoid severe spinal flexion because it can decrease the epidural space and increase the possibility of puncturing the dura. The respiratory effect of obesity in pregnancy is minimal when placed in the sitting position (Roofthooft, 2009).
9. Alert the woman to normal sensations felt with skin preparation, taping, local injection stinging, and needle placement.	Use of sterile gloves is required by the anesthesia provider; however, a sterile gown is not necessary. Wearing a mask will decrease potential for droplet contamination of the sterile field. A 2% chlorhexidine in 70% alcohol skin prep is recommended (ASA, 2008).
10. Monitor for IV injection of local anesthetic during the test dose.	Signs of intravascular injection include: • Maternal tachycardia or bradycardia • Hypertension • Seizures • Dizziness • Restlessness • Tinnitus • Metallic taste in mouth • Perioral paresthesia • Difficulty speaking • Loss of consciousness

(continued)

Table 16–12. CARE OF PATIENTS RECEIVING NEURAXIAL ANALGESIA (*Continued*)

Nursing Care	Referenced Rationale
11. Monitor for signs of infusion of medication into the intrathecal space.	Signs of infusion into the intrathecal space leading to a high spinal block include: • Immediate upper thoracic sensory loss • Severe lower extremity motor blockade • Respiratory paralysis • Total autonomic blockage • Loss of consciousness
12. Monitor BP, pulse, respiration, and FHR every 5 min during the first 15 min following initiation or rebolus of regional analgesia to identify and manage side effects.	Women who have received neuraxial opioids should be observed for adequate ventilation by assessing respiratory rate, depth of respiration, level of consciousness, and pulse oximetry when appropriate (ASA, 2009a).
13. Temperature should be assessed according to hospital protocol and based on risk factors with ruptured membranes.	Use of labor epidural analgesia is associated with a clinically significant increase in the incidence of intrapartum fever (Yancey et al., 2001).
14. If maternal hypotension occurs (systolic <100 or a 20-mm Hg decrease from prior readings), initiate IV bolus, place in lateral position, administer oxygen at 10 L per nonrebreather facemask, stop oxytocin administration, notify obstetric and anesthesia service, and prepare for IV administration of ephedrine to improve maternal hypotension.	An indeterminate or abnormal FHR pattern associated with regional analgesia/anesthesia may respond to maternal position change, an IV fluid bolus, and/or oxygen supplementation (Simpson & James, 2005; Simpson, 2007). Maternal hypotension has been treated successfully with maternal position change, IV administration of 5–10 mg of ephedrine or 50–100 µg of phenylephrine, and an IV fluid bolus of non–glucose-containing solution (Skupski, Abramovitz, Samuels, Pressimone, & Kjaer, 2009).
15. Assess uterine activity following neuraxial placement and infusion. Following neuraxial analgesia, tachysystole or a decrease in uterine activity may occur requiring an oxytocin infusion to be initiated for augmentation of labor.	Tachysystole and uterine hypertonus may be noted after combined spinal epidural analgesia, epidural analgesia, or intrathecal opioids (Skupski et al., 2009; Reynolds, 2011). Uterine activity may slow in the first 30–60 min after regional block administration secondary to rapid preload of 500 mL or more of IV fluid. There is an increase in oxytocin use in the first stage of labor among women who receive epidural analgesia when compared to women who received parenteral opioids. The use of epidural analgesia was associated with a statistically significant longer duration of both first and second stages of labor among nulliparous (nearly 4 hr) and multiparous women (Cheng, Nicholson, Shaffer, Lyell, & Caughey, 2009).
16. Evaluate pain with each assessment of maternal vital signs or using a visual or verbal analog scale according to institutional policy. If pain continues to be felt on one side of the body, sometimes lying on that side will achieve increased relief. Request that the anesthesia care provider reevaluate the patient as needed for further pain management.	93% of women with labor epidurals, who reported a pain score >3 using a 0–10 numeric rating scale, wanted additional medication (Beilin, Hossain, & Bodian, 2003).
17. Encourage the woman to void frequently during labor. If the bladder is distended and the woman experiences decreased bladder sensation or is unable to use a bed pan to void, placement of an indwelling catheter eliminates the need for repeated catheterizations.	Inability to void and need for catheterization have been reported in up to two thirds of women after epidural analgesia during labor (Mayberry, Clemmens, & De, 2002).
18. Women who experience pruritus should be assured that this is usually a transitory symptom and should decrease within an hour on onset.	The most common side effect of intrathecal opioid administration is pruritus and is more frequently observed with intrathecal opioid administration compared to epidural administration (Wong, 2009).
19. Oral intake of modest amounts of clear liquids may be allowed for uncomplicated laboring women.	Oral liquid intake of clear liquids during labor does not increase maternal complications. Clear liquids include but are not limited to water, fruit juices without pulp, carbonated beverages, clear tea, black coffee, and sports drinks. Women with additional risk factors for aspiration (morbid obesity, diabetes, difficult airway) may have restricted intake based on the decision of the anesthesiologist (ACOG, 2009c).
20. Assist with second-stage management and prepare for possibility of operative vaginal delivery.	Regional anesthesia/analgesia diminishes the sensation of the urge to push in varying degrees, depending on the type of agents used and route of administration. Research has demonstrated that delaying pushing for various time intervals after complete cervical dilation vs. pushing immediately has been accomplished without lengthening the second stage of labor or negatively affecting birth outcome in women who received epidural analgesia (Brancato, Church, & Stone, 2008; Mayberry et al., 2002; Wong, 2009; Beilin, Mungall, Hossain, & Bodian, 2009). There may be an increased risk for vacuum-assisted delivery and labor dystocia with epidural analgesia (O'Hana et al., 2008).

BP, blood pressure; EFM, electronic fetal monitoring; FHR, fetal heart rate; HELLP, hemolysis, elevated liver enzymes, low platelet count; IV, intravenous.

LOCAL ANESTHETIC

During the second stage of labor, lidocaine hydrochloride or chloroprocaine hydrochloride, local anesthetics, may be injected into the perineum and posterior vaginal wall before performing an episiotomy. The duration of action is approximately 20 to 40 minutes for these medications (Briggs & Wan, 2006). This area may be reinjected after delivery of the placenta in preparation for perineal repair.

PUDENDAL BLOCK

A pudendal block during the second stage of labor using lidocaine hydrochloride or chloroprocaine hydrochloride anesthetizes the lower vagina, vulva, and perineum. An anesthetic is injected through the lateral vaginal walls into the area of the pudendal nerve. This technique provides adequate anesthesia for spontaneous vaginal birth, application of outlet forceps or vacuum, and perineal repair. Because it is possible for a pudendal block to be ineffective, it is frequently combined with local infiltration of the perineum. The potential risks for pudendal block are hematoma, infection, and nerve damage as well as local anesthetic toxicity and extension of the nerve block, but the complications are unusual (Volmanen et al., 2011).

PARACERVICAL BLOCK

The paracervical block was once a widely accepted technique for relief of labor pain. The historical deep injection and high-dose technique was found to have serious fetal adverse effects, an especially high rate of postparacervical block fetal bradycardia, and even fetal loss. However, a new, superficial injection method combined with the use of milder anesthetic solutions has decreased the risk of bradycardia to 2.2%, and these episodes were transient and did not lead to emergency cesarean birth (Volmanen et al., 2011; Palomaki, Huhtala, & Kirkinen, 2005).

SUMMARY

The perinatal nurse is an integral member of the healthcare team and, as such, works collaboratively with the obstetric and anesthesia healthcare providers to meet women's needs for pain management during labor and birth. Labor causes pain, which leads to a physiologic stress response. A woman should be given options regarding both nonpharmacologic and pharmacologic choices for pain management, which maintains her sense of control and allows participation of her birthing partner. None of the methods described constitute the ideal analgesic for labor—all have pros and cons. A combination of techniques is often more effective than reliance on a single plan of action. Nurses should encourage women in labor to utilize a variety of techniques to decrease the pain perception and sustain her coping. Pharmacologic pain management strategies represent one aspect of intrapartum pain management and may be used to augment, not substitute for, nonpharmacologic strategies. The nurse must remember that a woman who has been given intravenous pain medication or received neuraxial anesthesia may still need, and can benefit from, all of the available nonpharmacologic nursing interventions. Labor pain is a unique, individual, and multifaceted phenomenon compounded by various contributing physiologic, emotional, social, and cultural components.

REFERENCES

Abenhaim, H. A., & Fraser, W. D. (2008). Impact of pain level on second-stage delivery outcomes among women with epidural analgesia: Results from the PEOPLE study. *American Journal of Obstetrics & Gynecology, 199,* 500e1–500e6. doi:10.1016/j.ajog.2008.04.052

Althaus, J., & Wax, J. (2005). Analgesia and anesthesia in labor. *Obstetrics and Gynecology Clinics of North America, 32*(2), 231–244. doi:10.1016/j.ogc.2005.01.002

American Academy of Pediatrics & American College of Obstetricians and Gynecologists. (2007). *Guidelines for Perinatal Care* (6th ed.). Elk Grove Village, IL: Author.

American Academy of Pediatrics and American Heart Association; Kattwinkel J., Ed. (2011). *Neonatal Resuscitation* (6th ed). Washington, DC: Author.

American College of Obstetricians and Gynecologists. (2002). *Obstetric Analgesia and Anesthesia* (Practice Bulletin No. 36). Washington, DC: Author.

American College of Obstetricians and Gynecologists. (2004). *Pain Relief During Labor* (Committee Opinion No. 295). Washington, DC: Author.

American College of Obstetricians and Gynecologists. (2006). *Analgesia and Cesarean Delivery Rates* (Committee Opinion No. 339). Washington, DC: Author.

American College of Obstetricians and Gynecologists. (2009a). *Intrapartum Fetal Heart Rate Monitoring: Nomenclature, Interpretation, and General Management Principles* (Practice Bulletin No. 106). Washington, DC: Author.

American College of Obstetricians and Gynecologists. (2009b). *Optimal Goals for Anesthesia Care in Obstetrics* (Committee Opinion No. 433). Washington, DC: Author.

American College of Obstetricians and Gynecologists. (2009c). *Oral Intake During Labor* (Committee Opinion No. 441). Washington, DC: Author.

American College of Obstetricians and Gynecologists. (2009d). *Patient Safety in Obstetrics and Gynecology* (Committee Opinion No. 447). Washington, DC: Author.

American Society of Anesthesiologists. (2007a). *Guidelines for Regional Anesthesia in Obstetrics*. Park Ridge, IL: Author.

American Society of Anesthesiologists. (2007b). Practice guidelines for obstetric anesthesia: An updated report by the American Society of Anesthesiologists task force on obstetric anesthesia. *Anesthesiology, 106*(4), 843–863.

American Society of Anesthesiologists. (2008). *Optimal Goals for Anesthesia Care in Obstetrics*. Park Ridge, IL: Author.

American Society of Anesthesiologists. (2009a). Practice guidelines for the prevention, detection, and management of respiratory depression associated with neuraxial opioid administration: An updated report by the American Society of Anesthesiologists task force on neuraxial opioids. *Anesthesiology, 110*(2), 218–230. doi:10.1097/ALN.0b013e31818ec946

American Society of Anesthesiologists. (2009b). Statement on pain relief during labor. Approved by the ASA House of Delegates on October 13, 1999 and last amended on October 21, 2009. Retrieved from http://www.asahq.org/publicationsAndServices/standards/47.pdf

Armstrong, K. P., Kennedy, B., Watson, J. T., Morley-Forster, P. K., Yee, I., & Butler, R. (2002). Epinephrine reduces the sedative side effects of epidural sufentanil for labor analgesia. *Canadian Journal of Anesthesia, 49*(1), 72–80.

Association of Women's Health, Obstetric and Neonatal Nurses. (2000). *Professional Nursing Support of Laboring Women* (Policy Statement). Washington, DC: Author.

Association of Women's Health, Obstetric and Neonatal Nurses. (2007). *Role of the Registered Nurse (RN) in the Care of the Pregnant Woman Receiving Analgesia/Anesthesia by Catheter Techniques (Epidural, Intrathecal, Spinal, PCEA Catheters)* (Position Statement). Washington, DC: Author.

Association of Women's Health, Obstetric and Neonatal Nurses. (2008). *Nursing Care and Management of the Second Stage of Labor* (2nd ed.). Washington, DC: Author.

Association of Women's Health, Obstetric and Neonatal Nurses. (2009). *Standards for Professional Nursing Practice in the Care of Women and Newborns* (7th ed.). Washington, DC: Author.

Association of Women's Health, Obstetric and Neonatal Nurses. (2010). *Guidelines for Professional Nurse Staffing for Perinatal Units.* Washington, DC: Author.

Association of Women's Health, Obstetric and Neonatal Nurses. (2011). *Nursing Care of the Woman Receiving Regional Analgesia/Anesthesia in Labor.* Washington, DC: Author.

Atienzar, M. C., Palanca, J. M., Torres, F., Borras, R., Gil, S., & Esteve, I. (2008). A randomized comparison of levobupivacaine, bupivacaine, and ropivacaine with fentanyl, for labor analgesia. *International Journal of Obstetric Anesthesia, 17*(2), 106–111.

Bahasadri, S., Ahmadi-Abhari, S., Dehghani-Nik, M., & Habibi, G. R. (2006). Subcutaneous sterile water injections for labor pain: A randomized controlled trial. *Australia & New Zealand Journal of Obstetric & Gynecology, 46*(2), 102–106. doi:10.1111/j.1479-828X.2006.00536.x

Ballen, L. E., & Fulcher, A. J. (2006). Nurses and doulas: Complementary roles to provide optimal maternity care. *Journal of Obstetrics, Gynecologic, and Neonatal Nursing, 35*(2), 304–311. doi:10.1111/j.1552-6909.2006.00041.x

Beilin, Y., & Abramovitz, S. (2007). The anticoagulated parturient. *International Anesthesiology Clinics, 45*(1), 71–81.

Beilin, Y., Bodian, C. A., Weiser, J., Hossain, S., Arnold, I., Feierman, D. E., . . . Hotzman, I. (2005). Effect of labor epidural analgesia with and without fentanyl on infant breastfeeding: A prospective, randomized double-blind study. *Anesthesiology, 103*(6), 1211–1217.

Beilin, Y., Hossain, S., & Bodian, A. A. (2003). The numeric rating scale and labor epidural analgesia. *Anesthesia & Analgesia, 96*(6), 1794–1798.

Beilin, Y., Mungall, D., Hossain, S., & Bodian, C. A. (2009). Labor pain at the time of epidural analgesia and mode of delivery in nulliparous women presenting for an induction of labor. *Obstetrics & Gynecology, 114*(4), 764–769. doi:10.1097/AOG.0b013e3181b6beee

Benfield, R., Herman, J., Katz, V. L., Wilson, S. P., & Davis, J. M. (2001). Hydrotherapy in labor. *Research in Nursing & Health, 24*(1), 57–67. doi:10.1002/1098-240X(200102)24:1<57::AID-NUR1007>3.0.CO;2-J

Bergh, I., Stener-Victorin, E., Wallin, G., & Martensson, L. (2011). Comparison of the PainMatcher and the visual analogue scare for assessment of labour pain following administered pain relief treatment. *Midwifery, 27*, e134–e139. doi:10.1016/j.midw.2009.03.004

Berghella, V., Baxter, J. K., & Chauhan, S. P. (2008). Evidence-based labor and delivery management. *American Journal of Obstetrics & Gynecology, 199*(5), 445–454. doi:10.1016/j.ajog.2008.06.093

Brancato, R. M., Church, S., & Stone, P. W. (2008). A meta-analysis of passive descent versus immediate pushing in nulliparous women with epidural analgesia in the second stage of labor. *Journal of Obstetric, Gynecologic & Neonatal Nursing, 37*(1), 4–12. doi:10.1111/j.1552-6909.2007.00205.x

Briggs, G. G., & Wan, S. R. (2006). Drug therapy during labor and delivery, part 2. *American Journal of Health-System Pharmacy, 63*(12), 1131–1139. doi:10.2146/ajhp050265.p2

Browning, C. A. (2000). Using music during childbirth. *Birth, 27*(4), 272–276. doi:10.1046/j.1523-536x.2000.00272.x

Bryanton, J., Fraser-Davey, H., & Sullivan, P. (1994). Women's perceptions of nursing support during labor. *Journal of Obstetric, Gynecologic, and Neonatal Nursing, 23*(8), 638–644.

Bucklin, B. A., Hawkins, J. L., Anderson, J. R., & Ullrich, R. A. (2005). Obstetric anesthesia workforce survey: Twenty year update. *Anesthesiology, 103*(3), 645–653.

Camann, W. (2005). Pain relief during labor. *New England Journal of Medicine, 352*(7), 718–720.

Campbell, D. A., Lake, M. F., Falk, M., & Backstrand, J. R. (2006). A randomized control trial of continuous support in labor by a lay doula. *Journal of Obstetric, Gynecologic, and Neonatal Nursing, 35*(4), 456–464. doi:10.1111/j.1552-6909.2006.00067.x

Carlton, T., Callister, L. C., & Stoneman, E. (2005). Decision making in laboring women: Ethical issues for perinatal nurses. *Journal of Perinatal and Neonatal Nursing, 19*(2), 145–154.

Chandler, S., & Field, P. (1997). Becoming a father: First-time fathers' experience of labor and delivery. *Journal of Nurse-Midwifery, 42*(1), 17–24. doi:10.1016/s0091-2(96)00067-5

Chang, M. Y., Chen, C. H., & Huang, K. F. (2006). A comparison of massage effects on labor pain using the McGill Pain Questionnaire. *Journal of Nursing Research, 14*(3), 190–197. doi:10.1097/01.JNR.0000387577.51350.5f

Chang, M. Y., Wang, S. Y., & Chen, C. H. (2002). Effects of massage on pain and anxiety during labor: A randomized controlled trial in Taiwan. *Journal of Advanced Nursing, 38*(1), 68–73. doi:10.1046/j.1365-2648.2002.02147.x

Chapman, L. L. (1991). Searching: Expectant fathers' experience during labor and birth. *Journal of Perinatal and Neonatal Nursing, 4*(4), 21–29.

Chapman, L. L. (1992). Expectant fathers' roles during labor and birth. *Journal of Obstetric, Gynecologic, and Neonatal Nursing, 21*(2), 114–120. doi:10.1111/j.1552-6909.1992.tb01729.x

Chapman, L. L. (2000). Expectant fathers and labor epidurals. *MCN: The American Journal of Maternal Child Nursing, 25*(3), 133–139.

Cheng, Y., Nicholson, J., Shaffer, B., Lyell, D., & Caughey, A. (2009). The second stage of labor and epidural use: A larger effect than previously suggested. *American Journal of Obstetrics & Gynecology, 201*(6), S46. doi:10.1016/j.ajog.2009.10.097

Christiaens, W., Verhaeghe, M., & Bracke, P. (2010). Pain acceptance and personal control in pain relief in two maternity care models: A cross national comparison of Belgium and the Netherlands. *BMC Health Services Research, 10*, 268–280.

Cluett, E. R., & Burns, E. (2009). Immersion in water in labour and birth. *Cochrane Database of Systematic Reviews, 2.*

Cluett, E. R., Pickering, R., Getliffe, K., St. James, N., & Saunders, G. (2004). Randomised controlled trial of labouring in water compared with standard of augmentation for management of dystocia in first stage of labour. *British Medical Journal, 328*(7435), 314–320.

Cohen, S. (1997). Strategies for labor pain relief—past, present and future. *ACTA Anaesthesiologica Scandinavia, 110S*, 17–21. doi:10.1111/j.1399-6576.1997.tb05485.x

Cyna, A. M., McAuliffe, G. I., & Andrew, M. I. (2004). Hypnosis for pain relief in labour and childbirth: A systematic review. *British Journal of Anaesthesia, 93,* 505–511. doi:10.1093/bja/aeh225

daSilva, F. M., deOliveira, S. M., & Nobre, M. R. (2009). A randomised controlled trial evaluating the effect of immersion bath on labour pain. *Midwifery, 25*(3), 286–294. doi:10.1016/j.midw.2007.04.006

Declercq, E. R., Sakala, C., Corry, M. P., & Applebaum, S. (2007). Listening to mothers II: Report of the second national U.S. survey of women's childbearing experiences. *Journal of Perinatal Education, 16*(4), 15–17. doi:10.1624/105812407X244895

DiFranco, J. (2000). Relaxation: Music. In F. Nichols & S. Humernick (Eds.), *Childbirth Education: Practice, Research and Theory* (2nd ed.). Philadelphia: WB Saunders.

D'Onofrio, P., Novelli, A. M., Mecacci, F., & Scarselli, G. (2009). The efficacy and safety of continuous intravenous administration of remifentanil for birth pain relief: An open study of 205 parturients. *International Anesthesia Research Society, 109*(6), 1922–1924. doi:10.1213/ane.0b013e3181acc6fc

El-Wahab, N., & Robinson, N. (2011). Analgesia and anaesthesia in labour. *Obstetrics, Gynaecology & Reproductive Medicine, 21,* 137–141.

Eriksson, M., Ladfors, L., Mattsson, L. A., & Fall, O. (1996). Warm tub bath during labor: A study of 1385 women with prelabor rupture of the membranes after 34 weeks of gestation. *Acta Obstetricia et Gynecologica Scandinavica, 75*(7), 642–644. doi:10.3109/00016349609054689

Eriksson, M., Mattsson, L. A., & Ladfors, L. (1997). Early or late bath during the first stage of labour: A randomized study of 200 women. *Midwifery, 13*(3), 146–148. doi:10.1016/S0266-6138(97)90005-X

Escott, D., Slade, P., & Spiby, H. (2009). Preparation for pain management during childbirth: The psychological aspects of coping strategy development in antenatal education. *Clinical Psychology Review, 29*(7), 617–622. doi:10.1016/j.cpr.2009.07.002

Evron, S., & Ezri, T. (2007). Options for systemic labor analgesia. *Current Opinion in Anaesthesiology, 20*(3), 181–185. doi:10.1097/ACO.0b013e328136c1d1

Faucher, M. A., & Brucker, M. C. (2000). Intrapartum pain: Pharmacologic management. *Journal of Obstetric, Gynecologic, and Neonatal Nursing, 29*(2), 169–180. doi:10.1111/j.1552-6909.2000.tb02037.x

Field, T., Hemandez-Reif, M., Taylor, S., Quintino, O., & Burman, I. (1997). Labor pain is reduced by massage therapy. *Journal of Psychosomatic Obstetrics & Gynecology, 18*(4), 286–291. doi:10.3109/01674829709080701

Flink, I. K., Mroczek, M., Sullivan, M., & Linton, S. J. (2009). Pain in childbirth and postpartum recovery—the role of catastrophizing. *European Journal of Pain, 13*(3), 312–316. doi:10.1016/j.ejpain.2008.04.010

Florence, D. J., & Palmer, D. G. (2003). Therapeutic choices for the discomforts of labor. *Journal of Perinatal and Neonatal Nursing, 17*(4), 238–249.

Gale, J., Fothergill-Bourbonnais, F., & Chamberlain, M. (2001). Measuring nursing support during childbirth. *MCN: The American Journal of Maternal Child Nursing, 26*(5), 264–271.

Garland, D., & Jones, K. (1997). Waterbirth: Updating the evidence. *British Journal of Midwifery, 5,* 6.

Gentz, B. A. (2001). Alternative therapies for the management of pain in labor and delivery. *Clinical Obstetrics and Gynecology, 44*(4), 704–732.

Gillesby, E., Burns, S., Dempsey, A., Kirby, S., Morgensen, K., Naylor, K., . . . Whelan, B. (2010). Comparison of delayed versus immediate pushing during second stage of labor for nulliparous women with epidural anesthesia. *Journal of Obstetrics, Gynecology, and Neonatal Nursing, 39*(6), 635–644. doi:10.1111/j.1552-6909.2010.01195.k

Gilliland, A. L. (2002). Beyond holding hands: The modern role of the professional doula. *Journal of Obstetric, Gynecologic, and Neonatal Nursing, 31*(6), 762–769. doi:10.1177/0884217502239215

Green, J. (1993). Expectations and experiences of pain in labor: Findings from a large prospective study. *Birth: Issues in Perinatal Care and Education, 20*(2), 65–72. doi:10.1111/j.1523-536X.1993.tb00419.x

Halpern, S., Muir, H., Breen, T. W., Campbell, D. C., Barrett, J., Liston, R., . . . Blanchard, J. W. (2004). A multicenter randomized controlled trial comparing patient-controlled epidural with intravenous analgesia for pain relief in labor. *Anesthesia & Analgesia, 99*(5), 1532–1538. doi:10.1213/01.ANE.0000136850.08972.07

Hawkins, J. (2010). Epidural analgesia for labor and delivery. *New England Journal of Medicine, 362*(16), 1503–1510.

Hawkins, J., Chang, J., Palmer, S. K., Gibbs, C. P., & Callaghan, W. M. (2011). Anesthesia-related maternal mortality in the United States: 1979-2002. *Obstetrics and Gynecology, 117*(1), 69–74. doi:10.1097/AOG.0b013e31820093a9

Hebl, J. R. (2006). The importance and implications of aseptic techniques during regional anesthesia. *Regional Anesthesia and Pain Medicine, 31*(4), 311–323.

Hinova A., & Fernando, R. (2009). Systemic remifentanil for labor analgesia. *Anesthesia & Analgesia, 109*(6), 1925–1929. doi:10.1213/ANE.0b013e3181c03e0c

Hodnett, E. D. (2002). Pain and women's satisfaction with the experience of childbirth: A systematic review. *American Journal of Obstetrics and Gynecology, 186*(5, Suppl.), S160–172.

Hodnett, E. D., Gates, S., Hafmeyr, G. I., & Sakala, C. (2012). Continuous support for women during childbirth. *Cochrane Database Systematic Review,* CD003766. doi:10.1002/14651858.CD003766.pub4

Hodnett, E. D., Lowe, N. K., Hannah, M. E., Willan, A. R., Stevens, B., Weston, J. A., . . . Stremler, R. (2002). Effectiveness of nurses as providers of birth labor support in North American hospitals: A randomized controlled trial. *Journal of the American Medical Association, 288*(11), 1373–1381. doi:10.1001/jama.288.11.1373

Hong, R. W. (2010). Less is more: The recent history of neuraxial labor analgesia. *American Journal of Therapeutics, 17*(5), 492–497. doi:10.1097/MJT.0b013e3181ea788

Horlocker, T. T., Wedel, D. J., Rowlingson, J. C., Enneking, F. K., Kopp, S. L., Benzon, H. T., . . . Yuan, C. S. (2010). Regional anesthesia in the patient receiving antithrombotic or thrombolytic therapy. American Society of Regional Anesthesia and Pain Medicine evidence-based guidelines (3rd edition). *Regional Anesthesia and Pain Medicine, 35*(1), 64–101. doi:10.1097/AAP.0b013e3181c15c70

Huntley, A. L., Coon, J. T., & Ernst, E. (2004). Complementary and alternative medicine for labor pain: A systematic review. *American Journal of Obstetrics and Gynecology, 191*(1), 36–44. doi:10.1016/j.ajog.2003.12.008

Ketterhagen, D., VandeVusse, L., & Berner, M. (2002). Self-hypnosis: Alternative anesthesia for childbirth. *MCN: American Journal of Maternal Child Nursing, 27*(6), 335–340.

Kiani, K. (2009). Effect of water birth on labor pain during active phase of labor. *International Journal of Gynecology & Obstetrics, 107S2,* S93–S96.

Kimber, L., McNabb, M., McCourt, C., Haines, A., & Brocklehurst, P. (2008). Massage or music for pain relief in labour: A pilot randomized placebo controlled trial. *European Journal of Pain, 12*(8), 961–969. doi:10.1016/j.ejpain.2008.01.004

King, T. L., & McCool, W. F. (2004). The definition and assessment of pain. *Journal of Midwifery & Women's Health, 49*(6), 471–472. doi:10.1016/j.jmwh.2004.09.010

Klaus, M. H., Kennell, J. H., & Klaus, P. H. (2002). *The Doula Book: How a Trained Labor Companion Can Help You Have a Shorter, Easier, and Healthier Birth.* Cambridge, MA: Perseus.

Kuczkowski, K. M., & Reisner, L. S. (2003). Anesthetic management of the parturient with fever and infection. *Journal of Clinical Anesthesia, 15*, 478–488. doi:10.1016/S0952-8180(03)00081-3

Labrecque, M., Nouwen, A., Bergeron, M., & Rancourt, J. F. (1999). A randomized controlled trial of nonpharmacologic approaches for relief of low back pain during labor. *Journal of Family Practice, 48*(4), 259–230.

Lally, J. E., Murtagh, M. J., Jacphail, S., & Thomson, R. (2008). More in hope than expectations: A systematic review of women's expectations and experience of pain relief in labour. *BMC Medicine, 6*, 1–10. doi:10.1186/1741-7015-6-7

Lavender, T., Walkinshaw, S. A., & Walton, I. (1999). A prospective study of women's views of factors contributing to a positive birth experience. *Midwifery, 15*(1), 40–46. doi:10.1016/S0266-6138(99)90036-0

Liu, E. H., & Sia, A. T. (2004). Rates of cesarean section and instrumental vaginal delivery in nulliparous women after low concentration epidural infusions or opioid analgesia: Systematic review. *British Medical Journal, 328*(7453), 410–415. doi:10.1136/bmj.38097.590810.7C

Lothian, J. (2005). Birth plans: The good, the bad, and the future. *Journal of Obstetric and Neonatal Nurses, 35*, 295–303. doi:10.1111/J.1552-6909.2006.00042.x

Lowe, N. (2002). The nature of labor pain. *American Journal of Obstetrics and Gynecology, 186*, S16–24. doi:10.1067/mob.2002.121427

Lytzen, T., Cederberg, L., & Moller-Nielsen, J. (1989). Relief of low back pain in labor by using intracutaneous nerve stimulation with sterile water papules. *Acta Obstetricia et Gynecologica Scandinavica, 68*(4), 341–343. doi:10.3109/00016348909028669

MacKenzie, I. Z., Xu, J., Cusick, C., Midwinter-Morten, H., Meacher, H., Mollison, J., & Brock, M. (2011). Acupuncture for pain relief during induced labor in nulliparae: a randomized controlled study. *BJOG, 118*(4), 440–447. doi:10.1111/j.1471-0528.2010.02825.x

Mackey, M. M. (2001). Use of water in labor and birth. *Clinical Obstetrics and Gynecology, 44*(4), 733–749.

Manning-Orenstein, G. (1998). A birth intervention: The therapeutic effects of doula support versus Lamaze preparation on first-time mother's working models of caregiving. *Alternative Therapeutic Health Medicine, 4*(4), 73–81.

Martensson, L., & Wallin, G. (1999). Labor pain treated with cutaneous injections of sterile water: A randomized controlled trial. *British Journal of Obstetrics and Gynecology, 106*(7), 633–637. doi:10.1111/j.1471-0528.1999.tb08359.x

Mayberry, L. J., Clemmens, D., & De, A. (2002). Epidural analgesia side effects, co-interventions, and care of women during childbirth: A systematic review. *American Journal of Obstetrics and Gynecology, 186*(5), S81–S94.

Mayberry, L. J., Wood, S. H., Strange, L. B., Lee, L., Heisler, D. R., & Nielsen-Smith, K. (2000). *Second Stage Labor Management: Promotion of Evidence-Based Practice and a Collaborative Approach to Patient Care.* (Symposium). Washington, DC: Author.

McCaffery, M., & Pasero, C. (1999). Practical nondrug approaches to pain. In M. McCaffery & C. Pasero (Eds.), *Pain: Clinical Manual for Nursing Practice* (2nd ed., pp. 399–427). St Louis, MO: Mosby.

Melzack, R. (1984). The myth of painless childbirth. *Pain, 19*(4), 321–327. doi:10.1016/0304(84)90079-4

Melzack, R. (1999). From the gate to the neuromatrix. *Pain, 82*(Suppl.), S121–126. doi:10.1016/s0304-3959(99)00145-1

Melzack, R., & Wall, P. D. (1965). Pain mechanisms: A new theory. *Science, 150*, 971–979.

Merson, N. (2001). A comparison of motor block between ropivacaine and bupivacaine for continuous labor epidural analgesia. *Journal of the American Association of Nurse Anesthetists, 69*(1), 54–58.

Miltner, R. S. (2002). More than support: Nursing interventions provided to women in labor. *Journal of Obstetric, Gynecologic, and Neonatal Nursing, 31*(6), 753–761. doi:10.1177/0884217502239214

Molina, F. J., Sola, P. A., Lopez, E., & Pires, C. (1997). Pain in the first stage of labor: Relationship with the patient's position. *Journal Pain Symptom Management, 13*(2), 98–103. doi:10.1016/50885-3924(96)00270-9

Mosallam, M., Rizk, D. E., Thomas, L., & Ezimokhai, M. (2004). Women's attitudes towards psychosocial support in labour in United Arab Emirates. *Archives of Gynecology and Obstetrics, 269*(3), 181–187. doi:10.1007/s00404-002-0448-7

Mussell, S. (1998). Narcotic analgesia during labor and birth: Maternal and newborn effects. *Mother-Baby Journal, 3*(6), 19–23.

National Institute for Clinical Excellence. (2008). *Antenatal care: Routine care for the healthy pregnant woman. Clinical guideline.* Retrieved from http://www.nice.org.uk/nicemedia/live/11947/40145/40145.pdf

Nikodem, V. C. (2004). Immersion in water in pregnancy, labour and birth. *Cochrane Database of Systematic Reviews, 2.*

Niven, C. A., & Gijsbers, K. J. (1989). Do low levels of labor pain reflect low sensitivity to noxious stimulation? *Social Science and Medicine, 29*(4), 585–588. doi:10.1016/0277-9536(89)90204-9

O'Hana, H. P., Levy, A., Rozen, A., Greemberg, L., Shapira, Y., & Sheiner, E. (2008). The effect of epidural analgesia on labor progress and outcome in nulliparous women. *The Journal of Maternal-Fetal and Neonatal Medicine, 21*(8), 517–521. doi:10.1080/14767050802040864

Osborne, L., Snyder, M., Villecco, D., Jacob, A., Pyle, S., & Crum-Cianflone, N. (2008). Evidence-based anesthesia: Fever of unknown origin in parturients and neuraxial anesthesia. *American Association of Nurse Anesthetists Journal, 76*(3), 221–226.

O'Sullivan, G. (2009). Epidural analgesia and labor. *European Journal of Pain Supplements, 3*, 65–70. doi:10.1016/j.eujps.2009.08.006

O'Sullivan, G. (2010). Non-neuraxial analgesia during labour. *Anaesthesia and Intensive Care Medicine, 11*(7), 270–273. doi:10.1016/j.mpaic.2010.04.009

Palomaki, O., Huhtala, H., & Kirkinen, P. (2005). A comparative study of the safety of 0.25% levobupivacaine and 0.25% racemic bupivacaine for paracervical block in the first stage of labor. *Acta Obstetricia et Gynecologica Scandinavica, 84*(10), 956–961. doi:10.1111/j.0001-6349.2005.00709.x

Polley, L. S., Columb, M. O., Naughton, N. N., Wagner, D. S., & van de Ven, C. J. (2002). Effect of epidural epinephrine on the minimum local analgesic concentration of epidural bupivacaine in labor. *Anesthesiology, 96*(5), 1123–1128.

Poole, J. (2003). Analgesia and anesthesia during labor and birth: Implications for mother and fetus. *Journal of Obstetrics, Gynecology, and Neonatal Nursing, 32*(6), 780–793. doi:10.1177/0884217503258498

Rayburn, W. F., Smith, C. V., Parriott, J. E., & Woods, R. E. (1989). Randomized comparison of meperidine and fentanyl during labor. *Obstetric & Gynecology, 74*(4), 604–606.

Reynolds, F. (2010). The effects of maternal labour analgesia on the fetus. *Best Practice & Research Clinical Obstetrics and Gynaecology, 24*(3), 289–302. doi:10.1016/j.bpobgyn.2009.11.003

Reynolds, F. (2011). Labour analgesia and the baby: Good news is no news; review article. *International Journal of Obstetric Anesthesia, 20*(1), 38–50. doi:10.1016/j.ijoa.2010.08.004

Roberts, L., Gulliver, B., Fisher, J., & Cloyes, K. G. (2010). The coping with labor algorithm: An alternate pain assessment tool for the laboring woman. *Journal of Midwifery & Women's Health, 55*(2), 107–116. doi:10.1016/j.jmwh.2009.11.002

Rosen, M. A. (2002). Nitrous oxide for relief of labor pain: A systematic review. *American Journal of Obstetrics and Gynecology, 186*(5), S110–126.

Roofthooft, E. (2009). Anesthesia for the morbidly obese parturient. *Current Opinion in Anaesthesiology, 22*(3), 341–346. doi:10.1097/ACO.0b013e328329a5b8

Royal College of Obstetricians and Gynaecologists. (2006). *Immersion in water during labor and birth. No. 1.* Retrieved from http://www.rcog.org.uk/files/rcog-corp/uploaded-files/Joint StatmentBirthInWater2006.pdf

Ruppen, W., Derry, S., McQuay, H., & Moore, R. N. (2006). Incidence of epidural hematoma, infection and neurologic injury in obstetric patients with epidural analgesia/anesthesia. *Anesthesiology, 105*(2), 394–399.

Russell, R., & Reynolds, F. (1996). Epidural infusion of low-dose bupivacaine and opioid in labor. *Anaesthesia, 51*(3), 266–273. doi:10.1111/j.1365-2044.1996.tb13645.x

Sanders, R. D., Weimann, J., & Maze, M. (2008). Biologic effects of nitrous oxide. *Anesthesiology, 109*(4), 707–722. doi:10.1097/ALN.0b013e3181870a17

Saravanakumar, K., Rao, S. G., & Cooper, G. M. (2006). The challenges of obesity and obstetric anesthesia. *Current Opinion in Obstetrics and Gynecology, 18*(6), 631–635.

Scott, K. D., Berkowitz, G., & Klaus, M. (1999). A comparison of intermittent and continuous support during labor: A meta-analysis. *American Journal of Obstetrics and Gynecology, 180*(5), 1054–1059.

Simkin, P. (1995). Reducing pain and enhancing progress in labor: A guide to nonpharmacologic methods for maternity caregivers. *Birth, 22*(3), 161–171. doi:10.1111/j.1523-536X.1995.tb00693.x

Simkin, P., & Bolding, A. (2004). Update on nonpharmacologic approaches to relieve labor pain and prevent suffering. *Journal of Midwifery and Women's Health, 49*(6), 489–504. doi:10.1016/j.jmwh.2004.07.007

Simkin P., & O'Hara, M. A. (2002) Nonpharmacologic relief of pain during labor: Systematic reviews of five methods. *American Journal of Obstetrics and Gynecology, 186*(5, Suppl.), S131–S159. doi:10.1067/mob.2002.122382

Simpson, K. R. (2007). Intrauterine resuscitation during labor: Review of current methods and supportive evidence. *Journal of Midwifery and Women's Health, 52*(3), 229–237. doi:10.1016/j.jmwh.2006.12.010

Simpson, K. R., & James, D. C. (2005). Efficacy of intrauterine resuscitation techniques in improving fetal oxygen status during labor. *Obstetrics and Gynecology, 105*(6), 1362–1368. doi:10.1097/01.AOG.0000164474.03350.7c

Skupski, D. W., Abramovitz, S., Samuels, J., Pressimone, V., & Kjaer, K. (2009). Adverse effects of combined spinal-epidural versus traditional epidural analgesia. *International Journal of Gynecology and Obstetrics, 106*(3), 242–245. doi:10/1016/j.ijgo.2009.04/019

Sleutel, M. R. (2000). Climate, culture, context, or work environment: Organizational factors that influence nursing practice. *Journal of Nursing Administration, 30*(2), 53–58.

Somers-Smith, M. J. (1999). A place for the partner? Expectations and experiences of support during childbirth. *Midwifery, 15*(2), 101–108. doi:10.1016/S0266-6138(99)90006-2

Stark, M. A., Rudell, B., & Haus, G. (2008). Observing position and movements in hydrotherapy: A pilot study. *Journal of Obstetric, Gynecologic, & Neonatal Nursing, 37*(1), 116–122. doi:10.1111/J1552*6909.2007.00212.x

Sun, L. S. (2011). Labor analgesia and the developing human brain. *Anesthesia & Analgesia, 112*(6), 1265–1267. doi:10.1213/ANE.0b013e3182135a4d

The Joint Commission on Accreditation of Healthcare Organizations. (2011). *National patient safety goals: Hospital.* Retrieved from http://www.jointcommission.org/assets/1/6/2011_NPSGs_HAP.pdf

Thorp, J. (1999). Epidural analgesia during labor. *Clinical Obstetrics and Gynecology, 42*(4), 785–801.

Touitou, Y., Dispersyn, G., & Pain, L. (2010). Labor pain, analgesia and chronobiology: What factor matters? *Anesthesia & Analgesia, 111*(4), 838–840. doi:10:1213/ANE.0b013e3181ee85d9

Tournaire, M., & Theau-Yonneau, A. (2007). Complementary and alternative approaches to pain relief during labor. *Evidenced Based Complimentary and Alternative Medicine, 4*(4), 409–417. doi:10.1093/ecam/nem012

Trolle, B., Moller, M., Kronborg, H., & Thomsen, S. (1991). The effect of sterile water blocks on low back labor pain. *American Journal of Obstetrics and Gynecology, 164*(5, Pt. 1), 1277–1281.

Ullman, R., Smith, L. A., Burns, E., Mori, R., & Dowswell, T. (2010). Parenteral opioids for maternal pain relief in labor (Review). *Cochrane Database of Systematic Reviews,* (9), CD007396. doi:10.1002/14651858.CD007396.pub2

Verani, J. R., McGee, L., & Schrag, S. J. (2010). Prevention of perinatal group B streptococcal disease—Revised guidelines from the CDC, 2010. *Morbidity and Mortality Weekly Report, 59*(RR-10), 1–36.

Vincent, R. D., & Chestnut, D. H. (1998). Epidural analgesia during labor. *American Family Physician, 58*(8), 1785–1792.

Volmanen, P., Palomaki, O., & Ahonen, J. (2011). Alternatives to neuraxial analgesia for labor *Current Opinion in Anesthesiology, 24*(3), 235–241. doi:10.1097/ACO.0b013e328345ad18

Wakefield, M. L. (1999). Systemic analgesia: Opioids, ketamine, and inhalational agents. In D. H. Chestnut (Ed.), *Obstetric Anesthesia: Principles and Practice* (pp. 340–353). St. Louis, MO: Mosby.

Wesselmann, U. (2008). Pain in childbirth. In M. C. Bushnell, D. V. Smith, G. K. Beauchamp, S. J. Firestein, P. Dallos, D. Oertel, . . . A. I. Basbaum (Eds.), *The Senses: A Comprehensive Reference* (pp. 579–583). St. Louis, MO: Elsevier.

Williams, M. S., Davies, J. M., & Ross, B. K. (2009). Medicolegal issues in obstetric anesthesia. In D. H. Chestnut, L. S. Polley, L. C. Tsen, & C. A. Wong (Eds.), *Chestnut's Obstetric Anesthesia: Principles and Practice* (4th ed., pp. 727–746). Philadelphia: Mosby.

Wiruchpongsanon, P. (2006). Relief of low back labor pain by using intracutaneous injections of sterile water: A randomized clinical trial. *Journal of the Medical Association of Thailand, 89*(5), 571–576.

Wong, C. A. (2009). Epidural and spinal analgesia/anesthesia for labor and vaginal delivery. In D. H. Chestnut, L. S. Polley, L. C. Tsen, & C. A. Wong (Eds.), *Chestnut's Obstetric Anesthesia: Principles and Practice* (4th ed., pp. 429–492). St. Louis, MO: Mosby.

Wong, C. A., McCarthy, R. J., & Hewlett, B. (2011). The effect of manipulation of the programmed intermittent bolus time interval and injection volume on total drug use for labor epidural analgesia: A randomized controlled trial. *Anesthesia & Analgesia, 112*(4), 904–911. doi:10.1213/ANE.0b013e31820e7c2f

Wong, C. A., Scavone, B. M., Peaceman, A. M., McCarthy, R. J., Sullivan, J. T., Diaz, N. T., . . . Grouper, S. (2005). The risk of cesarean delivery with neuraxial analgesia given early versus late in labor. *New England Journal of Medicine, 352*(7), 655–665.

Wright, M., McCrea, H., Stringer, M., & Murphy-Black, T. (2000). Personal control in pain relief during labor. *Journal of Advanced Nursing, 32*(5), 1168–1177. doi:10.1046/j.1365-2648.2000.01587.x

Yancey, M. K., Zhang, J., Schwatz, J., Dietrick, C. S., & Klebanoff, M. (2001). Labor epidural analgesia and intrapartum maternal hyperthermia. *Obstetrics & Gynecology, 98*(5, Pt. 1), 763–770. doi:PII S0029-7844(01)01537-X

Zwelling, E. (2010). Overcoming the challenges: Maternal movement and positioning to facilitate labor progress. *MCN: The American Journal of Maternal/Child Nursing, 35*(2), 72–78. doi:10.1097/NMC.0b013e3181caeab3

Zwelling, E., Johnson, K., & Allen, J. (2006). How to implement complimentary therapies for laboring women. *MCN: The American Journal of Maternal/Child Nursing, 31*(6), 364–370.

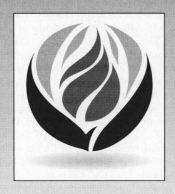

Dotti C. James

CHAPTER 17

Postpartum Care

A woman experiences significant alterations in physical and psychosocial status after childbirth. The postpartum period is a time of transition involving physiologic changes, adaptation to the maternal role, and modification of the family system by the addition of the baby. Nurses have a unique opportunity to promote and support maternal and family adaptation. Inpatient postpartum care routines are ideally focused on the needs of the mother, baby, and family, rather than on arbitrary rules and unit traditions. Postpartum nursing care should be as individualized and flexible as needed. The perinatal nurse recognizes women and their families as integral members of the healthcare team and encourages them to enter into decision-making processes and planning of care (Association of Women's Health, Obstetric and Neonatal Nurses [AWHONN], 2009). Open visiting and family interaction with the new mother and newborn are supported. The father of the baby and other support persons should be encouraged to be present, according to the desires of the woman, and actively involved in postpartum and newborn care. Family-centered maternity care is based on the philosophy that the physical, social, psychological, and spiritual needs of the family are included in all aspects of the nursing care provided (AWHONN, 2009).

Implementation of family-centered maternity care requires collaboration among childbearing women, families, and healthcare providers. The family is defined by the woman and frequently extends beyond traditional definitions. Cultural beliefs and values of the woman and her family should be respected and accommodated. Chapter 2 and the March of Dimes Nursing Module *Cultural Competence: An Essential Journey for Perinatal Nurses* (Moore, Moos, & Callister, 2010) provide a comprehensive review and discussion of various cultural and religious perspectives and can be helpful in developing nursing care for specific women.

A woman experiences significant changes in physical and psychosocial status following childbirth. Nurses have a unique opportunity to promote and support maternal and family adaptation during this time. The chapter begins with a discussion of planning the transition to parenthood, which ideally occurs during pregnancy. Physiologic changes during the postpartum period, appropriate nursing assessments, and interventions for healthy women, as well as common complication and care for these are reviewed as well. Physiologic and psychosocial adaptation are reviewed as well as educational needs and follow-up after discharge.

PLANNING FOR THE TRANSITION TO PARENTHOOD

According to current trends, length of stay (LOS) for childbirth is now more realistically in line with the physical and psychosocial needs of the new mother and her family rather than with the previous arbitrary mandates from health insurance companies in an effort to control costs. However, although LOS has slightly increased over the past several years, it is still relatively short in all settings. One observation of the effect of longer LOS is a significant decline in neonatal readmissions but not in 1-year mortality (Datar & Sood, 2006). Thus, discharge planning cannot be delayed until admission for childbirth. Women in active labor and women who have just given birth are not candidates for a discussion of learning needs or for typical classroom education about self-care or infant care. The woman's focus during the intrapartum period is on safe passage through labor and on a healthy, positive childbirth experience.

Rubin's (1961a) classic research suggests that during the immediate postpartum period, the new mother is not physically or emotionally ready to listen to extensive presentations of how to care for herself and her newborn. Postpartum women have transient deficits in cognition, particularly in memory function, the first day after giving birth. According to Rana, Lindheimer, Hibbard, and Pliskin (2006), normal pregnant women can temporarily develop mild cognitive defects during labor and after birth when compared with nonpregnant women. Women in their study reported problems with attention, concentration, and memory throughout pregnancy and in the early postpartum period (Rana et al., 2006). This decline was not attributed to depression, anxiety, sleep deprivation, or other physical changes associated with pregnancy. Causes suggested included the increased levels of pregnenolone and allopregnanolone that are correlated with negative effects on memory, as well as the high levels of endogenous and exogenous cortisol, which affect hippocampal integrity and, therefore, explicit memory (Rana et al., 2006). Based on available evidence, traditional discharge planning that includes verbal transmission of information or instruction in child care techniques immediately after birth or on the first postpartum day will be poorly remembered. These findings underscore the importance of providing the family with appropriate written material they can review after discharge. Priorities for most women in the first 24 hours postpartum are rest; time to touch, hold, and get to know their baby; and an opportunity to review and discuss their labor and birth (Rubin, 1961a).

New mothers recognize their babies by olfactory and/or tactile cues, senses that do not primarily require cognitive function. In a recent study, 90% of women tested identified their newborns by olfactory cues after only 10 minutes to 1 hour exposure to their babies. All of the women tested recognized their babies' odor after exposure periods greater than 1 hour. Interestingly, women holding nonrelated infants for at least 1 hour could also recognize the infant, suggesting that this may be a human trait (Jacob, 2006). The childbearing experience is very different today than it was nearly 50 years ago when Rubin (1961a, 1961b) began her research. Major changes include the availability of prenatal classes; women and families as active participants in all aspects of perinatal care; fathers, siblings, and other support persons present for labor and birth; epidural anesthesia/analgesia; open visiting; single-room maternity care; couplet care models; and shorter hospitalizations. However, despite the progress made toward a healthcare environment where childbearing women have more participation and control, much of Rubin's work about the taking-in and taking-hold phases of the postpartum period is still valid today.

The discharge planning process should be ongoing during pregnancy, labor, and the postpartum period.

Although education about maternal and infant care can occur during the inpatient stay, information should be offered during pregnancy and reinforced after discharge in many different settings using a variety of teaching methods. The prenatal period provides a window of opportunity to prepare families not only about pregnancy and birth but also about the postpartum and newborn periods. Prenatal visits to the primary healthcare provider are an ideal time for the perinatal nurse to assess family learning needs and concerns and to offer information, support, and resources in a personalized way. Prenatal classes should provide education about pregnancy, health promotion, labor and birth, postpartum, maternal and infant care, and the transition to parenthood. Critical concepts can then be reviewed and reinforced during the postpartum stay.

Follow-up home visits or visits to outpatient clinics and offices offer the perinatal nurse another opportunity to assess knowledge, skills, and learning needs, as well as to provide individualized education, support, and referrals (Ladewig, London, & Davidson, 2009). If home visits are not possible, follow-up phone calls after discharge provide the perinatal nurse an opportunity to clarify information and answer additional questions. Finally, classes and support groups for new parents are another way for families to continue learning about maternal and infant care, parenting, and how to nurture the couple relationship.

Healthcare providers continue to struggle to find innovative ways to provide safe, cost-effective, and comprehensive perinatal care in response to economic pressures. Although consumer pressures resulted in state and federal laws mandating minimal LOS coverage, costs remain a very real issue for institutions and individual healthcare providers. Prenatal education in healthcare provider offices and in the classroom combined with written materials and/or videos are some methods that prepare women and their families for discharge (Brown, 2006; Roudebush, Kaufman, Johnson, Abraham, & Clayton, 2006). Women feel more in control and express greater feelings of maternal confidence and competence when they have adequate knowledge about how to care for themselves and their newborns after discharge (Brown, 2006; Roudebush et al., 2006).

PRENATAL PATIENT DATABASE

Early identification and entry into the system can facilitate prenatal preparation for hospitalization and postpartum discharge. Successful programs require communication among primary healthcare providers, prenatal educators, community resources, and the perinatal center. A simple, user-friendly system that incorporates demographic data, estimated date of birth, significant clinical history, family assessment and learning needs, participation in prenatal education programs, and a mechanism to communicate all pertinent information to the inpatient unit is critical. A computerized database is ideal, but traditional file systems in addition to communication in person or by phone, facsimile (fax), and e-mail also work well for women with access to the Internet. Healthcare providers at each institution can develop a prenatal patient database to meet specific needs. For example, when a woman registers her intent to give birth at the institution early in pregnancy, demographic and insurance data can be entered into the system. Primary healthcare providers and those in community prenatal clinics that refer women for inpatient care can be encouraged to send notification about women who have selected the institution for childbirth.

Some hospitals have developed Internet Web sites where women can register for childbirth classes, seek prenatal care information, download patient education materials, and take a virtual tour of the facilities. Summaries of the educational and clinical backgrounds, services, office hours, and insurance plan participation of healthcare providers that have privileges at the institutions can offer valuable information to women who are in the process of selecting a healthcare provider and an institution for birth. Links to offices of obstetricians, family practice physicians, and nurse midwives on staff can be helpful as well. Information about financial criteria for eligibility to participate in programs such as Medicaid and the Special Supplemental Nutrition Feeding Program for Women, Infants, and Children (WIC) are useful for selected families. As more families of childbearing age gain access to the Internet, these Web sites will meet the needs of both patients and healthcare institutions.

Healthcare providers can provide mothers with a childbirth and parenting preparation book (or suggest one to be purchased) in early pregnancy, supply expectant families with information about the institution, and urge them to take a tour of the perinatal unit. Brochures describing all perinatal services available at the institution, including telephone numbers, are especially helpful and ideally should be available in the offices of all healthcare providers affiliated with the institution. Written materials should be available in the languages of the population served. Families should be informed about prenatal classes and encouraged to attend. Selected women and their families can be referred for case management, especially when the pregnancy and the social or economic situation are complex.

By the 36th week of pregnancy, a record of prenatal care should be sent by the primary healthcare provider to the perinatal institution to be available when the woman is admitted for labor and birth (American Academy of Pediatrics [AAP] & American College of Obstetricians and Gynecologists [ACOG], 2008). Specific individualized care plans or guides developed by the case manager, social worker, or perinatal nurse for the woman's inpatient stay also should be added to the patient database. With this type of system, when the woman is admitted for childbirth, the perinatal nurse has valuable information about current maternal–fetal health status, family learning needs, and the education programs the family attended. The quality and quantity of prenatal data about the childbearing family enhance the perinatal nurse's ability to provide individualized care and teaching.

PRENATAL CLASSES

In the past, most prenatal classes consisted of a series lasting 6 to 8 weeks in the last trimester of pregnancy focused primarily on preparation for labor and birth and, to a lesser extent, on pregnancy, infant care, and the transition to parenthood. For many working couples, making the time commitment to attend a series of six classes is often difficult. Multiple factors such as perceived knowledge, support systems, transportation issues, work schedules, childcare availability, and previous newborn and childbirth experience influence the decision to attend prenatal classes. Many institutions and perinatal educators have responded to consumer needs by streamlining content to decrease program length and offering alternatives such as weekend programs, flexible hours, informative Web sites, and antepartum home visits.

Information about health promotion should be presented early in pregnancy to have the opportunity to make a difference in pregnancy outcomes. Topics of early pregnancy classes may include:

- Fetal growth and development
- Expected physical changes during pregnancy
- Normal discomforts of pregnancy
- Lifestyle modifications
- Nutrition
- Activity and exercise
- Effects of smoking cigarettes, drinking alcohol, and using illegal drugs
- The need to ask primary healthcare providers about use of over-the-counter medications and medications prescribed by other healthcare providers prior to use
- Warning signs of pregnancy complications including a comprehensive discussion about preterm labor signs and symptoms and when to call their primary healthcare provider if these signs and symptoms should occur

Many hospitals have developed courses that cover early pregnancy content and have systems in place that prompt referral to these classes when women are seen for their first prenatal visit. Close partnerships with healthcare providers who are affiliated with the institution are essential to encourage women and their partners to attend classes that focus on early pregnancy health promotion.

Traditional prepared childbirth classes are offered during the third trimester when the mother and her partner are intent on learning about how to cope with labor pain and what to expect during labor and birth. Although the process of labor and birth is valuable content, information about parenthood and infant care is also important for expectant parents. (Display 17–1 displays course content for classes that include prepared childbirth and infant care information for a 6-week course.) For couples unable to meet the 6-week time commitment, classes that meet

DISPLAY 17–1

Prepared Childbirth and Infant Care Class Curriculum Overview

Prepared Childbirth	Infant Care
Class I	
Introduction	Selecting a pediatrician
Discomforts of pregnancy	Immunizations
Preterm labor	Child care
Exercises	Baby time
Relaxation and breathing patterns	
Slow-paced breathing and progressive relaxation	
Class II	
Preview of labor	Bathing video or bathing baby demonstration
Relaxation and breathing patterns	Changing or diapering
Favorite place, slow-paced, and bridged breathing	Holding baby
Position changes for labor	
Class III	
Birth video	Breastfeeding versus bottle-feeding
Goody bag	Burping
Relaxation and breathing patterns	Sleeping patterns
Transition	Pacifiers
Class IV	
Labor, birth, and nursery tour	Newborn characteristics
Medical interventions	
Class V	
Labor rehearsal	Infant CPR
Review breathing and relaxation	Choking demonstration
Emergency childbirth	Illness and when to call pediatrician
Cesarean birth video	Parents as teachers video
Medication, analgesia, anesthesia	
Class VI	
Postpartum discussion	Safety discussion
Postpartum care	Car seat safety
Party	

CPR, cardiopulmonary resuscitation.

Adapted from Harper, J. (2006). *Prenatal Class Content Outline*. St. Louis, MO: St. John's Mercy Medical Center.

less frequently can be designed. Options can include a 1-, 2-, or 3-week series covering critical content that is prioritized based on class time limitations. (Display 17–2 lists sample curricula for prenatal classes based on a 1-, 2-, or 3-week series.) Classes about parenting issues and infant care have been developed by many institutions. These classes are more commonly attended during pregnancy; however, some institutions have been successful in offering these classes to new parents during evening hours and inviting them to bring their newborn.

Although there is a significant need for information to assist in preparing couples for labor and birth, pregnant women and their partners can benefit from a comprehensive educational program that includes preconception health promotion, healthy behaviors during the prenatal period, breastfeeding, the postpartum period, and infant care content. (Display 17–3 shows suggested course content from early pregnancy to the postpartum period.)

Prenatal education classes should be designed to meet the needs of the population served and based on the knowledge of what information and skills are useful and relevant to expectant parents at various stages of pregnancy. Classes should be made available to a variety of women including teenagers, women who have previously given birth but desire a review class, women requesting private instruction, women who are hospitalized or on bed rest at home for much of their pregnancy, and women who speak a language other than English. Classes focusing on breastfeeding, sibling preparation, grandparents, car seat safety, exercise during pregnancy, labor preparation for women who desire a vaginal birth after cesarean birth (VBAC), and families expecting more than one baby complement the core curriculum.

A comprehensive education program developed by parent and childbirth educators in partnership with healthcare providers, perinatal nurses, and parents is ideal. An education curriculum designed using a team approach ensures that educators provide families with important information about pregnancy, childbirth, infant and postpartum care, and the transition to parenthood. Parent and birth educators play a significant role in preparing families for the postpartum period. It is important that their work is valued and that there is ongoing communication between the educators and the perinatal unit staff, especially if the educators are not formally affiliated with the institution. Disappointments and unmet expectations for the labor, birth, and postpartum experience can be avoided if childbirth educators are fully familiar with the policies of the perinatal unit. In some institutions, educators are invited to attend staff meetings and retreats and are offered the opportunity to spend time on the unit with a labor nurse periodically to maintain an awareness of the daily realities of the childbirth experience and unit routines.

Sample Curricula for Prenatal Classes

Class Content: One 3-Hour Prenatal Class

Essentials to bring to the hospital

Early signs of labor and when to come to the hospital

What to expect during labor and birth

Formulating a birth plan

Anesthesia and analgesia options

Visiting policies

How to anticipate length of stay (LOS), third-party payer issues, precertification, deductibles, and copayments

Choosing a pediatrician

Warning signs of pregnancy complications, including preterm labor and preeclampsia

Maternal care issues: episiotomy care, normal lochia, afterpains, incision care, breast care, nutrition, rest, "baby blues"

Newborn care issues: umbilical cord care, circumcision care, breastfeeding, formula feeding, diapering, bathing, behavioral and satiation cues, crying, comforting, car seats, sleep positioning, and other safety issues

Videotapes and booklets to reinforce class content

Parent hotline number for additional questions

Community and institutional resources

Class Content: Two 3-Hour Prenatal Classes

Class I

Essentials to bring to the hospital

Formulating a birth plan

Early signs of labor, relaxation, and breathing techniques

When to come to the hospital

The admission process

Ambulation in early labor

Electronic fetal monitoring and intermittent auscultation

Labor induction and augmentation

Amniotomy

Active labor

Transition

Second stage of labor

Anesthesia and analgesia options, review of pain relief and comfort measures, nonpharmacologic and pharmacologic

The unanticipated cesarean birth

Visiting policies

How to anticipate LOS, third-party payer issues, precertification, deductibles, and copayments

Warning signs of pregnancy complications, including preterm labor and preeclampsia

Class II

Choosing a pediatrician

Maternal care issues: episiotomy care, normal lochia, afterpains, incision care, breast care, nutrition, rest, baby blues, sexuality issues, contraception, and family planning

Newborn care issues: umbilical cord care, circumcision care, breastfeeding, formula feeding, diapering, bathing, behavioral and satiation cues, sleep–awake state, crying, comforting, car seats, sleep positioning, other safety issues

Videotapes and booklets to reinforce class content

Parent hotline number for additional questions

Community and institutional resources

Class Content: Three 3-Hour Prenatal Classes

Class I

Brief overview of fetal development

Changes during pregnancy

Nutrition and lifestyle modification

Sexuality during pregnancy

Formulating a birth plan

Relaxation and breathing techniques

Childbirth options

Visiting policies

How to anticipate LOS, third-party payer issues, precertification, deductibles, and copayments

Choosing a pediatrician

Tour of perinatal unit

Warning signs of pregnancy complications, including preterm labor and preeclampsia

Class II

Essentials to bring to the hospital

Early signs of labor and when to come to the hospital

The admission process

Ambulation in early labor

Electronic fetal monitoring and intermittent auscultation

Labor induction and augmentation

Amniotomy

Active labor

Transition

Second stage of labor

Anesthesia and analgesia options, review of pain relief and comfort measures, nonpharmacologic and pharmacologic

Reinforcement of relaxation and breathing techniques

The unanticipated cesarean birth

Class III

Maternal care issues: episiotomy care, normal lochia, afterpains, incision care, breast care, nutrition, rest, baby blues, sexuality issues, contraception, and family planning

Newborn care issues: umbilical cord care, circumcision care, breastfeeding, formula feeding, diapering, bathing, behavioral and satiation cues, sleep–awake state, crying, comforting, car seats, sleep positioning, other safety issues

Videotapes and booklets to reinforce class content

Parent hotline number for additional questions

Community and institutional resources

DISPLAY 17-3

Becoming Parents Course

The *Becoming Parents* course is designed to provide expectant families with the knowledge and skills needed to promote health during pregnancy and to prepare for childbirth and parenting. It reflects our philosophy that birth is one of life's most special events, and that the role of family maternity education is to enhance the joy of this experience by providing families with support and education throughout the childbearing years in partnership with healthcare providers and hospital staff.

Celebrating Your Pregnancy—First Trimester
This informative and entertaining evening seminar focuses on how to grow a healthy baby and have a healthy pregnancy. You will learn about fetal growth and development, optimal lifestyle choices for pregnancy, workplace and environmental hazards to avoid, common changes in family relationships during pregnancy, how to be an informed healthcare consumer, and resources for education and support at our hospital and in the community.
2-hour seminar

Growing the Baby of Your Dreams—Second Trimester
In the middle trimester, most families begin to imagine what their baby will look like and be like. You'll be amazed to discover the unique physical characteristics and capabilities of newborns and how able they are to respond to your love. We'll talk about what it means to be a parent and how becoming a parent affects your family relationships. You'll also learn about baby care and what supplies you'll need, and you will begin to master some of the labor coping skills such as relaxation and the first level of breathing. This series is also offered as *Christian Growing the Baby of Your Dreams*, with time to discuss the spiritual aspects of pregnancy, birth, and parenting.
Two 2-hour classes or one 4-hour class, small group

Breastfeeding Basics—Second or Third Trimester
This class is recommended for all expectant families. You will learn about the health benefits of breastfeeding for mothers and infants; how to get off to a good start; how fathers, partners, and family can support breastfeeding; and resources for support. A panel of families shares their breastfeeding experiences and valuable insights.
2-hour seminar

Breastfeeding and the 21st Century Family: Beyond the Basics—Second or Third Trimester (can be repeated after the birth)
Expectant mothers, fathers, partners, and family are encouraged to attend this class to learn about how breastfeeding fits into a busy lifestyle. You will learn how to express or pump breast milk, which pumps are best, how to store breast milk and for how long, and how to feed your baby when mother is away or at work. Tips for working mothers are provided. Breastfeeding Basics is a prerequisite.
2-hour seminar

CPR, cardiopulmonary resuscitation.

Sneak Peek: A Look at Postpartum—Early Third Trimester
Take a peek at the realities of life with a newborn baby—the joys and the challenges. You will learn about physical recovery from birth and self-care to enhance healing and increase comfort. Also discussed are emotional and lifestyle changes to expect after delivery and resources to help you cope. A new-parent panel offers suggestions for a smooth transition to parenthood.
2-hour seminar

Birth Basics—Middle to Late Third Trimester
This class prepares you for childbirth. What to expect in labor and birth, how to develop an individual approach to birth, the partner's role in labor, breathing and relaxation techniques, methods of pain management, medical procedures, common variations in childbirth, and cesarean birth will be discussed. Included in this class is a tour of the Family Maternity Center. This series is also offered as Christian, Spanish language, and Teen Birth Basics courses.
Four 2-hour classes or two 4-hour weekend classes, small group

OTHER CLASSES RELATED TO CHILDBIRTH AND EARLY PARENTING
During Pregnancy
Vaginal Birth After Cesarean (VBAC)
Labor and Birth Refresher
Becoming Grandparents
For Dads Only
Sibling Preparation
Car-Safe Kids
Maternity Fitness and Education
Yoga for Pregnancy
Family Maternity Center Tours
After Birth
    Parent–Baby Classes—a weekly class for parents and babies through the first year
    Yoga for New Moms
    Infant Massage
    Infant and Child CPR
    Early parenting seminars and series:
        Guiding Children's Behavior
        Toddler Development
        Parenting with Love and Logic
Breastfeeding the Older Baby
Starting Solids
Infant Sleep and the Conflict with American Culture
Young Moms Support Group
This Is Not What I Expected—emotional support for new families in postpartum
During Pregnancy or After
IMET: Keys for Couples—a weekend seminar to strengthen couple relationships
In Special Circumstances
Private classes for childbirth preparation are available.

EDUCATIONAL METHODS AND MATERIALS

Whether education is provided at the bedside, in a large auditorium, or in a small classroom, the teaching method must complement the information presented and must be appropriate for the learner. Skills such as comfort measures and pain relief during labor, infant bathing, or cord care are most effectively taught by demonstration and return demonstration. Feelings and beliefs are best addressed individually or in a small group setting. Consideration needs to be given to personal learning styles and basic education level and knowledge. Including parents as part of the prenatal education team enhances the likelihood that topics offered will be what parents want and need to know. Some institutions periodically hold new parent focus groups or use telephone or mailed surveys to validate the content of their educational materials and classes and to make sure they are consistent with the needs of their patients.

Written materials support and reinforce interactive learning. Books, pamphlets, brochures, and other handouts must have a consistent message and support the philosophy of the perinatal institution. There are a number of excellent resources in print, or the prenatal educators may develop their own education materials. Selection or development of written materials should be based on the education level of the population served and the financial resources available. The healthcare provider, educator, and representatives from the perinatal institution should collectively choose written materials and be familiar with the content. Parents should be asked to evaluate the usefulness and helpfulness of the written materials. Providing families with standardized written materials can be a timesaving and cost-effective strategy. If the institution chooses to use materials purchased from companies that specialize in developing childbirth and parenting educational materials, it is important to thoroughly review the content for accuracy before distributing to patients. Standardized materials (either purchased or developed by the institution) provide a ready resource for parents at any time and potentially decrease the volume of calls to the perinatal center and to the primary healthcare provider. Written materials should be developed or chosen with consideration to the basic language level of the family and to the language they speak. Families who do not speak English should be supplied with language-appropriate materials.

Some institutions use in-hospital television channels with programs on newborn bath, cord and circumcision care, and breastfeeding and formula feeding. Purchased videos or those produced by the institution are another method of providing important information. The videos can be given as gifts, loaned to families, or purchased in the hospital gift shop. As with written materials, television instruction and videos need to be evaluated for consistent, correct information that is learner appropriate and reflects the philosophy of the perinatal institution.

FAMILY PREFERENCE PLAN

Involving women and their families in decisions about their perinatal care increases satisfaction and promotes a collaborative relationship between healthcare providers and families. A preference plan helps to individualize the family's care (Display 17–4). Women who are asked about care preferences feel their unique needs will be met by nurses and other healthcare providers. Advantages of methods that encourage women and their families to define their individual approach to birth such as a birth plan or a list of family preferences include validation of the family's knowledge of available labor and birth options and perinatal center policies. The family preference plan can be given to all pregnant women registered for birth or given to families during prenatal classes. The preference plan provides the healthcare provider with information about the family's special needs, concerns, and requests and allows the healthcare provider to have a meaningful discussion with the family about their expectations. This discussion should occur during the pregnancy with the primary healthcare provider and with the perinatal nurse on admission to the unit for labor and birth.

Preference plans can be helpful in clarifying unit protocols and avoiding unmet expectations when women have plans for techniques or procedures that are not available on the unit. For example, the woman may have learned about the benefits of hydrotherapy in a Jacuzzi tub and wish to labor in the tub, but the unit may not have a Jacuzzi tub available; the woman may intend to use candles for aromatherapy; however, the unit may not allow burning candles for safety reasons; or the woman may plan to use a birthing ball during labor, but the unit may not have birthing balls. If these limitations are known in advance of admission, alternative plans can be made. In the examples described here, hydrotherapy can be provided in the shower, aromatherapy can be used with methods that do not include candles, and a birthing ball can be obtained on loan from a childbirth educator or purchased before admission.

The preference plan can be sent to the hospital with the prenatal care records or brought to the unit by the woman on admission for childbirth. It is important that any record-keeping process about childbirth preferences includes a system to ensure that it is available to all healthcare providers when the woman is admitted for labor and birth. The initial interaction during the admission process is used to develop rapport with the woman and her family and to get a sense of their expectations for their birth experience. Ideally, the amount of childbirth preparation and type of pain management anticipated during labor are covered prior to or during

DISPLAY 17-4

Family Preference Plan

My name: _____   My doctor's name: _____

1. I would like to have these persons visit during labor:
   _____   _____
   _____   _____

2. My main support person is:
   Relationship: _____

3. For pain control/positioning during labor and birth, I would like to:
   _____ walk in room/halls   _____ listen to special music
   _____ sit in recliner   _____ use special focal point
   _____ use shower   _____ use my own pillows
   _____ use Jacuzzi   _____ use squat bar
   _____ use heat/cold/massage   _____ use foot pads on bed

4. I would like to have these persons present during birth:
   _____   _____

5. I have these religious requests:
   _____ birth blessing by chaplain
   _____ Eucharist or communion
   _____ have visit by my own clergy
   _____ other: _____
   _____ none

6. After birth: I would like to:
   _____ place baby skin-to-skin
   _____ wrap baby in blanket before holding
   _____ breastfeed my baby
   _____ bathe my baby
   _____ have doctor circumcise my son
   _____ have pictures taken of my baby
   _____ keep baby in my room as long as he or she is stable

7. During my hospital stay, I would like to have my support person:
   _____ put baby skin-to-skin to him or her
   _____ assist with baby care
   _____ give the baby's first bath
   _____ spend the night in my room
   _____ take pictures of birth experience

8. I plan to attend, or have already attended, these classes/services during this pregnancy:
   _____ prenatal class
   _____ hospital OB tour
   _____ sibling class
   _____ exercise sessions
   _____ Lamaze

9. Child care has been arranged for other dependent children:
   _____ during the hospital stay
   _____ after mom and baby go home
   _____ not applicable
   _____ other: _____

10. I plan to have my other child(ren) come to visit:
    _____ during birth
    _____ in the first 2-hour recovery time
    _____ after I arrive in my postpartum room
    _____ not at all
    _____ not applicable

11. After going home, these persons will help out for the first 2 days:
    _____
    _____

12. Additional ideas:
    _____
    _____
    _____
    _____

the admission assessment. A review of preferences for childbirth, including reinforcement of options that are available at the institution, works best to facilitate a positive experience. Although some nurses and physicians have negative feelings about written birth plans, a birth plan helps the nurse meet the couple's expectations and indicates that the woman has given considerable thought to how she would like labor and birth to proceed. Every effort should be made to meet the expectations and wishes of the woman. The woman's desires for positioning, ambulation, and method of fetal assessment should be honored in ways that are consistent with safe care. If maternal and/or fetal status is such that the woman's wishes cannot be met within reason, a thorough discussion with adequate explanation of the rationale for the decision should occur. The woman should be allowed and encouraged to ask any questions and be given appropriate answers to those questions. It may be necessary for the primary healthcare provider to talk to the woman in person or by telephone about her concerns. The nurse should acknowledge the woman's disappointment and assure her that every attempt to meet her expectations will be made if the clinical situation changes.

Arbitrary rules prohibiting more than one support person during labor and birth are contrary to the philosophy that the birth experience belongs to the woman and her family rather than to those providing clinical care. Although healthcare providers are sometimes inclined to attempt to control this aspect of the birth process using various arguments for safety and convenience, when examined critically, these arguments have little scientific merit. Women should be able to choose who will be with them during this very special and unique life experience. Family-centered care supports the concept that the "family" is defined by childbearing women. Families should be free to take still pictures and record video and/or audiotapes during labor and birth. Policies restricting cameras are in conflict with the philosophy that the birth experience should be what the woman and her family desire within reason. Concerns about safety, liability, privacy, and space limitations can be adequately addressed without restrictive policies about visitors and use of cameras or filming during labor and birth if care providers are committed to meeting the needs of childbearing women and their support persons.

LEARNING NEEDS ASSESSMENT

Needs assessment tools, care paths, or teaching lists can assist nurses and families in identifying learning needs and in documentation of the type and timing of prenatal education (Brown, 2006). A learning needs assessment can be initiated at various times during the perinatal period depending on when a woman has first contact with the hospital system. Opportunities include prenatal classes, prenatal visits, hospital tours, and telephone contact with a case manager during admission to the hospital, following birth, and at the mother–infant follow-up visit or contact. Many families attending prenatal classes are first-time parents. A detailed assessment of individual learning needs discussed during the first prenatal class alerts prospective parents to information and skills they need to acquire by the time they are discharged from the hospital. The learning needs assessment tool or the defined curriculum and supporting written materials document the information, instruction provided, and the skills taught. When a formal needs assessment tool is used during pregnancy, the tool is forwarded to the perinatal unit from the prenatal instructor to be stored with the woman's prenatal data. Display 17–5 is an example of a tool that can be used on admission (if not in active labor) to assess learning needs and continued after birth to document teaching of self-care and baby care, and it then becomes the discharge teaching record. Content with an asterisk is reviewed with all women prior to hospital discharge. Referencing specific content to written materials provides reinforcement and promotes the use of materials as a reference for both families and perinatal nurses.

For women who have not attended prenatal classes or completed a learning needs assessment during a prenatal visit, the process begins on admission to the hospital. With the help of the labor nurse, families identify specific learning needs they want to address during the inpatient stay. Whether the needs assessment is completed prior to admission, during early labor, or after birth, the education process begins as soon as possible for each woman and family.

Primary responsibility for patient and family education varies with the institution. Patient education may be coordinated by the case manager, clinical nurse specialist, or perinatal educator; however, in any practice model, the perinatal staff nurse plays a key role. Critical concepts and essential information that families need have been identified. They are presented regardless of the family's past experience or self-assessment. Critical concepts include the following:

Maternal care
- Activity and rest
- Pain relief and comfort measures
- Care of the perineum and care of lacerations or episiotomy
- Breast care for breastfeeding women and lactation suppression for women who are formula feeding
- Postoperative cesarean birth instructions
- Expected emotional adaptations
- Signs of postpartum complications to report to the nurse in the hospital or to the healthcare provider after discharge

DISPLAY 17–5

Mother-Baby Discharge Record

M = Mother
S = Significant Other

Please go through the following list and check whether you understand each topic or need to know more.

Please read ...For Moms and Babies booklet given to you **after** the birth of your baby.

NURSES MUST DATE & INITIAL

I know this already		Doesn't apply to me		I need to know more			Booklet page #	Mother & family reviewed/ demonstrated	
M	S	M	S	M	S			Date	Initials
						POSTPARTUM			
						Activity – how much is OK	10		*
						Care of perineum and episiotomy	7,8		*
						Postoperative C-section instructions	9		*
						Signs of postpartum complications	11		*
						Changes in vaginal bleeding, return of my period	7		
						Comfort measures for afterpains, constipation, and hemorrhoids	7,9		
						Postpartum exercises for the first weeks	8		
						Postpartum "baby blues," depression, hormonal changes	9		
						How to minimize milk production if I'm not nursing			
						BABY CARE			
						What to do if baby is choking or gagging	14		*
						How to do skin care/cord care	14		*
						How to take care of the circumcision or genital area Type: Bell/Gomco	13		*
						How to know if my baby is sick and what to do	21		
						What is jaundice? What to look for: (Recieved Handout) • Increasing yellow color of baby's skin • Poor feeding/lethargy/irritability • Dark urine/light stool	15		
						Use and cleaning of bulb syringe	14,15		*
						How and when to burp baby	17		
						How to position baby after feeding	17		*
						Parents aware to never shake a baby			
						How to complete and obtain a birth certificate			
						BREASTFEEDING			
						I attended Breastfeeding class/watched Breastfeeding video ❑ YES ❑ NO			
						How to position baby for feeding	23		*
						How to get baby to latch onto my nipple properly	23		*
						Removal of baby from my nipple	24		*
						What is the supply and demand concept	23,24		*
						When does breast milk come in	25		
						Implications of supplementing for breastfeeding mothers	24		
						Prevention and comfort measures for sore nipples	24		
						Prevention and comfort measures for engorgement	25		
						How to express milk by hand/breast pump	25		
						BOTTLE FEEDING			
						How and when to feed my baby a bottle	16		*
						Reasons for NOT propping bottles	17		
						What formula should my baby drink	16		

STATE LAW REQUIRES USE OF INFANT CAR SEAT. I have a baby/infant car seat and know how to use it.   ❑ YES   ❑ NO

LEARNING EVALUATION   How do you like to learn new information? Check all that may apply.
[ ] Reading material handouts   [ ] Personal demonstration   [ ] Videotapes/TV   [ ] Hearing/audiotapes

Discharge weight ____lb ___oz   Discharge Transcutaneous Bilirubin ____
State Mandated Hearing Screen: Completed___ Refusal Form Signed: ____
__ Pass ___ Fail __ Repeat
Medications:
Mother: None____ Prescriptions:_____

Baby: None____ Prescriptions:_____
Discharge Instructions: _____

Follow-up doctor's appointment:
Mother: Date:_____
Baby: Date:_____ if <48 hrs of age call physician for an appt.
Please call your doctor if you have any questions or concerns.

❑ Patient has physician contact phone numbers.

My discharge instructions have been explained to me and I have received a copy.

Mother Signature:_____

Significant Other Signature (if applicable): _____

Person receiving infant: _____

Discharge Nurse:_____ Date:_____ Time:_____

Your baby is required by law to have testing done prior to discharge from the hospital for metabolic and genetic disorders (Including: PKU/Hypo-Thyroidism/ Galactosemia/Hemoglobin abnormalities). Testing will be done at least 24 hours after the initiation of feeding and prior to discharge. Colostrum is considered to be adequate feeding. Repeat testing will be required if initial testing was collected prior to 24 hours of feeding.
Criteria met - completed Metabolic Screen on: Date_____Time_____
(Repeat Not Needed)

Initial criteria not met - Repeat needed _____
Written physician order must accompany the baby at time of repeat collection and certain insurance companies may need pre-authorization. Bring your baby to the admitting lab on 2L (next to the escalators). The repeat metabolic test will require registration which will generate a fee for the service. Appropriate insurance information is necessary. The estimated time for the process is 1 hour. No appointment is necessary. For specific hours call 569-6814.

Nurses Signature(s) and Initials	

PATIENT IDENTIFICATION

MOTHER–BABY DISCHARGE RECORD

ST. JOHN'S MERCY MEDICAL CENTER/ST. LOUIS, MO

Newborn care

- Newborn adaptation to extrauterine life: need to be held, need for thermoregulation, need for comfort
- Newborn feeding cues
- Breastfeeding basics
- Formula feeding basics
- Care of an infant who is spitting up or choking
- Use of the bulb syringe
- Umbilical cord care
- Circumcision care and care of the uncircumcised penis
- Position for sleep: Back to Sleep campaign to reduce the risk of sudden infant death syndrome (SIDS)
- Information about immunizations and newborn screening tests
- Signs of newborn complications to report to the nurse in the hospital or to the healthcare provider after discharge and contact telephone numbers
- Safe use of infant and child car seats
- Appointment made for follow-up clinic or home visit offered by the hospital or community nursing agency
- When to schedule the first mother and newborn visits with their primary care provider

Written materials provided to the woman and her family should contain information about all critical concepts. Some institutions have adopted interactive documentation forms signed by the mother and the nurse providing the education (Brown, 2006; Roudebush et al., 2006).

Before discharge, knowledge and skills about self-care and infant care are validated. Validation can be accomplished by discussion with the new mother during which understanding is verbalized or by demonstration of critical skills such as feeding, sleeping position, or umbilical cord care. No one method of validation is superior; rather, nurses in each institution can develop a system with enough flexibility to meet the needs of the population served. Validation ensures that women who indicate they need no additional information are, in reality, prepared and knowledgeable. The goal is for all women to verbalize understanding or demonstrate skills related to all critical concepts. Women with special needs who have not demonstrated knowledge of critical concepts or have not acquired the skills to care for themselves or their infants are referred for follow-up support and care. Referrals are made to the clinical nurse specialist, lactation consultant, social worker, dietitian, and/or home care agency. Follow-up contacts to ensure that the critical concepts have been learned and to verify that the woman can safely care for her infant and herself can occur at a clinic or home visit, during a phone assessment, through involvement in support groups and community programs, or at healthcare provider office visits. Assessment of maternal knowledge and skills is documented on the discharge teaching record or other appropriate medical record form.

ANATOMIC AND PHYSIOLOGIC CHANGES DURING THE POSTPARTUM PERIOD

Perinatal nurses should have knowledge of normal anatomic and physiologic changes that occur during the postpartum period in order to plan comprehensive assessments and interventions for new mothers. Many changes are apparent immediately after birth and require inpatient nursing assessment and intervention. However, over the course of the first 12 weeks postpartum, there are ongoing alterations as the woman's body returns to its nearly prepregnant state.

UTERUS

Involution results from a decrease in myometrial cell size, not in the number of myometrial cells. This decrease is the result of ischemia, autolysis, and phagocytosis. Ischemia occurs when the retraction of uterine musculature necessary for hemostasis after placental separation results in decreased blood flow to the uterus. Proteolytic enzymes are released, and macrophages migrate to the uterus, resulting in autolysis or self-digestion and subsequent reduction in myometrial cell size. Some of the excess elastic and fibrous tissue is removed by phagocytosis, but the incomplete process results in a uterus that does not return to its nulliparous size. Within 24 hours, the uterus is approximately the size it was at 20 weeks' gestation (Cunningham et al., 2009). Immediately after birth, the uterus weighs approximately 1,000 g (2 lb, 4 oz). As involution occurs, the uterine weight continues to decrease to 500 g (1 week), 300 g (2 weeks), and by 6 weeks postpartum, it weighs 100 g or less. Immediately after birth, the uterine fundus can be palpated midway between the umbilicus and symphysis pubis. During the first 12 hours after birth, the muscles relax slightly, and the fundus returns to the level of the umbilicus. Beginning on postpartum day 2 or 3, the usual progression of uterine descent into the pelvis is 1 cm/day (Display 17–6).

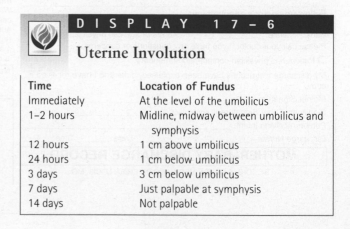

DISPLAY 17 – 6

Uterine Involution

Time	Location of Fundus
Immediately	At the level of the umbilicus
1–2 hours	Midline, midway between umbilicus and symphysis
12 hours	1 cm above umbilicus
24 hours	1 cm below umbilicus
3 days	3 cm below umbilicus
7 days	Just palpable at symphysis
14 days	Not palpable

During the first few days after birth, oxytocin secretion causes strong uterine contractions and a further reduction in size, especially after breastfeeding and in multiparas. Multiparity, multiple gestation, polyhydramnios, and bladder distention can influence uterine size and the progression of uterine involution.

PLACENTAL SITE AND LOCHIA

The placenta separates spontaneously from the uterus within 15 minutes of birth in 90% of women and within 30 minutes after birth in 95% of women. Separation of the placenta and membranes includes the spongy layer of the endometrium, leaving the decidua basalis in the uterus. This remaining layer reorganizes into basal and superficial layers. The superficial layer becomes necrotic and is sloughed in the lochia, and the basal layer becomes the source of new endometrium. The endometrium is regenerated by 2 to 3 weeks after birth, except at the site of placental attachment (Blackburn, 2012; Cunningham et al., 2009). Immediately after delivery of the placenta, the placental site is approximately 8 to 10 cm, and by end of the second week, it is about 3 to 4 cm. Exfoliation, the process of placental site healing, occurs over the first 6 weeks after birth by necrotic sloughing of the infarcted superficial tissues. A reparative process follows in which the endometrium regenerates from the margins and base. This process prevents the formation of a fibrous scar in the decidua. At 7 to 14 days' postpartum, the infarcted superficial tissue over the placental site sloughs. At this time, the woman may notice an episode of increased vaginal bleeding, which is usually self-limited. Bleeding lasting more than 1 to 2 hours should be evaluated for late postpartum hemorrhage (PPH). Ultrasonography can be useful in determining the presence of retained placental tissue (Thorpe, 2009).

Lochia is the postpartum uterine discharge. Although lochia varies in amount, the total volume lost usually is 150 to 400 mL. Initially, lochia rubra is reddish and continues for 3 to 4 days. Lochia serosa, a pinkish discharge,

continues from day 4 to day 10. Lochia alba, a yellow-white discharge, follows lochia serosa (Table 17–1). The choice of feeding method for the baby and the use of oral contraceptives do not affect duration of lochia (Cunningham et al., 2009).

CERVIX, VAGINA, AND PELVIC FLOOR

The cervix and lower uterine segment are thin and flaccid immediately postpartum. Cervical lacerations can occur during any birth; however, women with precipitous labor and operative procedures are at increased risk for lacerations. At 2 to 3 days, the cervix has resumed its customary appearance but remains dilated 2 to 3 cm. By the end of the first week, the cervical os narrows to a diameter of 1 cm. The external cervical os remains wider than its pregravid state, and bilateral depressions typically are seen at the site of lacerations. Cervical edema may persist for several months (Cunningham et al., 2009). The vagina and vaginal outlet are smooth walled and may appear bruised early in the puerperium. The apparent bruising, caused by pelvic congestion, disappears quickly after birth. Rugae reappear in the distended vagina by the third week. The voluntary muscles and supports of the pelvic floor gradually regain tone during the first 6 weeks postpartum. These changes occur in response to the reduced amount of circulating progesterone. For some women, vaginal tone may be improved by perineal tightening exercises, such as Kegel exercises (Ladewig et al., 2009; Weber & Richter, 2005). In the lactating woman, the hypoestrogenic state resulting from ovarian suppression may cause the vagina to appear pale and without rugae. This may result in dyspareunia.

OVARIAN FUNCTION AND RETURN OF MENSES

Although the return of menses and ovulation varies, the first menstrual period usually occurs within 7 to 9 weeks postpartum in nonnursing mothers. There are

Table 17–1. TYPES OF LOCHIA

	Rubra	Serosa	Alba
Normal color	Red	Pink, brown tinged	Yellowish-white
Normal duration	1–13 days	3–110 days	10–14 days, but not abnormal to last longer
Normal discharge	Bloody with clots; fleshing odor; increased flow on standing or breast-feeding, or during physical activity	Serosanguineous (blood and mucus) consistency; fleshy odor	Mostly mucus, no strong odor
Abnormal discharge	Foul smell; numerous and/or large clots; quickly saturates perineal pad	Foul smell; quickly saturates perineal pad	Foul smell; saturates perineal pad; reappearance of pink or red lochia; discharge lasts far too long (past 4 wk)

great variations in the return of menses for women who are nursing because of depressed estrogen levels. In nursing mothers, menstruation usually returns between months 2 and 18.

Estrogen and progesterone levels decrease suddenly after placental delivery. For the first 2 to 3 weeks after birth, there is minimal gonadotropin activity, possibly because of a transient pituitary insensitivity to luteinizing hormone–releasing factor. As sensitivity returns, hormonal function returns to normal levels. The first menstrual cycle is usually anovulatory, but 25% of women may ovulate before menstruation. The mean for the return of ovulation is 10 weeks postpartum for women who are not lactating and approximately 17 weeks postpartum for women who are breastfeeding. The delay in the resumption of menses in lactating women in part may result from elevated prolactin levels (Cunningham et al., 2009).

METABOLIC CHANGES

Prolactin, a pituitary hormone, is responsible for stimulating and sustaining lactation. Like estrogen and progesterone, prolactin levels decrease with placental delivery, although they remain elevated over nonpregnant levels. The decrease in estrogen and progesterone stimulates the anterior pituitary to produce prolactin. Between the third and fourth week postpartum, the prolactin level returns to normal in women who formula-feed their infants. For those who breastfeed, prolactin levels increase with each nursing episode (Cunningham et al., 2009).

Thyroid function returns to prepregnant levels within 4 to 6 weeks after birth. Because immunosuppression is a normal physiologic consequence of pregnancy, there is an increased risk of developing transient autoimmune thyroiditis, followed by hypothyroidism. This depression of thyroid function may cause depression, carelessness, and impairment of memory and concentration. There is a slightly increased risk of recurrence of autoimmune hypothyroidism or hyperthyroidism postpartum (Nader, 2009; Cunningham et al., 2009).

Low levels of placental lactogen, estrogen, cortisol, growth hormone, and the placental enzyme insulinase reduce their anti-insulin effect in the early puerperium. This results in lower glucose levels for women during this period and a reduction in insulin requirements for insulin-dependent diabetic women (Cunningham et al., 2009). Breastfeeding may precipitate hypoglycemic episodes in women with insulin-dependent diabetes. Women with gestational diabetes often have normal glucose levels immediately postpartum. Nutritional needs must be reassessed during this period. The basal metabolic rate (BMR) increases 20% to 25% during pregnancy because of fetal metabolic activity. The BMR remains elevated for 7 to 14 days after giving birth.

In the first 2 hours postpartum, plasma renin and angiotensin II levels (involved in blood pressure [BP] maintenance) fall to normal, nonpregnant levels and then rise again and remain elevated for up to 14 days (Roberts & Funai, 2009). BP should remain stable during the postpartum period, but lowered vascular resistance in the pelvis may result in orthostatic hypotension when a woman moves from a supine to a sitting position. An increase in BP, especially if accompanied by headaches or visual changes, may indicate postpartum preeclampsia and should be evaluated. In the past, an incremental increase of 30 mm Hg systolic or 15 mm Hg diastolic above baseline values was used as diagnostic criteria. This is no longer recommended, as research shows those women are not likely to have adverse outcomes; however, patients with BP increases should be closely observed, especially if the BP is above 140/90 mm Hg on two or more occasions at least 6 hours apart (Roberts & Funai, 2009; Cunningham et al., 2009).

KIDNEYS AND BLADDER

Mild proteinuria (1+) may exist for 1 to 2 days after birth in 40% to 50% of women. Nonpathology can be assumed only in the absence of the symptoms of infection or preeclampsia (Blackburn, 2012).

If a urine specimen is necessary, it should be obtained through catheterization or as a clean-catch technique. These methods avoid contamination by protein-laden lochia (Gilbert, 2011). Glycosuria of pregnancy disappears, and creatinine clearance is usually normal by 1 week postpartum. Pregnancy-induced hypotonia and dilation of the ureters and renal pelves return to the prepregnant state by 8 weeks postpartum. The catabolic process of involution causes an increase of the blood urea nitrogen (BUN). By the end of the first week postpartum, the BUN level rises to values of 20 mg/dL, compared with 15 mg/dL in the late third trimester (Cunningham et al., 2009). Glomerular filtration rate, renal blood flow, and plasma creatinine return to normal levels by 6 weeks postpartum.

Labor may result in displacement of the urinary bladder and stretching of the urethra. Other factors that interfere with normal micturition include the numbing effect of anesthesia and the temporary neural dysfunction of the traumatized bladder. These may cause decreased sensitivity. As a result, overdistension and incomplete emptying may occur. Signs of bladder distention include uterine atony reflected in increased lochia, displacement of the uterus to the right and significantly above the umbilicus, decreased urine output compared with oral and intravenous (IV) intake, and a "soft fullness," sometimes with a palpable margin, in the suprapubic area. Normal postpartum diuresis combined with the often large amount of IV fluids administered during labor can result in bladder filling in a relatively short time. The woman should be encouraged to void as soon as possible after birth to avoid bladder filling, which can inhibit uterine contraction, thus predisposing to PPH. Assistance to the bathroom or on a bedpan may be helpful in facilitating bladder emptying. Women may report an urge but inability to urinate. Spontaneous voiding, however, should resume by 6 to 8 hours after birth, and bladder tone usually returns to normal levels 5 to 7 days later. Each voiding should be at least 150 mL. Edema, hyperemia, and submucous extravasation of blood are frequently evident in the bladder postpartum (Cunningham et al., 2009). The effects of trauma from labor on the bladder and urethra diminish during the first 24 hours, unless a urinary tract infection (UTI) is present. Some women may require in-and-out catheterization to empty their bladder in the immediate postpartum period. Avoid rapid emptying of the bladder if catheterization is performed. No more than 800 mL of urine should be removed at one time. This can avoid a precipitous drop in intraabdominal pressure, which may result in splenetic engorgement and hypotension.

STRESS INCONTINENCE

Many women report transient stress incontinence during the first 6 weeks postpartum. Although there are conflicting data on the effect of vaginal birth on future urinary status, some researchers have estimated that two vaginal births increase the risk of developing urinary incontinence twofold and increase the risk of surgery for pelvic organ prolapse eightfold (Schaffer et al., 2005). Other researchers have suggested that pregnancy itself may be a predisposing factor for urinary incontinence and pelvic organ prolapse, thus cesarean birth may not be protective against these conditions (Nygaard, 2006; Richter, 2006). A review of literature through 2005 suggested that there may be differences by parity and after exclusion of instrumental delivery. The risk of severe stress urinary incontinence and urge urinary incontinence did not appear to differ by mode of birth. Short-term occurrence of any degree of postpartum stress urinary incontinence is decreased with cesarean section (CS), although severe symptoms are equivalent by mode of birth (Press, Klein, Kaczorowski, Liston, & von Dadelszen, 2007). Persistent stress incontinence may result from pregnancy, labor, operative birth, a large baby, and perineal tissue damage. The influences of obstetric factors diminish over 3 months. The length of the second stage of labor, infant head size, birth weight, and episiotomy correlate with the development of postpartum stress incontinence (Casey et al., 2005). Impairment of muscle function near and surrounding the urethra underlies stress incontinence. Prompt catheterization for urinary retention during the postpartum can prevent urinary difficulties (Cunningham et al., 2009). Schaffer et al. (2005) suggest that the pelvic floor is exposed to compression and

extreme pressures during vaginal delivery and maternal expulsive efforts. Uncoached (non-Valsalva) pushing, a response to the urge to push, is characterized by several short bearing-down efforts per contraction with breath holding for 6 to 8 seconds. In contrast, coached pushing begins as soon as a contraction is noted by the coach, and the mother is urged to push for 10 seconds, take a deep breath, and push again. Coached pushing may potentially increase the pressure on the pelvic floor with subsequent deleterious effects. See Chapter 14 for a comprehensive discussion of second-stage pushing techniques that can minimize risk of injuries to the perineum and pelvic floor. Knowledge about clinical factors implicated in stress incontinence allows anticipatory guidance and interventions for women at risk.

Fluid Balance and Electrolytes

The physiologic reversal of the extracellular or interstitial fluid accumulated during a normal pregnancy begins during the immediate postpartum period. Diuresis begins within 12 hours after birth and continues up to 5 days. Diuresis occurs in response to the decrease in estrogen that stimulated fluid retention during pregnancy, the reduction of venous pressure in the lower half of the body, and the decrease in residual hypervolemia (Cunningham et al., 2009). Urine output may be 3,000 mL or more each day. Additional fluid is lost through increased perspiration. Diuresis results in a decrease in body weight of 2 to 3 kg. Electrolyte levels return to nonpregnant homeostasis by 21 days or earlier. Fluid loss is greater in women who have experienced preeclampsia or eclampsia. By the third postpartum day, resolution of the vasoconstriction and additional extracellular fluid of gestational hypertension contribute to significant expansion of the vascular volume (Cunningham et al., 2009).

NEUROLOGIC CHANGES

Discomfort and fatigue are common concerns after birth. Afterpains or painful uterine contractions during the first 2 to 3 days after birth; discomfort associated with episiotomy, incisions, lacerations, or tears; muscle aches; and breast engorgement may contribute to a woman's discomfort during the postpartum period. Neurologic changes related to anesthesia and analgesia are transient and, if present, require attention to ensure the woman's safety. Deep tendon reflexes remain normal. Sleep disturbances contributing to fatigue are related to discomfort and the demands of newborn care. The presence of children or a lack of social support may limit the time available for rest. Natural or pharmacologic comfort measures should be offered. Psychosocial support is necessary, and referral to home care nursing may be appropriate.

The carpal tunnel syndrome that results from compression of the median nerve by the physiologic edema of pregnancy is relieved by postpartum diuresis. Headaches may result from fluid shifts in the first week after birth, leakage of cerebrospinal fluid into the extradural space during spinal anesthesia, fluid and electrolyte imbalance, gestational hypertension, or stress. Assessment of the quality and location of the headache and of the vital signs are necessary. Interventions such as environmental control of lighting, noise levels, and visitors and administration of analgesic medications may be effective for nonpathologic headaches. Postpartum eclampsia (i.e., seizures beginning >48 hours and <4 weeks after birth) is often preceded by severe headache or visual disturbances. Women may have a postpartum eclamptic seizure without a prenatal diagnosis of preeclampsia or hypertension. Because women may experience prodromal signs and symptoms after discharge from the hospital, information should be provided about these subjective signs and symptoms, which include a severe and persistent occipital headache, scotomata (i.e., spots before the eyes), blurred vision, photophobia, and epigastric or right upper quadrant pain. Women should be encouraged to notify their primary healthcare provider if any of these symptoms develop to facilitate immediate evaluation.

HEMODYNAMIC CHANGES

Changes in the cardiovascular system occur early in the postpartum period, with a variable rate of return to baseline levels that ranges from 6 to 12 weeks. Blood volume changes occur rapidly. Autotransfusion occurs as a result of elimination of blood flow to the placenta. The blood flow of 500 to 750 mL per minute, formerly flowing to the uteroplacental unit, is diverted to maternal systemic venous circulation immediately after birth. The blood loss with an uncomplicated vaginal birth is approximately 500 to 1,000 mL or more with a cesarean birth. Plasma volume is diminished by approximately 1,000 mL as a result of blood loss and diuresis. By the third day postpartum, blood volume has decreased 16% from peak pregnancy levels and returns to nearly prepregnant levels by 1 to 2 weeks postpartum.

Cardiac output after birth depends on use and choice of anesthesia or analgesia, mode of birth, blood loss, and maternal position. Cardiac output peaks immediately after birth to approximately 80% above the prelabor value in women who have received only local anesthesia. After reaching a maximum value at 10 to 15 minutes after birth, cardiac output begins to decline, reaching pre-labor values approximately 1 hour postpartum, although it remains elevated for 48 hours after birth (Blackburn, 2012). It returns to prepregnant levels by 2 to 3 weeks after birth. Because the heart rate (HR) is stable or slightly decreased, the cardiac output is most likely caused by an increased stroke volume from venous return. Cesarean birth before labor onset avoids the hemodynamic effect of contractions but not the rise in cardiac output immediately postpartum. It is thought that epidural anesthesia during labor moderates the increase in cardiac output after birth by decreasing pain and anxiety (Cunningham et al., 2009).

The pulse rate remains stable or decreases slightly after birth. If the pulse rate is above 100 beats per minute (bpm), the woman should be assessed for infection or delayed PPH. Some women may exhibit puerperal bradycardia, with a pulse rate of 40 to 50 bpm. No conclusive proof has been given for this phenomenon. Orthostatic hypotension may occur when a woman sits up from a reclining position. Preeclampsia should be suspected if BP values are 140/90 mm Hg on two or more occasions at least 6 hours apart.

HEMATOLOGIC AND LIVER CHANGES

The decrease in plasma volume is greater than the loss of red blood cells (RBCs) after birth, causing an increase in the hematocrit between day 3 and day 7. The hematocrit returns to normal levels 4 to 8 weeks later as RBCs reach the end of their normal life span (Cunningham et al., 2009; Kilpatrick & Laros, 2009; Monga, 2009). In assessing postpartum laboratory values, a 1.0- to 1.5-g decrease in hemoglobin levels or 2- to 3-point decrease in the hematocrit value reflects a 500-mL blood loss. During the first 48 hours after birth, the physiologic reversal of the extracellular fluid accumulated during a normal pregnancy and IV fluids given during labor make accurate blood loss assessment difficult because hemodilution occurs as this fluid enters the vascular system. This phenomenon is seen even in women who have lost 20% of their circulating blood volume during birth. Hemoconcentration may occur with minimal blood loss if a woman has preexisting polycythemia (AWHONN & Johnson & Johnson Consumer Products, 2006; Cunningham et al., 2009; Monga, 2009).

Normal serum iron levels are regained by the second week postpartum. A relative erythrocytosis is seen in women who have received iron supplementation during pregnancy and had an average blood loss during the birth process. In the absence of iron supplementation, iron deficiency develops in most women (Cunningham et al., 2009; Stotland, 2009). The serum ferritin level correlates closely with the body's iron stores and is predictive of iron deficiency anemia (Cunningham et al., 2009; Stotland, 2009). Changes in blood coagulation factors remain for variable periods postpartum. Plasma fibrinogen levels and sedimentation rate levels remain elevated for at least the first week.

Leukocytosis from the stress of labor and birth is seen in the postpartum period. A nonpathologic white blood cell (WBC) count may reach 25,000/μL to 30,000/μL, with the increase predominantly in granulocytes. Relative lymphopenia (i.e., lymphocyte deficiency) and absolute eosinopenia (i.e., decreased eosinophils) may also be seen. This phenomenon, coupled with the increase in the sedimentation rate, may confuse the interpretation or assessment of infections during this period. Pathology should be suspected, and further evaluation is indicated when the WBCs increase 30% over a 6-hour period (AWHONN & Johnson & Johnson Consumer Products, 2006; Cunningham et al., 2009; Kilpatrick & Laros, 2009).

The alterations in liver enzymes and lipids that occurred in response to increased estrogen levels and hemodilution during pregnancy are reversed and returned to normal levels within 3 weeks postpartum. Elevated levels of free fatty acids, cholesterol, triglycerides, and lipoproteins seen during pregnancy return to normal levels within 10 days. Alkaline phosphatase, derived from the placenta, liver, and bone during pregnancy, may remain elevated for 6 weeks. The previously atonic gallbladder demonstrates increased contractility as progesterone levels decrease (Cunningham et al., 2009; Williamson & Mackillop, 2009).

RESPIRATORY AND ACID–BASE CHANGES

The respiratory system quickly returns to its prepregnant state after the birth of the baby. These changes result from the decrease in progesterone levels, the decrease in intraabdominal pressure that accompanies emptying of the uterus, and the increased excursion of the diaphragm. This reduction of diaphragmatic pressure results in the immediate return of chest wall compliance to normal levels and partially relieves the dyspnea experienced during pregnancy. Residual volume (i.e., amount of air remaining in the lung after maximum expiration) and tidal volume (i.e., volume of air inhaled and exhaled during each breath) normalize soon after birth; the expiratory reserve volume (i.e., maximum amount of air that can be exhaled), however, may remain in the abnormal range for several months. Vital capacity, inspiratory capacity, and maximum breathing capacity decrease after birth. The response to exercise may therefore be affected in the early postpartum weeks (Cunningham et al., 2009; Whitty & Dombrowski, 2009).

Length and severity of the second stage of labor appear to contribute to an "oxygen debt" (i.e., extra oxygen required after strenuous exercise) that extends into the immediate postpartum period (Cunningham et al., 2009; Whitty & Dombrowski, 2009). The BMR remains elevated for 7 to 14 days into the postpartum period and is attributable to mild anemia, lactation, and psychological factors.

As progesterone levels fall, the P_aCO_2 rises to the normal prepregnant values (35 to 40 mm Hg) within the first 2 days after birth. During the postpartum period, the P_aO_2 should be normal at 95% or higher. Normal levels of pH and base excess gradually return by approximately 3 weeks postpartum.

SKIN, MUSCLE, AND WEIGHT CHANGES

Overdistention of the abdominal wall as a result of pregnancy can rupture collagen fibers of the dermis, resulting in striae, which can occur also on the breasts, buttocks, and thighs. Striae eventually become irregular white lines. Diastasis (i.e., separation) of the rectus muscles is common and usually is reapproximated by the late postpartum period. Evidence of diastasis can be assessed by asking the woman to lift her head while lying in a supine position. If diastasis has occurred, a tentlike protrusion in the lower abdomen is noticeable. Abdominal binders are not recommended, and mild exercise to restore tone may be started after 1 to 2 weeks. The joint instability that occurred during pregnancy may not resolve until 6 to 8 weeks postpartum.

A woman loses an average of 12 lb (5.5 kg) at birth. Additional weight is lost between 2 weeks and 6 months postpartum, especially if the woman is breastfeeding (Cunningham et al., 2009). Women who choose formula feeding can expect a loss of 0.5 to 1 kg/week when eating a balanced diet containing slightly fewer calories than their usual daily expenditure. Weight loss occurs more rapidly in women of lower parity, age, and prepregnancy weight.

GASTROINTESTINAL CHANGES

After birth, there is a decrease in gastrointestinal muscle tone and motility. When these changes are coupled with relaxation of abdominal muscles, gaseous distention can occur during the first 2 to 3 days postpartum. Decreased motility can result in postpartum ileus. Constipation may result from hemorrhoids, perineal trauma, dehydration, pain, fear of having a bowel movement, immobility, and medication (i.e., magnesium sulfate antenatally for tocolysis, iron supplementation, codeine for pain, anesthetics during labor or surgery). Constipation can be minimized by encouraging the woman to drink adequate fluids and eat foods high in fiber. Hemorrhoids that develop during pregnancy may increase in size during labor and result in significant discomfort during the postpartum period. If the woman has hemorrhoids, suggesting warm or cold sitz baths and applying topical anesthetics can decrease discomfort. Stool softeners and laxatives are sometimes given. Bowel movements typically resume 2 to 3 days after birth, and normal bowel elimination patterns resume by 2 weeks postpartum.

HERNIAS AND PERINEAL, PELVIC FLOOR, AND ANAL SPHINCTER DAMAGE

Approximately one fifth to one third of U.S. women have symptoms of urinary incontinence or pelvic organ prolapse (Chaliha, 2009; Leijonhufvud et al., 2011) Genital hernias (i.e., cystocele, rectocele, uterine prolapse, enterocele) may occur because of overstretching or tearing of the muscles or fascia during birth. There is limited evidence that women who perform perineal massage, beginning at 35 weeks' gestation, are less likely to have perineal trauma (episiotomy or tears) that requires suturing in association with vaginal birth (Beckmann & Garrett, 2006). Chaliha (2009) and Boyles, Li, Mori, Osterweil, and Guise (2009) suggest that because of the lack of clarity in current data as to causation, the focus should be on modification of potential risk factors for pelvic floor trauma, such as constipation and high body mass index (BMI) (more than 30). Controversy exists regarding the use of episiotomy. Some practitioners recommend minimizing the use of midline episiotomy and using mediolateral episiotomy when the risk for extension is increased (i.e., macrosomia, shallow perineal body, operative vaginal birth), but there is little supportive evidence for that practice (Christianson, Bovbjerg, McDavitt, & Hullfish, 2003). Episiotomy does not always prevent third- or fourth-degree lacerations. Risk factors for lacerations include nulliparity, increased gestational age, second-stage labor arrest, macrosomia, persistent occiput posterior positions, episiotomy, forceps assistance, and use of vacuum extractors (Landy et al., 2011). Routine episiotomy is not recommended by ACOG (2008a; see Chapter 14 for an in-depth discussion of episiotomy).

Obstetric trauma such as injury to the sphincter muscle or damage to the innervation of the pelvic floor is a leading cause of anal incontinence in healthy women (Garcia, Rogers, Kim, Hall, & Kammerer-Doak, 2005). Other associations with anal incontinence include prolonged second-stage labor, macrosomia, labor augmentation, and episiotomy (Jastrow et al., 2010; Casey et al., 2005). One half of women with third-degree tears experience anal incontinence. Disturbances in bowel function (i.e., fecal urgency and anal incontinence of stool and flatus) from mechanical or neurologic injury to the anal sphincter during vaginal birth may also be the result of damage from the large size of the baby's head in relation to the vaginal opening. Women who experience a third- or fourth-degree perineal laceration report a greater incidence of incontinence of flatus than those without anal sphincter rupture. Full thickness anal sphincter disruption is the most significant factor in later development of fetal incontinence (Chaliha, 2009; Landy et al., 2011). Women with a long second-stage of labor, a large newborn, or both have the greatest risk of nerve damage (Cunningham et al., 2009; Landy et al., 2011). Parity is associated with an increased risk for urinary incontinence. Vaginal delivery increases the risk for urinary incontinence, but labor and pushing alone, without subsequent vaginal birth, do not appear to increase risk (Boyles et al., 2009). Pelvic floor exercises have shown to reduce urinary incontinence and increase pelvic floor strength, and pregnant women should be encouraged to perform them during the antepartum period (Chaliha, 2009).

Embarrassment may prevent women from reporting symptoms of anal sphincter damage. One study has suggested that there may be 80,000 women, about 2% of U.S. births, who have persistent long-term anal incontinence, but only 8,000 will report it to their providers (Lo et al., 2010). Symptoms may disappear or worsen with time. An accurate history is helpful so that women with major sphincter defects can be offered a cesarean birth when appropriate. Aging, menopause, progression of neuropathy, and effects of subsequent births may contribute to long-term sphincter weakness. In addition, women report that anal incontinence results in negative emotional health and a decrease in their quality of life (Lo et al., 2010).

FLUID AND NUTRITIONAL NEEDS

After vaginal birth, there are no dietary restrictions for women without underlying medical conditions or pregnancy-induced complications. Oral fluids or IV fluid administration helps restore the balance altered by fluid loss during the labor and birth process. Women should be encouraged to drink 3,000 mL of water and other liquids every 24 hours. Nurses should encourage healthy food choices with respect for ethnic and cultural preferences. Snack trays should be available for women who give birth when regular food service is unavailable. After cesarean birth, women usually receive clear liquids until bowel sounds are present and then advance to solid foods. For each 20 mL of breast milk produced, the woman must consume an additional 30 calories. This results in a dietary increase of 500 to 1,000 calories each day for women who are maintaining body weight (Lawrence & Lawrence, 2009). By 6 weeks postpartum, decreased pressure and distortion of the stomach from the gravid uterus and the normalization of lower esophageal sphincter pressure and tone resolves the heartburn experienced by many pregnant women.

IMMEDIATE POSTPARTUM PERIOD

During the immediate postpartum period, the perinatal nurse focuses on maternal and newborn stabilization and recovery from the birth process. Maternal–newborn attachment and breastfeeding (if the woman desires) should be promoted and encouraged (Figs. 17–1 and 17–2). Nursing assessments and interventions should occur concurrently with activities celebrating the joy of childbirth and welcoming the new baby into the family. Family and visitor interactions, including holding the new baby and taking video and still pictures of the first hours of life, should be supported as much as possible based on the condition of the mother and

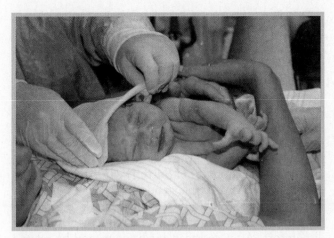

FIGURE 17–1. Promoting mother–baby attachment at birth.

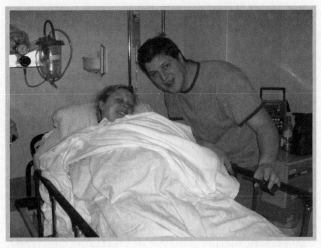

FIGURE 17–3. Support person with mother in the obstetric (OB) post-anesthesia care unit (PACU).

newborn. Every effort should be made to accommodate the wishes of the woman and her family.

When regional analgesia or anesthesia or general anesthesia has been used for vaginal or cesarean birth, the woman should be observed in an appropriately staffed and equipped labor/delivery/recovery room or post-anesthesia care unit (PACU) until she has recovered from the anesthetic (AAP & ACOG, 2008; American Society of Anesthesiologists [ASA], 2007). The patient's desires for support persons to be with her during the post-anesthesia care period should be honored as much as possible. At a minimum, at least one support person should be encouraged and allowed (Fig. 17–3). The woman should be discharged from post-anesthesia care only at the discretion of and after communication among the attending physician or a certified nurse midwife, anesthesiologist, and certified registered nurse anesthetist (AAP & ACOG, 2008; ASA, 2007). See Chapter 14 for an in-depth discussion of post-anesthesia care.

According to the wishes and condition of the woman, she and the newborn should be kept together as much as

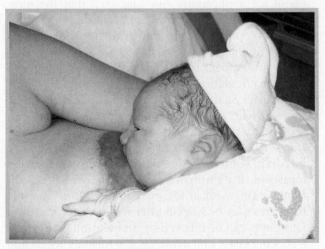

FIGURE 17–2. Promoting breastfeeding immediately after birth.

possible during the inpatient stay. Most perinatal units have models of care that support maternal–newborn attachment. Mother–baby or couplet care in which one nurse is responsible for both patients facilitates optimal interaction between the mother and baby and coordination of appropriate nursing assessments and interventions. Opportunities for rest for the new mother should be promoted, although this may be challenging for the nurse because of the number of congratulatory telephone calls and visitors and because of the unit routines that interrupt sleep. Nursing care should be planned so that necessary interventions and medication administration (if needed) can be grouped together, minimizing the need to wake the woman during daytime naps or during the night. A plan for rest designed collaboratively with the new mother and her family works well. Ambulation as soon as the mother feels able should be encouraged, but the woman should be instructed not to get out of bed on her own without assistance the first time after birth (AAP & ACOG, 2008). In the absence of complications or surgical recovery, a regular diet should be resumed as soon as the woman desires. Education for the new mother and her family about maternal postpartum care and newborn care should focus on easing the transition from hospital to home.

During the immediate postpartum period, maternal BP and pulse should be monitored at least every 15 minutes for the first hour or more often as indicated (AAP & ACOG, 2008). Most institutions have protocols that include comprehensive maternal assessments at least every 15 minutes for the first hour, then every 30 minutes for 1 hour, and then every 4 hours (or more frequently if complications are present) for 12 to 24 hours. If the mother is stable, some institutions defer the 4-hour assessments after the first 12 hours when the mother is sleeping. There are no data from prospective clinical trials to determine how often maternal status should be assessed during the postpartum period to promote safety and optimal outcomes. Each institution should develop protocols that are reasonable and based on the condition of the mother. A sample medical form for documentation of the immediate postpartum assessment is included in Chapter 14, Appendix 14–B. The following clinical parameters are included in a comprehensive assessment during the immediate postpartum period:

- Assess BP and pulse (AAP & ACOG, 2008).
- Assess the uterine fundus for tone and position. Uterine massage is indicated if the uterus is not firmly contracted.
- Support the lower uterine segment during massage to prevent uterine prolapse or inversion (Fig. 17–4). Uterine inversion is an obstetric emergency associated with hemorrhage and shock.
- Assess the amount of lochia on the perineal pad and under buttocks.
- Assess the condition of the perineum.
- Assess the condition of episiotomy after assisting the woman into lateral position with upper leg flexed; use the acronym REEDA (redness, edema, ecchymosis, discharge, approximation of edges of episiotomy) to guide assessment.
- Assess the temperature at least every 4 hours (AAP & ACOG, 2008).

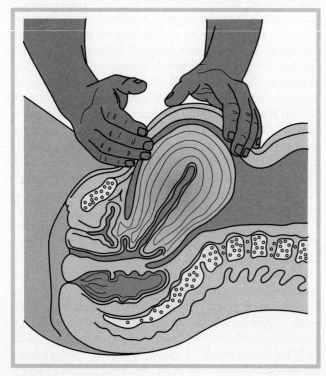

FIGURE 17–4. Fundal massage. The nurse uses two hands for fundal massage. One hand anchors the lower uterine segment just above the symphysis. The other gently massages the fundal area.

- Decisions about post-anesthesia status and readiness for discharge from the recovery area are made at the discretion of the attending physician, nurse midwife, anesthesiologist, or certified registered nurse anesthetist (AAP & ACOG, 2008; ASA, 2007).

PAIN MANAGEMENT

Pain during the postpartum period may be caused by the episiotomy, lacerations, perineal trauma, incisions, uterine contractions after birth, hemorrhoids, breast engorgement, and nipple tenderness. Nursing assessments, such as fundal assessment, may also result in discomfort. Some strategies can reduce the level of discomfort. After cesarean birth, pain may be related to the incision and intestinal gas. Pain causes stress and interferes with the woman's ability to interact with and care for her infant. Evidence for the effectiveness of topically applied local anesthetics for treating perineal pain is not compelling (Hedayati, Parsons, & Crowther, 2005). While manufactured ice packs may provide increased comfort, ice-filled gloves or zip-locked bags are considerably less expensive. Petersen (2011) recommends that if a community ice machine is used to fill these, consideration should be given to conducting cultures to determine the presence of harmful bacteria.

The following interventions are included in a comprehensive assessment during the immediate postpartum period:

- Ask about type and severity of pain.
- Explain rationale for uterine massage and periodic assessments. Encourage slow, deep breathing during the assessment.
- Gentle palpation with warm hands can enhance comfort and encourage participation in the procedure.
- Apply ice pack to perineum during the first 24 to 48 hours to reduce edema (some women may prefer an ice pack to the perineum intermittently for more than 48 hours). Peterson (2011) reviewed the literature about ice applications and suggested that the most benefit is received when the ice packs are applied for 10- to 20-minute intervals rather than leaving them in place continually.
- Apply moist heat (i.e., sitz bath) after 24 hours to increase circulation and promote healing.
- Administer analgesic medication as ordered.
- Women who have cesarean birth may or may not require uterine massage to stimulate uterine contraction. If the amount of lochia indicates excessive bleeding, combine palpation and pain management measures. If pain management is inadequate, additional pain medication, reassurance, and comfort measures may be helpful after necessary procedures.
- Gas pains can be relieved by ambulation, rocking in a rocking chair, and avoiding gas-forming foods and carbonated beverages.

PSYCHOSOCIAL STATUS

Ongoing assessment of the psychosocial status should be personalized during the postpartum period to promote the development of healthy mother–infant relationships and maternal confidence (AAP & ACOG, 2008).

The following interventions are included in a comprehensive assessment during the immediate postpartum period:

- Determine the level of emotional lability and level of social support.
- Identify actual and potential sources of support.
- Assess the fatigue level.
- Ascertain educational needs and the level of confidence.
- Assess the teaching needs based on interview and observation.
- Use interactions with mothers as potential teaching moments.
- Use assessment of the fundus as an opportunity to provide information about involution.
- During perineal care, explain cleansing the vulva from front to back to avoid contamination, changing the pad at least four times each day or after each voiding or bowel movement, and washing hands before and after changing pads.
- Use bathing of the newborn at mother's bedside as an opportunity to discuss basic techniques of newborn care such as feeding, clothing, holding, and safety.
- Assess the interaction with the newborn and attachment behaviors.
  - Note whether the mother looks directly at the infant and maintains eye contact (i.e., en face position).
  - Note whether the mother touches and talks to the infant.
  - Note whether the mother interprets the infant's behaviors positively.
- Provide an early opportunity to hold the infant after birth, and keep the infant with the parents as much as possible.
- Ensure flexibility in visiting policies and opportunities for privacy.
- Demonstrate acceptance of expression of maternal feelings and reinforce parenting behaviors.
- Be a role model for infant-care activities.
- Assist parents in interpreting infant cues.
- Offer appropriate educational materials (i.e., consider age, educational level, resources).
- Identify risk factors for parenting (i.e., lack of economic or psychosocial resources) and assist in obtaining appropriate referrals and assistance.

PHYSICAL STATUS

Physical assessment is an essential component of comprehensive nursing care during the postpartum period. Changes in the breasts, uterus, lochia, bladder, abdomen, perineum, legs, and feet should be assessed periodically and appropriate nursing interventions initiated as needed. The following interventions are included in a comprehensive assessment during the immediate postpartum period:

- Assess breasts for redness, pain, engorgement, and, if nursing, correct latch-on and removal of the newborn from the breast.
- Assess the uterus and lochia as described previously.
- Note any foul-smelling lochia.
- Assess the bladder for fullness before and after voiding.
- Measure amount of the first void (repeat if an insufficient amount).
- Assess for burning, frequency, and flank tenderness.
- Assess the abdomen for muscle tone, and check the incision site if applicable.
- Assess bowel sounds in all four quadrants.
- Assess the perineum, labia, and anus for edema, redness, pain, bruising, and hematoma.
- Assess the episiotomy or abdominal incision for approximation and drainage.
- Assess for the presence, size, and condition of hemorrhoids.
- Assess dietary intake and elimination patterns.
- Assess legs and feet for edema and varicosities.
- Assess for the Homans' sign if agency protocol requires (i.e., positive if the woman reports pain in calf muscles when the foot is dorsiflexed), and measure the width of the calf if thrombophlebitis is suspected; the Homans' sign has not been found to be consistently predictive of the presence of deep vein thrombosis [DVT]).
- Assess activity tolerance.
- Assess the comfort level and response to pain medication.
- Assess breath sounds if the woman has received magnesium sulfate, other tocolytics, or oxytocin; has been on bed rest; has an infection; or had a multiple birth (i.e., greater risk for pulmonary edema, especially if the patient received large amounts of IV therapy).
- Use the acronym BUBBLERS (breasts, uterus, bladder, bowel, lochia, episiotomy or incision, emotional response) to guide this assessment.

POSTPARTUM HEMORRHAGE

PPH is the leading cause of maternal mortality, averaging 1% to 5% of all births (Jacob, 2012). In industrialized countries, it ranks in the top three causes of maternal mortality, together with embolism and hypertension (Smith & Rivlin, 2010). Healthy People 2020 includes an objective to reduce maternal illness and complications due to pregnancy during hospitalized labor and delivery (U.S. Department of Health and Human Services [DHHS], 2011). The baseline of pregnant females who suffered complications during hospitalized labor and delivery in 2007 was 31.1%. The target for 2020 is 28%. In January 2010, The Joint Commission (TJC) issued a Sentinel Event Alert: *Preventing Maternal Death*. It identified the most preventable errors as the following:

- Failure to adequately control BP in hypertensive women
- Failure to adequately diagnose and treat pulmonary edema in preeclamptics
- Failure to pay attention to vitals following cesarean section (CS)
- Hemorrhage following CS

The physiologic changes that occur during pregnancy are in anticipation of natural blood loss at birth. These changes include a plasma volume increase of approximately 40% and a red cell mass increase of approximately 25% (ACOG, 2008b). Uterine bleeding after birth is controlled by the contraction of the myometrium, which constricts blood vessels supplying the placenta, and local decidual hemostatic factors such as tissue factor, type-1 plasminogen activator inhibitor, and systemic coagulation from platelets and circulating clotting factors (Jacob, 2012). Some women experience a greater than normal blood loss evolving into PPH. The acute anemia resulting from PPH interferes with oxygen delivery to tissue. Acute blood loss leads to tissue hypoxia, with subsequent vasodilation of vascular beds in an attempt to bring more blood to the area. Tissue hypoxia then results in anaerobic metabolism and production of lactate with resultant lactic acidosis. The effects of hypovolemia are outlined in Figure 17–5.

PPH is diagnosed clinically as excessive bleeding that makes the patient symptomatic (e.g., pallor, lightheadedness, weakness, palpitations, diaphoresis, restlessness, confusion, air hunger, syncope) and/or results in signs of hypovolemia (e.g., hypotension, tachycardia, oliguria, low oxygen saturation [<95%]) (Jacob, 2012). Clinical

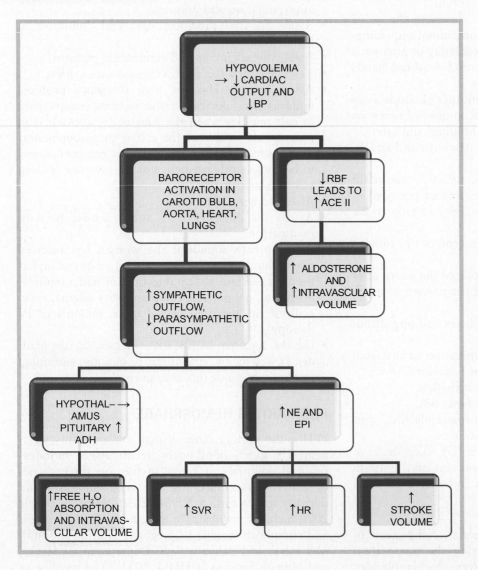

FIGURE 17–5. Physiology of blood loss. ACE-II, angiotensin-converting enzyme II; ADH, antidiuretic hormone; BP, blood pressure; EPI, epinephrine; HR, heart rate; NE, norepinephrine; RBF, renal blood flow; SVR, systemic vascular resistance. (From Mercy Hospital St. Louis Perinatal Service, 2011. Used with permission.)

signs and symptoms such as hypotension, dizziness, pallor, and oliguria do not occur until blood loss is PPH hemorrhage occurs in about 2% to 6% of women who have a vaginal birth (Cunningham et al., 2009; Karpati et al., 2004). It can occur early (first 24 hours) or secondary (>24 hours and <6 weeks after birth). Early or primary PPH is caused by uterine atony in 80% or more of cases (ACOG, 2008b). Display 17–7 lists factors associated with PPH etiology and clinical factors predisposing women to risk. The term *postpartum hemorrhage* is a description of an event, not a diagnosis. Estimates of blood loss after birth are notoriously inaccurate, with significant underreporting most common (ACOG, 2008b; Cunningham et al., 2009). PPH has traditionally been defined as blood loss of 500 mL or more after completion of the third stage of labor, as more than 500 mL after vaginal birth, more than 1,000 mL during cesarean birth, or more than 1,500 mL during a repeat cesarean birth. This definition is not considered reasonable or realistic because nearly half of women giving birth vaginally lose that amount or more.

During birth, a normal, healthy woman tolerates blood loss equal to the volume of blood added during pregnancy without any significant decrease in the postpartum hematocrit. Hematocrit and hemoglobin levels are often used to estimate blood loss after birth; however, laboratory values may not always reflect current hematologic status, especially when blood is drawn soon after the event before equilibrium has occurred and large amounts of rapid volume expanders have been administered intravenously (ACOG, 2008b). Within the clinical context of these limitations, blood loss is often estimated at 500 mL for every 3% drop in hematocrit values when comparing the admission hematocrit with the postpartum hematocrit (Cunningham et al., 2009). For example, a decrease in hematocrit from 38% on admission to 32% postpartum would represent an approximate blood loss of 1,000 mL. Hemoglobin values can be used similarly. The hemoglobin value can be assumed to decrease 1 to 1.5 g/dL for each 500 mL of blood loss (ACOG, 2008b; AWHONN & Johnson & Johnson Consumer Products, 2006; Cunningham et al., 2009). Acute blood loss can be classified as mild, moderate, or severe (Table 17–2).

Acute Blood Loss

The greatest risk for early PPH is during the first hour after birth because large venous areas are exposed after placental separation. According to ASA (2007), the following resources should be available in the event of an obstetric hemorrhagic emergency: large-bore IV catheters; IV fluid warmer; forced-air body warmer; an available blood blank; and equipment for infusing IV fluids or blood products rapidly, such as hand-squeezed fluid chambers, hand-inflated pressure bags, and automatic infusion devices. The frontline treatment for the management of PPH is uterotonic agents (oxytocin, methylergonovine, 15-methyl-prostaglandin (PG)$F_{2\alpha}$, dinoprostone, misoprostol) when atony is the cause of the bleeding (ACOG, 2008b). If these medications fail, an exploratory laparotomy is the next step. Maintaining uterine contraction by using fundal massage (Fig. 17–4) and IV oxytocin administration (20 U/L) reduces the incidence of hemorrhage from uterine atony (AAP & ACOG, 2008; ACOG, 2008b; Thorpe, 2009; Cunningham et al., 2009). Late postpartum bleeding most commonly occurs between day 6 and day 14.

DISPLAY 17–7

Factors Associated with Postpartum Hemorrhage

Etiology

Early or primary postpartum hemorrhage

Uterine atony (most common)

Retained placenta

Placenta accreta

Defects in coagulation

Uterine inversion

Genital tract hematomas

Late or secondary postpartum hemorrhage

Infection

Subinvolution of placental site

Retained placenta

Inherited coagulation defects

Risk Factors

History of uterine atony or postpartum hemorrhage

Trauma, lacerations, or hematoma of cervix and/or birth canal

Precipitous labor and birth

Prolonged labor

Induced or augmented labor

Difficult third stage (i.e., use of aggressive fundal manipulation or cord traction)

Operative vaginal birth (e.g., use of forceps or vacuum)

Cesarean birth

Uterine overdistension (e.g., large infant, multiple gestation, polyhydramnios)

Multiparity

Sepsis

Coagulopathies

Uterine rupture

Drugs (large dosages of oxytocin, magnesium sulfate, beta-adrenergic tocolytic agents; diazoxide [potent antihypertensive agent]; calcium channel blockers, such as nifedipine; and halothane [anesthetic agent])

Table 17–2. HEMORRHAGE AND PHYSICAL FINDINGS

	MILD	MODERATE	SEVERE	
Volume	900–1,000 mL	1,200–1,500 mL 20%–25% blood volume	2,000 mL 30%–35% blood volume	>2,400 mL 40% blood volume
Vital signs	Class 1 Normal or ↑ diastolic BP	Class 2 Mild tachycardia Narrowed pulse pressure Orthostatic hypotension	Class 3 Tachycardia–120 ↓ BP/systolic 90–100 Tachypnea ↓ urine output	Class 4 Shock
Exam	Normal	Delayed capillary refill Anxiety	Restless Cool, pale skin	Oliguria Anuria

BP, blood pressure.
Adapted from Estimated Blood Loss Presentation. Mercy Hospital St. Louis Perinatal Service, 2011. Used with permission.

Preexisting risk factors for PPH include:

- High parity
- Previous PPH
- Previous uterine surgery
- Coagulation defects or medical disorders of clotting

Current pregnancy risk factors for PPH include:

- Antepartal hemorrhage
- Uterine overdistension (macrosomia, multiple gestation, or polyhydramnios)
- Chorioamnionitis/intraamniotic infection
- Placental abnormality (succenturiate lobe, placenta previa, placenta accreta, abruptio placentae, hydatidiform mole)
- Fetal death

Risk factors for PPH associated with labor and birth include:

- Rapid or prolonged labor
- Use of tocolytic or halogenated anesthetic agents
- Large episiotomy
- Operative vaginal birth
- Cesarean birth
- Abnormally located or attached placenta
- Inversion of uterus

When PPH occurs, the perinatal team must work together to treat the underlying condition, manage the blood loss, and minimize the risk to the mother (Display 17–8).

The California Maternal Quality Care Collaborative (CMQCC) developed a toolkit to improve healthcare providers' response to maternal hemorrhage (Lyndon et al., 2010). Their recommendations include the following:

- Every hospital has a protocol outlining the steps for activation and response to maternal hemorrhage. Charge nurses triage and designate staff to respond to specific protocol steps; and all phone numbers of potentially needed personnel are included.
- Either physicians or nursing staff can activate an emergency maternal hemorrhage protocol.

- Develop a collaborative policy/procedure with the blood bank for issue of a specified "OB emergency hemorrhage pack" that includes RBCs, fresh frozen plasma (FFP), cryoprecipitate, and platelets.
- Identify a local expert with experience in hemorrhage and disseminated intravascular coagulation (DIC) treatment for contact as needed.
- Post medicine doses and suture techniques in labor and delivery and operating room (OR) suites for reference.
- Perform scheduled hemorrhage protocol drills and assessments for both physicians and registered nurses.

DISPLAY 17 – 8

Management of Postpartum Hemorrhage

Goals

Stop hemorrhage

Correct hypovolemia

Return of hemostasis

Identification of risk factors

Early recognition and treatment of hemorrhage

Treatment of underlying cause of hemorrhage

Medical–Surgical Management

Medications

Oxytocin

Ergot

Prostaglandins (15-methyl prostaglandin $F_{2\alpha}$, prostaglandin E_2, misoprostol)

Fundal massage

Bladder management

Mast trousers

Bimanual compression

Uterine packing

Curettage

Ligation of blood vessels (uterine, ovarian, hypogastric arteries)

Arterial embolization

The following assessments and interventions are included in comprehensive care during PPH based on the individual clinical situation:

- Plan for care and assessment to ensure early recognition of hemorrhage.
- Packed red blood cells (PRBCs) should be typed and cross-matched if excessive blood loss is anticipated (AAP & ACOG, 2008).
- Assess blood loss. Tips include assessing spill on floor:
  - 24 inches is about 500 mL
  - 34 inches is about 1,000 mL
  - 45 inches is about 1,500 mL
- Weigh peripads or Chux dressing (1 g = 1 mL). (Keep a gram scale on unit.)
- Assess excessive bleeding, which is defined as one perineal pad saturated within 15 minutes.
- Look for severe loss that may occur with steady, slow seepage.
- Assess vital signs at least every 15 minutes or more often if indicated.
- Mean arterial pressure (MAP), which is the mean BP in arterial circulation, should be assessed because the first BP response to hypovolemia may be a pulse pressure decreased to 30 mm Hg or less (Cunningham et al., 2009). MAP in nonpregnant women is normally 86.4 ± 7.5 mm Hg, with a slightly higher value for pregnant women, 90.3 ± 6 mm Hg (Martin & Foley, 2009; Cunningham et al., 2009). MAP can be calculated with this formula:

$$MAP = systolic\ BP + (2 \times diastolic\ BP)\ /\ 3$$

- Assess for tachypnea and tachycardia, which may occur while the BP is constant or slightly lowered.
- Assess for shock. Normal vital signs do not mean that the woman is not in shock. Traditional signs of hypovolemic shock are not evident until 10% to 30% of the total blood volume is lost due to the pregnancy-induced hypervolemia that accounts for the 30% to 70% increase in blood volume (an additional 1 to 2 L) that prevents symptoms with the typical 500 mL blood loss (ACOG, 2008b; Martin & Foley, 2009; Magann & Lanneau, 2005). The initial response of vasoconstriction shunts blood to vital organs to maintain their function and viability.
- Maintain accurate measurements of intake and output.
- Ensure large-bore (14-, 16-, or 18-gauge) needle IV access.
- Replace volume with crystalloid (normal saline [NS] or lactated Ringer's [L/R] solution) 1:3 or colloid (Hespan or albumin) 1:1 while waiting for blood or deciding on transfusion. Goal is to produce at least 30 mL/hr of urine output and hematocrit values of 30% (Cunningham et al., 2009).
- Draw blood for hemoglobin and hematocrit (compare with prenatal or admission values), type and cross-match, coagulation studies (i.e., fibrinogen, prothrombin time [PT], partial thromboplastin time [PTT], fibrin split products, and fibrin degradation products), and blood chemistry. The blood bank should be notified that transfusion may be necessary.
- The clot observation test provides a simple measure of fibrinogen. A volume of 5 mL of the patient's blood can be placed into a clean red-topped tube and observed frequently. Normally, blood will clot within 8 to 10 minutes and will remain intact. If the fibrinogen concentration is low, generally less than 150 mg/dL, the blood in the tube will not clot, or if it does, it will undergo partial or complete dissolution in 30 to 60 minutes (ACOG, 2008b).
- Arterial blood may be drawn for blood gas determinations.
- If blood transfusion is necessary, each unit of PRBCs (240 mL is the usual volume of 1 unit) can be expected to increase hematocrit 3% and hemoglobin by 1 g/dL. PRBCs contain RBCs, WBCs, and plasma (ACOG, 2008b).
- Transfusion can be withheld with adequate urine output and no appreciable postural hypotension or tachycardia (AAP & ACOG, 2008).
- Deficits in clotting factors may necessitate cryoprecipitate (i.e., for fibrinogen deficiency), recombinant activated factor VII, or FFP (i.e., for decreased levels of clotting factors) (AAP & ACOG, 2008; ACOG, 2008b; Bouwmeester, Jonhoff, Verheijen, & van Geijn, 2003). Each unit of 50 mL of platelets can be expected to increase platelet count 5,000 to 10,000/μL. Platelets contain platelets, RBCs, WBCs, and plasma. Each unit of 250 mL of FFP can be expected to increase fibrinogen by 10 mg/dL. FFP contains fibrinogen, antithrombin III, and factors V and VIII. Each unit of cryoprecipitate can be expected to increase fibrinogen by 10 mg/dL. Cryoprecipitate contains fibrinogen, factors VII and XIII, and von Willebrand factor (ACOG, 2008b).
- Use correct uterine massage to avoid ligament damage and potential uterine inversion (Fig. 17–4). Place one hand pointing toward the woman's head with thumb resting on one side of the uterus and fingers along the other side. Use the other hand to massage with *only the force needed to effect contraction or expulsion of clots*. Overaggressive uterine massage may tire muscle fibers and contribute to further atony.
- Early recognition minimizes blood loss and potential sequelae such as anemia, puerperal infection, thromboembolism, and necrosis of the anterior pituitary (i.e., Sheehan's syndrome).
- Anticipate pain management needs for fundal massage and uterotonic medications for treatment of hemorrhage.
- Urine should be sent to the laboratory as indicated.
- Insert a Foley catheter to empty the bladder and allow accurate measurement of output. A full bladder can impede complete uterine contraction.

- Administer prescribed medication. Labor and birth units should have the following pharmacologic agents available: oxytocin, methylergonovine, ergot alkaloids, 15-methyl-PGF$_{2\alpha}$, PGF$_{2\alpha}$, misoprostol, and dinoprostone (AAP & ACOG, 2008; ACOG, 2008b):

Oxytocin (Pitocin)	10 to 40 units in 500 to 1,000 mL of NS or L/R solution at 50 mU/min Vasodilation with decrease in BP and increase in HR Intramuscular: 10 units—avoid undiluted rapid IV infusion, which causes hypotension
Methylergonovine (Methergine)	0.2 mg intramuscular (IM) q 2 to 4 hours maleate (×5 dose maximum) 0.2 mg PO q 6 to 12 hours (IV administration not recommended) Avoid if patient is hypertensive
Ergonovine maleate	0.2 mg IM q 2 to 4 hours (×5 dose maximum) 0.2 mg PO q 6 to 12 hours (IV administration not recommended)
15-methyl-PGF$_{2\alpha}$	IM 250 mcg 15 to 90 minutes (eight doses maximum)
(Carboprost/ Hemabate)	Physician may administer by intramyometrial route Avoid in asthmatic patients; relative contraindication if patient has hepatic, renal, or cardiac disease; can cause diarrhea, fever, and tachycardia
Misoprostol (Cytotec)	800 to 1,000 mcg rectally
Dinoprostone (Prostin E$_2$)	Suppository (vaginally or rectally) 20 mcg every 2 hours Avoid if patient is hypotensive; fever is common; stored frozen—must be thawed to room temperature

- Apply pulse oximeter and administer oxygen according to unit protocol. This is usually accomplished with a nonrebreather face mask at 10 to 12 L/min.
- Continuous electrocardiographic monitoring may be indicated for hypotension, continuous bleeding, tachycardia, or shock.
- Elevate the legs to a 20- to 30-degree angle to increase venous return.
- Prepare for additional interventions if the situation does not resolve. These include packing the uterus with gauze or using a balloon tamponade, dilatation and curettage, exploratory laparotomy, bilateral uterine artery ligation, arterial embolization, and other surgical techniques. In some cases, PPH may require a transfer or return to the surgical suite. The surgical team should be notified that they may be needed.
- Provide emotional support and explanations for the woman and her family.

Following an interdisciplinary collaboration, the CMQCC (Lyndon et al., 2010) suggest a methodology for blood and fluid replacement following a PPH.

- Use a ratio of PRBCs to FFP to platelets that is 6 units PRBC: 4 units FFP: 1 unit pheresis platelets.
  - If bleeding continues after initial treatment, strong consideration should be given to increasing the amount of FFP to a ratio of 4 units PRBC: 4 units of FFP: 1 unit of pheresis platelets.
- STAT LABS
  - If bleeding exceeds expected volume for routine delivery and there is no response to initial therapy, request stat laboratory analysis for the following:
    - Complete blood count (CBC) with platelets
    - PT/PTT
    - Fibrinogen
    - Repeat labs one to three times every 30 minutes until patient is stable
- A glass red-topped tube without additives should be collected and taped to the wall and checked after 10 minutes; if the red-topped blood is not clotted at 10 minutes, assume patient has DIC until laboratory test(s) show otherwise. *Note that per the Occupational Safety and Health Administration (OSHA) regulations, many hospitals are now using plastic red-topped tubes, which contain an additive to induce clotting; in glass tubes, clotting was induced by the negative surface charge of glass. Reliable with the use of glass tubes, but not with plastic.*
- PBRCs
  - Initial request: 4 to 6 units of RBCs
  - O-negative or type-specific blood initially until cross-match units are released
- FFP
  - RBCs to FFP ratio not to exceed 3:2
  - Infuse FFP to maintain international normalized ratio <1.5
- Platelets
  - Single donor apheresis platelet pack
  - Infuse to maintain platelet count >50,000 to 100,000/uL in the face of ongoing hemorrhage
- Cryoprecipitate
  - Initial request: 10 units cryoprecipitate if fibrinogen is less than 100 mg/dL
  - Additional units to maintain fibrinogen concentration ≥100 to 125 mg/dL

- Recombinant activated factor VII (rVII)
  - If available, use when there is continued hemorrhage AND all other blood replacement therapies have failed (i.e., after the use of 10 to 12 units PRBC, 6 to 12 units FFP, and 2 to 3 units platelets).

Once the patient is stable, replacement of RBC mass is an important clinical intervention. The patient should be instructed to continue prenatal vitamins that contain about 60 mg of elemental iron and 1 mg of folate during the hospitalization and at least until the first postpartum office visit. Additional iron should be encouraged (two tablets of 300 mg ferrous sulfate) to maximize red cell production and restoration (ACOG, 2008b).

In July 2004, The Joint Commission (TJC) recommended conducting periodic drills for obstetric emergencies such as PPH. Although there are few data supporting improved outcomes in units where PPH birth drills are routine, it would seem likely that when all members of the perinatal team know their roles and responsibilities,

the location of key medications and equipment, and whom to call, the chances of the chaotic environment often associated with a significant PPH would be minimized (Simpson, 2005). During PPH, immediate access to required medications can be challenging. Common medications used to treat PPH such as oxytocin, Methergine, Prostin, and misoprostol are kept in locked drug-dispensing systems often remote from the labor room. IV fluids required for rapid volume expansion also may not be available in the labor room. Development of a clinical algorithm for interventions during PPH in addition to drills to evaluate the feasibility of getting necessary medications and IV fluids quickly may be helpful. Documenting interventions is important to keep both the drill and actual response organized (Display 17–9).

An interdisciplinary team at Mercy Hospital St. Louis developed a PPH protocol for mild, moderate, and severe (stable and unstable) PPH (Figs. 17–6 to 17–9) and a PPH team. To prepare for a drill,

---

DISPLAY 17–9

Flow Sheet for Postpartum Hemorrhage Documentation

POSTPARTUM HEMORRHAGE FLOWSHEET

Time	Temp	Heart Rate	Resp Rate	Blood Pressure	O₂ Sat	Fundus	Oxytocin (dose)	Methergine (dose)	Hemabate (dose)	Cytotec (dose)	Interval Blood Loss (ml)	Total Blood Loss (ml)	Interval Urine (ml)	Total Urine (ml)	Crystalloid (ml)	Colloid (ml)	PRBC Unit #	FFP Unit #	Platelet Unit #	Cryoprecipitate Unit #	Hgb/Hct	PT/INR/PTT	Fibrinogen	Other Labs

NOT A PART OF THE OFFICIAL PATIENT RECORD

FFP, fresh frozen plasma; Hct, hematocrit; Hgb, hemoglobin; INR, international normalized ratio; PRBC, packed red blood cell; PT, prothrombin time.

MILD PPH
EBL >500ml for vag del or >100ml for CS *OR* HR>110
OR BP ↓15% with ONGOING BLOOD LOSS

Primary RN	☐ **Notify Intern** ☐ **Notify Charge Nurse** ☐ **Administer uterotonics as directed** ☐ **Administer O2** ☐ **Send CBC, Type and Screen if not already done.** ☐ **Evaluate ongoing EBL**
Charge RN	☐ **Notify Chief Resident** ☐ **Notify Anesthesia Attending**
OB MD/Intern	☐ **Order uterotonics** ☐ **Evaluate and treat causes of hemorrhage (atony, retained POC, lacerations)**

If continued bleeding despite these maneuvers, proceed to MODERATE. If bleeding stops, initiate high level postpartum surveillance

FIGURE 17–6. Mild postpartum hemorrhage protocol. (From Mercy Hospital St. Louis Perinatal Service, 2011. Used with permission.)

develop a list of roles and responsibilities for each team member. Some have found it helpful to use a scribe or a video recording of the drill so that the organization of events and interventions can be analyzed retrospectively. Using a volunteer staff member as a surrogate for the patient can make the drill seem more realistic.

POSTPARTUM INFECTIONS

A puerperal infection should be suspected when a woman has an oral temperature higher than 38°C (100.4°F) on two occasions that are 6 hours apart during the first 10 days postpartum, exclusive of the first 24 hours. The cardinal symptoms of a postpartum infection are elevated temperature, tachycardia, and pain. The nursery should be notified of these findings, although the newborn need not be separated from the mother (AAP & ACOG, 2008; Cunningham et al., 2009; Duff, Sweet, & Edwards, 2009).

Endometritis

Postpartum endometritis occurs in 1% to 3% of vaginal births and is 10 times more common in cesarean births (Cunningham et al., 2009; Duff et al., 2009). Postpartum uterine infections, called *endometritis* (i.e., inflammation of endometrium), *endomyometritis* (i.e., inflammation of endometrium and myometrium), or *endomyoparametritis* (i.e., inflammation of endometrium and parametrial tissue), are the most commonly identified causes of puerperal morbidity. One of the most effective methods of prevention of infection is hand washing.

The most common cause of uterine infection tends to be polymicrobial, including aerobic and anaerobic organisms that have ascended to the uterus from the lower genital tract. Isolated organisms include streptococci A and B, enterococci, *Staphylococcus aureus*, *Gardnerella vaginalis*, *Escherichia coli*, *Enterobacter*, *Proteus mirabilis*, *Klebsiella pneumoniae*, *Bacteroides* species, *Peptostreptococcus* species, *Ureaplasma urealyticum*, *Mycoplasma hominis*, and

MODERATE PPH
EBL 1500-2000ml with ONGOING BLOOD LOSS

Primary RN	☐ Cycle BP every 5 mins ☐ Start 2nd IV (blood tubing, NS) ☐ Bolus NS wide open ☐ Draw CBC, T&C (if not already) ☐ Evaluate ongoing EBL
Charge RN	☐ Set up blood administration tubing ☐ Place SCD's and foley ☐ Assign secondary RN ☐ Assess ongoing EBL ☐ Update Anesthesia Attending ☐ Notify In-Hourse OB MD ☐ Get PPH cart
OB MD	☐ Evaluate ongoing EBL/patient condition ☐ Repeat uterotonics if appropriate ☐ Consider move to OR (if not already there ☐ Consider D&C, Bakri balloon, packing, uterine artery embo ☐ If CS consider B-lynch, Bakri balloon, UA embo/ligation, hysterectomy
Anesthesia MD	☐ Evaluate ongoing EBL/patient condition ☐ Assist with IV/blood draw ☐ Consider Hespan ☐ Call Blood Bank 1-6398 ☐ Order 2u PRBC and 6 FFP (if ongoing blood loss) ☐ Obtain fluid warmer and heating blanket

If EBL >2000ml or patient unstable proceed to SEVERE (STABLE or UNSTABLE). If bleeding stops, initiate high level postpartum surveillance.

FIGURE 17–7. Moderate postpartum hemorrhage protocol. (From Mercy Hospital St. Louis Perinatal Service, 2011. Used with permission.)

Chlamydia trachomatis. C. trachomatis has been specifically associated with late-onset postpartum endometritis (Cunningham et al., 2009; Duff et al., 2009). Blood cultures are positive in about 10% of women. Endometrial cultures may have limited value because of cervicovaginal contamination of the specimen, yet they may provide useful information if the woman does not respond to initial antibiotic therapy (Cunningham et al., 2005; Duff et al., 2009). If the infection does not respond to antibiotic therapy, an antiviral regimen should be considered for

pathogens such as herpes simplex virus (HSV) or cytomegalovirus (Giraldo-Isaza, Jaspan, & Cohen, 2011).

Parenteral broad-spectrum antibiotic therapy is promptly initiated when postpartum endometritis is diagnosed. Treatment continues until the woman has been afebrile for 48 hours. A common treatment regimen is a combination of clindamycin and gentamicin, with ampicillin in refractory cases, which is a cost-effective therapy. Women usually respond rapidly (48 to 72 hours) to antibiotic therapy. Occasional complications include pelvic

SEVERE PPH (stable)
EBL >2000ml, VS stable, no evidence DIC, bleeding stopped

Primary RN	☐ Evaluate ongoing EBL/patient condition ☐ Help check blood products
Secondary RN	☐ Enter orders in computer if needed ☐ Assist as needed
Charge RN	☐ Evaluate ongoing EBL/patient condition
OB MD	☐ Evaluate ongoing EBL/patient condition ☐ Continue to assess and attempt to treat primary cause of hemorrhage (consider uterine artery embo/ligation vs hysterectomy
Anesthesia MD	☐ Evaluate ongoing EBL/patient condition ☐ Tranfuse 2-4u PRBC ☐ Consider transfuse 2 FFP (if clinically indicated ☐ CBC, DIC, BMP now and 4 hours later

If bleeding stops, initiate high level post-partum surveillance. Otherwise proceed to SEVERE (unstable)

FIGURE 17–8. Severe postpartum hemorrhage (stable) protocol. (From Mercy Hospital St. Louis Perinatal Service, 2011. Used with permission.)

abscesses, septic pelvic thrombophlebitis, persistent fever, and retained infected placenta (AAP & ACOG, 2008).

Other causes of postpartum infection include wound and UTIs, pneumonia (usually related to general anesthesia), mastitis, pelvic thrombophlebitis, and necrotizing fasciitis, an uncommon but serious localized infection of the deep soft tissues.

Risk factors for endometritis include:

• Operative birth
• Prolonged labor or rupture of membranes
• Use of invasive procedures (i.e., internal monitoring, amnioinfusion, fetal scalp sampling, lacerations)
• Multiple pelvic examinations

• Excessive blood loss
• Pyelonephritis or diabetes
• Socioeconomic and nutritional factors compromising host defense mechanisms
• Anemia and systemic illness
• Smoking
• Diabetes

The following assessments and interventions are included in comprehensive nursing care for postpartum infections:

• Fever occurring about the third postnatal day is the most important finding.

SEVERE PPH (unstable) – OB MASSIVE HEMORRHAGE
EBL >2000ml, VS unstable, suspicion of DIC, and
continued bleeding after 2-4 units of blood

Primary RN	☐ **Evaluate ongoing EBL/patient condition** ☐ **Help check blood products**
Secondary RN	☐ **Record events on flowsheet** ☐ **Enter orders in computer if needed** ☐ **Assist as needed**
Charge RN	☐ **Evaluate ongoing EBL/patient condition** ☐ **Arrange for ICU bed**
OB MD	☐ **Evaluate ongoing EBL/patient condition** ☐ **Continue to assess and attempt to treat primary cause of hemorrhage (consider uterine artery embo/ligation vs hysterectomy** ☐ **Consider Gyn-Onc if needed (see list)**
Anesthesia MD	☐ **Evaluate ongoing EBL/patient condition** ☐ **If ongoing bleeding, call blood bank to activate OB Massive Hemorrhage Protocol 1-6398** ☐ **Consider trauma/MET team if needed** ☐ **Consider intubation, RIC line, art line** ☐ **CBC, DIC, BMP, ABG q30-60 mins until stable** ☐ **Give report to ICU physician**

Aggressively treat coagulopathy.
If fibrinogen <100, give 10 pack cryo
Keep patient warm and avoid acidemia
Consider rFactor VIIa after 10u PRBC's

FIGURE 17–9. Severe postpartum hemorrhage (unstable) protocol. (From Mercy Hospital St. Louis Perinatal Service, 2011. Used with permission.)

- Observe for tachycardia (rise of 10 bpm for every degree Celsius).
- Determine possible causes of malaise.
- Assess lower abdominal pain.
- Assess uterine tenderness on palpation (extending laterally) and slight abdominal distention.
- Determine cause of foul-smelling lochia (if organism is anaerobic).
- Obtain urinalysis to rule out UTI.
- Assess leukocytosis (WBC count >20,000/μL with increased neutrophils or polymorphonuclear leukocytes).
- Blood cultures are positive in about 10% of women.

- Endometrial cultures may have limited value because of cervicovaginal contamination of the specimen, but they may provide useful information if the woman does not respond to initial antibiotic therapy (Cunningham et al., 2009; Duff et al., 2009).
- Parenteral broad-spectrum antibiotic therapy is promptly initiated when postpartum endometritis is diagnosed. Treatment continues until the woman has been afebrile for 48 hours. A common treatment regimen is a combination of clindamycin and an aminoglycoside such as gentamicin, with ampicillin added in refractory cases. A protocol including activity against the *Bacteroides fragilis* group and

other penicillin-resistant anaerobic bacteria is better than one without. No one regimen is associated with fewer side effects, with the exception of cephalosporins, which are associated with less diarrhea.
- Women usually respond rapidly (48 to 72 hours) to antibiotic therapy. Occasional complications include pelvic abscesses, septic pelvic thrombophlebitis, persistent fever, and retained infected placenta (AAP & ACOG, 2008).
- Increase fluid intake and encourage adequate nutrition.
- Encourage intake of a minimum of six to eight glasses (1,500 to 2,000 mL) of water, milk, or juices; 3,000 mL is the preferred amount.
- Encourage intake of at least 1,800 to 2,000 calories daily if lactating and 1,500 calories if not lactating.
- Encourage the woman to eat a varied diet, with representation of foods from all food groups, that is high in protein and vitamin C to promote wound healing.
- Ensure adequate output (30 mL/hr) because renal toxicity can occur with antibiotic therapy.
- Provide comfort through meeting the woman's personal hygiene needs. Cool compresses, linen changes, massage, and positioning may enhance comfort.
- Assess vital signs every 4 hours or every 2 hours if her temperature is elevated.
- Use a semi-Fowler's position, ambulation, or both to promote uterine drainage.
- Administer oxytocics as ordered to promote uterine contraction and drainage.
- Observe for signs of septic shock: tachycardia (>120 bpm), hypotension, tachypnea, changes in sensorium, and decreased urine output (i.e., oliguria) (Cunningham et al., 2009). If septic shock develops, increase the frequency of obtaining vital signs and other assessments depending on the clinical situation.

Wound Infections

Wound infections can be classified as early onset (within 48 hours) or late onset (within 6 to 8 days). Early-onset wound infections are usually treated with antibiotic therapy and excision of necrotic tissue. Late-onset infections are treated with incision and drainage, and they may not require antibiotics unless there is extensive cellulitis (Cunningham et al., 2009; Duff et al., 2009). The following are risk factors for wound infections:

- History of chorioamnionitis or intraamniotic infection
- Hemorrhage or anemia
- Obesity
- Underlying medical problems such as diabetes and malnutrition
- Multiple vaginal examinations
- Corticosteroid therapy

- Immunosuppression
- Advancing age
- Malnutrition

The following assessments and interventions are included in comprehensive nursing care for wound infections:

- Observe for wound erythema, swelling, tenderness, and purulent discharge.
- Assess for localized pain and dysuria.
- Assess vital signs.
- Check for a low-grade temperature (38.3°C [101°F]).
- Acute cases may exhibit sudden chills and spikes in temperature to 40°C (104°F).
- The pulse usually is <100 bpm.
- Perform cultures as ordered.
- Assist with drainage, irrigation, and, occasionally, debridement procedures.
- Sitz baths are used for cleaning and promotion of increased circulation to the affected area.
- The wound may be packed. Treatment is directed toward cleaning the wound and promoting granulation.
- Change dressings and dispose appropriately of soiled dressings.
- Dressings may be continued after discharge. The patient and family will need instruction for dressing and wound care.
- Ensure frequent changes of peripads.
- Ensure pain management and appropriate administration of analgesia.
- Ensure adequate room ventilation prior to dressing changes.
- Continued hospitalization or readmission may be required.
- Provide explanations during this stressful period.
- Offer reassurance and encouragement.
- Encourage frequent visits by the family to help reduce anxiety.
- Assist breastfeeding women with pumping or lactation suppression.
- Administer antibiotic therapy as ordered (may be continued after discharge).
- Provide referrals for postpartum follow-up visits by home care nurses.
- Reduce anxiety and the incidence of rehospitalization by early identification and treatment of infections.

Necrotizing Fasciitis

Necrotizing fasciitis is a severe infection (polymicrobial more common) that is characterized by severe tissue necrosis, erythema, discharge, and severe pain. Partial liquefaction of fascia adjacent to the incision may also occur. Secondary healing may take 6 to 12 weeks (Cunningham et al., 2009; Duff et al., 2009).

Risk factors for necrotizing fasciitis include:

- Diabetes
- Obesity
- Hypertension

The following assessments and interventions are included in comprehensive nursing care for necrotizing fasciitis:

- Wound status (i.e., erythema, discharge)
- Pain
- Administration of broad-spectrum antibiotics, as ordered
- Surgical debridement

Mastitis

Both congestive and infectious mastitis are more commonly seen in primigravidas and nursing mothers. Symptoms usually appear between the third and fourth week after birth and are typically unilateral. Symptoms of mastitis may include fever; chills; localized tenderness; and a palpable, hard, reddened mass. Nipple trauma has been implicated in the development of mastitis. Trauma from incorrect latch-on or removal of the newborn from the breast permits the introduction of organisms from the newborn into the mother's breast. *S. aureus* is the most common causative organism. Administration of penicillinase-resistant antibiotics such as dicloxacillin for 7 to 10 days is recommended.

If a breast abscess develops, incision and drainage may be indicated. The decision to continue breastfeeding should be made jointly by the woman and the healthcare provider. If breastfeeding is delayed while purulent drainage continues, the woman may need assistance with breast pumping to reestablish lactation. If advised to discontinue breastfeeding, emotional support, reassurance, and comfort measures are important. Lactation consultant referral is indicated as a preventive or treatment measure when these services are available.

Risk factors for mastitis include:

- Infrequent breastfeeding
- Incomplete breast emptying
- Plugged milk duct
- Cracked and bleeding nipples (may be secondary to improper latch-on and removal)

The following assessments and interventions are included in comprehensive nursing care for mastitis:

- Assess fever and chills.
- Assess localized tenderness and a palpable, hard, reddened mass.
- Assess for tachycardia.
- Assess for purulent discharge.
- Offer education about preventive measures (i.e., hand washing, breast cleanliness, frequent breast-pad changes, exposure of the nipples to air, and correct infant latch-on and removal from the breast).
- Obtain a culture of the breast milk before initiating antibiotic therapy, if ordered.
- The infection usually resolves within 24 to 48 hours of antibiotic therapy.
- Suggest comfort measures, including warm or cold compresses, wearing a supportive bra, and analgesia as ordered.
- Offer education about completing the full regimen of antibiotic therapy.
- Encourage an increase in fluid intake from 2 to 2.5 L/day.
- Massage, positioning the newborn in the direction of the site, and frequent breastfeeding promote milk flow.
- Assist with the use of a breast pump or manual expression if indicated (Cunningham et al., 2009; Duff et al., 2009).

Urinary Tract Infections

UTIs are the most common medical complication occurring during pregnancy. They may be asymptomatic (i.e., bacteriuria) or symptomatic (i.e., cystitis, acute pyelonephritis). Asymptomatic UTIs occur in 4% to 7% of pregnant women. Diagnosis and treatment of bacteriuria can prevent the development of pyelonephritis, which places the fetus at increased risk for preterm birth or low birth weight. Women who develop UTIs during pregnancy are at increased risk for a UTI during the postpartum period (Cunningham et al., 2009; Duff et al., 2009).

Risk factors for UTIs include:

- A shorter urethra in women than men
- Contamination of the urethra with pathogenic bacteria from vagina and rectum
- High probability that women do not completely empty bladders
- Movement of bacteria into bladder during sexual intercourse
- Pregnancy-related changes (i.e., decreased ureteric muscle tone and activity from progesterone and pressure of gravid uterus, resulting in lower rate of urine passing through urinary collecting system)
- Urinary catheterization, frequent pelvic examinations, epidural anesthesia, genital tract injury, and cesarean birth

Asymptomatic Bacteriuria

The following assessments and interventions are included in comprehensive nursing care of asymptomatic bacteriuria:

- Evaluate urinalysis for bacteriuria (presence of 10^5 or more bacterial colonies per milliliter of urine on two consecutive, clean-catch, midstream voided specimens).

- *E. coli* is cultured in 60% to 90% of cases. (Other pathogens include *P. mirabilis, K. pneumoniae,* group B hemolytic streptococci, and *Staphylococcus saprophyticus.*)
- Educate women about the importance of repeat urinalysis to determine the effectiveness of antibiotics.
- Risk is associated with sickle cell trait, lower socioeconomic status, increased parity, and reduced availability of medical care.
- Administer or educate the woman to take antibiotics as ordered to eliminate bacteria in urine.
- Ampicillin and cephalosporins are used (no significant risk to the fetus); antibiotics are administered for 7 days.
- If continuous antimicrobial therapy is required, typically use a single daily dose of nitrofurantoin (100 mg), preferably after the evening meal (Duff et al., 2009).

Pyelonephritis and Cystitis

The following assessments and interventions are included in comprehensive nursing care for pyelonephritis and cystitis:

- Assess urinalysis for presence of untreated, asymptomatic bacteriuria.
  - High risk for pyelonephritis with untreated bacteriuria
  - Bacterial growth more than 100,000 colonies/mL
  - May have increased WBCs, protein, or blood in specimen
  - Most common bacteria: *E. coli* (80%), *Klebsiella, Enterobacter, Proteus*
  - First choice of therapy: cephalosporins for single-agent therapy
- Assess for symptoms of cystitis.
  - Urinary urgency, frequency, dysuria
  - Suprapubic pain without fever or tenderness at the costovertebral angle
  - Gross hematuria
- Assess for symptoms of pyelonephritis.
  - Shaking chills, fever, tachycardia, flank pain, nausea, vomiting
  - Urinary frequency, urgency, dysuria, and costovertebral angle tenderness
  - Possible endotoxin-mediated tissue damage (Duff et al., 2009)
- Administer antibiotics as ordered.
  - Short courses (1 to 3 weeks) of sulfonamides, ampicillin, or nitrofurantoin recommended for pyelonephritis
  - Recommended 7-day course of antibiotics for acute cystitis in pregnant women
- Monitor intake and output.
  - Maintain adequate hydration (at least 3,000 mL/day) with water and cranberry juice.
  - Measure urinary output for adequacy (at least 30 mL/hr).
- Administer antipyretics, antispasmodics, or urinary analgesics (Pyridium) and antiemetics as ordered.
- Encourage rest.
- Monitor vital signs every 4 hours.
- Educate the woman about monitoring temperature, bladder function, appearance of urine, importance of completing antibiotic therapy, proper perineal care (i.e., wiping front to back), wearing cotton underwear, adequate hydration, and balanced nutrition.

If readmission for treatment of a UTI is necessary, reassurance and family support are essential. Separation from the newborn is distressing to the mother and child. If the woman has been breastfeeding, interventions such as pumping and newborn visits can help to maintain lactation after antibiotic therapy has been initiated. If breastfeeding is temporarily contraindicated, the nurse can provide emotional support and offer strategies to maintain lactation (i.e., breast pump) until breastfeeding can be resumed (Cunningham et al., 2009; Duff et al., 2009).

THROMBOPHLEBITIS AND THROMBOEMBOLISM

Thrombophlebitis (inflammation of a vein after formation of a thrombus) is classified as superficial or deep. Superficial thrombophlebitis involves the superficial veins of the saphenous system. Deep vein thrombophlebitis affects the veins of the calf, thigh, or pelvis. Stasis is the most significant predisposing event to the development of DVT. Diagnosis of thrombophlebitis is based on objective and subjective signs and symptoms. Septic pelvic thrombophlebitis is a condition more common in women after a cesarean birth and occurs with infections of the reproductive tract. Ascending infection within the venous system results in thrombophlebitis. This condition should be suspected when the infection does not respond to antibiotics and is accompanied by abdominal or flank pain and guarding on the second or third postpartum day.

A more serious complication occurs when a thrombus forms in any of the dilated pelvic veins. Accompanied by thrombophlebitis, these formations can be a source of potentially fatal pulmonary emboli. In those cases, the clot becomes friable, and the pieces detach from the vessel wall and travel through the heart into the pulmonary circulation. Pulmonary embolism should be treated as a life-threatening event; interruption of blood flow to the pulmonary bed can result in cardiovascular collapse and death (Cunningham et al., 2009; Lockwood, 2009).

Risk factors for thrombophlebitis and thromboembolism include:

- Normal changes in coagulation status during pregnancy

- Increasing concentrations of coagulation factors and fibrinogen
- Decreasing natural anticoagulants protein S and activated protein C
- Shift of coagulation and fibrinolytic systems to hyper-coagulability (Jackson, Curtis, & Gaffield, 2011)
- History of thromboembolic disease or varicosities
- Increased parity
- Obesity
- Advanced maternal age (≥30 years)
- Immobility associated with extended antepartum bed rest
- Use of forceps
- Cesarean birth
- Blood vessel and tissue trauma
- Prolonged labor with multiple pelvic examinations
- Sepsis/trauma
- Blood type other than type O
- Dehydration

Thrombus formation can potentially be prevented by these interventions:

- Early ambulation or leg exercises for women on bed rest
- Education about correct posture
- Avoiding crossing legs
- Avoiding extreme flexion of legs at the groin
- Positioning without pressure on the backs of knees
- Use of support hose by women with a history of thrombophlebitis
- Padding of pressure points during birth while in the lithotomy position

Thrombophlebitis

The following assessments and interventions are included in comprehensive nursing care of thrombophlebitis:

- Evaluate the woman's physical status.
- A superficial vein (usually varicose) is reddened, hard, and tender.
- Apply a supportive bandage or antiembolic support stockings.
- Apply a soothing agent (i.e., glycerin and Ichthyol).
- Apply warm packs to the affected area.
- Slightly elevate the involved leg.
- Permit ambulation as indicated and ordered.
- Perform serial measurements of the circumferences of the calves; a circumference difference of more than 2 cm is classified as leg swelling.
- Monitor vital signs every 4 hours; there may be a slight increase in temperature.
- Compare pulses in both extremities, which may reveal decreased venous flow to the affected area.
- Heparin anticoagulation therapy may be ordered.

- If Homans' sign is part of the assessment protocol, the assessment is performed with the knee slightly flexed. The nurse abruptly and forcibly dorsiflexes the ankle, observing for pain in the calf and popliteal area. Numerous studies have questioned the accuracy and utility of the Homans' sign. Accuracy estimates range from a positive result in 8% to 56% of documented cases of DVT to a positive result in more than 50% of patients without DVT. "Pain from muscular causes will be absent or minimal on dorsiflexion of the ankle with the knee flexed but maximal on dorsiflexion of the ankle with the knee extended or during straight-leg raising (Homans' sign); thus, this test is unreliable for DVT" (Beers & Berkow, 2006). Therefore, most authors conclude that Homans' sign is unreliable, insensitive, and nonspecific in the diagnosis of DVT (Rasavong, 2009).

Nursing interventions for DVT include all of the previously described care measures plus the following:

- Bed rest with elevation of involved extremity until swelling is reduced and anticoagulation therapy is effective (promote venous return and decreases edema).
- As soon as symptoms allow, ambulation is encouraged as bed rest can increase venous stasis.
- There is no evidence to support that bed rest prevents embolus detachment (Lockwood, 2009).
- Anticoagulation therapy with IV heparin, followed by oral warfarin.
  - Maintenance of activated PTT that is prolonged by one and one half to two times laboratory control value (Cunningham et al., 2009)
  - Dosing regimens (Cunningham et al., 2009):
    - 5,000-unit bolus of heparin and then continuous infusion to a total 24,000 to 32,000 units/day
    - Intermittent IV injections of 5,000 units every 4 hours or 7,500 units every 6 hours
    - Subcutaneous heparin at dose of 10,000 units every 8 hours or 20,000 units every 12 hours
  - Monitor coagulation laboratory values.
- Carefully assess unusual bleeding. Heavy vaginal bleeding, generalized petechiae, bleeding from the mucous membranes, hematuria, or oozing from venipuncture sites should be reported to the physician. The heparin antidote protamine sulfate should be readily available.
- Educate and prepare women for diagnostic testing.
  - Physical assessments look for muscle pain, palpable deep linear cord, tenderness, swelling, and dilated superficial veins.
  - Doppler ultrasonography provides more sensitivity and is more specific for the diagnosis of popliteal and femoral vein thrombosis than for calf

vein thrombosis. It can evaluate venous flow and possible occlusion.

- Venography is a more specific test, but it is invasive, expensive, and difficult to interpret. Contrast material may cause chemical phlebitis.
- Impedance plethysmography has had little research to support its efficacy during pregnancy, but coupled with ultrasound, the reliability increases. A thigh cuff is inflated, resulting in temporary occlusion of venous return. Release results in a rapid decrease in volume as blood drains proximally. Volume changes are detected by measurement of electrical resistance in the calf.
- Blood studies can determine the formation of intravascular fibrin; results are positive in cases of thrombosis. Results are also positive in presence of hematomas or inflammatory exudates containing fibrin.

Septic Pelvic Thrombophlebitis

The following assessments and interventions are included in comprehensive nursing care of septic pelvic thrombophlebitis:

- Assess the woman for physical symptoms.
  - Fever and tachycardia
  - Spiking fever persisting despite antibiotic therapy
  - Abdominal and flank pain (paralytic ileus may develop)
  - Prepare and support the woman during examination (i.e., parametrial mass found on bimanual examination).
- Obtain appropriate laboratory testing.
  - CBC
  - Blood chemistry
  - Coagulation profile
  - Chest radiography, computed tomography, magnetic resonance imaging
- Administer medications as ordered.
  - Heparin regimen initiated with diagnosis
  - Coumarin agent substituted and continued for total course of anticoagulation of 3 to 6 weeks

Pulmonary Embolism

The following assessments and interventions are included in comprehensive nursing care of pulmonary embolism:

- The most common signs are dyspnea, chest pain, hemoptysis, and abdominal pain.
- The most serious signs are sudden collapse, cyanosis, and hypotension.
- Prepare the woman for diagnostic testing.
  - Ventilation/perfusion (VQ) scan
  - Blood gas studies
  - Radiography
  - Pulmonary angiography

- Elevate the head of the bed to facilitate breathing.
- Administer oxygen 10 L/min using a nonrebreather face mask; use pulse oximetry.
- Maintain the $P_aO_2 \geq 70$ mm Hg.
- Monitor arterial blood gases.
- Frequently assess vital signs.
- Provide for IV fluids (e.g., pulmonary artery catheter may be placed).
- Administer salt-poor or hypertonic IV fluids as ordered.
- Administer medications as ordered to counteract symptoms.
  - Medium dose of IV heparin (continued subcutaneous heparin or oral anticoagulant therapy for 6 months)
  - Total daily heparin dose of 30,000 to 40,000 units (Cunningham et al., 2009)
  - Dopamine to maintain BP
  - Morphine for analgesia
- Maintain adequate staffing.
  - Personnel who have completed an Advanced Cardiac Life Support (ACLS) course should be available for full resuscitation support, if needed. Since ongoing care may occur in an intensive care unit (ICU) setting, collaboration between the ICU staff and perinatal staff is essential. Maternal transport should be considered if the level of care and supportive staff necessary are unavailable.

DISPLAY 17-10

Clinical Signs and Symptoms to Report to the Primary Healthcare Provider

- Uterine atony or large/excessive clots; passage of placental tissue
- Excessive bleeding
- Continued bleeding in the presence of a firm uterus (suggests lacerations)
- Perineal pain greater than expected (suggests hematoma)
- Foul-smelling lochia (suggests endometritis)
- Temperature elevated to >100°F (38°C) (suggests dehydration in first 24 hours; thereafter, after 24 hours, suggests infection [i.e., thrombophlebitis or systemic infection])
- Bladder distention and/or inability to void
- Diminished urinary output (<30 mL/hr)
- Enlarging hematomas
- Restlessness; pallor of skin or mucous membranes; cool, clammy skin; tachycardia; thready pulse; fearfulness; vertigo; shaking; visual disturbances (symptoms of shock)
- Pain, redness, warmth, firm area in the calf area (although pain may be absent in deep vein thrombosis [DVT])
- Dyspnea, tachypnea, tachycardia, chest pain, cough, apprehension, hemoptysis, change in skin/mucous membrane color (paleness and/or cyanosis): symptoms of pulmonary embolism or amniotic fluid embolism

Although most women have a normal postpartum course, complications can occur. Comprehensive, frequent nursing assessments contribute to early identification and prompt treatment. Collaboration between the perinatal nurse and the primary healthcare provider is essential. Display 17–10 lists the clinical signs and symptoms suggesting postpartum complications that warrant communication with the primary healthcare provider.

INDIVIDUALIZING CARE FOR WOMEN WITH SPECIAL NEEDS

CESAREAN BIRTH

The cesarean birth rate in the United States in 2009 was 32.9% and has continued to rise each year since these data began to be collected from certificates of live birth (Hamilton, Martin, & Ventura, 2010). Both the primary and the repeat cesarean birth rates have steadily increased. Elective labor induction for nulliparous women is one factor that has had an impact on the rise in primary cesarean births. As vaginal birth after cesarean birth has fallen out of favor with many providers and patients, once a woman has a cesarean birth, it is likely that she will have another with a future pregnancy. When labor ends in cesarean birth, there is risk of lowered self-esteem related to failure to achieve the planned vaginal birth. The desired outcome of birth is for each couple to verbalize a positive birth experience and to feel happiness and excitement about a healthy baby, even if labor and birth do not go as planned. Nurses can assist in achieving this outcome for women experiencing a cesarean birth by involving the couple as much as possible in the decision-making process, keeping the couple informed, supporting the coach and family, encouraging verbalization, and providing reassurance that a cesarean birth is not a failure. If the cesarean birth was unexpected and/or emergent (Fig. 17–10)

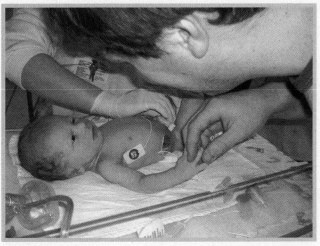

FIGURE 17–11. Promoting father visiting baby in the neonatal intensive care unit after emergent cesarean birth.

with minimal time to prepare the couple, time should be allocated as soon as possible after birth to discuss what occurred and why the provider felt cesarean birth was the safest option at that time for the mother and baby. Efforts should be made to allow the father of the baby to see the baby as soon as possible if the emergent birth resulted in the baby's admission to the special care nursery (SCN) or neonatal intensive care unit (NICU); thus, the baby has been separated from the couple during post-anesthesia care (Fig. 17–11). Some nurseries have cameras available to take pictures of the baby to immediately share with the mother until she is able to go to the nursery to see the baby herself.

Nurses caring for women after a cesarean birth should stress that the woman is a new mother with the same needs as other new mothers; however, she also requires supportive postoperative care. It is important to provide that extra level of care and include consideration of women in the postoperative period when planning nurse staffing. The woman who has experienced a cesarean birth usually has increased levels of fatigue, activity intolerance, and incisional pain. Women who have cesarean birth after a long labor may be especially fatigued. Women who are in the postoperative recovery period and during the first day or two postoperatively should have a support person with them to help care for the baby while rooming in (see Figs. 17–8, 17–12). Policies that require rooming in for these patients are not appropriate if the mother does not have a support person available to stay with her continuously until she can assume newborn care on her own. Mothers who have a cesarean birth stay longer in the hospital and require more intensive nursing care than for women who have a vaginal birth. The average length of inpatient stay for cesarean birth is 3.6 days as compared to 2.2 days for vaginal birth (DHHS, 2010). Chapter 14 provides a full discussion of cesarean birth and the immediate postoperative recovery period.

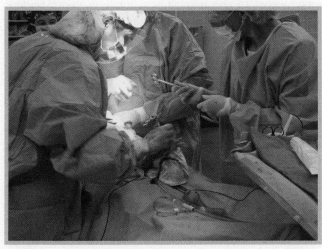

FIGURE 17–10. Emergent cesarean birth.

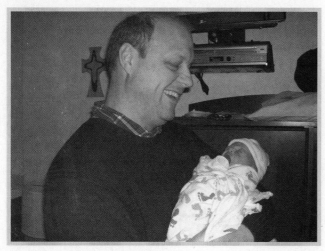

FIGURE 17–12. Support person in attendance to help mother care for baby after cesarean birth.

ANTEPARTUM BED REST AND POSTPARTUM RECOVERY

Approximately 20% of pregnant women will spend at least 1 week on bed rest (Dunn, Handley, & Carter, 2006). Bed rest has not been supported as an effective treatment for preterm labor or prolonging multifetal pregnancy and is not recommended by ACOG (2011). Despite lack of evidence to support bed rest therapy as contributing to positive outcomes, it has been prescribed routinely for women with high-risk pregnancies. Women with bleeding, preterm labor, and pregnancy-induced hypertension are frequently encouraged to maintain modified or strict bed rest in the hope of prolonging the pregnancy. Some research suggests that modified rest or some level of activity restriction at home, rather than strict bed rest, is an acceptable form of treatment for women with pregnancy-induced hypertension remote from term and women at risk for preterm labor and birth (ACOG, 2010, 2011).

Complete bed rest causes physiologic and psychosocial changes, including cardiovascular deconditioning; muscle loss, especially in the gastrocnemius muscle (used in ambulation); diuresis with fluid, electrolyte, and weight loss; bone demineralization; increased HR and blood coagulation; heartburn and reflux; constipation; glucose intolerance; and sensory disturbances, including depression, fatigue, and inability to concentrate (Maloni & Park, 2005). Isometric and isotonic conditioning exercises, Kegel exercises, pelvic tilts, and range-of-motion exercises can be used during hospitalization for the woman on bed rest. Deep breathing and coughing are added to exercise abdominal muscles and promote venous return.

After birth, the woman requires additional time, support, and education to prepare for safe and progressive levels of activity. Postpartum recovery may be prolonged. Ambulation after prolonged bed rest requires the continued presence of the perinatal nurse. Women should be alerted to the possibility of weakness, dizziness, shortness of breath, and muscle soreness and be reassured that these are normal physiologic consequences of prolonged bed rest that will reverse over time after resumption of normal activity (Dunn et al., 2006).

PRETERM BIRTH

After a long period of increase, the U.S. preterm birth rate (birth at less than 37 completed weeks of gestation) declined for the second year in 2008 to 12.3% from 12.8% in 2006, marking the first 2-year decline in the preterm birth rate in nearly three decades. The preterm birth rate has risen 20% since 1990 (Martin, Osterman, & Sutton, 2010). The low-birth-weight rate (babies weighing less than 2,500 g) decreased to 8.2% in 2007, down from 8.3% in 2006 (DHHS, 2009). Women who have experienced a preterm birth may have special needs related to a long period of antepartum bed rest and/or a cesarean birth as previously described. In addition, based on the gestational age and condition of the baby, they may be worried about their baby's survival. The day-to-day fluctuations in the baby's status can be emotionally draining for the woman and her family (Vargo & Trotter, 2006). Even if the preterm baby is healthy with no apparent life-threatening conditions, the woman and her family will likely be spending time visiting the baby in the NICU. Travel to and from the hospital and NICU observation can be physically exhausting. The mother is likely not to get adequate rest and nutrition for recovery. Nursing education prior to the mother's discharge should include an explanation of the importance of rest and proper diet to promote postpartum recovery. Some hospitals provide hospitality rooms for mothers and their families after discharge when the baby has to remain in the NICU. These accommodations can be helpful in avoiding maternal exhaustion and offer easy access to the baby. For a more in-depth review of nursing care for women who experience preterm birth and the implications for postpartum recovery, see Chapter 7.

MULTIPLE BIRTH

There has been a dramatic increase in the number of multiple births over the past two decades, mostly related to advances in assisted reproductive technologies and ovulation-inducing drugs (Russell, Petrini, Damus, Mattison, & Schwartz, 2003). Women of advanced age, especially those aged 30 to 34, 35 to 39, and 40 to 44 had the greatest increases (62%, 81%, and 110%, respectively) (Russell et al., 2003). Women who have a multiple birth have special needs during the postpartum period for multiple reasons. They may have experienced antepartum bed rest and/or a cesarean birth and are likely to have preterm babies admitted to the NICU. As compared to singleton births (10%), multiple birth babies are much more likely to be born preterm (twins: 57%, triplets: 93%, quadruplets: 99.9%) and are more likely to need NICU care (Keith & Oleszczuk, 2002). After the babies are discharged, mothers of multiples have additional responsibilities related to the condition and number of babies (Bowers & Gromada, 2006). Although there are often many offers of help for some families, as time goes on, the burden of ongoing care falls to the mother. A recent meta-analysis of qualitative research about mothers of multiples revealed five themes that can help increase understanding of what the mother experiences caring for multiples during the first year of life. These themes include "bearing the burden," "riding an emotional roller coaster," "lifesaving support," "striving for maternal justice," and "acknowledging individuality" (Beck, 2002). The mother's experiences are helpful for nurses when reviewing realistic expectations with patients with multiple births for postpartum recovery and newborn care. For a complete discussion of the nursing care of women with multiple births, see Chapter 11. Additional information can be found in the March of Dimes Nursing Module *Care of the Multiple-Birth Family: Pregnancy and Birth* (Bowers & Gromada, 2006).

PERINATAL LOSS

Not all pregnancies end in a healthy baby. Some women experience a pregnancy loss, stillbirth, or a neonatal death. Postpartum nursing care for these women can be a challenging and humbling experience. Nurses must examine their own thoughts, feelings, and assumptions about the death of a baby and the bereaved family. This self-examination covers preconceived ideas, judgments, and experiences of loss (Gemma & Arnold, 2002). To provide effective nursing care, the nurse must display an open and caring attitude expressed through appreciation and acceptance of validation of the experiences of the mother and her family (Gemma & Arnold, 2002). Sensitivity to the mother's wishes is critical. Some women who experience a perinatal loss may prefer a room on another unit away from the nursery and postpartum area. Other women prefer to be with nurses in labor and delivery or postpartum who are more comfortable with this type of loss. Ideally, the nursing unit is situated so these families do not have to come in contact with newborn infants. It is important to allow the woman and her family as much time as they need to be with their baby. The woman and her family's desires should guide postpartum nursing care. A comprehensive guide to caring for women who experience a perinatal loss is the March of Dimes Nursing Module *Loss and Grieving in Pregnancy and the First Year of Life: A Caring Resource for Nurses* (Gemma & Arnold, 2002).

POSTPARTUM LEARNING— NEEDS ASSESSMENT AND EDUCATION

Planning for education during the postpartum period begins as soon as possible after inpatient admission. Ideally, women have had opportunities during the prenatal period to learn about postpartum and baby care by attending classes and reading appropriate materials, but this may not be true for all pregnant women because of access to care issues, complications of pregnancy, unavailability of resources, language barriers, literacy issues, or lack of knowledge about existing programs. During the hospital stay, there are limited opportunities for assessment and education of new mothers. Access, availability, and acceptability must be considered when providing postpartum education. All available resources may not be able to be integrated within the hospital stay. Closed-circuit educational television and printed materials collaboratively developed by obstetric and pediatric professionals are helpful to new parents. Individual and group educational sessions held regularly during the postpartum period are beneficial. Baby care and normal infant behaviors and expected maternal physical and psychological changes should be included in the educational plans for each mother. New mothers should be aware of available community and healthcare resources (AAP & ACOG, 2008).

SELECTED POSTPARTUM TEACHING TOPICS

Pelvic Floor Exercises

Patient education should include pelvic muscle exercises according to the institutional protocol. Kegel exercises help the woman to regain muscle tone lost as pelvic tissues are stretched. Research suggests that few women who learn Kegel exercises perform them correctly and may increase their risk of later incontinence (Weber & Richter, 2005). Each contraction should be held at least 10 seconds, with a 10-second or longer rest between contractions for muscular recovery. Women with third- or fourth-degree lacerations, a long second stage of labor, a large newborn, or a combination of these factors should be taught to report potential anal sphincter symptoms, such as incontinence of flatus or stool, to the primary healthcare provider.

Postpartum Exercise

Exercise may begin soon after birth with simple exercises such as arm raises, leg rolls, and buttock lifts and proceed as the woman feels beneficial. Walking works well to get back to prepregnancy shape. After cesarean birth, abdominal exercises should be postponed for 4 weeks. Exercise benefits the mood, self-image, and energy level and improves or maintains muscular endurance, strength, and tone, but only if the exercise is stress relieving rather than stress provoking (ACOG, 2009). Women who exercise vigorously demonstrate better scores on measures of postpartum adaptation and are more likely to engage in social activities, hobbies, and entertainment. Research suggests that postpartum exercise has the capacity to improve aerobic fitness, high-density lipoprotein cholesterol level, insulin sensitivity, and psychological well-being, but no conclusive evidence was seen that postpartum exercise itself promotes greater body weight or body fat loss after childbirth (Larson-Meyer, 2002). Discharge instructions should include written information regarding activity, rest, and exercise for women who have given birth vaginally or by cesarean. Women should be instructed to listen to their bodies and avoid fatigue and pain.

Sexuality

Sexuality is one of the least understood and most superficially discussed topics by healthcare providers during a woman's postpartum experience. Sexuality encompasses physical capacity for sexual arousal and pleasure (i.e., libido), personalized and shared social meanings attached to sexual behavior, and formation of sexual and gender identities. Sexuality and gender attitudes and behaviors carry profound significance for women and men in every society. Sexuality is a vital component of physical and emotional well-being for men and women. Display 17–11 lists the factors contributing to decline in sexual interest during the postpartum period.

Nurses must assume responsibility for anticipatory guidance, reassurance, and counseling or referral. Research about dyspareunia (i.e., painful intercourse) suggests that some nontraditional forms of therapy,

DISPLAY 17–11

Factors Contributing to a Decline in Sexual Interest or Activity during the Postpartum Period

- Fatigue
- Fear of not hearing the infant
- Emotional distress on a continuum from baby blues to postpartum depression
- Adjustments to role change
- Hormonal changes
- Physical discomfort related to changes of vulva, vagina, perineum, and breasts
- Breastfeeding
- Decreased sense of attractiveness

such as acupuncture and ultrasound, may be helpful. Information about sexuality can be provided to the couple prenatally and after birth. Knowledge about normal physiologic and emotional changes allows the couple to discuss coping mechanisms and alternate means of maintaining intimacy during this challenging period. Education about sexuality during the postpartum period should include the following information:

- Sexual intercourse may be resumed approximately 3 to 4 weeks after the birth, although this should be individualized based on the woman's condition (i.e., a woman with a third- or fourth-degree laceration or other significant perineal trauma may not be comfortable resuming sexual intercourse until 6 to 8 weeks or more after birth).
- Sexual intercourse should be avoided until vaginal bleeding has stopped.
- A water-soluble gel may be necessary for additional lubrication.

Contraception

The infant feeding method and the involution process influence the woman's choice and use of postpartum contraception. Ideally, the primary healthcare provider has discussed the choice, use, advantages, and disadvantages of a variety of contraceptive methods with both partners during prenatal care. The nurse should encourage the woman to ask questions regarding contraception prior to discharge from the hospital. Although many couples wait 4 to 6 weeks after birth to resume sexual relations, some couples choose earlier resumption; thus, it is important to have this discussion while still in the hospital and to not wait until the first postpartum office or clinic visit. Consideration of the couple's needs and preferences is important when selecting a contraceptive method that is acceptable and effective for their unique situation. This approach allows sharing of responsibility, an opportunity to discuss advantages and disadvantages of methods, clarification of misconceptions, and discussion of prevention of sexually transmitted diseases (STDs). Information about contraception should include effectiveness, acceptability, and safety. Some of the available options for women and their partners are described in the following sections. This list is not all-inclusive. Although it is not the responsibility of the postpartum nurse to provide in-depth counseling to women regarding contraception, some basic knowledge is necessary if women have questions and if these types of discussions are not discouraged because of the institution's religious affiliation.

Depo-Provera

- Injections are given four times each year (150 mg given IM in the deltoid or gluteus maximus).
- The effectiveness rate is 99.7%.

- Advantages include long-lasting action, unimpaired lactation, and independence from coitus.
- Disadvantages include prolonged amenorrhea or uterine bleeding, weight gain, increased risk of venous thrombosis and thromboembolism, no STD protection, need for continued injections, fluid retention or edema, abdominal discomfort, and glucose intolerance.

Implanon

- The subdermal implant is inserted surgically and provides up to 3 years of contraception.
- The effectiveness rate is 99%.
- Advantages include long-lasting and reversible action.
- Disadvantages include menstrual irregularities, need for surgical removal, headaches, weight gain, breast pain, nervousness, nausea, skin changes, vertigo, no STD protection, and raised area on the arm.

Oral Contraceptives—Combined Estrogen–Progestin

- Dosage is one pill each day.
- The effectiveness rate is 96.8%.
- Advantages include coitus independent; decreased menstrual blood loss; decreased incidence of dysmenorrhea and premenstrual syndrome; reduction in endometrial adenocarcinoma, ovarian cancer, and benign breast disease; improvement in acne; protection against development of functional ovarian cysts; and decreased risk of ectopic pregnancy (Ladewig et al., 2009).
- Disadvantages include contraindications for women with a history of thromboembolic disorders; cerebrovascular or coronary artery disease; breast cancer; estrogen-dependent tumors; pregnancy; impaired liver function or tumors; hypertension; or diabetes of 20 years' duration; and for women who smoke (if older than 35 years), are lactating, or have had a period of immobilization (Ladewig et al., 2009). The drug can cause libido changes, breast tenderness, weight gain, nausea, and a delay in return of fertility.

Oral Contraceptives—Progestin Only

- Dosage is one pill each day.
- The effectiveness rate is 95%.
- In addition to the advantages of oral contraceptives listed previously, lactation is not impaired by this formulation, which is less likely to cause cardiovascular complications, headaches, or hypertension.
- In addition to the disadvantages of oral contraceptives listed previously, drug interactions are more likely, and irregular bleeding, amenorrhea, and functional ovarian cysts can occur. The pill must be taken at the same time each day.

Barrier Methods

- Device must be used at the time of sexual act.
- The effectiveness rate is 78% to 86%, depending on the device.

- Advantages include prevention of pregnancy, STDs, or both (used in combination with spermicides to achieve maximal protection); newer male condoms have various lengths, shapes, and adhesives.
- Tactylon, approved by the U.S. Food and Drug Administration (FDA) in 1991, is a hypoallergenic, synthetic polymer that is impervious to sperm and virus and is not degraded by oxidation or oil-based lubricants; it is used in male and female condoms.
- Reality vaginal pouch, approved by the FDA in 1992, is a female condom with two rings connected by a polyurethane sheath. The inner ring is fitted like a diaphragm; the outer ring protects the vulva and prevents slipping. It has a 15% failure rate.
- A diaphragm covers the cervix and requires fitting by healthcare professional. Its effectiveness is increased with the use of spermicide. It must be refitted after weight loss or gain greater than 22 kg and after birth. It has an 18% failure rate.
- A male condom is a latex or synthetic sheath placed over the erect penis before coitus. It must be applied before penile–vulvar contact and removed before the penis becomes flaccid to prevent sperm leakage at withdrawal. It has a 12% failure rate.

Chemical Methods (Spermicidal Creams, Jellies, Foams, Suppositories, and Vaginal Film Containing Nonoxynol-9)

- Agent must be used at the time of the sex act.
- The effectiveness rate is 50% to 95%.
- Advantages include ease of application, safety, low cost, no prescription required, and help in lubrication.
- Disadvantages include a maximum effect that lasts no longer than 1 hour, required reapplication for repeat intercourse, possibility of an allergic response or irritation, and messiness.

Intrauterine Devices (IUDs)

- No action is required at time of intercourse.
- Two types are approved for use in United States: Progestasert, which is T shaped with a progesterone reservoir in the stem and must be replaced yearly, and Copper T380, which is T shaped, wrapped with copper, and effective for 8 years.
- The effectiveness rate is 97% to 98%.
- Advantages include use for postpartum and breastfeeding women, long-term and continuous use requiring minimal effort, and no continual expense.
- Disadvantages include contraindications for women with a history of pelvic inflammatory disease or STDs; need for professional insertion; and generation of cramping, pain, and bleeding, which should be evaluated.

Postpartum Tubal Ligation/Vasectomy (Sterilization)

- It requires no additional effort after surgical procedure.

- The effectiveness rate is 99.5% (female) to 99.9% (male).
- Advantages include no need for additional contraception (should be considered permanent although reversal is technically possible).
- Its disadvantage is no STD protection.
- Before surgery, appropriate counseling is necessary regarding risks of failure, surgical risks, and potential psychosocial reactions to the procedure. A signed consent form according to institutional protocol is required.

Natural Family Planning

- It relies on fertility awareness, observations, and abstinence during the fertile portion of a woman's menstrual cycle.
- It requires an understanding of the changes occurring in a woman's ovulatory cycle.
- The fertile period is calculated with a set formula, basal body temperature, cervical mucus assessment, symptothermal techniques (i.e., combines body temperature and cervical mucus assessment), or over-the-counter ovulation test kit (e.g., Creighton Model, Billings Method, Sympto-Thermal).
- Advantages include a couple-centered method, low cost, lack of harm to fertility, no side effects, usefulness in diagnosing gynecologic disorders and infertility, and use in achieving pregnancy when desired.
- Disadvantages include no STD protection, difficult application during irregular cycles postpartum, need to begin charting 3 weeks after birth, and ovulation possibly occurring before the first postpartum menses (Ladewig et al., 2009).

PSYCHOLOGICAL ADAPTATION TO THE POSTPARTUM PERIOD

POSTPARTUM MOOD AND ANXIETY DISORDERS

Postpartum mood disorders have finally been given the attention they deserve by healthcare providers, unfortunately because of high profile cases of both maternal and child deaths. In 2001, a woman in Chicago committed suicide by drowning in Lake Michigan after weeks of bed rest to prolong her pregnancy and after giving birth to quadruplets (while they were still in the NICU). In another 2001 case, a woman in Texas drowned her five children several months after giving birth to a much wanted daughter after four sons. Numerous women suffering from postpartum psychosis, a severe and progressive form of postpartum depression, have killed themselves and/or their children before they were able to get the medical help they desperately needed. Prominent women, such as Marie

Osmond and Brooke Shields, have admitted suffering from postpartum depression and written of their experience with the disorder. Some of the attention is helpful to women who have suffered in the past and are currently struggling with postpartum depression. These women know they are not alone and that the feelings they are experiencing have been experienced by other new mothers who were successfully treated. Women with postpartum depression report feeling very alone and helpless. Although family members notice abnormal changes in the woman's mood and behavior, they frequently underestimate the extent of the illness. Women are told by well-meaning others that they just have the "baby blues" and they should snap out of it and take care of their beautiful baby. Women suffering from postpartum depression wish it could be that easy. Prompt diagnosis and treatment is needed for postpartum depression. Nurses can be helpful in identifying women who could benefit from referral and treatment.

During the postpartum hospital stay, the new mother has to move quickly from self-concern to other concern: her baby. It is important that her physical and psychological needs be met so that she will be better able to focus on her newborn's care. She may become intensely focused on the cognitive learning needs related to newborn feeding and physical care. The new mother may verbalize anxiety and concern. If so, she needs to be heard, and her concerns must be validated. The newly evolving relationship between the mother and her newborn is based on connection and care. If the woman has difficulty with these beginning skills, it may alter her self-esteem and maternal development. Postpartum depression can negatively affect the mother–infant interaction during the first 12 months after birth (Beck, 2008; McCoy, 2011). The nurse can assist the mother in this attachment process by establishing a responsive, nurturing environment; maximizing mother–infant contact; and assisting the mother to understand the newborn's behaviors (Karl, Beal, O'Hare, & Rissmiller, 2006). The woman brings with her many performance expectations that need to be discussed and clarified. Mercer (1986) described maternal role attainment as a process that takes a period of about 10 months to develop. During this postpartum phase, the new mother attaches to her newborn, gains competence as a mother, and should express gratification in the mother–baby interaction. This adaptation can be delayed or altered if the woman's health and mental status are less than optimal. The reality of the current healthcare delivery system is that much of the work of the postpartum maternal adjustment and role attainment is done after discharge. Thus, referral to community resources and discharge planning are imperative in the total care plan.

Emotionally, the early days after giving birth can be disconcerting. It is supposed to be such an exciting time; but in reality, the new mother may be experiencing alternating periods of crying and joy, irritability, anxiety, headaches, confusion, forgetfulness, depersonalization, and fatigue. These are characteristics of the "baby blues." It has been estimated that up to 50% of new mothers experience this transitory mood disorder (Miller, 2002). Unfortunately, this phenomenon occurs so frequently that it is often considered normal and therefore does not get the attention that it deserves. The causes of postpartum depression may be biologic, psychological, situational, or multifactorial (Beck, 2002; Beck & Indman, 2005). It is felt that this disorder is related to the normal physiologic and psychosocial changes that occur in the process of becoming a new mother. The rapid decrease in the levels of female reproductive hormones after birth may dysregulate the complex balance of neurotransmitters, stress hormones, and reproductive hormones (Driscoll, 2006). Having the "baby blues" can greatly affect the new mother and her family, especially if they are unaware of the possibility or what to do about it.

Women and their families need information about normal mood changes after childbirth. They should be aware that with a lot of support, reassurance, rest, and good nutrition, these labile moods usually balance out, and the woman will begin to feel better and feel more organized and confident. However, if the moods do not stabilize, referral should be made to the psychiatric/mental health team specialists in postpartum mood and anxiety disorders (Driscoll, 2008). Inpatient perinatal nurses interact with women during the first days after birth and are in the position to make initial assessments of mother–baby interactions and mood alterations. An important aspect of this nursing assessment is determining when the mother's behaviors are beyond normal "baby blues" and are pathologic, such as during postpartum depression (Beck, 2006). This is challenging, because alterations in mood are common during the immediate hours after labor and birth. An awareness of the risk factors for postpartum depression facilitates prompt diagnosis, treatment, and early recovery (Display 17–12). Because most postpartum LOSs are 1 to 4 days, there is a greater likelihood of mood disorders occurring at home rather than in the hospital environment. If a follow-up appointment with a healthcare provider occurs at 4 to 6 weeks after birth, then the woman experiences these conditions alone, without medical or nursing support. Thus, women and their families need anticipatory information about postpartum mood disorders so that prompt identification and early treatment can be initiated. A heightened awareness among perinatal healthcare providers about the incidence of postpartum mood and anxiety disorders, knowledge of common signs and symptoms, and the prospects for recovery can contribute to successful outcomes for affected women and their families.

DISPLAY 17–12

Risk Factors for Postpartum Depression

- Prenatal depression
- Low self-esteem
- Stress of child care
- Prenatal anxiety
- Life stress
- Lack of social support
- Marital relationship problems
- History of depression
- "Difficult" infant temperament
- Postpartum blues
- Single status
- Low socioeconomic status
- Unplanned or unwanted pregnancy
- Young maternal age

Adapted from Beck, C. (2001). Predictors of postpartum depression: An update. *Nursing Research, 50*(5), 275–282; Beck, C. (2002). Revision of the Postpartum Depression Predictors Inventory. *Journal of Obstetric, Gynecologic, and Neonatal Nursing, 31*(4), 394–402. doi:10.1111/j.1552-6909.2002.tb00061.x; McCoy, S. J. B. (2011). Postpartum depression: An essential overview for the practitioner. *Southern Medical Journal, 104*(2), 128–132. doi:10.1097/SMJ.0b013e318200c221

Each woman should be routinely assessed for maternal mental status and adjustment and mood disorders as a standard part of postpartum clinical nursing assessments (Driscoll, 2006, 2008; Logsdon, Wisner, & Pinto-Foltz, 2006). This assessment is facilitated by a professional nurse who is willing to listen to the woman's birth experience, observant of mother–baby interactions, and knowledgeable about the normal physiologic adaptations that are similar to symptoms of depression such appetite fluctuations, fatigue, and decreased libido. Prior to discharge from the hospital, the woman should be given a list of telephone numbers of her care providers as well as any emergency services that she may need. It is important to go over the key support people with the new mother and her partner during discharge teaching. When home visits by skilled perinatal nurses are available, the nurse should include a thorough assessment of the psychological adaptation of the new mother.

Psychiatric professionals have several instruments available for assessing women for postpartum depression (Display 17–13). These assessments require careful planning and knowledge about the instruments themselves and appropriate referral options. If perinatal care providers are knowledgeable about the woman's psychological well-being, appropriate referral and early identification of these disorders can be made, thus potentially preventing a crisis. Preparation for appropriate assessments and interventions can result from interdisciplinary efforts involving physicians,

DISPLAY   17 – 13

Instruments Developed by Nurse Researchers for Assessing Postpartum Depression, Mood Disorders, and Psychosis

- Edinburgh Postnatal Depression Scale (EPDS) (Cox, Holden, & Sagovsky, 1987)
- Postpartum Depression Predictors Inventory-Revised (PDPI-R) (Beck, 2001, 2002)
- Postpartum Depression Checklist (PDC) (Beck, 1995, 2001, 2002; Beck, Records, & Rice, 2006)
- Brisbane Postnatal Depression Index (Webster, Pritchard, Creedy, & East, 2003)
- Schedule for Affective Disorders And Schizophrenia (SADS) (Beck & Gable, 2005)
- Postpartum Depression Screening Scale (PDSS) (Beck & Gable, 2005)

nurse practitioners, nurse midwives, nurses, perinatal educators, lactation consultants, and support services such as social services and counselors. Educational programs sponsored by experts in postpartum mood disorders can be helpful to increase awareness and lead to appropriate, timely referral. Educational programs should also be offered within the community to increase public awareness and knowledge of available resources.

Validating the woman's experience as normal may provide needed reassurance. Talking with the woman in a familiar, comfortable environment about the stresses and challenges of new motherhood provides opportunities for early interventions, such as counseling, referrals to support services, and pharmacologic assistance. Help with infant and self-care, coupled with support from family members, promotes recovery. Providing appropriate interventions and therapy has far-reaching effects—improving the health of the women, their infants, and the family itself. These interventions become an investment in the future.

Psychosocial adaptation to pregnancy and postpartum is a dynamic process. The nurse plays a significant role in the promotion and facilitation of this experience in a healthy way. It is a time when the woman is open to great psychological growth and relies on the healthcare team for information and support. The nurse needs to be aware of the normal process in order to identify those that are abnormal. It is helpful in the assessment of mood, anxiety, and emotional states to remember three words: *frequency, duration,* and *intensity.* If the woman describes that she is having difficulty functioning in her activities of daily living and having a tough time coping due to emotional, mood, and/or anxiety changes, referral is necessary. The referral process needs to be managed in an empowering, supportive way. Letting her know that she is valued and her concerns and feelings are important is a way for the perinatal nurse to give the woman the message that she deserves good care. Appropriate healthcare provider attitudes support the referral process. Due to the rapid changes in the healthcare delivery system and decreasing LOSs, it is imperative for the perinatal nurse to actively pursue, nurture, and promote collaborative relationships with colleagues in the community. It is this active communication and relational approach to the care of this new mother and her family that will promote, facilitate, and encourage healthy maternal and paternal psychosocial adaptation and adjustment.

FATIGUE

The first 6 weeks after giving birth are a time of change and adjustment for the woman and the family. Fatigue, stress, depression, and infection are interrelated in postpartum mothers. These variables change over time, possibly placing mothers and infants in a psycho-neuroimmunologically vulnerable group (Groer et al., 2005). The variables reinforce one another and make it difficult to determine which occurs first—fatigue causing depression and stress or the reverse. Their alteration of immune function in new mothers may result in increased vulnerability to infection. In the breastfeeding woman, fatigue is associated with increased levels of melatonin in the mother's milk, which is transferred to the infant and influences the sleep/wake cycle. Fatigue affects emotional adjustment and adaptation to the maternal role, and it may cause feelings of inadequacy in meeting the needs of other family members and in assuming household responsibilities. Anticipatory guidance in identifying rest opportunities and organizing new responsibilities and tasks are important for the new mother. Education about the causes of fatigue and possible community and family resources enables the new mother to assume control and promotes problem-solving behaviors. Together, the nurse and the woman can develop strategies for requesting help with newborn care, household chores, and sibling care. Listing daily and weekly tasks provides an organizational framework and may serve as a readily available wish list that can be used when family and friends offer to help. Identification of family members and friends available to help provides an initial supportive structure for the new family.

FAMILY TRANSITION TO PARENTHOOD

After birth, the woman experiences psychological changes as well as physiologic reversal of the physical changes of pregnancy. For the woman, adoption of a maternal role begins during pregnancy as she develops an attachment to the fetus. This role evolution continues postpartum with the birth separation of the mother–infant pair, or polarization (Rubin, 1977). As the mother develops her style of parenting, she considers her behavior in relation to the infant and notices familial characteristics in the infant. These changes in the mother are referred to as maternal role attainment (Mercer, 1995). Mercer identified four stages in this process: anticipatory, formal, informal, and personal. The anticipatory stage, occurring during pregnancy, involves the observation of role models for mothering behaviors. During the formal stage, the new mother tries to perform infant care tasks as expected by others. The mother begins to make personal choices about mothering during the informal stage and attains comfort with the role during the personal stage. The final stages, informal and formal, correspond to the taking-in and taking-hold stages identified by Rubin (1961a). During the taking-in phase (first 24 hours or longer), the woman relives the birth experience, clarifies her understanding of the experience, and focuses on food and sleep. The taking-hold phase (second to fourth day) centers on concern with bodily functions, and the woman focuses on regaining control over her life and succeeding in infant-care responsibilities. Rubin (1961b) includes the letting-go phase to describe the new mother's letting go of who she was and full participation in the mothering role. Nurses can foster success in these processes by meeting the woman's needs during each stage and providing a supportive environment for listening and educating the new mother.

Paternal satisfaction with the birth experience and its associated stresses influences marital happiness and family life. For most women, being comfortable as a mother occurs during the first 3 to 10 months after birth. Nursing assessments about the quality of parenting behaviors during the postpartum period can guide the educational plan for the new couple. Display 17–14 lists adaptive and maladaptive parenting behaviors. Evidence of maladaptive parenting behaviors should prompt nursing communication with the primary healthcare provider and appropriate referral.

Nurses caring for women and families during the postpartum period must consider their cultural expectations and norms when planning care. This requires an open-minded, sensitive, and creative approach. Knowledge about various traditions and services within ethnic groups and a willingness to give up control demonstrate respect and encourage a collaborative approach to providing these women with a positive and satisfying birth experience. We must accept that maternity care system has a culture that may class with the cultures of our clients (Lewallen, 2011).

The changes that occur within the family are not limited to the woman. The family, however it is defined, experiences changes in structure and process. Parents adapt to these changes more easily when they are involved with a support network. This network may include family, friends, and institutional components. New parents often report a change in their immediate social network. This change typically involves increased contact with other new parents or with families facing similar challenges. For new parents living without immediate access to family, referral to support groups sponsored by hospitals or community centers may provide an opening into a circle of new parents and friends. New parents may place increased importance on family and the traditions they include. For other couples, increased familial contacts may result in an increased level of stress as the new family attempts to meet the external demands placed on them by enthusiastic or demanding family members. If the new mother decides not to return to a work environment outside the home, she may face the challenge of redefining herself. Individuals respond differently to life changes; other areas that may prove stressful to certain individuals include physical changes and complications, role-adaptation conflicts, newborn needs, relationship changes, returning to the work, and/or selecting a child care setting.

Nurses caring for families during this time can provide anticipatory guidance about possible areas of stress and options for stress reduction. Providing this information in a written format enables the couple to review the information as situations develop.

POSTPARTUM DISCHARGE FOLLOW-UP

In response to the current LOS, many perinatal centers now offer postdischarge follow-up home visits, clinic visits, or telephone calls. The AAP *Committee on the Fetus and Newborn* (2010) recommends in-person follow-up by an experienced healthcare professional occur within 48 hours of discharge following a maternity stay of 48 hours or less. The optimal time for assessing mothers and their infants is between 3 and 4 days after birth when infections, poor infant feeding, excessive weight loss, jaundice, and other problems become evident (Brown, 2006; Roudebush et al., 2006).

In-person follow-up visits afford the perinatal nurse an opportunity to carefully assess maternal and infant well-being and provide the family with continuing education and support (Brown, 2006). In some institutions, the primary staff nurse may see the family for their follow-up visit. The family may return to the hospital and be seen in a room set aside for outpatient follow-up visits, or the primary nurse may make a follow-up visit at the family's home. In other institutions, the volume of visits is large enough to require a separate nursing staff for follow-up visits (Brown, 2006; Ladewig et al., 2009; Roudebush et al., 2006).

DISPLAY 17-14

Adaptive and Maladaptive Parenting Behaviors

	ADAPTIVE	MALADAPTIVE
Feeding	Provides an appropriate amount and type of food	Makes inappropriate types or inadequate amounts of food available
	Burps the child both during and after feeding	Does not burp the baby, although she or he knows it is necessary to do so
	Prepares the meal appropriately	Prepares the meal inappropriately
	Feeds the infant regularly and as frequently as necessary	Rushes or delays feeding the child
Rest	Provides a quiet and relaxed environment for the resting baby	Does not provide a quiet and relaxed environment
	Schedules rest periods	Does not schedule rest periods
Stimulating caring for infant	Speaks to the child and makes other appropriate sounds	Speaks aggressively or not at all to the infant
	Provides tactile stimulation at a variety of times and not only when the baby is hungry or in danger	Plays aggressively with the baby or does not touch her or him
	Provides age-appropriate toys	Provides inappropriate toys
	Positions infant comfortably while holding the child	Does not hold the baby or ignores child's discomfort when being held
	The baby seems satisfied with the way it is being handled	The baby seems frustrated with the way it is handled
	Sees that the baby is dry, warm, and not hungry	Does not care for the baby who is hungry, cold, or soiled
	Exhibits initiative in trying to find how to deal with the baby's problems	Lacks initiative and does not try to meet the baby's needs
Self-perception/emotional state of parent	Usually maintains a realistic perception of and realistic expectations for the baby	Develops distorted perceptions of and unrealistic expectations for the baby
	Exhibits a realistic perception of her or his own mothering and fathering abilities	Holds unrealistic expectations of her or his own parenting abilities
	Shows some interest in understanding and/or discussing the childbirth	Is unable or unwilling to discuss the childbirth
	Exhibits friendly or neutral behavior with other children	Exhibits hostility/aggression toward other children
	Appears generally satisfied to be a parent	Appears dissatisfied to be a parent
	Is able or willing to turn to other people for social support when necessary	Is unable to provide adequately for relaxation and own emotional needs
		Is isolated and without adequate social support
		Is depressed

Medical complications identified during the visit are immediately referred to the primary healthcare provider. Other issues or concerns are addressed during the visit or referred to an appropriate resource. This assessment visit can take place in a home or clinical setting as long as the nurse examining the infant is competent in newborn assessment and the results of the follow-up visit are reported to the infant's physician or his or her designees on the day of the visit. The visit should include:

- Infant weight, general health, hydration, and degree of jaundice (if present)
- Identification of any new problems

- Review of feeding patterns and technique, including observation of breastfeeding for adequacy of position, latch on, and swallowing
- Historical evidence of adequate urination and stool patterns
- Assess quality of mother–infant interaction and infant behavior
- Reinforce maternal or family education in infant care, particularly regarding infant feeding
- Review of outstanding results of laboratory tests performed before discharge
- Performance of screening tests in accordance with state regulations and other tests that are clinically indicated, such as serum bilirubin

DISPLAY 17–15

Postpartum Follow-Up Telephone Call

Mother: Age _____ G/P_____   Vag Birth _____ C/Birth _____
Marital status: S   M   W   Discharge date: _____
Baby: Sex: M   F   Gestational age: _____
Newborn birth weight _____   Discharge weight: _____
Breast _____ Formula _____   Person making call: _____

BABY CARE	NO CONCERNS	PROBLEM IDENTIFIED	SUGGESTION MADE
Circumcision assessment			
Cord assessment			
Jaundice			
Changes in newborn:			
Behavior			
Feeding			
Temperature			
Breastfeeding:			
# wet diapers			
# & character of stools			
Latch-on/positioning			
Frequency of feeding/24 hours			
Breast & nipple assessment:			
Sore nipples			
Cracked nipples			
Breast fullness			
Suck/swallow assessment			
Other concerns			
Formula Feeding:			
# wet diapers			
# & characteristics of stools			
Ounces/feedings			
Frequency of feedings			
Skin appearance			
Sleep patterns			
Ability to care for newborn			
MATERNAL CARE	NO CONCERNS	PROBLEM IDENTIFIED	SUGGESTION MADE
Lochia			
Episiotomy			
Incision			
Discomforts:			
Breast			
Perineal			
Incisional			

Cramping			
Calf/leg tenderness			
Hemorrhoids			
Voiding:			
Frequency			
Dysuria			
Bowel movement			
Emotional:			
Weepy			
Fatigue			
Sadness			
Onset of feelings			
Adequate rest:			
Taking naps			
Sleeps well when baby sleeps			
Other			
Ability to care for self			
REFERRALS	**DATE**	**PROBLEM IDENTIFIED**	**SUGGESTION MADE**
Lactation Consultant			
Social Services			
Physician			
Clinical Specialist			
Home Health Care			
WIC			
Other			

- Verification of the plan for healthcare maintenance, including a method for obtaining emergency services, preventive care and immunizations, periodic evaluations and physical examinations, and necessary screenings (AAP, 2010)

When in-person follow-up visits are not offered, a postdischarge phone call gives families another opportunity to ask questions and receive important information and referrals. The perinatal nurse can use a standardized assessment tool to ask the family about infant feeding and elimination patterns, cord care, infant appearance and behavior, maternal comfort, lochia flow, perineal care, breast care, and maternal emotional well-being (Display 17–15). The nurse should ask the mother if she has any concerns about herself or her infant and reminds the mother about specific situations that would warrant a telephone call to the healthcare provider. The nurse should refer the mother to the written materials provided by the institution for further information.

Ideally, all women should receive a postdischarge visit or telephone call. If resources are limited, the following criteria define circumstances where postdischarge follow-up is essential:

- LOS less than 24 hours after a vaginal birth
- LOS less than 48 hours after a cesarean birth
- Limited or no prenatal care
- Infant feeding problems identified during hospital stay
- Infant gestational age less than 37 completed weeks
- Multiple birth
- Risk factors for developing hyperbilirubinemia
- Maternal or infant health conditions putting mother or infant at risk for complications
- Lack of adequate support system
- Women who express or show they feel overwhelmed, very anxious, or depressed
- Discharge evaluation indicates need for further teaching

The nurse providing postdischarge follow-up should have access to essential patient information including maternal age, health history, birth information, newborn assessment, infant weight, method of infant feeding, and name of the infant's and mother's healthcare providers. The nurse's assessment is documented and maintained as part of the permanent medical record.

EVALUATION OF POSTPARTUM SERVICES

An essential first step in program evaluation is the identification of goals and expected outcomes. Primary outcome criteria include family knowledge about maternal–newborn care, ability to identify support persons and community resources, and familiarity with signs and symptoms of complications that warrant a call to the primary healthcare provider. Criteria met both at discharge and in the immediate postpartum period should be included in the evaluation process. Both quantitative and qualitative approaches to data collection are useful.

It is important that nursing care as well as patient use of services following discharge are tracked to ensure that resources are available that are beneficial for new families. Quantitative evaluation may be a concurrent or retrospective review of medical record data, tracking readmissions, and/or keeping a log of parent phone calls to the nursery or maternity unit. Variance data provide information about maternal–newborn teaching and care completed within suggested time frames during the inpatient stay. Primary healthcare providers can participate in data collection by tracking phone calls, commonly asked questions, and nonroutine office visits. Data collected from postdischarge follow-up assessment tools can be used to identify topics of maternal and newborn care that suggest perinatal education was effective and to identify areas for improvement. In addition, results of individual follow-up contacts can be compared with learning needs assessments completed prior to discharge. If data analyses suggest specific topics should be covered in more depth in the inpatient setting, nurses can make appropriate revisions in patient teaching strategies.

Qualitative methods of evaluation such as patient interviews, focus groups, written surveys, letters, or phone calls from parents who have used programs and services are additional valuable sources of data. Women and their families frequently identify important issues not addressed on surveys or evaluation tools. Tracking data trends and adjusting discharge plans accordingly lead to improvements in the system. For example, if analysis of the parents' phone call log indicates many calls about a particular issue such as umbilical cord care, parent teaching plans can be redesigned to include comprehensive coverage of that topic. Childbearing family surveys may suggest a need to offer more flexibility in class schedules. Prenatal class evaluations provide information about class content and teaching methods that parents find useful. Prenatal classes can be revised based on consistent themes in participant feedback.

An additional benefit of soliciting patient feedback about services provided is the ability to share with perinatal educators and staff nurses' positive remarks about their individual contributions. Often, women will take time to write lengthy comments about their prenatal educator and the nurses who cared for them during the inpatient stay or at the outpatient home or clinic visit. Although perinatal nurses many times feel rushed to accomplish all there is to do in the limited time available, it is gratifying to know we can still make a positive difference. Conversely, a complaint or criticism offered by the mother or her family about a staff member, the education program, or the hospital stay is always valuable. Complaints can increase the nurse's understanding of how the family perceived their interactions with the nurse and the care provided. With this insight, the nurse has the opportunity to make improvements in clinical or interpersonal skills. Complaints also provide the institution with an opportunity to change or revise existing programs to meet consumer expectations. A well-designed postpartum discharge-planning program can be cost effective if unnecessary calls and return visits to the healthcare provider or institution are decreased, and readmissions to the hospital are decreased or stabilized. As healthcare dollars become scarcer, increased sophistication in linking positive outcomes (both clinical and financial) to perinatal education and discharge planning programs will be critical.

SUMMARY

The postpartum period is a time of transition and change for the new mother and her family. Physiologic and psychological changes occur immediately and over time, necessitating careful planning to meet the needs of the new family. Timely, frequent assessments and appropriate interventions require clinical skills and adequate knowledge about these processes. Supportive care that includes education for the woman and her family about what to expect in the first few weeks facilitates the transition from the inpatient setting to home. Being present during this period is a responsibility and a privilege that can affect society as a whole, one family at a time.

REFERENCES

American Academy of Pediatrics. (2010). Hospital stay for healthy term newborns. *Pediatrics, 125*(2), 405–409. doi:10.1542 /peds.2009-3119

American Academy of Pediatrics & American College of Obstetricians and Gynecologists. (2008). *Guidelines for Perinatal Care* (6th ed.). Elk Grove Village, IL: Author.

American College of Obstetricians and Gynecologists. (2008a). *Episiotomy* (Practice Bulletin No. 71). Washington, DC: Author.

American College of Obstetricians and Gynecologists. (2008b). *Postpartum Hemorrhage* (Practice Bulletin No. 76). Washington, DC: Author.

American College of Obstetricians and Gynecologists. (2009). *Exercise During Pregnancy and the Postpartum Period* (Committee Opinion No. 267). Washington, DC: Author.

American College of Obstetricians and Gynecologists. (2010). *Diagnosis and Management of Preeclampsia and Eclampsia* (Practice Bulletin No. 33). Washington, DC: Author.

American College of Obstetricians and Gynecologists. (2011). *Management of Preterm Labor* (Practice Bulletin No. 43). Washington, DC: Author.

American Society of Anesthesiologists. (2007). *Practice Guidelines for Obstetrical Anesthesia: An Updated Report by the American Society of Anesthesiologists Task Force on Obstetrical Anesthesia*. Park Ridge, IL: Author.

Association of Women's Health, Obstetric and Neonatal Nurses. (2009). *Standards and Guidelines for Professional Nursing Practice in the Care of Women and Newborns* (7th ed.). Washington, DC: Author.

Association of Women's Health, Obstetric and Neonatal Nurses & Johnson & Johnson Consumer Products. (2006). *Compendium of Postpartum Care* (2nd ed.). Washington, DC: Author.

Beck, C. T. (2001). Predictors of postpartum depression: An update. *Nursing Research, 50*(5), 275–282.

Beck, C. T. (2002). Revision of the Postpartum Depression Predictors Inventory. *Journal of Obstetric, Gynecologic, and Neonatal Nursing, 31*(4), 394–402. doi:10.1111/j.15526909.2002 .tb00061.x

Beck, C. T. (2006). Postpartum depression: It isn't just the blues. *American Journal of Nursing, 106*(5), 40–50.

Beck, C. T. (2008). State of the science on postpartum depression. *MCN: American Journal of Maternal Child Nursing, 33*(3), 151–156. doi:10.1097/01.NMC.0000318349.70364.1c

Beck, C. T., & Gable, R. K. (2005). *Postpartum Depression Screening Scale Manual*. Los Angeles: Western Psychological Services.

Beck, C. T., & Indman, P. (2005). The many faces of postpartum depression. *Journal of Obstetric, Gynecologic, and Neonatal Nursing, 34*(5), 569–576. doi:10.1177/0884217505279995

Beck, C. T., Records, K., & Rice, M. (2006). Further development of the Postpartum Depression Predictors Inventory revised. *Journal of Obstetrics, Gynecologic, and Neonatal Nursing, 35*(6), 735–745. doi:10.1111/j.1552-6909.2006.00094.x

Beckmann, M. M., & Garrett, A. J. (2006). Antenatal perineal massage for reducing perineal trauma. *Cochrane Database of Systematic Reviews, 1*, CD005123.

Beers, M. H., & Berkow, R. (Eds.). (2006). Venous thrombosis. *The Merck manual of diagnosis and therapy* (18th ed.) Retrieved from http://www.merck.com/mrkshared/mmanual/section16 /chapter212/212g.jsp

Blackburn, S. T. (2012). *Maternal, Fetal, & Neonatal Physiology: A Clinical Perspective* (4th ed.). Philadelphia: Saunders.

Bouwmeester, F. W., Jonhoff, A. R., Verheijen, R. H., & van Geijn, H. P. (2003). Successful treatment of life-threatening postpartum hemorrhage with recombinant activated factor VII. *Obstetrics and Gynecology, 101*(6), 1174–1176.

Bowers, N., & Gromada, K. K. (2006). *Care of the Multiple-Birth Family: Pregnancy and Birth* (Nursing Module). White Plains, NY: The March of Dimes Birth Defects Foundation.

Boyles, S. H., Li, H., Mori, T., Osterweil, P., & Guise, J. M. (2009). Effect of mode of delivery on the incidence of urinary incontinence in primiparous women. *Obstetrics and Gynecology, 113*(1), 134–141. doi:10.1097/AOG.0b013e318191bb37

Brown, S. E. (2006). Tender beginnings program: An educational continuum for the maternity patient. *Journal of Perinatal and Neonatal Nursing, 20*(3), 210–219.

Casey, B. M., Schaffer, J. I., Bloom, S. K., Heartwel, S. F., McIntire, D. D., & Leveno, K. J. (2005). Obstetric antecedents for postpartum pelvic floor dysfunction. *American Journal of Obstetrics and Gynecology, 192*(5), 1655–1662. doi:10.1016/j .ajog.2004.11.031

Chaliha, C. (2009). Postpartum pelvic floor trauma. *Current Opinion in Obstetrics and Gynezcology, 21,* 474–479.

Christianson, L. M., Bovbjerg, V. E., McDavitt, E. C., & Hullfish, K. L. (2003). Risk factors for perineal injury during delivery. *American Journal of Obstetrics and Gynecology, 189*(1), 255–260. doi:10.1067/mob.2003.547

Cox, J.L., Holden, J.M., and Sagovsky, R. (1987). Detection of postnatal depression. Development of the 10-item Edinburgh Postnatal Depression Scale. *British Journal of Psychiatry, 150*: 782-786.

Cunningham, F. G., Leveno, K. J., Bloom, S. K., Hauth, J. C., Rouse, D. J., & Spong, C. Y. (Eds.). (2009). The puerperium. In *Williams Obstetrics* (23rd ed., pp. 646–704). New York: McGraw-Hill.

Datar, A., & Sood, N. (2006). Impact of postpartum hospital stay legislation on newborn length of stay, readmission and mortality in California. *Pediatrics, 118*(1), 63–72. doi:10.1542/peds.2005 -3044

Driscoll, J. W. (2006). Postpartum depression: The state of the science. *Journal of Perinatal and Neonatal Nursing, 20*(1), 40–42.

Driscoll, J. W. (2008). Postpartum depression: How nurses can identify and care for women grappling with this disorder. *AWHONN Lifelines, 10*(5), 401–409.

Duff, W. P., Sweet, R. L., & Edwards, R. K. (2009). Maternal and fetal infections. In R. K. Creasy, R. Resnick, J. D. Iams, C. J. Lockwood, & T. R. Moore (Eds.), *Maternal-Fetal Medicine: Principles and Practice* (6th ed., pp. 739–796). Philadelphia: Saunders.

Dunn, L. L., Handley, M. C., & Carter, M. R. (2006). Antepartal bedrest: Conflicts, costs, controversies and ethical considerations. *Online Journal of Health Ethics, 3*(1). Retrieved from http://www.ojhe.org/index.php/ojhe/article/viewArticle/49/56

Garcia, V., Rogers, R. G., Kim, S. S., Hall, R. J., & Kammerer-Doak D. N. (2005). Primary repair of obstetric and anal sphincter laceration: A randomized trial of two surgical techniques. *American Journal of Obstetrics and Gynecology, 192*(5), 1697–1701. doi:10.1016/j.ajog.2004.11.045

Gemma, P. B., & Arnold, J. (2002). *Loss and Grieving in Pregnancy and the First Year of Life: A Caring Resource for Nurses* (Nursing Module). White Plains, NY: The March of Dimes Birth Defects Foundation.

Gilbert, E. S. (2011). *Manual of High Risk Pregnancy & Delivery* (5th ed.). St. Louis, MO: Mosby.

Giraldo-Isaza, M. S., Jaspan, D., & Cohen, A. W. (2011). Postpartum endometritis caused by herpes and cytomegaloviruses. *Obstetrics and Gynecology, 117*(2), 466–467. doi:10.1097 /AOG.0b013e3181f73805

Groer, M., Davis, M., Casey, K., Short, B., Smith, K., & Groer, S. (2005). Neuroendocrine & immune relationships in postpartum fatigue. *MCN: The American Journal of Maternal/Child Nursing, 30*(2), 133–138.

Hamilton, B. E., Martin, J. A., & Ventura, S. J. (2010). Births: Preliminary data for 2005. *National Center for Health Statistics.* Retrieved from http://www.cdc.gov.nchs/products/pubs/pubd/hestats/prelimbirths05/prelimbirths05.html

Hedayati, H., Parsons, J., & Crowther, C. A. (2005). Topically applied anaesthetics for treating perineal pain after childbirth. *Cochrane Database of Systematic Reviews, 18*(2), CD004223.

Jacob, A. G. (2012). Overview of postpartum hemorrhage. Diaphragmatic pacing. In C. J. Lockwood (Ed.), UpToDate. Retrieved from http://www.uptodateonline.com.

Jacob, T. (2006). *Smell.* Retrieved from http://www.cf.ac.uk/biosi/staff/jacob/teaching/sensory/olfact1.html

Jackson, E., Curtis, K. M., & Gaffield, M. E. (2011). Risk of venous thromboembolism during the postpartum period: A systematic review. *Obstetrics and Gynecology, 117*(3), 691–703.

Jastrow, N., Roberge, S., Gauthier, R. J., Laroche, L., Duperron, L., Brassard, N., & Bujold, E. (2010). Effect of birth weight on adverse obstetric outcomes in vaginal birth after cesarean delivery. *Obstetrics and Gynecology, 115*(2), 338–343. doi:10.1097/AOG.0b013e3181c915da

Karl, D. J., Beal, J. A., O'Hare, C. M., & Rissmiller, P. N. (2006). Reconceptualizing the nurse's role in the newborn period as an attacher. *MCN: The American Journal of Maternal/Child Nursing, 31*(4), 257–262.

Karpati, P. C., Rossignol, M., Pirot, M., Cholley, B., Vicaut, E., Henry, P., . . . Mebazaa, A. (2004). High incidence of myocardial ischemia during postpartum hemorrhage. *Anesthesiology, 100*(1), 30–36.

Keith, L. G., & Oleszczuk, J. J. (2002). Triplet births in the United States: An epidemic of high-risk pregnancies. *Journal of Reproductive Medicine, 47*(4), 259–265.

Kilpatrick, S. J., & Laros, R. K. (2009). Maternal hematologic disorders. In R. K. Creasy, R. Resnick, J. D. Iams, C. J. Lockwood, & T. R. Moore (Eds.), *Maternal-Fetal Medicine: Principles and Practice* (6th ed., pp. 125–142). Philadelphia: Saunders.

Ladewig, P. A., London, M. L., & Davidson, M. R. (2009). *Contemporary Maternal-Newborn Nursing Care* (7th ed.). Upper Saddle River, NJ: Prentice Hall.

Landy, H. J., Laughon, S. K., Bailit, J. L., Kominiarek, M. A., Gonzalez-Quintero, V. H., Ramirez, M., . . . Zhang, J. (2011). Characteristics associated with severe perineal and cervical lacerations during vaginal delivery. *Obstetrics and Gynecology, 111*(3), 627–635. doi:10.1097/AOG.0b013e31820afaf2

Larson-Meyer, D. E. (2002). Effect of postpartum exercise on mothers and their offspring: A review of the literature. *Obesity Research, 10*(8), 841–853. doi:10.1038/oby.2002.114

Lawrence, R. M., & Lawrence, R. A. (2009). The breast and the physiology of lactation. In R. K. Creasy, R. Resnick, J. D. Iams, C. J. Lockwood, & T. R. Moore (Eds.), *Maternal-Fetal Medicine: Principles and Practice* (6th ed., pp. 125–142). Philadelphia: Saunders.

Leijonhufvud, A., Lundholm, C., Cnattingius, S., Grannath, F., Andolf, E., & Altman, D. (2011). Risks of stress urinary incontinence and pelvic organ prolapse surgery in relation to mode of childbirth. *American Journal of Obstetrics & Gynecology, 204*(1), 70e1–70e7. doi:10.1016/j.ajog.2010.08.034

Lewallen, L. P. (2011). The importance of culture in childbearing. *Journal of Obstetric, Gynecologic, and Neonatal Nursing, 40*(1), 4–8. doi:10.1111/j.1552-6909.2010.01209.x

Lo, J., Osterweil, P., Li, H., Mori, T., Eden, K. B., & Guise, J. M. (2010). Quality of life in women with postpartum anal incontinence. *Obstetrics and Gynecology, 115*(4), 809–814. doi:10.1097/AOG.0b013e3181d4160d

Lockwood, C. J. (2009). Thromboembolic disease. In R. K. Creasy, R. Resnick, J. D. Iams, C. J. Lockwood, & T. R. Moore (Eds.), *Maternal-Fetal Medicine: Principles and Practice* (6th ed., pp. 855–858). Philadelphia: Saunders.

Logsdon, M. C., Wisner, K. L., & Pinto-Foltz, M. D. (2006). The impact of postpartum depression on mothering. *Journal of Obstetric, Gynecologic, and Neonatal Nursing, 35*(5), 652–661. doi:10.1111/j.1552-6909.2006.00087.x

Lyndon, A., Lagrew, D., Shields, L., Melsop, K., Bingham, B., & Main, E. (Eds.). (2010). *Improving Health Care Response to Obstetric Hemorrhage.* (California Maternal Quality Care Collaborative Toolkit to Transform Maternity Care). Developed under contract #08-85012 with the California Department of Public Health; Maternal, Child and Adolescent Health Division. Stanford, CA: California Maternal Quality Care Collaborative.

Magann, E. F., & Lanneau, G. S. (2005). Third stage of labor. *Obstetrics and Gynecology Clinics of North America, 32*(2), 323–332. doi:10.1016/j.ogc.2005.01.006

Maloni, J. A., & Park, S. (2005). Postpartum symptoms after antepartum bedrest. *Journal of Obstetric, Gynecologic, and Neonatal Nursing, 34*(2), 163–171. doi:10.1177/0884217504274416

Martin, A. R., & Foley, M. R. (2009). Intensive care monitoring of the critically ill pregnant patient. In R. K. Creasy, R. Resnick, J. D. Iams, C. J. Lockwood, & T. R. Moore (Eds.), *Maternal-Fetal Medicine: Principles and Practice* (6th ed., pp. 1167–1196). Philadelphia: Saunders.

Martin, J. A., Osterman, M. J. K., & Sutton, P. D. (2010). Are preterm births on the decline in the United States? Recent data from the National Vital Statistics System. *NCHS Data Brief, 36.*

McCoy, S. J. B. (2011). Postpartum depression: An essential overview for the practitioner. *Southern Medical Journal, 104*(2), 128–132. doi:10.1097/SMJ.0b013e318200c221

Mercer, R. (1986). *First-Time Motherhood: Experiences from Teens to Forties.* New York: Springer Publishing.

Mercer, R. T. (1995). *Becoming a Mother.* New York: Springer Publishing.

Miller, L. J. (2002). Postpartum depression. *Journal of the American Medical Association, 287*(6), 762–765. doi:10.1001/jama.287.6.762

Monga, M. (2009). Maternal cardiovascular, respiratory, and renal adaptation to pregnancy. In R. K. Creasy, R. Resnick, J. D. Iams, C. J. Lockwood, & T. R. Moore (Eds.), *Maternal-Fetal Medicine: Principles and Practice* (6th ed., pp. 101–110). Philadelphia: Saunders.

Moore, M. L., Moos, M. K., Callister, L. C., & Freda, M. C. (2010). *Cultural Competence: An Essential Journey for Perinatal Nurses.* (Nursing Module). White Plains, NY: The March of Dimes Birth Defects Foundation.

Nader, S. (2009). Thyroid disease and pregnancy. In R. K. Creasy, R. Resnick, J. D. Iams, C. J. Lockwood, & T. R. Moore (Eds.), *Maternal-Fetal Medicine: Principles and Practice* (6th ed., pp. 995–1014). Philadelphia: Saunders.

Nygaard, I. (2006). Urinary incontinence: Is cesarean delivery protective? *Seminars in Perinatology, 30*(5), 267–271. doi:10.1053/j.semperi.2006.07.007

Petersen, M. R. (2011). Review of interventions to relieve postpartum pain from perineal trauma. *MCN: The American Journal of Maternal Child Nursing, 36*(4), 241–245. doi:10.1097/NMC.0b013e3182182579

Press, J. Z., Klein, M. C., Kaczorowski, J., Liston, R. M., & von Dadelszen, P. (2007). Does cesarean section reduce postpartum urinary incontinence? A systematic review. *Birth, 34*(3), 228–237. doi:10.1111/j.1523-536X.2007.00175.x

Rana, S., Lindheimer, M., Hibbard, J., & Pliskin, N. (2006). Neuropsychological performance in normal pregnancy and preeclampsia. *American Journal of Obstetrics and Gynecology, 195*(1), 186–191. doi:10.1016/j.ajog.2005.12.051

Rasavong, C. (2009). Reliability and validity for Homan's sign for the detection of deep vein thrombosis. Retrieved from http://www.cyberpt.com/homansign.asp

Richter, H. E. (2006). Cesarean delivery on maternal request versus planned vaginal delivery: Impact on development of pelvic organ prolapse. *Seminars in Perinatology, 30*(5), 272–275. doi:10.1053/j.semperi.2006.07.008

Roberts, J. M., & Funai, E. F. (2009). Pregnancy-related hypertension. In R. K. Creasy & R. Resnick (Eds.), *Maternal-Fetal Medicine: Principles and Practice* (5th ed., pp. 651–690). Philadelphia: Saunders.

Roudebush, J. R., Kaufman, J., Johnson, B. H., Abraham, M. R., & Clayton, S. P. (2006). Patient and family centered perinatal care: Partnerships with childbearing women and families. *Journal of Perinatal and Neonatal Nursing, 20*(3), 201–209.

Rubin, R. (1961a). Puerperal change. *Nursing Outlook, 9,* 753–755.

Rubin, R. (1961b). Puerperal change. *Nursing Outlook, 11,* 828–831.

Rubin, R. (1977). Binding-in in the postpartum period. *Maternal-Child Nursing Journal, 6,* 67–75.

Russell, R. B., Petrini, J. R., Damus, K., Mattison, D. R., & Schwartz, R. H. (2003). The changing epidemiology of multiple births in the United States. *Obstetrics and Gynecology, 101*(1), 129–135.

Schaffer, J. I., Bloom, S. L., Casey, B. M., McIntire, D. D., Nihira, M. A., & Leveno, K. J. (2005). A randomized trial of the effects of coached vs uncoached maternal pushing during the second stage of labor on postpartum pelvic floor structure and function. *American Journal of Obstetrics and Gynecology, 192*(5), 1692–1696. doi:10.1016/j.ajog.2004.11.043

Simpson, K. R. (2005). Emergency drills in obstetrics. *MCN: The American Journal of Maternal Child Nursing, 30*(2), 220.

Smith, J. R., & Rivlin, M. E. (2010). Postpartum hemorrhage. Retrieved from http://emedicine.medscape.com/article/275038 -overview

Stotland, N. E. (2009). Maternal nutrition. In R. K. Creasy, R. Resnick, J. D. Iams, C. J. Lockwood, & T. R. Moore (Eds.), *Maternal-Fetal Medicine: Principles and Practice* (6th ed., pp. 143–150). Philadelphia: Saunders.

The Joint Commission. (2010). *Preventing Maternal Death* (Sentinel Event Alert No. 44). Oakbrook Terrace, IL: Author.

The Joint Commission on Accreditation of Healthcare Organizations. (2004). *Preventing Infant Death and Injury During Delivery* (Sentinel Event Alert No. 30). Oakbrook Terrace, IL: Author.

Thorpe, J. M. (2009). Clinical aspects of normal and abnormal labor. In R. K. Creasy, R. Resnick, J. D. Iams, C. J. Lockwood, & T. R. Moore (Eds.), *Maternal-Fetal Medicine: Principles and Practice* (6th ed., pp. 691–724). Philadelphia: Saunders.

U. S. Department of Health and Human Services (2009). *Child health USA 2008–2009.* Retrieved from http://mchb.hrsa.gov /chusa08/hstat/hsi/pages/202lbw.html

U.S. Department of Health and Human Services. (2010). National Hospital Discharge Survey: 2006 annual summary. *Vital and Health Statistics, 13*(168), 48.

U.S. Department of Health and Human Services. (2011). *Healthy People 2020.* Retrieved from http://healthypeople.gov/2020 /topicsobjectives2020/pdfs/HP2020objectives.pdf

Vargo, L. E., & Trotter, C. W. (2006). *The Premature Infant: Nursing Assessment and Management* (Nursing Module, 2nd ed.). White Plains, NY: The March of Dimes Birth Defects Foundation.

Weber, A. M., & Richter, H. E. (2005). Pelvic organ prolapse. *Obstetrics and Gynecology, 106*(3), 615–634. doi:10.1097/01 .AOG.0000175832.13266.bb

Webster, J., Pritchard, M.A., Creedy, D., and East, C. (2003). A simplified predictive index for the detection of women at risk for postnatal depression. *Birth, 30*(2): 101-108.

Whitty, J. E., & Dombrowski, M. P. (2009). Respiratory diseases in pregnancy. In R. K. Creasy & R. Resnick (Eds.), *Maternal-Fetal Medicine: Principles and Practice* (5th ed., pp. 927–952). Philadelphia: Saunders.

Williamson, C., & Mackillop, L. (2009). Diseases of the liver, biliary system, & pancreas. In R. K. Creasy, R. Resnick, J. D. Iams, C. J. Lockwood, & T. R. Moore (Eds.), *Maternal-Fetal Medicine: Principles and Practice* (6th ed., pp. 1059–1078). Philadelphia: Saunders.

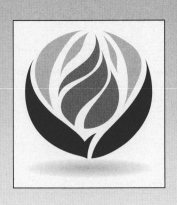

CHAPTER 18

Debbie Fraser

Newborn Adaptation to Extrauterine Life

Transition from fetal to newborn life is a critical period involving diverse physiologic changes. The newborn must move from an organism completely dependent on another for life-sustaining oxygen and nutrients to an independent being, a task that requires intense adjustment carried out over a period of hours to days. In addition to the normal physiologic tasks of transition, some neonates have congenital abnormalities, birth injury, or underlying disease processes. Careful assessment and nursing care is needed during the period of transition to ensure that the neonate who is experiencing problems with transition is recognized and appropriate interventions are initiated.

This chapter focuses on those factors influencing adaptation and physiologic changes during the early newborn period. These factors include the maternal history and medical and obstetric conditions, intrapartum status, delivery issues, and nursing assessment and interventions during transition, such as resuscitative needs and interventions facilitating maternal–newborn attachment.

MATERNAL MEDICAL AND OBSTETRIC CONDITIONS INFLUENCING NEWBORN ADAPTATION

A thorough review of the mother's prenatal and intrapartum history is essential to identify factors with the potential to compromise successful transition. Table 18–1 lists maternal risk factors and associated fetal and neonatal complications. In addition to identification of current pregnancy complications, it is important to review prior obstetric history. Conditions that predispose the newborn to risk may recur in subsequent pregnancies (Display 18–1). Intrapartum risk factors may also influence adaptation (Table 18–2).

Intrapartum fetal assessment provides important data about the fetal response to labor. Electronic fetal heart rate (FHR) monitoring or intermittent auscultation provides documentation of fetal well-being. Requisite perinatal nursing skills include knowledge of the physiologic basis for monitoring, an understanding of FHR patterns, and the initiation of appropriate nursing interventions based on data from the monitor or from auscultation. The FHR reflects the fetal response to labor. The perinatal nurse focuses on discriminating between reassuring and nonreassuring patterns. If the FHR pattern is nonreassuring, intrauterine resuscitation procedures such as maternal position change, oxygen therapy, and intravenous fluids are initiated. Oxytocin should be decreased or discontinued if infusing, or the next dose of cervical ripening agents should be delayed. Safe passage through the labor and birth process sets the stage for successful transition to extrauterine life.

UNIQUE MECHANISMS OF NEWBORN PHYSIOLOGIC ADAPTATION

The respiratory, cardiovascular, thermoregulatory, and immunologic systems undergo significant physiologic changes and adaptations during the transition from fetal to neonatal life. Successful transition requires a complex interaction among these systems.

RESPIRATORY ADAPTATIONS

Critical to the neonate's transition to extrauterine life is the ability to clear fetal lung fluid and establish

Table 18–1. MATERNAL RISK FACTORS AND POTENTIAL FETAL AND NEONATAL COMPLICATIONS

Risk Factors	Potential Complications
Maternal substance abuse	
Drug addiction	SGA, neonatal abstinence syndrome, neonatal HIV, hepatitis B and C
Alcohol use	Fetal alcohol spectrum disorder
Smoking	SGA, polycythemia
Maternal nutritional status	
Maternal weight <100 lb	SGA
Maternal weight >200 lb	SGA, LGA, neonatal hypoglycemia
Maternal medical complication	
Hereditary CNS disorders	Inherited CNS disorder
Seizure disorders requiring medication	Congenital anomalies (e.g., result of medication [Dilantin] use)
Chronic hypertension	IUGR, asphyxia, SGA
Congenital heart disease with congestive heart failure	Preterm birth, inherited cardiac defects
Hemoglobin <10 g/dL (100g/L)	Preterm birth, low birth weight
Sickle cell disease	IUGR, fetal demise
Hemoglobinopathies	IUGR, inherited hemoglobinopathies
ITP	Transient ITP, intracranial hemorrhage
Chronic glomerulonephritis, renal insufficiency	IUGR, SGA, preterm birth, asphyxia
Recurrent urinary tract infection	Preterm birth
Uterine malformation	Preterm birth, fetal malposition
Cervical incompetence	Preterm birth
Diabetes	LGA, hypoglycemia & hypocalcemia, anomalies, respiratory distress syndrome
Thyroid disease	Hypothyroidism, CNS defects, hyperthyroidism, goiter
Current pregnancy complications	
Pregnancy-induced hypertension	IUGR, SGA
TORCH infections	IUGR, SGA, active infection, anomalies
Sexually transmitted diseases	Ophthalmia neonatorum, congenital syphilis, chlamydial pneumonia
Hepatitis	Hepatitis
AIDS or HIV seropositive	Neonatal HIV
Multiple gestation	Preterm birth, asphyxia, IUGR, SGA, twin-to-twin transfusion, birth trauma
Fetal malposition	Prolapsed cord, asphyxia, birth trauma
Maternal blood group antibodies	Anemia, hyperbilirubinemia, immune-mediated hydrops fetalis
Prolonged pregnancy	Postmaturity, meconium aspiration, IUGR, asphyxia
Intraamniotic infection	Newborn sepsis, preterm birth
Group B streptococcal infection	Newborn sepsis, preterm birth

CNS, central nervous system; HIV, human immunodeficiency virus; ITP, idiopathic thrombocytopenic purpura; IUGR, intrauterine growth restriction; LGA, large for gestational age; SGA, small for gestational age; TORCH, *Toxoplasma gondii*, other agents, rubella virus, cytomegalovirus, herpes virus.

DISPLAY 18–1

Previous Pregnancy Complications that May Recur in Subsequent Pregnancies

Fetal loss beyond 28 weeks' gestation

Preterm birth

Abnormal fetal position or presentation

Previous neonate with group B streptococcal infection

Rh sensitization

Fetal compromise of unknown origin

Birth of newborn with anomalies

Birth of newborn weighing more than 10 lb

Birth of postterm newborn

Neonatal death

---

respirations, allowing the lungs to become the organ of gas exchange after separation from maternal uteroplacental circulation. Pulmonary fluid, secreted by the lung epithelium, is essential to the normal growth and development of alveoli (Helve, Pitkänen, Janér, & Andersson, 2009). Toward the end of gestation, production of lung fluid gradually diminishes. The catecholamine surge that occurs just before the onset of labor has been shown to correspond to a more rapid drop in fetal lung fluid levels (Katz, Bentur, & Elias, 2011). Those infants who do not experience labor, those born by elective cesarean section, are more likely to develop transient tachypnea of the newborn (TTN) because of lower levels of serum catecholamine (Jain & Dudell, 2006).

Initiation of breathing is a complex process that involves the interplay of biochemical, neural, and

Table 18–2. INTRAPARTUM RISK FACTORS AND POTENTIAL FETAL AND NEONATAL COMPLICATIONS

Risk Factors	Potential Complications
Umbilical cord	
Prolapsed umbilical cord	Asphyxia
True knot in cord	Asphyxia
Velamentous insertion	Intrauterine blood loss, shock, anemia
Vasa previa	Intrauterine blood loss, shock, anemia
Rupture or tearing of cord	Blood loss, shock, anemia
Membranes	
Premature rupture of membranes	Infection, respiratory distress syndrome, prolapsed cord, asphyxia
Prolonged rupture of membranes	Infection
Amnionitis	Infection
Amniotic fluid	
Oligohydramnios	Congenital anomalies, pulmonary hypoplasia
Polyhydramnios	Congenital anomalies, prolapsed cord
Meconium-stained fluid	Asphyxia, meconium aspiration syndrome
Placenta	
Placenta previa	Preterm birth, asphyxia
Abruptio placenta	Preterm birth, asphyxia
Placental insufficiency	Intrauterine growth restriction, SGA, asphyxia
Abnormal fetal presentations	
Breech birth	Asphyxia, birth injuries (CNS, skeletal)
Face or brow presentation	Asphyxia, facial trauma
Transverse lie	Asphyxia, birth injuries, cesarean birth, umbilical cord prolapse
Birth complications	
Forceps-assisted birth	CNS trauma, cephalohematoma, asphyxia, facial trauma
Vacuum extraction	Cephalohematoma, subgaleal hemorrhage
Manual version or extraction	Asphyxia, birth trauma, prolapsed cord
Shoulder dystocia	Asphyxia, brachial plexus injury, fractured clavicle
Precipitous birth	Asphyxia, birth trauma (CNS)
Undiagnosed multiple gestation	Asphyxia, birth trauma
Administration of drugs	
Oxytocin	Complications of uterine hyperstimulation (asphyxia)
Magnesium sulfate	Hypermagnesemia, CNS and respiratory depression
Analgesics	CNS and respiratory depression
Anesthetics	CNS and respiratory depression, bradycardia

CNS, central nervous system; SGA, small for gestational age.

mechanical factors, some of which have yet to be clearly identified (Alvaro & Rigatto, 2005). Pulmonary blood flow, surfactant production, and respiratory musculature also influence respiratory adaptation to extrauterine life. Establishment of independent breathing and oxygen–carbon dioxide exchange depends on these physiologic factors.

Chemical Stimuli

A number of factors have been implicated in the initiation of postnatal breathing: decreased oxygen concentration, increased carbon dioxide concentration, and a decrease in pH, all of which may stimulate fetal aortic and carotid chemoreceptors, triggering the respiratory center in the medulla to initiate respiration. Some researchers have questioned the influence of these factors and suggest instead that factors secreted by the placenta may inhibit breathing, and that regular breathing is initiated with the clamping of the umbilical cord (Alvaro & Rigatto, 2005).

Mechanical Stimulation

In utero, the fetal lungs are filled with fluid. Mechanical compression of the chest during vaginal birth forces approximately one third of this fluid out of fetal lungs. As the chest is delivered through the birth canal, it reexpands, creating negative pressure and drawing air into the lungs. This passive inspiration of air replaces fluid that previously filled the alveoli. Further expansion and distribution of air throughout the alveoli occurs when the newborn cries. Crying creates positive intrathoracic pressure that keeps alveoli open and forces the remaining fetal lung fluid into pulmonary capillaries and the lymphatic circulation.

Sensory Stimuli

The newborn is exposed to numerous tactile, visual, auditory, and olfactory stimuli during and immediately after birth. Tactile stimulation begins in utero as the fetus experiences uterine contractions and descent through the pelvis and birth canal. Stimulation to initiate breathing continues after birth as the neonate is exposed to stimuli such as light, sound, touch, smell, and pain. Vigorously drying the newborn immediately after birth is a significant tactile stimulation.

Contributing Factors

Pulmonary Blood Flow

In utero, the placenta is the organ of gas exchange for the fetus. Oxygenated blood is delivered from the placenta through the umbilical vein, through the ductus venosus into the inferior vena cava, and then to the left and right side of the fetal heart for distribution to the fetal body. Oxygenated blood is diverted away from pulmonary circulation in utero and instead flows through the foramen ovale and ductus arteriosus to the fetal body.

The fluid-filled lungs of the fetus create a state of alveolar hypoxia. Fetal pulmonary arterioles, which are very sensitive to oxygen, have thick musculature because of low oxygen tension in utero (Steinhorn, 2011). This results in constriction of pulmonary arterioles, which causes increased pulmonary vascular resistance (PVR) and decreased pulmonary blood flow. After birth, pulmonary vasodilatation occurs when oxygen enters the lungs as oxygen is a potent pulmonary vasodilator. This significantly decreases PVR. Increased pulmonary blood flow is established as PVR decreases with normal changes in arterial PO_2, alveolar PO_2, acid–base status, and absence of vasoactive substances such as prostaglandin and bradykinin. Adequate pulmonary blood flow is crucial for newborn gas exchange and successful transition. After the onset of breathing, fluid in the lungs is replaced by air.

Surfactant Production

Pulmonary surfactant is necessary to maintain expanded alveoli. Surfactant lowers surface tension, preventing alveolar collapse during inspiration and expiration. By approximately 34 to 36 weeks' gestation, there is adequate surfactant production to support respiration and to protect against development of respiratory distress syndrome (Gardner, Enzman-Hines, & Dickey, 2011). Surfactant deficiency results in atelectasis and requires greater than normal breathing efforts. Oxygen and metabolic needs increase as the newborn must use more energy to maintain respirations. Preterm newborns are at high risk for surfactant deficiency, which may significantly jeopardize respiratory adaptation to extrauterine life.

Respiratory Musculature

Intercostal muscles support the rib cage and assist with inspiration by creating negative intrathoracic pressure. Intercostal muscles may not be fully developed at birth, increasing the risk of respiratory compromise by increasing breathing effort.

CARDIOVASCULAR ADAPTATIONS

Transition from fetal to neonatal circulation is a major cardiovascular change and occurs simultaneously with respiratory system adaptation. To appreciate hemodynamic changes, an understanding of structural and blood flow differences between fetal and neonatal circulation is necessary. Figure 18–1 illustrates fetal circulation. Also influencing the cardiovascular system are physiologic changes in the vasculature, which include decreased PVR, resulting in increased pulmonary blood flow, and increased systemic vascular resistance (SVR).

Fetal Circulation

In utero, oxygenated blood flows to the fetus from the placenta through the umbilical vein. Although a small amount of oxygenated blood is delivered to the liver, most blood bypasses the hepatic system through the ductus venosus. The ductus venosus is a vascular structure that forms a connection between the umbilical vein and the inferior vena cava. Oxygenated blood from the inferior vena cava enters the right atrium, and most of it is directed through the foramen ovale to the left atrium, then to the left ventricle, and on to the ascending aorta, where it is primarily directed to the fetal heart and brain. The foramen ovale is a flap-like structure between the right and left atria. Blood flows through the foramen ovale because pressure in the right atrium is greater than that in the left atrium. In addition, the superior vena cava drains deoxygenated blood from the head and upper extremities into the right atrium, where it mixes with oxygenated blood from the placenta. This blood enters the right ventricle and pulmonary artery where again, increased resistance in the pulmonary vessels causes 60% of this blood to be shunted across the ductus arteriosus and into the descending aorta. This mixture of oxygenated and deoxygenated blood continues through the descending aorta, oxygenating the lower half of the fetal body and eventually draining back to the placenta through the two umbilical arteries. The remaining 40% of the blood coming from the right ventricle perfuses lung tissue to meet metabolic needs. The blood that actually reaches the lungs represents about

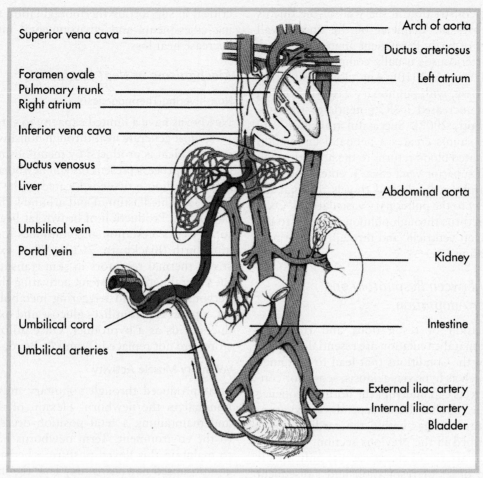

Superior vena cava
Foramen ovale
Pulmonary trunk
Right atrium
Inferior vena cava
Ductus venosus
Liver
Umbilical vein
Portal vein
Umbilical cord
Umbilical arteries

Arch of aorta
Ductus arteriosus
Left atrium
Abdominal aorta
Kidney
Intestine
External iliac artery
Internal iliac artery
Bladder

FIGURE 18–1. Fetal circulation.

8% to 10% of fetal cardiac output (Blackburn, 2012; Steinhorn, 2011).

Neonatal Circulation

During fetal life, the placenta is an organ of low vascular resistance. Clamping the umbilical cord at birth eliminates the placenta as a reservoir for blood, causing increased SVR, an increase in blood pressure, and increased pressures in the left side of the heart. Removal of the placenta also eliminates the need for blood flow through the ductus venosus, causing functional elimination of this fetal shunt. Systemic venous blood flow is then directed through the portal system for hepatic circulation. Umbilical vessels constrict, with functional closure occurring immediately. Fibrous infiltration leads to anatomic closure during the first week of life (Alvaro & Rigatto, 2005).

Several other significant events must take place for successful transition to neonatal circulation. With the infant's first breath and exposure to increased oxygen levels, the pulmonary blood flow must increase, allowing the lungs to become the organ for exchange

of oxygen and carbon dioxide; the foramen ovale must close (this occurs because left atrial pressures exceed right atrial pressures due to the increased pulmonary venous return of blood flow from the lungs) (Goldsmith, 2011); and the ductus arteriosus must close. In utero, shunting of blood from the pulmonary artery through the ductus arteriosus to the aorta occurs as a result of high PVR. After birth, SVR rises and PVR falls, causing a reversal of blood flow through the ductus. The mechanism of closure of the ductus arteriosus is not completely clear; however, it is known that rising arterial oxygen concentrations in the blood plays an important role (Freed, 2006). As the P_aO_2 level increases after birth, the ductus arteriosus begins to constrict. In utero, elevated prostaglandin levels helped maintain ductal patency. Removal of the placenta decreases prostaglandin levels, further influencing closure (Alvaro & Rigatto, 2005; Bagwell, 2007). Constriction of the ductus arteriosus is a gradual process, permitting bidirectional shunting of blood after birth. PVR may be higher than the SVR, allowing some degree of right-to-left shunting, until the SVR rises above PVR and blood flow is directed left to right.

Smooth muscle constriction in the wall of the ductus arteriosus narrows the diameter of the ductal wall within 18 hours of birth. Permanent anatomic closure of the ductus arteriosus is usually complete within 10 to 21 days (McDaniel, 2010). Any clinical situation that causes hypoxia, with pulmonary vasoconstriction and subsequent increased PVR, potentiates right-to-left shunting (Lott, 2007). Successful transition and closure of fetal shunts creates a neonatal circulation where deoxygenated blood returns to the heart through the inferior and superior vena cava. It enters the right atrium to the right ventricle and travels through the pulmonary artery to the pulmonary vascular bed. Oxygenated blood returns through pulmonary veins to the left atrium, the left ventricle, and through the aorta to systemic circulation.

Relationship between Respiratory and Cardiovascular Adaptation

Successful initiation of respirations and transition from fetal to neonatal circulation are essential to maintain life after birth. Conditions that lead to sustained elevated PVR such as hypoxia, acidosis, sepsis, or congenital heart defects can interrupt the normal sequence of events. Closure of fetal shunts depends on oxygenation and pressure changes within the cardiovascular system as described in the previous section. Foramen ovale and ductus arteriosus closure occurs only if PVR drops with the onset of respiration and subsequent oxygenation. The pulmonary vascular bed is very reactive to low oxygen levels. If the neonate experiences significant hypoxia, PVR will remain elevated with resultant decreased pulmonary blood flow and right-to-left shunting across the foramen ovale and ductus arteriosus. These events may induce a state of hypoxia as deoxygenated blood bypasses the lungs through the patent fetal shunts to be mixed with oxygenated blood entering the systemic circulation. The result is persistent pulmonary hypertension of the newborn (PPHN) requiring aggressive cardiorespiratory support.

THERMOREGULATION

The newborn's ability to maintain temperature control after birth is determined by external environmental factors and internal physiologic processes. Characteristics of newborns that predispose them to heat loss include a large body surface area in relation to body mass and a limited amount of subcutaneous fat. Newborns attempt to regulate body temperature by nonshivering thermogenesis, increased metabolic rate, and increased muscle activity. Peripheral vasoconstriction also decreases heat loss to the skin surface. Mechanisms of heat loss including evaporation, conduction, convection, and radiation play an integral part in newborn adaptation to extrauterine life. Nursing care is critical in supporting thermoregulation through ongoing assessments and environmental interventions to decrease heat loss.

Mechanisms of Heat Production

Nonshivering Thermogenesis

Newborns have a limited capacity to shiver and, therefore, must generate heat through nonshivering thermogenesis. Heat is produced by metabolism of brown fat, a unique process present only in newborns. This highly vascular adipose tissue is located in the neck, scapula, axilla, and mediastinum and around kidneys and adrenal glands. Production of brown fat begins around 26 to 28 weeks' gestation and continues for 3 to 5 weeks after birth (Blackburn, 2012). When exposed to cold stress, thermal receptors in skin transmit messages to the central nervous system, activating the sympathetic nervous system and triggering metabolism of brown fat, a process that utilizes glucose and oxygen and produces acids as a byproduct. Once utilized, brown fat stores are not replaced (Brand & Boyd, 2010).

Voluntary Muscle Activity

Heat produced through voluntary muscle activity is minimal in the newborn. Flexion of the extremities and maintaining a fetal position decreases heat loss to the environment. Term newborns have the ability to maintain this flexed posture, whereas preterm and compromised newborns may lack the muscle tone for this posturing, making them more vulnerable to cold stress (Bagwell, 2007).

Mechanisms of Heat Loss

Evaporation

Evaporation and heat loss occur as amniotic fluid on skin is converted to a vapor. Drying the newborn immediately after birth and removing wet blankets decreases evaporative losses and prevents further cooling. The amount of insensible water loss from the skin is inversely related to gestational age. Skin of a preterm newborn is more susceptible to evaporative losses because the keratin layer of the skin has not matured. Absence or greater permeability of this skin layer allows increased heat loss (Brown & Landers, 2011; Bagwell, 2007). Because the newborn's head is the largest surface area of the body, covering the head with a knit cap after birth when not under the radiant warmer greatly conserves heat. Under the radiant warmer, use of a cap prevents heat from reaching the newborn's head and may contribute to cold stress. Adding humidity to the environment may also decrease evaporative heat loss. To avoid hypothermia, it is recommended that low-birth-weight infants be placed directly in a sterile food or medical grade plastic bag or wrapped with occlusive wrap after delivery (Kattwinkel et al., 2010a).

Conduction

Conductive heat loss occurs when two solid objects of different temperatures come in contact. Heat loss occurs if the newborn is placed in direct contact with a cold scale, mattress, X-ray plate, or blanket. Mechanisms for preventing conductive heat loss in the birthing room immediately after birth include using preheated radiant warmer, warm blankets for drying, and covering scales and X-ray plates with warm blankets. Preheating the radiant warmer is necessary, because it may take 15 to 30 minutes to warm the mattress.

Providing skin-to-skin contact between mother and newborn after birth helps prevent conductive heat loss and enhances maternal–newborn attachment (Brown & Landers, 2011; Bohnhorst, Heyne, Peter, & Poest, 2001). Skin-to-skin contact has been shown to reduce the risk of mortality, decrease the length of hospital stay, increase feeding vigor, and improve growth (Conde-Agudelo, Belizán & Diaz-Rossello, 2011). Preterm newborns provided with opportunities for skin-to-skin contact with their mothers maintained normal oxygen saturation levels and thermal stability (Conde-Agudelo et al., 2011).

Convection

Convection is the transfer of heat from a solid object to surrounding air. Heat is lost from newborn skin as cooler air passes over it. Convection heat loss depends on the amount of exposed skin surface, temperature of air, and amount of air turbulence created by drafts. Interventions that prevent convection heat loss in the newborn include clothing, eliminating source of drafts, and, when necessary, providing heated, humidified oxygen through a face mask or hood (Blackburn, 2012).

Radiation

Radiation heat loss occurs when heat is transferred between two objects not in contact with each other. The newborn loses heat by radiation to nearby cooler surfaces such as those of the crib, Isolette, windows, or other objects. Some of the more common and efficient methods for preventing radiant heat loss are use of a radiant warmer after birth, moving the crib or Isolette away from a cold window, and use of a double wall or heat shield inside an incubator (for small, preterm newborns), creating an additional warmer barrier between skin and incubator wall.

Effects of Cold Stress

Thermal management of the newborn during the first few hours of life is critical to prevent detrimental effects of cold stress and hypothermia. Table 18–3 summarizes nursing interventions that support the newborn and prevent cold stress. Because heat production requires oxygen consumption and glucose use, persistent hypothermia may deplete these stores, leading to metabolic acidosis, hypoglycemia, decreased surfactant production, increased caloric requirements, and, if chronic, impaired weight gain (Blackburn, 2012; Bissinger & Annibale, 2010). This process is illustrated in Figure 18–2.

IMMUNE SYSTEM ADAPTATION

Newborns are vulnerable to infection because of their immature immune system and lack of exposure to organisms. Neonates depend on passive immunity acquired from their mother through active transport via the placenta of immunoglobulin (Ig) G during the third trimester (van den Berg, Westerbeek, van der Klis,

Table 18–3. MECHANISMS OF HEAT LOSS AND NURSING INTERVENTIONS THAT PREVENT COLD STRESS

Type of Heat Loss	Nursing Interventions
Evaporation	Dry late preterm or term infant thoroughly Place low–birth-weight infants in a food-grade plastic bag immediately after delivery Remove wet linen Place knit cap on infant's head when not under radiant warmer Bathe infant under radiant heat source after temperature stabilizes
Convection	Move infant away from drafts, open windows, vents, and traffic patterns When necessary, use humidified, warmed oxygen Avoid using ceiling fans in birthing room Move infant in prewarmed transport Isolette Place low-birth-weight infants in an incubator
Conduction	Preheat radiant warmer Place infant skin-to-skin with mother Use warmed blanket Warm stethoscope and your hands Place cover between infant and metal scale or X-ray plate
Radiation	Place stabilizing unit on an interior wall of the birthing room (away from cold windows) Use a double-walled incubator Preheat radiant warmer or transport incubator

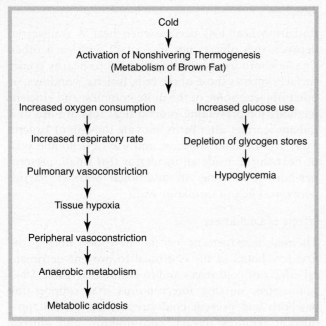

FIGURE 18-2. Effects of cold stress in the newborn.

Berbers, & van Elburg, 2011). Preterm newborns are at greater risk for infection because they may not have received this passive immunity and because the immaturity of the immune system is even more pronounced than in term infants (Strunk, Currie, Richmond, Simmer, & Burgner, 2011).

Immunity is conferred through immunoglobulins, antibodies secreted by lymphocytes, and plasma cells. There are three main classes of immunoglobulins responsible for immunity: IgG, IgA, and IgM. Because of their small molecular size, only IgG antibodies are capable of crossing the placenta. Maternally transmitted IgG provides protection for the newborn against bacterial and viral infections for which the mother already has antibodies (e.g., diphtheria, tetanus, smallpox, measles, mumps, poliomyelitis).

IgM and IgA immunoglobulins do not cross the placenta. If elevated levels of IgM are found in the newborn, it may indicate the presence of an intrauterine infection such as one organism traditionally known by the acronym TORCH (i.e., *Toxoplasma gondii* [toxoplasmosis]; other agents such as *Treponema pallidum* [syphilis], varicella virus, human immunodeficiency virus, and *Chlamydia*; rubella virus; cytomegalovirus; and herpes virus). IgA, found in colostrum, is thought to contribute to passive immunity for breast-fed newborns and may also play an important role in the development of the neonate's immune system (Brandtzaeg, 2010).

Immature leukocyte function in the newborn inhibits the ability to destroy pathogens. Deficiency in response prevents mature processes of chemotaxis (i.e., movement of leukocytes toward site of infection), opsonization (i.e., altering or preparing the cells for ingestion), and phagocytosis (i.e., ingestion of cells) from occurring. Low levels of immunoglobulin and complement components (i.e., plasma proteins that assist the immune system) leave newborns, especially preterm newborns, vulnerable to infection (Strunk et al., 2011).

Lymphocytes are responsible for the specific response in the immune system that involves antibody production. When lymphocytes are exposed to pathogens, they become sensitized to them. If repeated exposure occurs, lymphocytes will attempt to destroy the pathogen. Because newborns lack exposure to most common organisms, any action by lymphocytes is delayed.

Weak newborn defenses against infection make it imperative for the perinatal nurse and anyone coming in contact with newborns to follow careful hand washing practices and use of aseptic technique. Promoting skin integrity is essential for preventing neonatal infections. Newborn skin is thin and delicate, making it susceptible to alterations in integrity. Fetal scalp electrodes, fetal scalp pH sampling, and skin abrasions create portals for the entry of organisms. Umbilical cord and circumcision sites are also potential sites of infection.

Preterm newborns, with more fragile skin, are at a greater risk for infection. Invasive procedures, performed during the early hours after birth, further challenge the immune system. Treatments such as vitamin K injection, suctioning, and heel-stick blood samples predispose newborns to infection if the proper aseptic technique is not maintained.

Although most births result in a healthy newborn making the transition to extrauterine life without difficulty, perinatal nurses must anticipate and prepare for complications. This includes ensuring immediate availability of functioning resuscitation equipment and knowledge of equipment operation. The International Liaison Committee on Resuscitation (ILCOR) and the American Academy of Pediatrics (AAP) recommend that someone trained in neonatal resuscitation be available for all births (Kattwinkel et al., 2010b). Display 18-2 identifies equipment that should be available in every birthing room.

The Neonatal Resuscitation Program developed by the American Heart Association (AHA) and the AAP (Kattwinkel et al., 2010b) has become the standard for educating healthcare providers involved in newborn stabilization. Figure 18-3 illustrates steps used to evaluate and establish airway, breathing, and circulation as a basis for stabilization of the newborn immediately after birth. Although most newborns respond successfully to oral suctioning and tactile stimulation, 5% to 10% may require additional interventions, including ventilation by bag and mask or endotracheal

DISPLAY 18-2

Equipment Needed for Neonatal Resuscitation

Clock with second hand

Preheated radiant warmer

Firm, padded resuscitation surface

Warmed blankets

Neonatal stethoscope

Bulb syringe

Gloves and appropriate personnel protection

Pulse oximeter and probe

Mechanical suction with manometer and tubing

Oxygen source, flowmeter (flow rate up to 10 L/min), tubing, and blender

Resuscitation bag capable of delivering 90%–100% oxygen and pressure gauge

Face masks (newborn and preemie size)

Laryngoscope with sizes 0 and 1 blades (extra batteries; extra laryngoscope bulbs)

Endotracheal tubes (sizes 2.5, 3.0, 3.5, and 4.0 mm)

CO_2 detector or capnograph

Laryngeal mask airway (optional)

Suction catheters (sizes 5 Fr, 8 Fr, 10 Fr, 12 Fr, or 14 Fr)

Meconium aspirator device

8-Fr feeding tube and 20-mL syringe

Syringes (sizes 1, 3, 5, 10, 20, and 50 mL)

Needles 25-, 21-, 18-gauge, or puncture device for needleless system

Umbilical vessel catheterization supplies

Cord clamp

Tape

Scissors

Resuscitative drugs

   Epinephrine 1:10,000 concentration

   Naloxone hydrochloride (1 mg/mL or 0.4 mg/mL)

   Volume expanders

      Normal saline solution

      Lactated Ringer's solution 100 mL or 250 mL

Normal saline for flushes

---

intubation, chest compressions, and administration of resuscitative medications (Kattwinkel et al., 2010b).

Good communication among health team members is essential in anticipating and preparing for high-risk births. Communicating the details of the maternal and family history that will affect the resuscitation and treatment of the newborn is particularly important. In addition to undergoing dramatic physical changes to adapt to extrauterine life, newborns must handle the events and procedures they are subjected to after birth. After airway, breathing, and circulation have been established, a thorough assessment of the newborn is performed. This assessment includes Apgar scoring, evaluation of vital signs, physical examination, and measurements. Ideally, all aspects of transitional assessments are performed in the presence of parents in the birthing room. Only if significant maternal or newborn complications occur should parents and newborns be separated.

APGAR SCORE

The Apgar score was introduced in 1952 by Dr. Virginia Apgar, an anesthesiologist. It provides a simple method to evaluate the condition of the newborn at 1 and 5 minutes after life (Apgar, 1966). Five assessment criteria (i.e., heart rate, respiratory rate, muscle tone, reflex irritability, and color) are scored from 0 to 2. The highest total possible score is 10. The AAP and the American College of Obstetricians and Gynecologists (ACOG) recommend continuing the assessment every 5 minutes until the Apgar score is greater than 7 (AAP & ACOG, 2007). When used to evaluate preterm newborns, the Apgar score may have less validity. Findings common in the preterm newborn such as irregular respirations, decreased muscle tone, and decreased reflex irritability affect the overall score (Paxton & Harrell, 1991). The Apgar score should not be used as an indication for resuscitation (AHA & AAP, 2010). The Apgar score by itself is not an accurate predictor of long-term outcome; however, some studies have shown an increase of cerebral palsy in infants with low 5-minute Apgar scores (Kent, 2011; Lie, Grøholt, & Eskild, 2010).

PHYSICAL ASSESSMENT

A care provider skilled in newborn assessment should perform a physical assessment within the first 2 hours after birth (AAP & ACOG, 2007). This examination gives the perinatal nurse an opportunity to evaluate overall newborn well-being and transition to extrauterine life. Chapter 19 describes a comprehensive physical examination, including normal and abnormal findings. During the initial examination in the birthing room, all systems are evaluated using inspection, auscultation, and palpation. During the transitional period after birth, temperature, heart rate, rate and character of respirations, skin color, level of consciousness, muscle tone, and activity level are evaluated and documented at least once every 30 minutes until the newborn's condition has remained stable for 2 hours (AAP & ACOG, 2007).

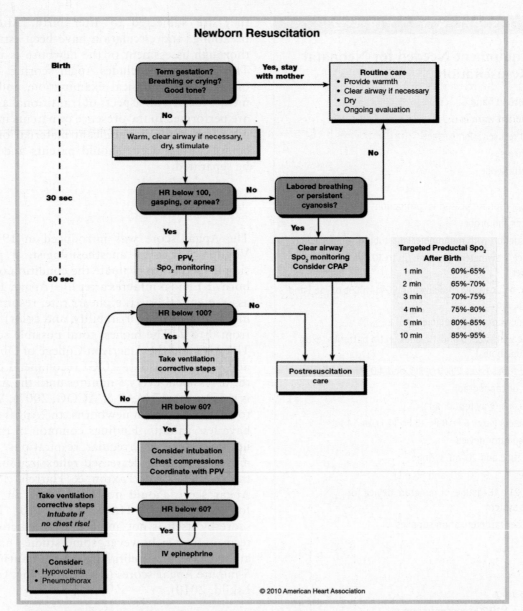

Newborn Resuscitation

FIGURE 18–3. Resuscitation in the birthing room. CPAP, continuous positive airway pressure; HR, heart rate; IV, intravenous; PPV, positive pressure ventilation. (From Kattwinkel, J., Perlman, J. M., Aziz, K., Colby, C., Fairchild, K., Gallagher, J., . . . Zaichkin, J. [2010b]. 2010 American Heart Association guidelines for cardiopulmonary resuscitation and emergency cardiovascular care science: Part 15: Neonatal resuscitation. *Circulation*, 122[18, Suppl. 3], S909–S919. Reprinted with permission.)

SKIN

An overall visual assessment of the newborn is performed, noting any obvious defects (e.g., neural tube defects, abdominal wall defects, extra digits) or trauma (e.g., bruising, petechiae, puncture wound from fetal scalp electrode). Skin is observed for color, texture, birthmarks, rashes, jaundice, and meconium staining. The newborn's back is inspected, noting a closed vertebral column or presence of abnormalities, such as masses and dimple or tuft of hair along the spine.

HEAD AND NECK

Symmetry of the head and face is noted, as well as the presence of molding, caput succedaneum, and bruising.

Fontanelles are palpated. Although it is not uncommon for eyelids to be edematous, drainage from the eye is not normal during this period. Subconjunctival hemorrhage, although not normal, is sometimes seen and resolves spontaneously. The neck is palpated for masses and full range of motion. The examiner assesses the position of the ears and looks for skin tags or evidence of a sinus on or around the ears. While assessing the mucous membrane of the mouth for a normal pink color, the lips and palate are inspected for a cleft.

RESPIRATORY SYSTEM

Inspection of the chest includes observing the shape, symmetry, and equality of chest movement. Asymmetry in chest movement may indicate pneumothorax or congenital defect. Respirations are nonlabored at a rate of 30 to 60 breaths per minute. Retractions, grunting, and nasal flaring are abnormal findings indicating respiratory distress. Breath sounds should be equal bilaterally. Initially, moist sounds may be heard as fluid is cleared from the lungs by absorption through pulmonary capillaries and by drainage through the nose and mouth. Special attention is paid to newborns when meconium-stained amniotic fluid is present. If meconium-stained amniotic fluid is noted prior to delivery, personnel capable of intubating the nonvigorous infant and clearing the trachea of meconium must be present at the delivery (AHA & AAP, 2010). Because meconium aspiration is a risk, careful assessment of the respiratory rate, quality of breath sounds, and color determines the need for interventions such as suctioning and supplemental oxygen. In the absence of meconium-stained amniotic fluid and respiratory depression, the newborn's mouth and nose are suctioned with a bulb syringe after delivery.

CARDIOVASCULAR SYSTEM

Inspection of the cardiovascular system includes observation of the color of the skin and mucous membranes and location of the point of maximal impulse (PMI). Although acrocyanosis (blueness of the hands and feet) is a normal finding, central cyanosis indicates inadequate oxygenation and the need for supplemental oxygen. Heart rate, rhythm, and normal heart sounds and murmurs are best identified when auscultated using a newborn stethoscope.

Cardiovascular assessment also includes palpation for the presence and equality of femoral pulses. Pulses should be equal and nonbounding. Bounding pulses may indicate patent ductus arteriosus, whereas absent or decreased pulses may occur with coarctation of the aorta (Vargo, 2009). Depending on the condition of the newborn, a baseline blood pressure may be recorded. Taking the blood pressure in all four extremities is usually reserved for a newborn showing signs of distress. Routine blood pressure screening for newborns in the absence of risk factors and without complications is not recommended by the AAP Committee on Fetus and Newborn (1993).

ABDOMEN

The examiner assesses the shape, symmetry, and consistency of the abdomen. The umbilical cord stump is inspected for the presence of three vessels (i.e., two arteries and one vein). The umbilical cord of a newborn exposed to meconium in utero for an extended period has a yellowish-brown discoloration. The abdomen is auscultated to detect bowel sounds.

MUSCULOSKELETAL SYSTEM

Extremities are assessed for symmetry, range of motion, and the presence of extra or missing digits. While moving the newborn's arm, clavicles are palpated for crepitus, which may indicate a fracture. The newborn's hips are evaluated for "clunks," which may indicate dislocation. Normal muscle tone is noted during this part of the examination and while evaluating the Apgar score.

GENITALIA

The presence of normal male or female genitalia is evaluated. Male newborns are assessed for location of the urethral meatus and presence of a hydrocele. The scrotum is palpated to detect the testes.

NEUROLOGIC SYSTEM

A complete neurologic assessment is usually reserved for newborns who are born with or develop complications. A brief neurologic assessment is performed by evaluating reflexes such as Moro, grasp, and suck.

In addition to ongoing physical assessments of the newborn, procedures such as newborn identification, instillation of eye prophylaxis, administration of vitamin K, and cord care are performed soon after birth. Ideally, each perinatal unit develops policies and procedures outlining expected newborn care. *Guidelines for Perinatal Care* (AAP & ACOG, 2007) is a resource for developing unit standards.

NEWBORN IDENTIFICATION

One of the first procedures after birth is newborn identification. Perinatal nurses must be meticulous when recording the identification band number and applying identification bands to mothers and newborns (AAP & ACOG, 2007). Some hospitals use a four-band system that includes a band for the support person or father of the newborn in addition to the band for the mother and two bands for the newborn, with one placed on an ankle and one on a wrist. Newborn footprinting and fingerprinting are not adequate methods of identification (AAP & ACOG, 2007). Some hospitals have abandoned these practices altogether as a form of identification. Other hospitals continue to do footprinting and fingerprinting but give the prints to the parents as a birth souvenir.

According to the National Center for Missing and Exploited Children (NCMEC; 2011), statistics for newborn abductions from hospital facilities may underrepresent the number of actual abductions from healthcare facilities (Table 18–4). Abductions and attempted abductions remain a significant threat to infant safety. Between 1983 and 2011, there were 128 hospital abductions reported (NCMEC, 2011). Infant abductions can

Table 18–4. REPORTED INFANT ABDUCTIONS FROM HEALTHCARE FACILITIES 1983–2011

Abductions = 128	Located = 123
	Missing = 5
From mother's room	74 (58%)
From nursery	17 (13%)
From pediatrics	17 (13%)
From "on premises"	20 (16%)
With violence to mother/caregiver	10 (8%)
(8 "on premises"; 2 nursery to RN)	

RN, registered nurse. (From National Center for Missing and Exploited Children. [2011].) *Newborn/infant abductions.* Retrieved from http://www.missingkids.com/en_US/documents/InfantAbductionStats.pdf)

be successfully prevented through a comprehensive safety program that may include alarm systems, video surveillance, and education of both staff and parents (Miller, 2007; Vincent, 2009). NCMEC (2009), in cooperation with the Association of Women's Health, Obstetric and Neonatal Nurses and the National Association of Neonatal Nurses, offer *Guidelines on Prevention of and Response to Infant Abductions.* Staff education should be combined with the development and testing of critical incident response procedures including mock infant abductions.

Newborn safety and security, including unit visiting policies, should be discussed with parents and family members. Parents should be made aware of what the hospital is doing to ensure the safety of every newborn and increasing their awareness of the need for vigilance. Parents need to understand what they can do to increase safety. An important part of any newborn security program is a discussion with the parents, including directions not to leave their newborn unattended and information about identification of caregivers who may transport the newborn to and from the nursery or other hospital department.

The efficacy of electronic newborn security systems in preventing newborn abductions remains controversial. No one method is superior; the key issue is that there must be some systematic newborn safety program in place known to the parents and perinatal healthcare providers to decrease the risk of newborn abduction. Nothing replaces vigilance on the part of parents, perinatal nurses, and other hospital employees.

VITAMIN K

One of the most important causes of a bleeding syndrome in an otherwise healthy newborn is hemorrhagic disease caused by vitamin K deficiency (Manco-Johnson, Rodden, & Hays, 2011). During the first week of life, newborns are at risk for bleeding disorders because of an immature liver that is unable to produce several coagulation factors and a sterile gastrointestinal tract that has not begun producing vitamin K. Consumption of breast milk and formula causes colonization of bacteria in the gastrointestinal tract, which is necessary for vitamin K production. Vitamin K stimulates the liver to synthesize coagulation factors II, VII, IX, and X (DeMarini & Rath, 2007). A single dose of 0.5 mg for newborns weighing less than 1.5 kg and 1 mg for newborns weighing more than 1.5 kg is administered intramuscularly within the first hour of life (AAP Committee on Fetus and Newborn, 2003 [reaffirmed 2009]).

EYE PROPHYLAXIS

Most states in the United States mandate that every newborn receive prophylaxis against eye infections. Erythromycin ointment is the drug of choice because of its effectiveness against gonococcal and chlamydial infections. To facilitate breastfeeding, ointment application can be delayed up to 1 hour after birth (AAP & ACOG, 2007). After the agent for prophylaxis is chosen, care should be taken to instill the ointment throughout the conjunctival sac. Excessive medication can be wiped away with a sterile cotton ball 1 minute after instillation (AAP & ACOG, 2007).

UMBILICAL CORD CARE

As part of the initial newborn assessment in the birthing room, the umbilical cord is examined for the presence of two arteries and a vein. Because a moist cord is vulnerable to pathogens, measures should be taken to promote drying of the cord, including exposing the cord to air. Over the years, a variety of methods of cord care have been used including alcohol, triple dye, and other antimicrobial agents. Research has shown that use of sterile water or air drying results in cords separating more quickly than those treated with alcohol (Dore et al., 1998; Hsu et al., 2010). The cord should be observed for the presence of serous, purulent, or sanguineous drainage.

PSYCHOLOGICAL ADAPTATION

After addressing physiologic adaptation to extrauterine life, the focus of nursing interventions is psychological adaptation. Perinatal nurses are in a position to promote early maternal–newborn attachment. Early and extended contact between mother and newborn facilitates development of a positive relationship (Bystrova et al., 2009). In a Cochrane review, Moore, Anderson, and Bergman (2007) identified positive benefits of early skin-to-skin contact on breastfeeding duration, infant crying, and early mother–infant attachment. The perinatal nurse assists in the attachment process by encouraging parents to see, touch, and hold their newborn. Providing uninterrupted time for them to be together gives parents the opportunity to recognize and identify unique behavioral and physical characteristics of their newborn.

Practices used to promote attachment usually do not interfere with transition to extrauterine life. The perinatal nurse can make a positive contribution to enhancing the attachment process by modifying practices that separate mothers and newborns immediately after birth. Newborn treatments can be performed in the birthing room, decreasing separation time between the mother and the newborn. The mother may immediately hold the newborn if the newborn is dried and covered with a warm blanket. The newborn could also be placed skin-to-skin with the mother. If both are covered with a blanket, neonatal thermoregulation is not interrupted. Application of ophthalmic antibiotics may safely occur within the first hour of life, enhancing maternal–newborn eye contact (AAP & ACOG, 2007). Maternal attachment is also supported when women are provided the opportunity to breastfeed immediately after birth. Breastfeeding is more than a feeding method; it is an intimate relationship between a mother and her newborn. Early suckling and opportunities for uninterrupted contact between mother and newborn increases breastfeeding duration (Bramson et al., 2010).

COMPLICATIONS AFFECTING TRANSITION

Infection with group B streptococci (GBS) was one of the leading causes of morbidity and mortality in newborn infants before labor prophylaxis was instituted (Verani & Schrag, 2010). It is estimated that 10% to 30% of women are GBS carriers (Verani, McGee, & Schrag, 2010). Pregnant women colonized with GBS are mostly asymptomatic but may experience urinary tract infections and amnionitis. The incidence of early-onset GBS infection is 0.3 to 0.4 cases per 1,000 live births when prenatal screening and a program of intrapartum antibiotic prophylaxis are in place compared to a rate of 1.7 cases per 1,000 live births prior to the introduction of universal screening and treatment (Verlani & Schrag, 2010).

Early-onset GBS infection can occur in the first 7 days of life but most commonly manifests in the first 24 hours after delivery. Early-onset infection presents as bacteremia, meningitis, or pneumonia. The mortality rate associated with each of these presentations is 4% to 6% (Verlani & Schrag, 2010). Risk factors for the development of GBS infection include gestational age less than 37 weeks, rupture of membranes more than 18 hours before birth, intrapartum fever of 38°C (99.4°F) or higher, a previous GBS-infected newborn, and GBS bacteriuria during pregnancy.

Late-onset GBS infections occur between 1 week and 3 months of age. Sepsis is the most common manifestation of both early and late onset GBS; however, meningitis is more common in late-onset than in early-onset disease. The mortality rate for late-onset GBS is 4% to 6% (Verani & Schrag, 2010).

Guidelines issued by the Centers for Disease Control and Prevention (CDC) in 1996 offered two approaches for the screening and treatment of GBS: screening cultures done at 35 to 37 weeks with treatment of positive results or treatment of women with risk factors without screening cultures. Studies examining these approaches found that the culture-only approach was much more effective than the risk factor approach in preventing GBS infection in the newborn (Schrag et al., 2002). In 2002, the CDC, ACOG, and AAP issued revised guidelines for prevention of perinatal invasive GBS disease, recommending universal screening of pregnant women at 35 to 37 weeks' gestation. This change resulted in a further decrease of early-onset GBS disease in the newborn by 31% from 2000 to 2001. Updated guidelines issued in 2010 (Verani et al., 2010) continue to support screening of all pregnant women at 35 to 37 weeks' gestation and administering intrapartum antimicrobial prophylaxis (IAP) to carriers (Fig. 18–4).

Cases of early-onset GBS disease continue to occur despite the new guidelines, and affected infants incur significant morbidity and mortality. Inaccurate screening results, improper implementation of intrapartum antibiotic prophylaxis, or antibiotic failure all may contribute to persistent disease. This highlights the importance of continued vigilance for signs of infection in the newborn. The assessment and care of a newborn after birth should be based on knowledge of maternal risk factors for GBS sepsis, maternal GBS status if known, and the timing and number of doses of antibiotic administered during labor. After delivery, it is important to evaluate the newborn for signs and symptoms of infection, including respiratory distress, apnea, tachycardia, hypotension, pallor, temperature instability, lethargy, and hypotonia. Asymptomatic newborns older than 35 weeks' gestation whose mothers received appropriate intrapartum chemoprophylaxis should be managed as healthy newborns. Symptomatic newborns should receive a diagnostic workup and prophylactic

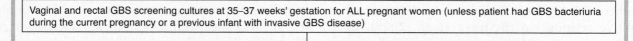

Vaginal and rectal GBS screening cultures at 35–37 weeks' gestation for ALL pregnant women (unless patient had GBS bacteriuria during the current pregnancy or a previous infant with invasive GBS disease)

Intrapartum prophylaxis indicated

- Previous infant with invasive GBS disease

- GBS bacteriuria during current pregnancy

- Positive GBS screening culture during current pregnancy (unless a planned cesarean delivery in the absence of labor or amniotic membrane rupture is performed)

- Unknown GBS status (culture not done incomplete or results unknown) and any of the following:
  - Delivery at <37 weeks' gestation*
  - Amniotic membrane rupture ≥18 hours
  - Intrapartum temperature ≥100.4∞F (≥38.0∞C)†

Intrapartum prophylaxis not indicated

- Previous pregnancy with a positive GBS screening culture (unless a culture was also positive during the current pregnancy)

- Planned cesarean delivery performed in the absence of labor or membrane rupture (regardless of maternal GBS culture status)

- Negative vaginal and rectal GBS screening culture in late gestation during the current pregnancy regardless of intrapartum risk factors

* If onset of labor or rupture of amniotic membranes occurs at <37 weeks' gestation and there is a significant risk for preterm delivery (as assessed by the clinician), a suggested algorthim for GBS prophylaxis management is provided (Figure 3).
† If amnionitis is suspected broad-spectrum antibiotic therapy that includes an agent known to be active against GBS should replace GBS prophylaxis.

FIGURE 18–4. Indications for antibiotic prophylaxis to prevent perinatal group B streptococci (GBS) disease. (From Verani, J. R., McGee, L., & Schrag, S. J. [2010]. Prevention of perinatal group B streptococcal disease–Revised guidelines from CDC. *MMWR Recommendations and Reports, 59*[RR-10], 1–36.)

treatment with antibiotics. Figure 18–5 provides an algorithm for management of the newborn born to a GBS-colonized mother.

HEPATITIS B

Each year in the United States, about 24,000 infants are born to hepatitis B virus (HBV)–positive women (U.S. Preventative Services Task Force, 2010). Universal vaccination and prenatal testing for HBV have decreased the incidence rate of acute HBV infections from more than 3 out of 100,000 to 0.34 out of 100,000 in all children (Slowik & Jhaveri, 2005).

Prior to routine use of HBV vaccinations in the United States, perinatal or early childhood transmission of HBV accounted for 30% to 40% of chronic infections (Mast et al., 2005). The spectrum of HBV infection ranges from asymptomatic seroconversion through general malaise, anorexia, nausea, and jaundice to fetal hepatitis. Development of a chronic infection is inversely proportional to the age at which the infection was acquired. Ninety percent of newborns infected in utero or at the time of birth develop chronic infection and become persistently positive for the hepatitis B surface antigen (HBsAg) (Lam, Gotsch, & Langan, 2010). In contrast, only 2% to 6% of older children, adolescents, and adults develop chronic HBV infection after acute illness (AAP Committee on Infectious Diseases, 2009). The immunologic response to infection leads to the development of cirrhosis, liver

failure, or hepatocellular carcinoma (HCC) in up to 40% of patients (Wright, 2006). Routine screening of pregnant women for HBsAg should be carried out when the hepatitis status is unknown. HBsAg can be detected in individuals with acute or chronic HBV infection.

The AAP recommends universal HBV immunization for all newborns. Newborns born to HBsAg-negative mothers should receive the first dose of vaccine at birth (before hospital discharge), with the second dose 1 to 2 months later, and the third dose by 6 to 18 months of age. An alternative schedule of vaccinations gives the HBV vaccine at 2, 4, and 6 months of age concurrently with other childhood vaccines (AAP Committee on Infectious Diseases, 2009). Babies born to HBsAg-positive mothers should receive one dose of hepatitis vaccine within 12 hours of birth, and hepatitis immunoglobulin (HBIG) should be given concurrently at a different site (AAP Committee on Infectious Diseases, 2009). HBIG provides temporary protection in postexposure situations, and HBV vaccine provides long-term protection. Newborns born to women with unknown HBsAg status should receive the first dose of HBV vaccine within 12 hours of birth (AAP & ACOG, 2007; AAP Committee on Infectious Diseases, 2009). Because the vaccine is highly effective in preventing infection in this population, further prophylaxis with HBIG can be delayed up to 7 days while awaiting maternal laboratory results.

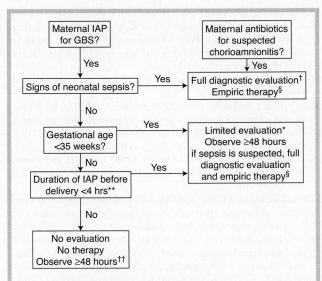

* If no maternal intrapartum prophylaxis for GBS was administered despite an indication being present, data are insufficient on which to recommend a single management strategy.

† Includes complete blood cell count and differential, blood culture, and chest radiograph if respiratory abnormalities are present. When signs of sepsis are present, a lumbar puncture, if feasible should be performed.

§ Duration of therapy varies depending on results of blood culture, cerebrospinal fluid findings, if obtained, and the clinical course of the infant. If laboratory results and clinical course do not indicate bacterial infection, duration may be as short as 48 hours.

** Applies only to penicillin, ampicillin, or cefazolin and assumes recommended dosing regimens

†† A healthy-appearing infant who was ≥38 weeks' gestation at delivery and whose mother received ≥4 hours of intrapartum prophylaxis before delivery may be discharged home after 24 hours if other discharge criteria have been met and a person able to comply fully with instructions for home observation will be present. If any one of these conditions is not met, the infant should be observed in the hospital for at least 48 hours and until criteria for discharged are achieved.

FIGURE 18–5. Management of a neonate born to a mother who received intrapartum antimicrobial prophylaxis (IAP) for prevention of early-onset group B streptococcal (GBS) disease. (From Verani, J. R., McGee, L., & Schrag, S. J. [2010]. Prevention of perinatal group B streptococcal disease—Revised guidelines from CDC. *MMWR Recommendations and Reports, 59*[RR-10], 1–36.)

SUMMARY

Most newborns need minimal support to make the transition to extrauterine life. Diverse and complex system adaptations make it a critical time for newborns. Strong desires to interact with their newborn make this a significant time for parents. The perinatal nurse must be knowledgeable about normal physiologic changes during the period of newborn transition from extrauterine life. Caring for newborns during this time requires the ability to recognize alterations from normal and becoming proficient at the skills necessary for conducting a newborn resuscitation.

REFERENCES

Alvaro, R. E., & Rigatto, H. (2005). Cardiorespiratory adjustments at birth. In *Avery's Neonatology Pathophysiology & Management of the Newborn* (6th ed., pp. 285–303). Philadelphia: Lippincott Williams & Wilkins.

American Academy of Pediatrics Committee on Fetus and Newborn. (1993). Routine evaluation of blood pressure, hematocrit, and glucose in newborns. *Pediatrics, 92*(3), 474–476.

American Academy of Pediatrics Committee on Fetus and Newborn. (2003). Controversies concerning vitamin K and the newborn. *Pediatrics, 112*(1), 191–192.

American Academy of Pediatrics Committee on Infectious Diseases. (2009). *2009 Red Book* (28th ed.). Elk Grove Village, IL: Author.

American Academy of Pediatrics & American College of Obstetricians and Gynecologists. (2007). *Guidelines for Perinatal Care* (6th ed.). Elk Grove Village, IL: Author.

American Heart Association & American Academy of Pediatrics. (2010). *Textbook of Neonatal Resuscitation* (6th ed.). Elk Grove Village, IL: American Heart Association.

Apgar, V. (1966). The newborn Apgar scoring system: Reflections and advice. *Pediatric Clinics of North America, 13*(3), 645–650.

Bagwell, G. A. (2007). Resuscitation and stabilization of the newborn and infant. In C. Kenner & J. W. Lott (Eds.), *Comprehensive Neonatal Care: An Interdisciplinary Approach* (4th ed., pp. 666–677). Philadelphia: Elsevier Saunders.

Bissinger, R. L., & Annibale, D. J. (2010). Thermoregulation in very low-birth-weight infants during the golden hour: Results and implications. *Advances in Neonatal Care, 10*(5), 230–238.

Blackburn, S. T. (2012). *Maternal, Fetal, & Neonatal Physiology. A Clinical Perspective* (4th ed.). Philadelphia: Elsevier Saunders.

Bohnhorst, B., Heyne, T., Peter, C., & Poest, C. (2001). Skin-to-skin (kangaroo) care, respiratory control and thermoregulation. *Journal of Pediatrics, 138*(2), 193–197.

Bramson, L., Lee, J. W., Moore, E., Montgomery, S., Neish, C., Bahjri, K., . . . Melcher, C. L. (2010). Effect of early skin-to-skin mother—infant contact during the first 3 hours following birth on exclusive breastfeeding during the maternity hospital stay. *Journal of Human Lactation, 26*(2), 130–137.

Brand, M. C., & Boyd, H. (2010). Thermoregulation. In T. Verklan & M. Walden (Eds.), *Core Curriculum for Neonatal Intensive Care Nursing* (4th ed., pp. 110–120). St. Louis, MO: Elsevier Saunders.

Brandtzaeg, P. (2010). The mucosal immune system and its integration with the mammary glands. *Journal of Pediatrics, 156* (2 Suppl), S8–S15.

Brown, V. D., & Landers, S. (2011). Heat balance. In G. B. Merenstein & S. L. Gardner (Eds.), *Handbook of Neonatal Intensive Care* (7th ed., pp. 113–133). St. Louis, MO: Mosby.

Bystrova, K., Ivanova, V., Edhborg, M., Matthiesen, A. S., Ransjö-Arvidson, A. B., Mukhamedrakhimov, R., . . . Widström, A. M. (2009). Early contact versus separation: Effects on mother-infant interaction one year later. *Birth, 36*(2), 97–109.

Centers for Disease Control and Prevention. (1996). Prevention of perinatal group B streptococcal disease: A public health perspective. *Morbidity and Mortality Weekly Report, 45*(RR-7), 1–24.

Centers for Disease Control and Prevention. (2005). Early-onset and late-onset neonatal group B streptococcal disease—United States, 1996–2004. *Morbidity and Mortality Weekly Report, 54*(47), 1205–1208.

Conde-Agudelo, A., Belizán, J. M., & Diaz-Rossello, J. (2011). Kangaroo mother care to reduce morbidity and mortality in low birthweight infants. *Cochrane Database of Systematic Reviews, 3*, CD002771. doi:10.1002/14651858.CD002771.pub2

DeMarini, S., & Rath, L. L. (2007). Fluids, electrolytes, vitamins, and minerals. In C. Kenner & J. W. Lott (Eds.), *Comprehensive Neonatal Care: An Interdisciplinary Approach* (4th ed., pp. 333–349). Philadelphia: Saunders.

Dore, S., Buchan, D., Coulas, S., Hamber, L., Stewart, M., Cowan, D., . . . Jamieson, L. (1998). Alcohol versus natural drying for newborn cord care. *Journal of Obstetric, Gynecologic, and Neonatal Nursing, 27*(6), 621–627.

Freed, M. D. (2006). Fetal and transitional circulation. In J. K. Keane, J. E. Lock, & D. C. Eyler (Eds.), *Nada's Pediatric Cardiology.* St. Louis, MO: Elsevier.

Gardner, S. L., Enzman-Hines, M., & Dickey, L. A. (2011). Respiratory diseases. In S. L. Gardner, B. S. Carter, M. I. Enzman-Hines, & J. A. Hernandez (Eds.), *Merenstein and Gardner's Handbook of Neonatal Intensive Care* (7th ed., pp. 581–677). St. Louis, MO: Mosby Elsevier.

Goldsmith, J. (2011). Delivery room resuscitation of the newborn. In R. J. Martin, A. A. Fanaroff, & M. C. Walsh (Eds.), *Fanaroff and Martin's Neonatal-Perinatal Medicine: Diseases of the Fetus and Infant* (9th ed.). St. Louis, MO: Elsevier Mosby.

Helve, O., Pitkänen, O., Janér, C., & Andersson, S. (2009). Pulmonary fluid balance in the human newborn infant. *Neonatology, 95*(4), 347–352.

Hsu, W. C., Yeh, L. C., Chuang, M. Y., Lo, W. T., Cheng, S. N., & Huang, C. F. (2010). Umbilical separation time delayed by alcohol application. *Annals of Tropical Paediatrics, 30*(3), 219–223.

Jain, L., & Dudell, G. G. (2006). Respiratory transition in infants delivered by cesarean section. *Seminars in Perinatology, 30*(5), 296–304.

Kattwinkel, J., Perlman, J. M., Aziz, K., Colby, C., Fairchild, K., Gallagher, J., . . . Zaichkin, J. (2010a). Neonatal resuscitation: American Heart Association guidelines for cardiopulmonary resuscitation and emergency cardiovascular care. *Pediatrics, 126*(5), e1400–1413.

Kattwinkel, J., Perlman, J. M., Aziz, K., Colby, C., Fairchild, K., Gallagher, J., . . . Zaichkin, J. (2010b). 2010 American Heart Association guidelines for cardiopulmonary resuscitation and emergency cardiovascular care science: Part 15: Neonatal resuscitation. *Circulation, 122*(18, Suppl. 3), S909–S919.

Katz, C., Bentur, L., & Elias, N. (2011). Clinical implication of lung fluid balance in the perinatal period. *Journal of Perinatology, 31*(4), 230–235.

Kent, A. (2011). Apgar scores and cerebral palsy. *Reviews in Obstetrics and Gynecology, 4*(1), 33–34.

Lam, N. C., Gotsch, P. B., & Langan, R. C. (2010). Caring for pregnant women and newborns with hepatitis B or C. *American Family Physician, 15*(10), 1225–1229.

Lie, K. K., Grøholt, E. K., & Eskild, A. (2010). Association of cerebral palsy with Apgar score in low and normal birthweight infants: Population based cohort study. *BMJ, 341*, 4990.

Lott, J. W. (2007). Cardiovascular system. In C. Kenner & J. W. Lott (Eds.), *Comprehensive Neonatal Care: An Interdisciplinary Approach* (4th ed., pp. 32–64). Philadelphia: Saunders.

Manco-Johnson, M., Rodden, D. J., & Hays, T. (2011). Newborn hematology. In G. B. Merenstein & S. L. Gardner (Eds.), *Handbook of Neonatal Intensive Care* (7th ed., pp. 503–530). St. Louis, MO: Mosby.

Mast, E. E., Margolis, H. S., Fiore, A. E., Brink, E. W., et al. (2005). A comprehensive immunization strategy to eliminate transmission of hepatitis B virus infection in the United States: Recommendations of the Advisory Committee on Immunization Practices (ACIP) part 1: Immunization of infants, children, and adolescents. *MMWR Recomm Rep, 23;54*(RR-16):1–31.

McDaniel, N. L. (2010) Alterations of cardiovascular function in children. In K. L. McCance, S. E. Huether, V. L. Brashers, & N. S. Rote (Eds.), *Pathophysiology: The Biologic Basis for Disease in Adults and Children* (6th ed., pp. 1209–1241). Maryland Heights, MS: Mosby Elsevier.

Miller, R. S. (2007). Preventing infant abduction in the hospital. *Nursing, 37*(10), 20–22.

Moore, E. R., Anderson, G. C., & Bergman, N. (2007). Early skin-to-skin contact for mothers and their healthy newborn infants. *Cochrane Database of Systematic Reviews, 18*(3), CD003519.

National Center for Missing and Exploited Children. (2009). *Guidelines on prevention of and response to infant abductions.* Retrieved from http://www.missingkids.com/en_US/publications/NC05.pdf

National Center for Missing and Exploited Children. (2011). *Newborn/infant abductions.* Retrieved from http://www.missingkids.com/en_US/documents/InfantAbductionStats.pdf

Paxton, J. M., & Harrell, H. (1991). Delivery room management of the asphyxiated neonate. *NAACOG's Clinical Issues in Perinatal and Women's Health Nursing, 2*(1), 35–47.

Schrag, S. J., Zell, E. R., Lynfield, R., Roome, A., Arnold, K. E., Craig, A. S., . . . Schuchat A. (2002). A population-based comparison of strategies to prevent early-onset group B streptococcal disease in neonates. *New England Journal of Medicine, 347*(4), 233–239.

Slowik, M. K., & Jhaveri, R. (2005). Hepatitis B and C viruses in infants and young children. *Seminars in Pediatric Infectious Diseases, 16*(4), 296–305.

Steinhorn, R. H. (2011). The cardiovascular system: Part 2 pulmonary vascular development. In R. J. Martin, A. A. Fanaroff, & M. C. Walsh (Eds.), *Fanaroff and Martin's Neonatal-Perinatal Medicine: Diseases of the Fetus and Infant* (9th ed., pp. 1216–1221). St. Louis, MO: Elsevier Mosby.

Strunk, T., Currie, A., Richmond, P., Simmer, K., & Burgner, D., (2011). Innate immunity in human newborn infants: Prematurity means more than immaturity. *Journal of Maternal Fetal &Neonatal Medicine, 24*(1), 25–31.

U. S. Preventive Services Task Force. (2010). Screening for hepatitis B virus infection in pregnancy: Reaffirmation recommendation statement. *American Family Physician, 81*(4), 502.

van den Berg, J. P., Westerbeek, E. A., van der Klis, F. R., Berbers, G. A., & van Elburg, R. M. (2011). Transplacental transport of IgG antibodies to preterm infants: A review of the literature. *Early Human Development, 87*(2), 67–72.

Vargo, L. (2009). Cardiovascular assessment. In E. P. Tappero & M. E. Honeyfield (Eds.), *Physical Assessment of the Newborn* (4th ed., pp. 87–105). Santa Rosa, CA: NICU INK.

Verani, J. R., McGee, L., & Schrag, S. J. (2010). Prevention of perinatal group B streptococcal disease—Revised guidelines from CDC. *MMWR Recommendations and Reports, 59*(RR-10), 1–36.

Verani, J. R., & Schrag, S. J. (2010). Group B streptococcal disease in infants: Progress in prevention and continued challenges. *Clinical Perinatology, 37*(2), 375–392.

Vincent, J. L. (2009). Infant hospital abduction: Security measures to aid in prevention. *MCN: American Journal of Maternal Child Nursing, 34*(3), 179–183.

Wright, T. L. (2006). Introduction to chronic hepatitis B infection. *American Journal of Gastroenterology, 101*(1, Suppl.), S1–S6.

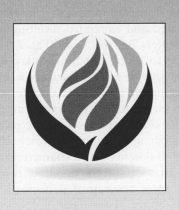

Lyn Vargo

CHAPTER 19

Newborn Physical Assessment

Perinatal and neonatal nurses frequently perform the first head-to-toe physical assessment of the newborn. Ideally, this examination occurs in the presence of the parents. Conducting the examination while parents observe allows the nurse to use this time to identify and discuss normal newborn characteristics and note variations. It also provides an opportunity for parents to ask questions about the newborn's physical appearance and condition. The focus of this chapter is the physical assessment and findings that the perinatal nurse may observe during the time the newborn is in the hospital or birthing center. Home care nurses may also find the information pertinent during early postpartum home visits. Although some references are made to preterm newborns, that subject is not the intended focus of this chapter. It is also assumed that the reader has basic knowledge of physical assessment skills and terminology. Normal findings and common variations for each body system are identified in the text. Tables describe pathologic findings and their causes.

Physical assessment skills of observation, palpation, and auscultation are used frequently throughout the examination. Percussion is not commonly used in the newborn exam. When performing a physical assessment, the following equipment should be available: scale, tape measure, tongue blades, stethoscope with a neonatal diaphragm and bell, and an ophthalmoscope. The initial physical assessment may be conducted with the infant under a radiant warmer or in an open crib. Regardless of the location, attention should be given to avoiding hypothermia and cold stress. Adequate lighting is also essential.

The sequence in which the nurse conducts the physical assessment is a matter of personal preference and most often depends on the cooperation of the newborn. Although we present the newborn assessment as a sequential examination covering one system at a time, the exam can be appropriately conducted in a cephalocaudal fashion, system by system, and more than one system concurrently.

The physical assessment usually begins by observing the breathing pattern, overall skin color, general state or level of alertness, posture, and muscle tone. The newborn's *state* refers to general level of alertness and is a reflection of a group of characteristics that occur together. In the newborn, these characteristics include body activity, eye movement, facial movements, breathing pattern, and level of response to internal and external stimuli (Pearson, 1999). Understanding the differences in state provides information about how the newborn will respond to the nurse or parents and about the condition of the newborn's health, and it has implications for parent education. Appendix 19–A describes newborn states, deep sleep, light sleep, drowsy, quiet alert, active alert, and crying and the implications these states have for caregivers.

The newborn is weighed and measured. It is normal for newborns to lose up to 10% of their birth weight during the first few days of life. Figure 19–1 illustrates the technique for obtaining accurate measurements. Normal measurements are:

- Head circumference, 32 to 38 cm (13 to 15 inches)
- Chest circumference, 30 to 36 cm (12 to 14 inches)
- Length, 45 to 55 cm (18 to 22 inches)

GESTATIONAL AGE ASSESSMENT

The American Academy of Pediatrics (AAP) and American College of Obstetricians and Gynecologists (ACOG) (2007) recommend that the gestational age of newborns

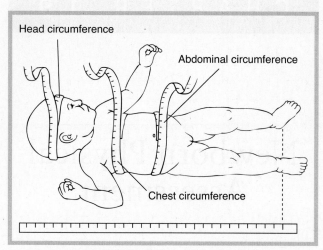

Head circumference

Abdominal circumference

Chest circumference

FIGURE 19–1. Newborn measurements. (Adapted from Wong, D. L. [Ed.]. [1997]. *Whaley & Wong's Nursing Care of Infants and Children* [6th ed., p. 139]. St. Louis, MO: Mosby-Year Book.)

be established by incorporating both obstetric and the initial physical and neurologic findings of the newborn. A gestational age assessment, evaluating physical and neuromuscular characteristics, is usually performed as part of the initial physical examination. Although some hospitals make gestational age assessment of all newborns a routine practice, other institutions have established criteria for performing gestational age assessment such as birth weight less than 2,500 g or more than 4,082 g, suspected intrauterine growth restriction (IUGR), gestation less than 37 weeks, and cesarean birth; and in some organizations, it is not part of the nursing assessment but instead determined during the primary care provider's assessment. Identifying newborns that are preterm, term, or postterm and those who are IUGR, small for gestational age (SGA), appropriate for gestational age (AGA), or large for gestational age (LGA) increases the likelihood of early identification and timely interventions for potential complications related to birth weight and gestational age during the immediate newborn period.

The original tool used for gestational assessment was the Dubowitz Scoring System. It contained 20 items combining neurologic and physical parameters that successfully estimated gestational age in infants older than 34 weeks (Dubowitz, Dubowitz, & Goldberg, 1970). The tool was revised in 1999, increasing the number of items on the neurologic exam. The test expanded the neurologic exam to include behavior states, tone, primitive reflexes, motility, and some aspects of behavior (Dubowitz, Ricci, & Mercuri, 2005).

The Ballard Maturational Score (BMS), developed in the late 1970s (Ballard, Novak, & Driver, 1979), is commonly used for determining gestational age. The original BMS contained 12 items based on the Dubowitz Scoring System. As more low-birth-weight infants were born and survived the initial neonatal period, an instrument that could accurately measure their gestational age was needed to plan initial care. In 1991, the BMS was reevaluated and expanded resulting in the development of a New Ballard Score (Fig. 19–2), which is what most organizations are using today. Criteria were broadened to provide greater accuracy when evaluating extremely premature neonates (Ballard et al., 1991).

The BMS is conducted by comparing the individual newborn's characteristics with the pictures on the form and assigning a number for each characteristic. Appendix 19–B describes each characteristic evaluated. Controversy exists about the timing of this assessment. The BMS is most accurate if performed between 10 and 36 hours of age. Assessment of newborns younger than 26 weeks' gestation is best conducted within the first 12 hours (Gagliardi, Brambilla, Bruno, Martinelli, & Console, 1993). The examination is separated into two parts: neuromuscular maturity assessment and physical maturity assessment. Scores from both sections are added together to determine gestational age.

SKIN ASSESSMENT

The newborn's entire body, as well as skin folds and scalp, should be inspected and palpated for changes in texture and the presence of masses that are not visible. Color, birth marks, rashes, skin lesions, texture, and turgor are noted. At birth, newborn skin may be covered with vernix, an odorless, white, cheesy, protective coating produced by sebaceous glands. Vernix develops during the third trimester and increases with gestational age. At about 37 weeks, the amount of vernix begins to decrease, and at term, it is present only in the creases of the arms, legs, and neck.

COLOR

Skin color reflects circulation, oxygenation, and hemoglobin saturation. Color is best observed in a well-lit room while the newborn is quiet. At birth, color ranges from pale to plethoric, depending on hematocrit and general perfusion. Skin pigmentation depends on ethnic origin and deepens over time. Caucasian newborns have pinkish red skin tones a few hours after birth, and African American newborns have a reddish-brown skin color. Hispanic and Asian newborns have an olive or yellow skin tone. Changes in the skin color of Caucasian newborns may be the first sign of illness such as sepsis, cardiopulmonary disorders, or hematologic diseases. Variations in skin color indicating illness are more difficult to evaluate in African American and Asian newborns.

Generalized or *central cyanosis* may be seen initially at the time of birth as the newborn transitions from fetal to neonatal circulation. Central cyanosis occurring beyond the initial minutes following birth refers to bluish color of the tongue, skin, lips and nail beds in the newborn and, when seen, requires urgent attention by a

Neuromuscular Maturity

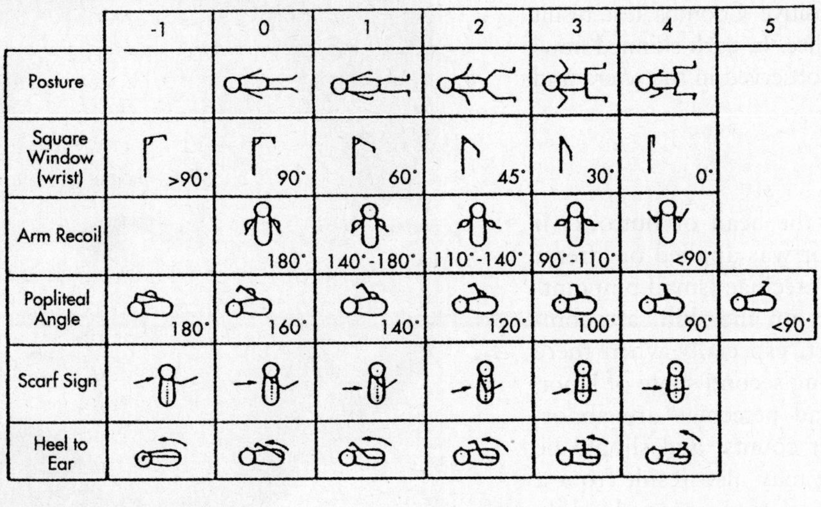

	-1	0	1	2	3	4	5
Posture							
Square Window (wrist)	>90°	90°	60°	45°	30°	0°	
Arm Recoil		180°	140°-180°	110°-140°	90°-110°	<90°	
Popliteal Angle	180°	160°	140°	120°	100°	90°	<90°
Scarf Sign							
Heel to Ear							

Physical Maturity

Skin	sticky friable transparent	gelatinous red, translucent	smooth pink visible veins	superficial peeling &/or rash few veins	cracking pale areas rare veins	parchment deep cracking no vessels	leathery cracked wrinkled
Lanugo	none	sparse	abundant	thinning	bald areas	mostly bald	
Plantar Surface	heel-toe 40-50 mm:-1 < 40 mm:-2	>50mm no crease	faint red marks	anterior transverse crease only	creases ant. 2/3	creases over entire sole	
Breast	imperceptible	barely perceptible	flat areola no bud	stippled areola 1-2mm bud	raised areola 3-4mm bud	full areola 5-10 mm bud	
Eye/Ear	lids fused loosely:-1 tightly:-2	lids open pinna flat stays folded	sl. curved pinna; soft; slow recoil	well-curved pinna: soft but ready recoil	formed & firm instant recoil	thick cartilage ear stiff	
Genitals male	scrotum flat, smooth	scrotum empty faint rugae	testes in upper canal rare rugae	testes descending few rugae	testes down good rugae	testes pendulous deep rugae	
Genitals female	clitoris prominent labia flat	prominent clitoris small labia minora	prominent clitoris enlarging minora	majora & minora equally prominent	majora large minora small	majora cover clitoris & minora	

Maturity Rating

score	weeks
-10	20
-5	22
-0	24
5	26
10	28
15	30
20	32
25	34
30	36
35	38
40	40
45	42
50	44

FIGURE 19–2. Gestational age assessment. (From Ballard, J. L., Khoury, J. C., Wedig, K., Wang, L., Ellers-Walsman, B. L., & Lipp, R. [1991]. New Ballard Score, expanded to include extremely premature infants. *Journal of Pediatrics, 119*[3], 417–423.)

physician or advanced practice nurse as it usually indicates a pathologic condition. It is the usually seen when there is less than 5 g of unsaturated hemoglobin per 100 mL of blood or a saturation of <85% (Hernandez & Glass, 2005). *Acrocyanosis*, the blue discoloration of newborn hands and feet, and *circumoral cyanosis*, a bluish color seen around the newborn's mouth, are normal findings and are often seen in the first 24 to 48 hours of life. Acrocyanosis is related to vasomotor instability and tends to worsen if the newborn becomes cold.

JAUNDICE

Jaundice, a bright yellow or orange discoloration of the skin, results from deposits of unconjugated bilirubin. Up to 60% of healthy term newborns develop some degree of jaundice (Kaplan, Wong, Sibley, & Stevenson, 2011). Jaundice results from the reduced ability of the newborn's liver to conjugate bilirubin. A mildly elevated indirect bilirubin level is considered normal in the first few days of life. An elevated direct bilirubin level that may occur as early as 24 hours of life is never normal and suggests some pathology involving the liver. The skin color change associated with an elevated direct bilirubin has a greenish hue (Gomella, Cunningham, & Eyal, 2009a). Jaundice progresses in a cephalocaudal fashion. Seen first on the head and face, jaundice progresses downward to the trunk and extremities and then to the sclera of the eye. When gentle pressure is applied to skin over cartilage or a bony prominence, skin blanches to a yellow hue on the face when bilirubin levels are 5 mg/dL, on the upper chest when levels are about 10 mg/dL, on the abdomen when levels are 12 mg/dL, and on the palms and soles of the feet when levels are greater than 15 mg/dL (Gomella et al., 2009b). Newborns with a positive Coombs test result almost certainly develop jaundice. In dark-skinned newborns, jaundice is more easily observed in the sclera and buccal mucosa.

BRUISING

Ecchymosis may occur over the head or buttocks if forceps or a vacuum extractor was applied or after a breech or face presentation. Petechiae (small pinpoint-sized reddish to purple spots on the skin) are common over the presenting part, especially when there has been a rapid descent during second stage of labor, but generalized or widespread petechiae are abnormal, may signify low platelet counts, and should be further investigated. Bruising may also result from a tight nuchal cord or an umbilical cord wrapped tightly around the upper body.

VARIATIONS RELATED TO VASOMOTOR INSTABILITY

Cutis marmorata, mottling, or a lacelike pattern on the skin is a vasomotor response to chilling. Parents should be aware that this may continue after discharge. The harlequin sign occurs when some newborns are positioned on their sides. The dependent side of the body becomes pink, and the superior half of the body is pale. This phenomenon is considered benign. The color change lasts 1 to 30 minutes and disappears gradually when the infant is placed on the abdomen or back (Witt, 2009).

Hemangiomas

Hemangiomas are vascular soft tissue tumors. They may be present at birth and may begin as a pale macule with threadlike markings and develop into a bright red elevated tumor that ranges in size. They can also develop in the first several weeks of life. One percent to 3% of newborns have hemangiomas, and they are more likely to occur in females than in males (Fig. 19–3). They are generally benign and self-limiting in that they often initially grow but then involute without treatment. However, they may ulcerate, become cavernous, and cause disfigurement or may require intervention (Hoath & Narendran, 2011).

NEVUS SIMPLEX

Commonly referred to as "stork bites" or salmon patches, these lesions composed of dilated capillaries are macular, irregularly shaped, reddish-colored patches that blanch with pressure and become darker when the newborn cries. Lesions may last 1 to 2 years or persist into adulthood. The most common newborn skin lesion, they are most often seen at the back of the neck, on the forehead,

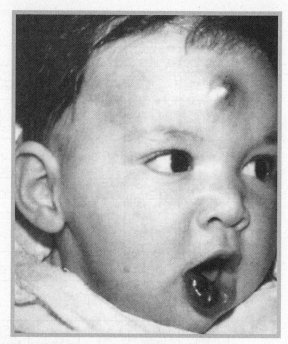

FIGURE 19–3. Hemangioma of the forehead and lip.

on eyelids, on the bridge of the nose, and over the base of the occipital bones. They may occur in up to 70% of newborns (Hoath & Narendran, 2011).

PORT-WINE STAIN

Port-wine stains are irregularly shaped, flat pink to reddish markings that are most often present at birth. Color varies from pink in Caucasian infants to black or deep purple in African American newborns or newborns of color. Most often seen on the head and neck, port-wine stains have discrete borders, do not blanch when pressure is applied, and do not lighten as the child ages (Witt, 2009). These lesions composed of dilated capillaries are generally benign unless they occur along the trigeminal nerve root, in which case they may be associated with glaucoma or optic atrophy, seizures, and mental retardation (Hoath & Narendran, 2011). Certain types of lasers effectively remove port-wine stains and can be used safely on infants.

MONGOLIAN SPOTS

Mongolian spots are large, nonblanching, blue-gray lesions resembling a bruise that are most often seen over the sacrum and flanks but may be present on the posterior thighs, legs, back, and shoulders (Fig. 19–4). They occur frequently in African American, Asian, and Native American infants but can be observed in Caucasian infants (Hoath & Narendran, 2011). Mongolian spots are caused by infiltration of melanin-forming cells into the dermal skin layer rather than the epidermis. Mongolian spots may persist into early childhood but usually fade.

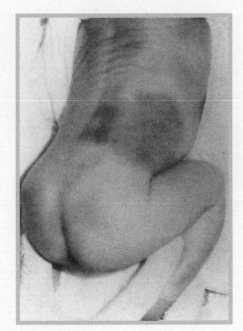

FIGURE 19–4. Mongolian spots.

newborns that are post–40 weeks. At term, lanugo is usually confined to the shoulders, ears, and forehead.

TURGOR

Skin turgor is the natural rebound elasticity of the skin. It can be assessed anywhere on the body by pinching the skin between the examiner's thumb and index finger and then quickly releasing it. Skin turgor is best assessed on the abdomen. Healthy, elastic tissue rapidly resumes its normal position without creases or tenting. Skin that remains tented indicates poor hydration and nutritional status. Table 19–1 identifies skin findings during the physical assessment that are abnormal and their related pathology.

ERYTHEMA TOXICUM

Erythema toxicum, also called newborn rash, is benign and generally occurs within 5 days of birth in approximately 50% of term newborn infants (Lund & Kuller, 2007). In preterm newborns, the rash may not develop for several days or weeks. Erythema toxicum is composed of small, yellow papules surrounded by an erythematous margin. The rash continues to appear and disappear over various parts of the body for several days. Most commonly seen on the face, trunk, and limbs, it may continue to appear up to 3 months of age (Witt, 2009).

MILIA

Milia are clogged sebaceous glands that appear as tiny, white, pinhead-sized papules presenting at birth over the chin, cheeks, forehead, and nose. They are benign and disappear during the first month of life (Lund & Kuller, 2007).

TEXTURE

Skin is evaluated for texture and the presence of lanugo during the physical examination and as part of the gestational age assessment. Texture ranges from smooth to cracked and peeling. Shortly after birth, most term newborns have dry, flaky skin. Peeling, leathery skin with deep cracks indicates postmaturity. Lanugo, a fine, downy hair that covers the body, begins to develop around 12 weeks and is abundant by 17 to 20 weeks' gestation (Moore & Persaud, 2008). It is seen in abundance on premature infants. However, it becomes less abundant as gestation increases and is rarely on

Table 19–1. INTEGUMENT

Assessment	Pathology
Pallor	Anemia Asphyxia Shock Sepsis Twin-to-twin transfusion Cardiac disease
Central cyanosis	Respiratory disorder Persistent pulmonary hypertension Neurologic disease Congenital heart disease Sepsis
Plethora	Polycythemia Overheated
Gray color	Sepsis Shock
Jaundice within 24 hr of birth	Liver disease Sepsis Maternal ingestion of drugs (e.g., aspirin) Blood incompatibilities
Generalized petechiae	Thrombocytopenia Clotting disorders Sepsis
Pustules	*Staphylococcus* Beta-hemolytic *Streptococcus* Varicella
Greenish, yellow vernix	Meconium staining Hemolytic disease
Generalized edema	Erythroblastosis fetalis Renal failure Turner syndrome
"Blueberry muffin" spots (purpura)	Congenital viral infection
Multiple tan or light brown macules (café au lait spots)	Neurofibromatosis
Cutis marmorata	Hypovolemia Sepsis Chromosomal abnormalities
Extensive Mongolian spots	Inborn errors of metabolism (Silengo, Battistoni, & Spada, 1999)

HEAD ASSESSMENT

The newborn head is examined using inspection and palpation and assessed for size, shape, and symmetry. The head of a term, AGA newborn has an occipital–frontal circumference (OFC) of 32 to 38 cm (12.5 to 14.5 inches). To measure the newborn's head, a tape measure is placed just above the eyebrows and continues around to the occipital prominence at the back of the skull (see Fig. 19–1). At birth, most skull deformities are the result of position in utero, decrease in space in utero due to multiple gestation, decreased amniotic fluid, or intrapartum events (AAP, 2003). Vaginal birth may cause the cranial bones to overlap (i.e., molding) as the fetus descends through the birth canal or as a result of the application of vacuum or forceps, giving the head an elongated, asymmetric appearance (Fig. 19–5). The overlapping cranial bones can be palpated along the suture lines. Molding may last several days and cause the head circumference to be smaller immediately after birth. The circumference returns to normal within 2 to 3 days after birth. Newborns delivered by cesarean section or in breech position have a more rounded, symmetric head.

Examination of the newborn head may reveal evidence of birth trauma such as bruising or swelling. A cephalhematoma is a common finding following vaginal delivery. It is a collection of blood between the skull and periosteum, which causes a distinct swelling on the newborn head. Cephalhematomas have clearly demarcated edges and are restricted by suture lines. Common

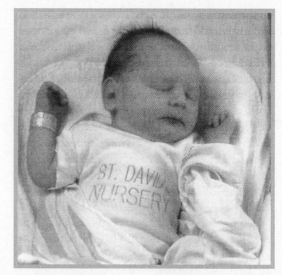

FIGURE 19–5. Molding. (From Pillitteri, A. [2003]. *Maternal and Child Health Nursing* [4th ed., p. 644]. Philadelphia: Lippincott Williams & Wilkins.)

locations for cephalhematomas are the occipital and parietal bones. If large, they can contribute to hyperbilirubinemia and jaundice but in general will resolve in several weeks or months.

Caput succedaneum, edema under the scalp, is caused by pressure over the presenting part of the newborn's head against the cervix during labor. Caput feels soft and spongy, crosses suture lines, and resolves within a few days. Figure 19–6 pictorially compares the location of caput succedaneum and cephalhematoma.

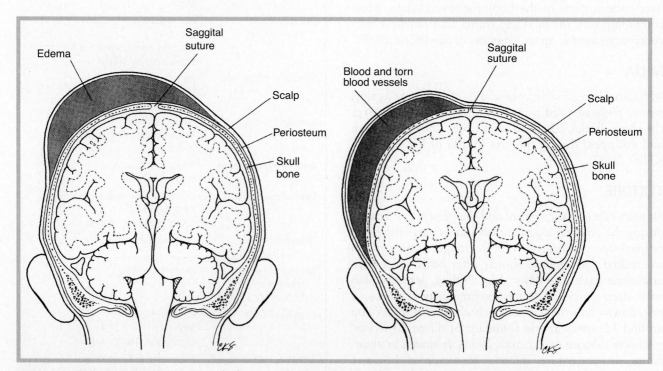

FIGURE 19–6. Comparison of caput succedaneum (*left*) and cephalhematoma (*right*).

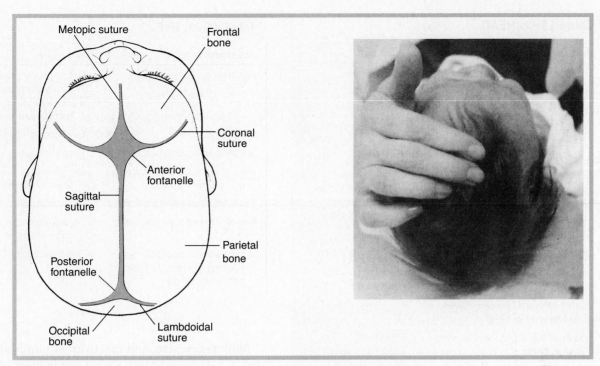

Metopic suture

Frontal bone

Coronal suture

Anterior fontanelle

Sagittal suture

Parietal bone

Posterior fontanelle

Occipital bone

Lambdoidal suture

FIGURE 19–7. Palpating the fontanelles.

The newborn's head is palpated for the presence of all suture lines (Fig. 19–7). Suture lines feel like soft depressions between the cranial bones. If instead a ridge of bone is felt, the examiner should determine whether it is the result of molding or premature closure of the suture. Normal mobility of the cranial bones is determined by placing each thumb on opposite sides of the suture and alternately pushing in slightly on each side. Lack of mobility of cranial bones indicates premature closure of the sutures (i.e., craniosynostosis). Craniosynostosis causes an abnormally shaped head, as the contents of the cranium enlarge, but the cranial bones do not. This abnormally shaped head may be apparent at birth or later in infancy.

The skull is palpated for masses and assessed for craniotabes. Craniotabes are a softening of cranial bones caused by pressure of the fetal skull against the bony pelvis. When pressure is exerted with the examiner's fingers at the margins of the parietal or occipital bones, a popping sensation similar to indenting a ping-pong ball is felt. Craniotabes is primarily seen in breech presentations and usually disappears within a few weeks.

Anterior and posterior fontanelles, the soft membranous coverings where two sutures meet, are palpated and measured (see Fig. 19–7). Fontanelles are measured diagonally from bone to bone rather than from suture to suture. They vary in size. The anterior fontanelle is diamond shaped, generally measures 1 to 4 cm, and closes around 18 months of age. The posterior fontanelle is triangular, generally measures less than a

fingertip, and closes between 2 and 4 months (Gardner & Hernandez, 2011). Fontanelles are best palpated when the newborn is quiet. The anterior area should be soft, often is depressed slightly, and may bulge with crying. Arterial pulsations may be felt over the anterior fontanelle. Molding may make it impossible to palpate fontanelles in the first few hours of life. Large fontanelles may be associated with various disorders (such as congenital hypothyroidism) and are a notable finding.

The scalp is examined for distribution, amount, and texture of hair. Hair is silky and may be straight, curly, or kinky, depending on ethnic origin. Bruising, lacerations, and bleeding are frequently seen as the result of the application of a scalp electrode or vacuum extractor. Table 19–2 identifies findings during the physical assessment of the head that are abnormal and their related pathology.

EYE ASSESSMENT

The newborn's eyes are assessed using inspection and an ophthalmoscope. This can be done early in the examination as part of the assessment of the head or whenever the newborn spontaneously opens his or her eyes. Although rarely accomplished, it is best done prior to insertion of prophylaxis. Eyes should be symmetric in size and shape. Lids may be edematous and puffy at birth. The distance between the eyes, measured from the inner canthus of each, is 1.5 to 2.5 cm

Table 19–2. HEAD

Assessment	Pathology
The following assessments may indicate increased intracranial pressure:	Hydrocephalus
Sutures separated more than 1 cm	Hypothyroidism
Bulging, tense anterior fontanelle	Tumor
Head circumference greater than 90th percentile for gestational age	Meningitis
Head circumference below 10th percentile for gestational age	Genetic disorder Congenital infection Maternal drug or alcohol ingestion
Depressed anterior fontanelle	Dehydration
Cephalhematoma: swelling due to bleeding between periosteum and skull bone; does not cross suture line; may not be evident until 1 day after birth and take several weeks to resolve (see Fig. 19–6)	Head trauma during birth
Texture of hair is fine, woolly, sparse, coarse, brittle	Prematurity Endocrine disorder Genetic disorder
Increased quantity of hair, low-set hairline	Genetic disorder
Limited forward growth of the skull; skull appears broad	Brachycephaly (fused coronal suture)
Limited lateral growth of the skull; skull appears long and narrow	Scaphocephaly (fused sagittal suture)

Table 19–3. EYE

Assessment	Pathology
Persistent purulent discharge	Ophthalmia neonatorum Chlamydial conjunctivitis Blocked lacrimal duct (dacryocystitis)
Blue sclera	Osteogenesis imperfecta
Sclera visible above iris (sunset eyes)	Hydrocephalus
Black or white spots on periphery of iris (Brushfield spots)	Benign or associated with Down syndrome
Pupils not equal, nonreactive, fixed	Neurologic insult
Keyhole-shaped pupil (coloboma)	Usually associated with other anomalies
Upward slant of palpebral fissures (opening between the upper and lower eyelids)	Down syndrome

Blink reflex, size, and reactivity of pupils are evaluated in a darkened room with a pen light or light from the ophthalmoscope. Pupils are equal and reactive to light (PERL). When a light is shined at an angle toward the eye, the lens should be clear. Equal color, intensity, and clarity of the red reflex in both eyes without opacities or white spots within either red reflex is considered a normal exam (AAP, 2008). Presence and clarity of the red reflex indicates an intact cornea and lens. Lack of a red reflex suggests congenital glaucoma or cataracts. Pale red reflexes are a normal variation in dark-skinned newborns.

Movement of the eye is observed. Strabismus, a cross-eyed appearance, is often seen in newborns because of weak eye musculature and lack of coordination. Nystagmus (i.e., constant, rapid, involuntary movement of the eye) may occur and usually disappears by 4 months of age. Newborns are nearsighted at birth and respond to bright or primary colors and to high contrast between colors such as black and white. They see objects clearly 8 to 10 inches in front of them. Table 19–3 identifies findings during the physical assessment of the eye that are abnormal and their related pathology.

EAR ASSESSMENT

The newborn ear is assessed by inspection and palpation. External structures are examined for position, presence of abnormal structures, and injury, which may have occurred during the birth process. The pinna normally lies on or above an imaginary line drawn from the inner to the outer canthus of the eye, back toward the ear (Fig. 19–8). Low-set ears, those that fall below this line, may be associated with genetic

(Hernandez & Glass, 2005). Eyes spaced closer (i.e., hypotelorism) or farther apart (i.e., hypertelorism) may be a variation of normal or associated with other anomalies. Eyes with small palpebral fissures (i.e., eye openings) may also be normal or associated with other anomalies.

The colors of eye structures are observed. The iris is usually slate gray, brown, or dark blue. Eye color becomes permanent at about 6 months of age. The normally blue-white sclera may contain subconjunctival hemorrhages, the result of ruptured capillaries during the birth process. Subconjunctival hemorrhages usually resolve within a week. A yellow sclera indicates hyperbilirubinemia. Years ago when silver nitrate was the standard of care for prophylaxis against ophthalmia neonatorum, the conjunctiva would frequently become inflamed. Today, most hospitals are using erythromycin ointment, which usually does not cause this complication.

Tears are usually absent in the newborn until the lachrymal duct becomes fully patent at about 4 to 6 months of age. Prominent epicanthal folds (i.e., Mongolian slant) is a normal finding in Asian infants but may suggest Down syndrome in other ethnic groups.

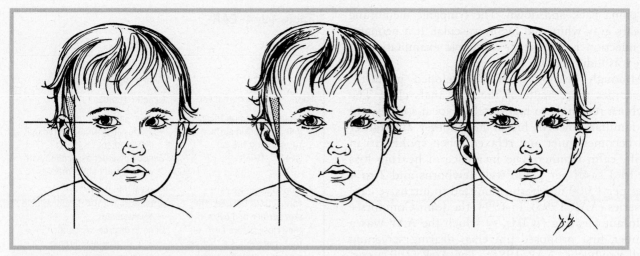

FIGURE 19–8. Normal ear position (*left*). Abnormally angled ear (*middle*). Low-set ears (*right*). (From Reeder, S. J., Martin, L. L., & Koniak-Griffin, D. [1997]. *Maternity Nursing: Family, Newborn and Women's Health* [18th ed., p. 706]. Philadelphia: Lippincott-Raven.)

syndromes. Temporary asymmetry of the ears can result from intrauterine position. Skin tags (Fig. 19–9) and small pits (Fig. 19–10) located anterior to the ear are usually benign, may be familial, but can also be associated with hearing loss and renal abnormalities. Malformation of the ears may be associated with renal abnormalities, chromosomal abnormalities, and other congenital problems (Gardner & Hernandez, 2011). Presence of ecchymosis, swelling, abrasions, or lacerations may be the result of pressure during the birth process, application of forceps or vacuum, or injury during cesarean section.

The ear is palpated as part of the gestational assessment to determine the presence and firmness of cartilage. By 38 to 40 weeks' gestation, the pinna is firm and well formed by cartilage, and incurving is present over two thirds of the ear. A soft pinna lacking cartilage is seen in premature newborns. At term, folding the pinna of the ear inward and releasing should result in brisk recoil. The more premature a newborn is, the slower the pinna will be to return to its normal position. The pinna of an extremely premature infant may remain folded.

The ear canal is inspected for patency. Use of the otoscope is limited because newborn ear canals contain vernix, mucus, and cellular debris. The ear canals clear spontaneously several days after birth. At this time, the tympanic membrane is visualized by pulling

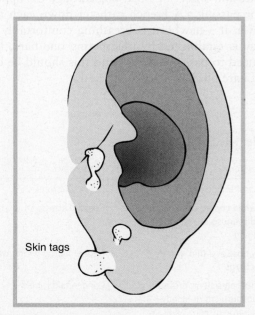

FIGURE 19–9. Preauricular skin tags.

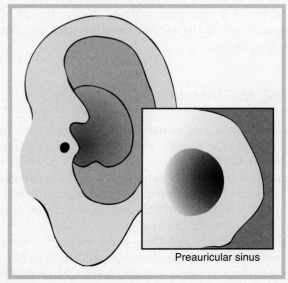

FIGURE 19–10. Preauricular sinus.

the pinna back and down. The tympanic membrane appears gray-white and highly vascular. If a neonatal ear infection is suspected, otoscopic examination of the ear is indicated.

Although hearing is well developed at birth, it becomes more acute as the ear canals clear. The newborn responds to high-pitched vocal sounds and the familiar voice of his or her mother and father and becomes quiet and relaxed when spoken to in a soft, calm manner. The incidence of hearing loss is 1 to 3 cases per 1,000 well newborns and 2 to 4 cases per 1,000 newborns admitted to intensive care nurseries (AAP, 1995). In 1994, the Joint Committee on Infant Hearing (JCIH), of which the AAP was a member, first proposed universal hearing screening of all newborns (AAP, 1995). The AAP (2007) currently recommends that all newborns should receive hearing screening using a physiologic measure by 1 month of age (preferably before hospital discharge). Two technologies are available for hearing screening: evoked otoacoustic emissions (OAE) and auditory brainstem response (ABR). Both methods are noninvasive, quick, and easy to perform. However, OAEs reflect only the status of the peripheral auditory system up to the cochlear outer hair cells, while ABRs can also detect neural dysfunction. It is for this reason that infants that have been hospitalized in the neonatal intensive care unit (NICU) for greater than 5 days are to have ABR screening rather than OAE screening, so that neural hearing loss can be identified (AAP, 2007).

Support for universal newborn hearing screening (UNHS) is based on the premise that if identification and intervention occur by 6 months of age for newborns that are hard of hearing or deaf, the infants will perform significantly higher on vocabulary, articulation, and other school-related measures because of the ability for language development (AAP, 2007).

Table 19–4 identifies findings during the physical assessment of the ear that are abnormal and their related pathology.

NOSE ASSESSMENT

The newborn's nose is assessed using inspection. The nose should be symmetric and midline but may be misshapen at birth because of the neonate's positioning in utero. If the septum cannot be easily straightened and the nose remains asymmetric, treatment may be required. A flattened or bruised nose may result from passage through the birth canal.

Nasal stuffiness and thin, white mucus is not an uncommon finding immediately after birth. Newborns sneeze to clear the upper respiratory tract. Nasal flaring, widening of the nares, is a compensatory mechanism

Table 19–4. EAR

Assessment	Pathology
Low-set ears	Genetic disorder Kidney abnormality
Poorly formed external ear	Genetic disorder
Skin tags located on the ear lobe or the skin surface surrounding the ear (see Fig. 19–9)	Familial variation Alteration in normal embryologic development Genetic disorder associated with urinary tract abnormalities
Preauricular sinuses are connections between the skin surface and cysts. If they close before birth, all that is present is a "pit" or pinpoint size indentation located in front of the ear (see Fig. 19–10).	Familial variation Alteration in normal embryologic development Genetic disorder associated with deafness and renal abnormalities
Absence of Moro reflex	Hearing loss—if sound was used to stimulate the Moro—if positional change was used, this would not be true
Microtia—abnormally small, underdeveloped external ear	Associated with inner ear malformations and hearing loss

that decreases upper airway resistance, allowing more air to enter the nasal passages. Nasal flaring is abnormal and one of the first symptoms observed when respiratory distress occurs. Table 19–5 identifies findings during the physical assessment of the nose that are abnormal and their related pathology.

Bilateral nasal patency should be established in all newborns as they are obligatory nose breathers. Patency should be determined by either obstructing one nare and observing breathing through the opposite nare or passing a 5 French catheter down each nare. However, if a newborn is breathing comfortably and patency is established by obstructing one nare, there is no need to pass a catheter, and this should be done only if nare obstruction is suspected.

Table 19–5. NOSE

Assessment	Pathology
Flat nasal bridge	Down syndrome
Pink when crying; chest retractions and cyanosis at rest; difficulty feeding	Choanal atresia
Stuffy nose and thin, watery discharge	Neonatal drug withdrawal
"Sniffles" persistent; profuse mucopurulent or bloody discharge (Green, 1998)	Congenital syphilis

MOUTH ASSESSMENT

The newborn mouth is assessed using inspection and palpation. In the sequence of the total examination, this assessment is frequently left until last. If the newborn's mouth is forced open, crying may result, altering aspects of the respiratory or cardiac assessments. The lips are observed for location, color, and symmetry. The mouth should be centrally located along the midline. At rest, the lips appear symmetric. Depending on skin color, the lips are pink or more darkly pigmented. Sucking blisters, centrally located on the upper lip, may be filled with fluid or have the consistency of a callus. Calluses may also be found on the hand as a result of vigorous sucking in utero or after birth. Muscle weakness or facial paralysis is best observed when the infant is sucking or crying; both conditions may be missed altogether if the infant is observed only in a quiet, alert state (Fig. 19–11). Rooting, suck, and gag reflexes are evaluated during this portion of the examination or during feeding.

The mucous membrane and internal structures of the mouth are inspected. If the mouth does not open spontaneously while the newborn cries, it can be gently opened by a downward pressure on the chin or with a pediatric tongue blade. In a healthy newborn, the mucous membrane is pink. Increased amounts of mucus during the first 1 to 2 days of life are removed with a bulb syringe. This is especially common in newborns born by elective cesarean section without labor because they do not benefit from the cessation of lung fluid production during labor. The tongue is mobile and

prominent within the mouth. Occasionally, the frenulum is short, causing a notch at the tip of the tongue. True congenital ankyloglossia (i.e., tongue tied) is rare.

Using adequate lighting, the hard and soft palates are examined. The uvula is midline and located at the posterior soft palate. Some practitioners use an index finger to palpate the hard and soft palates for the presence of clefts (Fig. 19–12). Whitish-yellow cysts (i.e., Epstein's pearls) containing epithelial cells may be present on the hard palate at birth, but they disappear within a few weeks. Some newborns are born with one or two natal teeth. These immature caps of enamel and dentin have poor root formation and are usually loose. These teeth may be aspirated if dislodged and make breastfeeding difficult or cause lacerations on the mucosa, lips, or tongue. They are usually removed during the neonatal period. Table 19–6 identifies findings during the physical assessment of the mouth that are abnormal and their related pathology.

NECK ASSESSMENT

Inspection and palpation are used to assess the neck. The neck is inspected for symmetry and range of motion. Newborns have short, thick necks with multiple skin folds. A predominant fat pad in the back of the neck, redundant skin, and webbing are findings associated with genetic syndromes.

Full range of motion is present at term. The newborn's head should be able to turn completely to face each shoulder. Torticollis, contraction of the neck muscles that pulls the head toward the affected side with the chin pointing toward the opposite shoulder and side, results from injury to the sternocleidomastoid muscle. More common on the right side, this injury may be congenital or occur during the birth process. A small mass at the site of the injury is palpated along the sternocleidomastoid muscle at birth or soon after. Parents are taught to perform stretching exercises to lengthen the muscle, and the newborn is followed by a physical therapist through the first year of life. If the contracture persists after 1 year, surgery may be necessary.

Cystic hygroma is one of the most common neck lesions (Fig. 19–13). This particular cystic structure occurs due to lymph channels that are sequestered and then dilate and become large cysts. Cystic hygroma most commonly occurs in the lateral neck (Johnson, 2009). The lesions vary in size from a few millimeters to large enough to deviate the trachea, cause respiratory distress, or interfere with feeding. A large cystic hygroma usually requires surgical excision.

The neck is palpated along the midline for the trachea and abnormal masses. The thyroid gland is difficult to palpate unless it is enlarged, an unusual finding during the newborn period. A potential for infection exists within all the cystic structures and abnormal sinuses

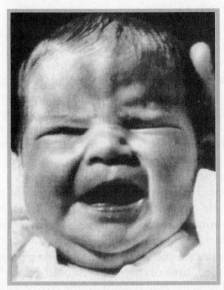

FIGURE 19–11. Facial nerve paralysis. Notice the asymmetry of the mouth during crying. (From Reeder, S. J., Martin, L. L., & Koniak-Griffin, D. [1997]. *Maternity Nursing: Family, Newborn and Women's Health* [18th ed., p. 1205]. Philadelphia: Lippincott-Raven.)

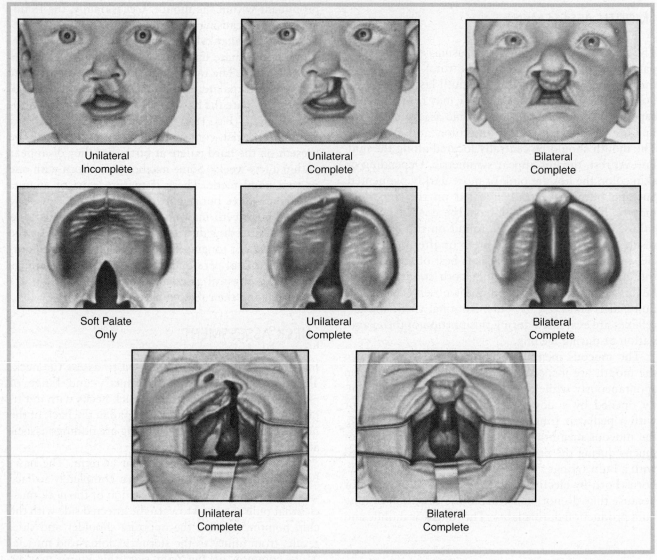

Unilateral
Incomplete

Unilateral
Complete

Bilateral
Complete

Soft Palate
Only

Unilateral
Complete

Bilateral
Complete

Unilateral
Complete

Bilateral
Complete

FIGURE 19–12. Cleft lip and cleft palate (redrawn from drawings by Ross Laboratories). (From Reeder, S. J., Martin, L. L., & Koniak-Griffin, D. [1997]. *Maternity Nursing: Family, Newborn and Women's Health* [18th ed., p. 1108]. Philadelphia: Lippincott-Raven.)

arising around the newborn's neck. Table 19–7 identifies additional findings during the physical assessment of the neck that are abnormal and their related pathology.

CHEST AND LUNG ASSESSMENT

Auscultation and inspection are used to assess the newborn's chest and respiratory status. The newborn's chest is cylindrical. Measured at the nipple line, its circumference is approximately 33 cm or 2 to 3 cm less than the infant's head (see Fig. 19–1). The xiphoid process is sometimes seen as a small protuberant area at the end of the sternum. Respirations are shallow and irregular. Chest movement should be symmetric and not labored. An accurate respiratory rate is obtained by counting for 1 full minute, preferably when the

newborn is quiet. Newborns have an average respiratory rate of 30 to 60 breaths per minute, and with each respiration, synchronous abdominal movement occurs. The color of the newborn's skin and mucous membranes is evaluated simultaneously. Presence of cyanosis may be a sign of respiratory distress or congenital cardiac disease.

Tachypnea (i.e., respiratory rate >60 breaths per minute) may be one of the first symptoms of morbidity in the newborn. If tachypnea is present, the respiratory rate may reach 120 breaths per minute. The primary healthcare provider should be notified when respiratory rates are increased, and oral feedings should be withheld if an infant is tachypneic because of the risk of aspiration.

Other signs of respiratory distress include retractions, nasal flaring, and grunting. Retractions are the drawing inward or shortening of small muscles in the chest wall.

Table 19–6. MOUTH

Assessment	Pathology
Mucous membranes dry	Dehydration
Cyanotic mucous membranes (central cyanosis)	Poor oxygenation, congenital heart disease or respiratory condition
Asymmetric movement of mouth	Facial nerve injury
Cleft lip and/or palate (see Fig. 19–12)	Teratogenic injury Genetic disorder Multifactorial inheritance
Hypertrophied tongue	Down syndrome Beckwith-Wiedemann syndrome Hypothyroidism
Protrusion of tongue	Genetic disorder
Weak, uncoordinated suck and swallow	Prematurity Neuromuscular disorder Asphyxia Maternal analgesia during labor Inborn error of metabolism
Frantic sucking	Infant of drug-addicted mother
Excessive drooling and salivating; unable to pass a nasogastric tube	Esophageal atresia
Circumoral cyanosis	Respiratory distress
Thin upper lip, smooth philtrum, short palpebral fissures	Fetal alcohol syndrome
Translucent, bluish swelling on either side of the frenulum under the tongue	Mucous or salivary gland retention cyst
Bifid uvula	Genetic disorder
Small lower jaw (micrognathia)	Pierre Robin syndrome Treacher Collins syndrome De Lange syndrome
Patches of white on tongue and mucous membrane	*Candida albicans*

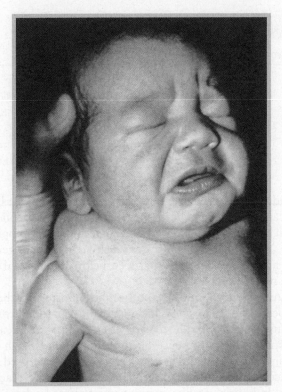

FIGURE 19–13. Cystic hygroma.

respiratory distress (Table 19–8). A score of 0 indicates no respiratory distress (Silverman & Andersen, 1956).

Inspection of the newborn's chest includes placement, shape, and amount of palpable breast tissue. Hypertrophy of breast tissue, with or without secretion of milky

Retractions occur when more energy is needed to assist respiratory effort. Retractions are seen between the ribs (intercostal), below the rib cage (subcostal), above the sternum (tracheal tug), below the xiphoid process, and surrounding the clavicles. Flaring of the nares occurs with inspiration. It is a compensatory mechanism used by the newborn in respiratory distress. Flaring of the nares widens the upper airway, decreasing airway resistance and making breathing easier. Grunting is a sound produced on expiration when air passes through a partially closed glottis. The partially closed glottis is a compensatory mechanism that traps air in the alveoli, increasing the time that gas exchange can occur. Grunting may be audible or heard only with a stethoscope. The Silverman-Anderson Index is a tool that can be used for systematically assessing and documenting newborn respiratory effort and the presence of physical symptoms of

Table 19–7. NECK

Assessment	Pathology
Multiple skin folds in the lateral, posterior region of the neck (webbing)	Down syndrome Turner syndrome
Enlarged thyroid	Hyperthyroidism Hypothyroidism
Absence of head control	Prematurity Genetic disorder Asphyxia Neuromuscular disorder
Abnormal opening along the anterior surface of the sternocleidomastoid muscle	
Brachial sinus leads to a blind pouch or communicates with deeper structures	
Mass high in the neck at midline extending to the base of the tongue; often, thyroglossal duct cyst appears after an upper respiratory infection	
Palpable cystic mass may open onto the skin surface or drain into the pharynx	
Brachial cleft cyst	

Table 19–8. SILVERMAN–ANDERSON INDEX

Score	Upper Chest	Lower Chest	Xiphoid	Nares	Grunt
0	Chest and abdomen rise together	No intercostal retractions	No xiphoid retractions	No nasal flaring	No expiratory grunt
1	Lag or minimal sinking of upper chest as abdomen rises	Minimal intercostal retractions	Minimal xiphoid retractions	Minimal nasal flaring	Expiratory grunt heard with stethoscope
2	Upper chest and abdomen move as a "seesaw"	Marked intercostal retractions	Marked xiphoid retractions	Marked nasal flaring	Audible expiratory grunt

fluid, may be present by the second or third day of life because of maternal hormones (Fig. 19–14). This condition lasts approximately 1 week. Supernumerary nipples (i.e., accessory nipples) are considered a benign congenital anomaly. They are often seen below and medial to the normal nipples.

Auscultation of the anterior and posterior chest proceeds in an orderly fashion from top to bottom, comparing from side to side for equality of breath sounds and the presence of abnormal sounds such as grunting and rales. The term *crackles* may be used in place of the traditional term *rales* for the fine cracking, bubbling, or fine rustling noises heard when air passes fluid. Rhonchi and wheezing are less common in the newborn period. These lower pitched sounds result from obstruction or narrowing of larger airways.

Newborns have a periodic breathing pattern resulting from the immaturity of their respiratory and central nervous systems. It is common to observe brief pauses in respiratory effort. Pauses lasting 20 seconds or longer and associated with color change or bradycardia are considered apneic periods and should be reported to the primary healthcare provider.

Apnea (i.e., pauses in respirations lasting 20 seconds or longer) or other signs of respiratory distress may occur in almost all illnesses in the newborn period. The list of differential diagnoses for respiratory distress and apnea in the newborn is extensive (Table 19–9). Table 19–10 identifies findings during the respiratory assessment that are abnormal and their related pathology.

CARDIOVASCULAR ASSESSMENT

The cardiovascular system is assessed using inspection, auscultation, and palpation. The examination begins with inspection of the newborn's color as one indication of oxygenation and perfusion. As the newborn transitions from intrauterine to extrauterine life, skin color changes occur. At birth, the newborn or neonate may be pale or cyanotic, becoming pink as respirations are established, fetal circulation is reversed, and blood is oxygenated by the lungs and circulated by the strength of the heart muscle.

The precordium (i.e., area on the anterior chest over the heart) is inspected and palpated for movement. In a term newborn, very little movement should be observed in this area (except during the first few hours of life as

Table 19–9. DIFFERENTIAL DIAGNOSIS OF RESPIRATORY DISTRESS IN THE NEWBORN

Respiratory	Extrapulmonary
Respiratory distress syndrome	Congenital heart disease
Transient tachypnea	Patent ductus arteriosus
Meconium aspiration	Hypothermia
Primary pulmonary hypertension	Metabolic acidosis Hypoglycemia
Pneumonia	Septicemia
Pulmonary hemorrhage	Ventricular hemorrhage
Pneumothorax	Edema
Airway obstruction	Drugs
Diaphragmatic hernia	Trauma
Hypoplastic lung	Hypovolemia Twin-to-twin transfusion

Adapted from Askin, D. F. (1997). *Acute Respiratory Care of the Newborn* (p. 32). Petaluma, CA: NICU INK.

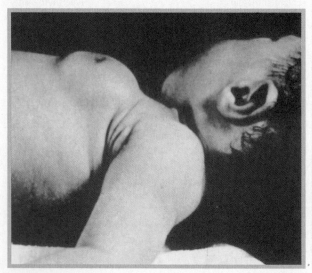

FIGURE 19–14. Neonatal breast hypertrophy.

Table 19–10. RESPIRATORY SYSTEM

Assessment	Pathology
Cessation of breathing for more than 20 sec (apnea)	Hypothermia/hyperthermia Infection Prematurity Respiratory disorders Cardiovascular disorders Neurologic disorders Maternal medications Metabolic disorders Gastroesophageal reflux Vigorous suctioning Passage of feeding tube Airway obstruction
Tachypnea	Retained lung fluid (transient tachypnea of the newborn) Meconium aspiration Respiratory distress syndrome Pneumonia Hyperthermia Pulmonary edema Sepsis Metabolic disorders
Decreased or absent breath sounds	Meconium aspiration Atelectasis Pneumothorax Diaphragmatic hernia Hypoplastic lungs Diaphragmatic hernia
Bowel sounds heard in place of breath sounds	Diaphragmatic hernia

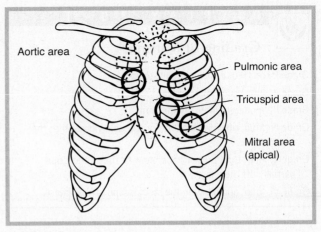

FIGURE 19–15. Auscultatory areas of the heart. (From Tappero, E. P., & Honeyfield, M. E. [Eds.]. [2009]. *Physical Assessment of the Newborn* [4th ed., p. 87]. Petaluma, CA: NICU INK.)

transition occurs). An active precordium could indicate patent ductus arteriosus or other left-to-right shunt lesions or occurs as a variation of normal in preterm or SGA newborns who are thin and have minimal subcutaneous tissue. After the first few hours or days of life, the point of maximal impulse (PMI) is normally auscultated or palpated in the third to fourth intercostal space at or just left of the midclavicular line. Displacement of the PMI can occur with cardiac enlargement, diaphragmatic hernia, dextrocardia, or pneumothorax. Three additional sensations—heave, tap, and thrill—may be felt as the chest is palpated. A heave is a diffuse pulsation that can occur with ventricular volume overload. A tap is a pronounced localized pulsation of the PMI. A thrill is a palpated vibration (similar to a purring cat) that is associated with a murmur.

Heart rate and rhythm are best auscultated using the bell and diaphragm of a small neonatal stethoscope while the newborn remains quiet. The diaphragm of the stethoscope can detect high-pitched murmurs, whereas the bell is better for detecting low-pitched murmurs. The stethoscope should be warmed before placement so the newborn is not startled. The apical rate is counted for 1 full minute. The normal heart rate is 100 to 160 beats per minute (bpm). In deep sleep, the heart rate

may be 80 to 110 bpm but should increase quickly if the newborn is disturbed. Auscultation begins at the mitral area (PMI) and proceeds systematically to the tricuspid, pulmonic, and aortic areas using the diaphragm of the stethoscope. The process is then repeated using the bell of the stethoscope (Fig. 19–15). Heart sounds are louder in newborn infants because of the thin chest wall.

Heart sounds become clearer over the first few hours of life as fetal circulation transitions to extrauterine circulation and the pulmonary vascular resistance lowers. Rapid heart rates often make it difficult to auscultate specific heart sounds. The first heart sound, S_1, is caused by the closure of the tricuspid and mitral valves at the beginning of systole. It is heard best at the apex of the heart, in the fourth intercostal space. S_1 is usually loudest at birth, decreasing in intensity over 24 to 48 hours. The second heart sound, S_2, is caused by the closure of the pulmonic and aortic valves and is heard best at the base of the heart. Splitting of S_2 with inspiration is common after the first 72 hours of life. Other forms of splitting, such as fixed or widely split heart sounds, may be considered pathologic and a sign of congenital heart disease.

Heart murmurs in newborns are common during the neonatal period and are caused by turbulence of blood flow. Murmurs are evaluated for loudness or intensity of sound (i.e., grade); timing in the cardiac cycle (i.e., systolic or diastolic); location of the murmur's maximum intensity, radiation, and pitch; or quality of sound. Most murmurs in the newborn are benign and transient in nature and are called innocent murmurs. These murmurs are usually grade I or II (Display 19–1), occur in the first 48 hours of life, and are not associated with any other abnormalities in the physical exam and evaluation. Pathologic murmurs are related to underlying cardiac problems. Pathologic murmurs are generally louder than grades I to II, may begin or persist after 48 hours of age, and may be associated with other symptoms (Vargo, 2009).

DISPLAY 19–1

Grading of Murmurs

Grade I: soft; requires extended listening

Grade II: soft; heard immediately

Grade III: moderate intensity; no thrill

Grade IV: loud; often with a thrill or palpable vibration at the murmur site

Grade V: loud; thrill present; audible with the stethoscope partially off the chest

Grade VI: loud; audible with the stethoscope off the chest

Peripheral pulses (i.e., brachial, radial, femoral, popliteal, and dorsalis pedis) are evaluated for presence, equality, and strength. Femoral pulses may be difficult to palpate but should be present in all infants. It is very important to note an absence or diminishment of the femoral pulses, and this should be further investigated by a physician or an advanced practice nurse.

Routine blood pressure (BP) screening is not recommended for all newborns (AAP & ACOG, 2007). Evaluating the BP is usually reserved for newborns with signs of distress, persistent murmurs, or abnormal pulses. BP varies depending on birth weight, gestational age, cuff size, and state of alertness. BP should be taken when the infant is quiet and reserved for the end of the assessment since the pressure of the cuff inflating may cause the newborn to cry. An appropriate size of BP cuff is necessary to ensure an accurate measurement. Cuffs that are too small will produce elevated BP values, and cuffs that are too large can produce values that are too low. Using limb length only to determine the cuff size used can be misleading. It is important to also consider cuff width when determining BP accurately. The width of the cuff should be 25% to 55% wider than the diameter of the extremity being measured, with the bladder entirely circling the extremity (but not overlapping) (Park, 2008). At term, the normal BP range is 65 to 95 mm Hg systolic and 30 to 60 mm Hg diastolic. BP in the lower extremities is usually higher than that in the upper extremities. When there is concern for a potential cardiac abnormality, BP should be measured in all four extremities. The primary caregiver should be notified if the systolic BP in the upper extremities is more than 20 mm Hg higher than that in the systolic BP in the lower extremities (Park, 2008). Table 19–11 identifies findings during the cardiovascular assessment that are abnormal and their related pathology.

ABDOMINAL ASSESSMENT

The abdomen is assessed using inspection, auscultation, and palpation. The abdomen is inspected for size and symmetry and is normally rounded, symmetric,

Table 19–11. CARDIOVASCULAR SYSTEM

Assessment	Pathology
Tachycardia (heart rate >160 bpm)	Anemia Congestive heart failure Shock or hypovolemia Respiratory distress Supraventricular tachycardia Sepsis Congenital heart anomalies Hyperthermia
Persistent bradycardia (heart rate <100 bpm)	Congenital heart block Sepsis Asphyxia Hypoxemia Increased intracranial pressure
Persistent murmurs	PPHN Congenital heart defects Peripheral pulmonic stenosis
Muffled heart sounds	Pneumothorax Pneumopericardium Diaphragmatic hernia Pneumomediastinum
Heart sound muffled on left side, loud on right side	Dextrocardia Pneumothorax with mediastinal shift
Decrease in intensity or absence of femoral pulses	Hip dysplasia Coarctation of the aorta
Bounding peripheral pulses; active precordium	Patent ductus arteriosus Fluid overload Congestive heart failure Ventricular septal defect
Difference of systolic blood pressure >20 mm Hg in upper extremities vs. systolic blood pressure in lower extremities	Coarctation of aorta
Central cyanosis	Congenital heart disease Hypertension Lung disease Sepsis
PPHN	
Cyanosis that does not improve with 100% oxygen	Congenital heart disease
Cyanosis that worsens with crying	Congenital heart disease

PPHN, persistent pulmonary hypertension.

protuberant, and soft because of weak abdominal musculature, with a slightly greater diameter above the umbilicus than below. The subcutaneous blood vessels in the abdomen may appear distended and blue (Hernandez & Glass, 2005). Abdominal movements correspond to respirations because newborns use the muscle of the diaphragm rather than intercostal muscles to assist with breathing. Movement of the diaphragm causes the abdomen to move. If abdominal distention is suspected, the circumference of the abdomen is periodically measured at the level of the

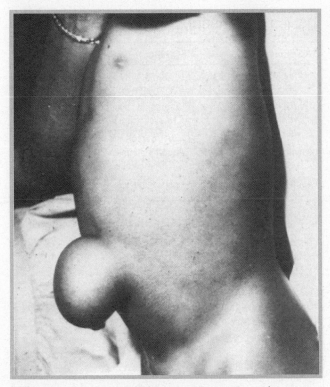

FIGURE 19–16. Umbilical hernia. (Courtesy of Dr. Mark Ravitch.)

umbilicus (see Fig. 19–1). The umbilical cord is examined for number of vessels, color, and condition. The cord should be opaque to white-blue and contain two thick-walled arteries and one thin-walled vein. Variations include a thin, dry cord associated with IUGR or a thick cord seen in LGA newborns. A greenish-yellow discoloration of the cord sometimes occurs with relaxation of the anal sphincter and subsequent passage of meconium prior to birth. The area surrounding the umbilical cord is observed for masses or the herniation of abdominal contents (Fig. 19–16). Umbilical hernias occur when the abdominal muscles do not close completely around the umbilicus during embryologic development. They are more common in low-birth-weight, African American, and male newborns. Some hernias are observable only when the newborn is crying. Separation of the abdominorectus muscle (i.e., diastasis recti) 0.5 to 2 inches wide may occur along the midline from the xiphoid to umbilicus, occasionally extending to the symphysis pubis. Separation of this muscle is not uncommon and is the result of the newborn's weak abdominal muscles.

The perianal region is inspected for the presence of a patent anus. Most newborns pass meconium within the first 24 hours of life but may go as long as 48 hours occasionally. Failure to pass meconium beyond this time may indicate a gastrointestinal obstruction and necessitates further evaluation.

Bowel sounds are normally present within the first hour of life as the newborn swallows air with crying and the sympathetic nervous system stimulates peristalsis. Bowel sounds are auscultated in all four quadrants.

Most perinatal/neonatal nurses conduct a limited assessment of the abdomen using light palpation for consistency and the presence of masses. A more detailed examination is conducted by the primary healthcare provider. The lower border of the liver is firm soft and palpated in the right upper quadrant 1 to 3 cm below the costal margin. The spleen, located in the left upper quadrant, may be palpable in preterm newborns but rarely in term newborns. The spleen should not be palpated more than 1 cm below the left costal margin (Goodwin, 2009). Kidneys are 4 to 5 cm long and are usually only palpable during the first 1 to 2 days of life (Hernandez & Glass, 2005). After this time, the bowel and stomach become distended with fluid and air, making this assessment difficult. With the newborn's legs flexed against the abdomen, kidneys are located using deep palpations at the level of the umbilicus, lateral to the midclavicular line (Fig. 19–17). The right kidney may be lower than the left.

FIGURE 19–17. Examiner demonstrating technique for palpation of the left kidney.

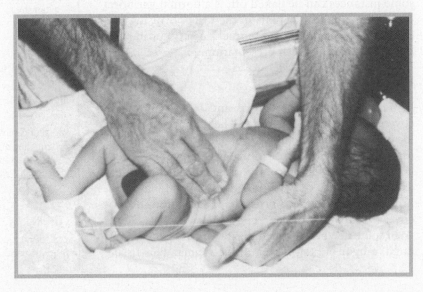

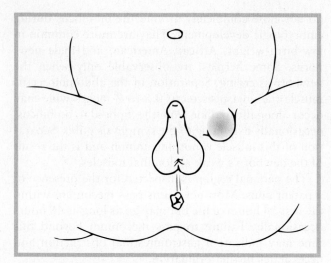

FIGURE 19–18. Left inguinal hernia producing a bulge in the groin of the affected side.

Inspection and palpation of the femoral region is conducted during this portion of the examination or as part of the cardiovascular assessment. A soft, compressible swelling in the groin may indicate an inguinal hernia in males or females, undescended testes, or an ovary within the hernia (Fig. 19–18). Bowel sounds can be auscultated in the testis if swelling is caused by herniation of the bowel. Table 19–12 identifies findings during the physical assessment of the abdomen that are abnormal and their related pathology.

GENITOURINARY SYSTEM

ASSESSMENT

The genitourinary system is assessed using inspection and palpation. External genitalia are evaluated as part of the physical examination and gestational age assessment. Newborns should void within 24 hours of birth. A rust-colored stain on the diaper, which in some instances can be flaked off, is a normal variation caused by uric acid crystals in the urine. Bruising and edema of the genitalia and buttocks can occur in newborns that had a breech presentation.

Female Newborns

In term newborns, the clitoris and labia minora are covered by the labia majora. The urinary meatus is located beneath the clitoris. The labia majora and clitoris are enlarged because of maternal hormones circulated to the fetus in utero. Bruising and swelling of the external genitalia may be present after a vaginal birth. In preterm female newborns, the labia majora do not cover the labia minora and clitoris.

In some newborns, when the introitus is gently separated, a hymenal tag is seen in the vagina. This tissue,

Table 19–12. ABDOMEN

Assessment	Pathology
Scaphoid	Diaphragmatic hernia Malnutrition
"Prune belly" flabby, wrinkled abdominal wall (see Fig. 19–20)	Congenital absence of abdominal musculature; associated with other GI or GU anomalies
Asymmetric abdomen	Abdominal mass GI/GU anomalies
Abdominal distention	Obstruction Masses Enlargement of abdominal organs Infection (Hernandez & Glass, 2005)
Distention in left upper quadrant	Pyloric stenosis Duodenal or jejunal obstruction
Ascites	Hydrops fetalis Viral infections (congenital)
Umbilical cord with one artery and one vein	Associated with GI/GU anomalies
Thin membrane covering herniation of abdominal contents through a defect in the umbilical ring	Omphalocele
Uncovered protrusion of abdominal contents, usually to the right of the umbilicus	Gastroschisis
Red, oozing, or foul-smelling cord	Infection (omphalitis)
Persistently moist umbilicus; clear discharge from umbilical cord stump	Granuloma of the umbilical cord (Hernandez & Glass, 2005) Umbilical urinary fistula—urachus, embryologic connection between the bladder and umbilicus remains patent Urachus cyst Omphalomesenteric duct—connection between the umbilicus and ileum (Goodwin, 2009)
Failure to pass meconium stool	Imperforate anus Meconium ileus Hirschsprung disease Meconium plug syndrome
Passage of sticky, thick, small plugs of meconium	Meconium ileus Cystic fibrosis
Bruit	Arteriovenous malformation (liver) Renal artery stenosis
Partial or complete herniation of the bladder through the abdominal wall	Bladder exstrophy—absence of muscle and connective tissue in the abdominal wall occurring during embryologic development
Hepatomegaly	Congenital heart disease Infection Hemolytic disease (Hernandez & Glass, 2005)

GI, gastrointestinal; GU, genitourinary.

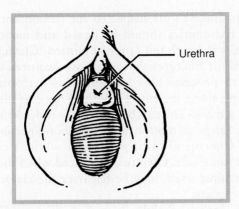

FIGURE 19–19. Imperforate hymen.

which developed from the hymen and labia minora, disappears within a few weeks (Cavaliere, 2009). A white mucous discharge from the vagina is not uncommon during the first week of life. Pseudomenstruation, caused by withdrawal of maternal hormones, is a pink-tinged mucous discharge lasting 2 to 4 weeks.

The labia majora are palpated for masses that could indicate a hernia or ectopic glands. Palpating a suprapubic mass or mass between the labia majora suggests an imperforate hymen. An imperforate hymen causes secretions to pool within the vagina (Fig. 19–19).

Male Newborns

In term male newborns, the external genitalia are observed for a normal penis, with a length of 2.5 to 5.0 cm (Shulman, Palmert, & Wherrett, 2011), the urethral opening located on the tip of the glans, and the glans covered by the prepuce or foreskin. The foreskin may need to be retracted slightly to accurately determine the location of the meatus. A physiologic phimosis (i.e., inability to retract the prepuce or foreskin) is present at birth. By 3 years of age, the foreskin usually can be retracted in 90% of uncircumcised males because adhesions between the prepuce and glans lyse and the distal phimotic ring loosen (Elder, 2007). Small, white cysts filled with epithelial cells may be transiently present on the distal portion of the prepuce. Smegma, a whitish-yellow, cheesy substance from sebaceous glands, collects between the glans and the prepuce.

The second most common genitourinary abnormality in male newborns is hypospadias, the placement of the urinary meatus on the ventral surface of the penis anywhere along a line extending from the tip of the penis, penile shaft, scrotum, or perineum. In more severe cases, the meatus opens on the lower penile shaft, junction of the penoscrotum, or perineum. Up to 15% of severe hypospadias are associated with endocrine problems, chromosomal problems, or intersex problems (Shulman et al., 2011). Because of the point

in embryologic development that the defect occurs, it is usually associated with some degree of failure of the foreskin to develop completely or excessive foreskin on the dorsal surface and absent foreskin on the ventral surface and chordee—the ventral curvature of the penis (Shulman et al., 2011). Circumcision is delayed when an abnormally located urinary meatus is observed, because if a surgery is necessary, the foreskin may be used for urethroplasty or penile shaft skin coverage. Surgical repair is ideally performed after 6 months of age by a skilled surgeon (Shulman et al., 2011).

The scrotum is more darkly pigmented than the skin surrounding it. This color variation is especially prominent in darker skinned newborns such a African American, Indian, and Hispanic newborns. The scrotum is palpated with the thumb and forefinger for the presence of the testes. Placing a finger between the scrotum and the inguinal canal area while palpating will minimize movement of the testes within the scrotum. Rugae (i.e., ridges or creases) begin to appear on the surface of the scrotum around 36 weeks' gestation, and by term, the entire surface of the scrotum is covered. The scrotum may be enlarged because of the effects of maternal hormones. Rugae and a pendulous scrotum usually indicate descent of the testes. Before 28 weeks' gestation, the testes lie within the abdomen. Migration through the inguinal canal to the scrotum occurs as a result of the effect of testosterone on the genitofemoral nerves. Stimulation of these nerves is postulated to cause the gubernaculum testis, a fetal ligament connecting the testes to the scrotum, to guide the movement of the testes to the scrotum (Moore & Persaud, 2008). Undescended testes (i.e., cryptorchidism) is the most common male genital abnormality. The condition may be unilateral or bilateral and occurs in about 3.7% of term newborns and up to 21% to 100% of preterm males depending on the gestation with very preterm infants approaching 100% (Shulman et al., 2011). Undescended testes are found along the normal path of descent between the abdomen and scrotum, most often below the external inguinal ring but not in the scrotum. They can also be within the inguinal canal or still in the abdomen. If undescended at birth, the testes usually descend by 9 months of age, 3 months of age in up to 75% of term males, and 90% of preterm males without intervention (Shulman et al., 2011). It is possible for one testis or both testes to migrate to an ectopic location, away from the normal path to the scrotum, if the gubernaculum ligament is in an abnormal location. Either or both of the testes can be classified as retractile. A testis is referred to as retractile if, when stimulated by palpation or cold, the cremasteric reflex causes it to move to the upper scrotum or as far as the external inguinal ring. This condition differs from the classification of undescended because gentle pressure can bring the testis completely down into the scrotum.

Table 19–13. GENITOURINARY SYSTEM

Assessment	Pathology
Ambiguous genitalia	Genetic disorder
Decreased or no urination within 24 hr of birth	Urinary tract obstruction Potter syndrome Polycystic kidney Hydronephrosis Renal failure
Female	
Urinary meatus near or just inside vagina (hypospadias)	Genitourinary anomaly
Fecal discharge from vagina	Fistula between rectum and vagina
Male	
Epispadias—meatus on dorsal surface of glans	Genitourinary anomaly
Hypospadias—meatus on ventral surface of glans	Genitourinary anomaly Congenital syndromes
Scrotal mass which does not transilluminate	Inguinal hernia (see Fig. 19–18)
Red to bluish-red scrotal sac; swelling or small mass palpable (Cavaliere, 2009)	Twisting of the testes and spermatic cord (testicular torsion)
Urinary stream not straight; weak urinary stream	Stenosis of the urethral meatus Urinary malformation

Arms and legs are inspected for flexion and symmetry. Extremities should be flexed and move symmetrically through full range of motion. Clavicles are assessed for fractures that may have occurred during the birth process. This assessment is performed by palpating along the entire length of the clavicle, feeling for a mass. The newborn's arm is moved through passive range of motion while the examiner uses his or her other hand to palpate the newborn's clavicle on that same side. Crepitus, produced when the bone slides against itself, may be felt over the clavicle if a fracture exists.

Legs appear slightly bowed with everted feet. A persistent breech presentation in utero may result in abducted hips and extended knees (Fig. 19–20). Positional deformities in the newborn period are often caused by intrauterine positioning and may continue to be present for a few days or weeks. Passive range of motion should correct positional deformities.

HIPS

The newborn's hips are evaluated for developmental dysplasia. Developmental dysplasia of the hip (DDH) describes the continuum of pathologic hip disorders in the newborn traditionally referred to as congenital dislocation of the hip. This terminology has been adapted

To prevent stimulation of the cremasteric reflex during examination, a finger can again be placed between the scrotum and the inguinal canal area while palpating to minimize movement of the testes within the scrotum. Surgical intervention for undescended or ectopic testes occurs when the child is 6 months to 1 year old.

An enlarged scrotum is evaluated for the presence of a hydrocele, which is an accumulation of fluid. Fluid accumulates during fetal development when sexual differentiation occurs. This fluid is usually reabsorbed in utero. If a hydrocele is present at birth, it should disappear within 3 months. The ability to transilluminate a hydrocele differentiates it from a solid or blood-filled mass. Table 19–13 identifies the findings of the physical assessment of male and female newborns that are abnormal and their related pathology.

MUSCULOSKELETAL ASSESSMENT

Inspection and palpation are used to assess the musculoskeletal system. Examination begins by observing the newborn at rest, noting position, symmetry, and presence of abnormal movements. The hands and feet are inspected for the number of digits. Nails are soft and cover the entire nail bed. In a newborn that is post–40 weeks, the nails may extend beyond the fingertips. Newborns exposed to meconium in utero have yellow discoloration of their nails.

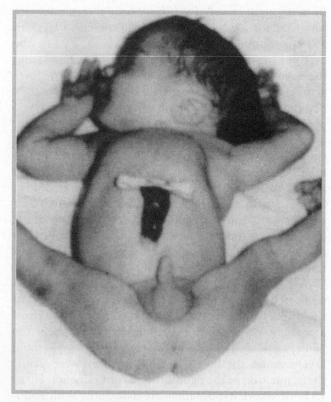

FIGURE 19–20. Result of a persistent breech position in utero. (Courtesy of Dr. David A. Clark, Louisiana State University Medical Center and Wyeth-Ayerst Laboratories, Philadelphia, PA.)

Factors Associated with Developmental Dysplasia of the Hip

- Family history of developmental dysplasia of the hip
- Oligohydramnios
- Breech presentation
- Foot deformities
- Primiparity
- Female sex
- Multiple pregnancy

by the AAP, the American Academy of Orthopaedic Surgeons, and the Pediatric Orthopaedic Society of North America (French & Dietz, 1999). The true incidence of DDH is unknown, but some newborn screening reports cite the incidence of 1 in 100 newborn infants with some degree of instability and 1 to 1.5 cases of dislocation per 1,000 infants (AAP, 2000). The exact cause of DDH is unknown. It is probably related to a variety of factors or situations interfering with the normal development of the acetabulum. Failure of the acetabulum to develop eventually allows the bell-shaped femoral head to migrate completely or partially out of normal position. Because of intrauterine position, DDH is more common in the left hip (AAP, 2000). Factors that put newborns at risk for DDH are listed in Display 19–2.

Evaluating the newborn's hips requires the infant to be in a quiet state. Crying causes increased muscle tone that could prevent the examiner from identifying an unstable hip. Assessing the newborn for DDH begins with inspection. Position the newborn on his or her back, with diaper off, hips and knees flexed at 90-degree angles, and feet level (Fig. 19–21). The presence of more skin folds on the medial aspect of the thigh or one knee noticeably lower than the other knee (Galeazzi sign) may indicate that the femoral head is dislocated or no longer positioned within the acetabulum.

To further determine the presence of an unstable or dislocated hip, the newborn's hips are put through three maneuvers. With the newborn's hips and knees still flexed at 90-degree angles, the hips are simultaneously abducted gently toward the examination table. Normal hips should abduct almost 90 degrees (i.e., thighs resting on the table). This is followed by the Ortolani and Barlow maneuvers. To perform the Ortolani maneuver, the examiner stabilizes one hip while the thigh of the hip being tested is abducted and gently pulled anteriorly. If the hip is dislocated, a palpable and sometimes audible "clunk" will be detected as the femoral head moves over the posterior rim of the acetabulum and back into position (Fig. 19–22).

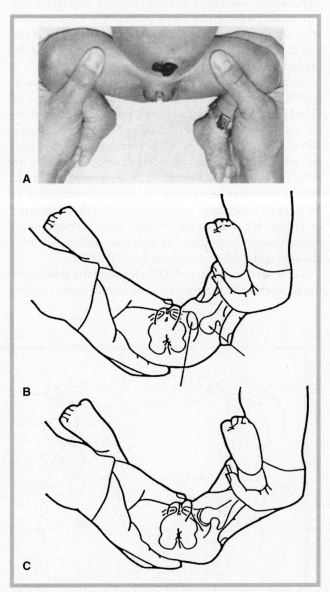

FIGURE 19–22. Ortolani maneuver. **A & B**, With the newborn's legs flexed, the thumb is over the femur and the fingers are on the trochanter. The femur is lifted forward as the thighs are abducted toward the bed. **C**, A "click" is heard or felt as the head of the femur moves into the acetabulum.

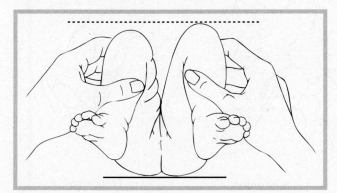

FIGURE 19–21. Asymmetry in number of thigh skin folds and uneven knee level. (From Ballock, R. T., & Richards, B. S. [1997]. Hip dysplasia: Early diagnosis makes a difference. *Contemporary Pediatrics, 14*[7], 110.)

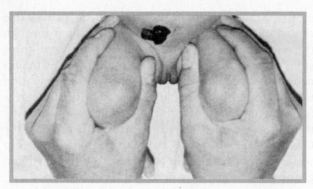

FIGURE 19–23. Barlow maneuver performed by adducting the thighs. If the head of the femur dislocates, it is felt and seen as it suddenly jerks over the acetabulum.

The Barlow maneuver is performed by adducting the hip while pushing the thigh posteriorly to determine whether the hip can be dislocated (Fig. 19–23). If the hip is dislocated by this maneuver, it is relocated by performing the Ortolani maneuver.

The continuum of DDH from dysplasia to dislocation is depicted in Figure 19–24. Only about 60% of DDH is identified clinically with initial newborn clinical assessment (Rosenberg, Bialik, Norman, & Blazer, 1998). In combination with ultrasound evaluation when DDH is suspected, identification increases to 90% (Donaldson & Feinstein, 1997; Rosenberg et al., 1998). However, ultrasound is only recommended as an adjunct to clinical evaluation and is the technique of choice for confirming an abnormal physical finding, assessment of infants at high risk, and monitoring changes of DDH as it is treated (AAP, 2000).

Early identification of DDH increases the possibility that conservative treatment can be initiated and surgery avoided (Ballock & Richards, 1997). Treatment then includes early and accurate diagnosis, use of a Pavlik harness, or closed reduction surgery (Cooperman & Thompson, 2011).

FEET

Feet are examined to determine whether deformities are positional abnormalities or structural malformations. Positional abnormalities are temporary, do not involve bone, and refer to alterations in shape and contour of a normally formed foot. Structural malformations usually involve bone and generally form during the fourth to eighth weeks of the embryonic period (Moore & Persaud, 2008). Feet are inspected for 10 digits.

Metatarsus adductus (i.e., inward turning of the front one third of the foot with a widening of the space between the first and second toe) is a common positional abnormality occurring in utero due to uterine positioning (Fig. 19–25). Treatment depends on the severity of the abnormality, which progresses along a continuum. The least severe is a foot that returns to the midline spontaneously by stroking the lateral side and usually requires no intervention. Moderately severe is where the examiner is able to easily manipulate the foot into correct position. Exercises performed by parents will usually correct this abnormality. The most severe is the foot that resists correction by the examiner and requires serial casting during infancy.

Talipes calcaneovalgus is a positional deformity caused by the sole of the foot being positioned against the uterine wall. Dorsiflexion of the ankle causes contact between the dorsal surface of the foot and the anterior aspect of the leg (tibia). The leg and foot form the shape of a check mark (✓) rather than the shape of an "L" (Fig. 19–26).

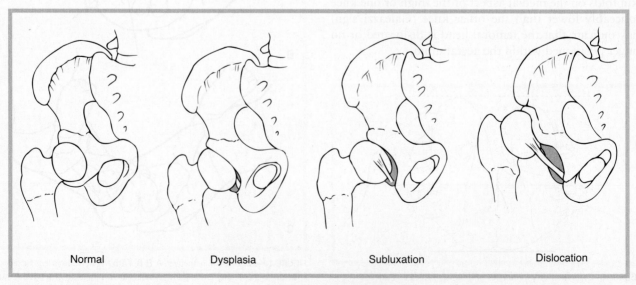

| Normal | Dysplasia | Subluxation | Dislocation |

FIGURE 19–24. Relationship of structures in developmental dysplasia of the hip. (Modified from Wong, D. L. [Ed.]. [1997]. *Whaley & Wong's Essentials of Pediatric Nursing* [5th ed., p. 1137]. St. Louis, MO: Mosby.)

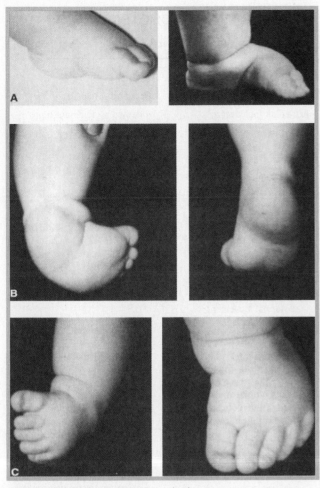

FIGURE 19–25. Comparison of clubfoot (*left*) and metatarsus adductus (*right*). **A,** Lateral view, showing the equinus (entire heel does not touch the flat surface); present only in clubfoot. **B,** Posterior view, showing the hindfoot varus in clubfoot but not in metatarsus adductus. **C,** Anterior view, showing adduction in both feet, with the varus also present in clubfoot.

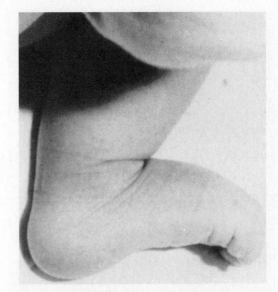

FIGURE 19–26. Talipes calcaneovalgus.

sacral area is inspected for the presence of a pilonidal dimple (Fig. 19–28), tuft of hair, skin lesion, or increased pigmentation that could indicate pathology. Table 19–14 identifies findings of the musculoskeletal assessment that are abnormal and their related pathology.

NEUROLOGIC ASSESSMENT

Assessment of the central nervous system is integrated throughout the physical examination and includes an evaluation of posture, cry, muscle tone, and movement; an evaluation of most cranial nerves; and an evaluation of all developmental reflexes. Findings during the

Talipes equinovarus or congenital clubfoot involves a deformity of the foot that involves the ankle bone and lower leg. In this pathologic deformity, the sole of the foot turns medially and the foot is inverted (see Fig. 19–25). There is also mild ankle atrophy. Because of the unusual position, the deformity does not allow weight bearing (Moore & Persaud, 2008). It develops more frequently in males and is bilateral in about half of the cases. Treatment may include serial casting; however, if clinical and radiologic correction is not achieved by casting at 3 months of age, surgery is indicated (Cooperman & Thompson, 2011).

BACK

In a prone position, the newborn's back is examined for asymmetric gluteal folds, indicating the presence of a congenital hip dislocation (Fig. 19–27). During this portion of the examination, the length of the spinal column is palpated for masses and abnormal curvatures. The

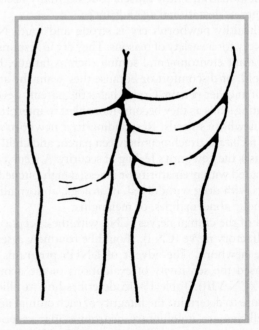

FIGURE 19–27. Asymmetric gluteal folds.

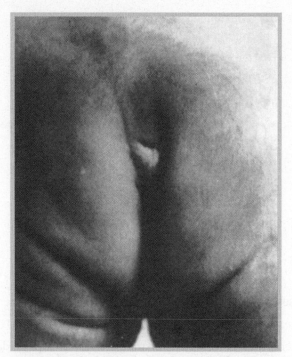

FIGURE 19–28. Pilonidal dimple. (Courtesy of Dr. David A. Clark, Louisiana State University Medical Center and Wyeth-Ayerst Laboratories, Philadelphia, PA.)

Table 19–14. MUSCULOSKELETAL SYSTEM

Assessment	Pathology
Weak or absent muscle tone	Neurologic disorder Prematurity Genetic disorder
Extra digit (polydactyly)	Inherited as dominant trait
Partial or complete fusion of digits, more often in feet than hands (syndactyly)	Inherited as dominant trait
Short fingers, incurving of fifth finger, fusion or palmar creases (simian crease), wide space between big toe and second toe	Down syndrome
Jitteriness	Hypoglycemia Hypocalcemia
Arm extended and limp, hand rotated inward, absence of normal movement, absent Moro reflex on affected side	Brachial plexus palsy
Club foot—sole of the foot pointed medially, toes pointed downward and heel pointing upward, upper third of the foot curved downward (can classify as congenital, teratologic, or positional)	Environmental factors in utero which decrease the ability of the fetus to move and/or increase the size of the fetus (i.e., oligohydramnios, maternal diabetes, maternal obesity may cause positional deformities) Exposure to teratogens and maternal smoking may cause teratologic deformities Genetic factors may cause congenital form (Furdon & Donlon, 2002)

neurologic assessment are influenced by the gestational age and physical health of the newborn.

At rest, a term newborn's posture is flexed, with extremities tight against the trunk. The neuromuscular portion of the gestational age assessment demonstrates the increasing muscle tone that the newborn develops as gestational age progresses. Scarf sign, popliteal angle, and heel-to-ear movements have less range of motion as gestational age increases. Leg and arm recoil also demonstrates how muscle tone normally becomes stronger as gestational age advances.

A healthy newborn's cry is strong and loud. Newborns cry for a variety of reasons. They cry in response to unpleasant environmental stimuli such as fatigue, hunger, cold, or discomfort or because they want the attention of another person. Crying helps the parents develop parenting skills as they become more alert to interpreting their newborn's needs. Responding to a newborn's cry helps facilitate attachment between parent and child and increases the newborn's feeling of security. A weak cry is associated with prematurity or illness; a high-pitched cry occurs with drug withdrawal, neurologic abnormalities, metabolic abnormalities, or meningitis.

All of the cranial nerves (CN), with the exception of the olfactory nerve (CN I), should be routinely assessed in the newborn. The advent of UNHS programs has increased the sensitivity of evaluations of the acoustic nerve (CN VIII). Table 19–15 describes how to illicit a response to determine the integrity of each cranial nerve.

Reflexes are involuntary neuromuscular responses that provide protection from harm. Whether a specific reflex is present depends on the gestational age of the newborn. Newborns demonstrate two types of reflexes. The first type is protective in nature (e.g., blink, cough, sneeze, gag). The second type, which disappears during the first year of life, is a result of the neurologic immaturity of newborns. These reflexes are sometimes referred to as developmental or primitive reflexes. Developmental reflexes are all present at birth in the healthy term newborn. Appendix 19–C describes how to elicit these reflexes, defines normal and abnormal responses, and explains at what age they disappear. Table 19–16 identifies findings during the neurologic assessment that are abnormal and their related pathology.

SUMMARY

A formal assessment of all body systems is completed by the perinatal nurse soon after birth and repeated at intervals established by institutional protocol

Table 19–15. ASSESSING THE INTEGRITY OF CRANIAL NERVES

Cranial Nerve (CN)	Method of Assessment
CN I, olfactory	Not assessed in the neonate
CN II, optic	Newborn follows brightly colored or contrasting object or face; blinks in response to light
CN III, oculomotor CN IV, trochlear CN VI, abducens	Pupils constrict equally in response to light; as newborn's head is moved to face one side or the other, eyes move in the opposite direction (dolls' eyes maneuver)
CN V, trigeminal	Presence of rooting and sucking reflexes; biting
CN VII, facial	Symmetry of facial movement while crying or smiling
CN VIII, acoustic	Positive Moro reflex or movement in the direction of sound; quiets to voice; hearing screening using brainstem auditory evoked response (BAER)
CN IX, glossopharyngeal CN X, vagus CN XII, hypoglossal	Coordination of suck and swallow; presence of gag reflex; tongue remains midline when mouth is open
CN XI, accessory	Head turns easily to either side; newborn attempts to move head back from side to midline; height of shoulders equal

throughout the newborn's hospitalization. Informal assessments are ongoing and occur during caregiving activities. Performing the physical assessment provides a picture of how the newborn is adapting to extrauterine life. The development of keen physical assessment skills allows the perinatal nurse to detect subtle changes in the newborn's condition, identify or anticipate the development of problems, and intervene immediately to prevent or minimize these problems.

Table 19–16. NEUROLOGIC SYSTEM

Assessment	Pathology
Persistent fisting	Brain lesions, asphyxia
Abnormal position of hands or feet	
Tremors	
Clonus	
Abnormal eye movements	
Poor suck	Neuromuscular disorders Basal ganglia or brainstem abnormalities
Altered state of consciousness and seizures	Asphyxia Perinatal infections Inborn error of metabolism

REFERENCES

American Academy of Pediatrics. (1995). Joint committee on infant hearing: 1994 position statement. *Pediatrics, 95*(1), 152–156.

American Academy of Pediatrics. (2000). Clinical practice guideline: Early detection of developmental dysplasia of the hip. *Pediatrics, 117,* 898–902.

American Academy of Pediatrics. (2003). Prevention and management of positional skull deformities in infants. *Pediatrics, 112*(1), 199–202.

American Academy of Pediatrics. (2007). Year 2007 position statement: Principles and guidelines for early hearing detection and intervention programs. *Pediatrics, 120*(4), 898–921.

American Academy of Pediatrics. (2008). Red reflex examination in neonates, infants & children. *Pediatrics, 122*(6), 1401–1404.

American Academy of Pediatrics & American College of Obstetricians and Gynecologists. (2007). *Guidelines for Perinatal Care* (6th ed.). Washington, DC: Author.

Ballard, J. L., Khoury, J. C., Wedig, K., Wang, L., Ellers-Walsman, B. L., & Lipp, R. (1991). New Ballard Score, expanded to include extremely premature infants. *Journal of Pediatrics, 119*(3), 417–423.

Ballard, J. L., Novak, K. K., & Driver, M. (1979). A simplified score for assessment of fetal maturation of newly born infants. *Journal of Pediatrics, 95*(5, Pt. 1), 769–774.

Ballock, R. T., & Richards, B. S. (1997). Hip dysplasia: Early diagnosis makes a difference. *Contemporary Pediatrics, 14*(4), 108–117.

Cavaliere, T. A. (2009). Genitourinary assessment. In E. P. Tappero & M. E. Honeyfield (Eds.), *Physical Assessment of the Newborn: A Comprehensive Approach to the Art of Physical Examination* (4th ed., pp. 115–132). Santa Rosa, CA: NICU INK.

Cooperman, D. R., & Thompson, G. H. (2011). Congenital abnormalities of the upper and lower extremities and spine. In R. J. Martin, A. A. Fanaroff, & M. C. Walsh (Eds.), *Neonatal-Perinatal Medicine: Diseases of the Fetus and Newborn,* (9th ed., pp. 1782–1801). St. Louis, MO: Elsevier.

Donaldson, J. S., & Feinstein, K. A. (1997). Imaging of developmental dysplasia of the hip. *Pediatric Clinics of North America, 44*(3), 591–614.

Dubowitz, L. M. S., Dubowitz, V., & Goldberg, C. (1970). Clinical assessment of gestational age in the newborn infant. *Journal of Pediatrics, 77*(1), 1–10.

Dubowitz, L., Ricci, D., & Mercuri, E. (2005). The Dubowitz neurological examination of the full-term newborn. *Mental Retardation and Developmental Disabilities Research Reviews, 11*(1), 52–60. doi:10.1002/mrdd.20048

Elder, J. S. (2007). Urologic disorders in infants and children. In R. E. Behrman, R. M. Kliegman, & H. B. Jenson (Eds.), *Nelson's Textbook of Pediatrics* (18th ed., pp. 2253–2260). Philadelphia: Saunders.

French, L. M., & Dietz, F. R. (1999). Screening for developmental dysplasia of the hip. *American Family Physician, 60*(1), 177–184.

Furdon, S. A., & Donlon, C. R. (2002). Examination of the newborn foot: Positional and structural abnormalities. *Advances in Neonatal Care, 2*(5), 248–258. doi: 10.1053/adnc.2002.35542Abstract

Gagliardi, L., Brambilla, C., Bruno, R., Martinelli, S., & Console, V. (1993). Biased assessment of gestational age at birth when obstetric gestation is known. *Archives of Disease in Childhood, 68*(1), 32–34. doi:10.1136/adc.68.1_Spec_No.32

Gardner, S. L., & Hernandez, J. A. (2011). Initial nursery care. In S. L. Gardner, B. S. Carter, M. Enzman-Hines, & J. A. Hernandez (Eds.), *Handbook of Neonatal Intensive Care* (7th ed., pp. 78–112). St. Louis, MO: Mosby/Elsevier.

Gomella, T. L., Cunningham, M. D., & Eyal, F. G. (Eds.). (2009a). Hyperbilirubinemia, direct (conjugated hyperbilirubinemia). In *Neonatology: Management, Procedures, On-Call Problems, Diseases and Drugs* (pp. 288–293). New York: McGraw-Hill.

Gomella, T. L., Cunningham, M. D., & Eyal, F. G. (Eds.). (2009b). Hyperbilirubinemia, indirect (unconjugated hyperbilirubinemia). In *Neonatology: Management, Procedures, On-Call Problems, Diseases and Drugs* (pp. 293–301). New York: McGraw-Hill.

Goodwin, M. (2009). Abdomen assessment. In E. P. Tappero & M. E. Honeyfield (Eds.), *Physical Assessment of the Newborn: A Comprehensive Approach to the Art of Physical Examination* (4th ed., pp. 105–114). Santa Rosa, CA: NICU INK.

Green, M. (1998). *Pediatric Diagnosis: Interpretation of Symptoms and Signs in Infants, Children and Adolescents* (6th ed.). Philadelphia: Saunders.

Hernandez, P. W., & Glass, S. M. (2005). Physical assessment of the newborn. In P. J. Thureen, J. Deacon, P. J. Hernandez, & D. M. Hall. (Eds.), *Assessment and Care of the Well Newborn* (pp. 119–172). Philadelphia: Saunders.

Hoath, S. B., & Narendran, V. (2011). The skin. In R. J. Martin, A. A. Fanaroff, & M. C. Walsh (Eds.), *Neonatal-Perinatal Medicine: Diseases of the Fetus and Newborn* (9th ed., pp. 1705–1736). St. Louis, MO: Elsevier.

Johnson, P. (2009). Head, eyes, ears, nose, mouth and neck assessment. In E. P. Tappero & M. E. Honeyfield (Eds.), *Physical Assessment of the Newborn: A Comprehensive Approach to the Art of Physical Examination* (4th ed., pp. 57–74). Santa Rosa, CA: NICU INK.

Kaplan, M., Wong R. J., Sibley, E., & Stevenson, D. K. (2011). Neonatal jaundice and liver disease. In R. J. Martin, A. A. Fanaroff, & M. C. Walsh (Eds.), *Neonatal-Perinatal Medicine: Diseases of the Fetus and Newborn* (9th ed., pp. 1443–1496). St. Louis, MO: Elsevier.

Lund, C. H., & Kuller, J. M. (2007). Integumentary system. In C. Kenner & J. W. Lott (Eds.), *Comprehensive Neonatal Care* (4th ed., pp. 65–91). St. Louis, MO: Saunders Elsevier.

Moore, K. L., & Persaud, T. V. N. (2008). *The Developing Human* (8th ed.). Philadelphia: Saunders/Elsevier.

Park, M. K. (2008). *Pediatric Cardiology for Practitioners* (5th ed.). Philadelphia: Mosby.

Pearson, J. (1999). Crying and calming: Important information and effective techniques to teach parents of full term newborns. *Mother-Baby Journal, 4*(5), 39–42.

Rosenberg, N., Bialik, V., Norman, D., & Blazer, S. (1998). The importance of combined clinical and sonographic examination of instability of the neonatal hip. *International Orthopedics, 22*(3), 431–434.

Shulman, R. M., Palmert, M. R., & Wherrett, D. K. (2011). Disorders of sex development. In R. J. Martin, A. A. Fanaroff, & M. C. Walsh (Eds.), *Neonatal-Perinatal Medicine: Diseases of the Fetus and Newborn* (9th ed., pp. 1584–1620). St. Louis, MO: Elsevier.

Silengo, M., Battistoni, G., & Spada, M. (1999). Is there a relationship between extensive Mongolian spots and inform errors of metabolism? *American Journal of Medical Genetics, 87*(3), 276–277. doi:10.1002/(SICI)1096-8628(19991126)

Silverman, W. A., & Andersen, D. H. (1956). A controlled clinical trial of water mist on obstructive respiratory signs, death rate, and necropsy findings among premature infants. *Pediatrics, 17*(1), 1–10.

Vargo, L. (2009). Cardiovascular assessment. In E. P. Tappero & M. E. Honeyfield (Eds.), *Physical Assessment of the Newborn: A Comprehensive Approach to the Art of Physical Examination* (4th ed., pp. 87–104). Santa Rosa, CA: NICU INK.

Witt, C. (2009). Skin assessment. In E. P. Tappero & M. E. Honeyfield (Eds.), *Physical Assessment of the Newborn: A Comprehensive Approach to the Art of Physical Examination* (4th ed., pp. 41–56). Santa Rosa, CA: NICU INK.

Wong, D. L. (Ed.). (1997). *Whaley & Wong's Nursing Care of Infants and Children* (6th ed.). St. Louis, MO: Mosby–Year Book.

APPENDIX 19 – A

Characteristics of Infant State

Infant States	Body Activity	Eye Movements	Facial Movements	Breathing Pattern	Level of Response	Implications for Caregiving
Sleep states						
Deep sleep (or quiet sleep)	Nearly still, except for occasional startle or twitch	None	Without facial movements, except for occasional sucking at regular intervals	Smooth and regular	Threshold to stimuli very high so that only very intense or disturbing stimuli will arouse infants	Caregivers trying to feed infants in deep sleep will probably find the experience frustrating. Infants will be unresponsive even if caregivers use disturbing stimuli (flicking feet) to arouse infants. Infants may arouse only briefly and then become unresponsive as they return to deep sleep. If caregivers wait until infants move to a higher, more responsive state, feeding or care giving will be much more pleasant.
Light sleep (or active sleep)	Some body movements	Rapid eye movements (REM); fluttering of eyes beneath closed eyelids	May smile and make brief fussy or crying sounds	Irregular	More responsive to internal and external stimuli. When stimuli occur, infant may remain in light sleep, return to deep sleep, or arouse to drowsy.	Light sleep makes up the highest proportion of newborn sleep and usually precedes wakening. The brief fussy or crying sounds made during this state may make caregivers who are not aware that these sounds occur normally think it is time for feeding, and they may try to feed infants before they are ready to eat.
Awake states						
Drowsy	Activity level variable, with mild startles interspersed from time to time; movement usually smooth	Eyes open and close occasionally and are heavy lidded with dull, glazed appearance	Some facial movements possible	Irregular	React to sensory stimuli although responses are delayed	From the drowsy state, infants may return to sleep or awaken further. To facilitate waking, caregivers can provide something for infants to see, hear, or suck. This may arouse them to a quiet alert state, a more responsive state. Infants left alone without additional stimulation from caregiver will progress to quiet alert state.
Quiet alert	Minimal	Brightening and widening of eyes	Face bright, shining, sparkling	Regular	Most attentive to environment, focusing attention on any stimuli that are present	Infants in quiet, alert state provide much pleasure and positive feedback for caregivers. Providing something for infants to see, hear, or suck will often maintain this state. In the first few hours after birth, most newborns commonly experience a period of intense alertness before going into a long sleeping period.
Active alert	Much body activity; periods of fussiness possible	Eyes open with less brightening	Much facial movement; face not as bright as quiet alert state	Irregular	Increasingly sensitive to disturbing stimuli (hunger, fatigue, noise, excessive handling)	Caregivers may intervene at this stage to console and to bring infants to a lower state.
Crying	Increased motor activity, with color changes	Eyes tightly closed or open	Grimaces	More irregular	Extremely responsive to unpleasant external or internal stimuli	Crying is the infant's communication signal. It is a response to unpleasant stimuli from the environment or from within (fatigue, hunger, discomfort). Crying tells us the infant's limits have been reached. Sometimes infants can console themselves and return to lower states. At other times, they need help from caregivers.

From Pearson, J. (1999). Crying and calming: Important information and effective techniques to teach parents of full-term newborns. *Mother Baby Journal, 4*(5), 39–42.

APPENDIX 19–B

Characteristics of the Ballard Gestation Age Assessment Tool

POSTURE

Observe the newborn lying quietly. Flexion of arms and legs increases with gestational age. The premature newborn lies with arms and legs extended. As gestational age increases, the more flexed the newborn's arms and legs are against the body.

SQUARE WINDOW (WRIST)

The angle that is created when the newborn's palm is flexed toward the forearm. A preterm newborn's wrist exhibits poor flexion and makes a 90-degree angle with the arm. An extremely preterm newborn has no flexor tone and cannot achieve even 90-degree flexion. A term newborn's wrist can flex completely against the forearm.

ARM RECOIL

After first flexing the arms at the elbows against the chest, then fully extending and releasing them, term newborns resist extension and quickly return arms to the flexed position. Very preterm newborns do not resist extension and respond with weak and delayed flexion.

POPLITEAL ANGLE

With the newborn supine and his or her pelvis flat, flex the thigh to the abdomen and hold it there while extending the leg at the knee. The angle at the knee is estimated. The preterm newborn can achieve greater extension.

SCARF SIGN

While the newborn is supine, move his or her arm across his or her chest toward the opposite shoulder. A term newborn's elbow does not cross midline. It is possible to bring the preterm newborn's elbow much farther.

HEEL TO EAR

Without holding the knee and thigh in place, move the newborn's foot as close to the ear as possible. A preterm newborn is able to get his or her foot closer to his or her head than a term baby.

SKIN

Assess for thickness, transparency, and texture. Preterm skin is smooth and thin with visible vessels. Extremely preterm skin is sticky and transparent. Term skin is thick, veins are difficult to see, and peeling may occur.

LANUGO

Fine hair seen over the back of premature newborns by 24 weeks' gestation. It begins to thin over the lower back first and disappears last over the shoulders.

PLANTAR CREASES

One or two creases over the pad of the foot at approximately 32 weeks' gestation. At 36 weeks, creases cover the anterior two thirds of the foot; at term, the whole foot. At very early gestations, the length from the tip of the great toe to the back of the heel is measured.

BREAST TISSUE

Examined for visibility of nipple and areola and size of bud when grasped between thumb and forefinger. The very premature newborn does not have visible nipples or areolae. These become more defined and then raised by 34 weeks, with a small bud appearing at 36 weeks and growing to 5 to 10 mm by term.

EAR FORMATION

Lack of cartilage in earlier gestation results in the ear folding easily and retaining this fold. As gestation progresses, soft cartilage provides increasing resistance to folding and increasing recoil. The pinnae are flat in very preterm newborns. Incurving proceeds from the top down toward the lobes as gestation advances.

GENITALIA

In males, rugae become visible at 28 weeks. By 36 weeks, the testes are in the upper scrotum, and rugae cover the anterior portion of the scrotum. At term, rugae cover the scrotum, and when postmature, the testes are pendulous. In preterm females, the clitoris is prominent, and the labia minora are flat. By 36 weeks, the labia majora are larger, nearly covering the clitoris.

APPENDIX 19-C

Developmental (Primitive) Reflexes

Reflex	How Elicited	Normal Response	Abnormal Response	Duration of Reflex
Rooting and sucking	Touch cheek, lip, or corner of mouth with finger or nipple.	Newborn turns head in direction of stimulus, opens mouth, and begins to suck. In the term newborn, suck is coordinated and strong.	Weak or absent response is seen with prematurity, neurologic deficit, or CNS depression from maternal drug ingestion.	Rooting disappears by 3–4 months; sucking disappears by 1 year.
Swallowing	Place fluid on back.	Newborn swallows in coordination with sucking.	Gagging, coughing, or regurgitation of fluid; possibly associated with cyanosis secondary to prematurity, neurologic deficit, or injury.	Does not disappear.
Extrusion	Touch tip of tongue with finger or nipple.	Newborn pushes tongue outward.	Continuous extrusion of tongue or repetitive tongue thrusting is seen with CNS abnormalities or seizures.	Disappears by 6 months.
Moro	Holding the newborn's head off the mattress slightly, let it drop quickly several inches into your hand.	Bilateral symmetric extension and abduction of all extremities, with thumb and forefinger forming characteristic "C," followed by adduction of extremities and return to relaxed flexion.	Asymmetric response is seen with peripheral nerve injury (brachial plexus), fracture of clavicle or long bone of arm or leg, or birth trauma such as skull fracture.	Disappears by 6 months.
Truck incurvature (Galant's reflex)	Use one hand to lift the prone newborn off a flat surface (ventral suspension). With a finger from the free hand, use some pressure to draw a line down the length of the back about an inch from the spinal column.	Newborn flexes pelvis toward the side stimulated.	Absence indicates spinal cord lesion or CNS depression.	Disappears by 4 months.
Tonic neck (fencing)	Turn the newborn's head to one side when infant is resting in the supine position.	Extremity on the side to which the head is turned extends and opposite extremities flex. Response may be absent or incomplete immediately after birth.	Persistent response after 4 months may indicate neurologic injury.	Diminishes by 4 months.
Moro	Expose the newborn to sudden movement or loud noise.	Newborn abducts and flexes all extremities and may begin to cry.	Absence of response may indicate neurologic deficit or deafness. Response may be absent or diminished during sleep.	Diminishes by 4 months.
Crossed extension	Place the newborn in the supine position and extend one leg while stimulating the bottom of the foot.	Newborn's opposite leg flexes and extends rapidly as if trying to deflect stimulus to the other foot.	Weak or absent response is seen with peripheral nerve injury or fracture of a long bone.	Disappears by 6 months.
Palmar grasp	Place a finger in the newborn's palm and apply slight pressure.	Newborn grasps finger; attempting to remove the finger causes newborn to tighten his or her grasp.	Weak or absent grasp is seen in the presence of CNS deficit or nerve or muscle injury.	Does not disappear.

CNS, central nervous system.

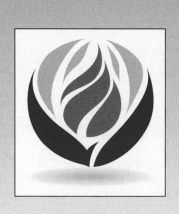

Jill Janke

CHAPTER 20

Newborn Nutrition

This chapter offers information and guidelines for the perinatal nurse caring for new mothers and infants during the initiation and early days of infant feeding. This chapter emphasizes that breast milk is the ideal food for the newborn and provides helpful information for nurses working with families who choose to breastfeed. In addition, guidelines are given for helping families who choose to formula-feed their newborn.

impact the infant feeding decision, including encouragement from the husband; significant others (AAFP, 2008; Bolling, Grant, Hamlyn, & Thornton, 2007; Kervin et al., 2010); extended family, including grandmothers (Anderson, Nicklas, Spence, & Kavanagh, 2009; Grassley & Eschiti, 2008; Ryan & Zhou, 2006); and peers (Anderson et al., 2009; Chapman, Morel, Anderson, Damio, & Perez-Escamilla, 2010).

INFANT FEEDING DECISION

The decision about what to feed a newborn is frequently made by the mother long before giving birth (American Academy of Family Physicians [AAFP], 2008; Labbock & Taylor, 2008; Swanson, Power, Kaur, Carter, & Shepherd, 2007). A woman's selection of an infant feeding method is more than just a lifestyle choice; it should be based on current scientific evidence. Perinatal nurses have the responsibility to make sure a woman has the needed information to make an informed decision. However, once an informed decision is made, the mother's choice should be respected by all healthcare professionals.

A mother's infant feeding decision is influenced by many factors, including her education (Callen & Pinelli, 2004; Labbock & Taylor, 2008; Phares et al., 2004), age (Labbock & Taylor, 2008; Phares et al., 2004), previous breastfeeding experience (Bailey & Wright, 2011), prenatal breastfeeding education (Dyson, Green, Renfrew, McMillan, & Woolridge, 2010; Kervin, Kemp, & Pulver, 2010), and the attitudes and knowledge of healthcare professionals (Britton, McCormick, Renfrew, Wade, & King, 2007; Kervin et al., 2010; Ryan & Zhou, 2006). Sources of personal support also

BENEFITS OF BREASTFEEDING

Human milk is a dynamic food, meeting the infant's needs to build an immune system, to grow and develop the brain, and to form attachments with other human beings. Research has produced compelling data about the short- and long-term health benefits of breastfeeding for the mother and newborn. Numerous economic advantages of breastfeeding have also been identified.

NEWBORN HEALTH BENEFITS

There is substantial scientific evidence that newborns who are breastfed, or who are given breast milk, are healthier than those who receive formula. An integrated review and meta-analysis (Ip et al., 2007) concluded that during the first year of life, breastfed infants have decreased their risk for severe respiratory illness by 72%, otitis media by 50%, gastrointestinal illness by 64%, necrotizing enterocolitis by 5%, and sudden infant death syndrome (SIDS) by 36%. The long-term neonatal health benefits of breastfeeding have also been identified. Table 20–1 lists long- and short-term medical problems that may be associated with not breastfeeding.

Table 20–1. RISK OF SPECIFIC MEDICAL CONDITIONS THAT MAY BE ASSOCIATED WITH NOT BREASTFEEDING

Disease or Condition	Study	Result
Asthma	Ip et al. (2007)	Meta-analysis found a significant association between breastfeeding and a 27% reduced risk of asthma in subjects without family history of asthma. Subjects under 10 yr of age who were breastfed and had positive family history of asthma also had reduced risk.
	Bener, Ehlayel, Alsowsidi, & Sabbah (2007)	Exclusive breastfeeding prevents development of asthma and allergic diseases in children.
	Ogbuanu, Karmaus, Arshad, Kurukulaaratchy, & Ewart (2009)	Using lung function as a measure of susceptibility to asthma, children breastfed for at least 4 mo had increased lung volume, suggesting a decreased susceptibility to asthma.
Otitis media	Ip et al. (2007)	Meta-analysis showed breastfeeding was associated with a significant reduction (50%) in the risk of otitis.
Respiratory conditions	Ip et al. (2007)	Meta-analysis found a 72% reduction in the risk of being hospitalized with a lower respiratory tract disease in infants who were exclusively breastfed for 4 mo or longer.
	Mihrshahi, Oddy, Peat, & Kabir (2008)	Exclusive or predominant breastfeeding can reduce rates of respiratory infection.
Gastrointestinal (GI) infection	Ip et al. (2007)	Evidence from three primary studies shows that breastfeeding was associated with 64% reduction in the risk for GI infection during first year of life.
	Mihrshahi et al. (2008)	Exclusive or predominant breastfeeding can reduce rates of diarrhea.
	Monterrosa et al. (2008)	Predominantly breastfed infants had lower risk for GI infection during the first 6 mo when compared to formula-fed and partially breastfed infants.
Cognitive development	Ip et al. (2007)	Meta-analysis included preterm and term infants. Results are inconclusive because no studies controlled for maternal IQ.
	Kramer et al. (2008)	Randomized controlled trial with 17,046 infants (81.5% were followed to age 6.5 yr). Reported strong evidence that prolonged and exclusive breastfeeding is associated with children's cognitive development.
	Bartels, van Beijsterveldt, & Boomsma (2009)	Significant positive effect of breastfeeding found on cognitive abilities after controlling for differences in maternal education.
	Rees & Sabia (2009)	A study of siblings concluded breastfeeding is associated with cognitive ability.
	Sloan, Stewart, & Dunne (2010)	A study of 137 infants concluded breastfeeding over 1 mo may have a beneficial effect on cognitive development.
Obesity	Ip et al. (2007)	Meta-analysis concluded there is an association between breastfeeding and reduced risk of obesity later in life.
	Butte (2009)	Breastfeeding had small but consistent protective effect against childhood obesity. Author noted that genetic and environmental variables may pose greater risk, such as socioeconomic status, parental obesity, parental smoking, birth weight, and rapid weight gain during infancy.
	Griffiths, Smeeth, Hawkins, Cole, & Dezateux (2009)	Initiating and prolonging breastfeeding may reduce excessive weight gain during the preschool years.
Diabetes	Ip et al. (2007)	Evidence suggests that breastfeeding for >3 mo is associated with reduced risk of developing type 1 and type 2 diabetes (39%).
	Taylor, Kacmar, Nothnagle, & Lawrence (2005)	Systematic review concluded that being breastfed for at least 2 mo might lower the risk of diabetes in children.
Necrotizing enterocolitis (NEC)	Ip et al. (2007)	Evidence supports an association between breastfeeding and reduced risk of NEC in preterm infants.
	Henderson, Craig, Brocklehurst, & McGuire (2007)	Subjects who did not develop NEC were significantly more likely to have received human breast milk when compared to those who did develop NEC (91% vs. 75%).
	Chauhan, Henderson, & McGuire (2008)	Concluded that feeding preterm infants human milk vs. formula can reduce the risk of NEC threefold.
Allergies	Ip et al. (2007)	Results equivocal, more research needed.
Sudden infant death syndrome (SIDS)	Ip et al. (2007)	Meta-analysis showed a significant reduction in the incidence of SIDS (36%) when infant breastfed.
Cardiovascular disease	Ip et al. (2007)	Results inconclusive on the relationship between breastfeeding and adult cholesterol and between breastfeeding and mortality from cardiovascular disease. However, there was a significant association between breastfeeding and a small reduction in adult blood pressure.
Childhood leukemia and lymphomas	Ip et al. (2007)	Meta-analysis concluded there was a significant association between breastfeeding for at least 6 mo and a reduced risk for acute lymphocytic leukemia (ALL) and acute myelogenous leukemia (AML).

MATERNAL HEALTH BENEFITS

Maternal health benefits also are associated with breastfeeding. In the immediate postpartum period, breastfeeding enhances mother–infant attachment. It also stimulates uterine involution resulting in less blood loss, thus reducing the risk for anemia and infection. Long-term maternal health benefits are also related with breastfeeding. Typically, the more breastfeeding a woman does during her lifetime, the greater the health benefits. Known benefits include a 28% risk reduction for developing breast cancer, a 21% risk reduction for ovarian cancer, and a 2% to 12% risk reduction for type II diabetes (Ip et al., 2007; Stuebe & Schwarz, 2010). In addition, breastfeeding is associated with a reduced risk for developing metabolic syndrome (Gunderson et al., 2010), hypertension, hyperlipidemia, and cardiovascular disease (Schwarz et al., 2009).

ECONOMIC BENEFITS

Exclusive use of formula and its consequent increased neonatal morbidity is responsible for substantial expenditures of healthcare dollars. Bartick and Reinhold (2010) estimated that there would be an annual healthcare cost savings of $13 billion if 90% of new mothers in the United States breastfed exclusively for the first 6 months. Employers also benefit when a woman breastfeeds. The U.S. Department of Health and Human Services (USDHHS; 2008) has published a toolkit, *The Business Case for Breastfeeding*, which includes reports from various companies that have implemented breastfeeding support programs in the workplace. One organization reported increased breastfeeding rates at 6 months (72.5%) after implementation of their support program. They also reported an annual savings of $240,000 in healthcare expenses for breastfeeding mothers and children, a 72% reduction in lost work time due to infant illness that resulted in an annual savings of $60,000, and lower pharmacy costs due to a 62% reduction in prescriptions.

CONTRAINDICATIONS TO BREASTFEEDING

The American Academy of Pediatrics (AAP; 2012) and AAFP (2008) maintain that with few exceptions, human milk is preferred for all infants, including premature and sick newborns. Contraindications to breastfeeding are rare and include a mother who has human T-cell lymphotropic virus type I or II infection; needs cancer treatment with antimetabolites, chemotherapeutic agents, or radiation; has untreated active tuberculosis; uses illicit drugs; has herpes simplex lesions on the breast; or who is seropositive for the human immunodeficiency virus (HIV). Breastfeeding is also contraindicated when infants have certain types of inborn errors of metabolism, such as galactosemia (AAP, 2012).

INCIDENCE OF BREASTFEEDING

HEALTHY PEOPLE GOALS

Given the importance of breast milk and breastfeeding to mothers, newborns, and society as a whole, one of the Healthy People 2020 national goals is to increase initiation and duration rates of breastfeeding. The target initiation and duration rates have been altered over the last three decades as more information about infant feeding practices is available. The Healthy People 2020 target for *any* breastfeeding is that 81.9% of women will initiate breastfeeding, 60.6% will be breastfeeding at 6 months, and 34.1% will still be breastfeeding until the infant is 12 months of age. The Healthy People 2020 target for *exclusive* breastfeeding is that 44.3% of women who initiated breastfeeding will exclusively breastfeed through the first 3 months and 25.5% will exclusively breastfeed for 6 months (USDHHS, 2011).

The AAP (2012) and the AAFP (2008) recommend that women continue to breastfeed longer than 12 months if mutually desired. The World Health Organization (WHO; 2011) extends that recommendation to 2 years or longer. There is no evidence of psychological or developmental harm from continued breastfeeding into the third year of life or longer. Researchers have reported distinct benefits to extending breastfeeding past the first year. The AAFP (2008) noted that children weaned before 2 years have an increased risk of illness. This was supported by an older study (Gulick, 1986) that reported toddlers between the ages of 16 and 30 months who continued to breastfeed had fewer illnesses and, when they did get sick, their illness was of shorter duration when compared to nonnursing toddlers.

While breastfeeding rates have steadily increased since the 1990s, more work is needed to meet the Healthy People 2020 goals. According to a national survey conducted on 2007 data, 75% of mothers in the United States initiated breastfeeding; of those, 33% were exclusively breastfeeding at 3 months. At 6 months, 43% continued to do some breastfeeding, with 13.3% breastfeeding exclusively. At 1 year, 22.4% of women continued doing some breastfeeding, and at 18 months, 7.4% were still breastfeeding (Centers for Disease Control and Prevention [CDC], 2010a). Although no Healthy People 2020 goal has been set for breastfeeding beyond 1 year, the Breastfeeding Report Card published by the CDC (2010a) noted that breastfeeding at 18 months ranged from 5.5% to 7.4% between 2000 and 2007.

Despite research identifying the benefits of giving breast milk to preterm infants, no national goal has been set for this high-risk population. No national statistics were found on breastfeeding rates for preterm infants, but we do know they are much lower than for term infants. In one report, breastfeeding rates in the neonatal intensive care unit (NICU) ranged from 36.9% to 50%

Table 20–2 HEALTHY PEOPLE BREASTFEEDING GOALS

Goal	2010 Target	2020 Target	National Immunization Study 2007 (CDC, 2010a)	
			Overall U.S. Average	Range (State Disparity)
Initiate any breastfeeding	75%	81.9%	75.0%	52.5%–89.8%*
At 6 mo, any breastfeeding	50%	60.6%	43.0%	20.2%–62.2%†
At 12 mo, any breastfeeding	25%	34.1%	22.4%	8.0%–39.7%†
At 3 mo, exclusive breastfeeding	40%	44.3%	33.0%	15.2%–50.8%**
At 6 mo, exclusive breastfeeding	17%	25.5%	13.3%	6.5%–23.7%

* Thirteen states have exceeded Healthy People 2020 goal for initiating any breastfeeding.
† One state has exceeded Healthy People 2020 goal for any breastfeeding at 6 mo.
† Four states have exceeded Healthy People 2020 goal for any breastfeeding at 12 mo.
** Nine states have exceeded Healthy People 2020 goal for exclusive breastfeeding at 3 mo.

(Castrucci, Hoover, Lim, & Maus, 2007). It is important to note that the higher rate was associated with hospitals that used lactation consultants. Among late preterm infants (34 0/7 to 36 6/7 weeks' gestation), breastfeeding initiation was reported between 59% and 70%, with a significant reduction in breastfeeding duration and exclusivity (Radtke, 2011).

Although the overall breastfeeding rates have improved, the CDC (2010a) reported great disparity in breastfeeding initiation and duration between geographic areas and various population groups, with some states reporting much higher rates than others. See Table 20–2 for a comparison of Healthy People 2010 and 2020 goals, the average U.S. breastfeeding rates, as well as the range disparities in rates between states.

PROFILE OF WOMEN WHO BREASTFEED

Knowing the characteristics of women who are less likely to initiate and continue breastfeeding can help the perinatal nurse target at-risk populations for more education and support. Researchers have reported consistently that breastfeeding is lowest among women who are African American, had less than or equal to a high school education, were single and younger than 20 years of age, lived in the southern United States, and were enrolled in the Women, Infants, and Children (WIC) program (CDC, 2010a; Labbock & Taylor, 2008; Ziol-Guest & Hernandez, 2010). In contrast, women who are more likely to initiate and continue breastfeeding tend to be Caucasian or Hispanic, at least 30 years of age, married, college educated, not enrolled in the WIC program, and not living in the southeastern part of the United States (CDC, 2010a; Labbock & Taylor, 2008).

It is anticipated that rates of breastfeeding initiation, duration, and exclusivity in WIC women will improve in the future. In 2009, federal regulations were passed that offered incentives to WIC women who exclusively breastfed. Examples of incentives included receiving larger maternal food packages over a longer period of time (1 year). By comparison, mothers who used formula received free formula and a smaller maternal food package for a shorter period of time (6 months). These incentives, in addition to the breastfeeding education and support from WIC counselors, should positively impact breastfeeding rates in WIC women (USDHHS, 2011).

BARRIERS TO BREASTFEEDING

Researchers have identified barriers to breastfeeding that are responsive to interventions (Display 20–1). The Healthy People 2020 national plan addresses several of those interventions, including increased worksite support, reduced hospital supplementation rates, and improved hospital practices (USDHHS, 2011).

It is well documented that hospital policies can adversely impact breastfeeding. In 1991, the WHO and the United Nations International Children's Emergency Fund (UNICEF) published the *Baby-Friendly Hospital Initiative* (WHO/UNICEF Joint Statement, 1989). This document included the *Ten Steps to Successful Breastfeeding*, which was designed to eliminate counterproductive hospital practices (Display 20–2). Researchers have reported that implementation of the *Ten Steps* facilitates successful breastfeeding by all women (Abrahams & Labbock, 2009; Bartick, Stuebe, Shealy, Walker, & Grummer-Strawn, 2009; DiGirolamo, Grummer-Strawn, & Fein, 2008; Forster & McLachlan, 2007; Murray, Rickets, & Dellaport, 2007; Rosenberg, Stull, Adler, Kasehagen, & Crivelli-Kovach, 2008). Some hospitals have sought official "Baby-Friendly Hospital" certification. In 2006, there were 52 Baby-Friendly hospitals and birthing centers in the United States. This increased to 108 in 2011. While not all hospitals have sought Baby-Friendly certification, many have modeled their policies and protocols after the *Ten Steps* with similar improvements in breastfeeding rates.

Perinatal nurses need to understand their role in promoting breastfeeding. The Association of Women's Health, Obstetric and Neonatal Nurses (AWHONN; 2007a) identifies the professional responsibilities of perinatal nurses who care for breastfeeding women

DISPLAY 20–1

Barriers to Breastfeeding that Are Responsive to Interventions

Healthcare Professionals
- Apathy
- Misinformation
- Professional education that lacks information on breastfeeding
- Outdated clinical practices

Hospital Practices
- Failing to provide skilled support (i.e., lactation experts)
- Routine separation of mother–infant dyad
- Delay of first feeding
- Routine formula or water supplementation
- Use of pacifiers
- Lack of staff training
- Lack of a breastfeeding policy
- Inappropriate interventions (i.e., supplemental feeding, pacifiers, overuse of nipple shields)
- Disruptions of breastfeeding
- Discharge packs that include formula samples and/or coupons for formula
- Lack of discharge policy
- Lack of follow-up after discharge

Lack of Support
- From partner, peers, and family
- From workplace
- From healthcare professionals

Societal Attitudes
- Media portrayal of bottle-feeding as normal
- Commercial pressures on mothers to bottle-feed or supplement with formula
- Formula club sign-up sheets in obstetric offices and clinics
- Prenatal formula starter kits
- Coupons for free formula
- Formula ads in parent magazines
- Formula ads on Internet sites of interest to parents
- Discounted formula available through the Internet

DISPLAY 20–2

Ten Steps to Successful Breastfeeding

1. Have a written breastfeeding policy that is routinely communicated to all healthcare staff (see *Model Breastfeeding Policy* [Academy of Breastfeeding Medicine [ABM], 2010b]).
2. Educate healthcare providers in skills necessary to implement this policy.
3. Inform all pregnant women about the benefits and management of breastfeeding.
4. Help mothers initiate breastfeeding within 1 hour of birth.
5. Show mothers how to breastfeed and how to maintain lactation even when they are separated from their newborns.
6. Give newborns no food or drink other than breast milk, unless medically indicated.
7. Practice "rooming-in"; allow mothers and newborns to remain together 24 hours each day.
8. Encourage unrestricted breastfeeding.
9. Give no artificial nipples or pacifiers to breastfeeding newborns.
10. Foster the establishment of breastfeeding support groups and refer mothers to them on discharge from the hospital or clinic.

From World Health Organization/United Nations International Children's Emergency Fund Joint Statement. (1989). *Protecting and supporting breastfeeding: The special role of maternity services.* Geneva, Switzerland: World Health Organization. Retrieved from http://www.babyfriendlyusa.org/eng/index.html

and newborns in the prenatal and postpartum periods (Display 20–3). Many of those responsibilities are aimed at reducing barriers to breastfeeding.

BREASTFEEDING PROMOTION

Several systematic reviews were published on interventions designed to increase breastfeeding initiation, exclusivity, and duration in term infants (Chapman et al., 2010; Chung, Raman, Trikalinos, Lau, & Ip, 2008; Hannula, Kaunonen, & Tarkka, 2008). They concluded that multiple interventions, using a variety of educational methods and sources of professional and peer support, were more effective over any single intervention. In addition, programs that spanned the prenatal,

intrapartal, and postpartal time periods were more successful than interventions that focused on a single time period. A systematic review on breastfeeding promotion in the NICU found the following interventions to be effective at promoting preterm breastfeeding: skin-to-skin contact, peer support, breast milk pumping on both breasts simultaneously, staff training across all disciplines, and Baby-Friendly accreditation (Renfrew et al., 2009). The authors concluded it was unlikely any single intervention made a difference; rather, it was the combination of multiple interventions.

PHYSIOLOGY OF MILK PRODUCTION

Perinatal nurses need to understand the science of milk production. This knowledge is essential to help women breastfeed successfully.

MAMMOGENESIS

Mammogenesis refers to growth of the mammary glands. It occurs in two stages as the gland responds to the hormones of puberty and later during the first half of pregnancy. During pregnancy, estrogen and progesterone prepare the breasts for lactation. Numerous external changes occur. The breasts enlarge; the skin stretches and appears thinner, making veins more visible. The nipples enlarge, and the Montgomery glands

DISPLAY 20-3

Breastfeeding and the Role of the Nurse in the Promotion of Breastfeeding

- Attain knowledge about the benefits of breastfeeding, including anatomy and physiology of lactation, initiation of lactation, and management of common concerns and problems.
- Provide preconception and antenatal counseling on the benefits of breastfeeding.
- Provide breastfeeding education to all women during prenatal period, including exploration of concerns, fears, and myths that may inhibit successful breastfeeding.
- Work in collaboration with lactation specialists and other healthcare providers to optimize the breastfeeding experience for the mother and infant.
- Integrate culturally appropriate and sensitive information into all breastfeeding education.
- Ensure that breastfeeding is initiated in the immediate postpartum period whenever possible.
- Promote nonseparation of mother and baby during the postpartum period.
- Provide information about breastfeeding resources in the community at the time of hospital or birthing center discharge.
- Use and conduct research related to breastfeeding.

From Association of Women's Health, Obstetric and Neonatal Nurses. (2007a). *Breastfeeding and the Role of the Nurse in the Promotion of Breastfeeding*. Washington, DC: Author.

become prominent and start to secrete a substance that lubricates and protects the nipples and areola. The areola grows in diameter and darkens. Internal changes in the breast also occur and include growth and differentiation of the mammary ducts as well as development of the lobules and alveoli. Sometime in the second trimester, lactogenesis I begins (Lauwers & Swisher, 2011; Lawrence & Lawrence, 2011).

LACTOGENESIS I

Lactogenesis I starts around midpregnancy and lasts until 1 to 2 days postpartum. During this time, further cell differentiation occurs, and the lactocytes that are capable of secreting milk components proliferate. Prolactin levels rise during pregnancy and stimulate production of colostrum, which is present from midpregnancy forward (Lauwers & Swisher, 2011; Lawrence & Lawrence, 2011).

LACTOGENESIS II

Lactogenesis II is defined as the onset of copious milk production that occurs 48 to 72 hours after the birth (Hurst, 2007). Prolactin levels rise higher in the postpartum period when levels of progesterone drop after the placenta is expelled. The higher prolactin levels, along with infant suckling, stimulate the breast to

synthesize and secrete milk (Lauwers & Swisher, 2011; Lawrence & Lawrence, 2011).

Delayed onset of lactogenesis II can occur. In one study, 44% of the 431 subjects experienced delayed onset of lactation (Nommsen-Rivers, Chantry, Peerson, Cohen, & Dewey, 2010). It is important that perinatal nurses know the risk factors for delayed onset and monitor and intervene accordingly. Common risk factors for delayed onset of lactogenesis II are listed in Display 20–4.

LACTOGENESIS III

Lactogenesis III is the phase when a woman has established a mature milk supply. Production of milk changes from the hormonal endocrine control that exists in the first few days after birth to autocrine control when the milk supply is more established. With autocrine control, prolactin continues to be produced in response to infant suckling and emptying of the breasts. Oxytocin is also released in response to suckling. This occurs numerous times during a feeding. Oxytocin stimulates the cells around the alveoli to contract and eject milk down the ducts, making it accessible when the newborn suckles. The sensation that accompanies the release of oxytocin on breast tissue is referred to as the letdown reflex or the

DISPLAY 20-4

Common Risk Factors for Delayed Onset of Lactogenesis II

Primiparity

Maternal age ≥30 years

Cesarean birth

Prolonged labor

Obesity

High levels of stress during the birth

Premature delivery (including late preterm)

Insulin dependent diabetes mellitus

Birth weight >3,600 g

Retained placenta

Surgical procedures on breast

Insufficient mammary tissue

Breast hypoplasia

Delay with first feeding

Hypothyroid

Hypertension

Data from Hurst, 2007; Nommsen-Rivers, L. A., Chantry, C. J., Peerson, J. M., Cohen, R. J., & Dewey, K. G. (2010). Delayed onset of lactogenesis among first-time mothers is related to maternal obesity and factors associated with ineffective breastfeeding. *American Journal of Clinical Nutrition, 92*(3), 574–584; Scott, J. A., Binns, C. W., & Oddy, W. H. (2007). Predictors of delayed onset of lactation. *Maternal & Child Nutrition, 3*(3), 186–193. doi:10.1111 /j.1740-8709.2007.00096.x

milk-ejection reflex. Some mothers feel this as a heaviness or tingling sensation in the breast. Other mothers never feel the milk let down but observe milk leaking from the other breast or hear the newborn swallowing milk (Riordan & Wambach, 2010; Walker, 2011).

Oxytocin also stimulates uterine contractions that control postpartum bleeding and promote involution. Mothers, especially multiparous women, feel these "after-birth pains" during feedings for several days after the birth. The discomfort can create a distraction that inhibits milk letdown. It is important to make the mother comfortable prior to and during the feeding. To minimize discomfort from afterpains, mothers should be encouraged to keep their bladder empty, since a full bladder contributes to cramping. An analgesic prior to feeding should be considered. Ibuprofen is often effective, but in some cases, a mother might need something stronger. Nurses should reassure the mother that afterpains are normal and help limit blood loss; they are also self-limiting, lasting a few days (Riordan & Wambach, 2010; Walker, 2011).

Oxytocin-producing neurons throughout the brain are thought to be associated with social behavior and attachment. In addition to being released in the maternal brain tissue, oxytocin is released into the newborn brain by means of milk transfer and is thought to modulate attachment behaviors between mother and newborn (Insel, 1997; Nelson & Panksepp, 1998). Oxytocin also is partially responsible for the calmness women exhibit while breastfeeding and has been linked to a decreased response to stressors and pain in the breastfeeding woman (Goer, Davis, & Hemphill, 2002).

Milk production is a supply-and-demand system; as milk is removed from the breast, prolactin triggers the breast to produce more milk. For most women, milk production closely matches the needs of the newborn. The more efficiently the newborn nurses, the faster the rate of milk synthesis (Lawrence & Lawrence, 2011).

Leaving milk in the breasts for long periods can contribute to slower and lower amounts of milk production. A whey protein, feedback inhibitor of lactation (FIL), inhibits milk secretion as alveoli become distended and milk is not removed. The longer the period of time milk is left in the breast, the greater the concentrations of FIL. This mechanism works independently, and each breast will synthesize milk at different rates depending on the frequency and degree of drainage (Lawrence & Lawrence, 2011).

BIOSPECIFICITY OF HUMAN MILK

Human milk is a species-specific fluid. The composition is not static or uniform. Breast milk is designed to meet the needs of newborns to grow and develop a brain, protect the immature gut, be a substitute for an immature immune system, and assist in developing attachment behavior. The composition of human milk changes over time. Colostrum (1 to 5 days postpartum) evolves to transitional milk (6 to 13 days postpartum) and then into mature milk (14 days and beyond). During any given feeding, foremilk changes to hindmilk the longer the infant breastfeeds. Milk composition also fluctuates over the course of the entire lactation. Milk of preterm mothers differs from that of term mothers in order to meet the nutritional needs based on gestational age. For example, during the first 3 to 5 days after birth, term milk contains 1.85 g/dL of protein, whereas preterm milk contains 3.00 g/dL (Walker, 2011).

Colostrum is present in the breast from about 12 to 16 weeks of pregnancy. This first milk is thick and has a yellowish color. Average energy value is about 18 kcal/oz, compared with mature milk, which contains 21 kcal/oz (AAP Committee on Nutrition, 2009). The volume of colostrum is low (measured in teaspoons), which ensures the infant will want to nurse frequently. This frequent nursing is what stimulates the transition to milk. Compared with mature milk, colostrum is higher in protein, sodium, chloride, potassium, and fat-soluble vitamins. It is rich in antioxidants, antibodies, interferon, fibronectin, and immunoglobulins, especially secretory immunoglobulin (Ig) A. Secretory IgA is antigen specific. When mothers come in contact with microbes, antibodies are synthesized in their milk, targeting pathogens in the newborn's immediate environment. These antibodies are passed to the newborn. Separating the mother and newborn interferes with this defense mechanism. Colostrum begins the establishment of normal bacterial flora in the newborn's gastrointestinal tract and exerts a laxative effect that begins elimination of meconium, decreasing the potential reabsorption of bilirubin (Riordan & Wambach, 2010; Walker, 2011).

Mature milk composition changes during the feeding. Foremilk is produced initially; it is more watery and has lower fat content. Later in the feeding on a given breast, cell membranes release fat globules and protein, which forms hindmilk (Lawrence & Lawrence, 2011). Hindmilk is high in calories and fat and is critical to growth and brain development. To make sure infants get adequate hindmilk, the baby should be allowed to completely finish on one side before offering the other breast. Babies are done feeding on a breast when the baby lets go of the nipple, falls asleep, or ceases to actively suck and swallow (Lawrence & Lawrence, 2011).

NUTRITIONAL COMPONENTS

WATER

Human milk is composed of 87.5% water, in which all other components are dissolved, dispersed, or in suspension (Riordan & Wambach, 2010; Walker, 2011).

Infants receiving adequate amounts of breast milk do not need additional water, even in hot climates (Almroth, 1978; Ashraf, Jalil, Aperia, & Lindblad, 1993).

FAT (LIPIDS)

Fat content of human milk ranges from 3.5% to 4.5% and contributes 50% of the calories (Walker, 2011). It varies during a feeding; hindmilk has almost double the fat content when compared to levels in foremilk (Saarela, Kokkonen, & Koivisto, 2005). Fat content increases over the first days of lactation and shows diurnal rhythms. Total fat content is reduced in mothers who smoke (Agostoni et al., 2003; Vio, Salazar, & Infante, 1991) and increases when women breastfeed more frequently. The long-chain polyunsaturated fatty acids docosahexanoic acid and arachidonic acid contained in breast milk are found in the brain, retina, and central nervous system of newborns and are necessary for the growth of these structures during the first year of life (Riordan & Wambach, 2010). The absence of these fatty acids in formula may contribute to differences in cognitive development that has been reported in the literature (Anderson, Johnstone, & Remley, 1999; Ip et al., 2007; Walker, 2011).

PROTEIN

Protein concentration is high in colostrum and settles to 0.8% to 1.0% in mature milk. The whey-to-casein ratio in human milk changes from 90:10 in the early milk to 60:40 in mature milk and 50:50 in late lactation (AAP Committee on Nutrition, 2009; Walker, 2011). The whey protein that predominates in human milk forms soft curds that are easily digested and supply the infant with most of the nutrients in human milk. One of the components of the whey protein, lactoferrin, is important in the immunologic effects of human milk. The bacteriostatic effect of lactoferrin makes iron unavailable to pathogens that require the mineral to proliferate (Riordan & Wambach, 2010).

CARBOHYDRATE

The principal carbohydrate in human milk is lactose. Lactose supports colonization of the gut with microflora that increases the acidity of the intestine. The increased acidity decreases growth of pathogens and ensures a supply of galactose and glucose, which are necessary for brain development. Calcium absorption is also enhanced in the acidic environment (Riordan & Wambach, 2010; Walker, 2011).

VITAMINS AND MINERALS

Breast milk contains all of the vitamins and minerals needed by most infants for about the first 6 months of life. In the event that iron stores need additional support in the first 6 months, oral iron drops may be needed. After 6 months of exclusive breastfeeding, infants require supplementary food rich in iron and zinc (AAP, 2012). Vitamin D deficiency is a risk factor for some breastfed children, and due to scattered reports of rickets in the United States, the AAP now recommends all infants receive a vitamin D supplement of 400 IU/day beginning at hospital discharge (AAP, 2012; Wagner & Greer, 2008). It is important to note that human milk does have vitamin D, estimated to average 26 IU/mL. While adequate for some infants, this quantity is inadequate in cases where infants lack sun exposure (due to climate or use of sunscreen) or when the mother is deficient in vitamin D during pregnancy.

PRETERM MILK AND LACTATION

DIFFERENCES BETWEEN PRETERM AND TERM MILK

Like milk produced by mothers of term infants, milk produced by mothers of preterm infants changes to meet the infant's growth needs. Composition differs from term milk with higher levels of immune factors, energy, lipids, protein, nitrogen, and fatty acids (Riordan & Wambach, 2010; Walker, 2011).

BENEFITS OF HUMAN MILK FOR PRETERM INFANTS

The preterm infant benefits from receiving human milk with lower rates of infection, necrotizing enterocolitis, and hospital readmissions. In addition, preterm infants who receive breast milk have improved feeding tolerance, enhanced neurodevelopment, increased scores on cognitive and developmental tests, and closer family attachment. Given the extensive benefits of human milk, the AAP (2012) indicated all preterm infants should receive human milk, ideally the mother's own milk; if mother's milk is not available, pasteurized donor milk can substitute. Mothers who breastfeed or provide breast milk for their preterm infants demonstrated increased self-esteem and maternal role attainment. Although these benefits are similar for term infants, they have far greater impact on the vulnerable preterm infant (British Columbia Reproductive Care Program, 2001; Merewood, Brooks, Bauchner, MacAuley, & Mehta, 2006).

PRETERM BREASTFEEDING BARRIERS

Mothers of preterm infants face the same barriers to breastfeeding as do mothers of term infants. They also have unique barriers, such as the need to use hand expression or a breast pump for a prolonged period of time and possible limited contact with their infant. Reduced mother–infant contact may be due to the infant's condition or due to the mother being discharged from the hospital. In some large regional centers, mothers may live a distance from the facility. Stress is known to inhibit milk production (Walker, 2011). The NICU environment contributes to maternal stress with all its

DISPLAY 20-5

Resources and Guidelines for Preterm Breastfeeding

Association of Women's Health, Obstetric and Neonatal Nurses (AWHONN) (http://www.awhonn.org)

March of Dimes (http://www.modimes.org)

Oklahoma Infant Alliance (http://www.oklahomainfantalliance.org /lpi_guidelines.html)

Cochrane Database of Systematic Reviews (http://www.thecochrane library.com)

California Perinatal Quality Care Collaborative (http://www.cpqcc .org/quality_improvement/qi_toolkits/nutritional_support_of _the_vlbw_infant_rev_december_2008)

Academy of Breastfeeding Medicine (ABM) Protocols (http://www.bfmed.org/Resources/Protocols.aspx)

Breastfeeding Support: Prenatal Care Through the First Year Guideline, Second Edition. (AWHONN, 2007b)

Assessment & Care of the Late Preterm Infant Guideline (AWHONN, 2010)

Prematurity Awareness Campaign

Caring for the Late Preterm Infant: A Clinical Practice Guideline (Oklahoma Infant Alliance, 2010)

"Cup Feeding versus Other Forms of Supplemental Enteral Feeding for Newborn Infants Unable to Fully Breastfeed" (Flint, New, & Davies, 2008)

Nutrition support of the VLBW infant (revised) (California Perinatal Quality Care Collaborative, 2008)

ABM Clinical Protocol #10: "Breastfeeding the Late Preterm Infant" (ABM, 2011)

ABM Clinical Protocol #16: "Breastfeeding the Hypotonic Infant" (ABM, 2007b)

ABM Clinical Protocol #22: "Guidelines for Management of Jaundice in Breastfeeding Infant Equal to or Greater than 35 Weeks' Gestation" (ABM, 2010a)

---

machines, monitoring devices, and alarms (AAFP, 2008). Other sources of stress for NICU mothers often include fear for their infant, separation from their infant, or concerns about the cost of intensive care.

PROMOTING PRETERM BREASTFEEDING

Nurses play a major role in promoting breastfeeding for preterm infants. Certain practices have been proven helpful: early discussion of breastfeeding; written materials; promotion of hand expression along with simultaneous pumping of both breasts with a hospital grade electric pump; breast massage; encouraging skin-to-skin contact (kangaroo care) to facilitate attachment, milk production, and subsequent establishment of breastfeeding; and use of an alternate feeding method, such as cup feeding, instead of an artificial nipple (AAFP, 2008). Mothers also need to learn about storage methods for expressed milk. Display 20–5 provides a list of guidelines and resources for preterm breastfeeding.

BREASTFEEDING PROCESS

PREPARATION FOR BREASTFEEDING

Physical Preparation

There is no research supporting physical preparation of the breasts during pregnancy. Prenatal nipple rolling, application of creams, and expression of colostrum have not been shown to decrease pain or nipple trauma during the postpartum period. Use of methods to improve nipple erectility, such as Hoffman exercises and breast shells, may actually decrease a woman's desire and motivation to breastfeed by conveying the message that her nipples are inferior and need correcting (Centuori et al., 1999; Riordan & Wambach, 2010).

Prenatal Education

Women should be encouraged to attend prenatal breastfeeding classes. The short postpartum hospital stay puts pressure on the nurse, the mother, and the newborn to demonstrate effective breastfeeding before some mother–baby couples are ready. The fast learning pace in the inpatient setting and the mother's cognitive sluggishness for verbal instructions during the first 24 hours postpartum suggest that there would be a benefit in providing breastfeeding information before birth. Prenatal breastfeeding education programs have been shown to increase the knowledge levels of pregnant women and their partners, increase the support women perceive from their partners around the decision to breastfeed, and increase breastfeeding initiation and duration rates (Guise et al., 2003; Lauwers & Swisher, 2011; Riordan & Wambach, 2010; Sikorski, Renfrew, Rindoria, & Wade, 2002; U.S. Preventive Services Task Force [USP-STF], 2008). The Academy of Breastfeeding Medicine (ABM; 2009) has a clinical protocol for breastfeeding promotion (see Display 20–5 for resources).

POSITIONING FOR BREASTFEEDING

A variety of positions are used for breastfeeding. It is important that the mother assume a relaxed, comfortable position with her back and arms well supported. If she is seated in a chair, placing a footstool beneath her feet decreases strain on her back and may discourage her from leaning forward over the baby. Some mothers benefit from a pillow on the lap or use of a commercially available nursing pillow. These can be especially helpful when nursing twins. If the mother is lying on her side, a pillow behind her back will help with support (Riordan & Wambach, 2010; Walker, 2011).

The newborn and the mother should face each other while breastfeeding. The mother should not lean forward over the newborn but instead concentrate on bringing the baby toward her. The newborn should be loosely wrapped or not wrapped at all so the nurse and the mother can clearly see the infant's position on the breast. There is no need to be concerned about keeping the newborn warm because mother and baby generate body heat during breastfeeding. Skin-to-skin contact is useful for increasing a low temperature in a newborn during the transitional period. As the feeding progresses, if necessary, a light blanket may be placed over both for privacy (Riordan & Wambach, 2010; Walker, 2011).

Cradle Hold

With the mother comfortably seated, the newborn is held in a side-lying position with his or her entire body completely facing the mother. Held on a slight incline, the newborn's lower arm is tucked around the outside of the breast. The newborn's body is in complete contact with the mother; the newborn's legs are wrapped around her waist. If the newborn is wrapped in a blanket, loosen it to permit the newborn to freely move its arms and legs. Avoid covering the infant's hands with the undershirt cuffs. The newborn's head rests on the mother's forearm, which along with her wrist and hands, supports the baby's back and bottom (Fig. 20–1). Specially designed L-shaped pillows fit around the mother's waist and help to elevate and support her arm. Use of this pillow has been associated with increased length of breastfeeding at 2 and 8 weeks (Humenick, Hill, & Hart, 1998). Regular bed pillows may also be used.

Cross-Cradle Hold

The cradle position can be modified by having the woman alter the position of her arms, using what is called the cross-cradle hold. This is a good position to use for preterm infants and infants with fractured clavicles. The newborn is placed in the same position

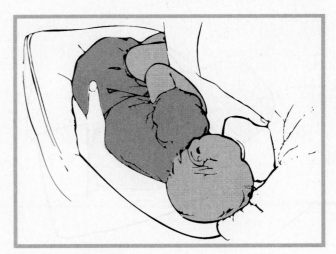

FIGURE 20–1. Cradle hold.

as in the cradle hold but held with the opposite arm such that the head is in the mother's hand and her forearm is supporting the back. This gives the mother much more control over positioning and, along with the clutch hold, may be easier to learn (Fig. 20–2).

Clutch Hold

The clutch position (i.e., football hold) is useful for feeding preterm infants or twins and for mothers who have had a cesarean birth. The newborn is positioned to the mother's side. Placing a pillow under the newborn raises the infant slightly and decreases the weight the mother needs to lift. The newborn's head is in her hand, and its feet are positioned toward her back. Care should be taken to ensure that the full weight of the breast does not rest on the newborn's chest (Fig. 20–3).

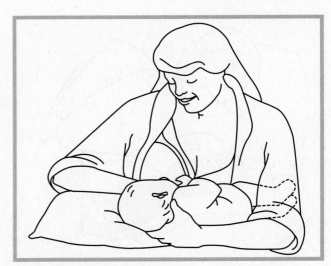

FIGURE 20–2. Cross-cradle hold.

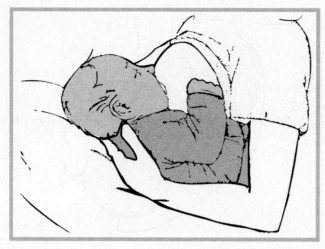

FIGURE 20–3. Clutch hold.

Side Lying

The side-lying position works well after a cesarean birth or for a woman with a painful perineum. In this position, the newborn and the mother lay on their sides facing each other. A small rolled blanket can be placed behind the newborn's back, or the mother can support the infant with her free arm (Fig. 20–4).

Laid-Back Breastfeeding

Laid-back breastfeeding is based on the concept of biologic nurturing (BN). Central to BN is the assumption that breastfeeding initiation is intrinsic for both mother and baby and not something they need to learn. BN stresses the fact that no one posture is right for everyone. Women are capable of finding a position of comfort, and positions can change and evolve over time (Colson, Meek, & Hawdon, 2008).

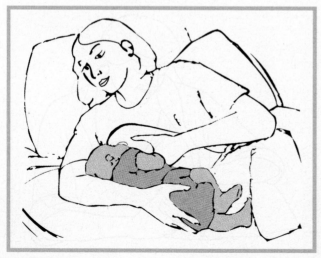

FIGURE 20–4. Side lying.

Many women choose a semireclined position. Once the mother is comfortable, the baby is placed prone on the mother's front with the baby's face near the breast. Skin-to-skin should be optional based on the mother's preference. While the traditional positions (see previous) may work for some women, the BN approach allows women more options and is much less prescriptive. More information on BN can be found at http://www.biologicalnurturing.com (Colson et al., 2008).

SUPPORTING THE BREAST

Historically, mothers have been encouraged to support their breasts using a variety of techniques (scissor hold, C-hold, etc.). The current approach is to let the mother decide what works best for her. In some cases and in some positions, there is no need to hold the breast. In the event the breast is being held, a variety of techniques could be used as long as the mother's fingers do not impede the infant from a correct latch or compress ducts (Colson et al., 2008).

Figure 20–1 shows the commonly used C-hold. With this technique, the mother supports her breast with her thumb on top and fingers below and against the chest wall. The thumb and fingers are away from the areola. This hold makes it easy for the mother to direct her nipple toward the center of the mouth during latch on. Mothers are encouraged to use whichever hand is more comfortable. Pressure should not be applied to the breast with the thumb. The newborn's pug-shaped nose allows breathing through the grooves along the sides of the nares during breastfeeding, even when the nose is touching the breast. In all breastfeeding positions, pulling the newborn's buttocks closer to the mother's body or gently lifting the breast causes the newborn's head to drop back slightly, providing room for breathing (Riordan & Wambach, 2010; Walker, 2011).

LATCH ON

Proper attachment of the newborn at the breast is necessary for pain-free and effective milk transfer. Once positioned comfortably, the mother moves the newborn's lips to the nipple; when the newborn's mouth is wide open, she draws the newborn forward toward her. The lower lip and chin contact the breast first. The newborn should grasp the nipple and areola, pulling it as a unit forward and deep into his mouth. The tongue is cupped and thrust forward over the lower gum. When the jaw lowers and creates negative pressure, milk moves into the trough of the tongue and is channeled to the back of the mouth, where the swallow reflex is triggered. Display 20–6 lists observations made when the newborn is latched on to the breast correctly.

For women with very large breasts, a rolled receiving blanket or small towel can be placed under the breast so the baby does not drag down on the nipple. Care

DISPLAY 20-6

Observations Indicating Correct Latch On

- Lips are rolled outward (flared).
- Clicking or smacking sounds are absent.
- Dimpled cheeks are absent.
- Muscles above and in front of the ear move.
- Both cheeks are equally close to the breast.
- Chin and nose are touching the breast.
- All of the nipple and part of the areola is covered by the newborn's mouth.
- More of the areola is visible above the upper lip than below it.
- Angle at the corner of the mouth is wide.
- When the lower lip is gently pulled away from the breast, the tongue is visible over the lower gum line.

Data from Lauwers, J., & Swisher, A. (2011). *Counseling the Nursing Mother: A Lactation Consultant's Guide* (5th ed.). Sudbury, MA: Jones & Bartlett; Lawrence, R. A., & Lawrence, R. M. (2011). *Breastfeeding: A Guide for the Medical Profession* (7th ed.). Philadelphia: Saunders; Riordan, J. M., & Wambach, K. (2010). *Breastfeeding and Human Lactation* (4th ed.). London, England: Jones & Bartlett.

DISPLAY 20-7

Signs that Milk Transfer Is Occurring

- Proper latch on.
- Baby moves from short, rapid sucks to slow, deep sucks early in feeding.
- Vibration on the occipital region of the head.
- Deep jaw excursion.
- No dimpling or puckering of baby's cheeks.
- Mother verbalizes a drawing sensation on the breast.
- Breast tissue does not slide in and out of baby's mouth when baby sucks or pauses.
- No smacking or clicking sounds with sucking, which indicate that the tongue has lost contact with the nipple and areola.
- Mother notices letdown.
- Audible swallows (usually heard after onset of copious milk production).
- Mother's breast softens (noted after stage II lactogenesis).
- Baby spontaneously unlatches and is satiated.
- Mothers nipple does not appear blanched or compressed.
- Adequate newborn weight gain of 4–6 oz/week.
- Baby stooling and voiding appropriate for age.
- Baby content between most feedings.

Data from Lauwers, J., & Swisher, A. (2011). *Counseling the Nursing Mother: A Lactation Consultant's Guide* (5th ed.). Sudbury, MA: Jones & Bartlett; Lawrence, R. A., & Lawrence, R. M. (2011). *Breastfeeding: A Guide for the Medical Profession* (7th ed.). Philadelphia: Saunders; Riordan, J. M., & Wambach, K. (2010). *Breastfeeding and Human Lactation* (4th ed.). London, England: Jones & Bartlett.

should be taken to avoid pushing the newborn's head into the breast. Pressure on the occipital region of the head causes extension of the neck. Tilting, squeezing, or distorting the nipple or areola should also be avoided because doing so can cause pain and skin damage. If the mother feels a pinching or biting sensation while nursing, she should be instructed to pull down gently on the newborn's chin. This causes his mouth to open wider so that more of the areola is drawn into his mouth. If this does not work, have the mother insert her little finger into the side of the newborn's mouth to release the suction (Riordan & Wambach, 2010; Walker, 2011). She should begin again to achieve a better latch on.

MILK TRANSFER

When the newborn suckles effectively, the breast releases milk and milk transfer occurs. Even though a newborn may suck at the breast for 15 minutes with its jaw moving up and down, it does not mean that there has been a transfer of milk. Display 20–7 lists the signs that are observed when milk transfer occurs.

SIGNS OF ADEQUATE INTAKE

Evaluating the newborn for adequate intake is based on elimination patterns, behavioral observations, moist mucous membranes, and weight gain. Table 20–3 outlines elimination patterns for the early days of life. If the number of wet diapers or bowel movements is below what is expected based on age, parents should be instructed to notify their primary care provider.

Wet diapers can be used to assess hydration, and the number of bowel movements provide evidence that milk

transfer has occurred. Urine should be clear and pale yellow. Because urine contains an abundance of uric acid crystals during the first week of life, occasionally, a pink or rust-colored stain is seen on the diaper. After the first week, presence of this pink stain is an indicator of insufficient intake. Super absorbent diapers make it difficult for some parents to tell when the diaper is wet. Parents can place a soft, dry paper towel, tissue, or square of toilet paper inside the diaper with each change to more easily tell when the diaper is wet. Other signs that the newborn is sufficiently hydrated include moist mucous membranes and skin that does not remain tented when lightly pinched.

Table 20–3. ELIMINATION PATTERN DURING THE FIRST WEEK OF LIFE

Age (days)	Number of Wet Diapers	Number of Bowel Movements
1	1–2	1
2	2–3	2
3	3–4	3–4
4	4–5	3–4
5	4–5	3 or more
6	6–8	3 or more
7	8 or more	3 or more

Stools change from meconium to transitional stools to yellow, seedy liquid. Yellow stool should be present by the end of the first week. Some infants pass stool as frequently as every feeding for the first 4 to 6 weeks. Shrago, Reifsnider, and Insel (2006) reported that less weight loss has a positive association with the number of bowel movements a newborn has per day during the first 5 days. Other indications of adequate intake is earlier transition to yellow bowel movements, earlier return to birth weight, and increased weight at 14 days of life (Riordan & Wambach, 2010; Walker, 2011).

Observation of newborn behaviors also provide clues regarding adequacy of intake. The newborn should demonstrate a range of behaviors during the day, including being alert, acting hungry, being fussy, and acting satisfied after feeding (Riordan & Wambach, 2010; Walker, 2011).

Newborns should regain their birth weight by 2 weeks of age and continue to gain 4 to 7 oz weekly or at least a pound per month (Lawrence & Lawrence, 2011). According to the AAP (2012), all breastfed newborns should be assessed by a healthcare provider 3 to 5 days after birth (or sooner if indicated) to assure there is adequate intake. An infant who has lost more than 7% of his or her birth weight may have breastfeeding problems that need addressing (Riordan & Wambach, 2010; Walker, 2011). Researchers are currently looking at iatrogenic neonatal weight loss that is unrelated to breastfeeding problems. In 2011, Chantry, Nommensen-Rivers, Cohen, and Dewey reported that excessive neonatal weight loss was associated with mothers who received large quantities of intravenous (IV) fluids in labor. They hypothesized that the IV fluids resulted in fetal volume expansion, which increased birth weight. They reported that newborns of mothers who had large amounts of IV fluids had more voids when compared to newborns of mothers who did not receive large amounts of IV fluids. While these are preliminary findings, the authors proposed that increased number of voids resulted in greater weight loss (Chantry et al., 2011).

BREASTFEEDING MANAGEMENT

GETTING STARTED

Early and frequent breastfeeding along with skin-to-skin contact promotes optimal breastfeeding (Merten, Dratva, & Ackermann-Liebrich, 2005; Riordan & Wambach, 2011). Breastfeeding should be initiated within an hour of birth. This is an ideal time since the infant demonstrates sucking movements that peak 45 minutes after birth and decline over the next 2 hours. Early feedings are associated with mothers who breastfeed for a longer duration (Anderson, Moore, Hepworth, & Bergman, 2007; Chaves, Lamounier, & Cesar, 2007; Ekstrom, Widstrom, & Nissen, 2003; Hake-Brooks & Anderson, 2008; Moore, Anderson, & Bergman, 2007).

Skin-to-skin contact following the birth has been correlated with exclusive breastfeeding. A dose-response relationship was found with the odds of exclusive breastfeeding, increasing the longer the initial skin-to-skin contact lasted. Women who experienced skin-to-skin contact for 15 minutes were 1.3 times more likely to exclusively breastfeed, whereas those who had skin-to-skin contact for an hour or longer were 3.15 times more likely to exclusively breastfeed (Bramson et al., 2010).

It is recommended that the healthy newborn be placed on the mother's chest and given the opportunity to seek and find the nipple. Nonsedated babies follow a predictable pattern of prefeeding behavior when held on the mother's chest immediately after birth. This enhances bonding and elicits newborn feeding behavior such as bringing hands to mouth, nuzzling, and licking the breast (Colson et al., 2008; Righard, 2008). Successful latch on and suckling at this time greatly reduces sucking disorganization or dysfunction later on and contributes to increased breastfeeding duration (Chaves et al., 2007; Wiklund, Norman, Uvnäs-Moberg, Ransjö-Arvidson, & Andolf, 2009). It also lowers the risk of hypothermia (Galligan, 2006), hyperbilirubinemia, and hypoglycemia, all of which can adversely impact breastfeeding initiation and duration (Anderson et al., 2007; McCall, Alderdice, Halliday, Jenkins, & Vohra, 2008; Walker, 2009; Walters, Boggs, Ludington-Hoe, Price, & Morrison, 2007).

Some analgesics given during labor (such as nalbuphine [Nubain] or butorphanol [Stadol]) have the potential to interfere with the early development of breastfeeding behaviors, especially if given within 1 hour of birth (Jordan, Emery, Bradshaw, Watkins, & Friswell, 2005; Ransjo-Arvidson et al., 2001). These drugs can also negatively influence breastfeeding in the long term (Henderson, Dickinson, Evans, McDonald, & Paech, 2003; Jordan, 2006; Torvaldsen, Roberts, Simpson, Thompson, & Ellwood, 2006). DiGirolamo and colleagues (2008) reported mothers who did not receive any pain medication during labor were more likely to breastfeed beyond 6 weeks.

One group of researchers reported that mothers who received epidurals were less likely to initiate breastfeeding in the first 4 hours, and, subsequently, their infants were more likely to receive formula and not be fully breastfeeding at discharge (Wiklund et al., 2009). Researchers reported labor epidurals had no adverse effects on breastfeeding, although it was acknowledged that confounding variables such as postnatal support may have influenced the results (Wieczorek, Guest, Balki, Shah, & Carvalho, 2010). It has been suggested that with the trend toward lower dosed epidurals, the adverse impact on breastfeeding is negated (Chang & Heaman, 2005; Devroe, DeCoster, & Van de Velde, 2009). The perinatal nurse may be able to offset some of the side effects of labor medications by placing the infant skin-to-skin and helping the mother initiate breastfeeding early. It is important to keep the mother and the newborn together and to teach the mother to recognize hunger cues (Lauwers & Swisher, 2011).

SUSTAINED MATERNAL–NEWBORN CONTACT

Twenty-four–hour rooming-in supports breastfeeding and is an integral component of family-centered maternity care. However, the practice of rooming-in needs to be flexible and its implementation needs to be respectful of the needs and desires of new mothers. Rooming-in enables a woman to recognize and respond to her newborn's needs and begin to develop confidence in her mothering role. The mother learns to recognize hunger cues and to respond with a feeding (American College of Obstetricians & Gynecologists [ACOG], 2007). If the mother and the newborn are together when the newborn demonstrates early hunger cues (Display 20–8), she can begin feeding. If the newborn is in a nursery, feeding is delayed until a healthcare professional witnesses the hunger cues and transports the newborn to the mother's room. During this delay, the newborn may become increasingly agitated, may self-console and return to sleep, or become exhausted from crying and return to sleep. By the time the newborn reaches his mother, the optimal feeding opportunity is missed.

Hunger cues can be observed for up to 30 minutes before the newborn begins a sustained cry for food. Feeding is most successful if initiated while the newborn is in a quiet, alert state. Crying is a late hunger cue and may interfere with effective breastfeeding. It is often necessary to console the newborn before he will settle and feed well. Feeding before the newborn begins a sustained cry reduces stress and some of the accompanying

undesirable physiologic side effects such as glycogen depletion, increased intracranial pressure, resumption of fetal circulation within the heart, disorganized sucking, and poor feeding (Riordan & Wambach, 2010; Walker, 2011).

Extended contact with the newborn may facilitate a feeding pattern that includes clustered feedings (i.e., 5 to 10 feedings over 2 to 3 hours, followed by 4 to 5 hours of deep sleep). Parents need to understand that cluster feedings are normal and that they often occur in the evenings. Many mothers interpret the increased feeding demands as an inadequate supply of breast milk and it undermines their confidence. In reality, cluster feedings often occur in the evening (6 pm to 10 pm), which results in the deep sleep occurring when parents also want to sleep. Despite the many benefits of rooming-in, DiGirolamo and colleagues (2008) reported that only 57% of U.S. hospitals allowed 24-hour rooming-in (Riordan & Wambach, 2010; Walker, 2011).

FEEDING FREQUENCY AND DURATION

Historically, fixed breastfeeding schedules were thought to be more scientific, safer because the stomach had to be emptied before allowing a refill, a way to prevent sore nipples, less disruptive for the family if the newborn was on a schedule, and more efficient on a maternity unit. Current understanding of this practice is that restricting breastfeeding in the early days after birth can increase the incidence of sore nipples, engorgement, and perceived need to supplement. In addition, more women may discontinue breastfeeding by 6 weeks postpartum (Renfrew, Lang, Martin, & Woolridge, 2000). Breastfeeding patterns, however, vary widely between mother and baby pairs, over each 24-hour period, and during the course of the lactation. When no artificial time limits are placed on breastfeeding, the number of feedings during each 24 hours ranges from 8 to 12. The number of feedings depends on age, physiologic capacity of the stomach, ability of the newborn, and storage capacity of the breasts (Riordan & Wambach, 2010; Walker, 2011).

Frequency and duration of feedings is different for breastfed and formula-fed newborns. Formula-fed infants have a mean gastric half-emptying time of 65 minutes, with a range of 27 to 98 minutes; breastfed infants have a mean gastric half-emptying time of 47 minutes, with a range of 16 to 86 minutes (Van den Driessche et al., 1999). The shorter emptying time means breastfed newborns can be hungry 30 to 60 minutes after a feeding, and parents need to know this is normal and expected. They also need to know that newborns who nurse frequently are learning to feed and that the amount of colostrum available for initial feedings is ideal to meet the current physiologic stomach capacity of the newborn. In a typical feeding, the newborn should feed on the first breast until satiated. The feeding ends when the newborn comes

---

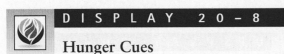

DISPLAY 20 - 8

Hunger Cues

- Rapid eye movements under the eyelids
- Sucking movements of the mouth and tongue
- Hand-to-mouth movements
- Body movements
- Small sounds (soft cooing or sighing sounds)
- Rooting
- Mouth opening in response to tactile stimulation
- Smacking of lips
- Wide-open eyes; quiet, alert state
- Restlessness

Crying is a late feeding cue and may interfere with effective breastfeeding. Data from Lauwers, J., & Swisher, A. (2011). *Counseling the Nursing Mother: A Lactation Consultant's Guide* (5th ed.). Sudbury, MA: Jones & Bartlett; Lawrence, R. A., & Lawrence, R. M. (2011). *Breastfeeding: A Guide for the Medical Profession* (7th ed.). Philadelphia: Saunders; Riordan, J. M., & Wambach, K. (2010). *Breastfeeding and Human Lactation* (4th ed.). London, England: Jones & Bartlett.

off the breast on its own after swallowing for most of the feeding. If the mother is uncertain whether the newborn is satisfied, she can use hand/manual expression (Display 20–9) and/or alternate massage (Display 20–10). Alternate massage is recommended when infant's swallowing is slowing down. This technique increases the volume and fat content of the milk. There are no time limits on the duration of feedings. In the first days after birth, some newborns nurse from only one breast at a feeding. The other side is offered at the next feeding, usually within 1 or 2 hours. Feeding frequently encourages an abundant milk supply, minimizes engorgement and sore nipples, enhances weight gain, reduces jaundice and hypoglycemia, and

---

DISPLAY 20-9

Manual Expression Technique

Preparation
Wash hands.
Have a clean container to collect expressed milk (or a towel if not saving the milk).
Promote flow of milk, for example.
Gently massage breasts prior to and throughout manual expression.
Take warm shower or bath.
Apply warm moist cloth before expressing milk, or take a shower.
Try relaxation techniques, picture of baby, etc.
Find comfortable position, nipple aimed at collection container.

Technique*
Position hands on breast:
1. Place thumb behind areola, above nipple, usually 2–3 cm behind areola.[†]
2. Place index finger behind areola, usually 2–3 cm behind areola.[†]
3. Some women choose a two-handed technique, especially if hands are small relative to breast size.

Expression
1. Press thumb and index finger directly back toward chest wall.
2. Then gently compress ducts with thumb and finger together.
3. Maintain compression while moving thumb and finger back toward the nipple in a milking action (this is a rolling motion; caution the mother not to slide the thumb or fingers along the skin, which will quickly make her sore).
4. Repeat steps 1 through 3 while rotating fingers around the breast (e.g., think of the nipple as a clock, begin with thumb at 12 and finger at 6, then move to 1 and 7, 2 and 8, 3 and 9, etc.)

---

* Many mothers find a variation of the previous method that works equally well or better. Encourage experimentation until they find what works best for them. There is no one correct way.
[†] This is the same position where baby's gums should be during efficient latch on.
Data from Lauwers, J., & Swisher, A. (2011). *Counseling the Nursing Mother: A Lactation Consultant's Guide* (5th ed.). Sudbury, MA: Jones & Bartlett; Lawrence, R. A., & Lawrence, R. M. (2011). *Breastfeeding: A Guide for the Medical Profession* (7th ed.). Philadelphia: Saunders; Riordan, J. M., & Wambach, K. (2010). *Breastfeeding and Human Lactation* (4th ed.). London, England: Jones & Bartlett.

DISPLAY 20-10

Alternate Massage Technique

Purpose
• Encourages sucking in a sleepy baby or poor feeder
• Increases volume of fat content per feeding
• Increases the volume of milk ingested

Technique
• Massage when infant pauses between sucking bursts; massage should be downward and inward to deliver milk into baby's mouth.
• Compress milk ducts with thumb above and your fingers below.
• Or gently massage breast with flat surface of middle fingers.
• Rotate massage around breasts.

Data from Lauwers, J., & Swisher, A. (2011). *Counseling the Nursing Mother: A Lactation Consultant's Guide* (5th ed.). Sudbury, MA: Jones & Bartlett; Lawrence, R. A., & Lawrence, R. M. (2011). *Breastfeeding: A Guide for the Medical Profession* (7th ed.). Philadelphia: Saunders; Riordan, J. M., & Wambach, K. (2010). *Breastfeeding and Human Lactation* (4th ed.). London, England: Jones & Bartlett.

---

increases breastfeeding duration. Display 20–11 lists behavioral signs that indicate the newborn is satiated after feeding. Observing these cues provides new parents with positive feedback that increases their confidence (Riordan & Wambach, 2010; Walker, 2011).

ASSESSMENT

Nursing History

Breastfeeding assessments may be brief or comprehensive, depending on where in the perinatal period the mother is encountered and on whether she or the newborn is having problems. An initial assessment includes

---

DISPLAY 20-11

Satiation Cues

• Gradual decrease in number of sucks over course of feeding
• Pursed lips followed by pulling away from the breast and releasing the nipple
• Relaxed body
• Legs extended
• Absence of hunger cues
• Sleep
• Small amount of milk drools from mouth
• Contented state

Data from Lauwers, J., & Swisher, A. (2011). *Counseling the Nursing Mother: A Lactation Consultant's Guide* (5th ed.). Sudbury, MA: Jones & Bartlett; Lawrence, R. A., & Lawrence, R. M. (2011). *Breastfeeding: A Guide for the Medical Profession* (7th ed.). Philadelphia: Saunders; Riordan, J. M., & Wambach, K. (2010). *Breastfeeding and Human Lactation* (4th ed.). London, England: Jones & Bartlett.

a thorough history. Information should be elicited about any surgery or breast trauma as well as previous experiences with breastfeeding such as problems with latch on, sore nipples, engorgement, and newborn weight gain. Other information that may be useful includes the amount and quality of social support, the mother's knowledge regarding the mechanics of breastfeeding, how long the mother exclusively breastfed other children, when or if she introduced pacifiers and/or bottles, how satisfied she was with the feeding experience, and how long she plans to breastfeed this newborn. It is also important to review a list of all current medications to determine what effect, if any, they may have on lactation. This comprehensive history provides insight into potential problem areas. Without proper evaluation, the wrong nursing interventions may be utilized.

Physical Assessment

A thorough physical assessment should be performed at the time breastfeeding is initiated. Some abnormal physical findings are risk factors for breastfeeding difficulties and should alert the nurse of the need for more help with breastfeeding initiation. Some observations to be aware of include inverted nipples, hypoplastic breasts, and scars.

Women with inverted nipples are able to breastfeed successfully but may need extra help from a lactation expert. Protraction of the nipple often increases with breastfeeding and becomes more pronounced with subsequent pregnancies (Riordan & Wambach, 2010; Walker, 2011).

Another finding indicative of potential breastfeeding problems is hypoplastic breasts. Hypoplastic breasts appear tubular, flat or empty, small, and are usually spaced far from each other. The nipple and areola appear enlarged and bulging at tip. Women with hypoplastic breasts may have difficulty producing milk due to the diminished breast tissue. Initiation of lactation will require frequent, on demand feedings as well as pumping or hand expression (Display 20–9) in between feedings to stimulate milk production. When milk supply is still inadequate to meet the neonate's needs, referral to a lactation expert should be made and other feeding options should be considered, such as a supplementary feeding device (Riordan & Wambach, 2010; Walker, 2011).

Presence of scars on the breasts should be explored to determine their origin, whether surgical or traumatic. Many factors determine if a woman with a history of trauma or surgery can breastfeed. In most cases, they are encouraged to initiate breastfeeding. With the nurses' help and support, many are quite successful in fully or partially breastfeeding.

Assessment Tools

Common methods of documenting breastfeeding interactions do not always provide useful information. Subjective words such as well, fair, and poor do not capture the data needed to assess adequate intake or effectively identify problem areas. Similarly, the phrase "breastfeeding well" does not capture information regarding latch on, audible swallow, time frames, or satiation. Numerous breastfeeding assessment tools assist the perinatal nurse by providing consistent guidelines for evaluating individual feeding events, ensuring continuity of care and communication between healthcare professionals, and providing a clear record in the chart of breastfeeding progress. One example of a breastfeeding assessment tool, the LATCH tool, is displayed in Table 20–4 (Jensen, Wallace, & Kelsey, 1994).

Table 20–4. LATCH: BREASTFEEDING CHARTING SYSTEM

System Component	0	1	2
L = Latch	Too sleepy or reluctant No latch achieved	Repeated attempts Hold nipple in mouth Stimulate to suck	Grasps breast Tongue down Lips flanged Rhythmic sucking
A = Audible swallowing	None	A few with stimulation	Spontaneous and intermittent <24 hr old Spontaneous and frequent >24 hr old
T = Type of nipple	Inverted	Flat	Everted (after stimulation)
C = Comfort (breast/nipple)	Engorged Cracked, bleeding, large blisters or bruises Severe discomfort	Filling Reddened small blisters or bruises Mild or moderate discomfort	Soft Nontender
H = Hold (positioning)	Full assist (staff holds infant at breast)	Minimal assist (i.e., place pillows for support, elevate head of bed) Teach one side; mother does other Staff holds and then mother takes over	No assist from staff Mother able to position and hold baby

From Jensen, D., Wallace, S., & Kelsey, P. (1994). LATCH: A breastfeeding charting system and documentation tool. *Journal of Obstetric, Gynecologic, and Neonatal Nursing, 23*(1), 27–32.

Similar to an Apgar score, this tool assists the perinatal nurse to perform and document a thorough assessment and to identify areas where assistance and support are needed. Another clinical instrument, the Preterm Infant Breastfeeding Behavior Scale (PIBBS) was developed specifically for assessment of preterm infants. The instrument measures rooting, alveolar grasp, duration of latch, sucking, and swallowing (Hedberg & Ewald, 1999; Nyqvist, Rubertsson, Ewald, & Sjoden, 1996). Selection of an assessment tool should be based on what it measures and whether it is appropriate for a given population. Many facilities use a combination of tools. It is important to monitor the literature, as new instruments are being developed and there is ongoing refinement of existing ones. See Table 20–5 for a list of tools currently in use.

SUPPLEMENTAL FEEDINGS

Supplemental feedings for term, healthy, breastfed newborns are seldom necessary except for medical indications (AAP Committee on Nutrition, 2009). If supplementation is being considered, a thorough assessment of the mother and infant should be conducted by a lactation expert. Illnesses in the mother or newborn that may require supplementation include inborn errors of metabolism, very low-birth-weight infants, preterm infants, and certain medications being taken by the mother. Use of supplements without a medical indication is associated with decreased rates of breastfeeding duration and exclusivity (Asole, Spinelli, Antinucci, & DiLallo, 2009; Chezem, Friesen, & Boettcher, 2003; Forde & Miller, 2010; Hauck, Fenwick, Dhaliwal, & Butt, 2010; Pincombe et al., 2008; Rodriguez-Garcia & Acosta-Ramirez, 2008). Placing formula or water bottles in the bassinet or at the bedside of a breastfeeding mother sends a negative message about her ability to successfully breastfeed. Despite the known adverse effect of routine supplementation, 24% of 2,687 birth facilities in the United States reported over half of their healthy full-term breastfed newborns received supplementation while in the hospital (CDC, 2008).

Once the supplement is chosen, a decision must be made about its delivery. It is better to avoid using an artificial nipple since it requires a different sucking technique when compared to breastfeeding and may create problems when the infant is transitioned back to the breast (Rodriguez-Garcia & Acosta-Ramirez, 2008). Using other devices may be preferable to avoid nipple confusion. Some options include tube feeding, cup feeding, finger feeding, spoon feeding, or using a dropper or syringe. All of these methods have strengths and limitations that must be considered (Walker, 2011).

USE OF PACIFIERS AND ARTIFICIAL NIPPLES

Artificial nipples and pacifiers have been associated with incorrect sucking techniques at the breast (Righard, 1998), decreased total duration of breastfeeding (Howard et al., 2003; Kramer et al., 2001; Kronborg & Vaeth, 2009; Nelson, Yu, & Williams, 2005), and fewer feeds in 24 hours (Aarts, Hornell, Kylberg, Hofvander, & Gebre-Medhin, 1999; Howard et al., 1999; Victora, Behague, Barros, Olinto, & Weiderpass, 1997). Use of the artificial nipple may not be the cause of breastfeeding problems; rather, their use may be an indicator of breastfeeding difficulties (Benis, 2002; Kramer et al., 2001; Kronborg & Vaeth, 2009; Schneller, 2010). Mothers who request bottles or pacifiers may be doing so because they lack appropriate knowledge about the effects of artificial nipples and pacifiers and lack confidence in their ability to successfully breastfeed. These women may benefit from contact with a skilled perinatal nurse or lactation consultant to assess the situation and provide appropriate support and education for the breastfeeding mother–infant dyad (Riordan & Wambach, 2010; Walker, 2011).

While there is evidence that early and regular use of a pacifier decreases breastfeeding duration, other researchers reported pacifier use at bedtime resulted in a 36% reduction in the incidence of SIDS (Ip et al., 2007). The exact mechanism of protection is unknown, although some speculate it may be due to the pacifier protecting the airway, or perhaps it lessens the likelihood of sleep apnea. The AAP Task Force on Sudden Infant Death Syndrome (2005) recommends that parents consider offering a pacifier at nap and at bedtime. However, for breastfed infants, they recommend pacifier introduction be delayed until breastfeeding is well established (at least 1 month). Since SIDS typically occurs in infants over 2 months of age, delaying introduction of the pacifier 1 month should not pose a risk. At no time should an infant be forced to take a pacifier. To decrease risk of infection, pacifiers should be cleaned often and replaced regularly. It is also recommended to avoid pacifiers made out of latex, given the risk of allergies (Riordan & Wambach, 2010; Walker, 2011).

MILK EXPRESSION AND BREAST PUMPS

In some situations, a woman may not be able to breastfeed early and frequently enough to stimulate and sustain lactation. When there is a delay, perinatal nurses should teach hand expression (Display 20–9) and advise the mother to use a breast pump. A Cochrane systematic review (Becker, McCormick, & Renfrew, 2008)

Table 20-5. BREASTFEEDING ASSESSMENT INSTRUMENTS

Name of Instrument	Assessment Parameters	Reference
Infant Breastfeeding Assessment Tool (IBFAT)	Readiness to feed Rooting Fixing (latch on) Sucking pattern	Matthews, 1988
Latch Assessment Documentation Tool	Baby's gum line placement Flanged lips Complete jawbone movement Tongue under areola Adequate suction	Jenks, 1991
Systematic Assessment of the Infant at Breast (SAIB)	Alignment Areolar grasp Areolar compression Audible swallowing	Shrago & Bocar, 1990
Mother-Baby Assessment (MBA)	Signaling Positioning Fixing Milk transfer Ending	Mulford, 1992
Latch-on Assessment Tool/ Lactation Assessment Tool (LAT)	The latching process Angle of infant's mouth opening Infant's lip position Infant's head position Infant's cheek line Height at the breast Body rotation Body relationship Breastfeeding dynamic Rhythm of mother's breast while breastfeeding	Healthy Children Project, 2000 Grey Bruce Health Services-Owen Sound (2007) adapted the LAT for clinical use. This can be viewed at: (http://www.gbhn.ca/ebc/documents/LatchToolMarch2007.pdf)
LATCH Scoring System	Latch Audible swallowing Type of nipple Comfort (breast/nipple) Hold	Jensen et al., 1994
Breastfeeding Assessment Score	Maternal age Previous breastfeeding experience Latching difficulty Breastfeeding interval Number of bottles of formula	Hall et al., 2002
H & H Lactation Scale	Maternal confidence/commitment to breastfeeding Perceived infant breastfeeding satiety Maternal/infant breastfeeding satisfaction	Hill & Humenick, 1996
Neonatal Oral-Motor Assessment Scale	29 characteristics of sucking Diagnoses disorganized and dysfunctional sucking	Palmer, 1993
Preterm Infant Breastfeeding Behavior Scale (PIBBS)	Rooting Areolar grasp Duration of latch while sucking Longest sucking episode Swallowing Scores range from 1 to 20	Nyqvist et al., 1996
Mother-Infant Breastfeeding Progress Tool	Mother responds to feeding cues Mother goes ≤3 hr between feeding attempts Mother independently positions self for feeding Mother independently latches infant onto breast No nipple trauma is present No negative comments about breastfeeding	Johnson, Mulder, & Strube, 2007
Protocol to transition breastfeeding/ breast milk–fed premature infant from NICU to home	ABM Clinical Protocol #12: Transitioning the Breastfeeding/ Breast Milk–Fed Premature Infants from the Neonatal Intensive Care Unit to Home	Academy of Breastfeeding Medicine, 2004

NICU, neonatal intensive care unit.

on milk expression notes a greater volume of milk is obtained with the use of simultaneous pumping on a hospital-grade breast pump. While the hospital-grade breast pump is effective, greater output will result when the mother combines the breast pump with hand expression (Morton et al., 2009).

Nurses should know how to correctly size the shield/flange of the breast pump. Shields that are too big or too small can lead to nipple soreness, cracks, and excoriation. A shield that is too big can result in a loss of suction, which leads to inadequate stimulation and lower milk volume (Jones & Hilton, 2008). One author estimated that 30% to 50% of mothers using a breast pump need a larger shield (Jones, Dimmock, & Spencer, 2001; Jones & Spencer, 2007).

Women need education on the correct use of breast pumps and the storage of breast milk. An aseptic technique should be used, starting with clean hands and clean equipment. Many women begin a pumping session by massaging the breasts and expressing a few drops of milk. This does a better job at stimulating letdown than starting immediately with the pump. To stimulate lactation, women should pump at least 8 to 12 times every 24 hours, no matter how high the milk volume. Pumping at night may produce larger quantities of milk because of the higher prolactin levels at that time of day, and mothers should be encouraged to pump at least once during the night. Based on the circumstances, a mother may pump to stimulate initiation of lactation, in place of a missed feeding, between feedings, on one breast while feeding the baby on the other breast, or at the end of a feeding. Table 20–6 describes proper breast milk storage.

HOSPITAL DISCHARGE

Birth facilities should have a discharge protocol to ensure ongoing successful breastfeeding after mothers go home. General recommendations include formal documentation of breastfeeding effectiveness prior to discharge; identification of possible breastfeeding problems based on maternal and/or infant risk factors and a plan of action to address them; ongoing encouragement to breastfeed exclusively for 6 months, followed by ongoing breastfeeding combined with appropriate complimentary foods through the first year of life and preferably for the first 2 years; and the provision of noncommercial breastfeeding educational materials. Additional discharge recommendations can be found in the *Guidelines for Hospital Discharge* (ABM, 2007a).

Many women in the United States come to the hospital expecting to receive some type of discharge "gift bag." The dilemma for perinatal nurses who support breastfeeding is that frequently, these packs contain formula samples. It has been established that receipt of these formula samples has an adverse impact on breastfeeding duration and exclusivity (Rosenberg, Eastham, Kasehagen, & Sandoval, 2008). Despite the scientific evidence about the negative relationship between breastfeeding and formula samples at discharge, many hospitals continue to feel pressure from patients and manufacturers to distribute some type of discharge

Table 20–6. PROPER HANDLING AND STORAGE OF HUMAN MILK FOR HEALTHY TERM INFANTS

Cautions	Do not add fresh milk to already frozen milk.
	Do not save milk from a used bottle for use at another feeding.
	Do not refreeze breast milk once it is thawed.
	Milk should be labeled with date and time.
	Store in 1–4 oz portions to avoid waste and allow faster thawing; you can add portions together (always using oldest milk first).
Thawing	Transfer to refrigerator or thaw in warm water.
	Do not use microwave: heats unevenly and could scald baby or damage milk (heat will destroy up to 30.5% of IgA).
Milk storage for term infants (CDC, 2010b)	Human milk can be kept in the back of the refrigerator for 3–5 days (less temperature fluctuation).
	Milk can be stored in a refrigerator freezer for 6 mo (do not store near ice maker or on door since temperature fluctuates).
	Milk can be stored in deep freezer for up to 1 yr.
Storage containers	Plastic bags designed specifically for freezing human milk. These bags are sturdier than those used in baby bottles and have self-closures that are easier to seal and label. Avoid using ordinary plastic storage bags or formula bottle bags, as these could easily leak or spill.
	Glass or clear hard plastic bottles with single component top (cloudy plastic bottles may have been made with BPA, which can leach into the milk).
Labeling	Clearly label the milk with the date it was expressed to facilitate using the oldest milk first.
	If delivering breast milk to a child care provider, clearly label the container with the child's name and date.

BPA, bisphenol A; IgA, immunoglobulin A.
Data from Centers for Disease Control and Prevention. (2010b). *Proper handling and storage of human milk.* Retrieved from http://www.cdc.gov/breastfeeding/recommendations/handling_breastmilk.htm; Riordan, J. M., & Wambach, K. (2010). *Breastfeeding and human lactation* (4th ed.). London, England: Jones & Bartlett.

pack. A recent national survey found 70% of the birth facilities were giving out discharge packs with formula samples (CDC, 2008). Ideally, a discharge pack given to breastfeeding women would not contain formula samples or coupons but have products that support breastfeeding, such as a manual pump, instructions for manual expression, chemical cold packs, and breast pads.

POTENTIAL BREASTFEEDING PROBLEMS

RELUCTANT NURSER

Newborns are described as reluctant nursers when they latch on only after many attempts, move their head from side to side without latching on, fall asleep or aggressively push away from the breast and arch their back, have a preference for nursing only on one side, do not latch on, or latch on but feed ineffectively. Numerous factors can contribute to a newborn being reluctant to nurse (Display 20–12). Managing this situation requires that the nurse and parents be very patient and not give up on the newborn's ability to eventually latch on correctly and nurse efficiently. Table 20–7 identifies interventions that the nurse can use to encourage the newborn to latch on successfully (Lauwers & Swisher, 2011; Walker, 2011).

Newborns should demonstrate at least one effective breastfeed before discharge. If the newborn has not latched on at all by 24 hours, the mother should begin

to express colostrum manually and feed with a syringe, spoon, or cup (depending on the circumstances, this may need to be started sooner). If the woman is unable to manually express colostrum, an electric or hand pump can be used as an alternative. These mothers should be referred to a lactation consultant for home follow-up and the primary care physician notified of the feeding difficulty. Care should be taken to ensure early follow-up after discharge, within 24 hours (Lauwers & Swisher, 2011).

ANKYLOGLOSSIA (TONGUE TIE)

Ankyloglossia refers to a lingual frenulum that is excessively short and restricts movement of the tongue. The incidence of ankyloglossia in newborns ranges from 3.2% (Ballard, Auer, & Khoury, 2002) to 11% (Hogan, Westcott, & Griffiths, 2005) with a male-to-female ratio of 2:1. In some cases, it can lead to breastfeeding difficulties such as problems with latch on, nipple pain, trauma, and ultimately to premature weaning (Geddes et al., 2008). In one study, frenuloplasty (clipping the frenulum) of 35 newborns diagnosed with ankyloglossia and having breastfeeding difficulties resulted in improved latch on and less pain. At follow-up, 31 out of 35 of the mothers were still breastfeeding and reported satisfaction with the results (Ballard et al., 2002). Other studies have also found that those infants with breastfeeding difficulties and a short frenulum demonstrated improved breastfeeding after a frenulotomy (Geddes et al., 2008; Hong et al., 2010; Klockars & Pitkaranta, 2009). Perinatal nurses should routinely assess the frenulum at birth and reassess should problems with latch on and pain develop. Specifically, they should look for a tongue that does not extrude past the lips, a tongue tip that cannot touch the roof of the mouth, a tongue that cannot be moved sideways, a tongue tip that may look flat or square instead of pointy when the tongue is extruded, or a tongue tip that may be notched or heart shaped.

NIPPLE PAIN

Sore nipples are common during the early days of breastfeeding. Pain can range from mild tenderness to major discomfort. Nipple pain is one of the primary reasons women stop breastfeeding, and nurses should routinely assess for sore nipples. Pain or tenderness may occur in the following situations:

- When the newborn first latches on, disappearing after the newborn begins swallowing
- Periodically during the feeding
- Throughout an entire feeding
- After and/or in between feedings

Obtaining a thorough history of the pain characteristics, observing a feeding, and doing a physical assessment

---

DISPLAY 20–12

Factors Contributing to a Reluctant Nurser

- Poor position at the breast
- Interruption of the organized sequence of prefeeding behaviors immediately after birth
- Use of medications during labor that may prolong the period of state disorganization
- Hypertonia (i.e., jaw clenching, pursed lips, neck and back hyperextension, and tongue retraction or elevation)
- Infrequent feeds leading to an overly hungry newborn baby
- Excessive or prolonged crying, resulting in behavioral disorganization
- Interference with imprinting on the breast from separation, artificial nipples, pacifiers, or inappropriate use of nipple shields
- Excessive pressure on the occipital region of the baby's head from pushing the head forward into the breast
- Vigorous or deep suctioning or intubation causing swelling or pain in the mouth or throat
- Ankyloglossia (tongue tie)

Data from Lauwers, J., & Swisher, A. (2011). *Counseling the nursing mother: A lactation consultant's guide* (5th ed.). Sudbury, MA: Jones & Bartlett; Riordan, J. M., & Wambach, K. (2010). *Breastfeeding and human lactation* (4th ed.). London, England: Jones & Bartlett.

Table 20–7. TECHNIQUES TO ENCOURAGE LATCH ON

Management	Rationale
Keep the mother and baby together.	
After birth, allow the newborn time to seek and find the nipple.	This approach provides the opportunity for the prefeeding sequence of behaviors to occur, which increases the likelihood of proper attachment to the breasts.
Place baby skin-to-skin on mother's chest.	This approach reestablishes or repatterns the initial sucking sequence that may not have occurred immediately after birth. It often calms the baby.
Try laid-back breastfeeding (biologic nursing).	Encourages mothers and babies to do what they know how to do instinctually. Stresses that mother positions for her comfort, often in a semireclined position. Mother places baby "tummy down" on chest and lets gravity keep baby in position. Infant's cheek is rested somewhere near the breast. The baby can lie across the mother in many positions (e.g., vertical, horizontal, at an angle). Using skin-to-skin while doing laid-back nursing also helps.
Help mother recognize feeding cues.	
Instruct the mother to feed her baby on cue (see Display 20–8).	The mother who recognizes and responds to early feeding cues by offering the breast is more likely to achieve successful latch on.
Check positioning at the breast.	
Newborn should completely face the mother with head, neck, and spine aligned.	Poor positioning increases the number of latch attempts needed before obtaining milk, which can frustrate the mother and the newborn.
Mother reclined back comfortably and not leaning forward.	Incorrect position increases the chances that the newborn will not latch correctly, leading to sore nipples, engorgement, insufficient milk production, and slow weight gain.
Mother stabilizes breast if needed and avoids doing so in a way that interferes with milk flow (e.g., scissor hold, fingers touching areola).	Compressing the breast may block ducts, slowing or preventing milk flow.
If the newborn needs help with attachment: • Support head by putting your palm behind baby's shoulders and your index finger and thumb behind the ear. • Cradle head in hand and direct newborn toward breast with heel of hand. • Use forearm to support shoulders.	Avoid pushing on the back of the head; this can stimulate some newborns to arch away.
Bring newborn's nose near nipple with chin touching breast under areola.	Gentle touch of chin on breast triggers reflex to open wide (~140-degree angle).
With mouth open wide, bring newborn onto breast chin first; lower lip should cover more of the areola than upper lip.	This places the nipple at the back of the mouth and allows the tongue and jaw to work smoothly to remove the milk.
Provide latch and sucking incentives.	
Place newborn skin-to-skin.	Helps to calm newborn. Stimulates instinctive feeding efforts.
Have mother express colostrum into a spoon and let newborn lap it up.	Provides nutrients and calms newborn if hungry.
A syringe or soft clinic dropper with expressed colostrum can be used to elicit sucking and guide baby to breast.	
After crying hard for a while, the newborn may not be able to organize himself to feed.	
Place skin-to-skin.	These interventions can calm the newborn and allow him to have a little food in his stomach so he is not so hungry.
Allow newborn to suck on a finger.	
Try spoon, cup, or finger feeding with a little colostrum.	

can help identify the cause of nipple pain and guide interventions. Physical findings include vertical or horizontal red or white lines on the breast; fissures, cracks, or bleeding from the nipple; and blisters or scabs on one or both nipples. Display 20–13 outlines factors that contribute to nipple pain. Transient nipple pain usually peaks between postpartum days 3 and 6. Prolonged or severe soreness beyond the first week requires intervention (Lauwers & Swisher, 2011; Lawrence & Lawrence, 2011; Riordan & Wambach, 2010).

Various interventions can be used by the perinatal nurse to assist a woman experiencing nipple pain continuously or intermittently with feedings. One common misconception is that limiting time on the breast will prevent sore nipples. In reality, it only delays the onset of soreness and causes additional feeding complications such as delay in lactogenesis II, insufficient milk for the baby, increased nipple soreness due to breaking the suction to remove the baby from the breast, and inadequate emptying of the breast

DISPLAY 20-13

Factors Contributing to Sore Nipples

- Poor latch
- *Candida* pain (yeast infection of breast) causes a burning or stabbing pain that continues during the feeding
- Vasospasm caused by infant compressing the nipple so that blood flow is interrupted
- Natural oils being removed from nipple or keratin layers broken down by drying agents (e.g., soap)
- Nipples not being allowed to dry
- Delayed letdown resulting in unrelieved negative pressure
- Manipulation of the nipple and areola such as squeezing it, tilting or pointing it up or down, or pushing it into the mouth
- Mother leaning over to "insert" the breast into the newborn's mouth instead of bringing the baby to the breast
- Not enough of the nipple and areola in the mouth
- Lips curled under rather than flared out
- Tongue behind lower gum and pinching or biting of the nipple
- Breast pushed sideways into the mouth rather than centered over where the nipple points naturally
- Nipple confusion (i.e., mouth configured for feeding on an artificial nipple or pacifier)
- Disorganized or dysfunctional sucking pattern
- Flat or retracted nipples
- Mouth not opened wide enough to encompass areola
- Ankyloglossia (tongue tie)
- Incorrect use of breast pump or shield/flange not correct size for breast

Data from Lauwers, J., & Swisher, A. (2011). *Counseling the Nursing Mother: A Lactation Consultant's Guide* (5th ed.). Sudbury, MA: Jones & Bartlett; Lawrence, R. A., & Lawrence, R. M. (2011). *Breastfeeding: A Guide for the Medical Profession* (7th ed.). Philadelphia: Saunders; Riordan, J. M., & Wambach, K. (2010). *Breastfeeding and Human Lactation* (4th ed.). London, England: Jones & Bartlett.

(Lauwers & Swisher, 2011; Lawrence & Lawrence, 2011; Riordan & Wambach, 2010).

A systematic review of the literature concluded the most important way to prevent sore nipples was to provide prenatal and early postnatal education related to proper breastfeeding techniques and latch on, as well as anticipatory guidance (Joanna Briggs Institute, 2009; Morland-Schultz & Hill, 2005). A variety of topical treatments to reduce nipple pain have been studied, and warm water compresses significantly decreased pain in several studies (Joanna Briggs Institute, 2009). There is anecdotal support for other treatments; however, the scientific evidence is inconclusive for the use of expressed breast milk, breast shells, breast shields, aerosol spray, hydrogel dressing, film dressing, modified lanolin, collagenase, peppermint water/gel, tea bag compresses, and dexpanthenol. The only treatment found to be detrimental was a glycerin-based hydrogel dressing, which was associated with infection in one study (Lochner, Livingston, & Judkins, 2009; Melli et al., 2007; Morland-Schultz & Hill, 2005). Perinatal nurses need to closely monitor the literature on this topic as more research is being conducted on the older treatments as well as some new treatments.

Once the skin is broken around the nipple, there is increased risk of infection. It has been suggested that putting expressed colostrum/breast milk on the nipple helps to prevent infection and assist healing. This is based on knowledge of its bacteriostatic qualities, the antibodies, and anti-inflammatory factors present in colostrum and breast milk. Antibiotic ointment has also been used to prevent bacterial infection once the integrity of the skin is broken. Oral antibiotics are recommended if there is an active infection (Schanler & Enger, 2012). Using a thin silicone nipple shield when the skin is broken to prevent further damage may also help; a lactation expert should be consulted whenever a shield is considered to ensure its proper use (Riordan & Wambach, 2010).

ENGORGEMENT

Women experience a sense of full breasts during the transition to full milk production. This is a physiologic process that is expected and normal. Engorgement is different and results in painful swelling that occurs when the breasts become overfull (Lauwers & Swisher, 2011). Three elements contribute to breast engorgement: congestion and vascularity, accumulation of milk, and edema caused by the swelling and obstruction of drainage of the lymphatic system. Engorgement can involve the areola, the body of the breast, or both areas (Lawrence & Lawrence, 2011).

Areolar Engorgement

Areolar engorgement may reflect edema from large amounts of IV fluids infused during labor or may be due to distension from milk production. If IV fluids cause areolar engorgement, the areola may appear puffy and is responsive to cold-pack application. If distended with milk, the areola may envelop the nipple, and the whole unit becomes difficult for the newborn to grasp. When this occurs, the mother should hand express (Display 20–10) some milk before putting the baby to the breast to avoid tissue damage and pain (Lawrence & Lawrence, 2011).

Peripheral Engorgement

Peripheral engorgement usually does not develop until 2 to 3 days after birth. Some swelling of the entire breast is normal; but if the breasts become hard, red, hot, shiny, and throbbing physiologic engorgement has changed to pathologic engorgement. This can be extremely painful, and the mother needs to breastfeed frequently using gentle, alternate massage (see

Display 20–10). Hand expression (see Display 20–9) may provide relief, and some women are made more comfortable by using cold packs wrapped around the breast (a bag of frozen peas works well). It is important to nurse even when engorged because milk stasis can increase the risk of mastitis; is a major cause of insufficient milk production; and contributes to sore nipples, poor latch on, reduced milk transfer, and slow weight gain by the infant. Separating mothers and babies, especially at night, giving unnecessary supplements, skipping night feedings, and long intervals between feedings exacerbates the problem of engorgement. It is vital to maintain frequent and thorough drainage of the breasts when the breasts become engorged since back pressure in the ducts can lead to atrophy of the milk-secreting cells (Lawrence & Lawrence, 2011; Mangesi & Dowswell, 2010).

HYPOGLYCEMIA

Hypoglycemia in a term newborn usually refers to a blood glucose level below 40 mg/dL. This is a common and usually transient occurrence in the immediate postbirth period. Routine monitoring of blood glucose in healthy term newborns is unnecessary (Committee on Fetus and Newborn & Adamkin, 2011). For at-risk newborns, specific protocols for screening and treatment are recommended (Committee on Fetus and Newborn & Adamkin, 2011).

Hypoglycemia in breastfed newborns can be prevented or greatly reduced by hospital policies that support breastfeeding (Committee on Fetus and Newborn & Adamkin, 2011):

- Breastfeeding within 30 to 60 minutes of birth
- Skin-to-skin contact between mother and newborn to prevent cold stress and use of glucose stores
- Breastfeeding 8 to 12 times per day
- Feeding in response to readiness cues and not on a predetermined schedule
- Not leaving the newborn to cry since prolonged crying rapidly depletes glycogen stores and can contribute to a steep drop in blood sugar levels

Hypoglycemia that recurs or persists longer than 48 to 72 hours may be caused by hyperinsulinemia, an underlying medical condition that is not related to feeding. Hypoglycemia in an asymptomatic newborn that does not respond to oral feeding or in a symptomatic newborn usually necessitates IV glucose infusions. The mother should be encouraged to pump or hand express colostrum into a spoon or cup for the newborn who is unable or reluctant to suckle at the breast. This will help stimulate and maintain the milk supply. If the medical condition permits, the newborn should be fed colostrum every 1 to 2 hours until able to feed effectively at the breast (Riordan & Wambach, 2010).

JAUNDICE

Clinical signs of hyperbilirubinemia are present in up to 60% of all term newborns in their first week and in nearly all preterms (Watson, 2009). There are several types of jaundice, and the perinatal nurse should be able to differentiate between them since the treatment depends on the etiology.

Physiologic Jaundice

Physiologic jaundice, also known as normal newborn jaundice, appears after 24 hours of age, peaks on the third or fourth day of life, and steadily declines through the first month to normal levels. It occurs when bilirubin production exceeds the liver's ability to process it. This results in unbound, unconjugated bilirubin circulating in the bloodstream and then being deposited in the skin (AAP Subcommittee on Hyperbilirubinemia, 2004; Lauwers & Swisher, 2011; Maisels et al., 2009).

Breastfeeding-Associated Jaundice

Breastfeeding-associated jaundice results from iatrogenic causes such as maternal–newborn separation, delayed or scheduled feedings, pacifier use, labor medications resulting in sleepy babies, and unnecessary supplementation. Elevated bilirubin in breastfeeding-associated jaundice is due to inadequate caloric intake and subsequent decreased stooling that allows the high levels of bilirubin in meconium to be reabsorbed. Hospital policies based on the *Ten Steps to Successful Breastfeeding* (see Display 20–2) helps eliminate practices that lead to this type of jaundice (ABM, 2010a; DiGirolamo et al., 2008; Merewood et al., 2006; Lauwers & Swisher, 2011).

Prolonged Physiologic Jaundice (Breast Milk Jaundice; Late-Onset Jaundice)

Prolonged physiologic jaundice is also known as breast milk jaundice or late-onset jaundice. It usually occurs later than physiologic jaundice and is typically seen between the fourth and seventh days of life. Bilirubin levels peak during the second or third week and may persist for 6 to 15 weeks. The etiology is unknown; however, experts agree it is related to suboptimal feeding. Around 10% to 18% of exclusively breastfed infants in the United States lose more than 10% of their birth weight, and reduced caloric intake leads to increased concentrations of bilirubin (ABM, 2010a).

Optimal breastfeeding practices can decrease the incidence and severity of this type of jaundice. However, once identified, it is important to closely monitor bilirubin levels in the event it rises to toxic levels.

In a few cases, it might require treatment. Treatment can include phototherapy and/or short-term supplementation or replacement of breast milk with formula feedings. Supplementation is more supportive of breastfeeding but results in a slower drop in bilirubin levels. When supplementing breastfeeding, excessive amounts of formula should be avoided so the mother can maintain frequent breastfeeding. Another option is to stop breast milk totally for 24 hours and substitute formula. Mothers will need support to maintain breast milk production if they need to supplement or replace breast milk. Care needs to be taken to help mothers understand there is nothing wrong with their breast milk. Rather, it is thought formulas produced from cow's milk inhibit the intestinal absorption of bilirubin (Riordan & Wambach, 2010).

Jaundice Prevention

The following steps are recommended to prevent high levels of bilirubin (AAP Subcommittee on Hyperbilirubinemia, 2004; ABM, 2010a; Maisels et al., 2009; National Association of Neonatal Nursing [NANN], 2010):

- Early initiation of breastfeeding, within 1 hour of birth
- Frequent, on demand breastfeeding (8 to 12 times per day)
- Implementation of protocols for the identification and evaluation of hyperbilirubinemia
  - Assessment of jaundice at least every 8 to 12 hours
  - Provider education stressing that visual inspection is not reliable as the sole method for assessing jaundice
  - Giving nurses independent authority to obtain a TSB (total serum bilirubin) or TcB (transcutaneous bilirubin) level
- Exclusive breastfeeding (no test feedings or supplementation)
- Optimization of breastfeeding management from birth: position, latch, observation of feeding, presence of expert help (i.e., healthcare provider trained in breastfeeding management)
- Maternal education on early feeding cues
- Identification of at-risk infants (so close surveillance/early interventions occur)
- Parental education (written and verbal) on jaundice
- Follow-up care and screening based on time of discharge and risk assessment

INSUFFICIENT MILK

Real or perceived insufficient milk supply is the most common reason for premature weaning (Gatti, 2008; Li, Fein, Chen, & Grummer-Strawn, 2008). Gatti (2008) reported the early postpartum period is when mothers begin to develop a belief of perceived insufficient milk. This is an ideal time for perinatal nurses to educate the mother on ways to ensure adequate supply, to recognize infant hunger (see Display 20–8) and satiety cues (see Display 20–11) as well as signs of milk transfer (see Display 20–7), and signs of adequate intake. Mothers also need to know what "normal newborn behavior" is regarding infant feeding. Many women report they have insufficient milk when the infant wants to eat every 1 to 2 hours or will not sleep through the night, which is a normal and expected behavior. Anticipatory guidance should include the normality of cluster feeds and the sudden increased demand to feed during growth spurts, which typically occur around 2 to 3 weeks, 6 weeks, 3 months, and 6 months. The mother should understand that by feeding frequently, milk supply increases.

Qualitative research during the early postpartum period revealed that women became more confident and empowered by breastfeeding or that their confidence progressively diminished as they expressed concerns about the adequacy of their breast milk. The perception of breast milk inadequacy was related to the inability to determine how much breast milk the infant was getting, anxiety about the adequacy of their own diet, inadequate and conflicting advice from healthcare professionals, and unmet needs for support and nurturing for themselves (Dykes & Williams, 1999). A Bolivian study in 2006 reported women quit breastfeeding due to perceived insufficient breast milk. When asked what led them to the conclusion of insufficient milk, they indicated it was because the "baby cried." The authors of this study concluded that nurses need to go beyond the "breast is best" message and educate women to breastfeed more frequently as a first response to perceived insufficient milk supply (McCann & Bender, 2006).

A small percentage of women produce insufficient milk for psychological, physiologic, or pathologic reasons. These reasons can lead to decreased production and ejection of milk (Riordan & Wambach, 2010). Psychological factors include stress, embarrassment, and pain, all of which may increase production of epinephrine, which causes blood vessels to constrict, resulting in reduced milk synthesis. Epinephrine also decreases production of oxytocin, which is needed for letdown to occur. Physiologic factors include maternal illness such as diabetes, hypothyroidism, anemia, retained placenta, smoking over 15 cigarettes per day, severe postpartum bleeding, past breast surgery (i.e., reduction, augmentation), and some medications. Conditions that interfere with the early, effective, and consistent stimulation of the breasts may also result in insufficient milk. Examples include restrictions on frequency and duration of feedings, more than 3 hours between feedings, skipping night feedings, and use of supplements. Pathologic factors that negatively affect milk production are related to endocrine problems.

Mothers often describe perceived insufficient milk when they experience one or more of the following:

- Baby does not settle or fusses after a feeding.
- Baby wants to feed more frequently (usually associated with growth spurt).
- Baby takes formula from a bottle directly after breastfeeding (artificial nipples stimulate the sucking reflex even when the infant is satiated).
- Mother is unable to express much milk.
- Baby does not sleep through the night or is awake much of the day.
- Breasts are smaller and softer than they should be.
- Initial weight loss of a healthy term baby exceeds 7% (Lauwers & Swisher, 2011; Lawrence & Lawrence, 2011; Riordan & Wambach, 2010).

Strategies to handle real or perceived insufficient milk depend on the cause of the problem. Mismanagement of breastfeeding is the most common contributor to low milk production. This problem is usually revealed during a feeding history. Mothers should be breastfeeding 8 to 12 times each 24 hours with no supplements or pacifiers. A feeding observation is necessary to confirm whether the newborn is swallowing milk or simply engaging in nonnutritive sucking. Mothers should perform alternate massage (Display 20–10) and feed at closer intervals to increase milk production. Refer mothers to a lactation consultant for a thorough breastfeeding assessment and follow-up.

CANDIDA ALBICANS

If the mother complains of burning pain on the nipple or burning and shooting pains in the breast, a fungal infection (i.e., thrush) may be present. This is usually caused by *Candida albicans*. Positive predictive symptoms of *Candida* include complaints of soreness, burning, pain on nipple/areola, nonstabbing pain of the breast, stabbing pain in the breast, and/or skin changes of the nipple/areola that looks shiny and flaky. Common predisposing factors for mothers include women who tested positive for vaginal *C. albicans*, who used broad-spectrum antibiotics, who have nipple damage, whose infant has oral thrush, or whose infant uses a pacifier and/or bottle. Certain oral contraceptives and asthma medications are also risk factors, along with maternal conditions such as diabetes, obesity, or poor endocrine function (Riordan & Wambach, 2010; Walker, 2011). Treatment can be challenging because women often present with *Candida* and *Staphylococcus aureus*, especially if there are nipple fissures. Treatment can be topical or systemic. Every treatment plan should include both mother and infant. Early diagnosis and treatment for *Candida* infection of the nipple and/or breast are critical to supporting successful long-term breastfeeding (Riordan & Wambach, 2010; Walker, 2011; Wiener, 2006).

The newborn with *C. albicans* presents with white patches (i.e., "crumbling curds") on the buccal mucosa, gums, or tongue that can travel to the hard and soft palate and down to the tonsils. It may also appear as pearly white or gray patches. If a patch is removed, a bright red base may be seen as a painfully eroded area. Most babies with thrush in the mouth also have the infection in the intestines and stools, which contributes to a *Candida*-caused diaper rash. Some newborns' mouths are colonized with *C. albicans*, but it is not clinically apparent. Infected infants may be fussy, have a poor appetite, breastfeed poorly, and experience general discomfort (Riordan & Wambach, 2010; Walker, 2011).

The treatment of the fungal infection depends on the location and severity of the infection. Treatment of the mother and newborn simultaneously is important, even if only one has clinical symptoms. Women or infants with suspected *C. albicans* infection should be referred to their primary care provider.

PLUGGED DUCT

Plugged ducts are small, tender breast lumps, the size of a pea. Symptoms include tenderness, heat, possible redness, or a palpable lump with generalized fever. Sometimes the plug can be seen at the opening of the nipple duct (Riordan & Wambach, 2010). Milk stasis or a component of the milk may contribute to this. The application of hot packs and massaging the lump while the baby is sucking helps move this blockage. Other treatments include breast massage, altering infant's position for feeding, and avoiding constrictive clothing. Some women experience repeated plugging of ducts and describe fatty strings being expressed from the breast. Continued milk stasis increases the risk for mastitis (Riordan & Wambach, 2010).

MASTITIS

Mastitis is an inflammatory condition of the breast that may or may not lead to an infection. The incidence of mastitis is between 3% and 30%, and onset is typically in the first 6 weeks postpartum, although it can occur at anytime. The inflammation tends to be unilateral. Symptoms include fever (temperature >38°C [100.4°F]); aching, chills, swelling, and pain at the site which may also be red, hot, and hard; tenderness under the arm; and red streaks from lump toward axilla. Common risk factors include cracked or bleeding nipples, inefficient removal of milk, engorgement, stress or getting run down, missed feedings, longer intervals between feedings, rapid weaning, and pressure on the breast (i.e., tight bra).

Treatment of mastitis includes nursing frequently on both breasts (start on unaffected breast until letdown occurs and then switch), ensuring that the affected breast is emptied, and getting enough rest and adequate nutrition. If symptoms become severe, most clinicians treat with antibiotics. Although antibiotics treat the infection, they do not address the underlying cause of the mastitis. Antibiotic therapy must be accompanied by interventions to identify and correct the cause. Early identification of the cause and the use of appropriate interventions may halt the inflammatory process and prevent progression of an infection. Pain and inflammation at this point can be treated with a nonsteroidal anti-inflammatory drug such as ibuprofen. If there is no improvement within 8 to 24 hours and the mother has signs of a bacterial infection such as a discharge of pus from the nipple, continued fever, or a sudden spike of fever, she should contact her primary care provider immediately. Because *S. aureus* is most commonly associated with breast infections, choices of antibiotics are generally penicillinase-resistant penicillins or cephalosporins. These antibiotics are safe for the infant, and the mother should continue breastfeeding frequently from the affected side (Lawrence & Lawrence, 2011).

LATE PRETERM

Late preterm infants (34 0/7 to 36 6/7 weeks' gestation) are often treated the same as term infants. However, they have a high risk for breastfeeding problems. These infants tend to be sleepy, tire easily, have problems latching on, and may struggle with coordinating their suck-swallow-breathe pattern. In addition, they are at increased risk for dehydration, hypothermia, respiratory distress, hypoglycemia, and jaundice. These problems, along with possible separation of mother and infant secondary to the problems, increase the risk for delayed lactogenesis, which can lead to excessive weight loss (ABM, 2011; Ahmed, 2010; Hamilton, Martin, & Ventura, 2007; Meier, Furman, & Degenhardt, 2007). Interventions should concentrate on establishment of milk supply. The following actions are recommended for stable newborns:

- Have immediate and extended skin-to-skin contact at birth.
- Breastfeed within 1 hour of birth.
- Monitor closely in the first 12 to 24 hours for physiologic stability (temperature, apnea, tachypnea, hypoglycemia).
- Have mother room-in and use frequent skin-to-skin contact.
- Breastfeed on demand, at least eight times in 24 hours and preferably more.
- Offer breast if the newborn does not show feeding cues within 2 to 3 hours.
  - To wake a sleepy newborn who needs to feed, try some of the following: unwrap; place skin-to-skin,

dim the lights; talk to him and try to make eye contact; hold him upright; rub back in a circular motion from shoulder blades down and back up; stroke scalp in gentle but firm circles; change diaper; wipe face with a cool, damp cloth.
- Avoid dehydration or excessive weight loss (weight loss >3% by day 1 or >7% by day 3).
  - Begin using breast pump and/or hand expression if the newborn cannot sustain 15 minutes of effective sucking at least eight times per 24 hours OR within 4 to 6 hours of birth if not breastfeeding well; this provides needed stimulation for milk production. Pumping and hand expression can be after a feeding or in-between feedings.
  - If ineffective breastfeeding continues, may need to supplement with pumped milk using a supplemental feeding device, finger, or cup feeding (avoid bottles).
- Consider ultrathin silicone nipple shield if there is difficulty with latch or evidence of ineffective milk transfer.
- Assess and document breastfeeding at least three times per day by two different healthcare professionals using standardized tool (see Table 20–5).

There are numerous protocols and guidelines on breastfeeding preterm infants available to perinatal nurses. Some are specific to late preterm infants (see Display 20–5).

MEDICATIONS AND BREASTFEEDING

Interruption of breastfeeding for women who are taking medications is usually an unnecessary and potentially damaging recommendation. Most medications have few side effects because the dose received by the newborn is usually less than 1% of the maternal dose and may have low bioavailability to the newborn. Antimetabolites and therapeutic doses of radiopharmaceuticals are examples of medications where breastfeeding is contraindicated. If such medication is needed for a short time period, women can be assisted to pump and dispose of their milk until it is safe for the newborn to nurse. Ideally, newborns can be syringe fed or cup fed during this time (Hale, 2010). There are several excellent sources providing information on the safe use of medications for breastfeeding women (Display 20–14).

POSTPARTUM SURGERY AND BREASTFEEDING

Occasionally, a woman needs surgery while still breastfeeding. When this occurs, she may be advised to stop breastfeeding for a variety of reasons such as the mother's condition, the mother's medications, the lack of caregiver knowledge, or the inability to room-in with

DISPLAY 20-14

Resources for Medications and Breastfeeding

Publications

American Academy of Pediatrics Committee on Nutrition. (2009). *Pediatric Nutrition Handbook* (6th ed.). Elk Grove Village, IL: Author.

Briggs, G. G., Freeman, R. K., & Yaffee, S. J. (Eds.). (2011). *Drugs in Pregnancy and Lactation: A Reference Guide to Fetal and Neonatal Risk* (9th ed.). Philadelphia: Lippincott Williams & Wilkins.

Hale, T. (2010). *Medications and Mothers' Milk* (14th ed.). Amarillo, TX: Pharmasoft Medical.

Drug Information Services

InfantRisk Center. Provides up-to-date evidence-based information on the use of medications during pregnancy and breastfeeding. Calls answered M–F 8 am–5 pm CST (806) 352–2519. Executive director: Dr. Thomas Hale. Web site: http://www.infantrisk.com/

LactMed. Provides free online database with information on drugs and lactation. Part of the National Library of Medicine's TOXNET system, a Web-based collection of resources covering toxicology, chemical safety, and environmental health. Web site: http://toxnet.nlm.nih.gov/cgi-bin/sis/htmlgen?LACT

La Leche League. Offers free phone breastfeeding help 24 hours a day, 7 days a week. Call (877) 452–5324. Web site: http://breastfeedinghelpline.com/

University of Rochester Lactation Study Center. Rochester, NY. Computer database on drugs and human milk for health professionals. Center staffed M–F 10 am–3:30 pm EST. Call (585) 275–0088.

---

the infant. Ideally, everything should be done to help the woman continue breastfeeding if that is her choice. Lactating women admitted to a medical or surgical unit should be seen by a lactation consultant. The staff and the mother often need education on use of the breast pump and the recommended schedule for pumping. If the milk is still safe for the infant, additional education is needed on the storage of the milk. The perinatal nurse and lactation experts have the responsibility of letting other units and physicians know of their availability for consultation.

FORMULA FEEDING

Use of a commercially prepared, iron-fortified infant formula is another method of providing nutrition during the first year of life. Although there is formula available without iron, its use should be discouraged. Parents should be told that the amount of iron in formula is what the baby needs, and contrary to common belief, it does not cause stomach upset or constipation. Use of formula is indicated for newborns in the following situations (AAP Committee on Nutrition, 2009):

- When a mother chooses not to breastfeed or not to breastfeed exclusively
- In the presence of maternal infections caused by organisms that may be transmitted through human milk (such as HIV)
- If the newborn is diagnosed with an inborn error of metabolism causing intolerance to components of human milk, such as galactosemia
- When the mother has been exposed to foods, medications, or environmental agents that are excreted in human milk and may be harmful to the newborn (i.e., drugs of abuse, antineoplastics, mercury, lead)
- After exposure to radioactive compounds requiring temporary cessation of breastfeeding
- As supplementation to breast milk when the newborn does not demonstrate adequate weight gain

Parents may benefit from an understanding that newborns fed formula have a greater risk of acute and chronic illness in the immediate newborn period as well as later in life. Cow's milk; goat's milk; 1%, 2%, or fat-free milk; and evaporated milk are not recommended during the first year of life. These milk products do not contain adequate iron; they increase the renal solute load because of the amount of protein, sodium, potassium, and chloride; and may result in deficiencies in essential fatty acids, vitamin E, and zinc (AAP Committee on Nutrition, 2009). This important information should be provided to the women in an objective manner. The purpose of the discussion is not to make the women feel guilty about their choices but to make sure they have made an informed choice.

COMPOSITION OF FORMULA

Commercially prepared formula can never totally duplicate the hormones, immunologic agents, enzymes, and live cells found in human milk. In 1980, Congress passed the first Infant Formula Act, which was recently revised in 2010 and has addressed some of the differences between breast milk and formula (U.S. Food and Drug Administration [FDA], 2010). This legislation sets minimum and maximum levels of certain nutrients and requires that manufacturers analyze all batches of formula and state on the labels the concentration of specific nutrients.

The concentrations of nutrients in formula vary slightly between manufacturers and are usually slightly higher in formula than in breast milk to compensate for the possible lower bioavailability (AAP Committee on Nutrition, 2009). Although formula companies may be able to provide a rationale for their individual differences, large randomized clinical trials supporting their conclusions do not exist. Most formulas use cow's milk as the protein base. Because some newborns develop formula intolerance and some families are aware of existing milk intolerance, formula companies manufacture alternative formulas of special composition for newborns with gastrointestinal or metabolic disturbances.

Milk-Based Formula

Formula development and improvement is an ongoing challenge. Recent changes have been made to make the formulas more closely resemble breast milk. For example, there have been changes in the whey-to-casein ratio, the quantity of nucleotides, and the addition of long-chain polyunsaturated fatty acids (Schuman, 2003; Wright & Lo, 2007). Animal fat in cow's milk has been replaced with vegetable oils in order to improve digestibility and absorption, eliminate cholesterol, increase the concentration of essential fatty acids, and reduce environmental pollutants (AAP Committee on Nutrition, 2009). The major source of carbohydrate in human milk and formula is lactose. The presence of lactose in the bowel is responsible for proliferation of acidophilic bacterial flora necessary to prevent the growth of pathogenic organisms. Most formulas are fortified with iron, minerals, and electrolytes such as calcium, phosphorus, magnesium, sodium, potassium, and chloride. Cow's milk is the source of most minerals and electrolytes, although some are added as inorganic salts.

Milk-based formulas are available for newborns with special needs. Newborns requiring a lower renal solute load, such as those with cardiovascular or renal disease, can use formulas containing low levels of minerals and electrolytes. Newborns who experience lactose intolerance or have a family history of lactose intolerance can be given a lactose-free formula in which glucose rather than lactose is the carbohydrate source. Because this formula contains very small amounts of lactose, it should not be given to newborns with galactosemia. There are also milk-based formulas in which the fat content has been lowered for newborns with fat malabsorption, bile duct obstruction, or severe cholestasis. Newborns who cannot digest protein (i.e., cystic fibrosis, short gut syndrome, biliary atresia, cholestasis, and protracted diarrhea) or are severely allergic to cow's milk protein can receive formula in which the protein has been treated with heat and enzymes, decreasing the potential allergic response (Wright & Lo, 2007).

Soy Formulas

There are few indications for soy formula. According to the AAP (Bhatia & Greer, 2008), soy formula should be limited to infants with galactosemia or congenital lactase deficiency. Soy formulas may also be used by strict vegan families who want to avoid animal protein. Although the major source of protein is soy, it is possible for a newborn allergic to cow's milk protein to also demonstrate an allergic reaction to soy protein. The carbohydrate source in these formulas is sucrose. Preterm infants should not be given soy protein as there is significantly less weight gain with soy and an increase in osteopenia of prematurity (Bhatia & Greer, 2008).

Preterm Human Milk Modifiers

Preterm and very low-birth-weight infants may need to supplement breast milk with a human milk modifier (Schuman, 2003). The AAP (2005) policy statement, "Breastfeeding and the use of human milk" (2011), recommends the use of human milk fortifiers containing protein, minerals, and vitamins to ensure preterm human milk meets the nutritional needs for very low-birth-weight newborns.

MECHANICS OF FORMULA FEEDING

The perinatal nurse should ensure that parents who choose to use commercially prepared formula have sufficient information and are doing so safely. Unfortunately, this is not always done. In one study using the 2005 to 2007 Infant Feeding Practices Study II data, 77% of the participants reported that they had not received instruction from healthcare professionals on how to prepare formula, and 73% did not receive instruction on formula storage (Labiner-Wolf, Fein, & Shealy, 2008). Errors in formula preparation do occur. In one trial, less than half of the mothers mixed the feeding correctly, and 26% offered overly concentrated feedings, with the potential for serious consequence such as diarrhea (Lucas, Lockton, & Davies, 1992). Oral water intoxication can be the outcome of mixing too much water with the formula to stretch its availability or accidentally adding water to ready-to-feed formula. These babies may present to the emergency room with seizures and apnea (Keating, Schears, & Dodge, 1991). Parents need to carefully read labels for expiration dates and preparation instructions. This may be a problem if the adult cannot read or does not speak English (Lauwers & Swisher, 2011).

Types of Formula

Formula is available as ready-to-feed, liquid concentrate, or as a powder. Ready-to-feed is the most expensive but safest in terms of risk for contamination. No water is needed for dilution, and it is sterilized during manufacturing. Liquid concentrate is also sterilized during manufacturing but must be mixed with equal parts of water (1:1 ratio). Powdered formula requires one level scoop added to every 2 oz of water. Unlike the liquid forms of formula, powdered formula is not sterile and carries a small risk of being contaminated with *Enterobacter sakazakii*. The risk can be minimized when parents follow preparation and storage guidelines. Premature and low-birth-weight infants are more likely to become infected if exposed to *E. sakazakii,* and many providers recommend using ready-to-feed or concentrated formula with vulnerable populations, especially during the first 3 months of life (Lauwers & Swisher, 2011; WHO & Food and Agriculture Organization of the United Nations [FAO], 2007).

Formula Reconstitution

Water safety should be reviewed with parents (Pastore, 2010). Typically, water for reconstitution comes from the tap or is bottled. Parents should talk with their healthcare provider about the most appropriate source of water, as this may vary based on water source and locale.

Tap water from most municipal systems in the United States is safe because it must meet federal standards. However, water has to pass through various fixtures to get to the tap and can absorb lead, copper, or other contaminants from the fixtures and pipes, especially in older buildings. Most municipal water sources fluoridate the water. Too much fluoride (0.7 mg/L or higher) puts the baby at risk for enamel fluorosis, which can result in faint white lines or white areas on the permanent teeth. Parents can check with their water utility to find out how much fluoride is present. Parents can test their water for lead, arsenic, pesticides, and bacteria using a home test kit. They should read and follow the directions carefully to get accurate results.

Bottled water is filtered so impurities are removed, but it is not sterilized. By law, bottled water must meet the FDA's standard for water quality, which is at least as stringent as the U.S. Environmental Protection Agency's (EPA's) standards for tap water. Low-fluoride bottled water will be labeled as purified, deionized, demineralized, distilled, or prepared by reverse osmosis. Most grocery stores sell these types of low-fluoride water.

The AAP (2012) recommends that all water be boiled for 1 to 2 minutes in a covered pan and then cooled prior to mixing with formula. With tap water, higher levels of impurities are found in hot water and water that has sat in pipes for a while. Therefore, it is best to run cold water from the tap for a few minutes before filling the pan.

Bottles of reconstituted powder formula may be refrigerated for 24 hours; bottles of liquid concentrate or ready-to-feed formula are good for 48 hours in the refrigerator. Caution parents to follow directions on the formula container for proper storage.

New bottles, nipples, caps, and rings should be washed in warm soapy water and then sterilized by placing them in a pan of boiling water for 5 minutes. After initial sanitizing, subsequent cleaning can be done with warm soapy water using a bottle and nipple brush to remove dried formula (Alden, 2012; Murray & McKinney, 2010; USDHHS, n.d.). Dishwashers are usually safe; however, parents should follow their caregiver and manufacturer instructions before cleaning equipment in a dishwasher.

Frequency of Feeding

Standard commercially prepared formula contains 20 kcal/oz and can be offered to newborns on demand. During the first 3 months of life, intake is approximately 150 to 200 mL/kg each day (AAP Committee on Nutrition, 2009). This provides 100 to 135 kcal/kg/day. Weight gain should be approximately 25 to 30 g/day. Infants receiving formula do not need additional water in their diet.

Parents can begin feeding 0.5 to 1 oz of formula at each feeding during the first 24 hours of life. During the next 24 hours, the feedings can be increased by 0.5 oz increments, feeding the same volume for two to three feedings before increasing. Parents should not force the baby to finish the bottle and should feed on cue when the baby shows signs of hunger. The newborn should be burped halfway through the feeding. During a feeding, the infant should be held at about a 45-degree angle, and the bottle should be held so that the nipple is full of formula to avoid sucking air.

Once a bottle is prepared, it should be used or remain in the refrigerator until needed. Any formula remaining in the bottle when the infant is done eating should be discarded because it is an excellent medium for bacterial growth. To avoid waste, smaller amounts of formula should be prepared for the early postbirth period, gradually increasing until the infant is eating 6 to 8 oz per feeding. Formula should be fed at room temperature. A bottle from the refrigerator can be warmed by placing it in a pan or warm water. Microwaves should never be used to warm formula as it heats unevenly and the infant may get burned.

Hunger and Satiety Cues

Parents who formula feed need to recognize and respond to infant cues. The cues are the same as for infants who are breastfed (see Displays 20–8 and 20–11). Similar to breastfeeding, parents should watch for and respond to early signs of hunger and not wait until the infant is upset or crying. Some infants eat less than what is in the bottle. It is important that the infant not be forced to finish a bottle nor should the parents keep the bottle to use at the next feeding.

Feeding Positions

There is evidence that feeding position contributes to the increased incidence of otitis media in bottle-fed newborns. Supine feeding, positioning the newborn in a horizontal position, or propping the bottle for feeding has been associated with reflux of milk into the eustachian tubes. Researchers have identified a significant difference in the number of abnormal postfeeding tympanogram results when infants were fed in the supine position compared with those fed in the semiupright position (Tully, Bar-Haim, & Bradley, 1995). Propping bottles can also lead to dental caries (bottle mouth syndrome), choking, or aspiration. This information should be shared with parents choosing to bottle feed along with the following recommendations:

- Hold infant during feedings. The newborn needs human contact and this provides an ideal time for socialization and bonding. Avoid feeding while infant is in an infant seat.
- Sit in a comfortable armchair while feeding to reduce arm fatigue; use pillows to support arm as needed.
- Rest newborn's head in the crook of the elbow, with head slightly higher than the rest of his body so he faces caregiver's face (a position similar to the breastfeeding newborn).
- Keep upright after feeding for about 15 minutes before placing the infant in a supine position to sleep.
- Never put the newborn to bed with a bottle or prop bottles.
- Refrigerated bottles should be placed in warm water for no longer than 15 minutes. Prior to feeding, shake the bottle and test the temperature by sprinkling a few drops on the inside of the wrist. Never use a microwave as it does not heat evenly and there may be hot spots in the milk.

Equipment for Bottle Feeding

There are many different types of bottles and nipples. Each has advantages and disadvantages. Some parents may need to try several to find one that works best for their infant. If feeding does not go smoothly, some experimentation may be necessary. Consumer Reports (n.d.) has published a *Baby Bottle Guide* that can be accessed online at http://www.consumerreports.org/cro/babies-kids/baby-toddler/baby-bottles/baby-bottle-buying-advice/index.htm. This provides unbiased information on the pros and cons of various brands.

Nipple holes should allow a few drops to come out when the bottle is inverted. If holes are too big, formula flows too fast and, if too small, the infant gets frustrated and ingests air. Nipples come in three standard flow variations with different size holes. Typically, smaller babies prefer slower flows, while older babies prefer faster flow. Avoid latex nipples due to allergy risks; instead, use nipples made from silicone.

Bottles come in a variety of shapes: standard bottles (classic shape), angle-neck bottles, disposable liner bottles, and natural flow bottles. Several are designed to prevent air ingestion (angle neck, line bottles, and natural flow bottles). Caution parents about bisphenol A (BPA). BPA is used to harden plastics, keep bacteria from contaminating foods, and prevent cans from rusting. In 2008, concern was raised that it can leach into food. Bottles or bag inserts that have a recycle code of "7" and the letters "PC" or those that are certified or identified on the labeling as BPA free are safe options.

LACTATION SUPPRESSION

In postpartum women who are not breastfeeding, milk leakage and breast pain begins 1 to 3 days after the birth, and engorgement begins between 1 and 4 days after the birth. Considerable pain may be experienced during this time. Over the years, a variety of interventions have been suggested to decrease milk leakage and pain associated with lactation suppression, but few interventions are supported by randomized, controlled clinical research. Some techniques that may help include:

- Wearing a well-fitting bra or sport bra 24 hours each day until the breasts are soft and nontender.
- Applying cold packs to the breasts. These may be commercial cold packs or bags of frozen peas. If the woman does not want to use cold for cultural reasons, warmth may also provide comfort.
- Using mild over-the-counter analgesics, taken according to manufacturers' recommendations.
- Avoiding nipple or breast stimulation; however, when discomfort is severe, hand expressing or pumping a small amount of milk may provide relief; taking a warm shower and letting the water run over the breasts may stimulate milk leakage. This type of stimulation is not enough to prolong the time needed to stop producing milk.

Restricting fluids is neither necessary nor desirable. The breasts return to normal, and tenderness decreases within 48 to 72 hours after engorgement occurs.

SUMMARY

The abundance of research on breastfeeding and human lactation clearly shows the importance of breastfeeding, the adverse effects of newborn formula use, and the evidence that many traditional newborn feeding practices have no scientific or physiologic validity. Parents and health professionals should be aware of this information. Healthcare professionals have an obligation to support changes in practice that have been shown to remove institutional barriers to breastfeeding. Clinical nurse specialists, advance practice nurses, educators, nurse managers, lactation consultants, hospital administrators, and physicians can take steps to see that breastfeeding is supported in their community, clinic, and institution.

Many national organizations have policies that support breastfeeding. For example, AWHONN (www.awhonn.org) supports breastfeeding as the optimal method of feeding and challenges its membership to foster environments that support breastfeeding. In April 2010, The Joint Commission on the Accreditation of Health Care Facilities (2010) included exclusive breast milk feeding rates as part of its perinatal care core measures for maternity hospitals seeking accreditation.

The choice of infant feeding method has a significant effect on the health and development of the newborn, health of the mother, and cost of illness to the healthcare system. The perinatal nurse's interactions with families should reflect promotion, protection, and support of breastfeeding as the normal and natural way to feed a newborn. Perinatal nurses also are responsible to provide support and education for women who choose to formula feed. Making sure parents clearly understand formula preparation is critical to the health and well-being of the newborn.

REFERENCES

Aarts, C., Hornell, A., Kylberg, E., Hofvander, Y., & Gebre-Medhin, M. (1999). Breastfeeding patterns in relation to thumb sucking and pacifier use. *Pediatrics, 104*(4), E50.

Abrahams, S. W., & Labbock, M. H. (2009). Exploring the impact of the Baby-Friendly Hospital initiative on trends in exclusive breastfeeding. *International Breastfeeding Journal, 4*, 11. doi:10.1186/1746-4358-4-11

Academy of Breastfeeding Medicine. (2004). ABM clinical protocol #12: Transitioning the breastfeeding/breastmilk-fed premature infant from the neonatal intensive care unit to home. *Breastfeeding Medicine, 3*(2), 129–132. doi:10.1089/bfm.2008.9998

Academy of Breastfeeding Medicine. (2007a). ABM clinical protocol #2 (2007 revision): Guidelines for hospital discharge of the breastfeeding term newborn and mother: "The Going Home Protocol." *Breastfeeding Medicine, 2*(3), 158–165. doi:10.1089/bfm.2007.9990

Academy of Breastfeeding Medicine. (2007b). ABM clinical protocol #16: Breastfeeding the hypotonic infant. *Breastfeeding Medicine, 2*(2), 112–118. doi:10.1089/bfm.2007.9995

Academy of Breastfeeding Medicine. (2009). ABM clinical protocol #19: Breastfeeding promotion in the prenatal setting. *Breastfeeding Medicine, 4*(1), 43–45. doi:10.1089/bfm.2008.9982

Academy of Breastfeeding Medicine. (2010a). ABM clinical protocol #22: Guidelines for management of jaundice in breastfeeding infant equal to or greater than 35 weeks' gestation. *Breastfeeding Medicine, 5*(2), 87–93. doi:10.1089/bfm.2010.9994

Academy of Breastfeeding Medicine. (2010b). ABM clinical protocol #7: Model breastfeeding policy (revised). *Breastfeeding Medicine, 5*(4), 173–177. doi:10.1089/bfm.2010.9986

Academy of Breastfeeding Medicine. (2011). ABM clinical protocol #10: Breastfeeding the late preterm infant (34 0/7 to 36 6/7 weeks gestation). *Breastfeeding Medicine, 6*(3), 151–156. doi:10.1089/bfm.2011.9990

Agostoni, C., Marangoni, F., Grandi, F., Lammardo, A. M., Giovannini, M., Riva, E., & Galli, C. (2003). Earlier smoking habits are associated with higher serum lipids and lower milk fat and polyunsaturated fatty acid content in the first 6 months of lactation. *European Journal of Clinical Nutrition, 57*(11), 1466–1472.

Ahmed, A. H. (2010). Role of the pediatric nurse practitioner in promoting breastfeeding for late preterm infants in primary care settings. *Journal of Pediatric Health Care, 24*(2), 116–122.

Alden, K. R. (2012). Newborn nutrition and feeding. In D. L. Lowdermilk, S. E. Perry, K. Cashion, & K. R. Alden (Eds.), *Maternity and Women's Health Care* (10th ed., pp. 606–636). St. Louis, MO: Mosby.

Almroth, S. G. (1978). Water requirements of breastfed infants in a hot climate. *American Journal of Clinical Nutrition, 31*(7), 1154–1157.

American Academy of Family Physicians. (2008). *Breastfeeding policy statement*. Retrieved from http://www.aafp.org/online/en/home/policy/policies/b/breastfeedingpolicy.html

American Academy of Pediatrics. (2012). Breastfeeding and the use of human milk. *Pediatrics, 129*(2), e827-e841. doi:10.1542/peds211-3552

American Academy of Pediatrics Committee on Nutrition. (2009). *Pediatric Nutrition Handbook* (6th ed.). Elk Grove Village, IL: Author.

American Academy of Pediatrics Subcommittee on Hyperbilirubinemia. (2004). Clinical practice guideline: Management of hyperbilirubinemia in the newborn infant 35 or more weeks of gestation. *Pediatrics, 114*(1), 297–316.

American Academy of Pediatrics Task Force on Sudden Infant Death Syndrome. (2005). The changing concept of sudden infant death syndrome: Diagnostic coding shifts, controversies regarding the sleeping environment, and new variables to consider in reducing risk. *Pediatrics, 116*(5), 1245–1255.

American College of Obstetricians and Gynecologists. (2007). Breastfeeding: Maternal and infant aspects. *ACOG Clinical Review, 12*(1), 1s–16s.

Anderson, J. W., Johnstone, B. M., & Remley, D. T. (1999). Breastfeeding and cognitive development: A meta-analysis. *American Journal of Clinical Nutrition, 70*(4), 525–535.

Anderson, G. C., Moore, E., Hepworth, J., & Bergman, N. (2007 rev). Early skin-to-skin contact for mothers and their healthy newborn infants. *Cochrane Database of Systematic Reviews*, (1), CD003519.

Anderson, K. E., Nicklas, J. C., Spence, M., & Kavanagh, K. (2009). Roles, perceptions and control of infant feeding among low-income fathers. *Public Health Nutrition, 13*(4), 522–530.

Ashraf, R. N., Jalil, F., Aperia, A., & Lindblad, B. S. (1993). Additional water is not needed for breast-fed babies in a hot climate. *Acta Paediatrica, 82*(12), 1007–1011.

Asole, S., Spinelli, A., Antinucci, L. E., & DiLallo, D. (2009). Effect of hospital practices on breastfeeding: A survey in the Italian region of Lazio. *Journal of Human Lactation, 25*(3), 333–340.

Association of Women's Health Obstetric and Neonatal Nurses. (2007a). *Breastfeeding and the Role of the Nurse in the Promotion of Breastfeeding*. Washington, DC: Author.

Association of Women's Health Obstetric and Neonatal Nurses. (2007b). *Breastfeeding Support: Prenatal Care Through the First Year Guideline* (2nd ed.). Washington, DC: Author.

Association of Women's Health, Obstetric and Neonatal Nurses. (2010). *Assessment & Care of the Late Preterm Infant Guideline*. Washington, DC: Author.

Bailey, B. A., & Wright, H. N. (2011). Breastfeeding initiation in a rural sample: Predictive factors and the role of smoking. *Journal of Human Lactation, 27*(1), 33–40. doi:10.1177/0890334410386955

Ballard, J. L., Auer, C. E., & Khoury, J. C. (2002). Ankyloglossia: Assessment, incidence, and effect of frenuloplasty on the breastfeeding dyad. *Pediatrics, 110*(5), e63.

Bartels, M., van Beijsterveldt, C. E. M., & Boomsma, D. I. (2009). Breastfeeding, maternal education and cognitive function: A prospective study of twins. *Behavior Genetics, 39*(6), 616–622. doi:10.1007/s10519-009-9293-9

Bartick, M., & Reinhold, A. (2010). The burden of suboptimal breastfeeding in the United States: A pediatric cost analysis. *Pediatrics, 125*(5), e1048–e1056. doi:10.1542/peds.2009-1616

Bartick, M., Stuebe, A., Shealy, K. R., Walker, M., & Grummer-Strawn, L. M. (2009). Closing the quality gap: Promoting evidence-based breastfeeding care in the hospital. *Pediatrics, 124*(4), e793–e802.

Becker, G. E., McCormick, F. M., & Renfrew, M. J. (2008). Methods of milk expression for lactating women. *Cochrane Database of Systematic Reviews,* (4), CD006170. doi:10.1002/14651858 .CD006170.pub2

Bener, A., Ehlayel, M. S., Alsowsidi, A., & Sabbah, A. (2007). Role of breast feeding in primary prevention of asthma and allergic diseases in traditional society. *European Annals of Allergy and Clinical Immunology, 39*(10), 337–343.

Benis, M. M. (2002). Critically appraised topic: Are pacifiers associated with early weaning from breastfeeding. *Advances in Neonatal Care, 2*(5), 259–266.

Bhatia, J., & Greer, F. (2008). Use of soy protein-based formulas in infant feeding. *Pediatrics, 121*(5), 1062–1068.

Bolling, K., Grant, C., Hamlyn, B., & Thornton, A. (2007). *Infant feeding survey 2005.* London, England: BMBR Social Research. Retrieved from http://www.ic.nhs.uk/statistics-and-datacollections/health-and -lifestyles/infant-feeding/infant-feeding-survey–2005

Bramson, L., Lee, J. W., Moore, E., Montgomery, S., Neish, S., Neish, C., & Melcher, C. (2010). Effect of early skin-to-skin mother-infant contact during the first 3 hours following birth on exclusive breastfeeding during the maternity hospital stay. *Journal of Human Lactation, 26*(2), 130–137.

Briggs G. G., Freeman R. K., & Yaffee S. J. (Eds.) (2011). *Drugs in Pregnancy and Lactation: A Reference Guide to Fetal and Neonatal Risk* (9th ed.). Philadelphia: Lippincott Williams & Wilkins.

British Columbia Reproductive Care Program. (2001). *Breastfeeding the healthy preterm infant ≤ 37 weeks.* Retrieved from http://www .rcp.gov.bc.ca/guidelines/Master.Nutrition PartII.PremBreastfeeding. October.2001.pdf

Britton, C., McCormick, F. M., Renfrew, M. J., Wade, A., & King, S. E. (2007). Support for breastfeeding mothers. *Cochrane Database of Systematic Reviews,* (1), CD001141. doi:10.1002/14651858 .CD001141.pub3

Butte, N. F. (2009). Impact of infant feeding practices on childhood obesity. *Journal of Nutrition, 139*(2), 412s–416s.

California Perinatal Quality Care Collaborative. (2008). *Nutrition support of the VLBW infant* (revised). Retrieved from http:// www.cpqcc.org/quality_improvement/qi_toolkits/nutritional _support_of_the_vlbw_infant_rev_december_2008

Callen, J., & Pinnelli, J. (2004). Incidence and duration of breastfeeding for term infants in Canada, United States, Europe and Australia: A literature review. *Birth, 31*(4), 285–292.

Castrucci, B. C., Hoover, K. S., Lim, S., & Maus, K. C. (2007). Availability of lactation counseling services influences breastfeeding among infants admitted to neonatal intensive care units. *American Journal of Health Promotion, 21*(5), 410–415.

Centers for Disease Control and Prevention. (2008). Breastfeeding-related maternity practices at hospitals and birth center—United States 2007. *Morbidity and Mortality Weekly Report, 57,* 621–625.

Centers for Disease Control and Prevention. (2010a). *Breastfeeding report card, United States, 2010: Outcome indicators.* Retrieved from http://www.cdc.gov/breastfeeding/data/reportcard.htm

Centers for Disease Control and Prevention. (2010b). *Proper handling and storage of human milk.* Retrieved from http://www.cdc.gov /breastfeeding/recommendations/handling_breastmilk.htm

Centuori, S., Burmaz, T., Ronfani, L., Franiacomo, M., Quintero, S., Pavan, C., & Cattaneo, A. (1999). Nipple care, sore nipples, and breastfeeding: A randomized trial. *Journal of Human Lactation, 15*(2), 125–130.

Chang, Z. M., & Heaman, M. I. (2005). Epidural analgesia during labor and delivery: Effects on the initiation and continuation of effective breastfeeding. *Journal of Human Lactation, 21*(3), 305–314.

Chantry, C. J., Nommensen-Rivers, J. M. P., Cohen, R. J., & Dewey, K. G. (2011). Excess weight loss in first-born breastfed newborns related to maternal intrapartum fluid balance. *Pediatrics, 127*(1), e171–e179. doi:10.1542/peds.2009–2663.

Chapman, D. J., Morel, K., Anderson, A. K., Damio, G., & Perez-Escamilla, R. (2010). Breastfeeding peer counseling: From efficacy through scale-up. *Journal of Human Lactation, 26*(3), 314–326. doi:10.1177/0890334410369481

Chauhan, M., Henderson, G., & McGuire, W. (2008). Enteral feeding for very low birth weight infants: Reducing the risk of necrotizing enterocolitis. *Archives of Disease in Childhood: Fetal and Neonatal Edition, 93*(2), F162–F166. doi:10.1136 /adc.2007.115824

Chaves, R., Lamounier, J. A., & Cesar, C. C. (2007). Factors associated with duration of breastfeeding. *Journal of Pediatrics, 83*(3), 241–246.

Chezem, J., Friesen, C., & Boettcher, J. (2003). Breastfeeding knowledge, breastfeeding confidence, and infant feeding plans: Effects on actual feeding practices. *Journal of Obstetric Gynecologic and Neonatal Nursing, 32*(1), 241–246.

Chung, M., Raman, G., Trikalinos, T., Lau, J., & Ip, S. (2008). Interventions in primary care to promote breastfeeding: An evidence review to the U.S. Preventive Services Task Force. *Annals of Internal Medicine, 149*(8), 565–582.

Colson, S. D., Meek, J. H., & Hawdon, J. M. (2008). Optimal positions for the release of primitive neonatal reflexes stimulating breastfeeding. *Early Human Development, 84*(7), 441–449.

Committee on Fetus and Newborn & Adamkin, D. H. (2011). Clinical report: Postnatal glucose homeostasis in late-preterm and term infants. *Pediatrics, 127*(3), 575–579. doi:10.1542/peds.2010–3851

Consumer Reports. (n.d.). *Baby bottle guide.* Retrieved from http://www.consumerreports.org/cro/babies-kids/baby-bottle -buyingadvice/index.htm

Devroe, S., DeCoster, J., & Van de Velde, M. (2009). Breastfeeding and epidural analgesia during labour. *Current Opinion in Anesthesiology, 22*(3), 327–329.

DiGirolamo, A. M., Grummer-Strawn, L. M., & Fein, S. B. (2008). Effect of maternity-care practices on breastfeeding. *Pediatrics, 122,* S43–S49. doi:10.1542/peds.2008–1351e

Dykes, F., & Williams, C. (1999). Falling by the wayside: A phenomenological exploration of perceived breast milk inadequacy in lactating women. *Midwifery, 15*(4), 232–246.

Dyson, L., Green, J. M., Renfrew, M. J., McMillan, B., & Woolridge, M. (2010). Factors influencing the infant feeding decision for socioeconomically deprived pregnant teenagers: The moral dimension. *Birth, 37*(2), 141–149.

Ekstrom, A., Widstrom, A. M., & Nissen, E. (2003). Duration of breastfeeding in Swedish primiparous and multiparous woman. *Journal of Human Lactation, 19*(2), 172–178.

Flint, A., New, K., & Davies, M. W. (2008). Cup feeding versus other forms of supplemental enteral feeding for newborn infants unable to fully breastfeed. *Cochrane Database of Systematic Reviews,* (2), CD005092. doi:10.1002/14651858.CD005092.pub2

Forde, K. A., & Miller, L. J. (2010). North Metropolitan Perth breastfeeding cohort study: How long are mothers breastfeeding? *Breastfeeding Review, 18*(2), 14–24.

Forster, D. A., & McLachlan, H. S. (2007). Breastfeeding initiation and birth setting practices: A review of the literature. *Journal of Midwifery and Women's Health, 52*(3), 273–280.

Galligan, M. (2006). Proposed guidelines for skin-to-skin treatment of neonatal hypothermia. *Maternal Child Nursing, 31*(5), 298–304.

Gatti, L. (2008). Maternal perceptions of inadequate milk supply in breastfeeding. *Journal of Nursing Scholarship, 40*(4), 355–363.

Geddes, D. T., Langton, D. B., Gollow, I., Jacobs, L. A., Hartman, P. E., & Simmer, K. (2008). Frenulotomy for breastfeeding infants with ankyloglossia: Effect on milk removal and sucking mechanism as imaged by ultrasound. *Pediatrics, 122*(1), 3188–3194. doi:10.1542/peds.2007–2553

Goer, M. W., Davis, M. W., & Hemphill, J. (2002). Postpartum stress: Current concepts and the possible protective role of breastfeeding. *Journal of Obstetric Gynecologic and Neonatal Nursing, 31*(4), 411–417.

Grassley, J., & Eschiti, V. (2008). Grandmother breastfeeding support: What do mothers need and want. *Birth, 35*(4), 329–335.

Grey Bruce Health Services-Owen Sound. (2007). *Adapted LAT.* Retrieved from http://www.gbhn.ca/ebc/documents/LatchTool March2007.pdf

Griffiths, L. J., Smeeth, L., Hawkins, S. S., Cole, T. J., & Dezateux, C. (2009). Effects of infant feeding practices on weight gain from birth to 3 years. *Archives of Diseases in Childhood, 94*(8), 577–582.

Guise, J. M., Palda, V., Westhoff, C., Chan, B. K., Helfand, M., & Lieu, T. A. (2003). The effectiveness of primary care-based interventions to promote breastfeeding: Systematic evidence review and meta-analysis for the U.S. Preventive Services Task Force. *American Family Medicine, 1*(2), 70–78.

Gulick, E. E. (1986). The effects of breastfeeding on toddler health. *Pediatric Nursing, 12*(1), 51–54.

Gunderson, E. P., Jacobs, D. R., Chiang, V., Lewis, C. E., Feng, J., Quesenberry, C. P. Jr., & Sidney, S. (2010). Duration of lactation and incidence of the metabolic syndrome in women of reproductive age according to gestational diabetes mellitus status: A 20-year prospective study in CARDIA (Coronary Artery Risk Development In Young Adults). *Diabetes, 59*(2), 495–504.

Hake-Brooks, S. J., & Anderson, G. C. (2008). Kangaroo care and breastfeeding of mother-preterm infant dyads 0–18 months: A randomized, controlled trial. *Neonatal News, 27*(3), 151–159.

Hale, T. (2010). *Medications and Mothers' Milk* (14th ed.). Amarillo, TX: Pharmasoft Medical.

Hall, R. T., Mercer, A. M., Teasley, S. L., McPherson, D. M., Simon, S. D., Santos, S. R., & Hipsh, N. E. (2002). A breast-feeding assessment score to evaluate the risk for cessation of breast-feeding by 7 to 10 days of age. *Journal of Pediatrics, 141*(5), 659–664.

Hamilton, B. E., Martin, J. A., & Ventura, S. J. (2007). Births: Preliminary data for 2006. *National Vital Statistics Reports, 56*(7), 1–18.

Hannula, L., Kaunonen, M., & Tarkka, M. T. (2008). A systematic review of professional support interventions for breastfeeding. *Journal of Clinical Nursing, 17*(9), 1132–1143. doi:10.1111/j .1365–2702.2007.02239.x

Hauck, Y., Fenwick, J., Dhaliwal, S., & Butt, J. (2010). A Western Australian survey of breastfeeding initiation, prevalence and early cessation patterns. *Maternal and Child Health Journal, 15*(2), 260–268.

Healthy Children Project. (2000). *Latch-On Assessment Tool (LAT).* East Sandwich, MA: Author.

Hedberg, N. K., & Ewald, U. (1999). Infant and maternal factors in the development of breastfeeding behaviour and breastfeeding outcome in preterm infants. *Acta Paediatrica, 88*(11), 1194–1203.

Henderson, G., Craig, S., Brocklehurst, P., & McGuire, W. (2007). Enteral feeding regimens and necrotizing enterocolitis in preterm infants: A multicentre case-control study. *Archives of Disease in Childhood: Fetal and Neonatal Edition, 94*(2), F120–F123.

Henderson, J. J., Dickinson, J. E., Evans, S. F., McDonald, S. J., & Paech, M. J. (2003). Impact of intrapartum epidural analgesia on breastfeeding duration. *Australian and New Zealand Journal of Obstetrics and Gynecology, 43*(5), 372–377.

Hill, P., & Humenick, S. (1996). Development of the H & H Lactation Scale. *Nursing Research, 45*(3), 136–140.

Hogan, M., Westcott, C., & Griffiths, M. (2005). Randomized, controlled trial of division of tongue-tie in infants with feeding problems. *Journal of Pediatrics and Child Health, 41*(5–6), 246–250.

Hong, P., Lago, D., Seargeant, J., Pellman, L., Magit, A. E., & Pransky, S. M. (2010). Defining ankyloglossia: A case series of anterior and posterior tongue ties. *International Journal of Pediatric Otorhinolaryngology, 74*(9), 1003–1006.

Howard, C. R., Howard, F. M., Lanphear, B., deBlieck, E. A., Eberly, S., & Lawrence, R. A. (1999). The effects of early pacifier use on breastfeeding duration. *Pediatrics, 103*(3), E33.

Howard, C. R., Howard, F. M., Lanphear, B., deBlieck, E. A., Oakes, D., & Lawrence, R. A. (2003). Randomized clinical trial of pacifier use and bottle-feeding or cup feeding and their effect on breastfeeding. *Pediatrics, 111*(3), 511–518.

Humenick, S. S., Hill, P. D., & Hart, A. M. (1998). Evaluation of a pillow designed to promote breastfeeding. *Journal of Perinatal Education, 7*(3), 25–31.

Hurst, N. M. (2007). Recognizing and treating delayed or failed lactogenesis II. *Journal of Midwifery & Women's Health, 52*(6), 588–594.

Insel, T. R. (1997). A neurobiological basis of social attachment. *American Journal of Psychiatry, 154*(6), 726–735.

Ip, S., Chung, M., Raman, G., Chew, P., Magula, N., DeVine, D., & Lau, J. (2007). *Breastfeeding and Maternal and Infant Health Outcomes in Developed Countries* (Evidence Report/Technology Assessment No. 153) (AHRQ Publication No. 007–E007). Rockville, MD: Agency for Healthcare Research and Quality.

Jenks, M. (1991). Latch assessment documentation in the hospital. *Journal of Human Lactation, 7*(1), 19–20.

Jensen, D., Wallace, S., & Kelsey, P. (1994). LATCH: A breastfeeding charting system and documentation tool. *Journal of Obstetric, Gynecologic, and Neonatal Nursing, 23*(1), 27–32.

Joanna Briggs Institute. (2009). The management of nipple pain and/or trauma associated with breastfeeding. *Best Practice: Evidence Based Practice Information Sheets for Health Professionals, 13*(4), 1–4.

Johnson, T. S., Mulder, P. J., & Strube, K. (2007). Mother-infant breastfeeding progress tool: A guide for education and support of the breastfeeding dyad. *Journal of Obstetric Gynecologic and Neonatal Nursing, 36*(4), 319–327.

Joint Commission on the Accreditation of Health Care Facilities. (2010). *Specifications Manual for Joint Commission National Quality Measures* (v2011A). Retrieved from http://manual.joint commission.org/releases/TJC2011A/PerinatalCare.html

Jones, E., Dimmock, P. W., & Spencer, S. A. (2001). A randomized controlled trial to compare methods of milk expression after preterm delivery. *Archives of Disease in Childhood, 85*, F91–F95.

Jones, E., & Hilton, S. (2008). Correctly fitting breast shields are the key to lactation success for pump dependent mothers following preterm delivery. *Journal of Neonatal Nursing, 15*, 14–17. doi:10.1016/j.jnn.2008.07.011

Jones, E., & Spencer, S. A. (2007). The physiology of lactation. *Paediatric Child Health, 17*(6), 244–248.

Jordan, S. (2006). Infant feeding and analgesia in labour: The evidence is accumulating. *International Breastfeeding Journal, 1*(25). doi:10.1186/1746–4358–1–25

Jordan, S., Emery, S., Bradshaw, C., Watkins, A., & Friswell, W. (2005). The impact of intrapartum analgesia on infant feeding. *British Journal of Obstetrics & Gynecology, 112*(7), 927–934.

Keating, J. P., Schears, G. J., & Dodge, P. R. (1991). Oral water intoxication in infants. *American Journal of Diseases in Children, 145*(9), 985–990.

Kervin, B. E., Kemp, L., & Pulver, L. J. (2010). Types and timing of breastfeeding support and its impact on mothers' behaviours. *Journal of Paediatrics and Child Health, 46*(3), 85–91.

Klockars, T., & Pitkaranta, A. (2009). Pediatric tongue-tie division: Indications, techniques and patient satisfaction. *International Journal of Pediatric Otorhinolaryngology, 73*(10), 1399–1401. doi:10.1016/j.ijporl.2009.07.004

Kramer, M. S., Aboud, F., Mironova, E., Vanilovich, I., Platt, R. W., Matush, L., . . . Shapiro, S. (2008). Breastfeeding and child cognitive development: New evidence from a large randomized trial. *Archives of General Psychiatry, 65*(5), 578–584.

Kramer, M. S., Barr, R. G., Dagenais, S., Yang, H., Jones, P., Ciofani, L., & Jane, F. (2001). Pacifier use, early weaning, and cry/fuss behavior: A randomized controlled trial. *Journal of the American Medical Association, 286*(3), 322–326.

Kronborg, H., & Vaeth, M. (2009). How are effective breastfeeding technique and pacifier use related to breastfeeding problems and breastfeeding duration? *Birth, 36*(1), 34–42.

Labbock, M., & Taylor, E. (2008). *Achieving Exclusive Breastfeeding in the United States: Findings and Recommendations.* Washington, DC: United States Breastfeeding Committee.

Labiner-Wolfe, J., Fein, S. B., & Shealy, K. R. (2008). Infant formula handling education and safety. *Pediatrics, 122*, S85. doi:10.1542/peds.2008–1315k

Lauwers, J., & Swisher, A. (2011). *Counseling the Nursing Mother: A Lactation Consultant's Guide* (5th ed.). Sudbury, MA: Jones & Bartlett.

Lawrence, R. A., & Lawrence, R. M. (2011). *Breastfeeding: A Guide for the Medical Profession* (7th ed.). Philadelphia, PA: Saunders.

Li, R., Fein, S. B., Chen, J., & Grummer-Strawn, L. M. (2008). Why mothers stop breastfeeding: Mothers' self-reported reasons for stopping during the first year. *Pediatrics, 122*(Suppl. 2), S69–S76.

Lochner, J. E., Livingston, C. J., & Judkins, D. Z. (2009). Which interventions are best for alleviating nipple pain in nursing mothers? *The Journal of Family Practice, 58*(11), 612a–612c. Retrieved from http://www.jfponline.com

Lucas, A., Lockton, S., & Davies, P. S. (1992). Randomized trial of a ready-to-feed compared with powdered formula. *Archives of Diseases of Children, 67*(7), 935–939.

Maisels, M. J., Bhutani, V. K., Bogen, D., Newman, T. B., Stark, A. R., & Watchko, J. F. (2009). Hyperbilirubinemia in the newborn infant ≥ 35 weeks' gestation: An update with clarifications. *Pediatrics, 124*(4), 1193–1198.

Mangesi, L., & Dowswell, T. (2010). Treatments for breast engorgement during lactation. *Cochrane Database of Systematic Reviews,* (9), CD006946. doi:10.1002/14651858.CD006946.PUB2

Matthews, M. K. (1988). Developing an instrument to assess infant breastfeeding behavior in the early neonatal period. *Midwifery, 4*(4), 154–165.

McCall, E., Alderdice, F., Halliday, H. L., Jenkins, J. G., & Vohra, S. (2008). Interventions to prevent hypothermia at birth in preterm and/or low birthweight infants. *Cochrane Database of Systematic Reviews,* (1), CD004210.

McCann, M. F., & Bender, D. E. (2006). Perceived insufficient milk as a barrier to optimal feeding: Examples from Bolivia. *Journal of Biosocial Science, 38*(3), 341–364.

Meier, P. P., Furman, L. M., & Degenhardt, M. (2007). Increased lactation risk for late preterm infants and mothers: Evidence and management strategies to protect breastfeeding. *Journal of Midwifery & Women's Health, 52*, 579–587.

Melli, M. S., Rashidi, M. R., Nokohoodchi, A., Tagavi, S., Farzadi, L., Sadaghat, K., . . . Sheshvan, M. K. (2007). A randomized trial of peppermint gel, lanolin ointment, and placebo gel to prevent nipple crack in primiparous breastfeeding women. *Medical Science Monitor, 13*(9), CR406–CR411

Merewood, A., Brooks, D., Bauchner, H., MacAuley, L., & Mehta, S. D. (2006). Maternal birthplace and breastfeeding initiation among term and preterm infants: A statewide assessment for Massachusetts. *Pediatrics, 118*(4), e1048.

Merten, S., Dratva, J., & Ackermann-Liebrich, U. (2005). Do baby-friendly hospitals influence breastfeeding duration on a national level? *Pediatrics, 116*(5), e702–e708. doi:10.1542/peds.2005-0537

Mihrshahi, S., Oddy, W. H., Peat, J. K., & Kabir, I. (2008). Association between infant feeding patterns and diarrhoeal and respiratory illness: A cohort study in Chittagong, Bangladesh. *International Breastfeeding Journal, 3*(28). doi:10.1186/1746-4538-3-28

Monterrosa, E. C., Frongillo, E. A., Vasquez-Garibay, E. M., Romero-Velarde, E., Casey, L. M., & Willows, N. D. (2008). Predominant breast-feeding from birth to six months is associated with fewer gastrointestinal infections and increased risk for iron deficiency among infants. *Journal of Nutrition, 138*(8), 1499–1504.

Moore, E. R., Anderson, G. C., & Bergman, N. (2007). Early skin-to-skin contact for mothers and their healthy newborn infants. *Cochrane Database of Systematic Reviews,* (3), CD003519. doi:10.1002/14651858. CD 003519.pum2

Morland-Schultz, K., & Hill, P. (2005). Prevention of and therapies for nipple pain: A systematic review. *Journal of Obstetric Gynecologic and Neonatal Nursing, 34*(4), 428–443. doi:10.1177/0884217505276056

Morton, J., Hall, J. Y., Wong, R. J., Thairu, L., Benitz, W. E., & Rhine, W. D. (2009). Combining hand techniques with electric pumping increases milk production in mothers of preterm infants. *Journal of Perinatology, 29*(11), 757–764.

Mulford, C. (1992). The mother-baby assessment (MBA): An "Apgar score" for breastfeeding. *Journal of Human Lactation, 8*(2), 79–82.

Murray, E. K., Ricketts, S., & Dellaport, J. (2007). Hospital practices that increase breastfeeding duration: Results from a population-based study. *Birth, 34*(3), 202–211.

Murray, S., & McKinney, E. (2010). *Foundations of Maternal-Newborn Nursing* (5th ed.). St. Louis, MO: Saunders Elsevier.

National Association of Neonatal Nursing. (2010). *Prevention of acute bilirubin encephalopathy and kernicterus in newborns: Position statement #3049.* Retrieved from http://www.nann.org/pdf/PBE.pdf

Nelson, E. E., & Panksepp, J. (1998). Brain substrates of infant–mother attachment: Contributions of opioids, oxytocin, and norepinephrine. *Neuroscience and Biobehavioral Reviews, 22*(3), 437–452.

Nelson, E. A., Yu, L., & Williams, S. (2005). International child care practices study: Breastfeeding and pacifier use. *Journal of Human Lactation, 21*(3), 289–295.

Nommsen-Rivers, L. A., Chantry, C. J., Peerson, J. M., Cohen, R. J., & Dewey, K. G. (2010). Delayed onset of lactogenesis among first-time mothers is related to maternal obesity and factors associated with ineffective breastfeeding. *American Journal of Clinical Nutrition, 92*(3), 574–584.

Nyqvist, K. H., Rubertsson, C., Ewald, U., & Sjoden, P. O. (1996). Development of the preterm infant breastfeeding behavior scale (PIBBS): A study of nurse-mother agreement. *Journal of Human Lactation, 12*(3), 207–219.

Ogbuanu, I. U., Karmaus, W., Arshad, S. H., Kurukulaaratchy, R. J., & Ewart, S. (2009). Effect of breastfeeding duration on lung function at age 10 years: A prospective birth cohort study. *Thorax, 64*(1), 62–66.

Oklahoma Infant Alliance. (2010). *Caring for the late preterm infant: A clinical practice guideline.* Retrieved from http://www.oklahomainfantalliance.org/uploads/LPI_Clinical_Practice_Guideline_Sample.pdf

Palmer, M. M. (1993). Identification and management of the transitional suck pattern in premature infants. *The Journal of Perinatal & Neonatal Nursing, 7*(1), 66–75.

Pastore, R. (2010). Are you preparing your baby's bottles correctly? *AAP News, 31*(10). Retrieved from http://aapnews.aappublications.org

Phares, T. M., Morrow, B., Lansky, A., Barfield, W. D., Prince, C. B., Marchi, K. S., & Kinniburgh, B. (2004). Surveillance for disparities in maternal health-related behaviors—Selected states, Pregnancy Risk Assessment Monitoring Systems (PRAMS), 2000–2001. *Morbidity and Mortality Weekly Report, 53*(4), 1–13.

Pincombe, J., Baghurst, P., Antoniou, G., Peat, B., Henderson, A., & Reddin, E. (2008). Baby-Friendly Hospital Initiative practices and breast feeding duration in a cohort of first-time mothers in Adelaide, Australia. *Midwifery, 24*(1), 55–61.

Radtke, J. (2011). The paradox of breastfeeding-associated morbidity among late preterm infants. *Journal of Obstetric Gynecologic and Neonatal Nursing, 40*(1), 9–24.

Ransjo-Arvidson, A. B., Matthiesen, A. S., Lilja, G., Nissen, E., Widstrom, A. M., & Uvnas-Moberg, K. (2001). Maternal analgesia during labor disturbs newborn behavior: Effects on breastfeeding, temperature, and crying. *Birth, 28*(1), 5–12.

Rees, D. I., & Sabia, J. J. (2009). The effect of breastfeeding on educational attainment: New evidence from siblings. *Journal of Human Capital, 3*(1), 43–72.

Renfrew, M. J., Craig, D., Dyson, L., McCormick, F., Rice, S., King, S. E., . . .Williams, A. F. (2009). Breastfeeding promotion for infants in neonatal units: A systematic review and economic analysis. *Health Technology Assessment, 13*(40), 1–146.

Renfrew, M. J., Lang, S., Martin, L., & Woolridge, M. W. (2000). Feeding schedules in hospitals for newborn infants. *Cochrane Database of Systematic Review,* (2), CD000090.

Righard, L. (2008). The baby is breastfeeding—Not the mother. *Birth, 35*(1), 1105–1107.

Riordan, J. M., & Wambach, K. (2010). *Breastfeeding and Human Lactation* (4th ed.). London, England: Jones & Bartlett.

Rodriguez-Garcia, J., & Acosta-Ramirez, N. (2008). Factors affecting how long exclusive breastfeeding lasts. *Revista de Salud Publica (Bogata), 10*(1), 71–84.

Rosenberg, K. D., Eastham, C. A., Kasehagen, L. J., & Sandoval, A. P. (2008). Infant formula marketing through hospitals: The impact of commercial hospital discharge. *American Journal of Public Health, 98*(2), 290–295.

Rosenberg, K. D., Stull, J. D., Adler, M. R., Kasehagen, L. J., & Crivelli-Kovach, A. (2008). Impact of hospital policies on breastfeeding outcomes. *Breastfeeding Medicine, 3*(2), 110–116.

Ryan, A., & Zhou, W. (2006). Lower breastfeeding rates persist among the special supplemental nutrition program for Women, Infants, and Children participants, 1978–2003. *Pediatrics, 117*(4), 1136–1142.

Saarela, T., Kokkonen, J., & Koivisto, M. (2005). Macronutrient and energy content of human milk fractions during the first six months of lactation. *Acta Paediatrica, 94*(9), 1176–1181.

Schanler, R. J., & Enger, L. (2012). *Patient information: Common breastfeeding problems.* Retrieved from http://www.uptodate.com/

Schneller, L. E. (2010). Evidence summary: Pacifier use. *Joanna Briggs Institute Database of Evidence summaries.* Retrieved from http://www.jbiconnectplus.org/ViewDocument.aspx?0=4084

Schuman, A. J. (2003). A concise history of infant formula (twists and turns included). *Contemporary Pediatrics.* Retrieved from http://www.contemporarypediatrics.com/contpeds/article/articleDetail.jsp?id=111702

Schwarz, E. B., Ray, R. M., Stuebe, A. M., Allison, M. A., Ness, R. B., Freiberg, M. S., & Cauley, J. A. (2009). Duration of lactation and risk factors for maternal cardiovascular disease. *Obstetrics & Gynecology, 113*(5), 974–982.

Scott, J. A., Binns, C. W., & Oddy, W. H. (2007). Predictors of delayed onset of lactation. *Maternal & Child Nutrition, 3*(3), 186–193. doi:10.1111/j.1740-8709.2007.00096.x

Shrago, L., & Bocar, D. (1990). The infant's contribution to breastfeeding. *Journal of Obstetric Gynecologic and Neonatal Nursing, 19,* 209–215.

Shrago, L. C., Reifsnider, E., & Insel, K. (2006). The neonatal bowel output study: Indicators of adequate breastmilk intake in neonates. *Pediatric Nursing, 32*(3), 195–201.

Sikorski, J., Renfrew, M. J., Rindoria, S., & Wade, A. (2002). Support for breastfeeding mothers. *Cochrane Database of Systematic Reviews,* (2), CD001141.

Sloan, S., Stewart, M., & Dunne, L. (2010). The effect of breastfeeding and stimulation in the home on cognitive development in one-year-old infants. *Child Care in Practice, 16*(2), 101–110.

Stuebe, A. M., & Schwarz, E. B. (2010). The risks and benefits of infant feeding practices for women and children. *Journal of Perinatology, 30*(3), 155–162. doi:10.1038/jp.2009.107

Swanson, V., Power, K., Kaur, B., Carter, H., & Shepherd, K. (2007). The impact of knowledge and social influences on adolescent breastfeeding beliefs and intentions. *Public Health Nutrition, 9*(3), 297–305.

Taylor, J. S., Kacmar, J. E., Nothnagle, M., & Lawrence, R. (2005). A systematic review of literature associating breastfeeding with type 2 diabetes and gestational diabetes. *Journal of American College of Nutrition, 24*(5), 320–326.

Torvaldsen, S., Roberts, C. L., Simpson, J. M., Thompson, J. F., & Ellwood, D. A. (2006). Intrapartum epidural analgesia and breastfeeding: A prospective cohort study. *International Breastfeeding Journal, 1*(24). doi:10.1186/1746-4358-1-24

Tully, S. B., Bar-Haim, Y., & Bradley, R. L. (1995). Abnormal tympanography after supine bottle feeding. *Journal of Pediatrics, 126*(6), S105–S111.

U.S. Department of Health and Human Services. (n.d.) *Bisphenol A (BPA) information for parents.* Retrieved from http://www.hhs.gov/safety/bpa/

U.S. Department of Health and Human Services. (2008). *The business case for breastfeeding: Steps for creating a breastfeeding friendly workplace.* Retrieved from http://www.womenshealth.gov/breastfeeding/government-programs/business-case-for-breastfeeding/tool-kit.cfm

U.S. Department of Health and Human Services. (2011). *Healthy people 2020.* Retrieved from http://www.healthypeople.gov/2020

U.S. Food and Drug Administration. (2010). *Infant formula nutrient specifications (21 C.F.R. 107.100).* Washington, DC: Author. Retrieved from http://www.accessdata.fda.gov/scripts/cdrh/cfdocs/cfcfr/CFRSearch.cfm

U.S. Preventive Services Task Force. (2008). Primary care interventions to promote breastfeeding: U.S. Preventive Services Task Force Recommendation Statement. *Annals of Internal Medicine, 149*(8), 560–564.

Van den Driessche, M., Peeters, K., Marien, P., Ghoos, Y., Devlieger, H., & Veereman-Wauters, G. (1999). Gastric emptying in formula-fed and breastfed infants measured with the C-octanoic acid breath test. *Journal of Pediatric Gastroenterology and Nutrition, 29*(1), 46–51.

Victora, C. G., Behague, D. P., Barros, F. C., Olinto, M. T., & Weiderpass, E. (1997). Pacifier use and short breastfeeding duration: Cause, consequence, or coincidence? *Pediatrics, 99*(3), 445–453.

Vio, F., Salazar, G., & Infante, C. (1991). Smoking during pregnancy and lactation: Its effects on breast milk volume. *American Journal of Clinical Nutrition, 54*(6), 1011–1016.

Wagner, C. L., & Greer, F. R. (2008). Prevention of rickets and vitamin D deficiency in infants, children and adolescents. *Pediatrics, 122*(5), 1142–1152.

Walker, M. (2009). *Breastfeeding the Late Preterm Infant: Improving Care and Outcomes.* Amarillo, TX: Hale.

Walker, M. (2011). *Breastfeeding Management for the Clinician: Using the Evidence* (2nd ed.). Sudbury, MA: Jones & Bartlett.

Walters, M. W., Boggs, K. M., Ludington-Hoe, S., Price, K. M., & Morrison, B. (2007). Kangaroo care at birth of full term infants: A pilot study. *American Journal of Maternal Child Nurse, 32,* 375–381.

Watson, R. (2009). Hyperbilirubinemia. *Critical Care Nursing Clinics of North America, 21*(1), 97–120, vii.

Wieczorek, P. M., Guest, S., Balki, M., Shah, V., & Carvalho, J. C. A. (2010). Breastfeeding success rate after vaginal delivery can be high despite the use of epidural fentanyl: An observational cohort study. *International Journal of Obstetric Anesthesia, 19*(3), 273–277. doi:10.1016/j.ijoa.2010.02.001

Wiener, S. (2006). Diagnosis and management of Candida of the nipple and breast. *Journal of Midwifery & Women's Health, 51*(2), 125–128.

Wiklund, I., Norman, M., Uvnäs-Moberg, K., Ransjö-Arvidson, A. B., & Andolf, E. (2009) Epidural analgesia: Breast-feeding success and related factors. *Midwifery, 25*(2), e31–e38.

World Health Organization. (2011). *Exclusive breastfeeding for six months best for babies everywhere*. Retrieved from http:// www.who.int/mediacentre/news/statements/2011/breastfeeding _20110115/en/index.html

World Health Organization & Food and Agriculture Organization of the United Nations. (2007). *Safe preparation, storage and handling of powdered infant formula guidelines*. Retrieved from http:// www.who.int/foodsafety/publications/micro/pif_guidelines.pdf

World Health Organization/United Nations International Children's Emergency Fund Joint Statement. (1989). *Protecting and Supporting Breastfeeding: The Special Role of Maternity Services*. Geneva, Switzerland: World Health Organization. Retrieved from http:// www.babyfriendlyusa.org/eng/index.html

Wright, M., & Lo, C. (2007). Infant formulas: A practical guide. *Family Practice Recertification Online, 29*(10), 33-39.

Wright, N., & Marinelli, K. A. (2006). American academy of breastfeeding medicine protocols: Guidelines for glucose monitoring and treatment of hypoglycemia in breastfed neonates. *Breastfeeding Medicine, 1*(3), 178–184. Retrieved from http://www.bfmed .org/Resources/Download.aspx?filename=hypoglycemia.pdf

Ziol-Guest, K. M., & Hernandez, D. C. (2010). First and second trimester WIC participation is associated with lower rates of breastfeeding and early introduction of cow's milk during infancy. *Journal of the American Dietetic Association, 110*(5), 702–709. doi:10.1016/j.jada.2010.02.013

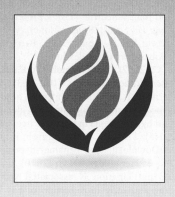

Joan Renaud Smith
Annette Carley

CHAPTER 21

Common Neonatal Complications

Most newborns with complications are identified and cared for in community hospitals or level II perinatal centers (American Academy of Pediatrics [AAP], 2012). Perinatal nurses must have a thorough understanding of pathophysiologic and clinical signs of illness during the immediate newborn period. The length of stay limits the time to identify behavioral cues or subtle changes that could potentially compromise newborn well-being.

Conditions discussed in this chapter include common complications such as respiratory distress, congenital heart disease (CHD), hypoglycemia, hyperbilirubinemia, and sepsis. Less common but important topics include neonatal resuscitation, perinatal HIV-1 exposure, neonatal substance exposure, and hypoxic ischemic encephalopathy (HIE). The target population is term and preterm newborn infants, including the late preterm infant born between 34 0/7 and 36 6/7 weeks' gestational age. This chapter concludes with a discussion of neonatal transport because, in some cases, the severity of the disease process necessitates transfer to a tertiary care center.

NEONATAL RESUSCITATION AND STABILIZATION

Most newborns transition from fetal to extrauterine life uneventfully. However, approximately 1 in 10 will require some assistance after delivery to initiate or sustain respiratory effort, and 1% will require extensive measures to survive. In keeping with the "ABCs" of resuscitation, providers must ensure that the airway is clear and unimpeded, breathing is spontaneous and unassisted, and that circulation is maintained to adequately perfuse tissues and organs. The AAP and

the American Heart Association (AHA) (2011) recommend that all births be attended by someone capable of initiating resuscitation and those resources for sustained resuscitation efforts be available as needed.

Prior to birth, the fetus receives oxygen by diffusion from the mother's blood across the placental membranes. Since the fetal lungs do not participate in oxygenation, only a small fraction of fetal blood passes through them. The fetal alveoli, although round and expanded, are fluid filled, and the surrounding arterioles are constricted. The increase in pulmonary vascular resistance (PVR) favors blood flow in a manner which bypasses the lungs through a series of fetal shunts, allowing delivery of optimally oxygenated blood through the ductus arteriosus to the body. After birth, the placenta no longer supports fetal needs, and the newborn must quickly establish ventilation, clear fluid from the alveoli, and dilate the pulmonary vasculature to support ongoing oxygenation. Failure to do so results in hypoxemia and acidosis. The newborn may respond briefly to hypoxia with compensatory tachypnea, although this is quickly followed by primary apnea and a fall in heart rate (HR). If breathing is not quickly established, secondary apnea occurs, and assisted ventilation must be provided to reverse the process (AAP & AHA, 2011).

Certain antepartum and intrapartum risk factors are associated with the need for resuscitation. Maternal factors may be chronic or acute and include such conditions as diabetes, hypertension, cardiopulmonary disease, substance exposure, late trimester bleeding, and infection. Intrapartum factors may also complicate fetal transition, including assisted delivery, cesarean delivery, abnormal fetal lie, presence of meconium, and placental complications. Newborns who are postterm, premature, or who have size-date discrepancies pose additional risks for poor transition. An anticipated compromised birth warrants the presence of personnel who can initiate and sustain resuscitation, including use of ventilatory support, chest compressions, and selected medications. However, risk factors are not always apparent, and providers must be able to anticipate and intervene quickly to support the compromised newborn. Three assessment prompts will assist with quick identification of newborns who will require support: Is the baby term? Is the baby breathing? Is there good muscle tone? (AAP & AHA, 2011).

The Neonatal Resuscitation Program (NRP) was developed in 1987 to provide a systematic method for managing the compromised newborn. It supports consistent and appropriate actions to address ventilation and circulation needs, which are continually evaluated using an algorithm containing action blocks. The resuscitation sequence begins with positioning the newborn infant on his back or side to open the airway, and then proceeding to drying and stimulating. It is important to ensure resuscitation occurs in a warm environment. Following this initial 30-second block ("A"), the infant is assessed. If the infant responds with a sustained heart rate above 100 beats per minute and sustained breathing or crying, additional measures are unnecessary. However, an infant who does not establish sustained breathing is presumed to be exhibiting secondary apnea, and the next block ("B") commences with assisted ventilation. The infant is continually assessed, and additional maneuvers are applied according to infant response (AAP & AHA, 2011).

Effective neonatal resuscitation for at-risk infants requires not only dexterity with maneuvers such as ventilation and compressions but also collaboration among a neonatal team to ensure timely and organized support. Poor communication and lack of teamwork have been identified as factors in poor outcomes following neonatal resuscitation, and the most recent edition updates recommendations to increase focus on team building and collaborating, and alternate learning strategies such as more effective use of simulation and debriefing (AAP & AHA, 2011; Perlman et al., 2010; Zaichkin & Weiner, 2011).

Some lingering controversies related to neonatal resuscitation and stabilization have prompted changes to the NRP guidelines, including the management of meconium exposure and the use of supplemental oxygen. Of the 13% of newborns born through meconium-stained amniotic fluid, less than 12% will go on to develop meconium aspiration syndrome (MAS). However, for many years, providers performed aggressive perineal and direct tracheal suctioning on all exposed infants in an attempt to prevent MAS. The latest recommendations for management of meconium-exposed infants include an assessment of infant behavior. For the meconium-exposed infant who is vigorous (e.g., with normal respiratory rate, tone, and HR), intrapartal suctioning and immediate neonatal tracheal suctioning are no longer recommended. However, for the meconium-exposed infant who is depressed, direct suctioning of the trachea before establishment of respirations is indicated (AAP & AHA, 2011; Bry, 2008).

Data regarding use of supplemental oxygen during neonatal resuscitation is evolving, and the ideal concentration of oxygen during resuscitation is unknown. Some evidence suggests enhanced risk for inadvertent oxidant injury across all gestational ages when supplemental oxygen is used. Until more definitive evidence is available, providers must attempt to avoid hypoxemia and hyperoxemia when supplemental oxygen is applied (Bry, 2008; Rabi, 2010), and the use of room air for initial resuscitation of the term infant is currently recognized as acceptable practice if well monitored. The most recent NRP guidelines recommend the use of pulse oximetry for neonatal resuscitations, especially of the preterm population, to more optimally titrate supplemental oxygen when used (Perlman et al., 2010; Zaichkin & Weiner, 2011).

An additional neonatal education program endorsed by the AAP is S.T.A.B.L.E., which reinforces key stabilization skills via an acronym: _Sugar, Temperature, Airway, Blood pressure, Lab work assessment, and Emotional support of families._ This program supports nursery staff who participate in postresuscitation stabilization and pretransport care of the neonate requiring intensive care and encourages a systematic approach to management (Taylor & Price-Douglas, 2008). Both S.T.A.B.L.E. and the NRP have been disseminated worldwide as stabilization programs for at-risk neonates.

RESPIRATORY DISTRESS

Respiratory distress is a major cause of neonatal morbidity and mortality despite significant technologic and pharmacologic advances during the past 30 years. Respiratory distress is one of the most common neonatal complications seen by the perinatal and neonatal nurse and is a principal indication for neonatal transfer to tertiary care units. The pathophysiology and etiology of respiratory distress varies, but the result is decreased ability to exchange the oxygen and carbon dioxide necessary to ensure delivery of well-oxygenated blood to vital organs. Respiratory distress may be an isolated finding or occur in association with other medical or systemic problems. It may be due to structural or functional abnormality or as a consequence of acute lung injury and result in prolonged transition to extrauterine life. Five of the most common respiratory diseases occurring during the neonatal period are respiratory distress syndrome (RDS), MAS, pneumonia, transient tachypnea of the newborn (TTNB), and persistent pulmonary hypertension of the newborn (PPHN).

RESPIRATORY DISTRESS SYNDROME

RDS primarily occurs in preterm newborns. In the United States, approximately 24,000 newborns develop RDS each year. The incidence of RDS is inversely related to gestational age: 60% of infants are born at less than 28 weeks, 30% of those are born at 28 to 34 weeks' gestation, and less than 5% of those born after 34 weeks are affected (Warren & Anderson, 2009). The mortality rate for RDS across all gestational ages is about 10%, attributable to improved prenatal and postnatal management (Dudell & Stoll, 2007; Warren & Anderson, 2009). RDS is caused by insufficient amounts of surfactant or delayed or impaired surfactant synthesis. Surfactant is a mixture of phospholipids and proteins synthesized, packaged, and excreted by alveolar type II cells that lowers surface tension in the alveoli and functions as a stabilizer to prevent atelectasis and alveolar collapse at end expiration (Cole, Nogee, & Hamvas, 2006). Without surfactant, atelectasis (alveolar collapse) occurs, resulting in a series of events that progressively increase disease severity. These events include hypoxemia (decreased concentration of oxygen), hypercapnia (increased concentration of carbon dioxide), mismatch of ventilation with perfusion, acidosis, pulmonary vasoconstriction, alveolar endothelial and epithelial damage, and subsequent protein-rich interstitial and alveolar edema. This cascade of events further decreases surfactant synthesis, storage, and release and leads to pulmonary failure (Dudell & Stoll, 2007; Warren & Anderson, 2009).

MECONIUM ASPIRATION SYNDROME

Passage of meconium in utero or perinatally is primarily seen in term and postterm infants and those experiencing stress such as growth-restricted infants or those with cord complications compromising uteroplacental circulation (Dudell & Stoll, 2007). Meconium passage occurs as a response to hypoxia, as relaxation of the anal sphincter allows passive escape of meconium into the amniotic fluid. Under normal intrauterine conditions, amniotic fluid does not enter the fetal lung. However, when the fetus experiences hypoxemia, gasping may result in aspiration of meconium-stained amniotic fluid. Of newborns, 8% to 20% are exposed to amniotic fluid stained by meconium; of these, 5% to 10% will go on to develop MAS (American College of Obstetricians and Gynecologists [ACOG], 2006; Dudell & Stoll, 2007; van Lerland & de Beaufort, 2009).

Preventive strategies have been evaluated for cases at risk for MAS, including amnioinfusion and direct tracheal suctioning of the neonate. Although amnioinfusion appears to be a reasonable treatment for repetitive variable decelerations, its sole use as a technique to prevent MAS is not warranted (ACOG, 2006; Xu, Wei, & Fraser, 2008). When aspirated by the fetus before or during birth, meconium can obstruct the airways, leading to severe hypoxia, inflammation, and infection and cause significant respiratory difficulties. Past evidence suggested that intrapartum suctioning before the first breath would decrease the risk of MAS; however, subsequent evidence from a large multicentered randomized trial did not show benefit from routine intrapartum oropharyngeal and nasopharyngeal suctioning (Velaphi & Vidyasagar, 2006; van Lerland & de Beaufort, 2009). Currently, the NRP no longer recommends that all meconium-stained babies routinely receive intrapartum suctioning (AAP & AHA, 2011; Vain, Szyld, Prudent, & Aguilar, 2009).

Pneumonitis is an inflammatory response likely secondary to bile salts present in aspirated meconium. Pneumonitis results in acute lung injury with protein-rich interstitial and alveolar edema. In situations where meconium only partially obstructs the airway, a ball-valve effect results. Air enters the lower airways on inspiration but cannot escape on expiration. This causes overdistension of alveoli, leading to alveolar rupture and pulmonary air leaks. Pneumonitis and airway obstruction result in hypoxemia and acidosis, which cause increased PVR and subsequent PPHN (Steinhom & Farrow, 2007).

PNEUMONIA

Pneumonia is acquired through vertical or horizontal transmission of a pathogenic organism and may present clinically as early-onset sepsis develops in the neonate. Vertical transmission occurs in utero in association with chorioamnionitis, intraamniotic infection, transplacental transmission of organisms, or aspiration of infected amniotic fluid. It may also occur following prolonged rupture of the membranes due to loss of the bacteriostatic protection of amniotic fluid. Horizontal transmission occurs in the nursery as pathogenic organisms spread from hospital personnel, equipment, or families or present as secondary infections as the result of some other primary infection. Pneumonia causes an inflammatory process, disrupting the normal barrier function of the pulmonary endothelium and epithelium, leading to abnormal protein permeability and edema of lung tissue. Hypoxemia and acidosis result, causing increased PVR and potential sequelae such as PPHN (Stoll, 2007a).

TRANSIENT TACHYPNEA OF THE NEWBORN

TTNB occurs in approximately 0.3% to 0.5% of newborns, although the exact incidence is unknown

(Yurdakok, 2010). Generally, TTNB is a mild, self-limiting disorder of term and near-term infants (NTIs), lasting from 12 to greater than 72 hours. Fetal lungs are fluid filled during gestation, although production of lung fluid decreases at birth with the onset of breathing and secondary to other influences of labor. Fluid is then absorbed from the air spaces through blood vessels, lymphatics, and the upper airways (Yurdakok, 2010).

In certain infants, however, the residual fluid in the alveoli persists, alters oxygen exchange, and increases work of breathing. Several pathophysiologic mechanisms have been suggested for TTNB. Historically, this condition was thought to be related to delayed reabsorption of lung fluid by the pulmonary lymphatic system. Retained fluid causes bronchiolar collapse with air trapping or hyperinflation of the alveoli. Hypoxia results when poorly ventilated alveoli are perfused, and hypercarbia results from mechanical interference with alveolar ventilation by fluid. Decreased lung compliance results in tachypnea and increased energy needed to do the work of breathing. It is known that stimuli during labor and at the time of birth cause active transport of chloride from plasma into the fetal lung fluid to cease. As the concentration of chloride becomes higher in the plasma, fetal lung fluid begins to be reabsorbed. Two thirds of the fetal lung fluid is absorbed before birth. Newborns without the benefit of labor and those born prematurely do not have the same amount of time to reabsorb lung fluid as those born after a normal course of labor. Infants delivered by elective cesarean section also have a higher incidence of TTNB (Jain & Eaton, 2006). Some also suggest that TTNB may result from mild immaturity of the surfactant system, which may explain cases of TTNB in late preterm infants (Yurdakok, 2010).

PERSISTENT PULMONARY HYPERTENSION OF THE NEWBORN

PPHN is defined as a failure of the pulmonary vasculature to relax at birth, resulting in delivery of unoxygenated blood to the systemic circulation. In fetal circulation, pulmonary blood vessels are constricted, causing most blood flow to bypass the lungs. This is appropriate for the fetus because the placenta rather than the fetal lung acts as the organ of gas exchange. PPHN is the result of a sustained elevation of the PVR after birth, preventing transition to the normal pattern of circulation. When the PVR remains elevated, blood bypasses the lungs by flowing through the foramen ovale or ductus arteriosus. This pattern of circulation is referred to as right-to-left shunting because blood is diverted from the venous circulation on the right side of the heart to the arterial circulation on the left side of the heart without going through the pulmonary vascular system. In approximately 1/500 to 1/1,500 live births, severe, prolonged hypoxemia (decreased oxygen in the blood) progresses to hypoxia (decreased oxygen in the tissues) and results in metabolic acidosis and worsening pulmonary vasoconstriction. A vicious cycle ensues. PPHN may be idiopathic, caused by abnormal development of pulmonary vessels, or may result from pathopysiologic events such as asphyxia, MAS, pneumonia, and RDS (Dudell & Stoll, 2007; Lapointe & Barrington, 2011; Stayer & Liu, 2010; Steinhom & Farrow, 2007). Infants with PPHN are typically labile and often require sedation to control competing respiratory effort, vasodilators to overcome pulmonary vasoconstriction, and vasopressors to support systemic blood pressure. A small percentage with refractory hypoxemia may require extracorporeal membrane oxygenation (ECMO) for survival (Dudell & Stoll, 2007).

ASSESSMENT OF RESPIRATORY DISTRESS

Clinical signs of respiratory distress may be present at birth or occur at any time in the early neonatal period. These signs include tachypnea, grunting, retractions, nasal flaring, and cyanosis. Tachypnea is defined as a sustained respiratory rate greater than 60 to 70 breaths per minute (Gardner, Enzman-Hines, & Dickey, 2011). Tachypnea develops when the newborn attempts to improve ventilation. Because of the very compliant chest wall, especially in the preterm newborn, it is more energy efficient for the newborn to increase the respiratory rate rather than the depth of respirations. However, persistent tachypnea results in muscular fatigue and, over time, further compromises pulmonary status.

On exhalation, a grunting sound is sometimes heard in newborns with respiratory distress. Grunting is the result of forceful closure of the glottis in an attempt to increase intrapulmonary pressure, keep alveoli open, and create residual lung gas volume (functional residual capacity). Keeping alveoli open during exhalation is a compensatory response to decreased partial pressure of oxygen (PO_2) and allows more time for gas exchange to occur (Gardner et al., 2011).

Retractions are depressions observed between the ribs, above the sternum, or below the xiphoid process during inhalation. Retractions are the result of a very compliant chest wall and noncompliant lung. Compliance refers to the stiffness or distensibility of the chest wall and lung parenchyma. As the amount of negative intrathoracic pressure increases on inspiration, the rib cage expands until the soft tissue of the thorax and weak intercostal muscles are pulled inward toward the spine. The result is worsening atelectasis with marked oxygenation and ventilation abnormalities (Cifuentes, Segars, & Carlo, 2003; Gardner et al., 2011).

Nasal flaring occurs with respiratory distress as the newborn attempts to decrease airway resistance and increase the inflow of air through dilation of the alae nasi (Gardner et al., 2011).

Cyanosis results from inadequate oxygenation caused by atelectasis, poor lung compliance, and right-to-left shunting. Although the newborn's color may be an indicator of oxygenation, variables such as skin temperature and perfusion affect the accuracy of this finding. Precise measurement of oxygen and acid–base status may be necessary for the management of respiratory distress using tools such as pulse oximetry and blood gases (Gardner et al., 2011; Rohan & Golembek, 2009).

INTERVENTIONS FOR RESPIRATORY DISTRESS

Care for newborns with respiratory distress focuses on oxygenation and ventilation as well as controlling factors that increase oxygen demands such as hypothermia or stress. Adequate oxygenation and ventilation requires supportive mechanisms ranging from supplemental oxygen only to application of assisted ventilation with techniques such as continuous positive airway pressure (CPAP) or mechanical ventilation. Pulse oximetry and direct arterial blood gas monitoring are methods used to ensure adequate gas exchange. In a preterm newborn, delivery of oxygen should be sufficient to maintain arterial oxygen tension at 50 to 70 mm Hg, corresponding to a pulse oximetry reading of approximately 85% to 95% (Dudell & Stoll, 2007). Because oxygen may be toxic to some tissue, care should be taken to avoid excessive tissue oxygenation, which might have toxic effects such as chronic lung disease or retinopathy of prematurity. In a term newborn at risk for PPHN, oxygen delivery should be sufficient to maintain normoxemia yet avoid hypoxia, which is a potent stimulus for vasoconstriction (Lapointe & Barrington, 2011). Infants with suspected PPHN will need to be transferred to a tertiary care center for further evaluation and management, including potential use of high-frequency ventilation (HFOV), inhaled nitric oxide (i-NO), or ECMO for severe hypoxemia (Stayer & Liu, 2010).

Select pharmacologic agents may be used in the prevention or management of neonatal respiratory distress. Prenatally, at-risk mothers may receive antenatal steroids to stimulate surfactant synthesis in an effort to prevent RDS. Postnatally, commonly used preparations include airway-instilled surfactant (for RDS prophylaxis or treatment), antibiotics (for pneumonia prophylaxis or treatment), and inhaled or vascularly delivered pulmonary vasodilators (for PPHN treatment) (Konduri & Kim, 2009; Warren & Anderson, 2009).

A neutral thermal environment (NTE) is crucial in the care of a newborn with respiratory distress. Hypothermia or hyperthermia both increase metabolic demands, leading to decreased oxygenation, metabolic acidosis, and worsening respiratory distress (Cifuentes et al., 2003). Newborns with respiratory distress are cared for under a radiant warmer or in an incubator.

Adequate nutrition frequently requires the administration of intravenous (IV) fluids during the early neonatal period. Care is taken to prevent hypoglycemia that may occur from respiratory distress and increased metabolic demands (Rohan & Golembek, 2009).

CONGENITAL HEART DISEASE

CARDIOVASCULAR SYSTEM

The cardiovascular system begins to develop in the third week of gestation and is fully developed by the end of the eighth week. It is the first major organ system to develop in the embryo. In the United States, an estimated 32,000 infants are expected to be affected with CHD annually. Of these, an approximate 25% require invasive treatment in the first year of life (AHA, 2012). Heart defects are among the most common birth defects and are the leading cause of birth defect-related deaths. However, the overall mortality has significantly declined over the past few decades (AHA, 2012). The cause of CHD cannot be ascribed to any single factor. Most cases are multifactorial, involving genetic predisposition, familial recurrence, and environmental factors. A family history of CHD is significant; if the mother has a history of a child with CHD, her risk of recurrence increases by threefold (Kenney, Hoover, Williams, & Iskersky, 2011). CHD can also be associated with chromosomal abnormalities (i.e., trisomies 21, 18, 13; chromosome deletion syndromes; DiGeorge deletion 22q; Turner syndrome; and Cornelia de Lange) and maternal–environmental factors, such as drugs (i.e., thalidomide, anticonvulsants, lithium, retinoic acid) and alcohol exposure, or diseases (e.g., insulin-dependent diabetes, maternal lupus erythematosus) and infections (e.g., rubella, Coxsackie B, and enteroviruses) (Kenney et al., 2011).

Cardiac lesions are classified as cyanotic, acyanotic, or according to the hemodynamic characteristics related to pulmonary blood flow. Five of the most commonly occurring cardiac lesions presenting in the early neonatal period include ventricular septal defect (VSD), tetralogy of Fallot (TOF), PDA, atrial septal defect (ASD), and d (dextro)-transposition of the great arteries (d-TGA).

The assessment to exclude CHD includes the following:

- Close observation of cardiorespiratory status
- Palpation of peripheral pulses
- Blood pressures of the four extremities
- Chest radiograph to evaluate heart size and pulmonary vascularity
- Blood gas determinations to evaluate oxygenation and metabolic status
- Evaluation of response to 100% oxygen (a hyperoxia test is used to differentiate respiratory disease from cyanotic heart disease)

The newborn with CHD or persistence of a fetal shunt may present shortly after birth or within the first weeks of life with cyanosis or symptoms of congestive heart failure (CHF). The newborn becomes cyanotic when gas exchange is impaired by pulmonary edema, blood flow to the lungs is restricted as a result of a structural abnormality, or blood flow is shunted away from the lungs. In the newborn with CHD, central cyanosis (bluish discoloration of the skin, nail beds, and mucous membranes) is one of the most common presenting signs and is generally not visible until there is 4 to 5 g/dL of deoxygenated hemoglobin in the arterial system (Mahle et al., 2009). Both the severity of hypoxemia and the hemoglobin concentration determine the degree of cyanosis (Kenney et al., 2011). It is important to differentiate central cyanosis from acrocyanosis (cyanosis of the extremities is commonly seen in newborns because of reduced blood flow through the small capillaries), which is considered a normal finding (Lott, 2007; Kenney et al., 2011).

When the heart is unable to meet the metabolic demands of the tissues, CHF ensues. Unlike infants with CHD, infants with CHF typically present with significant respiratory distress. Common clinical signs associated with CHF (Kenney et al., 2011; Lott, 2007):

- Tachypnea (due to pulmonary edema)
- Respiratory distress
- Gallop rhythm (caused by dilation of the ventricles)
- Decreased peripheral pulses and mottling of the extremities (decrease in peripheral tissue perfusion)
- Tachycardia (in an attempt to compensate for a decrease in cardiac output [CO], the heart either increases the rate or the stroke volume [SV])
- Hepatomegaly (right ventricle does not adequately empty, leading to an elevated right atrium pressure, resulting in hepatic venous congestion)
- Poor feeding (due to high respiratory rate and increases in basal metabolic rate demands)

A murmur, if present, varies in quality and intensity, depending on the particular cardiac lesion present. If a VSD or ASD is present, allowing mixing of oxygenated and unoxygenated blood, only mild cyanosis occurs. If there is no intracardiac shunt, severe cyanosis is observed. With the exception of cyanosis, the physical examination is often otherwise unremarkable. In the newborn with a large VSD or ASD, signs of CHF develop over time as the PVR falls and the pulmonary blood flow increases. In newborns without an intracardiac shunt, severe hypoxemia and metabolic acidosis develop, followed by a rapid demise if emergency measures are not instituted.

Routine newborn screening for critical congenital heart disease (CCHD) using pulse oximetry is recommended to prevent mortality and morbidity (Secretary's Advisory Committee on Heritable Disorders in Newborns and Children, 2011). Hypoplastic left heart syndrome, pulmonary atresia (with intact septum),

transposition of the great arteries, truncus arteriosus, tricuspid atresia, tetralogy of Fallot, and total anomalous pulmonary venous return are among the seven CCHDs that are primary targets for the routine screening in the well infant and intermediate nurseries (Mahle et al., 2009; Kemper et al., 2012).

VENTRICULAR SEPTAL DEFECT

Pathophysiology

The partitioning of the embryonic heart into chambers of the atria and ventricles begins near the fourth week of gestation and is completed by the end of the seventh week (Auckland, 2010). A VSD is present when there is an incomplete division of the right and left ventricles. VSDs are classified by their anatomic location; perimembranous and muscular are the two most common types. A perimembranous VSD is located just below the aortic valve and accounts for 80% of all VSDs. A muscular VSD is located in the muscular septum. Of membranous and muscular VSDs, 75% to 80% close spontaneously. A VSD is considered an acyanotic lesion with increased pulmonary blood flow. The size and location of the defect, as well as the pulmonary-to-systemic vascular resistance ratio, determine the degree of left-to-right shunt. The timing of the onset of symptoms is directly related to the normal fall in the PVR after birth (Kenney et al., 2011).

Assessment

The onset of symptoms resulting from a VSD is related to the size of the defect and PVR. A newborn with a small defect has minimal left-to-right shunting at the ventricular level and may appear well with few or no symptoms other than a holosystolic systolic murmur heard best at the lower left sternal border. The murmur develops as the PVR falls. A newborn with a large defect may present with symptoms of CHF but not until approximately 2 to 4 weeks of life. As with the smaller defects, the murmur is holosystolic and heard over the left lower sternal border. Preterm newborns with large VSDs may present sooner and be more symptomatic compared to their term counterparts because preterm infants have lower PVR at birth, resulting in greater left-to-right shunting (Kenney et al., 2011).

TETRALOGY OF FALLOT

Pathophysiology

TOF consists of a large perimembranous VSD, pulmonary artery stenosis, an overriding aorta, and right ventricle hypertrophy (Kenney et al., 2011). This lesion is a result of disordered embryonic cardiac functioning. TOF occurs during the embryonic stage of development, when some unknown factor influences functioning of the heart at the cellular level. This alteration in cellular function is partly responsible for determining development. TOF is generally considered a cyanotic lesion with decreased pulmonary blood flow, but the hemodynamics vary widely, depending on the severity of pulmonary stenosis, the size of the VSD, and the pulmonary and systemic vascular resistance. Most newborns with TOF present with cyanosis because of the right-to-left intracardiac shunt. However, if the intracardiac shunt is mainly left to right due to a mild or moderate right ventricular outflow obstruction, the infant will not be cyanotic (Kenney et al., 2011). Typically, the course worsens over the first year of life.

Assessment

TOF is the most common cyanotic heart disease seen in the first year of life. Newborns with TOF are most often diagnosed in the first few weeks of life due to either a loud murmur or cyanosis. Newborns with TOF often present with cyanosis, hypoxia, and dyspnea. However, newborns who are symptomatic typically have severe right ventricular outflow tract obstruction (Kenney et al., 2011). The timing and degree of cyanosis depend on the severity of the pulmonary stenosis and may not be noticed until closure of the ductus arteriosus. In the case of pulmonary atresia and hypoplasia of the pulmonary arteries, marked cyanosis may be observed immediately after birth. The clinical signs of right-sided heart failure, resulting from right ventricular outflow tract obstruction, include hepatomegaly, tricuspid valve regurgitation, and a grade II to IV/VI harsh systolic murmur best heard over the mid to upper left sternal border.

PATENT DUCTUS ARTERIOSUS

Pathophysiology

The ductus arteriosus is a normal pathway of fetal circulation. The ductus arteriosus connects the pulmonary artery to the aorta, allowing blood to bypass the lungs directly into the placenta. During fetal life, PVR is greater than systemic vascular resistance. After birth, with spontaneous respiration, the arterial oxygen level increases and PVR decreases, causing the ductus to close. Functionally, the PDA closes within hours to several days after birth, but closure is often delayed in premature infants. If the ductus arteriosus does not close, blood begins to flow left to right through the patent ductus as the PVR decreases. A PDA is an acyanotic lesion with increased pulmonary blood flow. It presents with signs and symptoms of CHF. It occurs much more commonly in preterm newborns, with the incidence inversely proportional to gestational age (Kenney et al., 2011).

Assessment

The manifestation of PDA depends on the gestational age and the degree of lung disease. Preterm newborns generally develop signs associated with CHF at 3 to 7 days of life, but it can develop sooner in the smaller preterm newborn treated with surfactant. The development of clinical signs is related to the normal fall in the PVR, resulting in increased blood flow to the pulmonary circulation and volume overload of the left ventricles. In newborns, a grade I through III systolic ejection murmur will likely develop; if left untreated, a classic machinerylike continuous murmur may result in older infants and children. PDA murmurs are best heard at the upper left sternal border (over the first and second intercostal spaces to the left of the sternum) and may radiate to the back, between the scapulae. However, with a right-to-left shunt, a murmur may be absent (Kenney et al., 2011).

ATRIAL SEPTAL DEFECT

Pathophysiology

The separation of the atrium begins near the middle of the fourth week of gestation and is completed by the sixth week, leaving the foramen ovale open between the two atria. An abnormality occurring during atrial separation can result in an ASD. An ASD is considered an acyanotic lesion with increased pulmonary blood flow. Approximately 10% of newborns with very large ASDs develop CHF as the PVR decreases and a left-to-right shunt develops with concomitant right ventricular volume overload and hypertrophy (Sadowski, 2010). Three major types of ASDs occur and are differentiated from each other by whether they involve other structures of the heart and how they are formed during fetal development (Lott, 2007). The first type is ostium secundum, the most common yet least serious type of ASD, and is caused when a part of the atrial septum fails to close completely while the heart is developing. The second type is an ostium primum defect, part of the spectrum of atrioventricular (AV) canal defects, which is often associated with a cleft in the leaflet of the mitral valve. The third type is the sinus venosus defect, which occurs at the superior vena cava and right atrium junction and is most often associated with partial anomalous pulmonary venous connection.

Assessment

Newborns with an uncomplicated ASD are generally asymptomatic. However, about 10% present with signs of CHF, poor feeding, and poor growth. These symptoms develop as the PVR falls over the first few weeks of life. Associated with an ASD is a soft, systolic murmur best heard over the second intercostal space at the left upper sternal border.

d–TRANSPOSITION OF THE GREAT ARTERIES

Pathophysiology

The truncus arteriosus begins to divide during the fifth week of gestation. As the cardiac tube folds, the vessel twists on itself and divides into two separate vessels. The exact etiology of transposition remains unknown. Historically, transposition was thought to occur because of a failure of the aorticopulmonary septum to grow in a spiral fashion, resulting in inappropriate migration of the vessels. However, additional causes continue to be explored (Sankaran & Brown, 2007). The d (dextro)-transposition of the great arteries (d-TGA) occurs when the aorta arises from the right ventricle and the pulmonary artery arises from the left ventricle, resulting in pulmonary and systemic circulations functioning in parallel. When these two arteries are transposed, unoxygenated blood returning from the body enters the right side of the heart and returns to the body, and oxygenated blood returning from the lung enters the left side of the heart and returns to the lungs. d-TGA is considered a cyanotic lesion with increased pulmonary blood flow. d-Transposition can occur in isolation or can be associated with other defects (e.g., PDA, ASD, VSD, pulmonary stenosis). The degree of cyanosis depends on the amount of mixing of oxygenated and unoxygenated blood between the parallel systemic and pulmonary circulations through the associated lesions (e.g., patent foramen ovale [PFO], VSD, ASD, PDA, or collateral circulation) (Kenney et al., 2011).

Assessment

d-TGA is the most common cyanotic heart lesion that presents in the newborn period and is more prevalent in males (Kenney et al., 2011). The newborn with d-TGA presents with cyanosis typically within the first hours of life, and the degree of cyanosis varies depending on the amount of intracardiac mixing. For instance, if the mixing occurs through a large VSD or PDA, the cyanosis may be mild. If the ventricular septum is intact or the PDA is closing, the cyanosis is profound since there is no intracardiac shunt. With the exception of cyanosis, the physical examination findings are often otherwise unremarkable. With a large VSD or ASD, signs of CHF develop over time as the PVR falls and the pulmonary blood flow increases. In the absence of an intracardiac shunt, severe hypoxemia and metabolic acidosis develop, followed by a rapid demise if emergency measures are not instituted.

INTERVENTIONS FOR CONGENITAL HEART DISEASE

Newborns with known or suspected CHD usually require transfer to a tertiary center for treatment and follow-up. The complete diagnostic workup and subsequent repairs or palliative surgery are performed in centers with pediatric cardiac capabilities. Before transport, close observation and supportive care and treatment are warranted. Nursing care for newborns with known or suspected CHD includes the following:

- Cardiorespiratory monitoring
- Pulse oximetry
- Blood work, including blood gas determinations
- Ongoing assessment of color, perfusion, and degree of respiratory distress
- Maintaining a neutral thermal environment
- IV hydration and nutrition
- Oxygen therapy, if appropriate, and mechanical ventilation, if required

Metabolic acidosis is treated with sodium bicarbonate, pulmonary edema with respiratory distress is treated with diuretics, and shock is treated with vasopressors and calcium gluconate. A lesion such as d-TGA without an intracardiac shunt is treated with prostaglandin E1 to maintain patency of the ductus arteriosus until surgical correction takes place (Kenney et al., 2011).

HYPOGLYCEMIA

During the neonatal period, transient low glucose levels are not only common but also likely a normal adaptation to extrauterine life (Williams, 2005). Blood glucose as low as 30 mg/dL may occur during the first hours following birth (Committee on Fetus and Newborn & Adamkin, 2011). One of the major difficulties associated with defining hypoglycemia is the lack of correlation between a given blood glucose level and clinical signs. Whether producing symptoms or asymptomatic, hypoglycemia can result in either normal neonatal outcome or serious neurologic sequelae, such as brain injury, learning disabilities, and cerebral palsy. The clinical effects of hypoglycemia remain poorly defined. Neuropathology is available in only a few infants who have died after severe hypoglycemia, although follow-up studies of high-risk infants suggest that adverse neurodevelopmental outcomes are more prevalent when there is a history of asymptomatic hypoglycemic in the newborn period (McGowan & Perlman, 2006). Although the exact incidence is elusive due to inconsistent definitions, hypoglycemia is estimated to occur in 1 to 3/1,000 live births and up to 15% of those who are born growth restricted (McGowan, Rozance, Price-Douglas, & Hay, 2011; Stoll, 2007b).

Rather than identifying strict definitions of hypoglycemia, most authors suggest the use of *operational thresholds*. There is no absolute threshold applicable to all babies, and there is no glucose concentration that absolutely determines clinical risk or predicts sequelae. A glucose value must be assessed in conjunction with other clinical data, and treatment should be based upon this integrated input (Cornblath et al., 2000).

PATHOPHYSIOLOGY

During fetal life, insulin is secreted by the fetal pancreas in response to glucose that readily crosses the placenta. At birth, the newborn's blood glucose level is approximately 70% to 80% that of the mother. After removal of placental circulation, the newborn must maintain glucose homeostasis. This requires initiation of various metabolic processes, including gluconeogenesis (e.g., forming glucose from noncarbohydrate sources such as protein and fat) and glycogenolysis (e.g., conversion of glycogen stores to glucose), as well as an intact regulatory mechanism and an adequate supply of substrate (Kayiran & Gurakan, 2010; Sperling & Menon, 2004). While this is effective for the well or term infant, the sick or preterm infant is constrained in effectively mobilizing or utilizing fuel sources.

Hypoglycemia can occur at variable times in neonatal life, depending on its cause. Hypoglycemia during the first few hours of life can be a transient result of developmental immaturity or perinatal stress and may occur in preterm or small-for-gestational-age (SGA) infants. Beyond the first few hours of life, hypoglycemia is more common due to hyperinsulinemia, as with the infant of a diabetic mother. Persistent hypoglycemia, a rare event, may represent inborn metabolic errors of metabolism or endocrine disorders (Sperling & Menon, 2004).

Early feeding will contribute to stabilization of newborn blood sugar. Breastfed term infants have lower blood glucose levels but higher concentrations of ketone bodies than formula-fed infants (Hawdon, Ward Platt, & Aynsley-Green, 1992). Utilization of this alternate fuel source may allow them to tolerate lower serum glucose levels without sequelae (Committee on Fetus and Newborn & Adamkin, 2011; Cornblath et al., 2000).

ASSESSMENT

Identification of those infants at risk for developing hypoglycemia facilitates planning and implementation of appropriate nursing care. This process begins with a review of maternal prenatal and intrapartum history for risk factors associated with neonatal hypoglycemia and a careful physical examination. Symptoms of hypoglycemia are nonspecific and not easily differentiated from many other common neonatal conditions (Display 21–1).

Universal blood glucose screening before clinical signs develop is not currently recommended by the AAP (Committee on Fetus and Newborn & Adamkin, 2011). Selective screening of at-risk newborns is more appropriate and does not appear to decrease quality of care or result in adverse outcomes.

Newborns at risk should be screened within 30 to 60 minutes after birth. Use of proper screening

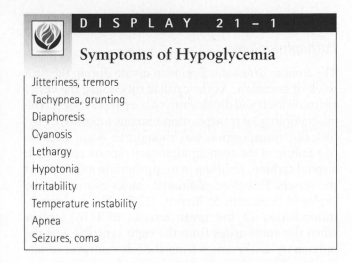

DISPLAY 21–1

Symptoms of Hypoglycemia

Jitteriness, tremors
Tachypnea, grunting
Diaphoresis
Cyanosis
Lethargy
Hypotonia
Irritability
Temperature instability
Apnea
Seizures, coma

techniques is one of the most important nursing functions. Point-of-care testing (POCT), performed using a bedside glucose oxidase stick method, will provide an expedient estimation of glucose values. Although glucose oxidase sticks are widely used, accuracy of the results from these screening tests depends on the hematocrit, blood source, and operator's skill. They have been shown to have considerable variance from actual blood glucose levels, which may be due to the source of blood used for testing. Venous blood samples have glucose levels that are approximately 10% less than capillary or arterial specimens (Deshpande & Ward Platt, 2005). Other factors limiting accuracy are improper storage, outdated shelf life of test strips, or contamination with isopropyl alcohol, which falsely elevates the glucose result. It is also important to remember that these POCT use whole blood, which will affect the ability to accurately detect glucose at extremes of hematocrit. The timing of glucose measurements may also result in inaccurate values, as failure to run the test promptly after sampling may result in red blood cell (RBC) oxidation of glucose and produce falsely low values. Blood samples should be transported on ice and analyzed quickly.

INTERVENTIONS

Newborns with asymptomatic hypoglycemia should be fed immediately and then retested. Invasive interventions on the basis of low values detected by screening are not warranted as long as infants are assessed and are found to be without clinical findings attributable to hypoglycemia. A low glucose in the asymptomatic newborn may initially be managed by offering breastfeeding or providing expressed breast milk or formula. The infant should be reassessed within 2 to 4 hours and, if the glucose remains low for a second measurement, should be fed again or have IV therapy started (Cornblath et al., 2000).

Newborns with symptomatic hypoglycemia, particularly those with neurologic signs and low POCT bedside blood glucose, should be treated immediately with an IV infusion of glucose, and a blood sample should be drawn and sent to the laboratory for glucose evaluation. Infusion rates should be similar to that expected with endogenous hepatic glucose production (approximately 5 mg/kg/min depending on maturity and weight for gestation—equivalent to 10% dextrose at approximately 70 to 80 mL/kg/day or 3 mL/kg/hr and titrated based on response) (Williams, 2005). Gradual increases in glucose infusion rate should not exceed 2 mg/kg/min each hour. Newborns who are unable to nipple feed and those whose blood glucose levels do not respond to oral feedings or have very low glucose levels (e.g., <20 mg/dL) should receive a 200 mg/kg (2 mL/kg) bolus of 10% dextrose in water intravenously over 1 minute, followed by a continuous infusion at the rates given previously until the blood glucose is stabilized (Cornblath et al., 2000; Rozance & Hay, 2010). Correction of hypoglycemia should result in resolution of the symptoms. IV administration is tapered off slowly, and the blood glucose level is monitored frequently, every 1 to 2 hours initially, and then intermittently before feedings until stable (Williams, 2005).

Newborns who experience persistent hypoglycemia may require an increased concentration of glucose, such as 12.5%, 15%, or 20%; dextrose solutions with concentrations greater than 12.5% require placement of a central line because of the risk of tissue extravasation. Other treatments for persistent or refractory hypoglycemia include glucagon, which promotes glycogenolysis and requires adequate stores, and corticosteroids, which induce gluconeogenic enzyme activity (Jain et al., 2010).

Hypoglycemia severe enough to warrant IV therapy, or which persists or recurs, requires further investigation to rule out underlying pathology, particularly infection or metabolic and endocrine disease (Deshpande & Ward Platt, 2005). The focus of nursing care is to prevent hypoglycemia when possible. Newborns should be fed within the first 2 hours of life. Care is taken to avoid cold stress and to recognize signs of respiratory distress and sepsis, which can increase the newborn's risk for developing hypoglycemia.

HYPERBILIRUBINEMIA

Hyperbilirubinemia resulting in clinical jaundice is detected in up to 60% of term and in 80% of preterm newborns (Juretschke, 2005; Piazza & Stoll, 2007). Typically, healthy newborns are discharged from the hospital before the usual peak of total serum bilirubin (TSB) (72 to 120 hours). Most jaundice is benign and

DISPLAY 21-2

Mechanisms Attributed to Physiologic Hyperbilirubinemia

Increased bilirubin related to relative polycythemia and short (80- to 90-day) life span of fetal red blood cells
Decreased uptake of bilirubin by the liver
Decreased enzyme activity and ability to conjugate bilirubin
Decreased ability to excrete bilirubin
Breastfeeding

resolves within 7 to 10 days in term newborns. However, severe hyperbilirubinemia may develop in 8% to 9% of all newborns during the first postnatal week (Kamath, Thilo, & Hernandez, 2011). Jaundice is a common indication for hospital readmission, affecting 1 in 100 term or late preterm infants (Alkalay, Bresee, & Simmons, 2010). Because of the potential for bilirubin toxicity, newborns require assessment to identify those at risk for severe hyperbilirubinemia or, in rare cases, bilirubin encephalopathy or kernicterus. Unconjugated hyperbilirubinemia results from physiologic mechanisms (Display 21–2) or pathologic causes (Display 21–3).

PATHOPHYSIOLOGY

Bilirubin is produced from the breakdown of heme-containing proteins (Juretschke, 2005). The major heme-containing protein is hemoglobin, which is the source of approximately 75% of the bilirubin produced. Heme is acted on by the enzyme heme oxygenase, releasing carbon monoxide and biliverdin. Biliverdin is then reduced to bilirubin through the activity of the enzyme biliverdin reductase. The degradation of every 1 g of hemoglobin produces 34 to 35 mg of bilirubin. Bilirubin binds with albumin for transport to the liver. Bilirubin, but not albumin, diffuses into the liver

DISPLAY 21-3

Causes of Pathologic Hyperbilirubinemia

Hemolytic disease of the newborn
Bruising, extravascular blood
Polycythemia
Intestinal obstruction
Metabolic conditions
Prematurity
Infection
Respiratory distress

cytoplasm, where it is transported to the endoplasmic reticulum for conjugation. Bilirubin combines with glucuronate with the help of glucuronyl transferase, the conjugating enzyme. Conjugated bilirubin is water soluble and excreted into bile and subsequently into the small intestine through the common bile duct. In the gut, conjugated bilirubin is excreted from the body through stool or converted to unconjugated bilirubin by a gut enzyme (beta-glucuronidase) that renders it reabsorbable. In fetal life, this reabsorption facilitates transport of bilirubin to the placenta for maternal excretion; however, postnatally, this pathway adds to the infant's bilirubin load (Kamath et al., 2011; Piazza & Stoll, 2007; Thilo, 2005).

Excretion of conjugated bilirubin is facilitated by bacteria in the gut. Meconium contains large amounts of bilirubin, but excretion is inhibited in the newborn because of the sterility of the gut. Normal colonization of bacteria occurs over time and is facilitated by early and frequent feeding. Feeding introduces bacteria into the gut. Lack of bacterial flora allows conversion of conjugated bilirubin back to an unconjugated form. This, along with greater red cell mass per kilogram in the newborn than in the adult and a shortened red cell life span, sets the stage for development of physiologic unconjugated hyperbilirubinemia. Newborns produce twice as much bilirubin as adults (Halamek & Stevenson, 2002; Piazza & Stoll, 2007; Thilo, 2005).

In a term newborn, physiologic unconjugated hyperbilirubinemia is characterized by a progressive increase in serum bilirubin to a peak of 6 to 8 mg/dL at 72 hours of age and a steady decline over the next week. In a preterm newborn, bilirubin continues to rise until the fourth to seventh postnatal day, reaching a peak of 8 to 12 mg/dL and decreasing thereafter as the processes of metabolism and excretion mature (Halamek & Stevenson, 2002). When jaundice is evident within the first 24 to 36 hours of life, bilirubin levels rise >5 mg/dL/day or peak in excess of 12 to 14 mg/dL; or if jaundice persists beyond 2 weeks of life, it is less likely to represent a physiologic process and warrants assessment (Burgos, Flaherman, & Newman, 2011; Piazza & Stoll, 2007).

Hyperbilirubinemia may result from three mechanisms: increased bilirubin production, increased bilirubin reabsorption, or decreased bilirubin excretion and may be attributed to *physiologic* or *pathologic* causes. Conditions contributing to physiologic, unconjugated hyperbilirubinemia include normal bilirubin load from a large fetal RBC mass with a shortened life span, as well as delayed stooling. Breastfed infants may experience exaggerated jaundice related to initial decreased caloric intake, decreased stooling with subsequent increase of enterohepatic circulation, or effects of substances within the milk, which interfere with conjugation and excretion (Kamath et al., 2011). Pathologic hyperbilirubinemia is most commonly associated

with conditions, which acutely increase the bilirubin load, such as isoimmune hemolytic disease in cases of Rh, ABO, or other minor blood group incompatibility between fetus and mother. Other causes contributing to excess bilirubin load or impaired excretion include extravascular blood, polycythemia, intestinal obstruction, prematurity, infection, infant of a diabetic mother, and rare metabolic or inherited conditions (Kamath et al., 2011; Juretschke, 2005; Thilo, 2005). Table 21–1 lists maternal and newborn risks for hyperbilirubinemia.

No absolute safe bilirubin level has been determined, and hyperbilirubinemia has the potential for leading to injury such as encephalopathy of kernicterus. Reports indicate that kernicterus, although rare, is still occurring and is almost always preventable (AAP, 2004a). The term *kernicterus* is used interchangeably with the acute and chronic findings of bilirubin encephalopathy. The AAP Subcommittee on Hyperbilirubinemia recommends acute bilirubin encephalopathy to be used when describing the acute manifestations of toxicity seen in the first weeks after birth and kernicterus reserved for the chronic and permanent clinical sequelae (AAP, 2004a; Schwartz, Haberman, & Ruddy, 2011). Permanent damage to the central nervous system (CNS) results from deposition of bilirubin in the brain, specifically in the basal ganglia, hippocampal cortex, subthalamic nuclei, and cerebellum (Juretschke, 2005).

During the early phase of acute bilirubin encephalopathy, severely jaundiced infants become lethargic and hypotonic and have a poor suck. The intermediate phase is characterized by moderate stupor, hypertonia,

Table 21–1. RISK FACTORS FOR HYPERBILIRUBINEMIA

Newborn	Maternal
Birth weight <1,500 g	Oxytocin, Valium
Preterm delivery	Forceps or vacuum delivery
Male sex	Diabetes
Hypothermia	East Asian heritage
Asphyxia	Native American heritage
Hypoalbuminemia	Pregnancy-induced hypertension
Sepsis	Family history of jaundice, liver
Meningitis	disease, anemia, or splenectomy
Polycythemia (Hct >65%)	Blood incompatibilities
Drugs that affect albumin binding	
Birth trauma (e.g., cephalhematoma, bruising)	
Congenital hypothyroidism	
Bruising	
Poor feeding	
Inborn error of metabolism	
Intestinal obstruction	
Erythrocyte disorders (e.g., G6PD deficiency)	

G6PD, glucose-6-phosphate dehydrogenase; Hct, hematocrit.

and irritability. The infant may also develop a fever and a high-pitched cry that alternates with drowsiness and hypotonia. The hypertonia is characterized by backward arching of the trunk (opisthotonos) and of the neck (retrocollis). CNS damage may, in some cases, be reversed during this phase with a combination of intensive phototherapy and an emergent exchange transfusion. The advanced phase is characterized by pronounced retrocollis and opisthotonos, shrill cry, inability to feed, apnea, fever, deep stupor to coma, seizures, and death. In the chronic form, kernicterus, surviving infants may develop severe athetoid cerebral palsy, auditory dysfunction, dental enamel dysplasia, paralysis of upward gaze, as well as intellectual and other handicaps (AAP, 2004a). There is no absolute level at which bilirubin encephalopathy occurs in all newborns. Gestational age, postnatal age, clinical condition, and the pathophysiologic process involved all play a part in determining what level of unconjugated bilirubin causes encephalopathy in a particular newborn (Juretschke, 2005).

ASSESSMENT

Clinical jaundice is apparent at serum bilirubin levels of 5 to 7 mg/dL (Juretschke, 2005; Kamath et al., 2011) and progresses cephalocaudally from head to the lower extremities. Visual recognition of jaundice is inaccurate, unreliable, and unsafe and varies with the experience and level of training of the observer (AAP, 2004a). A careful physical examination of any newborn presenting with jaundice aids in determining the cause of hyperbilirubinemia. The newborn should be assessed for risks including prematurity, low birth weight, indicators of bleeding or extravascular blood collections such as bruising, cephalhematoma or petechiae, and hepatosplenomegaly. In conjunction with the clinical examination, transcutaneous bilirubin (TcB) assessment and a number of laboratory tests including serum bilirubin may be done to quantify the bilirubin level and determine potential causes (Display 21–4). Any infant with jaundice presenting within the first 24 hours of life should have a bilirubin assessment (Burgos et al., 2011).

The AAP established new guidelines in 2004 for the management of hyperbilirubinemia in the newborn infant ≥35 weeks' gestation (AAP, 2004a). These guidelines stress the importance of universal systematic assessment while the newborn is hospitalized, close follow-up, and prompt intervention when indicated. The key elements of the recommendation suggest that the clinician should:

1. Promote and support successful breastfeeding.
2. Establish nursery protocols for the identification and evaluation of hyperbilirubinemia.
3. Measure the TSB or TcB level on infants jaundiced in the first 24 hours.
4. Recognize that visual estimation of the degree of jaundice can lead to errors, particularly in darkly pigmented infants.
5. Interpret all bilirubin levels according to the infant's age in hours.
6. Recognize that infants at less than 38 weeks' gestation, particularly those who are breastfed, are at higher risk of developing hyperbilirubinemia and require closer surveillance and monitoring.
7. Perform a systematic assessment on all infants before discharge for the risk of severe hyperbilirubinemia.
8. Provide parents with written and verbal information about newborn jaundice.
9. Provide appropriate follow-up based on the time of discharge and the risk assessment.
10. Treat newborns, when indicated, with phototherapy or exchange transfusion.

INTERVENTIONS

In supporting adequate breastfeeding, clinicians should instruct mothers to nurse their infants 8 to 10 times per day over the first several days (Thilo, 2005). This not only promotes adequate hydration and caloric intake but also decreases the likelihood of subsequent significant hyperbilirubinemia. Nurseries should have established protocols for the assessment of jaundice. Newborns should be assessed with vital signs but no less than every 8 to 12 hours. Assessment should be done in a well-lit room; however, it is important to remember that visual assessment of jaundice is unreliable and potentially unsafe (Piazza & Stoll, 2007). A low threshold should be used for assessing bilirubin. Noninvasive TcB devices have been proven to be very useful as screening tools. It has also been recommended that protocols allow nurses to access bilirubin testing, either TcB or TSB, without a physician's order.

DISPLAY 21–4

Laboratory Tests to Evaluate the Cause of Jaundice

Total and direct bilirubin
Blood type
Coombs test
Hematocrit
Peripheral smear for red blood cell morphology
Liver enzymes
Viral and/or bacterial cultures
pH
Serum albumin

Every newborn should be assessed for the risk of developing severe hyperbilirubinemia before discharge. As serum bilirubin rises >19 mg/dL, the risk of kernicterus increases incrementally (Smitherman, Stark, & Bhutani, 2006). In the Pilot Kernicterus Registry, the causes for kernicterus were attributed to the following three categories in equal proportions: hemolytic disorders (mostly ABO immunization), glucose-6-phosphate dehydrogenase (G6PD) deficiency (associated with hemolysis and impaired bilirubin conjugation), and idiopathic causes (presumably from delayed or impaired function of the glucuronyl transferase enzyme system), coupled with breastfeeding and inadequate nutritional intake (Bhutani, Johnson, & Shapiro, 2004). All nurseries should establish protocols for assessing this risk. This is particularly important if the infant is discharged before 72 hours of age. This risk can be assessed by predischarge measurement of bilirubin and/or assessment of clinical risk factors. Regardless of how risk is assessed, appropriate follow-up is essential. An hour-specific nomogram is a useful tool for determining the need for and appropriate timing of repeated TcB or TSB measurements. The assigned low-, intermediate-, or high-risk zone in which the individual bilirubin level falls (Fig. 21–1) will indicate the risk for developing clinically significant hyperbilirubinemia (Bhutani, Johnson, & Sivievri, 1999). Reassuring predischarge bilirubin levels do not eliminate the risk of developing significant hyperbilirubinemia, and careful follow-up of even "low risk" newborns is warranted (Bromiker, Bin-Nun, Schimmel, Hammerman, & Kaplan, 2012).

The risk factors most frequently associated with severe hyperbilirubinemia are predischarge TSB or TcB levels in the high-risk zone of the nomogram; jaundice within the first 24 hours of life, blood group incompatibility, or other known hemolytic disease with a positive direct antiglobulin test; gestational age of 35 to 36 weeks; previous sibling who received phototherapy; cephalhematoma or significant bruising; East Asian race; and exclusive breastfeeding, particularly if nursing is not going well and weight loss is excessive (AAP, 2004a; Burgos et al., 2011). Written and verbal information must be provided to parents at discharge. This should include an explanation of jaundice, the need to monitor infants for jaundice, and advice on how monitoring should be done. Newborn jaundice resource materials are available for parents in multiple languages (English, Spanish, Chinese, and Italian) and include a frequently asked question sheet from the AAP (2004b). All infants should be examined by a qualified healthcare professional in the first days after discharge, and those with jaundice should be evaluated within 24 hours (AAP, 2004a).

PHOTOTHERAPY

In the late 1940s, exchange transfusion was the only available treatment for newborns with hyperbilirubinemia. In the mid-1950s, an observant nurse noticed that newborns exposed to sunlight had less clinical jaundice over exposed areas and decreased serum bilirubin levels. This observation led to the use of phototherapy, which remains the primary treatment for hyperbilirubinemia. In nearly all newborns, phototherapy decreases or blunts the rise in serum-unconjugated bilirubin regardless of gestational age, race, or presence or absence of hemolysis. Phototherapy is used for treatment and prophylaxis of hyperbilirubinemia. No serious long-term side effects have been reported. Recommendations for treatment in infants born at ≥35 weeks' gestation are found in Figure 21–2. There is no consensus or recommendation regarding the discontinuation of phototherapy.

The goal of phototherapy is to decrease the level of unconjugated bilirubin. Phototherapy accomplishes this goal by means of the following:

- Absorption of light by bilirubin molecule
- Photoconversion of bilirubin by photochemical reaction, restructuring the molecule into an isomer
- Excretion of bilirubin through urine and bile, bypassing the conjugation process (Maisels & McDonagh, 2008; Schwartz et al., 2011).

Effectively used phototherapy can decrease bilirubin levels at a rate of 0.5 to 1.0 mg per hour (Kamath et al., 2011). For phototherapy to be effective, there must be illumination of an adequate area of exposed skin at a sufficiently short distance. Several types of phototherapy lamps are available: daylight, cool white fluorescent, fluorescent green, special blue fluorescent, quartz halogen, and high-intensity gallium nitride light-emitting diodes (AAP, 2004a). Phototherapy can also be delivered using a fiber-optic blanket (McFadden, 1991). Although any light source with irradiance between 400 and 500 nm can be used, the most effective light sources currently available are those that use special blue fluorescent tubes or a specially designed light-emitting diode light (AAP, 2004a). There is a direct relationship between the irradiance used and the rate of bilirubin decline with phototherapy. Irradiance should be monitored and is measured with a radiometer as $\mu W/cm^2/nm$. Standard phototherapy units deliver 8 to 10 $\mu W/cm^2/nm$ (AAP, 2004a). A fiber-optic blanket generally delivers irradiance of 15 to 20 $\mu W/cm^2/nm$ (McFadden, 1991). Intensive phototherapy requires >30 $\mu W/cm^2/nm$. Intensive phototherapy can be provided with special blue tubes placed 10 to 15 cm above the infant (AAP, 2004a). To expose the maximum surface area of the infant, overhead phototherapy can be used with a fiber-optic blanket. The newborn is placed naked under the phototherapy light and repositioned at least every 2 hours to ensure adequate light exposure to all areas. If a fiber-optic blanket is used, the blanket is wrapped around the newborn's trunk, and clothing is placed over the blanket.

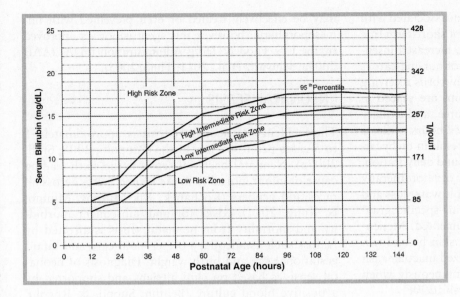

FIGURE 21–1. Nomogram for designation of risk of developing hyperbilirubinemia. (From Bhutani, V. K., Johnson, L. H., & Sivievri, E. M. [1999]. Predictive ability of a predischarge hour-specific serum bilirubin for subsequent significant hyperbilirubinemia in healthy term and near-term newborns. *Pediatrics, 103*[1], 6–14.)

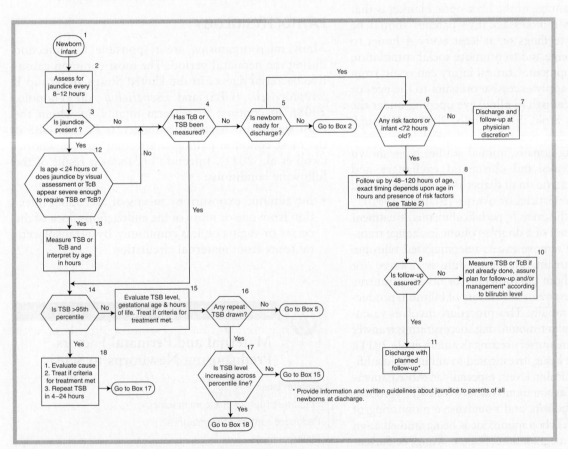

FIGURE 21–2. Algorithm for the management of jaundice in the newborn nursery. (From American Academy of Pediatrics Clinical Practice Guideline Subcommittee on Hyperbilirubinemia. [2004]. Management of hyperbilirubinemia in the newborn infant 35 or more weeks' gestation. *Pediatrics, 114*[1], 297–316.)

Although phototherapy has not been associated with any serious long-term effects, important short-term side effects include temperature instability, increased insensible fluid losses, and rash. The focus of nursing care is to prevent or minimize side effects. Newborns receiving phototherapy from phototherapy lamps are placed in a bassinet or under a radiant heat source, and axillary temperature is monitored at least every 2 hours to assess for hyperthermia. Hyperthermia can result in tachycardia and increased insensible water loss and dehydration. Loose stools are an unavoidable effect of phototherapy and can also result in increased insensible water loss and dehydration. Intake, output, and urine-specific gravity are measured accurately and documented. Meticulous skin care is necessary to prevent skin breakdown resulting from loose stools. A generalized macular rash frequently develops and resolves spontaneously when phototherapy is discontinued (Stokowski, 2006).

The newborn's eyes are covered at all times while under phototherapy lamps to prevent potential retinal damage. An advantage of the fiber-optic blanket is that eye protection is unnecessary. Eye patches should be removed during feedings or at least every 4 hours to observe for drainage and to promote social stimulation and visual development. Corneal injury can result from eye patches that apply excessive pressure to the eyes or which are loose enough to allow eye opening under the patch (Piazza & Stoll, 2007; Thilo, 2005). Although human studies have not confirmed irradiance effects on the developing gonads, animal studies have shown DNA strand breaks and chromatid exchanges and mutations. Diapers or small diaperlike devices are used as a shield for the testicles or ovaries (Maisels, 1990).

For infants with severe hyperbilirubinemia, treatment may also include use of a double-volume exchange transfusion to directly remove excess unconjugated bilirubin from the bloodstream. This procedure is reserved for severe cases in whom phototherapy or other treatments have proved ineffective or whose rate of bilirubin production is escalating rapidly. This procedure involves vascular access and vigilant monitoring, necessitating transfer to the intensive care nursery setting (Kamath et al., 2011).

Techniques are being investigated to aid in the identification of rising bilirubin levels, especially in those patients with hemolysis. Carbon monoxide is a known byproduct of bilirubin metabolism, and noninvasive monitoring of exhaled or serum carbon monoxide is being studied as an indicator of heme degradation (Cohen, Wong, & Stevenson, 2010; Juretschke, 2005). Another research focus is on replacing traditional treatment or augmenting therapy for those who do not respond to phototherapy. Metalloporphyrins, a family of compounds to which heme belongs, are known to interfere with heme degradation and bilirubin production. Two such compounds, tin-protoporphyrin and tin-mesoporphyrin, are potent inhibitors of heme oxygenase, an essential step in the degradation process. There is current evidence that hyperbilirubinemia may be effectively treated or even prevented with tin-mesoporphyrin; however, this agent is not yet approved by the U.S. Food & Drug Administration (FDA) (AAP, 2004a; Schwartz et al., 2011; Thilo, 2005).

NEONATAL SEPSIS

The incidence of neonatal sepsis is approximately 1 to 5 cases per 1,000 live births (Puopolo, 2008; Stoll, 2007a). Neonatal bacterial sepsis is the sixth leading cause of infant mortality in the United States across all races and genders (Kochanek, Xu, Murphy, Minino, & Kung, 2011). Risks for and subsequent morbidity and mortality from neonatal sepsis is affected by factors such as adequacy of perinatal care and infant gestational age and birth weight. Diagnosis of neonatal sepsis is based on clinical signs and supported by a positive blood culture (Bentlin, Suppo, & Rugolo, 2010). Display 21–5 identifies maternal and perinatal factors that may pose risks for neonatal sepsis.

PATHOPHYSIOLOGY

Many microorganisms are responsible for infection during the neonatal period. The most common causative bacterial agents in the United States are group B *Streptococcus* (GBS) and *Escherichia coli* (Puopolo, 2008). In contrast to preterm infants, in whom the most significant bacterial pathogen is *E. coli*, GBS is the most common pathogen affecting term newborns (Stoll et al., 2011). Infection occurs as a result of the following conditions:

- Intrauterine exposure by means of ascending infection from one or more of the endogenous flora of the cervix or vagina or, less commonly, by a transplacental route from maternal circulation

DISPLAY 21 – 5

Maternal and Perinatal Factors Predisposing Newborns to Sepsis

Preterm labor

Premature rupture of the membranes

Prolonged rupture of membranes

Maternal sepsis

Chorioamnionitis

Intraamniotic infection

Vaginal colonization with group B streptococci (GBS)

Perineal colonization with *Escherichia coli*

Prior birth of an infant with GBS

Chemical dependency or substance abuse

Urinary tract infection

Foul-smelling amniotic fluid

- Cutaneous transmission as the fetus passes through the birth canal
- Environmental contamination after the birth

Two presentations of infection, early versus late onset, are observed in neonates. Early-onset sepsis occurs within 7 days of life (Oh, 2013; Shane & Stoll, 2012). Frequently, inoculation occurred in utero. If symptoms are not present immediately after birth, most newborns become symptomatic within 12 hours with respiratory distress and nonspecific findings such as feeding intolerance, abdominal distension, apnea, or bradycardia (Ohlin, Bjorkqvist, Montgomery, & Schollin, 2010). Late onset sepsis may occur as early as 72 hours of age (Bentlin et al., 2010) but is more common after the first postnatal week. This presentation is likely due to exposure during the birth process or nosocomial transmission after birth from caregivers or invasive procedures and results in findings such as septicemia, pneumonia, and meningitis. Unrecognized sepsis may progress rapidly to hypotension and septic shock.

GBS is an important source of morbidity and mortality in the perinatal setting (Shane & Stoll, 2011). Of pregnant women, 20% to 30% are colonized with GBS; 50% of their infants will be colonized with GBS; and 1% to 2% will develop invasive disease (Oh, 2013; Puopolo, 2008). Most of these infections could be prevented by use of prophylactic antimicrobials in at-risk women. The CDC, AAP, the American College of Nurse Midwives, the American Academy of Family Physicians, the American Society for Microbiology, and ACOG endorse protocols to prevent early-onset infection (Verani, McGee, & Schrag, 2010). The 2010 recommendations state:

- All pregnant women should be screened at 35 to 37 weeks' gestation for vaginal and rectal colonization.
- Women with GBS bacteriuria during the current pregnancy should automatically receive chemoprophylaxis; no screening culture is needed. Bacteriuria is a marker for genital colonization.
- Women who have had a previous infant with invasive GBS disease should automatically receive intrapartum chemoprophylaxis; no screening culture is needed.
- At the onset of labor or rupture of membranes (ROM), chemoprophylaxis should be given to all women identified as GBS carriers.
- Chemoprophylaxis should be given at the onset of labor or ROM if the GBS status is unknown and there are risk factors and in women <37 weeks, with ROM ≥18 hours and/or temperature ≥38°C.

ASSESSMENT

As with all neonatal complications, early identification of newborns at risk and prompt recognition of developing signs decreases morbidity and increases the chances of survival. Recognizing multiple risk factors is the first step in identifying newborns whose early days may be complicated by infection. Risk factors can be categorized as maternal, neonatal, and environmental. A thorough review of antepartum and intrapartum history should specifically look for conditions that increase the risk of early-onset sepsis. If different nurses care for the mother and newborn, communication among healthcare team members is essential to ensure that maternal complications with potential impact on the newborn are not overlooked. The nurse caring for the mother during the postpartum period should notify the neonatal care provider if fever or other symptoms of infection develop.

The primary neonatal factors influencing development of sepsis are gestational age and birth weight. Gestational age and birth weight vary inversely with morbidity and mortality from sepsis. Preterm newborns may be exposed to the same organisms as term newborns, but their ability to fight infection is lessened. Other factors associated with increased risk of sepsis are resuscitation at birth and low Apgar scores. Congenital anomalies in which the skin or mucous membrane is not intact increase the risk of sepsis because a cutaneous port of entry is available for microorganisms. A history of a nonreassuring fetal HR pattern during labor, with or without meconium in the amniotic fluid, may identify fetuses at risk for infection. More male than female newborns develop sepsis, suggesting that the susceptibility may be sex linked (Stoll, 2007a). Maternal factors include premature rupture of membranes (PROM), chorioamnionitis, intrapartal fever, and GBS colonization (Puopolo, 2008; Shane & Stoll, 2012).

The most obvious environmental risk for developing sepsis is admission to a neonatal intensive care unit (NICU). Newborns in the NICU are compromised because of the original reason for admission along with being subjected to manipulation and invasive procedures that frequently puncture the skin, the first line of defense against infection. Environmental risks of nosocomial infection include use of equipment, indwelling catheters and chest tubes, inadequate hand washing or cleaning procedures, breaks in skin integrity, oxygen therapy, mechanical ventilation, surgical procedures, and possibly cohorting. Overcrowding in the nursery or inadequate attention to isolation precautions increases the risk of cross-contamination.

In addition to reviewing antepartum and intrapartum history, identifying the newborn with neonatal sepsis requires a thorough physical examination, evaluation of vital signs and laboratory data, and recognition of signs consistent with the diagnosis of sepsis. Like many conditions complicating the newborn period, the early signs of neonatal sepsis are vague and frequently nonspecific. Clinical indicators such as apnea, tachypnea, temperature instability, tachycardia, lethargy, and poor feeding may be early symptoms of sepsis.

A diagnostic evaluation includes a complete blood cell (CBC) count with a differential cell count, aerobic and anaerobic blood cultures, and supportive cultures such as tracheal aspirate, cerebrospinal fluid, or urine as clinically indicated. For best yield, cultures should be obtained before the initiation of antibiotic therapy from any newborn suspected of being septic. A positive blood culture remains the gold standard for the diagnosis of septicemia. Other studies may include evaluation of acute-phase reactants such as C-reactive protein (CRP). Acute-phase reactants increase in response to inflammation or tissue necrosis, which may indirectly support the diagnosis of infection (Shane & Stoll, 2012; Stoll, 2007a).

INTERVENTIONS

Many institutions have developed protocols for evaluations to exclude sepsis, including laboratory data and frequency of vital signs and clinical assessment. The CDC, AAP, and ACOG have also published certain

recommendations for the management of a neonate born to a mother who received intrapartum antimicrobial prophylaxis for GBS. If there are signs of sepsis, the newborn should receive a full diagnostic evaluation and antimicrobial therapy. If there are no signs of sepsis and the newborn is less than 35 weeks' gestation, a CBC and blood culture should be obtained and the newborn observed for 48 hours or longer. If the newborn is greater than or equal to 35 weeks' gestation and the mother received antibiotic prophylaxis less than 4 hours before delivery, a CBC and blood culture should also be obtained and the newborn observed for 48 hours or longer. If the mother received two or more doses of an antimicrobial agent, no evaluation or therapy is required, although the newborn must still be observed for 48 hours or longer. This approach would preclude an early discharge. Figure 21–3 is an algorithm for management of infants born to mothers who received intrapartum chemoprophylaxis for GBS infection.

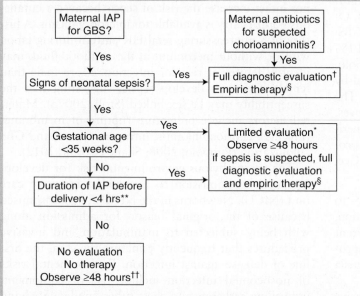

* If no maternal intrapartum prophylaxis for GBS was administered despite an indication being present, data are insufficient on which to recommend a single management strategy.

† Includes complete blood cell count and differential, blood culture, and chest radiograph if respiratory abnormalities are present. When signs of sepsis are present, a lumbar puncture, if feasible, should be performed.

§ Duration of therapy varies depending on results of blood culture, cerebrospinal fluid findings, if obtained, and the clinical course of the infant. If laboratory results and clinical course do not indicate bacterial infection, duration may be as short as 48 hours.

** Applies only to penicillin, ampicillin, or cefazolin and assumes recommended dosing regimens (Box 2).

†† A healthy-appearing infant who was ≥38 weeks' gestation at delivery and whose mother received ≥4 hours of intrapartum prophylaxis before delivery may be discharged home after 24 hours if other discharge criteria have been met and a person able to comply fully with instructions for home observation will be present. If any one of these conditions is not met, the infant should be observed in the hospital for at least 48 hours and until criteria for discharge are achieved.

FIGURE 21–3. Algorithm for infants of mothers who received antepartum antimicrobial agents for prevention of group B *Streptococcus* or suspected chorioamnionitis. GBS, group B *Streptococcus*; IAP, intrapartum antibiotic prophylaxis. (From Verani, J. R., McGee, L., & Schrag, S. [2010]. Prevention of perinatal group B streptococcal disease—Revised guidelines from CDC, 2010. *Morbidity & Mortality Weekly Report, 55*[RR-10], 1–36.)

After the diagnostic evaluation has been completed, antimicrobial agents are initiated. For early-onset sepsis, ampicillin, a broad-spectrum antimicrobial that is bactericidal for gram-positive and gram-negative bacteria, is used in combination with an aminoglycoside such as gentamicin. The usual dosage of ampicillin is 50 to 100 mg/kg every 8 to 12 hours for 7 to 10 days. When sepsis is complicated by meningitis, the dosage is increased and the duration of treatment is extended to 14 days. The choice of antibiotics is ultimately determined by the particular sensitivity of a recovered organism. If, however, after 48 to 72 hours, cultures are negative and the infant is clinically stable, antimicrobials may be discontinued (Stoll, 2007a).

PERINATAL HUMAN IMMUNODEFICIENCY VIRUS (HIV) INFECTION

Despite great strides in the prevention of perinatal and early childhood transmission of HIV infection, it remains an important source of mortality worldwide. Accounting for both developed and developing countries, it is estimated that 1,800 children will become infected with HIV daily, primarily from maternal-to-child transmission. In developed countries, however, the rate of maternal–child transmission has fallen from 15% to 30% to as low as 2%, attributable to the use of preventive strategies, including antiretroviral therapy (Committee on Obstetric Practice, 2008; Davis & Yawetz, 2012; Thorne & Newell, 2007).

ACOG and the CDC recommend offering all women of childbearing age the opportunity for preconception counseling and care as a component to routine medical care (ACOG, 2005; CDC, 2006a). ACOG, AAP, and the Canadian Paediatric Society recommend HIV testing and counseling, with consent, for all pregnant women in North America and advocate preconception counseling as part of a comprehensive healthcare program for all women (ACOG, 2005; CDC, 2006b; Davis & Yawetz, 2012; King, 2004; Public Health Service Task Force, 2006). HIV testing must be voluntary and free from coercion. No woman should be tested without her knowledge, and each woman has the option to decline or opt out of the HIV screening (CDC, 2006b). Early identification of the HIV-infected pregnant woman is essential for her health and that of her exposed infant (Panel on Antiretroviral Therapy and Medical Management of HIV-Infected Children, 2010). It has been demonstrated that rates of perinatal HIV transmission can be reduced significantly with prenatal testing and antiviral treatment (Davis & Yawetz, 2012).

Many women with HIV infection enter pregnancy with a known diagnosis and are already receiving antiretroviral therapy, although adjustment to their regimen may be necessary (Davis & Yawetz, 2012; Public Health Service Task Force, 2006). Decisions regarding therapy should be the same for pregnant and nonpregnant women with HIV infection, with the additional consideration of the potential impact of therapy on the fetus and infant. Discussions regarding the treatment of HIV should not be coercive, and the woman is ultimately responsible for the final decision. Staging of HIV infection and establishment of an appropriate management plan is essential to optimize both maternal and neonatal care. Assessment should include evaluation of prior HIV-related infections and need for prophylaxis against opportunistic infections. Prior antiretroviral therapy and past CD4-cell counts and plasma HIV viral load, as well as current antiretroviral agents, CD4-cell counts, and plasma HIV RNA copy numbers, will provide necessary data to craft a management plan (Panel on Antiretroviral Therapy and Medical Management of HIV-Infected Children, 2012).

Healthcare providers who treat HIV-infected pregnant women and their newborns are strongly advised to report all instances of prenatal exposure to antiretroviral drugs to the Antiretroviral Pregnancy Registry. This is an observational epidemiologic project assessing the potential teratogenicity of these drugs (Public Health Service Task Force, 2006).

Antiretroviral Pregnancy Registry
Research Park
1011 Ashes Dr.
Wilmington, NC 28405
1-800-258-4263
1-800-800-1052 (fax)
http://www.APRegistry.com

CHEMOPROPHYLAXIS FOR PERINATAL HIV TRANSMISSION

The patient who presents in labor without documented HIV status should receive rapid HIV antibody testing; and those with positive antibody results as well as those with pending HIV RNA copy number or CD4-cell count assessments should commence antiretroviral prophylaxis promptly. Repeat testing is recommended in the third trimester for the pregnant woman with a previous negative HIV antibody test if she remains in a high-risk category (e.g., engages in risky behavior or lives in a high prevalence area). For the patient in whom acute infection is suspected, virologic testing (e.g., plasma HIV RNA assay) should be obtained because serologic testing may be negative at early stages of infection (Davis & Yawetz, 2012; Panel on Antiretroviral Therapy and Medical Management of HIV-Infected Children, 2010, 2012).

Although intrapartum antiretroviral therapy will not prevent perinatal transmission that occurs before labor, most transmission occurs near or during labor and delivery. Therefore, preexposure prophylaxis is recommended to give antiretroviral drug levels in the fetus during the intensive exposure to HIV-1 in maternal genital secretions and blood during birth (Public Health Service Task Force, 2006).

MODE OF DELIVERY

Optimal medical management should focus on minimizing the risk of both perinatal transmission of HIV-1 and the potential for maternal and neonatal complications (Public Health Service Task Force, 2006). Use of instruments such as forceps or vacuum devices poses risks for HIV transmission and should be discouraged when possible. Previous data suggested that elective cesarean delivery at 38 weeks decreased perinatal transmission; however, as combination therapy has become more widely used, the added benefit of cesarean delivery became less clear. Current guidelines do not support routine cesarean delivery to prevent perinatal HIV transmission but rather recommend counseling patients regarding the potential benefits in cases where the HIV RNA is >1,000 copies/ml" (Davis & Yawetz, 2012).

CARE OF THE NEWBORN

HIV-exposed infants should be identified early. Viral diagnostic testing is recommended at birth for infants at high risk for HIV infection, including those born to HIV-positive mothers without prenatal care, those without prenatal antiretroviral prophylaxis, and those with an HIV viral load ≥1,000 copies per milliliter near the time of delivery. Repeated viral testing should occur at 14 to 21 days, 1 to 2 months, and 4 to 6 months postnatally (Panel on Antiretroviral Therapy and Medical Management of HIV-Infected Children, 2010).

Immediate care of the newborn should limit exposure to maternal fluids. A bath should be given once the infant's temperature is stable. Infants born to HIV-infected mothers should have an HIV DNA polymerase chain reaction (PCR) and CBC with manual differential as part of their admission labs (King, 2004; Public Health Service Task Force, 2006). Breastfeeding is a known risk for HIV transmission and is not recommended when suitable alternatives such as infant formula are available (Davis & Yawetz, 2012; King, 2004; Public Health Task Force, 2006).

Antiretroviral therapy has been shown to decrease seroconversion, and current recommendations support initiating treatment in newborns as close as possible to birth, but less than 12 hours of age. Once initiated, chemoprophylaxis should continue for 6 weeks. Zidovudine is currently recommended in infants, with a dose adjusted for gestational age. The dose for term newborns is 2 mg/kg twice daily, which can be given orally (Davis & Yawetz, 2012: Public Health Task Force, 2006).

Anemia is the primary complication of the 6-week course of zidovudine in the neonate. Therefore, at a minimum, a hemoglobin level should be obtained at the initiation and completion of the treatment course (Davis & Yawetz, 2012). Infants with negative virologic test results during the first 6 weeks of life should have a repeat HIV DNA PCR after completion of antiretroviral treatment. Routine infant immunizations should be administered to HIV-exposed infants utilizing specific *Red Book* guidelines when HIV infection is confirmed (King, 2004). To prevent *Pneumocystis carinii* pneumonia, all infants born to HIV-infected mothers should begin prophylaxis after completion of the ZDV prophylaxis regimen (Public Health Service Task Force, 2006).

NEONATAL SUBSTANCE EXPOSURE

Any drug that enters the mother's system has the potential for an effect on the fetus, and certain drugs (specifically opiates) may result in low birth weight or create effects such as neonatal intoxication or withdrawal. The incidence of neonatal abstinence syndrome (NAS) has been reported to be a range of 3% to 50%, depending on the population, community setting, and individual hospital sampling practices. Even though studies show that drug use among women of childbearing age is declining, a recent survey found that 5.5% of women use illicit drugs during pregnancy (Rosen & Bateman, 2002). Commonly abused drugs include alcohol, marijuana, cocaine and crack, heroin, amphetamine and methamphetamine, inhalants, and the "club drugs" (Rosen & Bateman, 2002). Drugs associated with NAS can be divided into four groups: CNS depressants, opioids, CNS stimulants, and hallucinogens.

PATHOPHYSIOLOGY

Maternal drug use in pregnancy has been associated with higher rates of fetal distress and demise, lower Apgar scores, growth retardation, adverse neurodevelopmental outcomes that may not manifest until later in infancy, and acute withdrawal during the neonatal period (Rosen & Bateman, 2002). It is difficult to know whether substance abuse alone or (more likely) the multifactorial influence of drug abuse and social problems is responsible. Many pregnant women who use illicit drugs also use tobacco and alcohol, which also pose risks to unborn babies, making it difficult to determine which health problems are caused by a specific substance. Drug abuse in pregnancy is frequently associated with poverty and family disruption, increasing the risk that women will place less value on seeking early and consistent prenatal care. The general health of these women may be poor, predisposing them to suboptimal weight gain and anemia.

Although addressed less extensively in substance abuse literature, there can be effects on the fetus and infant from tobacco exposure during pregnancy. Of pregnant women, 13% to 20% admit to smoking during pregnancy, which poses risks to the parturient as well. Some evidence suggests that tobacco exposure increases rates of placental pathology, ectopic pregnancy, and spontaneous abortion. Infants of smokers have smaller birth weights, are at risk for complications such as sudden infant death syndrome (SIDS), and may be at heightened risk for preterm birth or neurobehavioral effects due (at least partially) to the effects of multiple metabolites in tobacco smoke (Law et al., 2003; Rogers, 2008). It has been suggested that smoking cessation among childbearing women would reduce stillbirths more than 10% and newborn death by approximately 5% (Rogers, 2008).

Complete information on transmission of illicit drugs to the fetus is unavailable, but most appear to pass easily through the placenta. Based on animal studies, it is known that rates of transmission and metabolism vary from drug to drug and depend on fetal age. Increased maternal blood flow in later gestation appears to increase transport of substances to the fetus. The vasoconstricting effects of these substances cause abruptio placentae, elevated blood pressure, precipitous labor, inadequate contraction patterns, decreased fetal oxygenation, and decreased length and head circumference. Use of cocaine and heroin, amphetamine, and marijuana is associated with intrauterine growth restriction. Some studies have shown a higher incidence of genitourinary abnormalities in infants of cocaine-using mothers. Cocaine is also thought to increase fetal vasoconstricting hormones, leading to increased blood pressure and an elevated HR. These physiologic responses increase risk of cerebral ischemia and hemorrhagic lesions (Rosen & Bateman, 2002).

ASSESSMENT

NAS describes a range of symptoms the newborn experiences during withdrawal from exposure to a dependency-producing substance (Kuschel, 2007). It is often a multisystem disorder that frequently involves the central nervous and gastrointestinal (GI) systems. Although the most severe withdrawal symptoms are seen in the newborn exposed to opioids, symptoms can also occur after exposure to other drugs. Depending on the chemical agent the mother used, after several weeks or months, symptoms no longer represent withdrawal but rather the long-term effects of intrauterine drug exposure.

Clinical signs of opioid withdrawal usually begin 24 to 48 hours after birth, but they may not appear for as long as 10 days. Symptoms generally last for less than 2 weeks, but some infants show mild signs for up to 6 months (Fike, 2003). The severity of the abstinence syndrome is affected by the drug or combination of drugs used, although it may not correlate predictably with dose or duration of substance exposure (Burgos & Burke, 2009). Withdrawal symptoms are more severe when the drug exposure is closer to the time of birth. Methadone withdrawal is more severe than any other narcotic (Rosen & Bateman, 2002). Approximately 75% of newborns with prenatal exposure to methadone develop withdrawal symptoms. Time of onset is variable and is affected by last prenatal dose, gestational age, and mode of delivery (Liu, Jones, Murray, Cook, & Nanan, 2010). The newborn may have early withdrawal beginning at 24 to 48 hours or may have one or two types of late withdrawal, in which symptoms may appear shortly after birth, improve, and then reappear in 2 to 4 weeks, or there may be no symptoms until 2 to 3 weeks of age. Opioid withdrawal affects multiple systems including CNS (e.g., tremors, hypertonia, hyperreflexia, restlessness, irritability, high-pitched cry), GI (diarrhea, vomiting, poor feeding, or swallow), or autonomic nervous system (sweating, fever, nasal stuffiness, yawning, or mottling) (Burgos & Burke, 2009).

Heroin withdrawal begins within the first 2 weeks after birth, with an average onset at 72 hours. The incidence of withdrawal has been associated with maternal dosage of heroin, duration of maternal addiction, and time of the last maternal dose (Rosen & Bateman, 2002). Neonates who are exposed to barbiturates present with symptoms similar to opioids, although the onset is delayed until day 4 to 7 of life, and may persist up to 4 months of age (Burgos & Burke, 2009).

There is no clearly defined abstinence syndrome associated with in utero cocaine exposure (Fike, 2003); however, because it easily crosses the placenta, it may contribute to some neonatal behaviors. A significant perinatal effect of cocaine exposure is related to its potent vasoconstrictive activity, which may result in impaired placental blood flow to the fetus. This has been associated with findings such as growth restriction or asphyxia, which may be further complicated by polydrug exposure (Burgos & Burke, 2009). Several neurobehavioral abnormalities frequently occur after intrauterine cocaine exposure, including hypertonia, irritability, tremulousness, tachypnea, state disorganization, loose stools, and poor feeding. These findings usually occur on day 2 or 3 and are more consistent with the stimulant effect itself rather than withdrawal. Other stimulants such as methamphetamines less commonly create NAS, and fewer than 6% of exposed infants will require pharmacologic management for symptoms (Burgos & Burke, 2009).

Alcohol exposure in utero can be associated with a range of complications including growth restriction, birth defects, mental retardation, and lifelong behavioral problems. Fetal alcohol syndrome (FAS) and alcohol-related neurobehavioral disorders (ARND) refer to clustered findings attributed to in utero alcohol exposure and together affect approximately 0.9 per 100 live births (Langendoerfer, Johnson, & Thureen, 2005). Recently, an alcohol withdrawal syndrome has been described with onset at less than 12 hours after delivery, and findings include irritability, restlessness, inconsolability, and poor feeding (Burgos & Burke, 2009).

Preterm newborns may exhibit less severe or later onset effects from intrauterine substance exposure, either due to decreased risks from shorter term in utero exposure or their CNS immaturity and consequent decreased ability to manifest clinical signs (Kuschel, 2007). It is difficult to accurately assess the severity of abstinence in preterm newborns because the tools available were originally developed for use with term newborns. Many of the characteristics seen in neonatal drug withdrawal are common in preterm newborns, such as tremors, high-pitched cry, tachypnea, and poor feeding.

INTERVENTIONS

Appropriate care of drug-exposed newborns begins with early identification and recognition of maternal drug abuse. Careful prenatal and postnatal maternal screening for substance abuse is essential. All women, regardless of racial or social background and perceived risk status, should be asked directly in a nonjudgmental manner about drug and alcohol use during pregnancy. Illicit drug use should be considered as potentially complicating all pregnancies. The level of suspicion should increase when the pregnant woman:

- Has received little or no prenatal care
- Has a history of sexually transmitted diseases
- Insists on leaving the hospital shortly after birth
- Demonstrates signs of drug use such as needle marks and malnutrition
- Demands medication frequently and in large doses

Laws regulating toxicology screens without maternal consent vary regionally, and the perinatal nurse should be aware of local regulations. When indicated, a maternal urine toxicology screen can be included as part of laboratory tests routinely ordered during the hospital admission process. If results are positive or not obtained, a urine toxicology screen or meconium assay is performed with a sample collected from the newborn's first void or stool (Rosen & Bateman, 2002). The potential yield from newborn screening is affected by a limited diagnostic window following

exposure (Kuschel, 2007); thus, all newborns should be observed for signs of NAS.

Many withdrawal symptoms can be successfully treated with basic supportive care. These interventions increase the newborn's ability to regulate behavioral state, improve neuromotor control, and promote maternal newborn attachment. Minimal handling, swaddling, and a variety of positioning interventions have been used in an attempt to console and quiet the irritable, narcotic-withdrawn newborn. They can easily become overstimulated during the acute period of withdrawal (Fike, 2003). Using a neonatal abstinence scoring system (NASS), narcotic-withdrawn newborns placed in a prone position demonstrated lower scores than narcotic-withdrawn newborns placed in other positions (Fike, 2003). Display 21–6 depicts nonpharmacologic interventions to support the newborn experiencing withdrawal.

Newborns who do not respond to symptomatic treatment alone may need medication. Ideally, the decision to begin medication is based on an objective assessment of symptoms such as the NASS (Fig. 21–4). The newborn is assessed and scored every 2 hours for the first 48 hours and then every 8 hours while symptoms of withdrawal persist. Points are given for all behaviors or symptoms observed during the scoring interval. The newborn must be awake and calm to assess muscle tone, respirations, and Moro reflex. Observations should be made after feeding whenever possible because hunger can mimic withdrawal. Temperatures recorded on the scoring sheet should be obtained rectally, although an axillary temperature 2°F cooler may also indicate withdrawal. If the average of any three successive scores exceeds 8 points and is not reduced by nursing interventions, medications are initiated (Weiner & Finnegan, 1998). A simplified scoring system, the Neonatal Withdrawal Inventory (NWI), has been developed based on the NASS (Zahorodny et al., 1998).

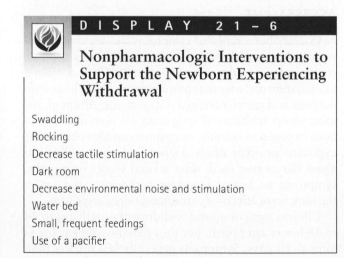

DISPLAY 21–6

Nonpharmacologic Interventions to Support the Newborn Experiencing Withdrawal

Swaddling

Rocking

Decrease tactile stimulation

Dark room

Decrease environmental noise and stimulation

Water bed

Small, frequent feedings

Use of a pacifier

CENTRAL NERVOUS SYSTEM DISTURBANCES													
SIGNS AND SYMPTOMS	SCORE	AM						PM					
Excessive High-Pitched Cry	2												
Continuous High-Pitched Cry	3												
Sleeps <1 Hour After Feeding	3												
Sleeps <2 Hours After Feeding	2												
Sleeps <3 Hours After Feeding	1												
Hyperactive Moro Reflex	2												
Markedly Hyperactive Moro Reflex	3												
Mild Tremors Disturbed	1												
Moderate–Severe Tremors Disturbed	2												
Mild Tremors Undisturbed	1												
Moderate–Severe Tremors Undisturbed	4												
Increased Muscle Tone	2												
Excoriation (Specify Area):	1												
Myoclonic Jerks	3												
Generalized Convulsions	5												
METABOLIC/VASOMOTOR /RESPIRATORY DISTURBANCES													
Sweating													
Fever <101(99–100.8°F/37.2–38.2°C)	1												
Fever >101(38.2°C and Higher)	2												
Frequent Yawning (>3–4 times/interval)	1												
Mottling	1												
Nasal Stuffiness	1												
Sneezing (>3–4 times/interval)	1												
Nasal Flaring	2												
Respiratory Rate >60/Min.	1												
Respiratory Rate >60/Min. with Retractions	2												
GASTROINTESTINAL DISTURBANCES													
Excessive Sucking	1												
Poor Feeding	2												
Regurgitation	2												
Projectile Vomiting	3												
Loose Stools	2												
Watery Stools	3												
TOTAL SCORE													

FIGURE 21–4. Neonatal abstinence scoring system. (From Cloherty, J. P., & Stark, A. R. [1998]. *Manual of Neonatal Care* [4th ed., pp. 26—27]. Boston: Little, Brown.)

A variety of medications are used to treat NAS, and the choice of medication varies with individual nurseries. In a recent Cochrane review, opiates (used with caution) are the preferred initial therapy for NAS, especially for infants of mothers who used opioids during pregnancy (Osborn, Cole, & Jeffery, 2005), and the AAP recommends diluted tincture of opium (Kuschel, 2007). Naloxone use is contraindicated in infants born to narcotic-addicted mothers due to the risk of seizures and/or the precipitation of severe signs and symptoms of withdrawal (Rosen & Bateman, 2002). Sedation is the most common potential complication related to treatment. Tapering and discontinuation of medications are best achieved using the NASS. After medication has been initiated, the newborn should be scored every 8 hours and reevaluated on a daily basis. If all scores are 8 or less, or the mean of any three successive scores is 7 or less, the dose should be maintained for 72 hours. If, after 72 hours, the scores are consistently 8 or less, or the mean of three successive scores is 7 or less, the dose should be decreased by 10%. This dose is maintained for 24 hours. If the mean score remains less than 8, the dose is decreased by 10% every 24 hours. After the medication has been discontinued, scoring continues until scores are 8 or less for 72 hours.

As symptoms of neonatal abstinence may not be completely resolved at the time of discharge, the parents need education to successfully care for the newborn. Parents should spend extended periods observing and interacting with their newborn in the presence of the nurse. These opportunities can be used by the nurse to observe parental interaction. Because drug-exposed newborns are discharged into an environment where drug use may still be a factor, families are followed after discharge to ensure that growth and development is adequate and that parents are aware of and receive available community resources. Breastfeeding is not contraindicated, unless there is evidence of ongoing use of agents such as heroin, cocaine, or amphetamines; methadone use is not a contraindication (Kuschel, 2007).

A component of perinatal substance exposure care is prevention, and evidence suggests that counseling should be directed early at all types of substances that can affect the health of mother and infant, both legalized and illicit. It has been shown that cessation interventions initiated during pregnancy can have a positive effect on both fetus and mother, but they must be sustained for optimal effect (Bailey, McCook, Hodge, & McGrady, 2011)

LATE PRETERM INFANTS

Prematurity is the major determinant of neonatal mortality and morbidity. In 2008, 12.3% of the births in the United States were premature (<37 completed weeks of gestation), representing a 3% decline from 2007 (12.7%) and a 4% decline from 2006 (12.8%). Despite the recent rate of decline, the premature rate has steadily increased by nearly 30% for more than two decades (Martin et al., 2010). This dramatic rise in prematurity has largely been due to the increase in the deliveries between 34 and 36 completed weeks of gestation. Nearly three fourths, or 8.8% of the total U.S. births in 2008, are between 34 and 36 completed weeks of gestation (Martin et al., 2010). There has been a shift from higher to lower gestational ages, leading to the most frequent length of gestation in the United States to shift from 40 to 39 weeks (Davidoff et al., 2006; Martin et al., 2010). These NTIs are often referred to as late preterm infants, the latter referring to the vulnerability of this unique population. This population of infants is often treated like full-term newborns. However, they have the same risk of complications as infants born prematurely. The magnitude of their morbidities and their impact on public health has not been well studied. Professional organizations including the Association of Women's Health, Obstetric and Neonatal Nurses (AWHONN), the National Institutes of Child Health and Human Development (NICHD) of the National Institutes of Health, and the AAP have led the way in defining and educating healthcare providers and the public on the distinct needs of the late preterm infant. In 2005, the NICHD convened a multidisciplinary task force, which summarized the current state of knowledge on late preterm births and published a special, two-part supplement summarizing the findings from the meetings in Seminars in Perinatology (NICHD Workshop, 2005; Raju, Higgins, Stark, & Leveno, 2006). This multidisciplinary team of experts discussed the definition and terminology, epidemiology, etiology, biology of maturation, clinical care, surveillance, and public health aspects of late preterm infants. Knowledge gaps were identified and research priorities listed. The NICHD panel recommended that births between 34 completed weeks (34 0/7 weeks or day 239) and less than 37 completed weeks (36 6/7 weeks or day 259) of gestation be referred to as late preterm (Raju et al., 2006). Also, in 2005, AWHONN (Medoff-Cooper, Bakewell-Sachs, Buus-Frank, & Santa-Donato, 2005) launched a multiyear initiative to address the unique physiologic and developmental needs of the late preterm infant that resulted in the development of a conceptual framework for optimizing the health of late preterm infant. In 2010, AWHONN released an evidence-based clinical practice guideline (EBG) to provide nurses and other healthcare professionals with state-of-the-science recommendations to accurately assess and manage this high-risk population. Additionally, in a clinical report defining and describing late preterm infants and their unique characteristics, the AAP has published guidelines for care of these at-risk infants (Engle, Tomashek, & Wallman, 2007).

OBSTETRIC AND NEONATAL ISSUES

Obstetricians face many challenges when managing a woman in preterm labor (Mi Lee, Cleary-Goldman, & D'Alton, 2006; Sibai, 2006; Hankins & Longo, 2006). Continuous assessment of anticipated risks for both the mother and the fetus is crucial. Although a baby born prematurely increases neonatal morbidity and mortality, a fetus left in a suboptimal intrauterine environment can lead to fetal demise. There are specific medical indications for delivering prior to 39 weeks' gestation (placental abruption, placenta previa, bleeding, infection, hypertension, preeclampsia, idiopathic preterm labor, preterm premature rupture of membranes [PPROM], intrauterine growth restriction, and multiple gestation); however, up to 15% of all births in the United States are currently performed electively (without identifiable medical or obstetric indication) (Clark et al., 2009; Clark et al., 2010; Clark, Knox, Simpson & Hankins, 2010). Early elective induction of labor and elective primary and repeat cesarean delivery resulting in late preterm births has contributed to the overall neonatal morbidity (Clark et al., 2009; Tita et al., 2009). ACOG (2009) have cautioned against elective delivery prior to 39 weeks' gestation. Nursing and medical leadership need to adopt strategies to reduce elective deliveries prior to 39 completed weeks. Specific evidence-based strategies and resources are available for clinicians to use in discouraging elective births prior to 39 completed weeks with the goal of improving both perinatal and infant mortality (March of Dimes Foundation, 2010a, 2010b).

PATHOPHYSIOLOGY

Late preterm infants are often referred to as great imposters because their initial size and presentation closely resemble the term newborn (Buus-Frank, 2005). Many times within hours of birth, the late preterm infant will appear to be functionally at term, allowing for management decisions to be made accordingly. Despite the fact that these infants are biologically and functionally premature by 3 to 8 weeks, they are often transferred to the regular nursery.

The third trimester is a critical period of rapid growth, development, and biologic maturation. The last few weeks of gestation are vital for fetal development and maturation including surfactant production, control and regulation of breathing, and brain maturation resulting in the infant's ability to coordinate sucking, swallowing, and breathing. Also, during the last trimester, dramatic growth ensues with an increase in body mass and fat stores, which enhance thermal and glucose regulation.

Late preterm infants, compared to term, have a higher frequency of respiratory distress, temperature instability, hypoglycemia, hyperbilirubinemia, kernicterus, apnea, seizures, feeding difficulties, symptoms prompting a sepsis evaluation, need for IV infusions, and higher rates of rehospitalization and a potential increase risk for long-term behavior and learning problems (Engle et al., 2007; Raju et al., 2006; Wang, Dorer, Fleming, & Catlin, 2004). Compared to term infants, late preterm infants have not only significantly more medical problems but also increased hospital costs (Bird et al., 2010; McLaurin, Hall, Jackson, Owens, & Mahadevia, 2009; Wang et al., 2004).

Hypothermia and Hypoglycemia

Late preterm infants are at risk for hypothermia and early hypoglycemia. Of the fetal energy consumption, 80% is provided by glucose. The fetus is solely dependent on maternal glucose that is supplied transplacentally by a process of facilitative diffusion (Garg & Devaskar, 2006). Once the cord is clamped, newborns are required to swiftly adapt to a life of independence and learn to produce endogenous glucose. The risk of hypoglycemia increases for late preterm infants because metabolic reserves are low, and further energy demands increase because of coexisting conditions of sepsis, birth asphyxia, or cold stress (Laptook & Jackson, 2006). Late preterm infants have less brown fat compared to term newborns, resulting in a higher risk of developing hypothermia. Cold stress and hypoglycemia are very common in late preterm infants, especially soon after birth during the early transitional period of adaptation (Engle et al., 2007; Laptook & Jackson, 2006; Vachharajani & Dawson, 2009).

Hyperbilirubinemia

Late preterm infants are more prone to developing hyperbilirubinemia and its sequelae and to require hospital readmission for treatment (Engle et al., 2007; Wang et al., 2004). These vulnerable infants are 2.4 times more likely to develop significant hyperbilirubinemia and to have significantly higher TSB levels. Elevated bilirubin levels are primarily due to immature liver function and diminished capacity for bilirubin conjugation. These physiologic risks, coupled with more difficult feeding patterns and lower oral intake, exacerbate increased enterohepatic recirculation of bilirubin and may explain the correlation among decreased postmenstrual age, hyperbilirubinemia, and the increased risk for kernicterus (Sarici et al., 2004). Although the incidence of kernicterus in late preterms is unknown, compared to term infants, these infants are at increased risk for bilirubin neurotoxicity and kernicterus (Bhutani et al., 2004; Sarici et al., 2004).

Respiratory Distress

Studies have shown the high incidence of respiratory distress and NICU admissions in late preterm infants (Clark, 2005; Consortium on Safe Labor, 2010; Escobar et al., 2005; Roth-Kleiner, Wagner, Bachmann, & Pfenninger, 2003). These infants have a higher incidence of TTNB, pneumonia, RDS, PPHN, and hypoxic respiratory failure than term infants (Consortium on Safe Labor, 2010). Nearly 50% of infants born at 34 weeks' gestation require intensive care; this number drops to 15% at 35 weeks' and 8% at 36 weeks' gestation (Dudell & Jain, 2006). The last few weeks of gestation are critical for fetal development and maturation specifically related to surfactant and lung maturity. Biochemical and hormonal changes that accompany spontaneous labor and vaginal delivery also play an important role in the newborn's ability to transition smoothly to an extrauterine environment (Dudell & Jain, 2006). For effective gas exchange to occur, alveolar spaces must be cleared of excess fluid and ventilated, and pulmonary blood flow must be increased to match ventilation with perfusion. Failure of either of these events may jeopardize neonatal transition and cause respiratory distress. A significant number of late preterm infants are delivered by cesarean section, and this number continues to rise steadily, reported at an all-time high in the United States at 32.3% in 2008 (Martin et al., 2010). A higher occurrence of respiratory morbidity in late preterm and term infants delivered by cesarean section has been observed (Jain & Dudell, 2006; Hansen, Wisborg, Uldbjerg, & Henriksen, 2007; Levine et al., 2001). These infants are known to develop PPHN and become seriously ill and require significant clinical interventions such as i-NO, HFOV, vasopressor support, and ultimately may progress to ECMO (Ramachandrappa & Jain, 2008). The inability to clear lung fluid, the relative deficiency of pulmonary surfactant, and birth in the absence of labor all contribute to pulmonary dysfunction (Jain & Eaton, 2006; Ramachandrappa & Jain, 2008).

Apnea of Prematurity

Late preterm infants are three times more likely to experience apnea than their term counterparts (Engle et al., 2007). Between 32 and 34 weeks of gestation, the fetus develops synchrony and control of breathing. This period of breathing pattern maturation decreases the risk of apnea of prematurity. The pathogenesis of apnea is multifactorial and includes immature lung volume and upper airway control, ventilatory responses to hypoxia and carbon dioxide, and feeding as well as physiologic and iatrogenic anemia (Darnall, Ariagno, & Kinney, 2006). It is important to remember that infants born between 33 and

38 weeks' gestation continue to have apnea and are at risk for the resulting periods of bradycardia and hypoxia and are at higher risk for SIDS (Hunt, 2006; Ramanathan et al., 2001).

Brain and Long-term Outcomes

Compared to term newborns, late preterm infants have a more immature brain. It is estimated that an infant at 35 weeks' gestation has fewer sulci and that the weight of the brain is approximately 65% that of the term infant. Periventricular leukomalacia is a known predictor of adverse neurologic outcomes in preterm infants. Late preterm infants are at risk for developing periventricular leukomalacia; however, the exact incidence is unknown (Kinney, 2006). Brainstem development of infants born between 33 and 38 weeks' gestation is less mature than that of a term newborn, although more research on this specific population of infants is needed (Darnall et al., 2006). There is a paucity of data on the long-term neurodevelopmental outcome in late preterm infants. Few studies have examined the long-term neurodevelopmental status of late preterm infants and the prevalence rates for subtle neurologic abnormalities, learning and behavioral difficulties, and scholastic achievement (Raju et al., 2006). However, there is a growing concern that these infants are more vulnerable to brain injury and long-term neurologic sequelae (Adams-Chapman, 2006; Morse, Zheng, Tang, & Roth, 2009; Petrini et al., 2009; Chyi, Lee, Hintz, Gould, & Sutcliffe, 2008) and are at more than a threefold increased risk for developing cerebral palsy compared to term newborns (Wang et al., 2004). In contrast to these studies, no significant differences in neurologic outcomes were found in school-aged children (between the ages of 4 and 15 years) who were born late preterm compared to children born at term (Gurka, LoCasale-Crouch, & Blackman, 2010).

Gastrointestinal Tract

The GI tract continues to develop throughout gestation, but the late preterm infant adapts quickly to enteral feedings, including the digestion and absorption of lactose, protein, and fats (Neu, 2006). However, peristaltic functions and sphincter controls in the esophagus, stomach, and intestines are less likely to be mature and fully functional in late preterm infants, which may lead to difficulty in coordinating suck and swallowing, gastroesophageal reflux, a delay in successful breastfeeding, poor weight gain, and dehydration during early postnatal weeks (Escobar et al., 2002; Neu, 2006; Tomashek et al., 2006).

The physiologic organization of sucking is almost fully organized by 36 weeks' gestation, whereas swallow rhythm is established by 32 weeks' gestation

(Gewolb, Vice, Schweiter-Kenney, Taciak, & Bosma, 2001). Precise timing for the activation of several upper airway muscles is critical for suck–swallow coordination, but unlike sucking, swallowing interrupts breathing, allowing protection of the airway and decreasing the risk for aspiration (Thach, 2005). It is likely that the etiology of the frequent feeding issues encountered by late preterm infants stems from the immaturity of the coordination of sucking, swallowing, and breathing (Darnall et al., 2006). It is important to remember that less energy is required to feed from the breast than from the bottle, as the peristaltic activity of the tongue provokes the peristaltic movement of the GI tract and stimulates swallowing (Aguayo, 2001).

Pharmacology and Drug Therapy

Few studies exist describing the drug clearance of a late preterm infant. Despite the limited evidence, many dosing guidelines used to treat late preterm infants are based on term data, allowing for inappropriate drug dosing because of the immaturity of the liver and kidney, which can reduce drug clearance in late preterm infants (Ward, 2006). Additional drug clearance studies are needed.

Immunologic System

Late preterm infants do have unique susceptibilities to infection including the closed setting of a NICU, and the immunologic immaturity of premature infants sets the stage for development of nosocomial infections (Benjamin & Stoll, 2006). Late preterm infants are more likely to be evaluated for sepsis and treated with a 7-day course of antibiotics compared to term newborns (Wang et al., 2004). There are little data on the host defense capabilities of late preterm infants. Recent advances provide a framework for understanding the mechanisms underlying the propensity of infections in this at-risk population. Compared with term and extremely preterm infants, late preterm infants are intermediate with regard to immunologic maturity (Clapp, 2006).

CARE ENVIRONMENT

Late preterm infants masquerade as term newborns, making it difficult to determine their potential immediately following delivery. Pathologic signs and symptoms of late preterm infants transitioning to extrauterine life may be subtle or may be considered normal transition. Depending on their presentation at delivery, an astute assessment of the late preterm infant is critical since many of these infants may be triaged to the newborn nursery and/or room in with their parents where policies, staffing, and care models focus on normal term newborns, resulting in little time for nurses to perform vigilant assessments, establish lactation, and provide detailed discharge instruction (Pappas & Walker, 2010)

PHYSIOLOGIC FUNCTION AND NURSING ASSESSMENT AND CARE

Until recently, EBGs for this vulnerable group of infants were nonexistent. However, new recommendations for assessment and care have emerged (AWHONN, 2010; Engle et al., 2007) along with discharge preparation criteria (Engle et al., 2007). AWHONN's (2010) clinical practice guideline provides a detailed systematic approach to assessing and managing late preterm infants and focuses on specific parent support and teaching recommendations. Table 21–2 outlines AWHONN's late preterm infant practice recommendations.

When managing these high-risk infants, it is important to focus on their gestational age and behavior rather than on weight and Apgar scores. Immediately following birth, late preterm infants need to be carefully assessed for respiratory issues and signs and symptoms related to *hypothermia or cold stress, hypoglycemia,* and *sepsis.* Following the initial resuscitation and stabilization, assessment of the late preterm infant needs to concentrate on *feeding challenges, jaundice* and *hyperbilirubinemia,* and *parent education for discharge teaching.* It is imperative for nurses to recognize the increased risks associated with breastfeeding late preterm mother–infant dyads, including hyperbilirubinemia, poor milk transfer, and rehospitalization. While more research is needed to examine the causes of poor breastfeeding establishment and associated outcomes among late preterm mother–infant dyads (Radtke, 2011), few published breastfeeding guidelines or recommendation exist to assist healthcare providers caring for the breastfed late preterm infant (Academy of Breastfeeding Medicine, 2008; Meier, Furman, & Degenhardt, 2007; Smith, Donze, & Schuller, 2007; Walker, 2008; Wight, Morton, & Kim, 2008).

Discharge teaching should include information about safe sleep environment that can reduce the risk of all sleep-related infant deaths, including SIDS. Compared to term infants, late preterm infants are at a twofold higher risk of developing SIDS (Darnall, Ariagno, & Kinney, 2006). Healthcare providers need to educate families about infants' increased risk for SIDS and demonstrate appropriate SIDS prevention strategies within the nurseries prior to discharge so families can mimic appropriate caregiving behaviors. The AAP Task Force on Sudden Infant Death Syndrome (2011) recommends:

- Infants be placed supine (wholly on the back) for every sleep
- The use of firm sleep surfaces (soft materials or objects should not be placed under a sleeping infant)

Table 21–2. ASSESSMENT AND CARE OF THE LATE PRETERM INFANT (LPI)

Goal	Nursing Assessment and Care Interventions
Determine accurate gestational age	• Review prenatal records to confirm gestational age from prenatal assessment • Perform postnatal gestational assessment within 12 hr of age (e.g., New Ballard Score) • Obtain infant's length, weight, and head circumference and plot on validated growth curve to determine size/dates (i.e., AGA, SGA, or LGA)
Cardiopulmonary stability	• VS within 30 min of age, every 30 min until 2 hr of age, then every 2–4 hr as stable • Assess respiratory rate (normal 30–60 breaths/min); note: LPI may exhibit periodic breathing or brief tachypnea during transition • Assess and document signs of respiratory distress; note: Normal newborns may exhibit grunting during the first 2 postnatal hours • If work of breathing is increased, implement appropriate interventions: Notify healthcare provider, apply pulse oximeter probe to determine saturation, consider supplemental oxygen (monitored and heated/humidified) to achieve pulse oximetry target of 85%–95% saturation • Assess heart rate (normal 120–160 bpm) and perfusion (normal capillary refill time up to 3 secs) • Assess muscle tone and overall activity as indicator of oxygenation • If infant is without distress, may initiate kangaroo care (KC)
Thermal stability	• Assess temperature within 30 min of age, followed by every 30 min until 2 hr of age, then every 2–4 hr as stable • Review perinatal history to identify risks for heat loss/cold stress • Thoroughly dry infant; provide prewarmed linens and dry cap for head • Preheat radiant warmer or incubator and utilize temperature controls • Target infant temperature: 97.7°–99.3°F (36.5°–37.4°C) • Avoid heat loss through conduction, convection, evaporation, and radiation • Initiate measures to support thermoneutrality, such as KC or swaddling • Postpone bath until thermal and cardiopulmonary stabilities are evident (typically 2–4 hr after birth), then bathe, incorporating measures such as short bath duration, sponge or swaddled bath, bath water temperature of 100°–104°F, minimized room drafts, room temperature set between 79° and 81°F, prewarmed towels for drying, immediate cap and wrap in warm blankets • If infant becomes hypothermic, place in KC, incubator, or under radiant warmer and monitor temperature every 30 min until normalized; review history for risk factors or other indicators of illness
Glucose stability	• Review antenatal/perinatal history to identify risks for glucose instability • Perform screening point-of-care glucose assessment within the first 2 hr of life and thereafter as indicated if infant is displaying symptoms suggesting hypoglycemia • Provide early, frequent feedings on demand, with interval between feedings no longer than 2–3 hr if breastfed and 3–4 hr if formula fed • If hypoglycemia is suspected, immediately assess glucose level; in general, for glucose <40–45 mg/dL (2.2–2.6 mmol/L), immediately send confirmatory serum glucose; note: No exact definition of hypoglycemia exists • For plasma glucose ≥40–45 mg/dL (2.2–2.6 mmol/L), establish frequent feedings and follow clinically • For plasma glucose <40–45 mg/dL, immediately feed per breast or formula per gavage or bottle and repeat glucose level within 30 min of feeding • If the infant exhibits signs of hypoglycemia and the glucose is <40–45 mg/dL and feedings are not tolerated, provide IV bolus of 10% dextrose in water (2 mL/kg) and establish IV maintenance at 4 to 6 mg/kg/min; repeat glucose testing within 30 min of bolus and thereafter every 1–2 hr until stabilized • For persistent hypoglycemia, consider transferring infant to a higher acuity unit or facility for supportive care
Feeding readiness and tolerance	• Assess readiness for feeding prior to initiating oral feedings, including infant's ability to coordinate sucking/swallowing and breathing; LPI may have weak suck, immature feeding pattern, and limited ability to display robust feeding cues • Monitor for stability during feedings; LPI may easily fatigue and lose stamina during feedings at bottle and breast • Evaluate maternal position for breastfeeding, latch, and milk transfer • Facilitate early and frequent breastfeeding (8–12 times/day) • Observe, educate, and validate maternal knowledge about feeding behaviors seen in the LPI, including need to wake before feedings, feeding frequently, and continually assessing coordination of sucking/swallowing/breathing • Encourage adequate milk supply and transfer with strategies such as prepumping breast prior to breastfeeding attempt and utilizing support of lactation consultant; extended lactation support, education, and frequent follow-up are warranted in this population to ensure successful lactation and to avoid potentially dangerous complications related to insufficient lactation (Radtke, 2011)

(continued)

Table 21–2. ASSESSMENT AND CARE OF THE LATE PRETERM INFANT (LPI) *(Continued)*

Goal	Nursing Assessment and Care Interventions

Recognition of potential complications	• Recognize that the late preterm is at increased risk for sepsis and identify maternal, perinatal, and neonatal risks
	  ○ Identify and address presenting signs of infection, including, but not limited to, temperature instability, behavioral changes, poor feeding, or cardiopulmonary instability
	• Recognize that the late preterm is at increased risk for significant hyperbilirubinemia and identify maternal and neonatal riskst
	  ○ Note presence of clinical jaundice within the first 24 hr of life and initiate immediate screening of total serum bilirubin if visible jaundice exists; plot bilirubin level on hour-specific nomogram and initiate phototherapy for levels above threshold
	  ○ Evaluate bilirubin level prior to discharge using serum or transcutaneous assessment
	• If the planned postdischarge primary provider visit does not coincide with the anticipated peak of bilirubin (e.g., 5–7 days of life), plan additional follow-up visit

Developing and supporting parental role	• Provide parent support to establish their new role • Encourage KC and prioritize care to support uninterrupted periods for parent/infant bonding • Help parents identify infant behaviors, especially alertness and hunger/satiety cues; develop and model appropriate responses to infant cues • Encourage parents to room-in prior to discharge • Assess level of emotional distress in parents, with attention to depression and post-traumatic stress symptoms and refer as needed • Ensure that parents identify primary care provider and community follow-up resources prior to discharge; first provider visit should occur within 24–48 hr of discharge • Document and clearly communicate all outpatient provider appointments
Discharge planning	• *Discharge should not be considered prior to 48 hr of age* • Conduct and document complete health assessment within 24 hr of discharge • Teach parents how to assess for signs of distress and intervene appropriately • Counsel parents about environmental risks, including secondhand smoke exposure • Reinforce supine positioning for sleep and avoidance of soft blankets, pillows, and crib toys • Assess for risks for respiratory syncytial virus (RSV) including <35 weeks' gestational age at birth, childcare attendance, preschool-aged siblings, exposure to environmental pollutants, male gender, household having more than five persons, SGA • Confirm pediatric care provider (PCP) follow-up visit is planned within 24–48 hr of discharge • Ensure that car seat safety test is performed prior to discharge • Confirm infant's ability to sustain normal temperature in open crib with appropriate clothing • Teach proper procedures for determining axillary temperature and performing bath • Complete teaching and assess learning about infant safety and indications for seeking assistance from PCP, including elevated temperature, signs of dehydration, poor feeding, lethargy, or irritability and provide supportive written information

AGA, appropriate for gestational age; IV, intravenous; LGA, large for gestational age; SGA, small for gestational age; VS, vital signs.
Adapted from Association of Women's Health, Obstetric and Neonatal Nurses. (2010). *Assessment and Care of the Late Preterm Infant. Evidence-Based Clinical Practice Guideline.* Washington, DC: Author.

• Breastfeeding
• Room-sharing without bed-sharing
• Routine immunizations
• Consideration of using a pacifier at naptime and bed time
• Supervised, awake tummy time to facilitate development and minimize development of positional plagiocephaly (e.g., asymmetrical skull)
• Healthcare professionals, newborn nursery and NICU staff, and childcare providers should endorse the SIDS risk-reduction recommendations from birth

In addition, the Task Force (AAP, 2011) recommends avoiding:

• Soft objects and loose bedding out of the crib
• Overheating
• Commercial devices marketed to reduce the risk of SIDS

• Exposure to tobacco smoke, alcohol, and illicit drugs
• Home cardiorespiratory monitors as a strategy for reducing the risk of SIDS

These recommendations were expanded to ensure a safe sleeping environment and ways to reduce the risks of all sleep-related infant deaths, including SIDS, suffocation, and other accidental deaths.

READMISSION RISK AND NEWBORN FOLLOW-UP

In general, late preterm infants are at greater risk of neonatal morbidity and are two to three times more likely to be readmitted to the hospital compared to term newborns (Burgos, Schmitt, Stevenson, & Phibbs, 2008; McLaurin et al., 2009; Tomashek et al., 2006). Hospital readmission risk factors include maternal complications during labor and delivery, families receiving support from a public payer, parents who are of Asian/Pacific Islander ethnicity, a firstborn infant, male gender, use of assisted ventilation, and an infant being breastfed at discharge (Escobar, Clark, & Green, 2006; Escobar et al., 2002; National Center for Health Statistics, 2005; Shapiro-Mendoza et al., 2006; Tomashek et al., 2006). Jaundice, proven or suspected infections, feeding and respiratory difficulties (including gastroesophageal reflux disease), sepsis, and failure to thrive were the most common diagnoses at readmission (Escobar et al., 2006; Jain & Cheng, 2006).

The AAP has established specific criteria for discharging late preterm infants (Engle et al., 2007). According to these guidelines, late preterm infants must be medically stable and able to spontaneously breathe room air without apnea, bradycardia, or episodes of significant desaturation prior to discharge. These infants must be able to maintain a normal body temperature without the use of adjunctive heating devices and should be assessed closely for immature feeding behaviors. Parents need to be confident and competent in their ability to care for their baby prior to discharge and need to be equipped and empowered with the knowledge to appropriately and effectively care for this population of infants and their potential risks after discharge. Specifically, parent education needs to include the increased risk that their child has hyperbilirubinemia, feeding difficulties, apnea, sepsis, respiratory problems, and hypothermia. It is imperative that a follow-up visit 24 to 48 hours after discharge is scheduled with an identified primary care provider prior to discharge.

SUMMARY

Research is still needed to understand the etiology of late preterm births. As the rate of preterm births increase, so does the impact on the burden of disease and the healthcare cost to society. The estimated economic burden caused by preterm births in the United States is $26.2 billion, or $51,600 per preterm infant (Berhman & Butler, 2006). Any decrease in the rate of prematurity, at any gestation, would reduce the burden of disease and lead to a significant cost savings. Late preterm infants require diligent evaluation, monitoring, referral, and early return appointments, not only for postneonatal evaluation but also for long-term follow-up (Raju et al., 2006).

HYPOXIC ISCHEMIC ENCEPHALOPATHY

HIE is the leading cause of neonatal encephalopathy (NE) in term and late preterm newborns and is a major cause of death and disability (Pfister & Soll, 2010). Typically, HIE ensues after a disruption in cerebral blood flow and oxygen delivery to the brain secondary to insufficient placental blood flow and gas exchange. The progression of HIE and degree of injury are dependent on the timing, duration, and severity of the insult (Pfister & Soll, 2010). The estimated incidence of HIE is 1.5 per 1,000 live births (Kurinczuk, White-Koning, & Badawi, 2010). Perinatal factors associated with the risk of HIE include maternal diabetes, fever, chorioamnionitis, placental abruption, umbilical cord prolapse, uterine rupture, tight nuchal cord, or an acute blood loss (Rutherford et al., 2005; Selway, 2010).

PATHOPHYSIOLOGY

Physiologic consequences of hypoxic ischemia evolve over hours to days, resulting in a biphasic pattern of energy failure leading to brain injury, separated by a brief recovery or "latent phase" (Gluckman & Williams, 1992). Primary cell death (necrosis) results if the oxygen deprivation is not corrected. In an effort to sustain functional ability, the neonate's brain converts to anaerobic metabolism leading to rapid depletion of adenosine triphosphate, accumulation of lactic acid, and failure of normal metabolic activity (Perlman, 2006; Selway, 2010). Loss of ionic homeostasis results in an accumulation of sodium, calcium, and water within brain cells. Once the cerebral blood flow and oxygenation are reestablished, the initial metabolic impairments resolve over 30 to 60 minutes. After reperfusion, during the "latent phase," complete recovery or development of a secondary phase may occur. The latent phase institutes the "therapeutic window." Whether injury reversal occurs depends on several factors (severity of the primary phase, body temperature, substrate availability, preconditioning, and simultaneous disease process), and some evidence suggests that it does not appear to extend more than 6 hours from the primary injury (Shankaran & Laptook, 2007).

In an attempt to restore brain function, the secondary phase of energy failure (apoptosis) begins about 6 to 15 hours after the initial injury and extends over several days (Williams, Gunn, & Gluckman, 1991). During this phase of energy failure, mitochondrial dysfunction results from excitatory neurotransmitters, an influx of calcium into the cells, oxygen free radicals, or nitric oxide formation (Cooper, 2011; Mathur, Smith, & Donze, 2008). This secondary phase is clinically associated with seizures, worsening neurologic examination, and is proportional to adverse neurodevelopmental outcomes at 1 and 4 years of age (Mathur et al., 2008; Roth et al., 1992, 1997). The degree of neuronal injury can be assessed using Sarnat and Sarnat's (1976) clinical staging of encephalopathy criteria. These criteria describe the evolution of the clinical encephalopathy over the first several days of life and emphasize that this encephalopathy is a dynamic clinical state that warrants close monitoring.

INTERVENTION

THERAPEUTIC HYPOTHERMIA

Until recently, supportive care and anticonvulsants for seizure control has been the management of choice for these infants. However, both large and small randomized controlled trials (RCTs) have demonstrated the efficacy and safety of instituting therapeutic hypothermia (whole body cooling or selective head cooling) to reduce death and disability in infants with moderate-to-severe HIE (Azzopardi et al., 2009; Eicher et al., 2005; Gluckman et al., 2005; Lin et al., 2006; Shankaran et al., 2005). Induced hypothermia initiated within 6 hours of birth is significantly associated with fewer deaths and less neurodevelopmental disability at 18-month follow-up in infants born at highest risk for brain injury (as defined by specific protocols) (Edwards et al., 2010). Both total body and selective head cooling methods have been shown to be effective (Jacobs, Hunt, Tarnow-Mordi, Inder, & Davis, 2007).

According to the AAP's and the AHA's NRP, therapeutic hypothermia is the treatment of choice in the delivery room for term or late preterm infants with evolving moderate encephalopathy (Perlman et al., 2010). Whole body or selective head cooling should be initiated and conducted in the context of rigorous and clearly defined protocols within NICUs with provisions for monitoring side effects and long-term follow-up.

Intervening with a neuroprotective intervention, such as therapeutic hypothermia (cooling), prior to the secondary phase of energy failure is the single most promising intervention for infants with HIE (Fairchild, Sokora, Scott, & Zanelli, 2010; Mathur et al., 2008; Pfister & Soll, 2010). Although the exact mechanism by which hypothermic neuroprotection works is unknown, it does seem to attenuate the secondary phase of neuronal injury. Most clinical trials have induced therapeutic hypothermia for hypoxic-ischemic neonates within 6 hours of birth. However, evidence that the duration of the latent phase is inversely proportional to the severity of the ischemic insult suggests that the therapeutic window for starting hypothermia therapy may be much shorter, within 2 hours of the suspected insult and no later than 6 hours (Iwata et al., 2007; Pfister & Soll, 2010). Therefore, early identification of hypoxic-ischemic neonates who meet the criteria for hypothermia therapy is critical. These infants have complex needs and are typically managed in tertiary centers with the availability of subspecialty evaluation and treatment. However, many of these at-risk infants are born in hospitals that do not provide neonatal intensive care, requiring transports that often take hours. Additionally, the timing of the onset of injury is often unclear, and since the therapeutic window for neuroprotection is limited, early initiation of cooling is

often warranted. Induced hypothermia should be only provided under strict protocols in nontertiary centers under guidance of the regional NICU and transport team. If a cooling protocol is not available, every effort to avoid overheating the infant should be made. Cooling protocols may vary; typically, passive cooling is initiated (if portable cooling equipment is unavailable) and achieved by turning off the radiant warmer, and the infant is cooled to a rectal temperature between 34°C and 35°C. Close monitoring of the rectal or esophageal temperature is required with the appropriate probe or low-reading thermometer (at least every 15 minutes or continuously, if possible) (Azzopardi et al., 2009; Fairchild et al., 2010; Kendall, Kapetanakis, Ratnavel, Azzopardi, & Robertson, 2010). Potential adverse effects of passive overcooling have been reported, highlighting the need for vigilant continuous or intermittent rectal temperature monitoring, ongoing education, and continuous collaboration among all members of the healthcare team (Hallberg, Olson, Bartocci, Edqvist, & Blennow, 2009; Thoresen, 2008).

Criteria for Cooling

Criteria for cooling should be discussed between the referring center and the neonatologist who is accepting the responsibility of the infant's care. Cooling criteria are fairly consistent among many of the RCTs for therapeutic hypothermia and include the following infants:

- Gestational age at least 36 weeks or more
- Weight of ≥1,800 g
- ≤6 hours of age at time of cooling
- pH ≤7 or base deficit >12 mEq/L within 1 hour following delivery
- Apgar score of ≤5 at 10 minutes following birth
- Moderate or severe encephalopathy as defined by Sarnat and Sarnat (1976)
- Moderate-to-severe electroencephalography (EEG) amplitude reduction (lower margin <5 microvolts and/or upper margin <10 microvolts) on a 20-minute amplitude-integrated EEG (aEEG) or evidence of seizures.

OR

- Evidence of perinatal metabolic compromise in the setting of a known event. Metabolic compromise is defined as at least two of the following:
  ○ Umbilical cord blood gas or blood gas within 1 hour of delivery showing a pH of 7.01 to 7.15 or base deficit of 10 to 15.9 mEq/L *or* no blood gas available within first hour; *and*
  ○ The need for respiratory support at 5 minutes of life or 10-minute Apgar score ≤ 5; *and*
  ○ Moderate or severe encephalopathy; *or*
  ○ Seizures

Exclusion criteria include infants with major congenital defects such as diaphragmatic hernia requiring ventilation, suspected chromosomal anomalies (e.g., trisomies 13 or 18), congenital disorders of the CNS, uncontrolled active bleeding, or parental refusal (Cooper, 2011; Mathur et al., 2008). It is extremely important to investigate other causes of NE, including infection and metabolic disorders, and institute specific treatment.

CARE AND ASSESSMENT

Nurses are key to the early identification of infants who are at risk for developing HIE as a result of an acute perinatal event. Nurses in the delivery room need to be knowledgeably astute of the clinical signs associated with neonatal asphyxia, seizures, and the criteria for therapeutic hypothermia. Utilizing a standard checklist for the neurologic examination provides optimal documentation of the stage and evolution of encephalopathy. Supportive nursing care is an essential element of cooling. Continuous monitoring of oxygenation, ventilation, perfusion, CO, strict intake and output, and glucose levels is essential to avoid additional adverse effects. Infants who are cooled typically have lower HRs (e.g., HR <100 bpm); however, prolonged bradycardia (e.g., HR <80 bpm) may indicate the need for slight warming (Selway, 2010). It is important to remember that vigilant monitoring and documentation of body temperatures are essential in these high-risk infants. Additionally, infants who are cooled need to be monitored and closely assessed for pain, and appropriate pharmacologic and nonpharmacologic therapies should be implemented (Cooper, 2011). Nurses are also key to providing emotional support to parents. Parents and family members need to know what to expect over the course of the next hours and days, the rationale for implementing therapeutic hypothermia, and the importance of further evaluation and management at a tertiary center with subspecialty availability.

TRANSPORT AND RETURN TRANSPORT

Many conditions complicating the neonatal period do not begin with dramatic clinical symptoms. Experience and well-developed assessment skills allow perinatal nurses to recognize subtle changes and intervene before the newborn's condition worsens. Occasionally, the condition of the newborn and services available at a particular perinatal center require transport to a level III/IV NICU. The goal of neonatal transport is to bring a sick newborn to a tertiary center in stable condition. The availability of neonatal intensive care has improved outcomes in high-risk newborns; although no standard definitions exist for graded levels of complexity of care that NICUs provide, thus making it difficult to compare outcomes (AAP, 2012). However, a uniform definition and classification of neonatal resources according to the different levels of care as recommended by AAP provides a framework for the development and implementation of consistent standards of service provided (AAP, 2012). Stabilization is an ongoing process, which begins with the referring hospital through consultation with the tertiary center as needed until the arrival and eventual departure of the transport team. Because of the diversity in the disease process and gestational age, stabilization takes on many forms. Basic care needs of newborns requiring transport to a tertiary center include adequate oxygenation, prevention of hypothermia, prevention of hypoglycemia, conservation of energy, and maintenance of physiologic integrity.

After the newborn's condition is no longer critical, in the event that an extended hospitalization is anticipated, the decision may be made to move the newborn back to the hospital in which he or she was born. This decision is made with input from neonatology staff at the level III/IV center, the newborn's primary care provider, the nursing staff in the level II hospital, and the parents. The decision also is influenced by the parents' insurance carrier or managed care providers. In order to make informed decision, the healthcare team and individual families need to consider the advantages and disadvantages associated with transporting convalescing infants back to their community hospital before return transport (Bowen, 2010). Return transport offers many advantages to family members of the high-risk newborn, although it requires involvement of personnel from the transferring and the receiving hospital as well as adequate parent preparation to be successful. Family involvement is essential to success of return transport. Ideally, the prospect of a return transport is introduced when the infant is initially transferred to the level III/IV center. Return transports should be celebrated as a milestone and a positive step toward discharge.

To provide newborns with the best care possible, healthcare professionals within the referring hospital and between the referring hospital and the tertiary center must communicate and work together as a team. The decision to transport back to the level II hospital first depends on whether the care needs of the newborn can be met at that institution. Communication between the level III/IV and the level II hospitals when a return transport is anticipated should begin several days before the actual transfer. This assists in preparing the parents, and the receiving hospital has time to anticipate staffing and equipment needs. Using a formal documentation system provides the receiving hospital with information about the current condition of the newborn.

SUMMARY

Most newborns are born in level II hospitals. They are healthy at birth, develop no complications during the neonatal period, and are discharged to their homes with their mothers. A small group of newborns are born with complications or develop complications immediately after birth. It is the newborn who develops complications that poses the challenge to the perinatal nurse. The nurse in a level II hospital must strive to identify complications in a timely fashion, care for the infant appropriately, stabilize the infant before transport to a level III/IV facility, and be prepared to accept the patient as a return transfer when he or she is no longer in need of intensive care.

REFERENCES

Academy of Breastfeeding Medicine. (2008). *Protocol #10: Breastfeeding the near-term infant (35 to 37 weeks gestation)*. Retrieved from http://www.bfmed.org/Resources/Protocols.aspx

Adams-Chapman, I. (2006). Neurodevelopmental outcome of the late preterm infant. *Clinics of Perinatology, 33*(4), 947–964. doi:10.1016/j.clp.2006.09.004

Aguayo, J. (2001). Maternal lactation for preterm newborn infants. *Early Human Development, 65*(Suppl.), S19–S29. doi:10.1016/s0378-3782(01)

Alkalay, A. L., Bresee, C. J., & Simmons, C. F. (2010). Decreased neonatal jaundice readmission rate after implementing hyperbilirubinemia guidelines and universal screening for bilirubin. *Clinical Pediatrics, 49*(9), 830–833. doi:10.1177/0009922810363728

American Academy of Pediatrics. (2004a). Management of hyperbilirubinemia in the newborn infant 35 or more weeks of gestation. *Pediatrics, 114*(1), 297–316. doi:10.1542/peds.114.1.297

American Academy of Pediatrics. (2004b). *Questions and Answers on Jaundice and Your Newborn*. Washington, DC: Author. Retrieved from http://www.aap.org/family/jaundicefaq.htm

American Academy of Pediatrics. (2008). Committee on pediatric AIDS. HIV testing and prophylaxis to prevent mother-to-child transmission in the United States. *Pediatrics, 122*(5), 1127–1134. doi:10.1542/peds.2008-2175

American Academy of Pediatrics (2012). Committee on fetus and newborn. Levels of neonatal care. *Pediatrics, 130*(3), 587–597. doi:10.1542/peds.2012-1999

American Academy of Pediatrics Task Force on Sudden Infant Death Syndrome. (2011). SIDS and other sleep-related infant deaths: expansion of recommendations for a safe infant sleeping environment. *Pediatrics, 128*(5), 1030–1039 doi:10.1542/peds.2011-2284

American College of Obstetricians and Gynecologists. (2003). *Scheduled Cesarean Delivery and the Prevention of Vertical Transmission of HIV Infection* (Committee Opinion No. 234). Washington, DC: Author.

American College of Obstetricians and Gynecologists. (2005). *The Importance of Preconception Care in the Continuum in Women's Health* (Committee Opinion No. 313). Washington, DC: Author.

American College of Obstetricians and Gynecologists. (2006). *Amnioinfusion Does Not Prevent Meconium Aspiration Syndrome* (Committee Opinion No. 346). Washington, DC: Author.

American Heart Association (2012). *Heart disease and stroke statistics—2012 update: A report from the American Heart Association Statistics Committee and Stroke Statistics Subcommittee*. Retrieved from http://circ.ahajournals.org/content/125/1/e2

American Academy of Pediatrics & American Heart Association. (2011). *Textbook of Neonatal Resuscitation* (6th ed.). Elk Grove Village, IL: Authors.

Association of Women's Health, Obstetric and Neonatal Nurses. (2010). *Assessment and Care of the Late Preterm Infant. Evidence-Based Clinical Practice Guideline*. Washington, DC: Author.

Auckland, A. K. (2010). Ventricular septal defects. In J. A. Drose (Ed.), *Fetal Echocardiography* (2nd ed., pp. 105–118). St. Louis, MO: Saunders.

Azzopardi, D. V., Strohm, B., Edwards, A. D., Dyet, L., Halliday, H. L., Juszczak, E., . . . Brocklehurst, P. (2009). Moderate hypothermia to treat perinatal asphyxial encephalopathy. *New England Journal of Medicine, 361*(14), 1349–1358.

Bailey, B. A., McCook, J. G., Hodge, A., & McGrady, L. (2011). Infant birth outcomes among substance using women: Why quitting smoking during pregnancy is just as important as quitting illicit drug use. *Maternal Child Health Journal*. Advance online publication.

Benjamin, D. K., & Stoll, B. J. (2006). Infection in late preterm infants. *Clinics in Perinatology, 33*(4), 871–882. doi:10.1016/j.clp.2006.09.005

Bentlin, M. R., Suppo, L. M., & Rugolo, S. (2010). Late-onset sepsis: Epidemiology, evaluation, and outcome. *NeoReviews, 11*(8), e426–e435.

Berhman, R. E., & Butler, A. S. (2006). *Preterm Birth: Causes, Consequences and Prevention*. Washington, DC: Institute of Medicine of the National Academies.

Bhutani, V. K., Johnson, L. H., & Shapiro, S. M. (2004). Kernicterus in sick and preterm infants (1999–2002): A need for an effective preventive approach. *Seminars in Perinatology, 28*(5), 319–325. doi:10.1053/j.semperi.2004.09.006

Bhutani, V. K., Johnson, L. H., & Sivievri, E. M. (1999). Predictive ability of a predischarge hour-specific serum bilirubin for subsequent significant hyperbilirubinemia in healthy term and near-term newborns. *Pediatrics, 103*(1), 6–14.

Bird, T. M., Bronstein, J. M., Hall, R. W., Lowery, C. L., Nugent, R., & Mays, G. P. (2010). Late preterm infants: Birth outcomes and health care utilization in the first year. *Pediatrics, 126*(2), e311–e319. doi:10.1542/peds.2009-2869

Bowen, S. L. (2010). Intrafacility and interfacility neonatal transport. In M. T. Verklan & M. Walden (Eds.), *Core Curriculum for Neonatal Intensive Care Nursing* (4th ed., pp. 415–433). St. Louis, MO: Saunders.

Bromiker, R., Bin-Nun, A., Schimmel, M. S., Hammerman, C., & Kaplan, M. (2012). Neonatal hyperbilirubinemia in the low-intermediate-risk category on the bilirubin nomogram. *Pediatrics, 130*(3), e470-e475. doi:10.1542/peds.2012-0005.

Bry, K. (2008). Newborn resuscitation and the lung. *NeoReviews, 9*(11), e506–e512. doi:10.1542/neo.9-11-e506

Burgos, A. E., & Burke, B. L. (2009). Neonatal abstinence syndrome. *NeoReviews, 19*(5), e222–e229.

Burgos, A. E., Flaherman, V. J., & Newman, T. B. (2011). Screening and follow-up of neonatal hyperbilirubinemia: A review. *Clinical Pediatrics, 5*(1), 7–16. doi:10.1177/0009922811398964

Burgos, A. E., Schmitt, S. K., Stevenson, D. K., & Phibbs, C. S. (2008). Readmission for neonatal jaundice in California, 1991–2000: Trends and implications. *Pediatrics, 121*(4), e864–e869. doi:10.1542/peds.2007-1214

Buus-Frank, M. (2005). The great imposter [Editorial]. *Advances in Neonatal Care, 5*(5), 233–236. doi:10.1016/j.adnc.2005.08.012

Centers for Disease Control and Prevention. (2006a). Preconception care for workgroup. Recommendations to improve preconception health and health care—United States. *Morbidity and Mortality Weekly Report, 55*(RR6), 1–30.

Centers for Disease Control and Prevention. (2006b). Revised recommendations for HIV testing of adults, adolescents, and pregnant women in health-care settings. *Morbidity and Mortality Weekly Report, 55*(RR14), 1–17.

Chyi, L. J., Lee, H. C., Hintz, S. R., Gould, J. B., & Sutcliffe, T. L. (2008). School outcomes of late preterm infants: Special needs and challenges for infants born at 32 to 39 weeks gestation. *Journal of Pediatrics, 153*(1), 25–31. doi:10.1016/j.jpeds.2008.01.027

Cifuentes, J., Segars, A. H., & Carlo, W. A. (2003). Respiratory system management and complications. In C. Kenner & J. W. Lott (Eds.), *Comprehensive Neonatal Nursing: A Physiologic Perspective* (3rd ed., pp. 348–375). St. Louis, MO: Saunders.

Clapp, D. W. (2006). Developmental regulation of the immune system. *Seminars in Perinatology, 30*(2), 69–72. doi:10.1053/j.semperi.2006.02.004

Clark, R. H. (2005). The epidemiology of respiratory failure in neonates born at an estimated gestational age of 34 weeks or more. *Journal of Perinatology, 25*(4), 251–257. doi:10.1038/sj.jp.7211242

Clark, S. L., Frye, D. R., Meyers, J. A., Belfort, M. A., Dildy, G. A., Kofford, S., . . . Perlin, J. A. (2010). Reduction in elective delivery at <39 weeks of gestation: Comparative effectiveness of 3 different approaches to change and the impact on newborn intensive care admissions and stillbirths. *American Journal of Obstetrics & Gynecology, 203*(5), 449.e1–449.e6. doi:10.1016/j.ajog.2010.05.036

Clark, S. L., Knox, E., Simpson, K. R., & Hankins, G. D. (2010). Quality improvement opportunities in intrapartum care. In *Toward Improving the Outcome of Pregnancy III* (pp. 66–74). New York: March of Dimes Foundation.

Clark, S. L., Miller, D. D., Belfort, M. A., Dildy, G. A., Frye, D. K., & Meyers, J. A. (2009). Neonatal and maternal outcomes associated with elective term delivery. *American Journal of Obstetrics and Gynecology, 200*(2), 156.e1–156.e4. doi:10.1016/j.ajog.2008.08.068

Cloherty, J. P., & Stark, A. R. (1998). *Manual of neonatal care* (4th ed., pp. 26–27). Boston, MA: Little, Brown.

Cohen, R. S., Wong, R. J., & Stevenson, D. K. (2010). Understanding neonatal jaundice: A perspective on causation. *Pediatrics & Neonatology, 51*(3), 143–148. doi:10.1016/S1875-9572(10)60027-7

Cole, F. S., Nogee, L. M., & Hamvas, A. (2006). Defects in surfactant synthesis: Clinical implications. *Pediatrics Clinics of North America, 53*(5), 911–927.

Committee on Fetus and Newborn & Adamkin, D. H. (2011). Clinical report: Postnatal glucose homeostasis in late-preterm and term infants. *Pediatrics, 127*(3), 575–579.

Committee on Obstetric Practice (2008). Prenatal and perinatal human immunodeficiency virus testing: Expanded recommendations. *Obstetrics & Gynecology, 112*(3), 739–742.

Consortium on Safe Labor. (2010). Respiratory morbidity in late preterm births. *Journal of the American Medical Association (JAMA), 304*(4), 419–425.

Cooper, D. J. (2011). Induced hypothermia for neonatal hypoxic-ischemic encephalopathy: Pathophysiology, current treatment, and nursing considerations. *Neonatal Network, 30*(1), 29–35.

Cornblath, M., Hawdon, J. M., Williams, A. F., Aynsley-Green, A., Ward-Platt, M. P., Schwartz, R., & Kalhan, S. C. (2000). Controversies regarding definition of neonatal hypoglycemia: Suggested operational thresholds. *Pediatrics, 105*(5), 1141–1145. doi:10.1542/peds.105.5.1141

Darnall, R. A., Ariagno, R. L., & Kinney, H. C. (2006). The late preterm infant and the control of breathing, sleep, and brainstem development: A review. *Clinics in Perinatology, 33*(4), 883–914. doi:10.1016/j.clp.2006.10.004

Davidoff, M. J., Dias, T., Damus, K., Russell, R., Bettegowda, V. R., Dolan, S., . . . Petrini, J. (2006). Changes in the gestational age distribution among U.S. singleton births: Impact on rates of late preterm birth, 1992–2002. *Seminars in Perinatology, 30*(1), 8–15. doi:10.1053/j.semperi.2006.01.009

Davis, J. A., & Yawetz, S. (2012). Management of HIC in the pregnant woman. *Clinical Obstetrics & Gynecology, 55*(2), 531–540.

Deshpande, S., & Ward Platt, M. W. (2005). The investigation and management of neonatal hypoglycaemia. *Seminars in Fetal and Neonatal Medicine, 10*(4), 351–361. doi:10.1016/j.siny.2005.04.002

Dudell, G. G., & Jain, L. (2006). Hypoxic respiratory failure in the late preterm infant. *Clinics in Perinatology, 33*(4), 803–830. doi:10.1016/j.clp.2006.09.006

Dudell, G. G., & Stoll, B. J. (2007). Respiratory tract disorders. In R. M. Kliegman, R. E. Behrman, H. B. Jensen, & B. F. Stanton (Eds.), *Nelson Textbook of Pediatrics* (18th ed., pp. 728–753). Philadelphia: Saunders Elsevier.

Edwards, A. D., Brocklehurst, P., Gunn, A. J., Halliday, H., Juszczak, E., Levene M., . . . Azzopardi, D. (2010). Neurological outcomes at 18 months of age after moderate hypothermia for perinatal hypoxic ischaemic encephalopathy: Synthesis and meta-analysis of trial data. *BMJ, 34*, 363. doi:10.1136/bmj.c363

Eicher, D. J., Wagner, C. L., Katikaneni, L. P., Hulsey, T. C., Bass, W. T., Kaufman, D. A., . . . Yager, J. Y. (2005). Moderate hypothermia in neonatal encephalopathy: Safety outcomes. *Pediatric Neurology, 32*(1), 18–24. doi:10.1016/j.pediatrneurol. 2004.06.015

Engle, W. A., Tomashek, K. M., & Wallman, C. (2007). Committee on fetus and newborn. Late-preterm infants: A population at risk. *Pediatrics, 120*(6), 1390–1401. doi:10.1542/peds.2007-2952

Escobar, G. J., Clark, R. H., & Green, J. D. (2006). Short-term outcomes of infants born at 35 and 36 weeks gestation: We need to ask more questions. *Seminars in Perinatology, 30*(1), 26–33. doi:10.1053/j.semperi.2006.01.005

Escobar, G. J., Gonzales, V. M., Armstrong, M. A., Flock, B. F., Xiong, B., & Newman, T. B. (2002). Rehospitalization for neonatal dehydration: A nested case-control study. *Archives of Pediatric and Adolescent Medicine, 156*(2), 155–161. doi:10-1001/pubs.Pediatr Adolesc Med.-ISSN-1072-4710-156-2-poa10396

Escobar, G. J., Greene, J. D., Hulac, P., Kincannon, E., Bischoff, K., Gardner, M. N., . . . France, E. K. (2005). Rehospitalisation after birth hospitalisation: Patterns among infants of all gestations. *Archives of Disease in Childhood, 90*(2), 125–131. doi:10.1136/adc.2003.039974

Fairchild, K., Sokora, D., Scott, J., & Zanelli, S. (2010). Therapeutic hypothermia on neonatal transport: 4-year experience in a single NICU. *Journal of Perinatology, 30*(5), 324–329. doi:10.1038/jp.2009.168

Fike, D. L. (2003). Assessment and management of the substance exposed newborn and infant. In C. Kenner & J. W. Lott (Eds.), *Comprehensive Neonatal Nursing: A Physiologic Perspective* (3rd ed., pp. 773–802). St. Louis, MO: Saunders.

Gardner, S. L., Enzman-Hines, M., & Dickey, L. A. (2011). Respiratory diseases. In S. L. Gardner, B. S. Carter, M. Enzman-Hines, & J. A. Hernandez (Eds.), *Merenstein & Gardner's Handbook of Neonatal Intensive Care* (7th ed.; pp. 581–677). St. Louis, MO: Mosby Elsevier.

Garg, M., & Devaskar, S. U. (2006). Glucose metabolism in the late preterm infant. *Clinics in Perinatology, 33*(4), 853–870. doi:10.1016/j.clp.2006.10.001

Gewolb, I. H., Vice, F. L., Schweiter-Kenney, E. L., Taciak, V. L., & Bosma, J. F. (2001). Developmental patterns of rhythmic suck and swallow in preterm infants. *Developmental Medicine and Child Neurology, 43*(1), 22–37. doi:10.1111/j.1469-8749.2001.tb00381.x

Gluckman, P. D., & Williams, C. E. (1992). When and why do brain cells die? *Developmental Medicine and Child Neurology, 34*(11), 1010–1014. doi:10.1111/j.1469-8749.1992.tb11407.x

Gluckman, P. D., Wyatt, J. S., Azzopardi, D., Ballard, R., Edwards, A. D., Ferriero, D. M., . . . Gunn, A. J. (2005). Selective head cooling with mild systemic hypothermia after neonatal encephalopathy: Multicentre randomized trial. *Lancet, 365*(9460), 663–670. doi:10.1016/S0140-6736(05)17946-X

Gurka, M. J., LoCasale-Crouch, J., & Blackman, J. A. (2010). Long-term cognition, achievement, socioemotional, and behavioral development of healthy late-preterm infants. *Archives of Pediatrics & Adolescent Medicine, 164*(6), 525–532. doi:10.1001/archpediatrics.2010.83

Halamek, L. P., & Stevenson, D. K. (2002). Neonatal jaundice and liver disease. In A. A. Fanaroff & R. J. Martin (Eds.), *Neonatal-Perinatal Medicine Diseases of the Fetus and Infant* (7th ed., pp. 1309–1350). St. Louis, MO: Mosby.

Hallberg, B., Olson, L., Bartocci, M., Edqvist, I., & Blennow, M. (2009). Passive induction of hypothermia during transport of asphyxiated infants: A risk of excessive cooling. *Acta Paediatrica, 98*(6), 942–946. doi:10.1111/j.1651-2227.2009.01303.x

Hankins, G. D. V., & Longo, M. (2006). The role of stillbirth prevention and late preterm (near-term) births. *Seminars in Perinatology, 30*(1), 20–23. doi:10.1053/j.semperi.2006.01.011

Hansen, A. K., Wisborg, K., Uldbjerg, N., & Henriksen, T. B. (2007). Elective caesarean section and respiratory morbidity in the term and near-term neonate. *Acta Obstetrica Gynecologica Scandinavica, 86*(4), 389–394. doi:10.1080/00016340601159256

Hawdon, J. M., Ward Platt, M. P., & Aynsley-Green, A. (1992). Patterns of metabolic adaptation for preterm and term infants in the first neonatal week. *Archives of Disease in Childhood, 67*(4, Spec No.), 357–365.

Hunt, C. E. (2006). Ontogeny of automatic regulation in late preterm infants born at 34–37 weeks postmenstrual age. *Seminars in Perinatology, 30*(2), 73–76. doi:10.1053/j.semperi.2006.02.005

Iwata, O., Iwata, S., Thornton, J. S., De Vita, E., Bainbridge, A., Herbert, L., . . . Robertson, N. J. (2007). "Therapeutic time window" duration decreases with increasing severity of cerebral hypoxia ischaemia under normothermia and delayed hypothermia in newborn piglets. *Brain Research, 1154*, 173–180. doi:10.1016/j.brainres.2007.03.083

Jacobs, S., Hunt, R., Tarnow-Mordi, W., Inder, T., & Davis, P. (2007). Cooling for newborns with hypoxic ischaemic encephalopathy. *Cochrane Database of Systematic Review*, (4), CD003311.

Jain, A., Aggarwal, R., Sankar, M. J., Agarwal, R., Deorari, A. K., & Paul, V. K. (2010). Hypoglycemia in the newborn. *Indian Journal of Pediatrics, 77*(1), 1137–1142. doi:10.1007/s12098-010-0176-0

Jain, S., & Cheng, J. (2006). Emergency department visits and rehospitalizations in late preterm infants. *Clinics in Perinatology, 33*(4), 935–945. doi:10.1016/j.clp.2006.09.007

Jain, L., & Dudell, G. G. (2006). Respiratory transition in infants delivered by cesarean section. *Seminars in Perinatology, 30*(5), 296–304. doi:10.1053/j.semperi.2006.07.011

Jain, L., & Eaton, D. C. (2006). Physiology of fetal lung fluid clearance and effect of labor. *Seminars in Perinatology, 30*(1), 34–43. doi:10.1053/j.semperi.2006.01.006

Juretschke, L. J. (2005). Kernicterus: Still a concern. *Neonatal Network, 24*(2), 7–19.

Kamath, B. D., Thilo, E. H., & Hernandez, J. A. (2011). Jaundice. In S. L. Gardner, B. S. Carter, M. Enzman-Hines, & J. A. Hernandez (Eds.), *Merenstein & Gardner's Handbook of Neonatal Intensive Care* (7th ed., pp. 531–552). St. Louis, MO: Mosby.

Kayiran, S. M., & Gurakan, B. (2010). Screening of blood glucose levels in healthy neonates. *Singapore Medical Journal, 51*(11), 853–855.

Kemper, A. R., Mahle, W. T., Martin, G. R., Cooley, W. C., Kumar, P., Morrow, W. R., Kelm, K., et al. (2011). Strategies for implementing screening for critical congenital heart disease. *Pediatrics, 128*(5):e1259–e1267. doi:10.1542/peds.2011–1317.

Kendall, G. S., Kapetanakis, A., Ratnavel, N., Azzopardi, D., & Robertson, N. J. (2010). Passive cooling for initiation of therapeutic hypothermia in neonatal encephalopathy. *Archives of Disease in Childhood. Fetal and Neonatal Edition, 95*(6), 408–412. doi:10.1136/adc.2010.187211

Kenney, P. M., Hoover, D., Williams, L. C., & Iskersky, V. (2011). Cardiovascular diseases and surgical interventions. In S. L. Gardner, B. S. Carter, M. Enzman-Hines, & J. A. Hernandez (Eds.), *Merenstein & Gardner's Handbook of Neonatal Intensive Care* (7th ed., pp. 678–716). St. Louis, MO: Saunders.

King, S. M. (2004). Evaluation and treatment of the human immunodeficiency virus-1-exposed infant. *Pediatrics, 114*(2), 497–505.

Kinney, H. C. (2006). The near-term (late preterm) human brain and risk for periventricular leukomalacia: A review. *Seminars in Perinatology, 30*(2), 81–88. doi:10.1053/j.semperi.2006.02.006

Kochanek, K. D., Xu, J., Murphy, S. L., Minino, A. M., & Kung, H. (2011). National Vital Statistics Reports, 59(4). Accessed at: www.cdc.gov/nchs/data/nvsr/ncsr59_04.pdf

Konduri, G. G., & Kim, U. O. (2009). Advances in the diagnosis and management of persistent pulmonary hypertension of the newborn. *Pediatric Clinics of North America, 56*(3), 579–600. doi:10.1016/j.pcl.2009.04.004

Kurinczuk, J. J., White-Koning, M., & Badawi, N. (2010). Epidemiology of neonatal encephalopathy and hypoxic-ischaemic encephalopathy. *Early Human Development, 86*(6), 329–338. doi:10/1016/j.earlhumdev.2010.05010

Kuschel, C. (2007). Managing drug withdrawal in the newborn infant. *Seminars in Fetal & Neonatal Medicine, 12*(2), 127–133. doi:10.1016/j.siny.2007.01.004

Langendoerfer, S., Johnson, J. J., & Thureen, P. J. (2005). Perinatal drug exposure. In P. J. Thureen, J. Deacon, J. A. Hernandez, & D. M. Hall (Eds.), *Assessment and Care of the Well Newborn* (2nd ed., pp. 279–292). St. Louis, MO: Elsevier.

Lapointe, A., & Barrington, K. J. (2011). Pulmonary hypertension and the asphyxiated newborn. *Journal of Pediatrics, 158* (2, Suppl.), e19–e24. doi:10.1016/j.jpeds.2010.11.008

Laptook, A., & Jackson, G. L. (2006). Cold stress and hypoglycemia in the late preterm ("near-term") infant: Impact on nursery of admission. *Seminars in Perinatology, 30*(1), 24–27. doi:10.1053/j.semperi.2006.01.014

Law, K. L., Stroud, L. R., LaGasse, L., Niaura, R., Liu, J., & Lester, B. M. (2003). Smoking during pregnancy and newborn neurobehavior. *Pediatrics, 111*(6), 1318–1323.

Levine, E. M., Ghai, V., Barton, J. J., & Strom, C. M. (2001). Mode of delivery and risk of respiratory disease in newborn. *Obstetrics & Gynecology, 97*(3), 439–442.

Lin, Z. L., Yu, H. M., Lin, J., Chen, S. Q., Liang, Z. Q., & Zhang, Z. Y. (2006). Mild hypothermia via selective head cooling as neuroprotective therapy in term neonates with perinatal asphyxia: An experience from a single neonatal intensive care unit. *Journal of Perinatology, 26*(3), 180–184. doi:10.1038/sj.jp.7211412

Liu, A. J., Jones, M. P., Murray, H., Cook, C. M., & Nanan, R. (2010). Perinatal risk factors for the neonatal abstinence syndrome in infants born to women on methadone maintenance therapy. *Australian & New Zealand Journal of Obstetrics & Gynaecology, 50*(3), 253–258.

Lott, J. W. (2007). Cardiovascular system. In C. Kenner & J. W. Lott (Eds.), *Comprehensive Neonatal Care: An Interdisciplinary Approach* (4th ed., pp. 32–64). St. Louis, MO: Saunders.

Mahle, W. T., Newburger, J. W., Matherne, G. P., et al. (2009). Role of pulse oximetry in examining newborns for congenital heart disease: a scientific statement from the AHA and AAP. *Pediatrics, 124*(2), 823–836. doi:10.1542/peds.2009 1397

Mahle, W. T., Newburger, J. W., Matherne, G. P., Smith, F. C., Hoke, T. R., Koppel, R., & Grosse, S. D. (2009). Role of pulse oximetry in examining newborns for congenital heart disease: A scientific statement from the AHA and AAP. *Pediatrics, 124*(2), 823–836.

Maisels, M. J. (1990). Gonad protection for phototherapy. *MCN, The American Journal of Maternal Child Nursing, 15*(4), 232.

Maisels, M. J., & McDonagh, A. F. (2008). Phototherapy for neonatal jaundice. *New England Journal of Medicine, 358*, 920–928.

March of Dimes Foundation. (2010a). *Elimination of non-medically indicated (elective) deliveries before 39 weeks gestational age.* Retrieved from http://www.marchofdimes.com/professionals /medicalresources_39weeks.html

March of Dimes Foundation. (2010b). *Toward Improving the Outcome of Pregnancy: Enhancing Perinatal Health Through Quality, Safety and Performance Initiatives* (TIOP III). White Plains, NY: Author.

Martin, J. A., Hamilton, B. E., Sutton, P. D., Ventura, S. J., Mathews, M. S., & Osterman, M. J. K. (2010). Births: Final data for 2008. *National Vital Statistics Reports, 59*(1), 1–105.

Mathur, A. M., Smith, J. R., & Donze, A. (2008). Hypothermia and hypoxic-ischemic encephalopathy: Guideline development using the best evidence. *Neonatal Network, 27*(4), 271–286.

McFadden, E. A. (1991). The Wallaby phototherapy system: A new approach to phototherapy. *Journal of Pediatric Nursing, 6*(3), 206–208.

McGowan, J. E., & Perlman, J. M. (2006). Glucose management during and after intensive delivery room resuscitation. *Clinics in Perinatology, 33*(1), 184–196. doi:10.1016/j.clp.2005.11.007

McGowan, J. E., Rozance, P. J., Price-Douglas, W., & Hay, W. W. (2011). Glucose homeostasis. In S. L. Gardner, B. S. Carter, M. Enzman-Hines, & J. A. Hernandez, *Merenstein & Gardner's Handbook of Neonatal Intensive Care* (7th ed., pp. 353–377). St. Louis, MO: Mosby Elsevier.

Medoff-Cooper, B., Bakewell-Sachs, S., Buus-Frank, M. E., & Santa-Donato, A. (2005). The AWHONN near-term infant initiative: A conceptual framework for optimizing health for near-term infants. *Journal of Obstetric, Gynecologic, and Neonatal Nursing, 34*(6), 666–671. doi:10.1177/0884217505281873

Meier, P. P., Furman, L. M., & Degenhardt, M. (2007). Increased lactation risk for late preterm infants and mothers: Evidence and management strategies to protect breastfeeding. *Journal of Midwifery & Women's Health, 52*(6), 579–587. doi:10.1016/j .jmwh.2007.08.003

Mi Lee, Y., Cleary-Goldman, J., & D'Alton, M. E. (2006). Multiple gestations and late preterm (near-term) deliveries. *Seminars in Perinatology, 30*(2), 103–112. doi:10.1053/j.semperi.2006.03.001

Morse, S. B., Zheng, H., Tang, Y., & Roth, J. (2009). Early school-age outcomes of late preterm infants. *Pediatrics, 123*(4), e622–e629. doi:10.1542/peds.2008-1405

National Center for Health Statistics. (2005). *Public Use Data Tapes. Natality Data Set: 1992–2002.* Hyattsville, MD: U.S. Department of Health and Human Services, Centers for Disease Control and Prevention.

National Institute of Child Health and Human Development Workshop. (2005). Optimizing care and long-term outcome of near-term pregnancy and near-term newborn infant. Workshop held July 18–19, 2005, Bethesda, MD.

Neu, J. (2006). Gastrointestinal maturation and feeding. *Seminars in Perinatology, 30*(2), 77–80.

Ohlin, A., Bjorkqvist, M., Montgomery, S. M., & Schollin, J. (2010). Clinical signs and CRP values associated with blood culture results in neonates evaluated for suspected sepsis. *Acta Paediatrica, 99*(11), 1635–1640. doi:10.1111/j.1651-2227.2010.01913.x

Osborn, D. A., Cole, M. J., & Jeffery, H. E. (2005). Opiate treatment for opiate withdrawal in newborn infants. *Cochrane Database of Systematic Review*, (3), CD002053.

Panel on Antiretroviral Therapy and Medical Management of HIV-Infected Children. (2010). *Guidelines for the use of antiretroviral agents in pediatric HIV infection.* Retrieved from http://aidsinfo .nih/gov/ContentFiles/PediatricGuidelines.pdf

Panel on Treatment of HIV-Infected Pregnant Women and Prevention of Perinatal Transmission. (2012). *Recommendations for Use of Antiretroviral Drugs in Pregnant HIV-1-Infected Women for Maternal Health and Interventions to Reduce Perinatal HIV Transmission in the United States.* Available at http://aidsinfo. nih.gov/contentfiles/lvguidelines/PerinatalGL.pdf.

Pappas, B. E., & Walker, B. (2010). Care of the late preterm infant. In M. T. Verklan & M. Walden (Eds.), *Core Curriculum for Neonatal Intensive Care Nursing* (4th ed., pp. 447–452). St. Louis, MO: Saunders.

Perlman, J. M. (2006). Intervention strategies for neonatal hypoxic-ischemic cerebral injury. *Clinical Therapeutics, 28*(9), 1353–1365. doi:10.1016/j.clinthera.2006.09.005

Perlman, J. M., Wyllie, J., Kattwinkel, J., Atkins, D. L., Chameides, L., Goldsmith, J. P., . . . Velaphi, S. (2010). Neonatal resuscitation: 2010 International consensus on cardiopulmonary resuscitation and emergency cardiovascular care science with treatment recommendations. *Circulation, 122*(Suppl. 2), S516–S538. doi:10.1161/CIRCULATIONAHA.110.971127

Petrini, J. R., Dias, T., McCormick, M. C., Massolo, M. L., Green, N. S., & Escobar, G. J. (2009). Increased risk of adverse neurological development for late preterm infants. *Journal of Pediatrics, 154*(2), 169–176. doi:10.1016/j.jpeds.2008.08.020

Pfister, R. H., & Soll, R. F. (2010). Hypothermia for the treatment of infants with hypoxic-ischemic encephalopathy. *Journal of Perinatology, 30*(S1), S82–S87. doi:10.1038/jp.2010.91

Piazza, A. J., & Stoll, B. J. (2007). Digestive system. In R. M. Kliegman, R. E. Berman, H. B. Jensen, & B. F. Stanton (Eds.), *Nelson Textbook of Pediatrics* (19th ed., pp. 753–766). Philadelphia: Saunders Elsevier.

Public Health Service Task Force. (2006). *Recommendations for use of antiretroviral drugs in pregnant HIV-1-infected women for maternal health and interventions to reduce perinatal HIV-1 transmission in the United States.* U.S. Public Health Service. Retrieved from http://www.aidsinfo.nih.gov, 1–65

Puopolo, K. M. (2008). Epidemiology of neonatal early-onset sepsis. *NeoReviews, 9*(12), e571–e579. doi:10.1542/neo.9-12-e571

Rabi, Y. (2010). Oxygen and resuscitation of the preterm infant. *NeoReviews, 11*(3), e130–e138. doi:10.1542/neo.11-3-e130

Radtke, J. V. (2011). The paradox of breastfeeding-associated morbidity among late preterm infants. *Journal of Obstetrics Gynecologic and Neonatal Nursing, 40*(1), 9–24. doi:10.1111 /j.1552-6909.2010.01211

Raju, T. N., Higgins, R. D., Stark, A. R., & Leveno, K. J. (2006). Optimizing care and outcome for late-preterm (near-term) infants: A summary of the workshop sponsored by the National Institute of Child Health and Human Development. *Pediatrics, 118*(3), 1207–1214. doi:10.1542/peds.2006-0018

Ramachandrappa, A., & Jain, L. (2008). Elective cesarean section: It's impact on neonatal respiratory outcome. *Clinics in Perinatology, 35*(2), 373–393. doi:10.1016/j.clp.2008.03.006

Ramanathan, R., Corwin, M. J., Hunt, C. E., Lister, G., Tinsley, L. R., Baird, T., . . . Keens, T. G. (2001). Cardiorespiratory events recorded on home monitors: Comparison of healthy infants with those at increased risk for SIDS. *The Journal of the American Medical Association, 285*(17), 2199–2207. doi:10.1001/jama.285 .17.2199

Rogers, J. M. (2008). Tobacco and pregnancy: Overview of exposure and effects. *Birth Defects Research, 84*(1), 1–15.

Rohan, A. J., & Golembek, S. G. (2009). Hypoxia in the term newborn: Part 1-cardiopulmonary physiology and assessment. *MCN, The American Journal of Maternal Child Nursing, 34*(2), 106–112. doi:10.1097/01.NMC.0000347304.70208.eb

Rosen, T. S., & Bateman, D. A. (2002). Infants of addicted mothers. In A. A. Fanaroff & R. J. Martin (Eds.), *Neonatal-Perinatal Medicine Diseases of the Fetus and Infant* (7th ed., pp. 661–673). St. Louis, MO: Mosby.

Roth, S. C., Baudin, J., Cady, E. B., Johal, K., Townsend, J. P., Wyatt, J. S., . . . Stewart, A. (1997). Relation of deranged neonatal cerebral oxidative metabolism with neurodevelopmental outcome and head circumference at 4 years. *Developmental Medicine and Child Neurology, 39*(11), 718–725. doi:10.1111/j.1469-8749.1997. tb07372.x

Roth, S. C., Edwards, A. D., Cady, E. B., Delpy, D. T., Wyatt, J. S., Azzopardi, D., . . . Reynolds, E. O. (1992). Relation between cerebral oxidative metabolism following birth asphyxia, and neurodevelopmental outcome and brain growth at one year. *Developmental Medicine and Child Neurology, 34*(4), 285–295. doi:10.1111/j.1469-8749.1992.tb11432.x

Roth-Kleiner, M., Wagner, B. P., Bachmann, D., & Pfenninger, J. (2003). Respiratory distress syndrome in near-term babies after caesarean section. *Swiss Medical Weekly, 133*(19–20), 283–288.

Rozance, P. J., & Hay, W. W. (2010). Describing hypoglycemia: Definition or operational threshold? *Early Human Development, 86*(5), 275–280. doi:10.1016/j.earlhumdev.2010.05.002

Rutherford, M. A., Azzopardi, D., Whitelaw, A., Cowan, F., Renowden, S., Edwards, A. D., & Thoresen, M. (2005). Mild hypothermia and the distribution of cerebral lesions in neonates with hypoxic-ischemic encephalopathy. *Pediatrics, 116*(4), 1001–1006. doi:10.1542/peds.2005-0328

Sadowski, S. L. (2010). Cardiovascular disorders. In M. T. Verklan & M. Walden (Eds.), *Core Curriculum for Neonatal Intensive Care Nursing* (4th ed., pp. 534–588). St. Louis, MO: Saunders.

Sankaran, V. G., & Brown, D. W. (2007). Congenital heart disease. In L. S. Lilly (Ed.), *Pathophysiology of Heart Disease* (4th ed., pp. 371–396). Baltimore, MD: Lippincott Williams & Wilkins.

Sarici, S. U., Serdar, M. A., Korkmaz, A., Erdem, G., Oran, O., Tekinalp, G., & Yigit, S. (2004). Incidence, course and prediction of hyperbilirubinemia in near-term and term newborns. *Pediatrics, 113*(4), 775–780.

Sarnat, H. B., & Sarnat, M. S. (1976). Neonatal encephalopathy following fetal distress: A clinical and electroencephalographic study. *Archives of Neurology, 33*(10), 696–705. doi:10.1001/archneur.1976.00500100030012

Schwartz, H. P., Haberman, B. E., & Ruddy, R. M. (2011). Hyperbilirubinemia: Current guidelines and emerging therapies. *Pediatric Emergency Care, 27*(9), 884–889.

Secretary's Advisory Committee on Heritable Disorders in Newborns and Children. (2011). *HHS Secretary adopts recommendation to add critical congenital heart disease to the Recommended Uniform Screening Panel. September 21, 2011.* Washington, DC: US Department of Health and Human Services. Retrieved from http://www.hrsa.gov/advisorycommittees/mchbadvisory/heritable disordes/recommendations/correspondence/cyanoticheartsecre 09212011.pdf on January 18, 2013.

Selway, L. D. (2010). State of the science: Hypoxic ischemic encephalopathy and hypothermic intervention for neonates. *Advances in Neonatal Care, 10*(2), 60–66. doi:10.1097/ANC.0b013e3181d54b30

Shane, A. L., & Stoll, B. J. (2012). Recent developments and current issues in the epidemiology, diagnosis, and management of bacterial and fungal neonatal sepsis. *American Journal of Perinatology.* doi:http://dx.doi.org/10.1055/s-0032-1333413

Shankaran, S., & Laptook, A. R. (2007). Hypothermia as a treatment for birth asphyxia. *Clinical Obstetrics and Gynecology, 50*(3), 624–635. doi:10.1097/GRF.0b013e31811eba5e

Shankaran, S., Laptook, A. R., Ehrenkranz, R. A., Tyson, J. E., McDonald, S. A., Donovan, E. F., . . . Jobe, A. H. (2005). Whole-body hypothermia for neonates with hypoxic-ischemic encephalopathy. *New England Journal of Medicine, 353*(15), 1574–1584.

Shapiro-Mendoza, C. K., Tomashek, K. M., Kotelchuck, M., Barfield, W., Weiss, J., & Evans, S. (2006). Risk factors for neonatal morbidity and mortality among "healthy," late preterm newborns. *Seminars in Perinatology, 30*(2), 54–60. doi:10.1053/j.semperi.2006.02.002

Sibai, B. M. (2006). Preeclampsia as a cause of preterm and late preterm (near-term) births. *Seminars in Perinatology, 30*(1), 16–19. doi:10.1053/j.semperi.2006.02.002

Smith, J. R., Donze, A., & Schuller, L. (2007). An evidence-based review of hyperbilirubinemia in the late preterm infant, with implications for practice: Management, follow-up, and breast-feeding support. *Neonatal Network, 26*(6), 395–405.

Smitherman, H., Stark, A. R., & Bhutani, V. K. (2006). Early recognition of neonatal hyperbilirubinemia and its emergent management. *Seminars in Fetal and Neonatal Medicine, 11*(3), 214–224. doi:10.1016/j.siny.2006.02.002

Sperling, M. A., & Menon, R. K. (2004). Differential diagnosis and management of neonatal hypoglycemia. *Pediatric Clinics of North America, 51*(3), 703–723. doi:10.1016/j.pcl.2004.01.014

Stayer, S. A., & Liu, Y. (2010). Pulmonary hypertension of the newborn. *Best Practices in Research in Clinical Anaesthesiology, 24*(3), 375–386. doi:10.1016/j.bpa.2010.02.021

Steinhom, R. H., & Farrow, K. N. (2007). Pulmonary hypertension in the neonate. *NeoReviews, 8*(1), e14–e21. doi:10.1542/neo.8-1-e14

Stokowski, L. A. (2006). Fundamentals of phototherapy for neonatal jaundice. *Advances in Neonatal Care, 6*(6), 303–312. doi:10.1016/j.adnc.2006.08.004

Stoll, B. J. (2007a). Infections of the neonatal infant. In R. M. Kliegmen, R. E. Behrman, H. B. Jensen, & B. F. Stanton (Eds.), *Nelson Textbook of Pediatrics* (18th ed., pp. 728–753). Philadelphia: Saunders Elsevier.

Stoll, B. J. (2007b). The endocrine system. In R. M. Kliegmen, R. E. Behrman, H. B. Jensen, & B. F. Stanton (Eds.), *Nelson Textbook of Pediatrics* (18th ed., pp. 782–786). Philadelphia: Saunders Elsevier.

Stoll, B. J., Hansen, N. I., Sanchez, P. J., Faix, R. G., Poindexter, B. B., Van Meurs, K. P., . . . Higgins, R. D. (2011). Early onset neonatal sepsis: The burden of group B streptococcal and E. coli disease continues. *Pediatrics, 127*(5), 817–826. doi:10.1542/peds.2010-2217.

Taylor, R. M., & Price-Douglas, W. (2008). The S.T.A.B.L.E. program: Postresuscitation-pretransport stabilization care of sick infants. *Journal of Perinatal & Neonatal Nursing, 22*(2), 159–165. doi:10.1097/01.JPN.0000319104.05346.b4

Thach, B. T. (2005). Can we breathe and swallow at the same time? *Journal of Applied Physiology, 99*(5), 1633. doi:10.1152/jappl-physiol.00715.2005

Thilo, E. H. (2005). Neonatal jaundice. In P. J. Thureen, J. Deacon, J. A. Hernandez, & D. M. Hall (Eds.), *Assessment and Care of the Well Newborn* (2nd ed., pp. 245–254). St. Louis, MO: Saunders Elsevier.

Thoresen, M. (2008). Supportive care during neuroprotective hypothermia in the term newborn: Adverse effects and their prevention. *Clinics in Perinatology, 35*(4), 749–763. doi:10.1016/j.clp.2008.07.018

Thorne, C., & Newell, M. (2007). HIV. *Seminars in Fetal & Neonatal Medicine, 12*(3), 174–181.

Tita, A. T., Landon, M. B., Spong, C. Y., Lai, Y., Leveno, K. J., Varner, M. W., . . . Mercer, B. M. (2009). Timing of elective repeat cesarean delivery at term and neonatal outcomes. *New England Journal of Medicine, 360*(2), 111–120.

Tomashek, K. M., Shapiro-Mendoza, C. K., Weiss, J., Kotelchuk, M., Barfield, W., Evans, S., . . . Declercq, E. (2006). Early discharge among late preterm and term newborns and risk of neonatal morbidity. *Seminars in Perinatology, 30*(2), 61–68.

Vachharajani, A. J., & Dawson, J. G. (2009). Short-term outcomes of late preterms: An institutional experience. *Clinical Pediatrics, 48*(4), 383–388. doi:10.1177/0009922808324951

Vain, N. E., Szyld, E. G., Prudent, L. M., & Aguilar, A. M. (2009). What (not) to do at and after delivery? Prevention and management of meconium aspiration syndrome. *Early Human Development, 85*(10), 621–626. doi:10.1016/j.earlhumdev.2009.09.013

van Lerland, Y., & de Beaufort, A. J. (2009). Why does meconium cause meconium aspiration syndrome? Current concepts of MAS pathophysiology. *Early Human Development, 85*(10), 617–620. doi:10.1016/j.earlhumdev.2009.09.009

Velaphi, S. V., & Vidyasagar, D. (2006). Intrapartum and postdelivery management of infants born to mothers with meconium-stained amniotic fluid: Evidence-based recommendations. *Clinics in Perinatology, 33*(1), 29–42. doi:10.1016/j.clp.2005.11.014

Verani, J. R., McGee, L., & Schrag, S. J. (2010). Prevention of perinatal group B streptococcal disease—Revised guidelines from CDC, 2010. *Morbidity & Mortality Weekly Report, 59*(RR-10), 1–36.

Walker, M. (2008). Breastfeeding the late preterm infant. *Journal of Obstetrics Gynecologic & Neonatal Nursing, 37*(6), 692–701. doi:10.1111/j.1552-6909.2008.00293.x

Wang, M. L., Dorer, D. J., Fleming, M. P., & Catlin, E. A. (2004). Clinical outcomes of near-term infants. *Pediatrics, 114*(2), 372–376.

Ward, R. M. (2006). Drug disposition in the late preterm ("near-term") newborn. *Seminars in Perinatology, 30*(1), 48–51. doi:10.1053/j.semperi.2006.01.013

Warren, J. B., & Anderson, J. M. (2009). Core concepts: Respiratory distress syndrome. *NeoReviews, 10*(7), e351–e361. doi:10.1542/neo.10-7-e351

Watchko, J. F., & Maisels, M. J. (2010). Enduring controversies in the management of hyperbilirubinemia in preterm neonates. *Seminars in Fetal & Neonatal Medicine, 15*, 136–140.

Weiner, S. M., & Finnegan, L. P. (1998). Drug withdrawal in the neonate. In B. B. Merenstein & S. L. Gardner (Eds.), *Handbook of Neonatal Intensive Care* (4th ed.). St. Louis, MO: Mosby.

Wight, N. E., Morton, J. A., & Kim, J. H. (2008). Breastfeeding the late preterm infant. In *Best Medicine: Human Milk in the NICU* (pp. 137–161). Amarillo, TX: Hale.

Williams, A. F. (2005). Neonatal hypoglycaemia: Clinical and legal aspects. *Seminars in Fetal and Neonatal Medicine, 10*(4), 363–368. doi:10.1016/j.siny.2009.12.003

Williams, C. E., Gunn, A., & Gluckman, P. D. (1991). Time course of intracellular edema and epileptiform activity following prenatal cerebral ischemia in sheep. *Stroke, 22*(4), 516–521. doi:10.1161/01.STR.22.4.516

Xu, H., Wei, S., & Fraser, W. D. (2008). Obstetric approaches to the prevention of meconium aspiration syndrome. *Journal of Perinatology, 28*(S3), S14–S18. doi:10.1038/jp.2008.145

Yurdakok, M. (2010). Transient tachypnea of the newborn: What is new? *Journal of Maternal-Fetal & Neonatal Medicine, 3*, S24–S26.

Zahorodny, W., Rom, C., Whitney, W., Giddens, S., Samuel, M., Maichuk, G., & Marshall, R. (1998). The neonatal withdrawal inventory: A simplified score of newborn withdrawal. *Journal of Developmental and Behavioral Pediatrics, 19*(2), 89–93.

Zaichkin, J., & Weiner, G. M. (2011). Neonatal resuscitation program (NRP) 2011: New science, new strategies. *Neonatal Network, 30*(1), 5–13. doi:10.1891/0710-0832.30.1.5

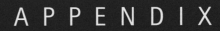
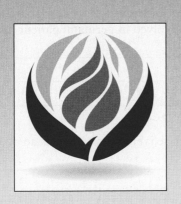

Item Bank Questions and Answer Key

QUESTIONS

CHAPTER 1 PERINATAL PATIENT SAFETY AND PROFESSIONAL LIABILITY ISSUES

Multiple Choice

1. Inpatient obstetric care results in approximately what percentage of malpractice claims in obstetrics and gynecology?

   a. 25%
   b. 50%
   c. 75%

2. Guidance for ethical nursing care is provided by the

   a. American Nurses Association *Code of Ethics for Nurses.*
   b. American Academy of Pediatrics (AAP) & American College of Obstetricians and Gynecologists (ACOG) *Guidelines for Perinatal Care*
   c. American Medical Association *Code of Medical Ethics.*

3. Disruptive clinician behavior

   a. is often directly linked to clinical practice issues.
   b. rarely involves clinical practice issues.
   c. should be handled separately from clinical practice issues.

4. The best approach for addressing disruptive clinician behavior is

   a. immediate intervention.
   b. monitoring trends.
   c. peer review.

5. Successful defense of malpractice claims is enhanced by following

   a. community standards.
   b. national professional standards.
   c. trends in practice.

6. When a sentinel event occurs, according to The Joint Commission (TJC),

   a. a root-cause analysis should be conducted.
   b. it must be reported to TJC within 60 days.
   c. those involved should be placed on administrative leave pending an investigation.

7. Based on TJC criteria, which of the following clinical situations is a sentinel event?

   a. Any unexplained adverse occurrence
   b. Birth of a baby with previously undiagnosed congenital abnormalities
   c. Unanticipated death of a full-term infant

8. The purpose of the root-cause analysis process is to

   a. determine fault of the healthcare provider or hospital.
   b. examine institutional liability.
   c. review potentially contributing systems.

9. Professional nursing liability is most commonly increased by the absence of

   a. adequate medical record documentation.
   b. annual competency validation.
   c. current unit policies and procedures.

10. An incident-management program will

    a. include "near misses" with potential for adverse outcomes.
    b. identify and discipline those at fault.
    c. increase institutional and nursing liability.

11. Nurse/physician difference of opinion about patient management should be

    a. considered unprofessional behavior.
    b. discussed with the patient's family.
    c. focused on the issue in question.

12. Despite repeated requests to a physician to come to the bedside to evaluate a deteriorating maternal condition, the physician has failed to respond. The nurse appropriately

    a. consults with another physician in the unit.
    b. institutes the chain of command/chain of consultation.
    c. provides the intervention indicated.

13. Outcome measures of patient safety include

    a. how care is delivered.
    b. policies and procedures.
    c. rates of maternal morbidity and mortality.

14. Structure measures of patient safety include

    a. the number of elective inductions of labor prior to 39 completed weeks' gestation.
    b. the rates of third- and fourth-degree lacerations.
    c. unit protocols.

15. Process measures of patient safety include

    a. how tachysystole is identified and treated.
    b. number of nurses who are certified in fetal monitoring.
    c. rates of cesarean birth for indeterminate fetal status.

16. Qualitative measures of patient safety include

    a. focus groups.
    b. number of sentinel events per year.
    c. policies and procedures consistent with national standards and guidelines.

Fill in the Blank

17. Essential criteria for safe care include

    _____

    _____

    _____

    _____

18. The areas of clinical practice that are most commonly involved in perinatal patient harm are

    _____

    _____

    _____

19. In a high-reliability unit, there is an agreement that

    _____

20. Standards and guidelines from professional organizations and regulatory agencies should guide clinical practice. These organizations and agencies include

    _____

    _____

    _____

    _____

21. According to ACOG (2009) misoprostol is not recommended for women _____.

22. Elective labor induction should not occur prior to _____.

23. According to ACOG (2009), the preferred method of fetal assessment during labor for women with high-risk conditions is _____.

24. Second-stage pushing should be initiated when _____ or when more than 2 hours have passed since complete dilation for _____ women or more than 1 hour has passed since complete dilation for _____ women.

25. ACOG and the Association of Women's Health, Obstetric and Neonatal Nurses (AWHONN) recommend use of the _____ definitions for fetal assessment during labor.

26. Triage for pregnant women who present for care should be based on guidelines from the _____.

27. Communication between patients and health-care providers can be protective against _____.

28. During clinical emergencies, the timing of medical record documentation is often _____.

29. The practice of duplicate documentation on the fetal monitoring strip and the medical record is _____, and it contributes to _____.

30. A serious adverse event is defined by TJC as a _____.

31. The recommended nurse-to-patient ratio during oxytocin administration is _____.

32. The recommended nurse-to-patient ratio in the second stage of labor is _____.

33. Notifying the charge nurse when the staff nurse remains concerned about a physician's plan of care after appropriate attempts to resolve the issues is an example of implementing the _____.

CHAPTER 2 INTEGRATING CULTURAL BELIEFS AND PRACTICES WHEN CARING FOR CHILDBEARING WOMEN AND FAMILIES

Multiple Choice

1. A 25-year-old Vietnamese woman admitted to the birthing unit requests that her husband stay in the waiting area until after she gives birth. The appropriate response is based on the nurse's knowledge that

   a. all husbands should be present during labor and birth.
   b. the husband may fear his response to his wife giving birth.
   c. the woman's request should be honored.

2. Wang Din Wah, a Laotian mother who is 24 hours postpartum, rejects the nurse's instructions to bring the newborn back to the clinic by the 7th day of life for a phenylketonuria test. Wang's reasons for this refusal are most likely based on

   a. her lack of recognition of appropriate health-care for the baby.
   b. the baby's early care being provided largely by the maternal grandmother.
   c. the first month after birth being considered a time for confinement and rest.

3. Berta Wolf Creek is 4 hours postpartum and requests permission to take her placenta home with her. Appropriate instruction by the nurse would include

   a. keeping the placenta in a leakproof container.
   b. requiring disposal of the placenta by internment (burial).
   c. keeping the placenta frozen until burial.

4. Maria Ochoa, a 23-year-old Filipino American, is 18 weeks pregnant. After receiving a prescription for prenatal vitamins, she tells the nurse that her mother has warned her to take only herbal medication during pregnancy. The nurse appropriately

   a. advises Maria that the pills are only vitamins and not considered medication.
   b. assesses the significance of Maria's mother's advice.
   c. reminds her that the vitamins were ordered by the nurse-midwife.

5. The percentage of the U.S. population who are African American or black is nearly

   a. 6%.
   b. 13%.
   c. 20%.

6. An African American/black woman who believes she should not swallow her saliva and carries a spit cup with her during pregnancy is most likely from

   a. Barbados.
   b. Haiti.
   c. West Indies.

7. A major cultural group of childbearing women at increased risk for alcoholism, heart disease, cirrhosis of the liver, and diabetes mellitus is the population of women who are

   a. African American/black.
   b. American Indian/Alaskan native.
   c. Asian American/Pacific Islander.

8. According to the hot/cold theory, pregnancy is thought to be which kind of a condition?

   a. cold
   b. hot
   c. lukewarm

9. Match the sacred day of worship with the religious group.

   a. Sunday

   b. Sunset Friday to sunset Saturday

   c. Sunset Thursday to sunset Friday

   1. Jewish or Seventh-Day Adventists

   2. Most Christians

   3. Muslims

10. Ethnocentrism is the belief that

    a. cultural values are major determiners of one's behavior.
    b. every cultural group has a core or center of common beliefs.
    c. values and practices of one's own culture are superior.

11. A woman whose discharge plan includes her mother-in-law caring for her and her newborn during the postpartum period by tradition is most likely from which of the following cultures?

    a. Korean
    b. Laotian
    c. Tongan

12. What percentage of nurses come from racial or ethnic minority backgrounds?

    a. 9%
    b. 13%
    c. 17%

13. Goals each nurse can set to increase cultural competence while caring for culturally diverse childbearing women and their families are described as

    a. culturally driven.
    b. externally based.
    c. self-generated.

Fill in the Blank

14. Identify three strategies to increase the cultural competence of the nurse.

    1) _____
    2) _____
    3) _____

CHAPTER 3 PHYSIOLOGIC CHANGES OF PREGNANCY

Multiple Choice

1. By 28 to 34 weeks' gestation in a normal pregnancy, blood volume has increased by approximately

   a. 10% to 20%.
   b. 30% to 50%.
   c. 60% to 80%.

2. During pregnancy, the position for optimum maternal cardiac output is

   a. lateral.
   b. semi-Fowler's.
   c. supine.

3. During labor, maternal cardiac output

   a. decreases slightly.
   b. increases progressively.
   c. remains the same.

4. An intravenous (IV) fluid bolus is given before epidural anesthesia to prevent

   a. hypotension.
   b. renal hypoperfusion.
   c. sympathetic blockade.

5. Normally during pregnancy, maternal sitting and standing diastolic blood pressure readings

   a. decrease, then increase.
   b. increase progressively.
   c. remain unchanged.

6. The volume of the maternal autotransfusion immediately after birth is approximately

   a. 600 mL.
   b. 800 mL.
   c. 1,000 mL.

7. What happens to maternal P_aO_2 and P_aCO_2 levels during pregnancy?

   a. Both decrease.
   b. Both increase.
   c. P_aO_2 increases and P_aCO_2 decreases.

8. The slight increase in pH that occurs during pregnancy is due to

   a. a decrease in hemoglobin and hematocrit.
   b. a decrease in renal excretion of bicarbonate.
   c. an increase in ventilatory rate.

9. During pregnancy, serum urea and creatine levels

   a. decrease.
   b. increase.
   c. remain constant.

10. Heartburn is common during pregnancy due primarily to

    a. decreased gastric motility.
    b. increased secretion of hydrochloric acid.
    c. relaxation of the lower esophageal sphincter.

11. A physical finding that may occur during pregnancy in response to normal cardiovascular changes is

    a. decreased heart rate.
    b. dependent edema.
    c. elevated blood pressure.

12. The average blood loss during vaginal birth is less than

    a. 300 mL.
    b. 500 mL.
    c. 700 mL.

13. The average blood loss during cesarean birth is less than

    a. 600 mL.
    b. 800 mL.
    c. 1,000 mL.

14. During pregnancy, cardiac output increases approximately

    a. 10% to 25%.
    b. 30% to 50%.
    c. 60% to 75%.

15. Cardiac output is greatest during which period of the birth process?

    a. First stage, active phase
    b. Immediately after birth
    c. Second stage

16. A cardiovascular parameter which normally decreases during pregnancy is

    a. heart rate.
    b. stroke volume.
    c. systemic vascular resistance.

17. An expected white blood cell count during labor and the early postpartum is

    a. 8,000 to 10,000 mm^3.
    b. 13,000 to 15,000 mm^3.
    c. 20,000 to 22,000 mm^3.

18. Which of the following coagulation factors does not increase during pregnancy?

    a. Fibrin
    b. Platelets
    c. Fibrinogen

19. Which of the following increases during pregnancy?

    a. Colloid oncotic pressure
    b. Glomerular filtration rate
    c. Serum osmolality

20. By term, blood flow to the uterus is approximately

    a. 200 mL/min.
    b. 500 mL/min.
    c. 800 mL/min.

21. During pregnancy, the pigmented line in the skin that traverses the abdomen longitudinally from the sternum to the symphysis is called the

    a. linea nigra.
    b. spider nevus.
    c. striae gravidarum.

22. Which of the following is a change occurring in the respiratory system during pregnancy?

    a. Oxygen consumption increases.
    b. Respiratory rate decreases.
    c. Tidal volume decreases.

23. A normal finding during pregnancy is

    a. glycosuria.
    b. hematuria.
    c. proteinuria.

24. The respiratory system parameter that decreases during pregnancy is the

    a. functional residual capacity.
    b. minute ventilation.
    c. vital capacity.

25. A metabolic change characteristic of late pregnancy is decreased

    a. blood free fatty acid levels.
    b. insulin sensitivity.
    c. serum glucose levels after meals.

Fill in the Blank

26. Metabolic changes are characterized by _____ during the first half of pregnancy and _____ during the second half.

27. The greater increase in plasma volume than in red blood cell volume results in _____.

28. Maternal weight gain during the first half of pregnancy is primarily due to changes in the weight of the _____.

29. Both maternal metabolic rate and thyroid hormone levels _____ during pregnancy.

30. The primary determinant of volume hemostasis is _____.

31. The renal clearance of many substances is increased during pregnancy due to the _____.

32. Normal stretching of the skin and hormonal changes during gestation may produce "stretch marks" that are called _____.

33. The hormone released from the anterior pituitary that is responsible for initiating lactation is _____.

34. The increased maternal intestinal absorption of calcium is due to increased _____.

35. Compared to nonpregnant women, a pregnant woman in the third trimester has a _____ initial fasting blood glucose.

36. The hormone responsible for maintaining progesterone and estrogen production by the ovaries until the placenta is established is _____.

37. Placental production of the hormone _____ requires interaction of the mother, fetus, and placenta.

38. Increases in plasma volume and red cell mass result in an increase in _____ during pregnancy.

39. Cardiac output progressively decreases postpartum and returns to nonpregnant levels by _____.

40. The _____ accommodates one third of the additional maternal blood volume at term.

41. The hormone _____ produces relaxation of smooth muscle and vasodilation.

42. Blood pressure reaches its lowest point at _____ weeks.

43. During pregnancy, the woman becomes resistant to the pressor effects of _____.

44. Pregnancy is considered a _____ state due to the increases of several essential coagulation factors.

45. The pregnant woman is at increased risk for venous thrombus formation due to _____ and _____.

46. _____ are potent vasodilators that affect smooth muscle contractility and play an important role in labor onset, myometrial contractility, and cervical ripening.

47. Irregularly shaped brown blotches on the face are known as _____, or the "mask of pregnancy."

48. The bluish discoloration of the cervix occurring during pregnancy is known as _____ sign.

CHAPTER 4 ANTENATAL CARE

Multiple Choice

1. Between 2009 and 2011, for the first time in 30 years, the preterm birth rate in the United States has

   a. declined.
   b. increased.
   c. remained the same.

2. An appropriate recommendation for weight gain for an underweight pregnant woman would be

   a. 20 lb.
   b. 25 lb.
   c. 30 lb.

3. The best time to encourage a woman to stop smoking is

   a. before pregnancy.
   b. as soon as she knows she is pregnant.
   c. by the end of the first trimester.

4. The time during pregnancy when blood pressure is lowest in the normotensive woman is the

   a. first trimester.
   b. second trimester.
   c. third trimester.

5. The time when measurement of fundal height in centimeters should correlate with gestational age is

   a. after 20 weeks' gestation.
   b. near term.
   c. before 20 weeks' gestation.

6. Planning culturally specific care includes

   a. making sure that a translator is available when requested.
   b. noting patterns of decision making in the family.
   c. using a translator at each visit.

7. A nonreactive nonstress test at 39 weeks' gestation is an indication for

   a. expedited birth.
   b. further testing.
   c. reassurance about fetal status.

8. Health promotion and education to improve pregnancy outcome in the next generation should begin when

   a. children are in elementary school.
   b. pregnancy occurs in the peer group.
   c. teens are sexually active.

9. An appropriate gestational age for a glucose screening test is at

   a. 23 weeks' gestation.
   b. 26 weeks' gestation.
   c. 29 weeks' gestation.

10. Risk assessment for all women during the initial prenatal visit should include

    a. a complete health history.
    b. a triple screen.
    c. an ultrasound for fetal anomalies.

11. Which of the following puts a woman at risk for nutritional problems during pregnancy?

    a. Advanced maternal age
    b. Cigarette smoking
    c. Gravida III, Term I, Preterm 0, Abortion I, Living Child I

12. An effect of cigarette smoking during pregnancy is increased incidence of

    a. low birth weight and prematurity.
    b. neonatal transient tachypnea of the newborn.
    c. pregnancy-induced hypertension.

13. Maternal serum alpha-fetoprotein specifically screens for

    a. heart defects.
    b. neural tube defects.
    c. placental defects.

14. If both parents are affected by sickle cell disease, the risk of their children being affected by sickle cell disease is

    a. 25%.
    b. 50%.
    c. 100%.

15. A primary method of fetal surveillance during pregnancy is

    a. fetal kick counts.
    b. nonstress testing.
    c. ultrasonography.

16. The most significant food shortages for low-income women occur

    a. at the end of the month, when federal/local resources diminish.
    b. before Women, Infants, and Children (WIC) eligibility is determined.
    c. postpartum, when fatigue prevents appointments with WIC.

17. A key component of preterm birth prevention education is

    a. discussing the hospital admission criteria.
    b. empowering the woman to act on her own instincts and self-knowledge.
    c. involving the significant other in the teaching.

True or False

18. True/False: With low income, the risk of perinatal morbidity increases after the age of 35 years, but with adequate income and healthcare, women have only a slight increase in gestational diabetes or pregnancy-induced hypertension.

Fill in the Blank

19. The monitoring of fetal activity by kick counts is initiated at _____ weeks' gestation.

20. It is recommended that every woman have an initial serology and gonorrhea culture and that the tests be repeated at _____ weeks.

21. The recommended weight gain for an obese woman during pregnancy is _____.

22. Approximately _____ % of human malformations are caused by genetic factors alone.

23. A _____ is an agent that causes congenital malformations.

24. A biophysical profile summative score of _____ or greater is considered a sign of fetal well-being.

25. Male and female genitalia are recognizable by _____ weeks' gestation.

26. Tay-Sachs disease is a recessive disorder common in families of _____ ancestry.

27. The anticoagulant drug _____ is a known teratogen.

28. Folic acid requirements are increased to _____ times normal during pregnancy.

29. List three basic components of prenatal care.

   1) _____
   2) _____
   3) _____

30. Moderate physical activity during an uncomplicated pregnancy maintains _____ and _____ fitness.

31. Diagnosis of gestational diabetes mellitus is made when a glucose tolerance test result has _____.

32. Maternal serum screening is offered between _____ and _____ weeks' gestation.

33. A healthy fetus usually has _____ perceivable movements in 1 hour.

34. List the five parameters assessed in the biophysical profile.

   1) _____
   2) _____
   3) _____
   4) _____
   5) _____

CHAPTER 5 HYPERTENSIVE DISORDERS OF PREGNANCY

Multiple Choice

1. A diagnosis of severe preeclampsia is consistent with a 24-hour urine showing protein excretion of

   a. 1 g/L.
   b. 3 g/L.
   c. 5 g/L.

2. An indication of impending magnesium sulfate toxicity in the patient being treated for preeclampsia is the absence of

   a. deep tendon reflexes.
   b. fetal movement.
   c. urine output.

3. The therapeutic range of serum magnesium during magnesium sulfate therapy to prevent eclamptic seizures is

   a. 1 to 4 mg/dL.
   b. 5 to 8 mg/dL.
   c. 9 to 12 mg/dL.

4. The first priority in the care of a patient during an eclamptic seizure is to

   a. administer an anticonvulsant agent.
   b. ensure a patent airway.
   c. establish IV access.

5. Diagnosis of preeclampsia requires the presence of hypertension and

   a. edema.
   b. headaches.
   c. proteinuria.

6. Severe preeclampsia can be diagnosed in the presence of

   a. excretion of 4,500 g protein in a 24-hour urine collection.
   b. serial diastolic blood pressures of at least 110 mm Hg.
   c. serum blood urea nitrogen of 10 mg/dL with a serum creatinine of 1 mg/dL.

Fill in the Blank

7. _____ disorders are the most common medical complication of pregnancy.

8. A diastolic blood pressure of _____ mm Hg on two occasions at least 6 hours apart is necessary for diagnosis of severe preeclampsia.

9. The blood pressure should be recorded with the pregnant woman in the _____ position.

10. _____ is the drug of choice to prevent seizure activity in the patient with preeclampsia.

11. Maternal morbidity from hypertension in pregnancy results from

    1) _____
    2) _____
    3) _____
    4) _____

12. The goals of antihypertensive therapy in the woman with preeclampsia are to _____ and to _____.

13. Laboratory markers for HELLP syndrome are _____, _____, and _____.

14. A leading cause of maternal morbidity following an eclamptic seizure is _____.

CHAPTER 6 BLEEDING IN PREGNANCY

Multiple Choice

1. Invasion of the trophoblastic cells into the uterine myometrium is termed *placenta*

   a. *accreta.*
   b. *increta.*
   c. *percreta.*

2. The incidence of placenta previa is increasing likely due to

   a. better diagnostic tools such as transvaginal ultrasound.
   b. increased rate of cesarean birth.
   c. more women delaying childbirth until they are older.

3. Painless, bright red vaginal bleeding at 28 weeks' gestation is most likely due to

   a. abruptio placentae.
   b. placenta previa.
   c. uterine rupture.

4. A clinical finding associated with a dehiscence of a uterine scar during a trial of labor after cesarean birth (TOLAC) is

   a. cessation of uterine contractions.
   b. fetal heart rate (FHR) with variable decelerations.
   c. sudden decrease of intrauterine pressure.

5. The initial drug of choice for excessive bleeding in the immediate postpartum period is

   a. Methergine IM.
   b. oxytocin IV infusion.
   c. prostaglandin 15-MF$_{2}\alpha$ suppository.

6. The most common cause of postpartum hemorrhage is

   a. an atonic uterus.
   b. a cervical laceration.
   c. a placenta accreta.

7. In the last 10 years in the United States, the maternal mortality rate has

   a. decreased.
   b. stabilized.
   c. increased.

8. Which group has the highest maternal mortality rate?

   a. African American women
   b. Hispanic women
   c. Native American women

9. Approximately two thirds of maternal trauma seen in the emergency department is related to

   a. domestic violence/intimate partner violence.
   b. falls at home or in the workplace.
   c. motor vehicle accidents.

10. The risk of uterine inversion is increased with

    a. a prior uterine scar.
    b. suprapubic pressure.
    c. traction applied to the cord.

11. Cervical laceration/s after birth should be suspected if

    a. estimated blood loss exceeds 500 mL.
    b. the mother reports severe cramping pain.
    c. the uterus is well contracted but frank bleeding continues.

Fill in the Blank

12. Vasa previa is the result of a _____ insertion of the cord.

13. For the fetus to maintain adequate oxygenation, the maternal oxygen saturation must be at least _____%.

14. _____ is a late sign of hypovolemia in the woman experiencing bleeding during pregnancy.

15. Active management of the third stage of labor involves

    1) _____
    2) _____
    3) _____
    4) _____

CHAPTER 7 PRETERM LABOR AND BIRTH

Multiple Choice

1. Which of the following is not a common symptom of preterm labor?

    a. Headache
    b. Menstrual-like cramps
    c. Pelvic pressure

2. One of the three most common risk factors predictive of preterm birth is

    a. low prepregnancy weight.
    b. smoking during pregnancy.
    c. history of preterm birth.

3. When considering nursing care of the woman in preterm labor, which of the following is true?

    a. Maternal transport to a high-risk center has improved outcome over neonatal transport to a special care nursery.
    b. The effect of antenatal glucocorticoid treatment is immediate.
    c. Tocolysis has great effectiveness in delaying preterm birth by 7 days.

4. A drug that is used for tocolysis but is not classified as a beta-mimetic is

    a. Procardia.
    b. ritodrine.
    c. terbutaline.

5. To accurately be considered preterm, an infant must be

    a. born at gestational age <37 weeks.
    b. <10th percentile in weight.
    c. small for gestational age.

6. Teaching pregnant women about the symptoms of preterm labor

    a. has been shown to prevent preterm birth.
    b. should be ongoing throughout pregnancy.
    c. should only be done on a one-to-one basis.

7. When administering IV fluids for a woman with preterm contractions, it is important to consider that

    a. IV hydration has not been shown to be an effective preventative measure for preterm birth.
    b. preterm labor contractions usually diminish within 1 hour of initiation of IV hydration.
    c. the first liter of IV fluid should be administered within the first hour of the admission.

8. Antenatal glucocorticoid administration for acceleration of fetal lung maturation is appropriate

    a. for all women who could give birth preterm before 37 weeks' gestation.
    b. for woman at 24 to 34 weeks' gestation at risk for preterm birth within 7 days
    c. once a week from the time of significant preterm symptoms until birth or 34 weeks' gestation, whichever comes first.

9. Research has shown that bed rest

    a. allows the pregnant woman to gain appropriate amounts of weight.
    b. causes bone demineralization.
    c. inhibits preterm labor contractions.

10. Smoking during pregnancy

    a. has been shown to decrease if cessation programs are offered.
    b. is best eradicated using the 2As program.
    c. is not a factor in risk of preterm birth.

Fill in the Blank

11. Preterm birth in the United States is _____ among African Americans than among whites.

12. During the past several years, rates of preterm birth have _____.

13. We now know that the term *Braxton-Hicks contractions* should be _____ from prenatal care teaching.

14. Early term births are often _____.

15. Signs and symptoms of preterm labor include

    _____

    _____

    _____

    _____

    _____

    _____

CHAPTER 8 DIABETES IN PREGNANCY

Multiple Choice

1. An indication to initiate insulin in a pregnant woman with gestational diabetes is

   a. fasting blood sugar (FBS) <85 mg/dL on two or more occasions.
   b. FBS = normal but 2-hour postprandial = >100 mg/dL.
   c. FBS = >95 mg/dL and 2-hour postprandial = >120 mg/dL.

2. Hypoglycemia is defined as a plasma blood glucose of

   a. less than 60 mg/dL.
   b. greater than 80 mg/dL.
   c. exactly 90 mg/dL.

3. To assist in controlling blood glucose, the recommendation for pregnant women with gestational diabetes is to exercise

   a. daily for less than 20 minutes.
   b. every other day for 45 minutes.
   c. at least three times a week for 20 minutes.

4. Women with a history of gestational diabetes with a normal postpartum follow-up test should be tested for overt diabetes

   a. every 3 years.
   b. before a subsequent pregnancy.
   c. a and b.

5. Intensive management of diabetes in women with pregestational diabetes should begin

   a. prior to conception.
   b. postpartum.
   c. only if planning to breast-feed.

6. In women with diabetes, medical nutrition therapy

   a. is not necessary.
   b. has no effect on glycemic control.
   c. is a vital component of care.

7. For women with diabetes, breastfeeding

   a. can prevent pregnancy.
   b. is contraindicated; a baby should be bottle-fed.
   c. has been associated with reduced incidence of childhood obesity and diabetes later in life.

8. Diagnostic testing for gestational diabetes is accomplished using a

   a. 2-hour 75-g oral glucose tolerance test.
   b. 3-hour 100-g oral glucose tolerance test.
   c. either a or b

9. Insulin dosage during periods of nausea and vomiting in pregnant women should be

   a. administered with no adjustment.
   b. based on a sliding scale.
   c. withheld until nausea is resolved.

10. Weekly nonstress testing should be initiated in women with vascular disease beginning at the gestational age of

    a. 28 weeks.
    b. 30 weeks.
    c. 32 weeks.

Fill in the Blank

11. _____ diabetes results due to an autoimmune reaction directed at the pancreas following an environmental trigger.

12. Metabolic changes during the first half of pregnancy characterized by fat storage is called the _____ phase.

13. List five diabetogenic hormones of pregnancy.

    1) _____
    2) _____
    3) _____
    4) _____
    5) _____

14. Preterm labor in women with diabetes should be treated with _____.

15. Three specific symptoms of hyperglycemia are

    1) _____
    2) _____
    3) _____

CHAPTER 9 CARDIAC DISEASE IN PREGNANCY

Multiple Choice

1. Congenital cardiac disease occurs in what approximate percentage of live births?

    a. 0.8%
    b. 1.5%
    c. 2.0%

2. Maternal outcomes in pregnancies of women with Marfan syndrome are related to

    a. cardiac dysrhythmias.
    b. degree of aortic root dilation.
    c. hypervolemia of pregnancy.

3. Symptoms indicative of heart disease in pregnancy include

    a. jugular venous distention, tachycardia, pedal edema, Grade II/VI systolic murmur.
    b. palpitations, exertional dyspnea, irregular syncope, third heart sound.
    c. severe dyspnea, diastolic murmurs, syncope with exertion, chest pain with exertion.

4. In a review of hospitalizations in the United States from 1995 to 2006, steady increases were seen in what conditions?

    a. Congenital heart disease, valvular disease from rheumatic fever, cardiomyopathy, and cardiac arrhythmias

    b. Acute myocardial infarction and peripartum cardiomyopathy
    c. Mitral valve prolapse, mitral stenosis, and acute myocardial infarction

5. The peak incidence of peripartum cardiomyopathy is during

    a. the third trimester of pregnancy.
    b. labor and birth.
    c. the second month postpartum.

6. A pregnant woman with New York Heart Association (NYHA) class II cardiac disease is symptomatic with

    a. bed rest.
    b. mild exertion.
    c. heavy exertion.

7. The drug of choice to treat epidural analgesia–related hypotension for a pregnant woman with a cardiac disorder would be

    a. dopamine.
    b. ephedrine.
    c. phenylephrine.

8. The time during labor and birth when cardiac output increases the most is during

    a. second stage with fetal descent.
    b. birth.
    c. the immediate postpartum period.

9. The physiologic changes of pregnancy that tend to be problematic for women with cardiac disease include

    a. decreased functional residual lung capacity, relaxation of the cardiac sphincter, and hypotension.
    b. increase in blood volume, decrease in systemic vascular resistance, the hypercoagulable state of pregnancy. and fluctuations in cardiac output.
    c. tachycardia and decreased blood volume.

10. An initial sign of inadequate cerebral perfusion is

    a. low pulse oximeter readings.
    b. restlessness.
    c. unequal pupil dilation.

Fill in the Blank

11. _____ regulate the distribution of extracellular fluid.

12. Mitral and aortic stenosis are examples of cardiac diseases caused by _____.

13. A diagnostic test often used for diagnosis of myocardial infarction is_____.

14. Current risk counseling for pregnant women with cardiac disease is based on the _____ and the _____.

15. The NYHA classification system for cardiac disease categorizes patients by _____.

CHAPTER 10 PULMONARY COMPLICATIONS IN PREGNANCY

Multiple Choice

1. During pregnancy, predicted values of peak expiratory flow rates are

   a. decreased.
   b. increased.
   c. unchanged.

2. The mainstay of asthma pharmacologic therapy is

   a. beta-2 agonists.
   b. corticosteroids.
   c. immunotherapy.

3. Moderate to severe asthma is apparent when respiratory rate is greater than

   a. 20 breaths per minute.
   b. 30 breaths per minute.
   c. 40 breaths per minute.

4. During an exacerbation of asthma, there is

   a. decreased functional residual capacity.
   b. increased expiratory airflow.
   c. increased peripheral vascular resistance.

5. A breath sound rarely auscultated in asthmatics is

   a. rales.
   b. rhonchi.
   c. wheezes.

6. The most commonly seen pneumonia of pregnancy is

   a. aspiration.
   b. bacterial.
   c. viral.

7. A complication seen in up to 26% of women with varicella pneumonia in the first 20 weeks of gestation is

   a. intrauterine infection.
   b. pneumothorax.
   c. small-for-gestational-age fetus.

8. When aspiration pneumonia occurs during pregnancy, it is most commonly a result of

   a. bronchitis.
   b. general anesthesia.
   c. smoking.

9. Initial arterial blood gases in the pregnant woman with pneumonia usually reflect significant

   a. acidosis.
   b. hypercapnia.
   c. hypoxia.

10. Hypoxia should be suspected when a pregnant woman is noted to have

    a. hypotension.
    b. increased urine output.
    c. restlessness.

Fill in the Blank

11. Exacerbations of asthma will occur during the intrapartum period _____ % of the time.

12. Maintaining oxygen saturation of greater than _____ % by pulse oximetry is vital for a pregnant woman with pneumonia.

13. After birth, _____ % of women will return to the prepregnancy status of their asthma.

14. A lifestyle risk factor that may increase a woman's risk of acquiring pneumonia during pregnancy is _____.

15. The most common bacterial pathogen in pneumonia during pregnancy is _____.

16. The maternal position that best supports maximum oxygenation is _____.

17. Common inhalation irritants for many asthmatics are _____.

18. Markers for potentially fatal asthma are _____.

19. Maternal complications of pneumonia during pregnancy are _____.

20. During pregnancy, _____% of women with asthma will experience worsening of symptoms.

CHAPTER 11 MULTIPLE GESTATION

Multiple Choice

1. Multiple birth rates have increased most dramatically in which maternal age group?

   a. 25 to 30 years
   b. 30 to 35 years
   c. 45 to 54 years

2. The likelihood of monozygotic twinning is affected by

   a. older maternal age.
   b. use of assisted reproductive technologies.
   c. black maternal race.

3. The lambda sign, a triangle-shaped ultrasound marker seen at the junction of the chorions and amnions, indicates

   a. monozygotic gestation.
   b. dizygotic gestation.
   c. trizygotic gestation.

4. An itching rash prominent in stretch marks in a woman pregnant with triplets is most likely

   a. pruritic folliculitis of pregnancy.
   b. herpes gestationis.
   c. pruritic urticarial papules and plaques of pregnancy syndrome.

5. The practice that has been shown to be ineffective in decreasing the risk of preterm labor and birth in multiples is

   a. 17-alpha-hydroxyprogesterone caproate.
   b. transvaginal ultrasound cervical assessment.
   c. use of a cervical pessary.

6. The greatest complication of tocolytic therapy for women with multiple gestations is

   a. pulmonary edema.
   b. maternal tachycardia.
   c. hyperreflexia.

7. The risk for fetal death in twin gestations is highest at

   a. 24 weeks.
   b. 35 weeks.
   c. 40 weeks.

8. The most appropriate treatment for severe twin-to-twin transfusion syndrome is

   a. expectant management.
   b. amniotic membrane septostomy.
   c. fetoscopic laser therapy.

9. The prenatal diagnostic screening test most accurate in multiple gestations is

   a. second trimester maternal serum testing.
   b. nuchal translucency.
   c. maternal age risk calculation.

10. Maternal weight gain has the greatest effect on fetal growth and birth weight when gains occur

    a. during the first 20 weeks.
    b. during the third trimester.
    c. evenly throughout pregnancy.

11. The complication that is most likely during the interdelivery interval for fraternal twins presenting as A, vertex and B, transverse is

    a. Shoulder dystocia
    b. Cord prolapse
    c. Maternal hypertension

12. The recommendation about cobedding at home for healthy fraternal boy twins born at 35 weeks' gestation is

    a. Only full-term twins can be cobedded at home.
    b. Only preterm twins that have cobedded in the neonatal intensive care unit should be cobedded at home.
    c. For safety reasons, each baby should have his own crib.

13. A sign of abnormal parent–infant interaction with multiples is

    a. initial unit attachment.
    b. ongoing preferential attention.
    c. alternating eye contact among infants.

14. After birth of multiples, breastfeeding or pumping should begin

    a. within 1 to 2 hours.
    b. by 24 hours.
    c. when the mother's milk comes in.

15. When part of a set of multiples dies, parents often

    a. begin grieving immediately.
    b. are able to bond effectively with the survivor.
    c. experience paradoxical feelings.

True or False

16. True/False: Hypertensive disorders in multiple gestations follow a classic pattern of signs and symptoms.

17. True/False: Prenatal education for parents expecting multiples should begin in the second trimester.

18. True/False: The increased prevalence of cerebral palsy in multiple birth infants is solely explained by the greater proportion of low birth weight and preterm births.

19. True/False: The increased prevalence of sudden infant death syndrome (SIDS) in multiple birth infants is explained by the greater proportion of low-birth-weight infants.

20. True/False: Mothers of multiples should begin simultaneous breastfeeding before hospital discharge.

Fill in the Blank

21. The greatest predictors of infant morbidity and mortality in multiples are _____ and _____.

22. The term for similarity in FHR accelerations, baseline oscillations, and periodic changes with contractions in healthy twins is _____ _____.

CHAPTER 12 OBESITY IN PREGNANCY

Multiple Choice

1. Based on the most recent data, what proportion of the U.S. population is estimated to be overweight?

    a. One third
    b. One half
    c. Two thirds

2. Based on the most recent data, what proportion of the women of childbearing age in the U.S. population is estimated to be overweight?

    a. One third
    b. One half
    c. Two thirds

3. Based on the most recent data, what proportion of the pregnant women in the U.S. population is estimated to be obese?

    a. One third
    b. One half
    c. Two thirds

4. When compared to women who are normal weight, obese women have an increased risk of

    a. ectopic pregnancy.
    b. spontaneous abortion.
    c. vaginal birth.

5. Multiple congenital anomalies have been associated with maternal obesity, such as

    a. cleft lip and palate.
    b. clubbing of the foot.
    c. extra digits on the hand.

6. Typically, a low transverse incision for cesarean birth is

    a. associated with less pain postoperatively.
    b. easier to accomplish on a mother who is extremely obese.
    c. preferred by most obstetricians for obese women.

7. A common complication of anesthesia encountered with obese pregnant women when compared to normal weight women is

    a. allergic reaction to anesthetic agents.
    b. excessive response to narcotic analgesia.
    c. difficulty with catheter placement.

8. Which of these ethnic groups has the highest rate of obesity in the United States?

    a. Mexican American women
    b. All Hispanic women
    c. Non-Hispanic white women

9. Fetal programming refers to the

   a. genetic predisposition of the fetus of an obese woman to develop obesity later in life despite healthy eating habits.
   b. inability of an obese pregnant woman with healthy lifestyle changes to pass these characteristics on to the developing fetus.
   c. process in which an in utero stimulus establishes a permanent fetal response that can lead to increased susceptibility to disease throughout life.

10. Patients are considered eligible for weight-loss surgery if they have a body mass index (BMI) of

    a. >30 kg/m^2 with other comorbid conditions
    b. >35 kg/m^2
    c. >35 kg/m^2 with other comorbid conditions

Fill in the Blank

11. According to the World Health Organization, obesity is defined as a body mass index of _____ kg/m^2.

12. A mother who is overweight should gain approximately _____ during her pregnancy.

13. The highest rate of obesity by ethnicity occurs in _____ women.

14. Approximately ____ % of women in the United States are obese.

15. Maternal morbidity and mortality _____ as BMI increases.

16. Extremely obese women have a _____ higher risk of stillbirth than a woman of normal weight.

17. After bariatric surgery, it is recommended that a woman postpone pregnancy for _____ months.

18. Women who are overweight or obese are _____ times more likely to develop gestational diabetes than a normal weight woman.

19. Uterine contractility may be _____ in overweight and obese women.

20. The amount of time from incision to birth may be _____ with obese women.

CHAPTER 13 MATERNAL–FETAL TRANSPORT

Multiple Choice

1. Which federal agency was responsible for developing the Emergency Medical Treatment and Active Labor Act (EMTALA)?

   a. Centers for Disease Control and Prevention (CDC)
   b. Centers for Medicare & Medicaid Services
   c. U.S. Public Health Service

2. The primary purpose of the EMTALA regulation is to ensure that

   a. all patients are provided medical treatment regardless of ability to pay or insurance status.
   b. pregnant women will not be transferred to another facility while in labor.
   c. reimbursement for medical services is provided on an equal basis to hospitals.

3. Which organization first recommended regionalization of perinatal care?

   a. AAP
   b. ACOG
   c. March of Dimes Foundation

4. Regionalization of perinatal care promotes

   a. closure of small perinatal services in rural areas.
   b. limitations on the number of level III neonatal services in each state.
   c. transfer of high-risk mothers to hospitals with appropriate level of care based on gestational age of fetus.

5. Which national organization recommended using *babies under 1,500 grams born at a hospital with the appropriate level of care* as a quality care indicator?

   a. National Quality Forum
   b. TJC
   c. Society for Maternal-Fetal Medicine

6. When compared to neonatal transport, maternal transport of babies in utero has been shown to

   a. cause a significant number of babies to be born during transport.
   b. improve neonatal outcomes.
   c. increase costs.

7. A common EMTALA violation is

   a. failure to document patient insurance status prior to transfer.
   b. inaccurate diagnosis by sending physician.
   c. lack of patient stabilization prior to transfer.

Fill in the Blank

8. Common modes of maternal transport include

1) _____

2) _____

3) _____

9. The following equipment is suggested regardless of the method of maternal transport:

1) _____

2) _____

3) _____

4) _____

5) _____

6) _____

7) _____

8) _____

CHAPTER 14 LABOR AND BIRTH

Multiple Choice

1. According to the ACOG, in the absence of risk factors, FHR should be assessed during second stage labor every

a. 5 minutes.
b. 15 minutes.
c. 30 minutes.

2. An appropriate lubricant to use for vaginal examinations during labor is

a. povidone-iodine gel.
b. sterile water.
c. water-soluble jelly.

3. According to the American Society of Anesthesiologists (ASA) *Guidelines For Obstetrical Anesthesia*, an elective cesarean could be done when the woman has been NPO for at least

a. 4 hours.
b. 5 hours.
c. 6 hours.

4. An involuntary urge to push is most likely a sign of

a. low fetal station.
b. occiput posterior fetal position.
c. transition.

5. An appropriate solution to use for amnioinfusion is

a. 5% dextrose in lactated Ringer's solution (D5L/R).
b. 5% dextrose in water (D5W).
c. lactated Ringer's solution.

6. An increased risk for shoulder dystocia is associated with

a. maternal diabetes.
b. post-date pregnancy.
c. TOLAC.

7. The primary factor that would allow second-stage labor to continue beyond 2 hours is that

a. epidural anesthesia is in place with level <T10.
b. the FHR, as the presenting part descends, does not suggest fetal compromise.
c. maternal pushing efforts result in progress.

8. Using the Zavanelli maneuver to resolve shoulder dystocia involves

a. assisting the woman to a knee–chest position.
b. elevating the fetal head back through the vagina.
c. sweeping an arm to deliver the posterior shoulder.

9. Included in ACOG (2009) definition of tachysystole is

a. contraction duration of >60 seconds.
b. contraction frequency of every 2 to 3 minutes.
c. more than five contractions in 10 minutes.

10. A high probability of successful induction of labor is associated with a Bishop score of

a. >4.
b. >6.
c. >8.

11. Appropriate treatment of tachysystole after dinoprostone administration is

a. IV bolus of D5W.
b. terbutaline 0.25 mg SQ.
c. vaginal irrigation with normal saline.

12. In the absence of complications, immediate postpartum maternal vital signs should be assessed every

a. 5 minutes for 30 minutes.
b. 15 minutes for 2 hours.
c. 30 minutes for 2 hours.

13. ACOG recommends a dosing interval for misoprostol of every

a. 1 to 2 hours.
b. 3 to 6 hours.
c. 7 to 12 hours.

14. The most common reason for hospital readmission following operative birth is

    a. endometritis.
    b. hemorrhage.
    c. wound infection.

15. Vacuum extractor cup placement on the fetal head should not exceed

    a. 5 minutes.
    b. 10 to 15 minutes.
    c. 20 to 30 minutes.

16. Anesthesia personnel are required to remain with a postanesthesia care unit (PACU) patient until the

    a. monitoring equipment has been applied.
    b. PACU nurse accepts responsibility for the patient.
    c. patient is alert and oriented.

17. The normal length of the pregravid cervix is

    a. 2.5 to 3.0 cm.
    b. 3.5 to 4.0 cm.
    c. 4.5 to 5.0 cm.

18. True labor is characterized by

    a. effacement and/or dilation of the cervix.
    b. painful uterine contractions.
    c. suprapubic discomfort at regular intervals.

19. One liter of D5L/R provides

    a. 150 calories.
    b. 180 calories.
    c. 250 calories.

20. Facilitating a family-centered birth experience involves

    a. allowing immediate family members to participate.
    b. providing a waiting area for siblings.
    c. supporting family as defined by the childbearing woman.

Fill in the Blank

21. Diastolic blood pressure measurements taken from an automatic blood pressure device are typically _____ than diastolic measurements utilizing a stethoscope and a mercury cuff.

22. The enzyme oxytocinase facilitates plasma clearance of oxytocin via the maternal _____ and _____.

23. During the second stage of labor, an alternative to squatting that provides the same benefits is _____.

24. Bearing down efforts accompanied by prolonged breath-holding typifies _____ pushing, which has associated negative maternal and fetal _____ effects.

25. AWHONN's second-stage labor nursing management protocol for a woman with epidural anesthesia encourages rest until the occurrence of _____.

26. The McRoberts maneuver is used to facilitate birth when there is an occurrence of _____.

27. Adverse outcomes associated with episiotomy include

    1) _____
    2) _____
    3) _____

28. Measures to aid perineal stretching and aid in the goal to avoid episiotomy include

    1) _____
    2) _____
    3) _____

29. Women who have a support person with them in labor have been found to have

    1) _____
    2) _____
    3) _____

30. Before the use of a cervical ripening or labor induction agent, the following should be assessed:

    1) _____
    2) _____
    3) _____

31. Normal latent phase labor of nulliparous women can last up to _____ hours

32. An interval of _____ hours is recommended between the final dose of dinoprostone and oxytocin administration.

33. Nursing documentation following amniotomy should include

    1) _____
    2) _____
    3) _____

34. A _____-degree laceration extends into the rectal lumen.

35. The maternal landmarks that must be identified to determine fetal stations are the _____.

36. With a physician or certified nurse midwife order, nurses with appropriate training may administer the cervical ripening agents _____ and _____.

37. _____ is a contraindication for the use of misoprostol and Cervidil.

38. A nursing measure to use before forceps application to help prevent maternal trauma is _____.

39. The recommendations for use of the vacuum extractor device state that the pressure should not exceed _____ mm Hg.

40. Requirements for postanesthesia recovery care include availability of

    1) _____
    2) _____
    3) _____
    4) _____
    5) _____
    6) _____
    7) _____

41. According to ACOG, selection criteria for women who are candidates for vaginal birth after cesarean (VBAC) include

    1) _____
    2) _____
    3) _____
    4) _____
    5) _____

42. _____ is a sign of impending uterine rupture in women experiencing a trial of labor after prior cesarean delivery.

43. Four maternal factors proposed as being responsible for initiation of labor are

    1) _____
    2) _____
    3) _____
    4) _____

44. If any of the following findings are present in a pregnant woman, the perinatal provider should be notified promptly:

    1) _____
    2) _____
    3) _____
    4) _____
    5) _____
    6) _____

45. The Bishop score evaluates these five parameters:

    1) _____
    2) _____
    3) _____
    4) _____
    5) _____

46. Unnecessary interventions during labor increase the risk of _____.

47. Informed consent for VBAC correctly includes discussion about

    1) _____
    2) _____
    3) _____

CHAPTER 15 FETAL ASSESSMENT DURING LABOR

Multiple Choice

1. When auscultation is used for fetal assessment during labor for a low-risk woman, the FHR should be auscultated in the first stage of labor every

   a. 5 minutes.
   b. 15 to 30 minutes.
   c. 60 minutes.

2. For a low-risk woman in the second stage of labor, the FHR should be auscultated every

   a. 5 to 15 minutes.
   b. 30 minutes.
   c. 60 minutes.

3. The normal FHR baseline

   a. decreases during labor.
   b. fluctuates during labor.
   c. increases during labor.

4. Bradycardia in the second stage of labor following a previously normal tracing may be caused by fetal

   a. hypoxemia.
   b. rotation.
   c. vagal stimulation.

5. A likely cause of fetal tachycardia with moderate variability is

   a. fetal hypoxemia.
   b. maternal fever.
   c. vagal stimulation.

6. Reduction in FHR variability can result from

   a. fetal scalp stimulation.
   b. medication administration.
   c. vaginal examination.

7. The primary goal in treatment for late decelerations is to

   a. correct cord compression.
   b. improve maternal oxygenation.
   c. maximize uteroplacental blood flow.

8. The most frequently observed type of FHR deceleration is

   a. early.
   b. late.
   c. variable.

9. Amnioinfusion may be useful in alleviating recurrent decelerations that are

   a. early.
   b. late.
   c. variable.

10. Findings indicative of progressive fetal hypoxemia are

    a. late decelerations, moderate variability, and stable baseline rate.
    b. prolonged decelerations recovering to baseline and moderate variability.
    c. loss of variability and recurrent late or variable decelerations.

11. Clinically significant fetal metabolic acidemia is indicated by an arterial cord gas pH of ≤7.10 and a base deficit of

    a. 3.
    b. 6.
    c. 12.

12. Fetal bradycardia can result during

    a. the sleep state.
    b. umbilical vein compression.
    c. vagal stimulation.

13. While caring for a 235-lb laboring woman who is HIV-seropositive, the external FHR tracing is difficult to obtain. An appropriate nursing action would be to

    a. apply a fetal scalp electrode.
    b. auscultate for presence of FHR variability.
    c. notify the attending midwife or physician.

14. FHR decelerations that are benign and do not require intervention are

    a. early.
    b. late.
    c. variable.

15. FHR decelerations that result from decreased uteroplacental blood flow are

    a. early.
    b. late.
    c. variable.

16. FHR decelerations that result from umbilical cord compression are

    a. early.
    b. late.
    c. variable.

17. An FHR pattern associated with severe fetal anemia is

    a. lambda.
    b. saltatory.
    c. sinusoidal.

18. A workup for maternal systemic lupus erythematosus would likely be ordered in the presence of

    a. complete fetal heart block.
    b. premature fetal ventricular contractions.
    c. fetal supraventricular tachycardia.

19. Which IV fluid is most appropriate for maternal administration for intrauterine resuscitation?

    a. Lactated Ringer's solution
    b. D5L/R
    c. Normal saline

20. The position/s that best promote/s maternal–fetal exchange is

    a. left lateral.
    b. right lateral.
    c. either right or left lateral.

21. Maternal oxygen for intrauterine resuscitation should be given at

    a. 8 L/min
    b. 10 L/min
    c. 12 L/min

22. The most appropriate equipment for administration of maternal oxygen for intrauterine resuscitation is a

    a. nasal cannula.
    b. simple face mask.
    c. nonrebreather face mask.

23. Accurate determination of baseline rate requires

    a. at least 2 contiguous minutes of FHR in a 10-minute window.
    b. evaluation of the FHR over at least a 10-minute window.
    c. averaging the FHR over 30 minutes.

24. An electronic fetal monitoring (EFM) tracing with moderate variability, no accelerations, and early decelerations would be classified as

    a. normal (category I).
    b. indeterminate (category II).
    c. abnormal (category III).

25. An EFM tracing with a sinusoidal pattern would be classified as

    a. normal (category I).
    b. indeterminate (category II).
    c. abnormal (category III).

26. An EFM tracing with marked variability would be classified as

    a. normal (category I).
    b. indeterminate (category II).
    c. abnormal (category III).

27. An EFM tracing with minimal variability and recurrent late decelerations would be classified as

    a. normal (category I).
    b. indeterminate (category II).
    c. abnormal (category III).

28. An EFM tracing with FHR 170 bpm and moderate variability would be classified as

    a. normal (category I).
    b. indeterminate (category II).
    c. abnormal (category III).

29. An EFM tracing with absent variability and no decelerations would be classified as

    a. normal (category I).
    b. indeterminate (category II).
    c. abnormal (category III).

30. An EFM tracing with absence of induced accelerations after fetal stimulation would be classified as

    a. normal (category I).
    b. indeterminate (category II).
    c. abnormal (category III).

31. An EFM tracing with absent variability and intermittent late decelerations would be classified as

    a. normal (category I).
    b. indeterminate (category II).
    c. abnormal (category III).

32. Interpretation and classification of FHR patterns are based on predictability of fetal status

    a. at birth.
    b. at the time the pattern is observed.
    c. over the previous hour.

33. Amnioinfusion is an appropriate measure for

    a. thick, meconium-stained fluid.
    b. oligohydramnios.
    c. recurrent variable decelerations unresolved by position changes.

34. Baroreceptors respond to changes in fetal

    a. blood pressure.
    b. oxygen status.
    c. acid–base status.

35. Fetal scalp stimulation is appropriate in the context of

    a. minimal variability.
    b. prolonged deceleration.
    c. bradycardia.

36. Maternal oxygen administration is appropriate in the context of

    a. recurrent variable decelerations/moderate variability.
    b. intermittent late decelerations/minimal variability.
    c. prolonged decelerations/moderate variability.

37. The preterm fetus

    a. is more susceptible to hypoxic insults during labor than the term fetus.
    b. requires internal monitoring if oxytocin is used for labor induction or augmentation.
    c. should be born via cesarean section unless there are maternal contraindications.

38. Oxygen is transferred from the mother to the fetus via the placenta through

    a. active transport.
    b. passive diffusion.
    c. facilitated diffusion.

39. Resting tone and intensity of uterine contractions cannot be assessed by

    a. external tocodynamometer.
    b. manual palpation.
    c. intrauterine pressure catheter.

40. The FHR characteristic most predictive of a well-oxygenated baby at the time observed is

    a. moderate variability.
    b. stable baseline rate.
    c. absence of decelerations.

41. In the context of hypoxemia, fetal blood flow is shifted to the

    a. brain.
    b. liver.
    c. lungs.

42. Baroreceptor-mediated decelerations are

    a. early.
    b. late.
    c. variable.

43. The primary goal in the treatment of variable decelerations is to

    a. correct umbilical cord compression.
    b. improve maternal oxygenation.
    c. maximize blood flow to the uterus.

44. Umbilical artery blood gas results reflect the status of the

    a. mother.
    b. fetus.
    c. placenta.

45. An appropriate initial treatment for recurrent late decelerations with moderate variability during first stage labor is

    a. amnioinfusion.
    b. maternal repositioning.
    c. oxygen at 10 L per nonrebreather facemask.

Fill in the Blank

46. Late decelerations are characterized by decelerations of the FHR that begin at the _____ of the contraction do not return to the baseline rate until _____ the contraction ends, and occur with every contraction.

47. Variable decelerations are characterized by decelerations that have _____ timing in relation to the contractions but always have a(n) _____ change in rate.

48. Early decelerations are characterized by a drop in FHR that begins at the _____ of a contraction and recovers to the _____ by the end of the contraction. Early decelerations are _____ and do not require intervention.

49. Nursing interventions for late decelerations include _____ the oxytocin if it is infusing.

50. Normal (category I) FHR tracings have an absence of late or variable decelerations, _____ variability, and may show accelerations.

51. When a woman presents with an FHR pattern that shows minimal or absent variability on admission, the possibility of a _____ or _____ should be also considered while making preparations to expedite birth.

52. Most fetal dysrhythmias are not life threatening except for _____, which may lead to fetal congestive heart failure.

53. Minimal baseline variability may be caused by multiple factors including _____, _____, and _____.

54. In the presence of variable decelerations, progressive hypoxemia may be characterized by an increasing _____ and loss of _____.

55. Late decelerations associated with acute conditions may be caused by uterine _____.

56. If the FHR tracing does not revert to a normal (category I) tracing following interventions for late decelerations, administration of a _____ to stop or decrease uterine activity may be indicated.

57. Uterine resting tone and the intensity of contractions are measured in millimeters of mercury only when a/an _____ is being used.

58. A sinusoidal pattern may develop in the Rh-sensitized fetus or the fetus who is _____.

59. In the absence of maternal and/or fetal risk factors, auscultation of the fetal rate should occur every _____ minutes in the active phase of the first stage of labor and every _____ minutes in the second stage of labor.

60. Moderate baseline variability is defined as _____ bpm.

61. Correcting variable decelerations can best be accomplished by _____.

62. In the presence of late or variable decelerations, two parameters that indicate adequate fetal oxygenation are _____ and _____.

63. Diminished variability was associated with fetal acidemia only ____% of the time in the literature reviewed by Parer et al. (2006).

64. In the presence of FHR accelerations greater than 15 bpm above baseline and lasting more than 15 seconds, the fetal condition is comparable to the fetal blood gas pH of at least _____ and is considered _____.

65. To correctly interpret a baseline FHR as tachycardic or bradycardic, the rate must persist for a minimum of _____ minutes.

66. In assessing fetal well-being, the most important characteristic of the FHR is _____.

67. Nursing interventions to maximize uteroplacental blood flow include

1) _____
2) _____
3) _____
4) _____
5) _____

68. The normal FHR baseline range is _____ bpm to _____ bpm.

69. The National Institute of Child Health and Human Development (NICHD, 2008) expert group recommended _____categories of FHR tracings.

70. FHR variability that is undetected from baseline is classified as _____.

CHAPTER 16 PAIN IN LABOR: NONPHARMACOLOGIC AND PHARMACOLOGIC MANAGEMENT

Multiple Choice

1. Pain during the first stage of labor is caused by

   a. cervical and lower uterine segment stretching and traction on ovaries, fallopian tubes, and uterine ligaments.
   b. pressure on the urethra, bladder, and rectum by the descending fetal presenting part.
   c. uterine muscle hypoxia, lactic acid accumulation, and distention of the pelvic floor muscles.

2. The release of maternal catecholamines during labor results in

   a. fetal tachycardia.
   b. decreased metabolic rate and oxygen consumption.
   c. uterine hypoperfusion and decreased blood flow to the placenta.

3. The purpose for administration of medications such as hydroxyzine hydrochloride (Vistaril) and propiomazine (Largon) during early labor is to

   a. decrease pain of contractions.
   b. potentiate effects of narcotics.
   c. provide sedation and relieve anxiety.

4. Intradermal injections of sterile water provide pain relief for up to

   a. 1 hour.
   b. 2 hours.
   c. 3 hours.

5. A medication commonly given to women who are experiencing prolonged latent labor to produce a period of sleep is

   a. butorphanol (Stadol).
   b. morphine.
   c. promethazine hydrochloride (Phenergan).

6. Neonatal respiratory depression could result from the maternal administration of IV opioids if birth occurs within

   a. 1 hour or after 4 hours following administration.
   b. 2 to 3 hours of administration.
   c. 12 hours of administration.

7. Ephedrine is used to correct which side effect of epidural anesthesia/analgesia?

   a. Hypotension
   b. Nausea and vomiting
   c. Pruritus

8. A medication given to reverse the symptom of a distended bladder during a continuous epidural infusion is

   a. bupivacaine.
   b. epinephrine.
   c. naloxone.

9. Touch/massage is thought to decrease or interrupt the pain of labor by

   a. activating large myelinated nerve fibers.
   b. activating the same type of nerve fibers that would transmit sensations of pain from the uterus.
   c. interrupting the habituation that occurs when labor is prolonged.

10. When pruritus occurs in the presence of an opioid in the epidural infusion, the nurse can correctly tell the patient that this symptom will most likely subside in about

    a. 15 minutes.
    b. 45 minutes.
    c. 1 to 2 hours.

11. Advantages of combined spinal epidural technique are

    a. decreased hypotension, decreased motor blockade, and increased maternal satisfaction.
    b. decreased hypotension, faster onset of pain relief, and decreased pruritus.
    c. faster onset of pain relief, decreased motor blockade, and increased maternal satisfaction.

12. Meperidine (Demerol) is used less frequently as an analgesia during labor because

    a. it cannot be given intravenously.
    b. it causes neonatal neurobehavioral depression, which may last for several days.
    c. most women receive epidural analgesia.

13. To decrease the transfer of medication to the fetus, IV push narcotics should be given when in relation to the time of uterine contractions?

    a. After
    b. Before
    c. During

14. The epidural catheter for labor pain management is generally placed between the

    a. 2nd and 3rd lumbar vertebrae.
    b. 3rd and 4th lumbar vertebrae.
    c. 4th and 5th lumbar vertebrae.

15. Epinephrine may be added to the epidural to

    a. decrease the amount of narcotic needed.
    b. lessen pruritus associated with epidural narcotic.
    c. prevent hypotension.

16. A test dose of a local anesthetic mixed with epinephrine may be injected to determine that the catheter is not in the epidural vein. Injection of epinephrine into an epidural vein causes almost immediate

    a. decreased blood pressure.
    b. increased blood pressure.
    c. increased heart rate.

17. When the epidural catheter is properly placed, a bolus of anesthetic medication is injected. Depending on the specific medications used, women begin to feel relief in

    a. 1 to 2 minutes.
    b. 5 to 10 minutes.
    c. 15 to 20 minutes.

18. Unlike the RN, the doula

    a. has minimal or no contact with the parents after the birth.
    b. meets the woman for the first time in labor.
    c. provides continuous labor support.

19. When a tub is used during labor, water should be maintained at a temperature of

    a. 34° to 35°C.
    b. 36° to 37°C.
    c. 38° to 39°C.

20. One of the contraindications to neuraxial analgesia is that the woman received her last dose of low-molecular-weight heparin within

    a. 1 hour.
    b. 6 hours.
    c. 12 hours.

21. The initial intervention for a woman experiencing pain on one side during a continuous epidural infusion is to

    a. maintain the woman in a lateral position, off the painful side.
    b. request that an anesthesiologist reevaluate the woman.
    c. turn the woman toward the side with pain.

22. The current recommendation from the ASA regarding nourishment during labor is that solid foods

    a. and liquids do not need to be avoided during labor because of superior anesthesia techniques available today, which do not increase the risk for complications should cesarean section become necessary.
    b. and liquids need to be avoided after the patient has reached 3 cm due to the potential for cesarean section and the potential risk of respiratory complications when any patient receives anesthesia.
    c. should be avoided, but clear liquids increase maternal comfort and satisfaction and do not increase maternal complications.

23. According to AWHONN, non-anesthetist registered nurses can

    a. increase/decrease the rate of a continuous epidural infusion.
    b. reinitiate an epidural infusion once it has been stopped.
    c. remove an epidural catheter after successfully completing an educational program.

24. Maintaining a horizontal position in labor promotes

    a. descent of the presenting part.
    b. increased perception of pain.
    c. maternal oxygenation and comfort.

Fill in the Blank

25. A major limitation for recommending most of the nonpharmacologic methods of pain relief for use in labor is the lack of large _____.

26. Women who labor with the baby's head in the occipitoposterior position report significantly less back pain when using _____ positioning.

27. Counterpressure requires application of enough force to meet the intensity of pressure from the fetal occipital bone against the _____.

28. _____ pressure equalizes the pressure exerted on all parts of the body below the water surface.

Questions 29 to 33 relate to the following statement:

Using the Gate Control Theory, explain how each nonpharmacologic pain management strategy interrupts the transmission of painful stimuli (options a–c).

a. auditory or visual stimulation of the cerebral cortex to prevent passage of painful stimuli
b. cutaneous stimulation to block or alter painful stimuli
c. supports the neuromatrix and ultimately how the individual perceives pain

29. _____ hydrotherapy

30. _____ focal point

31. _____ breathing techniques

32. _____ relaxation

33. _____ intradermal injections of sterile water

34. Following administration of an opioid during labor, frequency and duration of contractions and FHR variability may _____.

35. A fluid bolus should be administered before the initiation of regional analgesia/anesthesia to decrease the potential for maternal _____.

36. The advantage of bupivacaine (Marcaine) and ropivacaine (Naropin) over lidocaine (Xylocaine) and chloroprocaine (Nescaine) for use in epidural analgesia/anesthesia is less _____.

37. The failure to obtain complete pain relief despite proper placement of the epidural catheter may be due to the presence of _____ in the epidural space, which limit areas of the epidural space that can be reached by the medication infused.

38. _____ avoids continued pressure on one single area of the body and decreases the risk of unilateral blocks.

39. Supine position is associated with decreased _____ and _____.

CHAPTER 17 POSTPARTUM CARE

Multiple Choice

1. A normal hemodynamic/hematologic change occurring during the immediate postpartum period is

    a. decreased white blood cell count.
    b. elevated blood pressure.
    c. increased cardiac output.

2. During the postpartum period, normal respiratory and acid–base changes include

    a. decreased base excess.
    b. hypercapnia.
    c. increased PCO_2.

3. Postpartum teaching about sexual activity includes the information that

    a. interest in sexual activity may increase due to hormonal changes.
    b. lubricants will not be needed due to increased vaginal mucus.
    c. sexual intercourse should be avoided until vaginal bleeding has ceased.

4. A normal physiologic finding during the immediate postpartum period is

    a. dizziness when sitting up from a reclining position.
    b. saturation of the peripad every 15 minutes.
    c. urinary output of 25 mL/hour.

5. An appropriate nursing intervention for postpartum hemorrhage is

    a. bimanual pressure.
    b. bladder catheterization.
    c. continuous fundal massage.

6. On the second postpartum/postoperative day following her cesarean delivery, a woman exhibits hypotension, dyspnea, hemoptysis, and abdominal/chest pain. The nurse recognizes these as signs and symptoms of

    a. endometritis.
    b. pulmonary embolism.
    c. sepsis.

7. Normal metabolic changes during the postpartum period include increased levels of

    a. blood glucose.
    b. plasma renin and angiotensin II.
    c. prolactin.

8. The most significant factor influencing a woman's successful transition to motherhood is

    a. emotional support and physical involvement in child care by a significant other.
    b. regular attendance at parent support group meetings.
    c. resumption of a positive and satisfying sexual relationship with her partner.

9. Postpartum endometritis is

   a. associated with internal monitoring, amnio-infusion, prolonged labor, and prolonged rupture of membranes.
   b. effectively treated with a single dose of ampicillin or cephalosporin.
   c. less frequent following cesarean birth due to sterile technique used during surgery.

10. Disruptions in the integrity of the anal sphincter, third-degree tears, and sphincter weakness are

    a. associated with increased incidence of incontinence of flatus/stool.
    b. prevented through the judicious use of operative delivery.
    c. problems freely discussed by women with their healthcare providers.

11. The nurse can positively affect a new mother's self-concept and mothering abilities by encouraging

    a. establishment of a feeding schedule that the mother finds satisfying.
    b. supportive family and friends to participate in learning opportunities and infant care during the mother's hospitalization.
    c. the mother to provide as much of the infant care as possible.

12. Appropriate fundal massage for postpartum uterine atony involves using

    a. continuous two-handed pressure on the uterus until bleeding stops.
    b. firm one-handed pressure on the fundus until clots are expressed.
    c. two hands: one anchors the lower uterine segment and the other gently massages the fundus.

13. Stress incontinence during the postpartum period is more likely to be associated with the techniques used to manage which stage of labor?

    a. First
    b. Second
    c. Third

14. No more than 800 mL of urine should be removed during postpartum catheterization to minimize the potential for

    a. bladder spasm.
    b. hypertension.
    c. hypotension.

15. The most effective prevention of endometritis is

    a. use of early pericare.
    b. hand washing.
    c. use of intrapartum antibiotics.

16. The most likely cause of a decline in sexual interest/activity during the postpartum period is

    a. bleeding from the vagina.
    b. fatigue.
    c. vaginal dryness.

17. Initial treatment for postpartum hemorrhage is

    a. administration of blood products.
    b. exploratory laparotomy.
    c. uterotonic agents.

18. Peak cardiac output after birth occurs at

    a. 1 to 5 minutes.
    b. 10 to 15 minutes.
    c. 30 minutes.

19. A normal hematologic change during the postpartum period is a/an

    a. drop in hematocrit between days 2 and 4.
    b. increase in the sedimentation rate.
    c. leukocytosis of 25,000 to 30,000/μL.

20. Nutritional counseling for women who breast-feed should include increasing caloric intake by

    a. 300 calories.
    b. 400 calories.
    c. 500 calories.

Fill in the Blank

21. To increase venous return during postpartum hemorrhage, the woman should be positioned with _____.

22. A white blood cell count of 28,000/mm^3 on postpartum day 2 would be considered _____.

23. Vital signs within normal limits do not rule out hypovolemic shock in a woman who has experienced a postpartum hemorrhage because alterations in vital signs do not occur until there is _____.

24. _____ is an assessment technique for identification of deep vein thrombosis.

25. When a postpartum woman displays dyspnea and chest pain, the nurse most appropriately suspects _____.

26. The first blood pressure response to hypovolemia would be decreased _____.

27. Counseling regarding contraceptive methods must include information about the _____, _____, and _____.

28. Symptoms of postpartum blues include

    1) _____
    2) _____
    3) _____
    4) _____
    5) _____

29. During the initial postpartum period, the nurse should assess _____, _____, and _____ every 15 minutes for at least 1 hour, or more often if indicated.

30. Typically, postpartum blues occur at _____ days postpartum and continue for no more than a few days.

31. The normal postpartum physiologic diuresis begins within _____ hours of delivery and continues up to _____ days.

32. The acronym BUBBLERS, used to organize postpartum assessment, stands for

    1) _____
    2) _____
    3) _____
    4) _____
    5) _____
    6) _____
    7) _____
    8) _____

33. For each 500 mL of blood loss, the hematocrit will decrease _____% and the hemoglobin will decrease _____ g/dL.

34. Assessment findings suggesting the development of mastitis include

    1) _____
    2) _____
    3) _____
    4) _____

35. Essential topics to be discussed during postpartum teaching are

    1) _____
    2) _____
    3) _____
    4) _____

36. A major factor affecting emotional adjustment during the postpartum period in low-risk women is _____.

37. The first hour after birth is the time of greatest risk for postpartum hemorrhage because _____.

38. Symptoms indicating the development of postpartum preeclampsia are

    1) _____
    2) _____
    3) _____

39. It is important that the nurse has the drug _____ readily available when patients are receiving heparin therapy for thrombophlebitis.

40. Symptoms of impending postpartum eclamptic seizure are

    1) _____
    2) _____
    3) _____
    4) _____
    5) _____

CHAPTER 18 NEWBORN ADAPTATION TO EXTRAUTERINE LIFE

Multiple Choice

1. The newborn's metabolism of brown fat occurs

    a. immediately after birth.
    b. in response to cold stress.
    c. when oxygen saturation is below 90.

2. A 10-minute Apgar is assigned when the

    a. 1-minute Apgar is less than 8.
    b. 5-minute Apgar is less than 7.
    c. newborn has required resuscitation.

3. During the first week of life, newborns are at risk for bleeding because

   a. milk intake is inadequate to supply vitamin K requirements.
   b. several clotting factors are being under-produced by the spleen.
   c. the liver is immature and not yet producing several clotting factors.

4. According to the AAP, vitamin K should be administered

   a. after the infant is weighed and measured.
   b. after 2 hours of life.
   c. within 1 hour of birth.

5. After administration of eye prophylaxis, excess erythromycin ophthalmic ointment is correctly

   a. left in place until absorbed.
   b. removed using sterile water.
   c. wiped away after 1 minute.

6. According to research, there is an association between shorter separation time and umbilical cord care using

   a. alcohol.
   b. sterile water.
   c. triple antibiotic dye.

7. The key to infant abduction prevention is a

   a. carefully obtained set of newborn footprints.
   b. state-of-the-art electronic infant abduction alert.
   c. systematic infant safety program.

8. Vitamin K is produced by the newborn as

   a. a normal compensatory mechanism whenever bleeding occurs.
   b. a response to the parenteral administration of vitamin K.
   c. the gastrointestinal tract becomes colonized with bacteria following initiation of feeding.

9. As part of the algorithm for performing neonatal resuscitation, medications are administered when the

   a. code team physician orders them.
   b. heart rate is below 60 bpm after positive pressure ventilation (PPV) with 100% oxygen.
   c. heart rate is 60 to 80 bpm and not increasing.

10. Initiation of respirations is triggered in the brain by decreased concentration of

    a. carbon dioxide.
    b. oxygen.
    c. surfactant.

11. Fetal pulmonary vascular resistance is

    a. equal to neonatal.
    b. higher than neonatal.
    c. lower than neonatal.

12. In the fetus, blood is shunted into the inferior vena cava through the

    a. ductus arteriosus.
    b. ductus venosus.
    c. foramen ovale.

13. Clamping the umbilical cord at birth causes

    a. decreased blood pressure and decreased systemic vascular resistance.
    b. increased blood pressure and decreased systemic vascular resistance.
    c. increased blood pressure and increased systemic vascular resistance.

14. The major factor contributing to closure of the ductus arteriosus is sensitivity to

    a. decreasing arterial carbon dioxide concentration.
    b. decreasing left ventricular pressure.
    c. increasing arterial oxygen concentration.

15. In the majority of healthy newborns, the ductus arteriosus will have closed or will be closing by

    a. 1 to 6 hours of life.
    b. 12 to 24 hours of life.
    c. 48 to 72 hours of life.

16. The premature infant is more susceptible to evaporative heat loss because of

    a. decreased body surface area.
    b. decreased muscle tone.
    c. increased permeability of skin.

17. Hemorrhagic disease of the newborn is prevented by administration of

    a. vitamin A.
    b. vitamin D.
    c. vitamin K.

18. To protect newborns from infection with hepatitis B virus, all newborns

    a. born to mothers with unknown hepatitis B surface antigen (HBsAg) status should receive one dose of vaccine within 12 hours of birth.
    b. should be screened for HBsAg within 12 hours of birth.
    c. should receive the first dose of hepatitis vaccine within 12 hours of birth.

19. Intrauterine infection should be suspected when the newborn has elevated

    a. immunoglobulin (Ig) A.
    b. IgG.
    c. IgM.

20. An infant born to a group B streptococcus (GBS)–positive mother who did not receive antibiotics during labor is at risk for

    a. hyperbilirubinemia.
    b. hypoglycemia.
    c. pneumonia.

Fill in the Blank

For questions 21 to 24, the following nursing interventions support the newborn's transition to extrauterine life by interrupting what mechanism of heat loss (a–d)?

a. evaporation
b. convection
c. conduction
d. radiation

21. _____ Dry newborn thoroughly; remove wet linen.

22. _____ When necessary, use humidified, warmed oxygen.

23. _____ Place cover between newborn and metal scale.

24. _____ Preheat radiant warmer.

25. Maternal intrauterine transmission of _____ antibodies protects the newborn from bacterial and viral infections for which the mother has already produced antibodies.

26. The action that best protects newborns from infection is _____.

27. A 2,000-g infant should receive _____ mg of vitamin K.

28. Erythromycin ophthalmic ointment protects newborns from the organisms _____ and _____.

29. Immediately following birth, in the absence of spontaneous respirations, a nurse begins giving the newborn PPV. The second nurse should _____.

30. Respiratory adaptations during the transition to extrauterine life are dependent on _____, _____, and _____ stimuli to the brain.

31. In utero, oxygenated blood flows from the placenta to the fetus through the _____.

32. During fetal life, the placenta is an organ of _____ vascular resistance.

33. The vessels in the umbilical cord are two _____ and one _____.

34. The four main mechanisms of heat loss in the neonate are _____, _____, _____, and _____.

35. Nonshivering thermogenesis generates heat in the newborn through _____.

36. Hypothermia in the neonate increases _____ consumption.

37. The action of surfactant is to _____ in the alveoli.

38. In neonatal resuscitation, chest compressions should be initiated if the heart rate is below _____ bpm.

39. Women who are positive for GBS infection should be treated with _____ during labor.

40. Postpartum practices that increase breastfeeding duration include _____ and _____.

CHAPTER 19 NEWBORN PHYSICAL ASSESSMENT

Multiple Choice

1. In a newborn with hypospadias, the urinary meatus is located on the

   a. anterior surface of the glans.
   b. posterior surface of the glans.
   c. tip of the glans.

2. A nevus simplex "stork bite"

   a. is usually elevated, rough, and dark red.
   b. most often appears on the neck, forehead, and eyelids.
   c. will not blanch with pressure.

3. Tears are usually absent in a baby until the age of

   a. 2 to 4 weeks.
   b. 2 to 3 months.
   c. 4 to 6 months.

4. Newborn femoral pulses would characteristically be decreased or absent in

   a. congenital heart abnormalities.
   b. hip dysplasia.
   c. sepsis.

5. A persistent newborn heart rate of less than 100 bpm is consistent with

   a. congenital heart block.
   b. congestive heart failure.
   c. vagal stimulation.

6. In dark-skinned newborns, jaundice is more easily observed in the

   a. feet and hands.
   b. nail beds.
   c. sclera and buccal mucosa.

7. In the neonate, blood pressure in the lower extremities is usually

   a. higher than in the upper extremities.
   b. lower than in the upper extremities.
   c. no different than in the upper extremities.

8. The normal umbilical cord contains

   a. one artery and one vein.
   b. two arteries and one vein.
   c. two veins and one artery.

9. Jaundice within the first 24 hours of life may be related to

   a. asphyxia.
   b. cardiac disease.
   c. liver disease.

10. Edema over the presenting part of a newborn's head that feels spongy and resolves within a few days of life is characteristic of

    a. caput succedaneum.
    b. cephalhematoma.
    c. trauma during birth.

11. A gestational age assessment indicating the greatest degree of physical maturity is

    a. labia majora covering clitoris and labia minora.
    b. labia majora large and labia minora small.
    c. prominent clitoris and enlarging labia minora.

12. Newborn jaundice appears initially on the

    a. head and face.
    b. trunk and extremities.
    c. sclera.

13. To measure fontanelles accurately, a ruler or measuring tape is placed

    a. across the widest diameter.
    b. diagonally from bone to bone.
    c. from suture line to suture line.

14. A cross-eyed appearance in a newborn is called

    a. hypertelorism.
    b. nystagmus.
    c. strabismus.

15. Bowel sounds are expected to be present in the newborn

    a. after passage of first meconium stool.
    b. immediately after birth.
    c. within 1 hour of birth.

16. A prominent xiphoid process identified during a newborn physical assessment is

    a. a normal finding.
    b. associated with intrauterine growth retardation.
    c. indicative of respiratory distress.

17. The most common finding in assessment of the newborn's skin is a

    a. hemangioma.
    b. Mongolian spot.
    c. nevus simplex.

18. Permanent eye color is present by the age of

    a. 2 months.
    b. 4 months.
    c. 6 months.

19. In a newborn, the skin lesion that has discrete borders and does not blanch to pressure or lighten with age is a

    a. hemangioma.
    b. Mongolian spot.
    c. port wine stain.

20. The presence of the red reflex in the newborn indicates

    a. congenital cataracts.
    b. intact cornea and lens.
    c. weak eye musculature.

21. Umbilical hernias are more commonly seen in newborns who are

    a. African American.
    b. Native American.
    b. Southeast Asian.

22. Screening programs evaluating newborns at high risk for hearing loss will potentially miss what percentage of newborns with hearing loss?

    a. 25%
    b. 50%
    c. 75%

23. The most common abnormal neck finding in newborns is

    a. cystic hygroma.
    b. torticollis.
    c. webbing.

24. The Moro reflex should disappear by the age of

    a. 2 months.
    b. 4 months.
    c. 6 months.

25. A genitourinary finding in a gestational age assessment of a newborn male at 36 weeks' gestation is

    a. rugae becoming visible.
    b. pendulous scrotum.
    c. testes in the upper scrotum.

26. During the first few days of life, the percentage of newborns with developmental hip dysplasia that is identified during physical assessment is

    a. 40%.
    b. 60%.
    c. 80%.

27. A scrotal mass that does not transilluminate is a/an

    a. hydrocele.
    b. inguinal hernia.
    c. testis.

Fill in the Blank

28. When examining the clavicles, _____ is felt by the examiner if there is a fracture present.

29. At birth, newborns are covered with an odorless, white, cheesy substance called _____.

30. Epstein's pearls are composed of _____ cells.

31. Popping sensations (similar to indenting a ping-pong ball) felt when palpating the parietal or occipital bones of a newborn are called _____.

32. The anterior fontanelle normally closes at about _____ months.

33. The posterior fontanelle normally closes at about _____ months.

34. Apnea refers to pauses in respirations that last _____ seconds or longer.

35. Newborns can see an object clearly when the object is _____ inches away.

36. _____ describes the inability to completely retract the foreskin of the penis.

37. _____ is an asymmetric neck deformity in which the head is noted to be pulled toward the affected side, with the chin pointing toward the opposite shoulder, due to injury to the _____ muscle.

38. Acrocyanosis is the result of _____ and tends to worsen if the newborn becomes chilled.

39. _____ is a compensatory mechanism that decreases upper airway resistance, allowing more air to enter the nasal passages.

40. Newborn _____ are involuntary protective neuromuscular responses.

CHAPTER 20 NEWBORN NUTRITION

Multiple Choice

1. A woman who presents with a history of minimal increase in breast tissue during pregnancy should be informed that

    a. the amount of breast tissue influences milk production.
    b. breast growth during pregnancy does not influence milk production.
    c. breast tissue will increase as she nurses.

2. The onset of milk production in a postpartum woman is triggered by the

    a. periodic stimulation of oxytocin.
    b. rapid rise in prolactin.
    c. sudden decrease in progesterone.

3. A pregnant woman who asks what she should do to prepare her nipples for breastfeeding is correctly informed that nipple exercises

    a. do little to prevent nipple soreness.
    b. improve nipple erectility.
    c. reduce the incidence of engorgement.

4. Frequent breastfeeding during the first 24 hours postpartum increases newborn

    a. immunity.
    b. sleep cycles.
    c. weight gain.

5. Breast engorgement in the breastfeeding mother is minimized by

    a. avoiding unnecessary nipple stimulation.
    b. nursing without time limits.
    c. pumping after nursing.

6. As maternal prolactin levels decline over time, what is responsible for continued milk production?

    a. newborn sucking
    b. maternal ingestion of adequate fluids
    c. return of normal estrogen levels

7. During a home visit to a 4-day-old breastfeeding newborn, the nurse observes jaundice. Which of the following interventions should be suggested to the mother?

    a. increasing the frequency of breastfeeding
    b. supplementing breastfeeds with water
    c. temporarily pumping and discarding her breast milk

8. A newborn is reported to have breastfed very well during the first hour after birth. The baby is now 12 hours old and has not had a second successful feeding. The nurse should

    a. advise the mother to give water every 2 to 3 hours.
    b. review newborn sleep cycles and hunger cues.
    c. teach the mother to pump her breasts.

9. A woman calls the hospital asking what she should do for her 10-day-old breastfeeding newborn who wants to nurse "all the time." The nurse should recommend that the mother

    a. continue breastfeeding based on the newborn's cues.
    b. offer formula if the newborn is still hungry after breastfeeding.
    c. use other comforting techniques to space feedings at least 2 hours apart.

10. A bottle-feeding mother asks whether she should give her baby water. The nurse should instruct her to

    a. add a little extra water to the formula on hot days.
    b. feed the newborn properly mixed formula.
    c. give the newborn water between feedings if fussy.

11. The hormone responsible for milk ejection is

    a. oxytocin.
    b. progesterone.
    c. prolactin.

12. Mothers can encourage newborns to open their mouths wider while nursing by

    a. applying a small amount of downward pressure on the newborn's chin.
    b. guiding the newborn's head toward the breast.
    c. leaning forward toward the newborn.

13. Compared to mature milk, colostrum is higher in

    a. fat.
    b. IgG.
    c. protein.

14. As human milk matures, the concentration of Igs and proteins

    a. decreases.
    b. increases.
    c. remains the same.

15. A mother holds her breast with her thumb on top and fingers below; she is using the

    a. C hold.
    b. circle hold.
    c. cup hold.

16. Formula feeding is recommended for newborns with

    a. galactosemia.
    b. jaundice.
    c. thalassemia.

17. After opening a can or bottle of formula, the contents should be used within

    a. 24 hours.
    b. 48 hours.
    c. 72 hours.

18. The most economic formula preparation is

    a. concentrate.
    b. powder.
    c. ready-to-feed.

19. Methods to increase comfort while suppressing lactation include

    a. applying heat to the breast.
    b. limiting fluid intake for 48 hours.
    c. wearing a firm-fitting bra.

20. Which of the following breastfeeding positions is *most* useful for the mother recovering from a c-section?

    a. Cradle
    b. Cross cradle
    c. Clutch hold

21. Which of the following statements regarding supplementation of the breastfeeding infant is false?

    a. Mothers on a vegan diet, which excludes dairy products, may need supplemental vitamin B12.
    b. The AAP recommends breastfed infants receive a vitamin D supplement.
    c. Most infants need iron supplementation before 6 months of age.

22. Promotion of breastfeeding for preterm infants should include

    a. frequent pumping of both breasts simultaneously.
    b. skin-to-skin contact.
    c. all of the above.

23. Prenatal physical preparation of the breasts to prevent sore nipples should include

    a. nipple rolling.
    b. expression of colostrums.
    c. none of the above.

24. Breastfed infants may have inadequate intake if they

    a. have uric acid crystals during the first week.
    b. fail to regain birth weight by 2 weeks.
    c. have two to three wet diapers by day 2.

25. Which of the following is a true statement about pacifier use?

    a. They have been used effectively to correct sucking problems.
    b. Early introduction has been shown to prevent sore nipples.
    c. Introduction of a pacifier, after breastfeeding is well established, during sleep time may prevent SIDS.

26. Ankyloglossia can lead to

    a. yeast infections.
    b. nipple pain.
    c. a reliance on pacifiers.

Fill in the Blank

27. Healthy People 2010's target for percentage of women breastfeeding at discharge is _____.

28. A hard, tender area in the breast of a breastfeeding woman should be treated with _____ and _____.

29. When the breastfeeding baby is correctly latched onto the mother's breast, the tongue covers the _____.

30. Hunger cues can be observed for up to _____ minutes before the newborn begins sustained crying.

31. General guidelines for newborn weight gain during the first few weeks of life are regaining birth weight by _____ weeks and gaining _____ oz a week or at least _____ lb a month.

32. Current thinking is that newborns will lose _____% of their birth weight in their first few days of life.

33. The easiest, most economic treatments for nipple pain are _____.

34. Alternate breast massage is used to _____.

35. Instructions for alternate breast massage are to _____.

36. Feeding the infant in the _____ position may decrease the risk of otitis media.

CHAPTER 21 COMMON NEONATAL COMPLICATIONS

Multiple Choice

1. Transient tachypnea develops more often in the newborn who is born

   a. by cesarean section.
   b. after a prolonged first stage of labor.
   c. small for gestational age.

2. In a newborn, tachypnea is defined as a respiratory rate greater than

   a. 40 breaths per minute.
   b. 60 breaths per minute.
   c. 80 breaths per minute.

3. A cardiac lesion considered to be cyanotic is

   a. atrial septal defect (ASD).
   b. patent ductus arteriosus (PDA).
   c. transposition of great arteries (TGA).

4. A cardiac lesion which results in decreased pulmonary blood flow is

   a. ASD.
   b. TOF.
   c. PDA.

5. A medication used to maintain patency of the ductus arteriosus is

   a. caffeine.
   b. indomethacin.
   c. prostaglandin E_1.

6. Hypoglycemia in the infant born to an insulin-dependent diabetic mother occurs after birth between

   a. 1 and 3 hours.
   b. 5 and 7 hours.
   c. 8 and 10 hours.

7. One etiology of hypoglycemia is decreased production of glucose, which should be suspected in the newborn who is

   a. cold stressed.
   b. the infant of a diabetic mother.
   c. small for gestational age.

8. Clinical jaundice is first apparent at serum bilirubin levels of

   a. 1 to 3 mg/dL.
   b. 5 to 7 mg/dL.
   c. 9 to 11 mg/dL.

9. In a full-term newborn, physiologic hyperbilirubinemia is characterized by a progressive increase in serum bilirubin that peaks at

   a. 24 hours.
   b. 48 hours.
   c. 72 hours.

10. Gastrointestinal symptoms associated with neonatal abstinence syndrome include

    a. constipation.
    b. diarrhea.
    c. flatulence.

11. Which drug, when used alone, is responsible for the most severe withdrawal symptoms in the newborn?

    a. cocaine
    b. heroin
    c. methadone

12. When ruling out sepsis in the newborn, the broad-spectrum antimicrobial agents most commonly initiated after cultures have been obtained are

    a. ampicillin/cephalosporin.
    b. ampicillin/gentamicin.
    c. penicillin/gentamicin.

13. IV antibiotic treatment for neonatal sepsis should continue for

    a. 3 to 5 days.
    b. 7 to 10 days.
    c. 12 to 14 days.

14. Hypothermia can cause

    a. decreased metabolic demand.
    b. hypoglycemia.
    c. metabolic alkalosis.

15. A sign of hypoglycemia in the newborn is

    a. decreased skin turgor.
    b. increased appetite.
    c. temperature instability.

16. An indication to screen for hypoglycemia is an infant who is

    a. a second twin weighing 3,000 g.
    b. born at 38 weeks' gestation.
    c. small for gestational age.

17. In the newborn, physiologic hyperbilirubinemia is characterized by a progressive increase in serum bilirubin to a peak of

    a. 5 mg/dL at 72 hours of age.
    b. 8 mg/dL at 72 hours of age.
    c. 10 mg/dL at 48 hours of age.

18. Infants undergoing phototherapy should have axillary temperatures monitored at least every

    a. 30 minutes.
    b. 1 hour.
    c. 2 hours.

19. Infants born to cocaine-addicted mothers frequently exhibit

    a. constipation.
    b. feeding difficulties.
    c. lethargy.

20. Which of the following interventions is useful to support an infant experiencing abstinence syndrome?

    a. Massage
    b. Music
    c. Rocking

21. The diagnosis of neonatal sepsis is made in the presence of a positive culture of

    a. blood.
    b. both blood and urine.
    c. urine.

22. ACOG and the AAP recommend HIV testing and counseling with consent for

    a. pregnant women in at-risk populations.
    b. all pregnant teenagers.
    c. all pregnant women.

Fill in the Blank

23. Surfactant _____ surface tension in the alveoli functions as a stabilizer to prevent collapse during expiration.

24. When meconium only partially obstructs the airway, a _____ effect results in which air enters the lower airways on inspiration but cannot _____ on expiration.

25. The _____ is the first major organ system to function in the embryo.

26. A ventricular septal defect (VSD) is considered to be a(n) _____ lesion with _____ pulmonary blood flow.

27. The three pathophysiologic findings in tetralogy of Fallot are

    1) _____
    2) _____
    3) _____

28. The incidence of the congenital heart defect _____ is inversely proportional to gestational age.

29. An ASD is considered to be a(n) _____ lesion with _____ pulmonary blood flow.

30. With transposition of the great arteries in two _____ circulations, the degree of cyanosis present depends on the amount of mixing through the _____, if present, _____, or _____.

31. Glucose homeostasis requires the initiation of various metabolic processes, including _____, forming glucose from noncarbohydrate sources, and _____, conversion of glycogen stores to glucose.

32. As bilirubin levels rise, there is concern that bilirubin encephalopathy, also known as _____, will develop.

33. In nearly all newborns, phototherapy decreases or blunts the rise in serum _____ bilirubin regardless of gestational age, race, or presence or absence of hemolysis.

34. _____ is the one common side effect of all of the medications used to treat neonatal abstinence.

35. The two bacterial agents most commonly associated with neonatal sepsis are _____ and _____.

36. The primary neonatal factors influencing the development of sepsis are _____ and _____.

37. Intrapartum administration of prophylactic antibiotics has proven to be beneficial in preventing _____.

38. Heroin withdrawal in a newborn may last _____ weeks.

39. Skin care is important during phototherapy because the infant often has _____.

40. An infant born to a mother who received tocolytic therapy would be prone to _____.

41. Narcotics used to manage labor pain may result in _____ respiratory effort in the newborn.

42. The mortality rate associated with neonatal sepsis increases as birth weight _____.

43. Studies show a nearly _____ reduction in HIV-1 transmission in infants whose mothers received azidothymidine (ZDV) prophylaxis.

44. ACOG recommends considering an _____ for HIV-1 infected women with HIV-1 RNA levels >1,000 copies/mL near the time of delivery.

45. Newborn chemoprophylaxis should begin _____ hours after birth.

46. _____ is the primary complication of the 6-week course of ZDV in the neonate.

47. In the United States, women infected with HIV-1 are counseled not to _____ to avoid postnatal transmission.

ANSWER KEY

CHAPTER 1 PERINATAL PATIENT SAFETY AND PROFESSIONAL LIABILITY ISSUES ANSWERS

1. b
2. a
3. a
4. a
5. b
6. a
7. c
8. c
9. a
10. a
11. b
12. a
13. c
14. c
15. a
16. a
17. effective leadership, shared philosophy, professional behavior, excellence in key clinical practices
18. fetal assessment, labor induction, second-stage labor management
19. clinical practice will be based on the cumulative body of evidence and national standards and guidelines
20. AAP; American College of Nurse-Midwives (ACNM); ACOG; ASA; AWHONN; CDC; U.S. Food and Drug Administration (FDA); Joint Commission on Accreditation of Healthcare Organizations (JCAHO)
21. attempting VBAC
22. 39 completed weeks' gestation
23. electronic fetal monitoring
24. the woman feels the urge to push; nulliparous; multiparous
25. NICHD
26. EMTALA
27. lawsuits/litigation/"suits"
28. retrospective
29. outdated; error
30. sentinel event
31. 1:1
32. 1:1
33. chain of command/chain of consultation

CHAPTER 2 INTEGRATING CULTURAL BELIEFS AND PRACTICES WHEN CARING FOR CHILDBEARING WOMEN AND FAMILIES ANSWERS

1. c
2. c
3. a
4. b
5. b
6. b
7. b
8. b
9. a-2, b-1, c-3
10. c
11. a
12. a
13. c
14. enhance communication skills; develop linguistic skills; determine who the family decision makers are; understand that agreement may not indicate comprehension; utilize nonverbal communication; use appropriate names and titles; use culturally appropriate teaching techniques

CHAPTER 3 PHYSIOLOGIC CHANGES OF PREGNANCY ANSWERS

1. b
2. a
3. b
4. a
5. a
6. c
7. c
8. c
9. a
10. c
11. b
12. b
13. c
14. b
15. b
16. c
17. c
18. b
19. b
20. b
21. a
22. a
23. a
24. a
25. b
26. anabolism; catabolism
27. hemodilution

28. mother
29. increase
30. renal sodium
31. increased glomerular filtration rate
32. striae gravidarum
33. prolactin
34. vitamin D (or calciferol)
35. lower
36. human chorionic gonadotropin
37. estriol
38. blood volume
39. 6 to 12 weeks postpartum
40. uterus
41. progesterone
42. 24 to 32
43. angiotensin II
44. hypercoagulable
45. coagulation changes; venous stasis
46. prostaglandins
47. melasma
48. Chadwick's

CHAPTER 4 ANTENATAL CARE ANSWERS

1. a
2. c
3. a
4. b
5. a
6. b
7. b
8. a
9. b
10. a
11. b
12. a
13. b
14. c
15. a
16. a
17. b
18. True
19. 28
20. 36
21. 15 lb
22. 10
23. teratogen
24. 8
25. 12
26. Jewish
27. Coumadin
28. 5 to 10
29. 1) early and continuing risk assessment
    2) health promotion
    3) medical and psychosocial intervention

30. cardiorespiratory; muscular
31. two or more abnormally elevated values
32. 15; 20
33. 10
34. 1) fetal tone
    2) fetal reflex movement
    3) fetal breathing
    4) amniotic fluid volume
    5) nonstress test

CHAPTER 5 HYPERTENSIVE DISORDERS OF PREGNANCY ANSWERS

1. c
2. a
3. b
4. b
5. c
6. b
7. hypertensive
8. 110
9. semi-Fowler's
10. magnesium sulfate
11. 1) abruptio placentae
    2) disseminated intravascular coagulation
    3) hepatic failure
    4) acute renal failure
12. prevent maternal cerebral vascular accident; maintain uteroplacental perfusion
13. hemolysis; elevated liver enzymes; low platelets
14. aspiration

CHAPTER 6 BLEEDING IN PREGNANCY ANSWERS

1. b
2. b
3. b
4. b
5. b
6. a
7. c
8. a
9. c
10. c
11. c
12. velamentous
13. 95
14. hypotension
15. 1) administering oxytocin with delivery of the anterior shoulder
    2) clamping/cutting the umbilical cord by 2 to 3 minutes of birth

3) controlling traction of the umbilical cord, with the provider's hand supporting the uterus to prevent uterine inversion

4) performing vigorous fundal massage for at least 15 seconds

CHAPTER 7 PRETERM LABOR AND BIRTH ANSWERS

1. a
2. c
3. a
4. a
5. a
6. b
7. a
8. b
9. b
10. a
11. higher
12. stabilized
13. eliminated
14. elective
15. uterine cramping (menstrual-like cramps, intermittent or constant); uterine contractions every 10 to 15 minutes or more frequently; low abdominal pressure (pelvic pressure); dull, low backache (intermittent or constant); increase or change in vaginal discharge; feeling that the baby is "pushing down"; abdominal cramping with or without diarrhea

CHAPTER 8 DIABETES IN PREGNANCY ANSWERS

1. c
2. a
3. c
4. c
5. a
6. c
7. c
8. c
9. a
10. a
11. type 1
12. anabolic
13. 1) prolactin
    2) estrogen
    3) progesterone
    4) human placental lactogen
    5) cortisol
14. magnesium sulfate
15. 1) polyuria
    2) polyphagia
    3) polydipsia

CHAPTER 9 CARDIAC DISEASE IN PREGNANCY ANSWERS

1. a
2. b
3. c
4. a
5. c
6. c
7. c
8. b
9. b
10. b
11. capillaries
12. rheumatic fever
13. cardiac troponin I
14. type of cardiac disorder; secondary complications
15. functional ability

CHAPTER 10 PULMONARY COMPLICATIONS IN PREGNANCY ANSWERS

1. c
2. b
3. b
4. c
5. a
6. b
7. a
8. b
9. c
10. c
11. 10% to 20
12. 95
13. 75
14. illicit drug use; cigarette smoking; alcohol abuse
15. *Streptococcus pneumoniae*
16. high Fowler's
17. pollens, molds, dust mites, animal dander, cockroach antigens, air pollutants, strong odors, food additives, tobacco smoke
18. systemic steroid therapy >4 weeks; three visits for asthma recently; history of multiple hospitalizations for asthma; history of hypoxic seizure, hypoxic syncope, or intubation; history of admission to intensive care unit (ICU) for asthma
19. preterm labor, pericardial tamponade, bacteremia, pneumothorax, atrial fibrillation, respiratory failure
20. 30

CHAPTER 11 MULTIPLE GESTATION ANSWERS

1. c
2. b
3. b

4. c
5. a
6. a
7. c
8. c
9. b
10. a
11. b
12. c
13. b
14. a
15. c
16. False
17. True
18. False
19. True
20. False
21. low birth weight; preterm birth
22. fetal synchrony

CHAPTER 12 OBESITY IN PREGNANCY ANSWERS

1. c
2. a
3. a
4. b
5. a
6. a
7. c
8. a
9. c
10. c
11. greater than or equal to 30
12. 15 to 25 lb
13. non-Hispanic black
14. 30
15. increase
16. 40%
17. 12 to 24
18. six
19. decreased
20. increased

CHAPTER 13 MATERNAL–FETAL TRANSPORT ANSWERS

1. b
2. a
3. c
4. c
5. a
6. b
7. c

8. 1) ambulance
   2) airplane
   3) helicopter
9. 1) vital sign monitoring equipment
   2) Doppler for FHR assessment
   3) IV administration setup
   4) respiratory equipment
   5) medications
   6) emergency birth equipment
   7) infant resuscitation equipment (Bigelow, 1997).
   8) documentation method

CHAPTER 14 LABOR AND BIRTH ANSWERS

1. b
2. c
3. c
4. a
5. c
6. a
7. b
8. b
9. c
10. c
11. b
12. b
13. b
14. c
15. c
16. b
17. b
18. a
19. b
20. c
21. lower
22. kidneys; liver
23. sitting on the toilet
24. closed glottis; hemodynamic
25. spontaneous bearing-down efforts (urge to push)
26. shoulder dystocia
27. blood loss; infection; pain; third- and fourth-degree laceration; delayed healing; sexual dysfunction; scarring.
28. 1) open glottis—gentle pushing
    2) spontaneous rather than directed pushing
    3) upright position in second stage
29. 1) fewer perinatal complications
    2) shorter labors
    3) fewer NICU admissions
30. 1) maternal status
    2) fetal well-being
    3) cervical status
31. 18
32. 6 to 12

33. 1) color and amount of fluid
    2) FHR before procedure
    3) fetal response to procedure
34. fourth
35. ischial spines
36. misoprostol; Cervidil
37. prior cesarean birth or uterine scar
38. emptying the maternal bladder
39. 500 to 600
40. 1) oxygen delivery system
    2) continuous and intermittent suction
    3) blood pressure monitoring equipment
    4) ECG monitoring equipment
    5) pulse oximeter
    6) adjustable lighting
    7) means to ensure patient privacy
41. 1) one or two prior low transverse cesarean births
    2) clinically adequate pelvis
    3) no prior uterine surgery or rupture
    4) physician immediately available and capable of performing emergent cesarean birth
    5) surgical team and anesthesia personnel available for emergent cesarean birth
42. pain at the prior incision site
43. 1) stretching of uterine muscles
    2) pressure on the cervix
    3) endogenous oxytocin
    4) change in estrogen:progesterone ratio
44. 1) vaginal bleeding
    2) acute abdominal pain
    3) temperature of 100.4°F or higher
    4) preterm labor
    5) premature preterm rupture of membranes
    6) hypertension
45. 1) dilation
    2) effacement
    3) station
    4) consistency
    5) position
46. iatrogenic injuries to the mother and/or fetus
47. 1) risks
    2) benefits
    3) alternative approaches

CHAPTER 15 FETAL ASSESSMENT DURING LABOR ANSWERS

1. b
2. a
3. b
4. c
5. b
6. b
7. c
8. c
9. c
10. c
11. c
12. c
13. c
14. a
15. b
16. c
17. c
18. a
19. a
20. c
21. b
22. c
23. b
24. a
25. c
26. b
27. b
28. b
29. b
30. b
31. b
32. b
33. c
34. a
35. a
36. b
37. a
38. b
39. a
40. a
41. a
42. c
43. a
44. b
45. b
46. peak; after
47. variable; abrupt
48. beginning; baseline rate; benign
49. decreasing or discontinuing
50. moderate
51. previous hypoxic insult; congenital anomaly
52. supraventricular tachycardia
53. three of the following: medications, prematurity, fetal sleep, fetal dysrhythmia, anesthetic agents, cardiac anomaly
54. depth of decelerations; variability
55. tachysystole
56. tocolytic
57. intrauterine pressure catheter
58. anemic
59. 15 to 30; 5 to 15
60. 6 to 25
61. changing maternal position (amnioinfusion also acceptable)

62. moderate variability; normal baseline rate
63. 23
64. 7.19; adequately oxygenated
65. 10
66. variability
67. 1) increasing IV fluids
    2) maintaining lateral maternal position
    3) administering oxygen by nonrebreather facemask
    4) decreasing or discontinuing oxytocin
    5) delaying the next dose of Cervidil or Cytotec
68. 110; 160
69. three
70. absent

CHAPTER 16 PAIN IN LABOR: NONPHARMACOLOGIC AND PHARMACOLOGIC MANAGEMENT ANSWERS

1. a
2. c
3. c
4. b
5. b
6. a
7. a
8. c
9. a
10. b
11. c
12. a
13. c
14. c
15. a
16. c
17. b
18. c
19. b
20. c
21. c
22. c
23. c
24. b
25. randomized controlled clinical trials
26. hands and knees
27. sacrum
28. hydrostatic pressure
29. b
30. a
31. a
32. c
33. b
34. decrease
35. hypotension
36. motor block

37. connective tissue bands
38. turning
39. maternal cardiac output; lower fetal oxygen saturation

CHAPTER 17 POSTPARTUM CARE ANSWERS

1. c
2. c
3. c
4. a
5. b
6. b
7. b
8. a
9. a
10. a
11. c
12. c
13. b
14. c
15. b
16. b
17. c
18. b
19. c
20. c
21. legs elevated 20 to 30 degrees
22. nonpathologic leukocytosis
23. a loss of 15% to 20% of the total blood volume
24. measurement of the affected leg circumference
25. pulmonary embolism
26. pulse pressure to 30 mm Hg or less
27. advantages; disadvantages; prevention of sexually transmitted diseases
28. 1) insomnia
    2) weepiness
    3) anxiety
    4) irritability
    5) poor concentration
29. vital signs; lochia; uterine tone/position
30. 3 to 6
31. 12; 5
32. 1) breast
    2) uterus
    3) bladder
    4) bowel
    5) lochia
    6) episiotomy/incision
    7) emotional response
    8) Homans' sign
33. 2% to 4; 1 to 1.5
34. 1) fever and chills
    2) localized tenderness
    3) palpable, hard, reddened mass
    4) tachycardia

35. 1) pelvic floor exercises
    2) postpartum exercise
    3) sexuality
    4) contraception
36. fatigue
37. large venous areas are exposed after placental expulsion
38. 1) blood pressure of 140/90 mm Hg
    2) headache
    3) decreased urine output
39. protamine sulfate
40. 1) severe persistent headache
    2) scotomata
    3) blurred vision
    4) photophobia
    5) epigastric or right upper quadrant pain

CHAPTER 18 NEWBORN ADAPTATION TO EXTRAUTERINE LIFE ANSWERS

1. b
2. b
3. c
4. c
5. c
6. b
7. c
8. c
9. b
10. b
11. b
12. a
13. c
14. c
15. c
16. c
17. c
18. a
19. c
20. c
21. a
22. b
23. c
24. c
25. IgG
26. hand washing
27. 1
28. *Chlamydia*; gonococcus
29. evaluate the heart rate
30. chemical; mechanical; sensory
31. umbilical vein
32. low
33. arteries; vein

34. evaporation; convection; conduction; radiation
35. brown fat
36. oxygen
37. lower surface tension
38. 60
39. antibiotics
40. early suckling; uninterrupted contact between mother and newborn

CHAPTER 19 NEWBORN PHYSICAL ASSESSMENT ANSWERS

1. b
2. b
3. c
4. b
5. a
6. c
7. a
8. b
9. c
10. a
11. a
12. a
13. b
14. c
15. a
16. a
17. c
18. c
19. c
20. b
21. a
22. b
23. a
24. c
25. c
26. b
27. b
28. crepitus
29. vernix
30. epithelial
31. craniotabes
32. 18
33. 2 to 4
34. 20
35. 8 to 10
36. phimosis
37. torticollis; sternocleidomastoid
38. vasomotor instability
39. flaring
40. reflexes

CHAPTER 20 NEWBORN NUTRITION ANSWERS

1. b
2. c
3. a
4. c
5. b
6. a
7. a
8. b
9. a
10. b
11. a
12. a
13. c
14. a
15. a
16. a
17. a
18. b
19. c
20. c
21. c
22. c
23. c
24. b
25. c
26. b
27. 75%
28. warm compresses; frequent feedings
29. lower gum
30. 30 minutes
31. 2; 4 to 7; 1
32. 7
33. colostrum or breast milk on nipples after feeding; letting nipples air dry; warm, moist compresses
34. increase milk supply
35. massage the base of the breast when the infant stops sucking; alternate massaging of the breast between periods of sucking
36. semi-upright

CHAPTER 21 COMMON NEONATAL COMPLICATIONS ANSWERS

1. a
2. b
3. c
4. b
5. c
6. a
7. c
8. b
9. c
10. b
11. c
12. b
13. b
14. b
15. c
16. c
17. b
18. c
19. b
20. c
21. a
22. c
23. decreases
24. ball-valve; escape
25. cardiovascular system
26. acyanotic; increased
27. 1) VSD
    2) pulmonary stenosis
    3) overriding aorta and right ventricular hypertrophy
28. PDA
29. acyanotic; increased
30. parallel; VSD; PDA; patent foramen ovale (PFO)
31. gluconeogenesis; glycolysis
32. kernicterus
33. unconjugated or indirect
34. sedation
35. GBS; *E. coli*
36. gestational age; birth weight
37. early-onset GBS sepsis
38. 8 to 16
39. loose stools
40. hypoglycemia
41. poor
42. decreases
43. 70%
44. elective C-section
45. 8 to 12
46. anemia
47. breast-feed

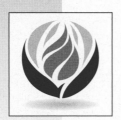

Index

Note: Page numbers followed by "*f*" indicate figures; "*t*" indicates tables; "*d*" indicates displays